Health Care State Rankings 2011

Other titles in the State Fact Finder series

City Crime Rankings

Crime State Rankings

Education State Rankings

State Rankings

Health Care State Rankings 2011
Health Care Across America

Kathleen O'Leary Morgan

and

Scott Morgan

Editors

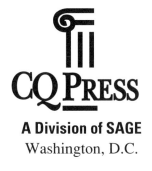

CQ PRESS

A Division of SAGE

Washington, D.C.

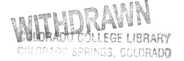

CQ Press
2300 N Street, NW, Suite 800
Washington, DC 20037

Phone: 202-729-1900; toll-free, 1-866-4CQ-PRESS (1-866-427-7737)

Web: www.cqpress.com

Cover design: Silverander Communications

⊗ The paper used in this publication exceeds the requirements of the American
National Standard for Information Sciences—Permanence of Paper for Printed
Library Materials, ANSI Z39.48-1992.

Printed and bound in the United States of America

15   14   13   12   11   1   2   3   4   5

ISBN: 978-1-60871-732-3
ISSN: 1065-1403

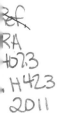

Contents

Detailed Table of Contents   vi

Introduction and Methodology   xiii

The 2011 Health Care State Rankings   xvi

Subject Rankings

    Births and Reproductive Health   3

    Deaths   90

    Facilities   189

    Finance   234

    Incidence of Disease   336

    Providers   413

    Physical Fitness   497

Appendix   532

Sources   537

Index   539

Detailed Table of Contents

I. BIRTHS AND REPRODUCTIVE HEALTH

Births in 2009 3
Birth Rate in 2009 4
Percent Change in Birth Rate: 2000 to 2009 5
Fertility Rate in 2009 6
Births to White Women in 2009 7
White Births as a Percent of All Births in 2009 8
Births to Black Women in 2009 9
Black Births as a Percent of All Births in 2009 10
Births to Hispanic Women in 2009 11
Hispanic Births as a Percent of All Births in 2009 12
Births in 2008 13
Birth Rate in 2008 14
Fertility Rate in 2008 15
Births to White Women in 2008 16
White Births as a Percent of All Births in 2008 17
Births to Black Women in 2008 18
Black Births as a Percent of All Births in 2008 19
Births to Hispanic Women in 2008 20
Hispanic Births as a Percent of All Births in 2008 21
Percent of Births That Are Pre-Term in 2008 22
Births of Low Birthweight in 2008 23
Births of Low Birthweight as a Percent of All Births
    in 2008 24
Births of Low Birthweight to White Women as a Percent
    of All Births to White Women in 2008 25
Births of Low Birthweight to Black Women as a Percent
    of All Births to Black Women in 2008 26
Births of Low Birthweight to Hispanic Women as a
    Percent of All Births to Hispanic Women in 2008 27
Births to Unmarried Women in 2008 28
Births to Unmarried Women as a Percent of All Births
    in 2008 29
Births to Unmarried White Women as a Percent of All
    Births to White Women in 2008 30
Births to Unmarried Black Women as a Percent of All
    Births to Black Women in 2008 31
Births to Unmarried Hispanic Women as a Percent of All
    Births to Hispanic Women in 2008 32

Births to Teenage Mothers in 2008 33
Births to Teenage Mothers as a Percent of All Births
    in 2008 34
Teenage Birth Rate in 2008 35
Percent Change in Teenage Birth Rate: 2007 to 2008 36
Births to White Teenage Mothers in 2008 37
White Teenage Birth Rate in 2008 38
Births to White Teenage Mothers as a Percent of All
    White Births in 2008 39
Births to Black Teenage Mothers in 2008 40
Black Teenage Birth Rate in 2008 41
Births to Black Teenage Mothers as a Percent of All
    Black Births in 2008 42
Births to Young Teenagers in 2008 43
Young Teen Birth Rate in 2008 44
Births to Women 35 to 54 Years Old in 2008 45
Birth Rate for Women 35 to 54 Years Old in 2008 46
Average Age of Woman at First Birth in 2006 47
Births by Vaginal Delivery in 2008 48
Percent of Births by Vaginal Delivery in 2008 49
Births by Cesarean Delivery in 2008 50
Percent of Births by Cesarean Delivery in 2008 51
Percent Change in Rate of Cesarean Births: 2005 to 2008 .. 52
Percent of Women Beginning Prenatal Care in First
    Trimester in 2008 53
Percent of White Women Beginning Prenatal Care in First
    Trimester in 2008 54
Percent of Black Women Beginning Prenatal Care in First
    Trimester in 2008 55
Percent of Hispanic Women Beginning Prenatal Care in
    First Trimester in 2008 56
Percent of Women Receiving Late or No Prenatal Care
    in 2008 57
Percent of White Women Receiving Late or No Prenatal
    Care in 2008 58
Percent of Black Women Receiving Late or No Prenatal
    Care in 2008 59
Percent of Hispanic Women Receiving Late or No
    Prenatal Care in 2008 60

Assisted Reproductive Technology Procedures in 2006 . . . 61
Infants Born from Assisted Reproductive Technology
    Procedures in 2006. 62
Percent of Assisted Reproductive Technology Procedures
    That Resulted in Live Births in 2006. 63
Percent of Total Live Births Resulting from Assisted
    Reproductive Technology Procedures in 2006 64
Percent of Assisted Reproductive Technology Procedure
    Infants Born in Multiple Birth Deliveries in 2006. 65
Pregnancy Rate in 2006 66
Teenage Pregnancy Rate in 2006 67
Reported Legal Abortions in 2006 68
Percent Change in Reported Legal Abortions:
    2002 to 2006. 69
Reported Legal Abortions per 1,000 Live Births in 2006 . . 70
Reported Legal Abortions per 1,000 Women 15 to
    44 Years Old in 2006. 71
Percent of Legal Abortions Obtained by Out-of-State
    Residents in 2006. 72
Percent of Reported Legal Abortions That Were
    First-Time Abortions: 2006 73
Percent of Reported Legal Abortions Obtained by White
    Women in 2006 74
Percent of Reported Legal Abortions Obtained by Black
    Women in 2006 75
Percent of Reported Legal Abortions Obtained by
    Hispanic Women in 2006. 76
Percent of Reported Legal Abortions Obtained by Married
    Women in 2006 77
Percent of Reported Legal Abortions Obtained by
    Unmarried Women in 2006 78
Reported Legal Abortions Obtained by Teenagers
    in 2006. 79
Percent of Reported Legal Abortions Obtained by
    Teenagers in 2006 80
Reported Legal Abortions Obtained by Teenagers
    17 Years and Younger in 2006. 81
Percent of Reported Legal Abortions Obtained by
    Teenagers 17 Years and Younger in 2006. 82
Percent of Teenage Abortions Obtained by Teenagers
    17 Years and Younger in 2006. 83
Reported Legal Abortions Performed at 12 Weeks or
    Fewer of Gestation in 2006 84
Percent of Reported Legal Abortions Performed at
    12 Weeks or Fewer of Gestation in 2006. 85
Reported Legal Abortions Performed at or after 21 Weeks
    of Gestation in 2006. 86
Percent of Reported Legal Abortions Performed at or after
    21 Weeks of Gestation in 2006 87

II. DEATHS

Deaths in 2009 90
Death Rate in 2009 91
Deaths in 2008 92
Death Rate in 2008 93
Age-Adjusted Death Rate in 2008 94
Percent Change in Death Rate: 1999 to 2008. 95

Deaths in 2007 96
Death Rate in 2007 97
Age-Adjusted Death Rate in 2007 98
Infant Deaths in 2007 99
Infant Mortality Rate in 2007 100
White Infant Mortality Rate in 2007. 101
Black Infant Mortality Rate in 2007. 102
Neonatal Deaths in 2007. 103
Neonatal Death Rate in 2007 104
White Neonatal Death Rate in 2007. 105
Black Neonatal Death Rate in 2007 106
Estimated Deaths by Cancer in 2010 107
Estimated Death Rate by Cancer in 2010. 108
Age-Adjusted Death Rate by Cancer for Males in 2006 . . 109
Age-Adjusted Death Rate by Cancer for Females
    in 2006 110
Estimated Deaths by Brain Cancer in 2010 111
Estimated Death Rate by Brain Cancer in 2010. 112
Estimated Deaths by Female Breast Cancer in 2010 113
Age-Adjusted Death Rate by Female Breast Cancer
    in 2006 114
Estimated Deaths by Colon and Rectum Cancer in 2010. . 115
Estimated Death Rate by Colon and Rectum Cancer
    in 2010 116
Estimated Deaths by Leukemia in 2010. 117
Estimated Death Rate by Leukemia in 2010. 118
Estimated Deaths by Liver Cancer in 2010 119
Estimated Death Rate by Liver Cancer in 2010 120
Estimated Deaths by Lung Cancer in 2010. 121
Estimated Death Rate by Lung Cancer in 2010 122
Estimated Deaths by Non-Hodgkin's Lymphoma
    in 2010 123
Estimated Death Rate by Non-Hodgkin's Lymphoma
    in 2010 124
Estimated Deaths by Ovarian Cancer in 2010 125
Estimated Death Rate by Ovarian Cancer in 2010. 126
Estimated Deaths by Pancreatic Cancer in 2010 127
Estimated Death Rate by Pancreatic Cancer in 2010 128
Estimated Deaths by Prostate Cancer in 2010 129
Age-Adjusted Death Rate by Prostate Cancer in 2006. . . . 130
Deaths by AIDS in 2007. 131
Death Rate by AIDS in 2007 132
Age-Adjusted Death Rate by AIDS in 2007. 133
Deaths by Alzheimer's Disease in 2007. 134
Death Rate by Alzheimer's Disease in 2007 135
Age-Adjusted Death Rate by Alzheimer's Disease
    in 2007 136
Deaths by Cerebrovascular Diseases in 2007. 137
Death Rate by Cerebrovascular Diseases in 2007 138
Age-Adjusted Death Rate by Cerebrovascular Diseases
    in 2007 139
Deaths by Chronic Liver Disease and Cirrhosis in 2007 . . 140
Death Rate by Chronic Liver Disease and Cirrhosis
    in 2007 141
Age-Adjusted Death Rate by Chronic Liver Disease and
    Cirrhosis in 2007 142
Deaths by Chronic Lower Respiratory Diseases in 2007 . . 143

Death Rate by Chronic Lower Respiratory Diseases in 2007 144
Age-Adjusted Death Rate by Chronic Lower Respiratory Diseases in 2007 145
Deaths by Diabetes Mellitus in 2007 146
Death Rate by Diabetes Mellitus in 2007 147
Age-Adjusted Death Rate by Diabetes Mellitus in 2007 . . 148
Deaths by Diseases of the Heart in 2007 149
Death Rate by Diseases of the Heart in 2007 150
Age-Adjusted Death Rate by Diseases of the Heart in 2007 151
Deaths by Malignant Neoplasms in 2007 152
Death Rate by Malignant Neoplasms in 2007 153
Age-Adjusted Death Rate by Malignant Neoplasms in 2007 154
Deaths by Nephritis and Other Kidney Diseases in 2007 . . 155
Death Rate by Nephritis and Other Kidney Diseases in 2007 156
Age-Adjusted Death Rate by Nephritis and Other Kidney Diseases in 2007 157
Deaths by Influenza and Pneumonia in 2007 158
Death Rate by Influenza and Pneumonia in 2007 159
Age-Adjusted Death Rate by Influenza and Pneumonia in 2007 160
Deaths by Injury in 2007 161
Death Rate by Injury in 2007 162
Age-Adjusted Death Rate by Injury in 2007 163
Deaths by Accidents in 2007 164
Death Rate by Accidents in 2007 165
Age-Adjusted Death Rate by Accidents in 2007 166
Deaths by Motor Vehicle Accidents in 2007 167
Death Rate by Motor Vehicle Accidents in 2007 168
Age-Adjusted Death Rate by Motor Vehicle Accidents in 2007 169
Deaths by Firearm Injury in 2007 170
Death Rate by Firearm Injury in 2007 171
Age-Adjusted Death Rate by Firearm Injury in 2007 172
Deaths by Homicide in 2007 173
Death Rate by Homicide in 2007 174
Age-Adjusted Death Rate by Homicide in 2007 175
Deaths by Suicide in 2007 176
Death Rate by Suicide in 2007 177
Age-Adjusted Death Rate by Suicide in 2007 178
Alcohol-Induced Deaths in 2007 179
Death Rate by Alcohol-Induced Deaths in 2007 180
Age-Adjusted Death Rate by Alcohol-Induced Deaths in 2007 181
Drug-Induced Deaths in 2007 182
Death Rate by Drug-Induced Deaths in 2007 183
Age-Adjusted Death Rate by Drug-Induced Deaths in 2007 184
Occupational Fatalities in 2009 185
Occupational Fatality Rate in 2009 186

III. FACILITIES

Community Hospitals in 2009 189
Rate of Community Hospitals in 2009 190
Community Hospitals per 1,000 Square Miles in 2009 . . . 191
Community Hospitals in Urban Areas in 2009 192
Percent of Community Hospitals in Urban Areas in 2009 193
Community Hospitals in Rural Areas in 2009 194
Percent of Community Hospitals in Rural Areas in 2009 . . 195
Nongovernment, Not-for-Profit Hospitals in 2009 196
Investor-Owned, For-Profit Hospitals in 2009 197
State and Local Government-Owned Hospitals in 2009 . . . 198
Beds in Community Hospitals in 2009 199
Rate of Beds in Community Hospitals in 2009 200
Average Number of Beds per Community Hospital in 2009 201
Admissions to Community Hospitals in 2009 202
Inpatient Days in Community Hospitals in 2009 203
Average Daily Census in Community Hospitals in 2009 . . . 204
Average Stay in Community Hospitals in 2009 205
Occupancy Rate in Community Hospitals in 2009 206
Outpatient Visits to Community Hospitals in 2009 207
Emergency Outpatient Visits to Community Hospitals in 2009 208
Medicare and Medicaid Certified Facilities in 2011 209
Medicare and Medicaid Certified Hospitals in 2011 210
Beds in Medicare and Medicaid Certified Hospitals in 2011 211
Medicare and Medicaid Certified Children's Hospitals in 2011 212
Beds in Medicare and Medicaid Certified Children's Hospitals in 2011 213
Medicare and Medicaid Certified Rehabilitation Hospitals in 2011 214
Beds in Medicare and Medicaid Certified Rehabilitation Hospitals in 2011 215
Medicare and Medicaid Certified Psychiatric Hospitals in 2011 216
Beds in Medicare and Medicaid Certified Psychiatric Hospitals in 2011 217
Medicare and Medicaid Certified Outpatient Surgery Centers in 2011 218
Medicare and Medicaid Certified Community Mental Health Centers in 2011 219
Medicare and Medicaid Certified Outpatient Physical Therapy Facilities in 2011 220
Medicare and Medicaid Certified Rural Health Clinics in 2011 221
Medicare and Medicaid Certified Home Health Agencies in 2011 222
Medicare and Medicaid Certified Hospices in 2011 223
Hospice Patients in Residential Facilities in 2011 224
Medicare and Medicaid Certified Nursing Care Facilities in 2011 225
Beds in Medicare and Medicaid Certified Nursing Care Facilities in 2011 226
Rate of Beds in Medicare and Medicaid Certified Nursing Care Facilities in 2011 227
Nursing Home Occupancy Rate in 2009 228
Nursing Home Resident Rate in 2009 229
Nursing Home Population in 2009 230
Health Care Establishments in 2008 231

IV. FINANCE

Average Medical Malpractice Payment in 2006. 234

Percent of Private-Sector Establishments That Offer
    Health Insurance: 2009 235

Percent of Private-Sector Establishments with Fewer
    Than 50 Employees That Offer Health Insurance:
    2009 236

Percent of Private-Sector Establishments with More Than
    50 Employees That Offer Health Insurance: 2009. 237

Average Annual Single Coverage Health Insurance
    Premium per Enrolled Employee in 2009 238

Average Annual Employee Contribution for Single
    Coverage Health Insurance in 2009. 239

Percent of Total Premiums for Single Coverage Health
    Insurance Paid by Employees in 2009. 240

Average Annual Family Coverage Health Insurance
    Premium per Enrolled Employee in 2009 241

Average Annual Employee Contribution for Family
    Coverage Health Insurance in 2009. 242

Percent of Total Premiums for Family Coverage Health
    Insurance Paid by Employees in 2009. 243

Persons Not Covered by Health Insurance in 2009 244

Percent of Population Not Covered by Health Insurance
    in 2009 245

Numerical Change in Persons Uninsured: 2005 to 2009 . . 246

Percent Change in Persons Uninsured: 2005 to 2009. 247

Change in Percent of Population Uninsured: 2005 to
    2009 248

Percent of Children Not Covered by Health Insurance
    in 2009 249

Persons Covered by Health Insurance in 2009. 250

Percent of Population Covered by Health Insurance
    in 2009 251

Percent of Population Covered by Private Health
    Insurance in 2009. 252

Percent of Population Covered by Employment-Based
    Health Insurance in 2009 253

Percent of Population Covered by Direct-Purchase
    Health Insurance in 2009 254

Percent of Population Covered by Government Health
    Insurance in 2009. 255

Percent of Population Covered by Military Health Care
    in 2009 256

Percent of Children Covered by Health Insurance
    in 2009 257

Percent of Children Covered by Private Health
    Insurance in 2009. 258

Percent of Children Covered by Employment-Based
    Health Insurance in 2009 259

Percent of Children Covered by Direct-Purchase Health
    Insurance in 2009. 260

Percent of Children Covered by Government Health
    Insurance in 2009. 261

Percent of Children Covered by Military Health Care
    in 2009 262

Percent of Children Covered by Medicaid in 2009 263

The Children's Health Insurance Program (CHIP)
    Enrollment in 2009. 264

Percent Change in the Children's Health Insurance
    Program (CHIP) Enrollment: 2008 to 2009. 265

Percent of Children Enrolled in the Children's Health
    Insurance Program (CHIP) in 2009 266

Expenditures for the Children's Health Insurance
    Program (CHIP) in 2009 267

Per Capita Expenditures for the Children's Health
    Insurance Program (CHIP) in 2009 268

Expenditures per Participant in the Children's Health
    Insurance Program (CHIP) in 2009 269

Health Maintenance Organizations (HMOs) in 2009. 270

Enrollees in Health Maintenance Organizations (HMOs)
    in 2009 271

Percent Change in Enrollees in Health Maintenance
    Organizations (HMOs): 2008 to 2009 272

Percent of Population Enrolled in Health Maintenance
    Organizations (HMOs) in 2009 273

Percent of Insured Population Enrolled in Health
    Maintenance Organizations (HMOs) in 2009 274

Medicare Enrollees in 2009 275

Percent Change in Medicare Enrollees: 2008 to 2009 276

Percent of Population Enrolled in Medicare in 2009 277

Percent of Medicare Enrollees in Managed Care
    Programs in 2009. 278

Percent of Physicians Participating in Medicare in 2010. . 279

Enrollees in Medicare Prescription Drug Program
    in 2010 280

Percent of Medicare Enrollees Participating in the
    Medicare Prescription Drug Program in 2010. 281

Medicare Program Payments in 2009. 282

Per Capita Medicare Program Payments in 2009. 283

Medicare Program Payments per Enrollee in 2009 284

Medicaid Enrollment in 2009. 285

Percent of Population Enrolled in Medicaid in 2009 286

Medicaid Managed Care Enrollment in 2009. 287

Percent of Medicaid Enrollees in Managed Care in 2009 . . 288

Estimated Medicaid Expenditures in 2010. 289

Estimated Per Capita Medicaid Expenditures in 2010. . . . 290

Estimated Medicaid Expenditures as a Percent of Total
    Expenditures in 2010 291

Percent Change in Medicaid Expenditures: 2009 to
    2010 292

Medicaid Expenditures in 2009 293

Per Capita Medicaid Expenditures in 2009 294

Medicaid Expenditures per Beneficiary in 2009. 295

Federal Medicaid Matching Fund Rate for 2011 296

State and Local Government Expenditures for Hospitals
    in 2008. 297

Per Capita State and Local Government Expenditures for
    Hospitals in 2008 298

Percent of State and Local Government Expenditures
    Used for Hospitals in 2008. 299

State and Local Government Expenditures for Health
    Programs in 2008. 300

Per Capita State and Local Government Expenditures for
    Health Programs in 2008 301

Percent of State and Local Government Expenditures
    Used for Health Programs in 2008. 302

Estimated Tobacco Settlement Revenues in Fiscal
    Year 2011 303
Annual Smoking-Related Health Costs in 2010 304
Personal Health Care Expenditures in 2004 305
Health Care Expenditures as a Percent of Gross State
    Product in 2004 306
Per Capita Personal Health Care Expenditures in 2004 . . . 307
Average Annual Growth in Personal Health Care
    Expenditures: 1991 to 2004 308
Expenditures for Hospital Care in 2004 309
Percent of Total Personal Health Care Expenditures
    Spent on Hospital Care in 2004 310
Per Capita Expenditures for Hospital Care in 2004 311
Expenditures for Physician and Clinical Services
    in 2004 312
Percent of Total Personal Health Care Expenditures
    Spent on Physician and Clinical Services in 2004 313
Per Capita Expenditures for Physician and Clinical
    Services in 2004 314
Expenditures for Dental Services in 2004 315
Percent of Total Personal Health Care Expenditures
    Spent on Dental Services in 2004 316
Per Capita Expenditures for Dental Care in 2004. 317
Expenditures for Other Professional Health Care
    Services in 2004 318
Percent of Total Personal Health Care Expenditures
    Spent on Other Professional Health Care Services
    in 2004 319
Per Capita Expenditures for Other Professional Health
    Care Services in 2004. 320
Expenditures for Nursing Home Care in 2004 321
Percent of Total Personal Health Care Expenditures
    Spent on Nursing Home Care in 2004 322
Per Capita Expenditures for Nursing Home Care in 2004. . 323
Expenditures for Home Health Care in 2004 324
Percent of Total Personal Health Care Expenditures
    Spent on Home Health Care in 2004 325
Per Capita Expenditures for Home Health Care in 2004 . . 326
Expenditures for Drugs and Other Medical Nondurables
    in 2004 327
Percent of Total Personal Health Care Expenditures
    Spent on Drugs and Other Medical Nondurables
    in 2004 328
Per Capita Expenditures for Drugs and Other Medical
    Nondurables in 2004 329
Expenditures for Durable Medical Products in 2004 330
Percent of Total Personal Health Care Expenditures
    Spent on Durable Medical Products in 2004 331
Per Capita Expenditures for Durable Medical Products
    in 2004 332
Projected National Health Care Expenditures in 2011 333

V. INCIDENCE OF DISEASE

Estimated New Cancer Cases in 2010 336
Estimated Rate of New Cancer Cases in 2010 337
Age-Adjusted Cancer Incidence Rates for Males in 2006. . 338
Age-Adjusted Cancer Incidence Rates for Females
    in 2006 339

Estimated New Cases of Bladder Cancer in 2010 340
Estimated Rate of New Bladder Cancer Cases in 2010 . . . 341
Estimated New Female Breast Cancer Cases in 2010 342
Age-Adjusted Incidence Rate of Female Breast Cancer
    Cases in 2006 343
Percent of Women 40 and Older Who Have Had a
    Mammogram in the Past Two Years: 2008 344
Estimated New Colon and Rectum Cancer Cases
    in 2010 345
Estimated Rate of New Colon and Rectum Cancer
    Cases in 2010 346
Percent of Adults Who Have Ever Had a Sigmoidoscopy
    or Colonoscopy Exam: 2008 347
Estimated New Leukemia Cases in 2010 348
Estimated Rate of New Leukemia Cases in 2010. 349
Estimated New Lung Cancer Cases in 2010. 350
Estimated Rate of New Lung Cancer Cases in 2010 351
Estimated New Non-Hodgkin's Lymphoma Cases
    in 2010 352
Estimated Rate of New Non-Hodgkin's Lymphoma
    Cases in 2010 353
Estimated New Prostate Cancer Cases in 2010 354
Age-Adjusted Incidence Rate of Prostate Cancer
    Cases in 2006 355
Percent of Males Receiving PSA Test for Prostate
    Cancer: 2008 356
Estimated New Skin Melanoma Cases in 2010 357
Estimated Rate of New Skin Melanoma Cases in 2010 . . . 358
Estimated New Cervical Cancer Cases in 2010 359
Estimated Rate of New Cervical Cancer Cases in 2010. . . 360
Percent of Women 18 Years Old and Older Who Have
    Had a Pap Smear in the Past Three Years: 2008 361
Estimated New Uterine Cancer Cases in 2010 362
Estimated Rate of New Uterine Cancer Cases in 2010. . . . 363
AIDS Cases Reported in 2008 364
AIDS Rate in 2008 365
AIDS Cases Reported through December 2008 366
AIDS Cases in Children 12 Years and Younger through
    December 2008 367
Chickenpox (Varicella) Cases Reported in 2010 368
Chickenpox (Varicella) Rate in 2010 369
E. Coli Cases Reported in 2010 370
E. Coli Rate in 2010 371
Hepatitis A and B Cases Reported in 2010. 372
Hepatitis A and B Rate in 2010 373
Hepatitis C Cases Reported in 2010 374
Hepatitis C Rate in 2010. 375
Legionellosis Cases Reported in 2010 376
Legionellosis Rate in 2010 377
Lyme Disease Cases Reported in 2010. 378
Lyme Disease Rate in 2010 379
Malaria Cases Reported in 2010. 380
Malaria Rate in 2010. 381
Meningococcal Infections Reported in 2010 382
Meningococcal Infection Rate in 2010. 383
Rabies (Animal) Cases Reported in 2010. 384
Rabies (Animal) Rate in 2010. 385
Spotted Fever Rickettsiosis Reported in 2010 386

Rocky Mountain Spotted Fever Rate in 2010. 387
Salmonellosis Cases Reported in 2010. 388
Salmonellosis Rate in 2010. 389
Shigellosis Cases Reported in 2010 390
Shigellosis Rate in 2010 391
West Nile Virus Disease Cases Reported in 2010 392
West Nile Disease Rate in 2010 393
Whooping Cough (Pertussis) Cases Reported in 2010. . . . 394
Whooping Cough (Pertussis) Rate in 2010. 395
Percent of Children Aged 19 to 35 Months Fully
    Immunized in 2009 396
Percent of Adults Aged 65 Years and Older Who
    Received Flu Shots in 2009 397
Percent of Adults Aged 65 Years and Older Who Have
    Had a Pneumonia Vaccine: 2009 398
Sexually Transmitted Diseases in 2009 399
Sexually Transmitted Disease Rate in 2009 400
Chlamydia Cases Reported in 2009 401
Chlamydia Rate in 2009 402
Gonorrhea Cases Reported in 2009 403
Gonorrhea Rate in 2009 404
Syphilis Cases Reported in 2009 405
Syphilis Rate in 2009 406
Percent of Adults Who Have Asthma: 2009. 407
Percent of Adults Who Have Been Told They Have
    Arthritis: 2009 408
Percent of Adults Who Have Been Told They Have
    Diabetes: 2009 409
Percent of Adults Reporting Serious Psychological
    Distress: 2007. 410

VI. PROVIDERS

Health Care Practitioners and Technicians in 2009 413
Rate of Health Care Practitioners and Technicians
    in 2009 414
Average Annual Wages of Health Care Practitioners and
    Technicians in 2009 415
Physicians in 2009 416
Rate of Physicians in 2009 417
Percent of Physicians Who Are Female: 2009 418
Percent of Physicians under 35 Years Old in 2009. 419
Percent of Physicians 65 Years Old and Older in 2009 . . . 420
Physicians in Patient Care in 2009 421
Rate of Physicians in Patient Care in 2009. 422
Physicians in Primary Care in 2009 423
Rate of Physicians in Primary Care in 2009. 424
Percent of Physicians in Primary Care in 2009 425
Percent of Population Lacking Access to Primary Care
    in 2011 426
Physicians in General/Family Practice in 2009 427
Rate of Physicians in General/Family Practice in 2009 . . . 428
Average Annual Wages of Family and General
    Practitioners in 2009 429
Percent of Physicians Who Are Specialists in 2009. 430
Physicians in Medical Specialties in 2009 431
Rate of Nonfederal Physicians in Medical Specialties
    in 2009 432
Physicians in Internal Medicine in 2009. 433

Rate of Physicians in Internal Medicine in 2009 434
Physicians in Pediatrics in 2009 435
Rate of Physicians in Pediatrics in 2009. 436
Physicians in Surgical Specialties in 2009 437
Rate of Physicians in Surgical Specialties in 2009. 438
Average Annual Wages of Surgeons in 2009. 439
Physicians in General Surgery in 2009. 440
Rate of Physicians in General Surgery in 2009 441
Physicians in Obstetrics and Gynecology in 2009 442
Rate of Physicians in Obstetrics and Gynecology
    in 2009 443
Physicians in Ophthalmology in 2009 444
Rate of Physicians in Ophthalmology in 2009 445
Physicians in Orthopedic Surgery in 2009 446
Rate of Physicians in Orthopedic Surgery in 2009. 447
Physicians in Plastic Surgery in 2009. 448
Rate of Physicians in Plastic Surgery in 2009 449
Physicians in Other Specialties in 2009 450
Rate of Physicians in Other Specialties in 2009. 451
Physicians in Anesthesiology in 2009 452
Rate of Physicians in Anesthesiology in 2009 453
Physicians in Psychiatry in 2009 454
Rate of Physicians in Psychiatry in 2009 455
Percent of Population Lacking Access to Mental Health
    Care in 2011 456
International Medical School Graduates in 2009 457
International Medical School Graduates as a Percent of
    Physicians in 2009 458
Osteopathic Physicians in 2010 459
Rate of Osteopathic Physicians in 2010 460
Podiatrists in 2009. 461
Rate of Podiatrists in 2009 462
Average Annual Wages of Podiatrists in 2009. 463
Doctors of Chiropractic in 2009 464
Rate of Doctors of Chiropractic in 2009. 465
Average Annual Wages of Chiropractors in 2009 466
Physician Assistants in Clinical Practice in 2008. 467
Rate of Physician Assistants in Clinical Practice in 2008 . . 468
Average Annual Wages of Physician Assistants in 2009. . 469
Registered Nurses in 2009 470
Rate of Registered Nurses in 2009 471
Average Annual Wages of Registered Nurses in 2009. . . . 472
Licensed Practical and Licensed Vocational Nurses
    in 2009 473
Rate of Licensed Practical and Licensed Vocational
    Nurses in 2009 474
Average Annual Wages of Licensed Practical and
    Licensed Vocational Nurses in 2009 475
Physical Therapists in 2009 476
Rate of Physical Therapists in 2009 477
Average Annual Wages of Physical Therapists in 2009. . . 478
Dentists in 2008 479
Rate of Dentists in 2008 480
Average Annual Wages of Dentists in 2009. 481
Percent of Population Lacking Access to Dental Care
    in 2011 482
Pharmacists in 2009 483
Rate of Pharmacists in 2009 484

Average Annual Wages of Pharmacists in 2009. 485
Optometrists in 2009. 486
Rate of Optometrists in 2009 487
Average Annual Wages of Optometrists in 2009 488
Emergency Medical Technicians and Paramedics
    in 2009 489
Rate of Emergency Medical Technicians and Paramedics
    in 2009 490
Average Annual Wages of Emergency Medical
    Technicians and Paramedics in 2009 491
Employment in Health Care Support Industries in 2009 . . 492
Rate of Employees in Health Care Support Industries
    in 2009 493
Average Annual Wages of Employees in Health Care
    Support Industries in 2009 494

VII. PHYSICAL FITNESS

Users of Exercise Equipment in 2009. 497
Participants in Golf in 2009 498
Participants in Running/Jogging in 2009 499
Participants in Swimming in 2009 500
Participants in Tennis in 2009. 501
Alcohol Consumption in 2007 502
Adult Per Capita Alcohol Consumption in 2007 503
Apparent Beer Consumption in 2007 504
Adult Per Capita Beer Consumption in 2007 505
Wine Consumption in 2007 506
Adult Per Capita Wine Consumption in 2007 507
Distilled Spirits Consumption in 2007 508
Adult Per Capita Distilled Spirits Consumption
    in 2007 509

Percent of Adults Who Do Not Drink Alcohol: 2009. 510
Percent of Adults Who Are Binge Drinkers: 2009 511
Percent of Adults Who Smoke: 2009 512
Percent of Men Who Smoke: 2009. 513
Percent of Women Who Smoke: 2009 514
Percent of Adults Who Are Former Smokers: 2009. 515
Percent of Adults Who Have Never Smoked: 2009 516
Percent of Population Who Are Illicit Drug Users: 2008. . 517
Percent of Adults Overweight: 2009. 518
Percent of Adults Obese: 2009 519
Percent of Adults Overweight or Obese: 2009 520
Percent of Adults Who Do Not Exercise: 2009 521
Percent of Adults Who Exercise Vigorously: 2009 522
Percent of Adults Who Are Disabled: 2009 523
Percent of Adults with High Blood Pressure: 2009 524
Percent of Adults with High Cholesterol: 2009 525
Percent of Adults Who Have Visited a Dentist or Dental
    Clinic: 2008 526
Percent of Adults 65 Years Old and Older Who Have
    Lost All Their Natural Teeth: 2008 527
Percent of Adults Who Average Five or More Servings
    of Fruits and Vegetables Each Day: 2009 528
Percent of Adults Rating Their Health as Fair or Poor
    in 2009 529
Safety Belt Usage Rate in 2009 530

APPENDIX

Population in 2009 532
Population in 2008 533
Male Population in 2009. 534
Female Population in 2009 535

Introduction and Methodology

Health Care State Rankings 2011 analyzes the latest health care data for each of the fifty states and the District of Columbia. This book provides state-by-state rankings of roughly five hundred health care factors in the following seven categories: births and reproductive health, deaths, facilities, finance, incidence of disease, providers, and physical fitness.

Purpose of This Book

The purpose of *Health Care State Rankings 2011* is to serve as a resource for researchers, health policy professionals, and the community. The book provides the means by which they can compare the status of their state's health care with that of other states and the nation as a whole.

These data and rankings can be used in a variety of ways, by a variety of audiences, including the following:

- Health care policymakers can use them to help identify health care problems for further study.
- State governments can determine whether their health care levels are on a par with those of the rest of the nation.
- The federal government can use this type of analysis to allocate grant funding (Bauer 2004).
- The media can rely on these results to compare health care rankings across states and years and to report to the public.

In addition to the data and rankings, this book offers numerous information-finding tools, including a detailed table of contents, a table of listings at the beginning of each chapter, and an index. A directory of data sources used by the editors is included, providing addresses, phone numbers, and Web sites. The appendix consists of four charts that look at the U.S. population in 2008 and 2009 and the male and female population in 2009.

The Data and Their Limitations

The data featured in *Health Care State Rankings 2011*, chosen specifically by the editors, come from a variety of government and private sector sources. They are more than a snapshot of the status of health care across the nation, but they do not include all the health care data that might be available.

Previous editions of this book have used the term *healthiest* when describing each state's place within the overall rankings. However, this term is no longer used because it is purely descriptive—at no time do we attempt to explain *why* a particular state is doing less well in health care than others, or against the national average. This explanation—which is currently sought by health policy experts and other social science researchers—is beyond the scope of this book.

Although our selection of factors clearly affects the rankings, we believe the rankings provide a solid measurement of how the fifty states and the District of Columbia are faring in health care. Researchers, practitioners, and others can confidently use the data to understand health care issues and to guide policy decisions.

Methodology

As noted earlier, the 2011 health care state rankings found on page xvi are based on seven overall categories (births and reproductive health, deaths, facilities, finance, incidence of disease, providers, and physical fitness), which are broken down into twenty-one factors that reflect access to health care providers, affordability of health care, and the general health of the population. These factors are then divided into two groups: those that are "negative" for which a high ranking would be considered troublesome for a state, and those that are "positive" for which a high ranking would be considered a good sign for a state. The negative factors are as follows:

- Births of Low Birthweight as a Percent of All Births in 2008
- Teenage Birth Rate in 2008
- Percent of Mothers Receiving Late or No Prenatal Care in 2008
- Age-Adjusted Death Rate in 2008
- Infant Mortality Rate in 2007
- Age-Adjusted Death Rate by Malignant Neoplasms in 2007
- Age-Adjusted Death Rate by Suicide in 2007
- Average Annual Family Coverage Health Insurance Premium per Enrolled Employee in 2009

- Percent of Population Not Covered by Health Insurance in 2009
- Percent of Children Not Covered by Health Insurance in 2009
- Estimated Rate of New Cancer Cases in 2010
- AIDS Rate in 2008
- Sexually Transmitted Disease Rate in 2009
- Percent of Population Lacking Access to Primary Care in 2011
- Percent of Adults Who Are Binge Drinkers: 2009
- Percent of Adults Who Smoke: 2009
- Percent of Adults Obese: 2009
- Percent of Adults Who Do Not Exercise: 2009

The positive factors are as follows:

- Rate of Beds in Community Hospitals in 2009
- Percent of Children Aged 19 to 35 Months Fully Immunized in 2009
- Safety Belt Usage Rate in 2009

The twenty-one factors involve a rate or percent of frequency, so that numbers are not biased toward population size, and the positive and negative nature of each factor is taken into account as part of the formula. Once we calculate the score for each individual factor, we add the scores to determine the overall ranking, with a positive score indicating a positive outlook for a state and one that is above the national average.

"Comparison Score" Methodology

The methodology for determining the health care state rankings involves multiple steps in which the rates for each of the twenty-one factors just listed are processed through a formula that measures how a state compares with the national average for a given category. The end result is that the further a state's health ranking is below the national average, the lower it ranks overall; the further a state's health ranking is above the national average, the higher it ranks overall. The methodology used for this edition of this book was also used for previous editions of *Health Care State Rankings* in which the editors subjectively determined which factors were "negative" and which were "positive," because negative and positive factors are treated differently in the formula.

The methodology for *Health Care State Rankings* is described here in detail, using the following formula for these calculations:

$$\frac{\text{State Rate} - \text{National Rate}}{\text{National Rate}} \times 100$$

The following are steps for the "comparison score" calculation and examples of the calculations:

1. Two factors are used for the state of Vermont as examples of positive and negative factors: Positive Factor: Percent of Children Aged 19 to 35 Months Fully Immunized in 2009—59.9; Negative Factor: Births of Low Birthweight as a Percent of All Births in 2008—7.0.

2. The percent difference between the state rate and the national rate for all twenty-one factors is then computed. For the positive factor of percent of fully immunized children, Vermont's rate of 59.9 is divided by the national rate of 70.5 for a percent difference of 0.8496. For the negative factor of low birthweight, Vermont's rate of 7.0 is divided by the national rate of 8.2 for a percent difference of 0.8537.

3. One is then subtracted from the percent difference for each factor so that states with the national average would equal 0 instead of 1. The results are then multiplied by 100 for a more manageable number. For the positive factor, 1 is subtracted from 0.8496 to equal (0.1504), which is then multiplied by 100 to equal (15.04). For the negative factor, 1 is subtracted from 0.8537 to equal (0.1463), which is then multiplied by 100 to equal (14.63).

4. These numbers are then scaled to be 1/21 of the index by multiplying each score by 4.76 percent (because there are twenty-one equally weighted factors, each factor is multiplied by 4.76 percent or 1/21). For the positive factor, (15.04) times 0.0476 equals (0.716). For the negative factor, (14.63) times 0.0476 equals (0.6963).

5. The negative factors are then multiplied by negative one (–1). Positive factors are not multiplied by anything. Therefore, Vermont's score for Percent of Children Aged 19 to 35 Months Fully Immunized in 2009 is (0.716). Its score for Births of Low Birthweight as a Percent of all Births in 2008 is 0.6963 or (0.6963) multiplied by –1 as this is a negative factor. A positive score illustrates that the state scored higher than the national average. Therefore, Vermont's score of (0.716) for the positive factor of Fully Immunized Children (a negative score of a positive factor) illustrates that Vermont has a score lower than the national average score for children fully immunized. Vermont's score of 0.6963 for the negative factor of Low Birthweight (a positive score of a negative number) illustrates that Vermont has a score lower than the national average score for babies born with a low birthweight.

6. The final comparison score for each state is the sum of the individual scores for the equally weighted twenty-one factors ("SUM" in the 2011 Health Care State Rankings table on p. xvi). This way, the states are assessed on how they stack up against the national average. In the case of Vermont, the SUM is 18.22 (note that the calculations of only two of the twenty-one factors are illustrated here). The interpretation of these scores is that the higher the state score, the further it is above the national score; the lower the score, the further it is below the national score; and a score of zero is equal to the national score. With a SUM of 18.22, Vermont is significantly above the national average.

The scores are then sorted to produce the rankings. The rankings do not indicate the actual difference between the scores, only their order, providing a means by which health care trends can be gauged in different communities.

For the tables in the rest of *Health Care State Rankings 2011* states are simply ranked from highest to lowest. For ties, the states are listed alphabetically for a given ranking. Negative numbers are reported in parentheses. Data reported as "NA" are not available or could not be calculated. In tables with national totals (as opposed to rates, per capita data, or the like), a separate column shows the percentage of the national total represented by each state. This "% of USA" column is particularly interesting when compared with a state's share of the national population for a particular year. Source information and other important notes are shown clearly at the bottom of each page.

Reference

Bauer, L. 2004. *Local Law Enforcement Block Grant Program, 1996–2004.* Technical Report. Washington, D.C.: Bureau of Justice Statistics.

The 2011 Health Care State Rankings

ALPHA ORDER

RANK	STATE	SUM	10 RANK	CHANGE
45	Alabama	(10.33)	40	-5
41	Alaska	(9.09)	42	1
32	Arizona	(2.75)	43	11
38	Arkansas	(6.97)	38	0
16	California	7.24	16	0
25	Colorado	2.69	27	2
10	Connecticut	10.16	12	2
37	Delaware	(5.64)	37	0
44	Florida	(10.30)	45	1
39	Georgia	(7.07)	39	0
6	Hawaii	17.12	4	-2
15	Idaho	7.46	19	4
30	Illinois	(0.51)	30	0
26	Indiana	2.43	28	2
8	Iowa	14.29	8	0
17	Kansas	6.76	18	1
35	Kentucky	(4.08)	35	0
50	Louisiana	(24.57)	49	-1
9	Maine	14.11	7	-2
31	Maryland	(1.26)	29	-2
2	Massachusetts	18.69	3	1
23	Michigan	3.68	23	0
3	Minnesota	18.52	2	-1
49	Mississippi	(24.03)	50	1
40	Missouri	(8.45)	34	-6
27	Montana	1.96	31	4
7	Nebraska	15.32	10	3
42	Nevada	(9.14)	48	6
1	New Hampshire	19.14	5	4
11	New Jersey	9.37	14	3
48	New Mexico	(15.81)	47	-1
28	New York	1.87	26	-2
33	North Carolina	(3.22)	32	-1
13	North Dakota	8.70	13	0
24	Ohio	2.81	21	-3
46	Oklahoma	(11.09)	44	-2
18	Oregon	6.31	17	-1
22	Pennsylvania	5.32	24	2
14	Rhode Island	8.53	9	-5
43	South Carolina	(10.07)	46	3
20	South Dakota	5.55	25	5
36	Tennessee	(4.88)	36	0
47	Texas	(11.70)	41	-6
5	Utah	17.83	6	1
4	Vermont	18.22	1	-3
21	Virginia	5.49	20	-1
12	Washington	9.32	11	-1
29	West Virginia	0.96	22	-7
19	Wisconsin	6.10	15	-4
34	Wyoming	(3.73)	33	-1

RANK ORDER

RANK	STATE	SUM	10 RANK	CHANGE
1	New Hampshire	19.14	5	4
2	Massachusetts	18.69	3	1
3	Minnesota	18.52	2	-1
4	Vermont	18.22	1	-3
5	Utah	17.83	6	1
6	Hawaii	17.12	4	-2
7	Nebraska	15.32	10	3
8	Iowa	14.29	8	0
9	Maine	14.11	7	-2
10	Connecticut	10.16	12	2
11	New Jersey	9.37	14	3
12	Washington	9.32	11	-1
13	North Dakota	8.70	13	0
14	Rhode Island	8.53	9	-5
15	Idaho	7.46	19	4
16	California	7.24	16	0
17	Kansas	6.76	18	1
18	Oregon	6.31	17	-1
19	Wisconsin	6.10	15	-4
20	South Dakota	5.55	25	5
21	Virginia	5.49	20	-1
22	Pennsylvania	5.32	24	2
23	Michigan	3.68	23	0
24	Ohio	2.81	21	-3
25	Colorado	2.69	27	2
26	Indiana	2.43	28	2
27	Montana	1.96	31	4
28	New York	1.87	26	-2
29	West Virginia	0.96	22	-7
30	Illinois	(0.51)	30	0
31	Maryland	(1.26)	29	-2
32	Arizona	(2.75)	43	11
33	North Carolina	(3.22)	32	-1
34	Wyoming	(3.73)	33	-1
35	Kentucky	(4.08)	35	0
36	Tennessee	(4.88)	36	0
37	Delaware	(5.64)	37	0
38	Arkansas	(6.97)	38	0
39	Georgia	(7.07)	39	0
40	Missouri	(8.45)	34	-6
41	Alaska	(9.09)	42	1
42	Nevada	(9.14)	48	6
43	South Carolina	(10.07)	46	3
44	Florida	(10.30)	45	1
45	Alabama	(10.33)	40	-5
46	Oklahoma	(11.09)	44	-2
47	Texas	(11.70)	41	-6
48	New Mexico	(15.81)	47	-1
49	Mississippi	(24.03)	50	1
50	Louisiana	(24.57)	49	-1

I. Births and Reproductive Health

Births in 2009 3
Birth Rate in 2009 4
Percent Change in Birth Rate: 2000 to 2009 5
Fertility Rate in 2009 6
Births to White Women in 2009 7
White Births as a Percent of All Births in 2009 8
Births to Black Women in 2009 9
Black Births as a Percent of All Births in 2009 10
Births to Hispanic Women in 2009 11
Hispanic Births as a Percent of All Births in 2009 12
Births in 2008 13
Birth Rate in 2008 14
Fertility Rate in 2008 15
Births to White Women in 2008 16
White Births as a Percent of All Births in 2008 17
Births to Black Women in 2008 18
Black Births as a Percent of All Births in 2008 19
Births to Hispanic Women in 2008 20
Hispanic Births as a Percent of All Births in 2008 21
Percent of Births That Are Pre-Term in 2008 22
Births of Low Birthweight in 2008 23
Births of Low Birthweight as a Percent of All Births
    in 2008 24
Births of Low Birthweight to White Women as a Percent
    of All Births to White Women in 2008 25
Births of Low Birthweight to Black Women as a Percent
    of All Births to Black Women in 2008 26
Births of Low Birthweight to Hispanic Women as a
    Percent of All Births to Hispanic Women in 2008 27
Births to Unmarried Women in 2008 28
Births to Unmarried Women as a Percent of All Births
    in 2008 29
Births to Unmarried White Women as a Percent of All
    Births to White Women in 2008 30
Births to Unmarried Black Women as a Percent of All
    Births to Black Women in 2008 31
Births to Unmarried Hispanic Women as a Percent of All
    Births to Hispanic Women in 2008 32
Births to Teenage Mothers in 2008 33

Births to Teenage Mothers as a Percent of All Births
    in 2008 34
Teenage Birth Rate in 2008 35
Percent Change in Teenage Birth Rate: 2007 to 2008 36
Births to White Teenage Mothers in 2008 37
White Teenage Birth Rate in 2008 38
Births to White Teenage Mothers as a Percent of All
    White Births in 2008 39
Births to Black Teenage Mothers in 2008 40
Black Teenage Birth Rate in 2008 41
Births to Black Teenage Mothers as a Percent of All
    Black Births in 2008 42
Births to Young Teenagers in 2008 43
Young Teen Birth Rate in 2008 44
Births to Women 35 to 54 Years Old in 2008 45
Birth Rate for Women 35 to 54 Years Old in 2008 46
Average Age of Woman at First Birth in 2006 47
Births by Vaginal Delivery in 2008 48
Percent of Births by Vaginal Delivery in 2008 49
Births by Cesarean Delivery in 2008 50
Percent of Births by Cesarean Delivery in 2008 51
Percent Change in Rate of Cesarean Births: 2005 to 2008 . . 52
Percent of Women Beginning Prenatal Care in First
    Trimester in 2008 53
Percent of White Women Beginning Prenatal Care in First
    Trimester in 2008 54
Percent of Black Women Beginning Prenatal Care in First
    Trimester in 2008 55
Percent of Hispanic Women Beginning Prenatal Care in
    First Trimester in 2008 56
Percent of Women Receiving Late or No Prenatal Care
    in 2008 57
Percent of White Women Receiving Late or No Prenatal
    Care in 2008 58
Percent of Black Women Receiving Late or No Prenatal
    Care in 2008 59
Percent of Hispanic Women Receiving Late or No
    Prenatal Care in 2008 60
Assisted Reproductive Technology Procedures in 2006 . . . 61

Infants Born from Assisted Reproductive Technology
 Procedures in 2006. 62
Percent of Assisted Reproductive Technology Procedures
 That Resulted in Live Births in 2006. 63
Percent of Total Live Births Resulting from Assisted
 Reproductive Technology Procedures in 2006 64
Percent of Assisted Reproductive Technology Procedure
 Infants Born in Multiple Birth Deliveries in 2006. 65
Pregnancy Rate in 2006 66
Teenage Pregnancy Rate in 2006 67
Reported Legal Abortions in 2006 68
Percent Change in Reported Legal Abortions:
 2002 to 2006. 69
Reported Legal Abortions per 1,000 Live Births in 2006 . . 70
Reported Legal Abortions per 1,000 Women 15 to
 44 Years Old in 2006. 71
Percent of Legal Abortions Obtained by Out-of-State
 Residents in 2006. 72
Percent of Reported Legal Abortions That Were
 First-Time Abortions: 2006 73
Percent of Reported Legal Abortions Obtained by White
 Women in 2006 74
Percent of Reported Legal Abortions Obtained by Black
 Women in 2006 75

Percent of Reported Legal Abortions Obtained by
 Hispanic Women in 2006. 76
Percent of Reported Legal Abortions Obtained by Married
 Women in 2006 77
Percent of Reported Legal Abortions Obtained by
 Unmarried Women in 2006 78
Reported Legal Abortions Obtained by Teenagers
 in 2006 79
Percent of Reported Legal Abortions Obtained by
 Teenagers in 2006 80
Reported Legal Abortions Obtained by Teenagers
 17 Years and Younger in 2006. 81
Percent of Reported Legal Abortions Obtained by
 Teenagers 17 Years and Younger in 2006. 82
Percent of Teenage Abortions Obtained by Teenagers
 17 Years and Younger in 2006. 83
Reported Legal Abortions Performed at 12 Weeks or
 Fewer of Gestation in 2006 84
Percent of Reported Legal Abortions Performed at
 12 Weeks or Fewer of Gestation in 2006. 85
Reported Legal Abortions Performed at or after 21 Weeks
 of Gestation in 2006. 86
Percent of Reported Legal Abortions Performed at or after
 21 Weeks of Gestation in 2006 87

Births in 2009

National Total = 4,131,019 Live Births*

ALPHA ORDER

RANK	STATE	BIRTHS	% of USA
24	Alabama	62,476	1.5%
47	Alaska	11,325	0.3%
13	Arizona	92,816	2.2%
32	Arkansas	39,853	1.0%
1	California	527,011	12.8%
22	Colorado	68,627	1.7%
34	Connecticut	38,896	0.9%
45	Delaware	11,562	0.3%
4	Florida	221,391	5.4%
8	Georgia	141,375	3.4%
40	Hawaii	18,888	0.5%
38	Idaho	23,731	0.6%
5	Illinois	171,255	4.1%
15	Indiana	86,698	2.1%
33	Iowa	39,700	1.0%
31	Kansas	41,396	1.0%
26	Kentucky	57,558	1.4%
23	Louisiana	64,988	1.6%
41	Maine	13,470	0.3%
19	Maryland	75,061	1.8%
18	Massachusetts	75,104	1.8%
10	Michigan	117,293	2.8%
21	Minnesota	70,648	1.7%
30	Mississippi	42,905	1.0%
17	Missouri	78,920	1.9%
43	Montana	12,261	0.3%
37	Nebraska	26,937	0.7%
35	Nevada	37,627	0.9%
42	New Hampshire	13,378	0.3%
11	New Jersey	110,324	2.7%
36	New Mexico	29,002	0.7%
3	New York	248,110	6.0%
9	North Carolina	126,846	3.1%
48	North Dakota	9,001	0.2%
7	Ohio	144,772	3.5%
27	Oklahoma	54,574	1.3%
29	Oregon	47,199	1.1%
6	Pennsylvania	146,432	3.5%
46	Rhode Island	11,443	0.3%
25	South Carolina	60,632	1.5%
44	South Dakota	11,935	0.3%
16	Tennessee	82,213	2.0%
2	Texas	402,011	9.7%
28	Utah	53,887	1.3%
50	Vermont	6,109	0.1%
12	Virginia	105,056	2.5%
14	Washington	89,284	2.2%
39	West Virginia	21,270	0.5%
20	Wisconsin	70,840	1.7%
49	Wyoming	7,884	0.2%

RANK ORDER

RANK	STATE	BIRTHS	% of USA
1	California	527,011	12.8%
2	Texas	402,011	9.7%
3	New York	248,110	6.0%
4	Florida	221,391	5.4%
5	Illinois	171,255	4.1%
6	Pennsylvania	146,432	3.5%
7	Ohio	144,772	3.5%
8	Georgia	141,375	3.4%
9	North Carolina	126,846	3.1%
10	Michigan	117,293	2.8%
11	New Jersey	110,324	2.7%
12	Virginia	105,056	2.5%
13	Arizona	92,816	2.2%
14	Washington	89,284	2.2%
15	Indiana	86,698	2.1%
16	Tennessee	82,213	2.0%
17	Missouri	78,920	1.9%
18	Massachusetts	75,104	1.8%
19	Maryland	75,061	1.8%
20	Wisconsin	70,840	1.7%
21	Minnesota	70,648	1.7%
22	Colorado	68,627	1.7%
23	Louisiana	64,988	1.6%
24	Alabama	62,476	1.5%
25	South Carolina	60,632	1.5%
26	Kentucky	57,558	1.4%
27	Oklahoma	54,574	1.3%
28	Utah	53,887	1.3%
29	Oregon	47,199	1.1%
30	Mississippi	42,905	1.0%
31	Kansas	41,396	1.0%
32	Arkansas	39,853	1.0%
33	Iowa	39,700	1.0%
34	Connecticut	38,896	0.9%
35	Nevada	37,627	0.9%
36	New Mexico	29,002	0.7%
37	Nebraska	26,937	0.7%
38	Idaho	23,731	0.6%
39	West Virginia	21,270	0.5%
40	Hawaii	18,888	0.5%
41	Maine	13,470	0.3%
42	New Hampshire	13,378	0.3%
43	Montana	12,261	0.3%
44	South Dakota	11,935	0.3%
45	Delaware	11,562	0.3%
46	Rhode Island	11,443	0.3%
47	Alaska	11,325	0.3%
48	North Dakota	9,001	0.2%
49	Wyoming	7,884	0.2%
50	Vermont	6,109	0.1%
	District of Columbia	9,044	0.2%

Source: U.S. Department of Health and Human Services, National Center for Health Statistics
"National Vital Statistics Reports" (Vol. 59, No. 3, December 21, 2010, http://www.cdc.gov/nchs/births.htm)
*Preliminary data by state of residence.

Birth Rate in 2009

National Rate = 13.5 Live Births per 1,000 Population*

ALPHA ORDER

RANK	STATE	RATE
25	Alabama	13.3
2	Alaska	16.2
17	Arizona	14.1
19	Arkansas	13.8
15	California	14.3
20	Colorado	13.7
46	Connecticut	11.1
33	Delaware	13.1
41	Florida	11.9
13	Georgia	14.4
9	Hawaii	14.6
4	Idaho	15.4
25	Illinois	13.3
21	Indiana	13.5
30	Iowa	13.2
7	Kansas	14.7
25	Kentucky	13.3
10	Louisiana	14.5
48	Maine	10.2
30	Maryland	13.2
45	Massachusetts	11.4
42	Michigan	11.8
23	Minnesota	13.4
10	Mississippi	14.5
30	Missouri	13.2
37	Montana	12.6
5	Nebraska	15.0
16	Nevada	14.2
49	New Hampshire	10.1
35	New Jersey	12.7
13	New Mexico	14.4
35	New York	12.7
21	North Carolina	13.5
18	North Dakota	13.9
38	Ohio	12.5
6	Oklahoma	14.8
40	Oregon	12.3
44	Pennsylvania	11.6
47	Rhode Island	10.9
25	South Carolina	13.3
7	South Dakota	14.7
33	Tennessee	13.1
2	Texas	16.2
1	Utah	19.4
50	Vermont	9.8
25	Virginia	13.3
23	Washington	13.4
43	West Virginia	11.7
38	Wisconsin	12.5
10	Wyoming	14.5

RANK ORDER

RANK	STATE	RATE
1	Utah	19.4
2	Alaska	16.2
2	Texas	16.2
4	Idaho	15.4
5	Nebraska	15.0
6	Oklahoma	14.8
7	Kansas	14.7
7	South Dakota	14.7
9	Hawaii	14.6
10	Louisiana	14.5
10	Mississippi	14.5
10	Wyoming	14.5
13	Georgia	14.4
13	New Mexico	14.4
15	California	14.3
16	Nevada	14.2
17	Arizona	14.1
18	North Dakota	13.9
19	Arkansas	13.8
20	Colorado	13.7
21	Indiana	13.5
21	North Carolina	13.5
23	Minnesota	13.4
23	Washington	13.4
25	Alabama	13.3
25	Illinois	13.3
25	Kentucky	13.3
25	South Carolina	13.3
25	Virginia	13.3
30	Iowa	13.2
30	Maryland	13.2
30	Missouri	13.2
33	Delaware	13.1
33	Tennessee	13.1
35	New Jersey	12.7
35	New York	12.7
37	Montana	12.6
38	Ohio	12.5
38	Wisconsin	12.5
40	Oregon	12.3
41	Florida	11.9
42	Michigan	11.8
43	West Virginia	11.7
44	Pennsylvania	11.6
45	Massachusetts	11.4
46	Connecticut	11.1
47	Rhode Island	10.9
48	Maine	10.2
49	New Hampshire	10.1
50	Vermont	9.8
	District of Columbia	15.1

Source: U.S. Department of Health and Human Services, National Center for Health Statistics
"National Vital Statistics Reports" (Vol. 59, No. 3, December 21, 2010, http://www.cdc.gov/nchs/births.htm)
*Preliminary data by state of residence.

Percent Change in Birth Rate: 2000 to 2009

National Percent Change = 6.3% Decrease*

ALPHA ORDER			RANK ORDER		
RANK	STATE	PERCENT CHANGE	RANK	STATE	PERCENT CHANGE
26	Alabama	(6.3)	1	North Dakota	15.8
7	Alaska	1.9	2	Wyoming	14.2
50	Arizona	(15.1)	3	South Dakota	7.3
13	Arkansas	(2.1)	4	Nebraska	4.2
41	California	(8.9)	5	Montana	4.1
43	Colorado	(9.9)	6	Oklahoma	2.8
47	Connecticut	(11.9)	7	Alaska	1.9
33	Delaware	(7.1)	8	West Virginia	1.7
32	Florida	(7.0)	9	Iowa	0.8
45	Georgia	(11.1)	10	Hawaii	0.7
10	Hawaii	0.7	11	Kansas	(0.7)
12	Idaho	(1.9)	12	Idaho	(1.9)
44	Illinois	(10.7)	13	Arkansas	(2.1)
26	Indiana	(6.3)	14	Minnesota	(2.2)
9	Iowa	0.8	14	Washington	(2.2)
11	Kansas	(0.7)	16	Pennsylvania	(2.5)
20	Kentucky	(4.3)	17	Wisconsin	(3.1)
21	Louisiana	(4.6)	18	Missouri	(3.6)
22	Maine	(4.7)	19	New Mexico	(4.0)
25	Maryland	(5.7)	20	Kentucky	(4.3)
46	Massachusetts	(11.6)	21	Louisiana	(4.6)
48	Michigan	(13.9)	22	Maine	(4.7)
14	Minnesota	(2.2)	23	South Carolina	(5.0)
29	Mississippi	(6.5)	23	Virginia	(5.0)
18	Missouri	(3.6)	25	Maryland	(5.7)
5	Montana	4.1	26	Alabama	(6.3)
4	Nebraska	4.2	26	Indiana	(6.3)
35	Nevada	(7.8)	28	Tennessee	(6.4)
49	New Hampshire	(14.4)	29	Mississippi	(6.5)
34	New Jersey	(7.3)	30	New York	(6.6)
19	New Mexico	(4.0)	31	Texas	(6.9)
30	New York	(6.6)	32	Florida	(7.0)
42	North Carolina	(9.4)	33	Delaware	(7.1)
1	North Dakota	15.8	34	New Jersey	(7.3)
40	Ohio	(8.8)	35	Nevada	(7.8)
6	Oklahoma	2.8	36	Oregon	(8.2)
36	Oregon	(8.2)	37	Rhode Island	(8.4)
16	Pennsylvania	(2.5)	37	Vermont	(8.4)
37	Rhode Island	(8.4)	39	Utah	(8.5)
23	South Carolina	(5.0)	40	Ohio	(8.8)
3	South Dakota	7.3	41	California	(8.9)
28	Tennessee	(6.4)	42	North Carolina	(9.4)
31	Texas	(6.9)	43	Colorado	(9.9)
39	Utah	(8.5)	44	Illinois	(10.7)
37	Vermont	(8.4)	45	Georgia	(11.1)
23	Virginia	(5.0)	46	Massachusetts	(11.6)
14	Washington	(2.2)	47	Connecticut	(11.9)
8	West Virginia	1.7	48	Michigan	(13.9)
17	Wisconsin	(3.1)	49	New Hampshire	(14.4)
2	Wyoming	14.2	50	Arizona	(15.1)

District of Columbia   12.7

Source: CQ Press using data from U.S. Department of Health and Human Services, National Center for Health Statistics
"National Vital Statistics Reports" (Vol. 59, No. 3, December 21, 2010, http://www.cdc.gov/nchs/births.htm) and
"VitalStats" (http://www.cdc.gov/nchs/nvss.htm)
*By state of residence.

Fertility Rate in 2009

National Rate = 66.7 Live Births per 1,000 Women 15 to 44 Years Old*

<table>
<tr><td colspan="3">ALPHA ORDER</td><td colspan="3">RANK ORDER</td></tr>
<tr><td>RANK</td><td>STATE</td><td>RATE</td><td>RANK</td><td>STATE</td><td>RATE</td></tr>
<tr><td>30</td><td>Alabama</td><td>65.7</td><td>1</td><td>Utah</td><td>88.4</td></tr>
<tr><td>2</td><td>Alaska</td><td>78.3</td><td>2</td><td>Alaska</td><td>78.3</td></tr>
<tr><td>12</td><td>Arizona</td><td>71.5</td><td>3</td><td>South Dakota</td><td>77.8</td></tr>
<tr><td>16</td><td>Arkansas</td><td>70.1</td><td>4</td><td>Texas</td><td>77.6</td></tr>
<tr><td>19</td><td>California</td><td>68.5</td><td>5</td><td>Idaho</td><td>77.4</td></tr>
<tr><td>24</td><td>Colorado</td><td>66.8</td><td>6</td><td>Nebraska</td><td>76.4</td></tr>
<tr><td>45</td><td>Connecticut</td><td>56.5</td><td>7</td><td>Hawaii</td><td>75.8</td></tr>
<tr><td>31</td><td>Delaware</td><td>65.4</td><td>8</td><td>Wyoming</td><td>75.0</td></tr>
<tr><td>39</td><td>Florida</td><td>63.6</td><td>9</td><td>Oklahoma</td><td>74.9</td></tr>
<tr><td>20</td><td>Georgia</td><td>67.7</td><td>10</td><td>Kansas</td><td>74.7</td></tr>
<tr><td>7</td><td>Hawaii</td><td>75.8</td><td>11</td><td>New Mexico</td><td>73.4</td></tr>
<tr><td>5</td><td>Idaho</td><td>77.4</td><td>12</td><td>Arizona</td><td>71.5</td></tr>
<tr><td>32</td><td>Illinois</td><td>64.7</td><td>13</td><td>Nevada</td><td>71.2</td></tr>
<tr><td>21</td><td>Indiana</td><td>67.6</td><td>14</td><td>Mississippi</td><td>70.9</td></tr>
<tr><td>18</td><td>Iowa</td><td>68.7</td><td>15</td><td>North Dakota</td><td>70.8</td></tr>
<tr><td>10</td><td>Kansas</td><td>74.7</td><td>16</td><td>Arkansas</td><td>70.1</td></tr>
<tr><td>25</td><td>Kentucky</td><td>66.6</td><td>17</td><td>Louisiana</td><td>69.8</td></tr>
<tr><td>17</td><td>Louisiana</td><td>69.8</td><td>18</td><td>Iowa</td><td>68.7</td></tr>
<tr><td>47</td><td>Maine</td><td>54.8</td><td>19</td><td>California</td><td>68.5</td></tr>
<tr><td>36</td><td>Maryland</td><td>63.8</td><td>20</td><td>Georgia</td><td>67.7</td></tr>
<tr><td>46</td><td>Massachusetts</td><td>55.4</td><td>21</td><td>Indiana</td><td>67.6</td></tr>
<tr><td>44</td><td>Michigan</td><td>59.8</td><td>22</td><td>Minnesota</td><td>67.5</td></tr>
<tr><td>22</td><td>Minnesota</td><td>67.5</td><td>23</td><td>Montana</td><td>67.3</td></tr>
<tr><td>14</td><td>Mississippi</td><td>70.9</td><td>24</td><td>Colorado</td><td>66.8</td></tr>
<tr><td>29</td><td>Missouri</td><td>66.2</td><td>25</td><td>Kentucky</td><td>66.6</td></tr>
<tr><td>23</td><td>Montana</td><td>67.3</td><td>26</td><td>Washington</td><td>66.4</td></tr>
<tr><td>6</td><td>Nebraska</td><td>76.4</td><td>27</td><td>North Carolina</td><td>66.3</td></tr>
<tr><td>13</td><td>Nevada</td><td>71.2</td><td>27</td><td>South Carolina</td><td>66.3</td></tr>
<tr><td>49</td><td>New Hampshire</td><td>51.9</td><td>29</td><td>Missouri</td><td>66.2</td></tr>
<tr><td>34</td><td>New Jersey</td><td>64.5</td><td>30</td><td>Alabama</td><td>65.7</td></tr>
<tr><td>11</td><td>New Mexico</td><td>73.4</td><td>31</td><td>Delaware</td><td>65.4</td></tr>
<tr><td>41</td><td>New York</td><td>61.7</td><td>32</td><td>Illinois</td><td>64.7</td></tr>
<tr><td>27</td><td>North Carolina</td><td>66.3</td><td>32</td><td>Tennessee</td><td>64.7</td></tr>
<tr><td>15</td><td>North Dakota</td><td>70.8</td><td>34</td><td>New Jersey</td><td>64.5</td></tr>
<tr><td>36</td><td>Ohio</td><td>63.8</td><td>35</td><td>Virginia</td><td>64.4</td></tr>
<tr><td>9</td><td>Oklahoma</td><td>74.9</td><td>36</td><td>Maryland</td><td>63.8</td></tr>
<tr><td>40</td><td>Oregon</td><td>62.5</td><td>36</td><td>Ohio</td><td>63.8</td></tr>
<tr><td>43</td><td>Pennsylvania</td><td>60.1</td><td>38</td><td>Wisconsin</td><td>63.7</td></tr>
<tr><td>48</td><td>Rhode Island</td><td>53.6</td><td>39</td><td>Florida</td><td>63.6</td></tr>
<tr><td>27</td><td>South Carolina</td><td>66.3</td><td>40</td><td>Oregon</td><td>62.5</td></tr>
<tr><td>3</td><td>South Dakota</td><td>77.8</td><td>41</td><td>New York</td><td>61.7</td></tr>
<tr><td>32</td><td>Tennessee</td><td>64.7</td><td>41</td><td>West Virginia</td><td>61.7</td></tr>
<tr><td>4</td><td>Texas</td><td>77.6</td><td>43</td><td>Pennsylvania</td><td>60.1</td></tr>
<tr><td>1</td><td>Utah</td><td>88.4</td><td>44</td><td>Michigan</td><td>59.8</td></tr>
<tr><td>50</td><td>Vermont</td><td>50.8</td><td>45</td><td>Connecticut</td><td>56.5</td></tr>
<tr><td>35</td><td>Virginia</td><td>64.4</td><td>46</td><td>Massachusetts</td><td>55.4</td></tr>
<tr><td>26</td><td>Washington</td><td>66.4</td><td>47</td><td>Maine</td><td>54.8</td></tr>
<tr><td>41</td><td>West Virginia</td><td>61.7</td><td>48</td><td>Rhode Island</td><td>53.6</td></tr>
<tr><td>38</td><td>Wisconsin</td><td>63.7</td><td>49</td><td>New Hampshire</td><td>51.9</td></tr>
<tr><td>8</td><td>Wyoming</td><td>75.0</td><td>50</td><td>Vermont</td><td>50.8</td></tr>
<tr><td></td><td></td><td></td><td></td><td>District of Columbia</td><td>60.0</td></tr>
</table>

Source: U.S. Department of Health and Human Services, National Center for Health Statistics
"National Vital Statistics Reports" (Vol. 59, No. 3, December 21, 2010, http://www.cdc.gov/nchs/births.htm)
*Preliminary data by state of residence.

Births to White Women in 2009

National Total = 2,211,960 Live Births to White Women*

<table>
<tr><td colspan="4">ALPHA ORDER</td><td colspan="4">RANK ORDER</td></tr>
<tr><td>RANK</td><td>STATE</td><td>BIRTHS</td><td>% of USA</td><td>RANK</td><td>STATE</td><td>BIRTHS</td><td>% of USA</td></tr>
<tr><td>24</td><td>Alabama</td><td>36,902</td><td>1.7%</td><td>1</td><td>California</td><td>146,392</td><td>6.6%</td></tr>
<tr><td>48</td><td>Alaska</td><td>6,018</td><td>0.3%</td><td>2</td><td>Texas</td><td>137,603</td><td>6.2%</td></tr>
<tr><td>23</td><td>Arizona</td><td>40,044</td><td>1.8%</td><td>3</td><td>New York</td><td>119,530</td><td>5.4%</td></tr>
<tr><td>32</td><td>Arkansas</td><td>26,998</td><td>1.2%</td><td>4</td><td>Ohio</td><td>109,698</td><td>5.0%</td></tr>
<tr><td>1</td><td>California</td><td>146,392</td><td>6.6%</td><td>5</td><td>Pennsylvania</td><td>103,302</td><td>4.7%</td></tr>
<tr><td>22</td><td>Colorado</td><td>41,169</td><td>1.9%</td><td>6</td><td>Florida</td><td>100,575</td><td>4.5%</td></tr>
<tr><td>33</td><td>Connecticut</td><td>22,798</td><td>1.0%</td><td>7</td><td>Illinois</td><td>90,964</td><td>4.1%</td></tr>
<tr><td>47</td><td>Delaware</td><td>6,183</td><td>0.3%</td><td>8</td><td>Michigan</td><td>81,218</td><td>3.7%</td></tr>
<tr><td>6</td><td>Florida</td><td>100,575</td><td>4.5%</td><td>9</td><td>North Carolina</td><td>70,428</td><td>3.2%</td></tr>
<tr><td>11</td><td>Georgia</td><td>61,732</td><td>2.8%</td><td>10</td><td>Indiana</td><td>66,345</td><td>3.0%</td></tr>
<tr><td>50</td><td>Hawaii</td><td>4,603</td><td>0.2%</td><td>11</td><td>Georgia</td><td>61,732</td><td>2.8%</td></tr>
<tr><td>37</td><td>Idaho</td><td>19,048</td><td>0.9%</td><td>12</td><td>Virginia</td><td>60,404</td><td>2.7%</td></tr>
<tr><td>7</td><td>Illinois</td><td>90,964</td><td>4.1%</td><td>13</td><td>Missouri</td><td>60,184</td><td>2.7%</td></tr>
<tr><td>10</td><td>Indiana</td><td>66,345</td><td>3.0%</td><td>14</td><td>Washington</td><td>56,543</td><td>2.6%</td></tr>
<tr><td>29</td><td>Iowa</td><td>33,381</td><td>1.5%</td><td>15</td><td>Tennessee</td><td>55,446</td><td>2.5%</td></tr>
<tr><td>31</td><td>Kansas</td><td>29,856</td><td>1.3%</td><td>16</td><td>Wisconsin</td><td>52,460</td><td>2.4%</td></tr>
<tr><td>20</td><td>Kentucky</td><td>48,059</td><td>2.2%</td><td>17</td><td>New Jersey</td><td>52,161</td><td>2.4%</td></tr>
<tr><td>26</td><td>Louisiana</td><td>34,591</td><td>1.6%</td><td>18</td><td>Minnesota</td><td>51,290</td><td>2.3%</td></tr>
<tr><td>39</td><td>Maine</td><td>12,504</td><td>0.6%</td><td>19</td><td>Massachusetts</td><td>50,411</td><td>2.3%</td></tr>
<tr><td>27</td><td>Maryland</td><td>34,014</td><td>1.5%</td><td>20</td><td>Kentucky</td><td>48,059</td><td>2.2%</td></tr>
<tr><td>19</td><td>Massachusetts</td><td>50,411</td><td>2.3%</td><td>21</td><td>Utah</td><td>42,388</td><td>1.9%</td></tr>
<tr><td>8</td><td>Michigan</td><td>81,218</td><td>3.7%</td><td>22</td><td>Colorado</td><td>41,169</td><td>1.9%</td></tr>
<tr><td>18</td><td>Minnesota</td><td>51,290</td><td>2.3%</td><td>23</td><td>Arizona</td><td>40,044</td><td>1.8%</td></tr>
<tr><td>34</td><td>Mississippi</td><td>21,510</td><td>1.0%</td><td>24</td><td>Alabama</td><td>36,902</td><td>1.7%</td></tr>
<tr><td>13</td><td>Missouri</td><td>60,184</td><td>2.7%</td><td>25</td><td>Oklahoma</td><td>34,734</td><td>1.6%</td></tr>
<tr><td>41</td><td>Montana</td><td>10,002</td><td>0.5%</td><td>26</td><td>Louisiana</td><td>34,591</td><td>1.6%</td></tr>
<tr><td>36</td><td>Nebraska</td><td>19,783</td><td>0.9%</td><td>27</td><td>Maryland</td><td>34,014</td><td>1.5%</td></tr>
<tr><td>38</td><td>Nevada</td><td>15,939</td><td>0.7%</td><td>28</td><td>South Carolina</td><td>33,985</td><td>1.5%</td></tr>
<tr><td>40</td><td>New Hampshire</td><td>11,955</td><td>0.5%</td><td>29</td><td>Iowa</td><td>33,381</td><td>1.5%</td></tr>
<tr><td>17</td><td>New Jersey</td><td>52,161</td><td>2.4%</td><td>30</td><td>Oregon</td><td>32,849</td><td>1.5%</td></tr>
<tr><td>43</td><td>New Mexico</td><td>8,081</td><td>0.4%</td><td>31</td><td>Kansas</td><td>29,856</td><td>1.3%</td></tr>
<tr><td>3</td><td>New York</td><td>119,530</td><td>5.4%</td><td>32</td><td>Arkansas</td><td>26,998</td><td>1.2%</td></tr>
<tr><td>9</td><td>North Carolina</td><td>70,428</td><td>3.2%</td><td>33</td><td>Connecticut</td><td>22,798</td><td>1.0%</td></tr>
<tr><td>44</td><td>North Dakota</td><td>7,319</td><td>0.3%</td><td>34</td><td>Mississippi</td><td>21,510</td><td>1.0%</td></tr>
<tr><td>4</td><td>Ohio</td><td>109,698</td><td>5.0%</td><td>35</td><td>West Virginia</td><td>19,962</td><td>0.9%</td></tr>
<tr><td>25</td><td>Oklahoma</td><td>34,734</td><td>1.6%</td><td>36</td><td>Nebraska</td><td>19,783</td><td>0.9%</td></tr>
<tr><td>30</td><td>Oregon</td><td>32,849</td><td>1.5%</td><td>37</td><td>Idaho</td><td>19,048</td><td>0.9%</td></tr>
<tr><td>5</td><td>Pennsylvania</td><td>103,302</td><td>4.7%</td><td>38</td><td>Nevada</td><td>15,939</td><td>0.7%</td></tr>
<tr><td>45</td><td>Rhode Island</td><td>6,979</td><td>0.3%</td><td>39</td><td>Maine</td><td>12,504</td><td>0.6%</td></tr>
<tr><td>28</td><td>South Carolina</td><td>33,985</td><td>1.5%</td><td>40</td><td>New Hampshire</td><td>11,955</td><td>0.5%</td></tr>
<tr><td>42</td><td>South Dakota</td><td>9,118</td><td>0.4%</td><td>41</td><td>Montana</td><td>10,002</td><td>0.5%</td></tr>
<tr><td>15</td><td>Tennessee</td><td>55,446</td><td>2.5%</td><td>42</td><td>South Dakota</td><td>9,118</td><td>0.4%</td></tr>
<tr><td>2</td><td>Texas</td><td>137,603</td><td>6.2%</td><td>43</td><td>New Mexico</td><td>8,081</td><td>0.4%</td></tr>
<tr><td>21</td><td>Utah</td><td>42,388</td><td>1.9%</td><td>44</td><td>North Dakota</td><td>7,319</td><td>0.3%</td></tr>
<tr><td>49</td><td>Vermont</td><td>5,803</td><td>0.3%</td><td>45</td><td>Rhode Island</td><td>6,979</td><td>0.3%</td></tr>
<tr><td>12</td><td>Virginia</td><td>60,404</td><td>2.7%</td><td>46</td><td>Wyoming</td><td>6,355</td><td>0.3%</td></tr>
<tr><td>14</td><td>Washington</td><td>56,543</td><td>2.6%</td><td>47</td><td>Delaware</td><td>6,183</td><td>0.3%</td></tr>
<tr><td>35</td><td>West Virginia</td><td>19,962</td><td>0.9%</td><td>48</td><td>Alaska</td><td>6,018</td><td>0.3%</td></tr>
<tr><td>16</td><td>Wisconsin</td><td>52,460</td><td>2.4%</td><td>49</td><td>Vermont</td><td>5,803</td><td>0.3%</td></tr>
<tr><td>46</td><td>Wyoming</td><td>6,355</td><td>0.3%</td><td>50</td><td>Hawaii</td><td>4,603</td><td>0.2%</td></tr>
<tr><td></td><td></td><td></td><td></td><td></td><td>District of Columbia</td><td>2,344</td><td>0.1%</td></tr>
</table>

Source: U.S. Department of Health and Human Services, National Center for Health Statistics
"National Vital Statistics Reports" (Vol. 59, No. 3, December 21, 2010, http://www.cdc.gov/nchs/births.htm)
*Preliminary data by state of residence. By race of mother. Does not include births to white Hispanic mothers.

White Births as a Percent of All Births in 2009

National Percent = 53.5% of Live Births*

RANK	STATE	PERCENT
30	Alabama	59.1
37	Alaska	53.1
45	Arizona	43.1
23	Arkansas	67.7
49	California	27.8
29	Colorado	60.0
31	Connecticut	58.6
35	Delaware	53.5
42	Florida	45.4
44	Georgia	43.7
50	Hawaii	24.4
10	Idaho	80.3
37	Illinois	53.1
12	Indiana	76.5
5	Iowa	84.1
19	Kansas	72.1
6	Kentucky	83.5
36	Louisiana	53.2
3	Maine	92.8
43	Maryland	45.3
25	Massachusetts	67.1
22	Michigan	69.2
18	Minnesota	72.6
39	Mississippi	50.1
14	Missouri	76.3
7	Montana	81.6
17	Nebraska	73.4
46	Nevada	42.4
4	New Hampshire	89.4
41	New Jersey	47.3
48	New Mexico	27.9
40	New York	48.2
34	North Carolina	55.5
8	North Dakota	81.3
15	Ohio	75.8
26	Oklahoma	63.6
21	Oregon	69.6
20	Pennsylvania	70.5
28	Rhode Island	61.0
33	South Carolina	56.1
13	South Dakota	76.4
24	Tennessee	67.4
47	Texas	34.2
11	Utah	78.7
1	Vermont	95.0
32	Virginia	57.5
27	Washington	63.3
2	West Virginia	93.9
16	Wisconsin	74.1
9	Wyoming	80.6

RANK	STATE	PERCENT
1	Vermont	95.0
2	West Virginia	93.9
3	Maine	92.8
4	New Hampshire	89.4
5	Iowa	84.1
6	Kentucky	83.5
7	Montana	81.6
8	North Dakota	81.3
9	Wyoming	80.6
10	Idaho	80.3
11	Utah	78.7
12	Indiana	76.5
13	South Dakota	76.4
14	Missouri	76.3
15	Ohio	75.8
16	Wisconsin	74.1
17	Nebraska	73.4
18	Minnesota	72.6
19	Kansas	72.1
20	Pennsylvania	70.5
21	Oregon	69.6
22	Michigan	69.2
23	Arkansas	67.7
24	Tennessee	67.4
25	Massachusetts	67.1
26	Oklahoma	63.6
27	Washington	63.3
28	Rhode Island	61.0
29	Colorado	60.0
30	Alabama	59.1
31	Connecticut	58.6
32	Virginia	57.5
33	South Carolina	56.1
34	North Carolina	55.5
35	Delaware	53.5
36	Louisiana	53.2
37	Alaska	53.1
37	Illinois	53.1
39	Mississippi	50.1
40	New York	48.2
41	New Jersey	47.3
42	Florida	45.4
43	Maryland	45.3
44	Georgia	43.7
45	Arizona	43.1
46	Nevada	42.4
47	Texas	34.2
48	New Mexico	27.9
49	California	27.8
50	Hawaii	24.4

| | District of Columbia | 25.9 |

Source: CQ Press using data from U.S. Department of Health and Human Services, National Center for Health Statistics
"National Vital Statistics Reports" (Vol. 59, No. 3, December 21, 2010, http://www.cdc.gov/nchs/births.htm) and
*Preliminary data by state of residence. By race of mother. Does not include births to white Hispanic mothers.

Births to Black Women in 2009

National Total = 609,552 Live Births to Black Women*

ALPHA ORDER				RANK ORDER			
RANK	STATE	BIRTHS	% of USA	RANK	STATE	BIRTHS	% of USA
15	Alabama	19,230	3.2%	1	Florida	50,723	8.3%
42	Alaska	409	0.1%	2	Georgia	46,242	7.6%
28	Arizona	4,136	0.7%	3	Texas	45,493	7.5%
21	Arkansas	7,649	1.3%	4	New York	40,982	6.7%
5	California	31,090	5.1%	5	California	31,090	5.1%
32	Colorado	3,120	0.5%	6	North Carolina	30,317	5.0%
27	Connecticut	4,971	0.8%	7	Illinois	29,947	4.9%
31	Delaware	3,178	0.5%	8	Louisiana	25,150	4.1%
1	Florida	50,723	8.3%	9	Maryland	24,992	4.1%
2	Georgia	46,242	7.6%	10	Ohio	23,834	3.9%
41	Hawaii	411	0.1%	11	Virginia	23,021	3.8%
47	Idaho	136	0.0%	12	Michigan	22,071	3.6%
7	Illinois	29,947	4.9%	13	Pennsylvania	21,482	3.5%
20	Indiana	10,076	1.7%	14	South Carolina	19,480	3.2%
34	Iowa	1,907	0.3%	15	Alabama	19,230	3.2%
33	Kansas	3,063	0.5%	16	Mississippi	19,043	3.1%
25	Kentucky	5,438	0.9%	17	Tennessee	17,405	2.9%
8	Louisiana	25,150	4.1%	18	New Jersey	17,131	2.8%
43	Maine	392	0.1%	19	Missouri	12,026	2.0%
9	Maryland	24,992	4.1%	20	Indiana	10,076	1.7%
23	Massachusetts	7,228	1.2%	21	Arkansas	7,649	1.3%
12	Michigan	22,071	3.6%	22	Wisconsin	7,288	1.2%
24	Minnesota	6,475	1.1%	23	Massachusetts	7,228	1.2%
16	Mississippi	19,043	3.1%	24	Minnesota	6,475	1.1%
19	Missouri	12,026	2.0%	25	Kentucky	5,438	0.9%
49	Montana	65	0.0%	26	Oklahoma	5,086	0.8%
35	Nebraska	1,759	0.3%	27	Connecticut	4,971	0.8%
30	Nevada	3,602	0.6%	28	Arizona	4,136	0.7%
45	New Hampshire	217	0.0%	29	Washington	4,083	0.7%
18	New Jersey	17,131	2.8%	30	Nevada	3,602	0.6%
40	New Mexico	513	0.1%	31	Delaware	3,178	0.5%
4	New York	40,982	6.7%	32	Colorado	3,120	0.5%
6	North Carolina	30,317	5.0%	33	Kansas	3,063	0.5%
46	North Dakota	162	0.0%	34	Iowa	1,907	0.3%
10	Ohio	23,834	3.9%	35	Nebraska	1,759	0.3%
26	Oklahoma	5,086	0.8%	36	Oregon	1,144	0.2%
36	Oregon	1,144	0.2%	37	Rhode Island	906	0.1%
13	Pennsylvania	21,482	3.5%	38	West Virginia	831	0.1%
37	Rhode Island	906	0.1%	39	Utah	548	0.1%
14	South Carolina	19,480	3.2%	40	New Mexico	513	0.1%
44	South Dakota	247	0.0%	41	Hawaii	411	0.1%
17	Tennessee	17,405	2.9%	42	Alaska	409	0.1%
3	Texas	45,493	7.5%	43	Maine	392	0.1%
39	Utah	548	0.1%	44	South Dakota	247	0.0%
48	Vermont	76	0.0%	45	New Hampshire	217	0.0%
11	Virginia	23,021	3.8%	46	North Dakota	162	0.0%
29	Washington	4,083	0.7%	47	Idaho	136	0.0%
38	West Virginia	831	0.1%	48	Vermont	76	0.0%
22	Wisconsin	7,288	1.2%	49	Montana	65	0.0%
50	Wyoming	56	0.0%	50	Wyoming	56	0.0%
					District of Columbia	4,720	0.8%

Source: U.S. Department of Health and Human Services, National Center for Health Statistics
 "National Vital Statistics Reports" (Vol. 59, No. 3, December 21, 2010, http://www.cdc.gov/nchs/births.htm)
*Preliminary data by state of residence. By race of mother. Does not include births to black Hispanic mothers.

Black Births as a Percent of All Births in 2009

National Percent = 14.8% of Live Births*

RANK	STATE	PERCENT
6	Alabama	30.8
38	Alaska	3.6
35	Arizona	4.5
12	Arkansas	19.2
32	California	5.9
35	Colorado	4.5
20	Connecticut	12.8
7	Delaware	27.5
9	Florida	22.9
4	Georgia	32.7
41	Hawaii	2.2
49	Idaho	0.6
14	Illinois	17.5
21	Indiana	11.6
33	Iowa	4.8
30	Kansas	7.4
26	Kentucky	9.4
2	Louisiana	38.7
39	Maine	2.9
3	Maryland	33.3
24	Massachusetts	9.6
13	Michigan	18.8
28	Minnesota	9.2
1	Mississippi	44.4
18	Missouri	15.2
50	Montana	0.5
31	Nebraska	6.5
24	Nevada	9.6
45	New Hampshire	1.6
17	New Jersey	15.5
43	New Mexico	1.8
15	New York	16.5
8	North Carolina	23.9
43	North Dakota	1.8
15	Ohio	16.5
27	Oklahoma	9.3
40	Oregon	2.4
19	Pennsylvania	14.7
29	Rhode Island	7.9
5	South Carolina	32.1
42	South Dakota	2.1
11	Tennessee	21.2
22	Texas	11.3
47	Utah	1.0
46	Vermont	1.2
10	Virginia	21.9
34	Washington	4.6
37	West Virginia	3.9
23	Wisconsin	10.3
48	Wyoming	0.7

RANK	STATE	PERCENT
1	Mississippi	44.4
2	Louisiana	38.7
3	Maryland	33.3
4	Georgia	32.7
5	South Carolina	32.1
6	Alabama	30.8
7	Delaware	27.5
8	North Carolina	23.9
9	Florida	22.9
10	Virginia	21.9
11	Tennessee	21.2
12	Arkansas	19.2
13	Michigan	18.8
14	Illinois	17.5
15	New York	16.5
15	Ohio	16.5
17	New Jersey	15.5
18	Missouri	15.2
19	Pennsylvania	14.7
20	Connecticut	12.8
21	Indiana	11.6
22	Texas	11.3
23	Wisconsin	10.3
24	Massachusetts	9.6
24	Nevada	9.6
26	Kentucky	9.4
27	Oklahoma	9.3
28	Minnesota	9.2
29	Rhode Island	7.9
30	Kansas	7.4
31	Nebraska	6.5
32	California	5.9
33	Iowa	4.8
34	Washington	4.6
35	Arizona	4.5
35	Colorado	4.5
37	West Virginia	3.9
38	Alaska	3.6
39	Maine	2.9
40	Oregon	2.4
41	Hawaii	2.2
42	South Dakota	2.1
43	New Mexico	1.8
43	North Dakota	1.8
45	New Hampshire	1.6
46	Vermont	1.2
47	Utah	1.0
48	Wyoming	0.7
49	Idaho	0.6
50	Montana	0.5
	District of Columbia	52.2

Source: CQ Press using data from U.S. Department of Health and Human Services, National Center for Health Statistics
"National Vital Statistics Reports" (Vol. 59, No. 3, December 21, 2010, http://www.cdc.gov/nchs/births.htm)
*Preliminary data by state of residence. By race of mother. Does not include births to black Hispanic mothers.

Births to Hispanic Women in 2009

National Total = 999,632 Live Births to Hispanic Women*

ALPHA ORDER					RANK ORDER			
RANK	STATE	BIRTHS	% of USA		RANK	STATE	BIRTHS	% of USA
30	Alabama	5,134	0.5%		1	California	270,239	27.0%
43	Alaska	695	0.1%		2	Texas	201,241	20.1%
6	Arizona	39,176	3.9%		3	Florida	61,987	6.2%
33	Arkansas	4,208	0.4%		4	New York	59,791	6.0%
1	California	270,239	27.0%		5	Illinois	40,425	4.0%
9	Colorado	20,680	2.1%		6	Arizona	39,176	3.9%
20	Connecticut	8,589	0.9%		7	New Jersey	29,003	2.9%
40	Delaware	1,648	0.2%		8	Georgia	24,595	2.5%
3	Florida	61,987	6.2%		9	Colorado	20,680	2.1%
8	Georgia	24,595	2.5%		10	North Carolina	20,171	2.0%
37	Hawaii	3,135	0.3%		11	Washington	17,189	1.7%
34	Idaho	3,681	0.4%		12	New Mexico	16,159	1.6%
5	Illinois	40,425	4.0%		13	Nevada	14,353	1.4%
21	Indiana	8,079	0.8%		14	Pennsylvania	14,115	1.4%
36	Iowa	3,210	0.3%		15	Virginia	13,688	1.4%
27	Kansas	6,795	0.7%		16	Massachusetts	11,021	1.1%
38	Kentucky	2,986	0.3%		17	Maryland	10,612	1.1%
35	Louisiana	3,558	0.4%		18	Oregon	9,701	1.0%
49	Maine	198	0.0%		19	Utah	8,773	0.9%
17	Maryland	10,612	1.1%		20	Connecticut	8,589	0.9%
16	Massachusetts	11,021	1.1%		21	Indiana	8,079	0.8%
22	Michigan	7,921	0.8%		22	Michigan	7,921	0.8%
28	Minnesota	5,625	0.6%		23	Tennessee	7,433	0.7%
41	Mississippi	1,514	0.2%		24	Oklahoma	7,273	0.7%
31	Missouri	4,290	0.4%		25	Wisconsin	6,934	0.7%
46	Montana	424	0.0%		26	Ohio	6,892	0.7%
32	Nebraska	4,265	0.4%		27	Kansas	6,795	0.7%
13	Nevada	14,353	1.4%		28	Minnesota	5,625	0.6%
44	New Hampshire	552	0.1%		29	South Carolina	5,562	0.6%
7	New Jersey	29,003	2.9%		30	Alabama	5,134	0.5%
12	New Mexico	16,159	1.6%		31	Missouri	4,290	0.4%
4	New York	59,791	6.0%		32	Nebraska	4,265	0.4%
10	North Carolina	20,171	2.0%		33	Arkansas	4,208	0.4%
47	North Dakota	312	0.0%		34	Idaho	3,681	0.4%
26	Ohio	6,892	0.7%		35	Louisiana	3,558	0.4%
24	Oklahoma	7,273	0.7%		36	Iowa	3,210	0.3%
18	Oregon	9,701	1.0%		37	Hawaii	3,135	0.3%
14	Pennsylvania	14,115	1.4%		38	Kentucky	2,986	0.3%
39	Rhode Island	2,508	0.3%		39	Rhode Island	2,508	0.3%
29	South Carolina	5,562	0.6%		40	Delaware	1,648	0.2%
45	South Dakota	476	0.0%		41	Mississippi	1,514	0.2%
23	Tennessee	7,433	0.7%		42	Wyoming	981	0.1%
2	Texas	201,241	20.1%		43	Alaska	695	0.1%
19	Utah	8,773	0.9%		44	New Hampshire	552	0.1%
50	Vermont	94	0.0%		45	South Dakota	476	0.0%
15	Virginia	13,688	1.4%		46	Montana	424	0.0%
11	Washington	17,189	1.7%		47	North Dakota	312	0.0%
48	West Virginia	231	0.0%		48	West Virginia	231	0.0%
25	Wisconsin	6,934	0.7%		49	Maine	198	0.0%
42	Wyoming	981	0.1%		50	Vermont	94	0.0%
						District of Columbia	1,510	0.2%

Source: U.S. Department of Health and Human Services, National Center for Health Statistics
   "National Vital Statistics Reports" (Vol. 59, No. 3, December 21, 2010, http://www.cdc.gov/nchs/births.htm)
*Preliminary data by state of residence. By race of mother. Persons of Hispanic origin may be of any race.

Hispanic Births as a Percent of All Births in 2009

National Percent = 24.2% of Live Births*

ALPHA ORDER				RANK ORDER		
RANK	STATE	PERCENT		RANK	STATE	PERCENT
34	Alabama	8.2		1	New Mexico	55.7
38	Alaska	6.1		2	California	51.3
4	Arizona	42.2		3	Texas	50.1
28	Arkansas	10.6		4	Arizona	42.2
2	California	51.3		5	Nevada	38.1
6	Colorado	30.1		6	Colorado	30.1
11	Connecticut	22.1		7	Florida	28.0
23	Delaware	14.3		8	New Jersey	26.3
7	Florida	28.0		9	New York	24.1
15	Georgia	17.4		10	Illinois	23.6
16	Hawaii	16.6		11	Connecticut	22.1
21	Idaho	15.5		12	Rhode Island	21.9
10	Illinois	23.6		13	Oregon	20.6
31	Indiana	9.3		14	Washington	19.3
35	Iowa	8.1		15	Georgia	17.4
17	Kansas	16.4		16	Hawaii	16.6
41	Kentucky	5.2		17	Kansas	16.4
39	Louisiana	5.5		18	Utah	16.3
48	Maine	1.5		19	North Carolina	15.9
24	Maryland	14.1		20	Nebraska	15.8
22	Massachusetts	14.7		21	Idaho	15.5
37	Michigan	6.8		22	Massachusetts	14.7
36	Minnesota	8.0		23	Delaware	14.3
45	Mississippi	3.5		24	Maryland	14.1
40	Missouri	5.4		25	Oklahoma	13.3
45	Montana	3.5		26	Virginia	13.0
20	Nebraska	15.8		27	Wyoming	12.4
5	Nevada	38.1		28	Arkansas	10.6
43	New Hampshire	4.1		29	Wisconsin	9.8
8	New Jersey	26.3		30	Pennsylvania	9.6
1	New Mexico	55.7		31	Indiana	9.3
9	New York	24.1		32	South Carolina	9.2
19	North Carolina	15.9		33	Tennessee	9.0
45	North Dakota	3.5		34	Alabama	8.2
42	Ohio	4.8		35	Iowa	8.1
25	Oklahoma	13.3		36	Minnesota	8.0
13	Oregon	20.6		37	Michigan	6.8
30	Pennsylvania	9.6		38	Alaska	6.1
12	Rhode Island	21.9		39	Louisiana	5.5
32	South Carolina	9.2		40	Missouri	5.4
44	South Dakota	4.0		41	Kentucky	5.2
33	Tennessee	9.0		42	Ohio	4.8
3	Texas	50.1		43	New Hampshire	4.1
18	Utah	16.3		44	South Dakota	4.0
48	Vermont	1.5		45	Mississippi	3.5
26	Virginia	13.0		45	Montana	3.5
14	Washington	19.3		45	North Dakota	3.5
50	West Virginia	1.1		48	Maine	1.5
29	Wisconsin	9.8		48	Vermont	1.5
27	Wyoming	12.4		50	West Virginia	1.1
					District of Columbia	16.7

Source: CQ Press using data from U.S. Department of Health and Human Services, National Center for Health Statistics
"National Vital Statistics Reports" (Vol. 59, No. 3, December 21, 2010, http://www.cdc.gov/nchs/births.htm)
*Preliminary data by state of residence. By race of mother. Persons of Hispanic origin may be of any race.

Births in 2008

National Total = 4,247,694 Live Births*

ALPHA ORDER

RANK	STATE	BIRTHS	% of USA
24	Alabama	64,546	1.5%
47	Alaska	11,442	0.3%
13	Arizona	99,442	2.3%
32	Arkansas	40,669	1.0%
1	California	551,779	13.0%
22	Colorado	70,031	1.6%
33	Connecticut	40,399	1.0%
44	Delaware	12,090	0.3%
4	Florida	231,445	5.4%
8	Georgia	146,603	3.5%
40	Hawaii	19,484	0.5%
38	Idaho	25,149	0.6%
5	Illinois	176,795	4.2%
15	Indiana	88,742	2.1%
34	Iowa	40,224	0.9%
31	Kansas	41,833	1.0%
26	Kentucky	58,375	1.4%
23	Louisiana	65,268	1.5%
42	Maine	13,609	0.3%
18	Maryland	77,289	1.8%
19	Massachusetts	77,022	1.8%
10	Michigan	121,127	2.9%
20	Minnesota	72,421	1.7%
30	Mississippi	44,947	1.1%
17	Missouri	80,963	1.9%
43	Montana	12,594	0.3%
37	Nebraska	26,989	0.6%
35	Nevada	39,506	0.9%
41	New Hampshire	13,683	0.3%
11	New Jersey	112,710	2.7%
36	New Mexico	30,173	0.7%
3	New York	250,383	5.9%
9	North Carolina	130,839	3.1%
48	North Dakota	8,938	0.2%
7	Ohio	148,821	3.5%
28	Oklahoma	54,781	1.3%
29	Oregon	49,096	1.2%
6	Pennsylvania	149,273	3.5%
46	Rhode Island	12,048	0.3%
25	South Carolina	63,071	1.5%
45	South Dakota	12,071	0.3%
16	Tennessee	85,560	2.0%
2	Texas	405,554	9.5%
27	Utah	55,634	1.3%
50	Vermont	6,339	0.1%
12	Virginia	106,686	2.5%
14	Washington	90,321	2.1%
39	West Virginia	21,501	0.5%
21	Wisconsin	72,261	1.7%
49	Wyoming	8,038	0.2%

RANK ORDER

RANK	STATE	BIRTHS	% of USA
1	California	551,779	13.0%
2	Texas	405,554	9.5%
3	New York	250,383	5.9%
4	Florida	231,445	5.4%
5	Illinois	176,795	4.2%
6	Pennsylvania	149,273	3.5%
7	Ohio	148,821	3.5%
8	Georgia	146,603	3.5%
9	North Carolina	130,839	3.1%
10	Michigan	121,127	2.9%
11	New Jersey	112,710	2.7%
12	Virginia	106,686	2.5%
13	Arizona	99,442	2.3%
14	Washington	90,321	2.1%
15	Indiana	88,742	2.1%
16	Tennessee	85,560	2.0%
17	Missouri	80,963	1.9%
18	Maryland	77,289	1.8%
19	Massachusetts	77,022	1.8%
20	Minnesota	72,421	1.7%
21	Wisconsin	72,261	1.7%
22	Colorado	70,031	1.6%
23	Louisiana	65,268	1.5%
24	Alabama	64,546	1.5%
25	South Carolina	63,071	1.5%
26	Kentucky	58,375	1.4%
27	Utah	55,634	1.3%
28	Oklahoma	54,781	1.3%
29	Oregon	49,096	1.2%
30	Mississippi	44,947	1.1%
31	Kansas	41,833	1.0%
32	Arkansas	40,669	1.0%
33	Connecticut	40,399	1.0%
34	Iowa	40,224	0.9%
35	Nevada	39,506	0.9%
36	New Mexico	30,173	0.7%
37	Nebraska	26,989	0.6%
38	Idaho	25,149	0.6%
39	West Virginia	21,501	0.5%
40	Hawaii	19,484	0.5%
41	New Hampshire	13,683	0.3%
42	Maine	13,609	0.3%
43	Montana	12,594	0.3%
44	Delaware	12,090	0.3%
45	South Dakota	12,071	0.3%
46	Rhode Island	12,048	0.3%
47	Alaska	11,442	0.3%
48	North Dakota	8,938	0.2%
49	Wyoming	8,038	0.2%
50	Vermont	6,339	0.1%
	District of Columbia	9,130	0.2%

Source: U.S. Department of Health and Human Services, National Center for Health Statistics
   "National Vital Statistics Reports" (Vol. 59, No. 1, December 2010, http://www.cdc.gov/nchs/births.htm)
*Final data by state of residence.

Birth Rate in 2008

National Rate = 14.0 Live Births per 1,000 Population*

ALPHA ORDER

RANK	STATE	RATE
25	Alabama	13.8
2	Alaska	16.7
5	Arizona	15.3
18	Arkansas	14.2
13	California	15.0
18	Colorado	14.2
46	Connecticut	11.5
25	Delaware	13.8
41	Florida	12.6
9	Georgia	15.1
9	Hawaii	15.1
4	Idaho	16.5
29	Illinois	13.7
22	Indiana	13.9
34	Iowa	13.4
16	Kansas	14.9
29	Kentucky	13.7
17	Louisiana	14.8
49	Maine	10.3
29	Maryland	13.7
44	Massachusetts	11.9
42	Michigan	12.1
22	Minnesota	13.9
5	Mississippi	15.3
29	Missouri	13.7
35	Montana	13.0
9	Nebraska	15.1
7	Nevada	15.2
48	New Hampshire	10.4
35	New Jersey	13.0
7	New Mexico	15.2
39	New York	12.8
18	North Carolina	14.2
22	North Dakota	13.9
35	Ohio	13.0
13	Oklahoma	15.0
35	Oregon	13.0
43	Pennsylvania	12.0
46	Rhode Island	11.5
21	South Carolina	14.1
13	South Dakota	15.0
25	Tennessee	13.8
2	Texas	16.7
1	Utah	20.3
50	Vermont	10.2
29	Virginia	13.7
25	Washington	13.8
45	West Virginia	11.8
39	Wisconsin	12.8
9	Wyoming	15.1

RANK ORDER

RANK	STATE	RATE
1	Utah	20.3
2	Alaska	16.7
2	Texas	16.7
4	Idaho	16.5
5	Arizona	15.3
5	Mississippi	15.3
7	Nevada	15.2
7	New Mexico	15.2
9	Georgia	15.1
9	Hawaii	15.1
9	Nebraska	15.1
9	Wyoming	15.1
13	California	15.0
13	Oklahoma	15.0
13	South Dakota	15.0
16	Kansas	14.9
17	Louisiana	14.8
18	Arkansas	14.2
18	Colorado	14.2
18	North Carolina	14.2
21	South Carolina	14.1
22	Indiana	13.9
22	Minnesota	13.9
22	North Dakota	13.9
25	Alabama	13.8
25	Delaware	13.8
25	Tennessee	13.8
25	Washington	13.8
29	Illinois	13.7
29	Kentucky	13.7
29	Maryland	13.7
29	Missouri	13.7
29	Virginia	13.7
34	Iowa	13.4
35	Montana	13.0
35	New Jersey	13.0
35	Ohio	13.0
35	Oregon	13.0
39	New York	12.8
39	Wisconsin	12.8
41	Florida	12.6
42	Michigan	12.1
43	Pennsylvania	12.0
44	Massachusetts	11.9
45	West Virginia	11.8
46	Connecticut	11.5
46	Rhode Island	11.5
48	New Hampshire	10.4
49	Maine	10.3
50	Vermont	10.2
	District of Columbia	15.4

Source: U.S. Department of Health and Human Services, National Center for Health Statistics
"National Vital Statistics Reports" (Vol. 59, No. 1, December 2010, http://www.cdc.gov/nchs/births.htm)
*Final data by state of residence.

Fertility Rate in 2008

National Rate = 68.6 Live Births per 1,000 Women 15 to 44 Years Old*

ALPHA ORDER

RANK	STATE	RATE
27	Alabama	68.5
3	Alaska	80.9
8	Arizona	77.4
15	Arkansas	72.1
17	California	71.0
26	Colorado	68.8
45	Connecticut	58.4
28	Delaware	68.4
33	Florida	66.7
18	Georgia	70.9
7	Hawaii	78.3
2	Idaho	83.4
34	Illinois	66.0
23	Indiana	69.3
21	Iowa	69.5
13	Kansas	75.6
32	Kentucky	67.7
18	Louisiana	70.9
48	Maine	54.5
37	Maryland	65.4
46	Massachusetts	56.7
44	Michigan	60.5
24	Minnesota	69.1
14	Mississippi	74.4
29	Missouri	68.3
21	Montana	69.5
9	Nebraska	76.9
10	Nevada	76.0
49	New Hampshire	52.8
38	New Jersey	65.1
11	New Mexico	75.9
43	New York	61.4
24	North Carolina	69.1
16	North Dakota	71.3
38	Ohio	65.1
11	Oklahoma	75.9
36	Oregon	65.6
42	Pennsylvania	61.8
47	Rhode Island	55.3
20	South Carolina	69.7
4	South Dakota	79.1
30	Tennessee	68.0
4	Texas	79.1
1	Utah	93.1
50	Vermont	52.4
34	Virginia	66.0
30	Washington	68.0
41	West Virginia	62.2
40	Wisconsin	64.9
6	Wyoming	78.4

RANK ORDER

RANK	STATE	RATE
1	Utah	93.1
2	Idaho	83.4
3	Alaska	80.9
4	South Dakota	79.1
4	Texas	79.1
6	Wyoming	78.4
7	Hawaii	78.3
8	Arizona	77.4
9	Nebraska	76.9
10	Nevada	76.0
11	New Mexico	75.9
11	Oklahoma	75.9
13	Kansas	75.6
14	Mississippi	74.4
15	Arkansas	72.1
16	North Dakota	71.3
17	California	71.0
18	Georgia	70.9
18	Louisiana	70.9
20	South Carolina	69.7
21	Iowa	69.5
21	Montana	69.5
23	Indiana	69.3
24	Minnesota	69.1
24	North Carolina	69.1
26	Colorado	68.8
27	Alabama	68.5
28	Delaware	68.4
29	Missouri	68.3
30	Tennessee	68.0
30	Washington	68.0
32	Kentucky	67.7
33	Florida	66.7
34	Illinois	66.0
34	Virginia	66.0
36	Oregon	65.6
37	Maryland	65.4
38	New Jersey	65.1
38	Ohio	65.1
40	Wisconsin	64.9
41	West Virginia	62.2
42	Pennsylvania	61.8
43	New York	61.4
44	Michigan	60.5
45	Connecticut	58.4
46	Massachusetts	56.7
47	Rhode Island	55.3
48	Maine	54.5
49	New Hampshire	52.8
50	Vermont	52.4

	District of Columbia	61.3

Source: U.S. Department of Health and Human Services, National Center for Health Statistics
"National Vital Statistics Reports" (Vol. 59, No. 1, December 2010, http://www.cdc.gov/nchs/births.htm)
*Final data by state of residence.

Births to White Women in 2008

National Total = 2,267,817 Live Births to White Women*

<table>
<thead>
<tr><th colspan="4">ALPHA ORDER</th><th colspan="4">RANK ORDER</th></tr>
<tr><th>RANK</th><th>STATE</th><th>BIRTHS</th><th>% of USA</th><th>RANK</th><th>STATE</th><th>BIRTHS</th><th>% of USA</th></tr>
</thead>
<tbody>
<tr><td>24</td><td>Alabama</td><td>38,169</td><td>1.7%</td><td>1</td><td>California</td><td>151,407</td><td>6.7%</td></tr>
<tr><td>45</td><td>Alaska</td><td>6,505</td><td>0.3%</td><td>2</td><td>Texas</td><td>139,389</td><td>6.1%</td></tr>
<tr><td>22</td><td>Arizona</td><td>42,202</td><td>1.9%</td><td>3</td><td>New York</td><td>120,581</td><td>5.3%</td></tr>
<tr><td>32</td><td>Arkansas</td><td>27,257</td><td>1.2%</td><td>4</td><td>Ohio</td><td>112,900</td><td>5.0%</td></tr>
<tr><td>1</td><td>California</td><td>151,407</td><td>6.7%</td><td>5</td><td>Pennsylvania</td><td>105,896</td><td>4.7%</td></tr>
<tr><td>23</td><td>Colorado</td><td>41,489</td><td>1.8%</td><td>6</td><td>Florida</td><td>105,710</td><td>4.7%</td></tr>
<tr><td>33</td><td>Connecticut</td><td>23,955</td><td>1.1%</td><td>7</td><td>Illinois</td><td>92,988</td><td>4.1%</td></tr>
<tr><td>46</td><td>Delaware</td><td>6,459</td><td>0.3%</td><td>8</td><td>Michigan</td><td>84,575</td><td>3.7%</td></tr>
<tr><td>6</td><td>Florida</td><td>105,710</td><td>4.7%</td><td>9</td><td>North Carolina</td><td>72,103</td><td>3.2%</td></tr>
<tr><td>11</td><td>Georgia</td><td>63,757</td><td>2.8%</td><td>10</td><td>Indiana</td><td>67,850</td><td>3.0%</td></tr>
<tr><td>50</td><td>Hawaii</td><td>4,812</td><td>0.2%</td><td>11</td><td>Georgia</td><td>63,757</td><td>2.8%</td></tr>
<tr><td>37</td><td>Idaho</td><td>19,868</td><td>0.9%</td><td>12</td><td>Virginia</td><td>61,454</td><td>2.7%</td></tr>
<tr><td>7</td><td>Illinois</td><td>92,988</td><td>4.1%</td><td>13</td><td>Missouri</td><td>61,385</td><td>2.7%</td></tr>
<tr><td>10</td><td>Indiana</td><td>67,850</td><td>3.0%</td><td>14</td><td>Tennessee</td><td>57,653</td><td>2.5%</td></tr>
<tr><td>30</td><td>Iowa</td><td>33,956</td><td>1.5%</td><td>15</td><td>Washington</td><td>57,060</td><td>2.5%</td></tr>
<tr><td>31</td><td>Kansas</td><td>30,196</td><td>1.3%</td><td>16</td><td>Wisconsin</td><td>53,812</td><td>2.4%</td></tr>
<tr><td>20</td><td>Kentucky</td><td>49,011</td><td>2.2%</td><td>17</td><td>New Jersey</td><td>53,540</td><td>2.4%</td></tr>
<tr><td>27</td><td>Louisiana</td><td>34,728</td><td>1.5%</td><td>18</td><td>Minnesota</td><td>52,684</td><td>2.3%</td></tr>
<tr><td>39</td><td>Maine</td><td>12,637</td><td>0.6%</td><td>19</td><td>Massachusetts</td><td>52,241</td><td>2.3%</td></tr>
<tr><td>25</td><td>Maryland</td><td>35,639</td><td>1.6%</td><td>20</td><td>Kentucky</td><td>49,011</td><td>2.2%</td></tr>
<tr><td>19</td><td>Massachusetts</td><td>52,241</td><td>2.3%</td><td>21</td><td>Utah</td><td>42,746</td><td>1.9%</td></tr>
<tr><td>8</td><td>Michigan</td><td>84,575</td><td>3.7%</td><td>22</td><td>Arizona</td><td>42,202</td><td>1.9%</td></tr>
<tr><td>18</td><td>Minnesota</td><td>52,684</td><td>2.3%</td><td>23</td><td>Colorado</td><td>41,489</td><td>1.8%</td></tr>
<tr><td>34</td><td>Mississippi</td><td>22,582</td><td>1.0%</td><td>24</td><td>Alabama</td><td>38,169</td><td>1.7%</td></tr>
<tr><td>13</td><td>Missouri</td><td>61,385</td><td>2.7%</td><td>25</td><td>Maryland</td><td>35,639</td><td>1.6%</td></tr>
<tr><td>41</td><td>Montana</td><td>10,328</td><td>0.5%</td><td>26</td><td>Oklahoma</td><td>35,172</td><td>1.6%</td></tr>
<tr><td>36</td><td>Nebraska</td><td>19,925</td><td>0.9%</td><td>27</td><td>Louisiana</td><td>34,728</td><td>1.5%</td></tr>
<tr><td>38</td><td>Nevada</td><td>16,228</td><td>0.7%</td><td>28</td><td>South Carolina</td><td>34,694</td><td>1.5%</td></tr>
<tr><td>40</td><td>New Hampshire</td><td>12,200</td><td>0.5%</td><td>29</td><td>Oregon</td><td>34,054</td><td>1.5%</td></tr>
<tr><td>17</td><td>New Jersey</td><td>53,540</td><td>2.4%</td><td>30</td><td>Iowa</td><td>33,956</td><td>1.5%</td></tr>
<tr><td>43</td><td>New Mexico</td><td>8,476</td><td>0.4%</td><td>31</td><td>Kansas</td><td>30,196</td><td>1.3%</td></tr>
<tr><td>3</td><td>New York</td><td>120,581</td><td>5.3%</td><td>32</td><td>Arkansas</td><td>27,257</td><td>1.2%</td></tr>
<tr><td>9</td><td>North Carolina</td><td>72,103</td><td>3.2%</td><td>33</td><td>Connecticut</td><td>23,955</td><td>1.1%</td></tr>
<tr><td>44</td><td>North Dakota</td><td>7,323</td><td>0.3%</td><td>34</td><td>Mississippi</td><td>22,582</td><td>1.0%</td></tr>
<tr><td>4</td><td>Ohio</td><td>112,900</td><td>5.0%</td><td>35</td><td>West Virginia</td><td>20,212</td><td>0.9%</td></tr>
<tr><td>26</td><td>Oklahoma</td><td>35,172</td><td>1.6%</td><td>36</td><td>Nebraska</td><td>19,925</td><td>0.9%</td></tr>
<tr><td>29</td><td>Oregon</td><td>34,054</td><td>1.5%</td><td>37</td><td>Idaho</td><td>19,868</td><td>0.9%</td></tr>
<tr><td>5</td><td>Pennsylvania</td><td>105,896</td><td>4.7%</td><td>38</td><td>Nevada</td><td>16,228</td><td>0.7%</td></tr>
<tr><td>49</td><td>Rhode Island</td><td>5,999</td><td>0.3%</td><td>39</td><td>Maine</td><td>12,637</td><td>0.6%</td></tr>
<tr><td>28</td><td>South Carolina</td><td>34,694</td><td>1.5%</td><td>40</td><td>New Hampshire</td><td>12,200</td><td>0.5%</td></tr>
<tr><td>42</td><td>South Dakota</td><td>9,193</td><td>0.4%</td><td>41</td><td>Montana</td><td>10,328</td><td>0.5%</td></tr>
<tr><td>14</td><td>Tennessee</td><td>57,653</td><td>2.5%</td><td>42</td><td>South Dakota</td><td>9,193</td><td>0.4%</td></tr>
<tr><td>2</td><td>Texas</td><td>139,389</td><td>6.1%</td><td>43</td><td>New Mexico</td><td>8,476</td><td>0.4%</td></tr>
<tr><td>21</td><td>Utah</td><td>42,746</td><td>1.9%</td><td>44</td><td>North Dakota</td><td>7,323</td><td>0.3%</td></tr>
<tr><td>48</td><td>Vermont</td><td>6,032</td><td>0.3%</td><td>45</td><td>Alaska</td><td>6,505</td><td>0.3%</td></tr>
<tr><td>12</td><td>Virginia</td><td>61,454</td><td>2.7%</td><td>46</td><td>Delaware</td><td>6,459</td><td>0.3%</td></tr>
<tr><td>15</td><td>Washington</td><td>57,060</td><td>2.5%</td><td>47</td><td>Wyoming</td><td>6,421</td><td>0.3%</td></tr>
<tr><td>35</td><td>West Virginia</td><td>20,212</td><td>0.9%</td><td>48</td><td>Vermont</td><td>6,032</td><td>0.3%</td></tr>
<tr><td>16</td><td>Wisconsin</td><td>53,812</td><td>2.4%</td><td>49</td><td>Rhode Island</td><td>5,999</td><td>0.3%</td></tr>
<tr><td>47</td><td>Wyoming</td><td>6,421</td><td>0.3%</td><td>50</td><td>Hawaii</td><td>4,812</td><td>0.2%</td></tr>
<tr><td></td><td></td><td></td><td></td><td></td><td>District of Columbia</td><td>2,364</td><td>0.1%</td></tr>
</tbody>
</table>

Source: U.S. Department of Health and Human Services, National Center for Health Statistics
"National Vital Statistics Reports" (Vol. 59, No. 1, December 2010, http://www.cdc.gov/nchs/births.htm)
*Final data by state of residence. By race of mother. Does not include births to white Hispanic mothers.

White Births as a Percent of All Births in 2008

National Percent = 53.4% of Live Births*

	ALPHA ORDER				RANK ORDER	
RANK	STATE	PERCENT		RANK	STATE	PERCENT
30	Alabama	59.1		1	Vermont	95.2
32	Alaska	56.9		2	West Virginia	94.0
45	Arizona	42.4		3	Maine	92.9
25	Arkansas	67.0		4	New Hampshire	89.2
49	California	27.4		5	Iowa	84.4
29	Colorado	59.2		6	Kentucky	84.0
28	Connecticut	59.3		7	Montana	82.0
35	Delaware	53.4		8	North Dakota	81.9
43	Florida	45.7		9	Wyoming	79.9
44	Georgia	43.5		10	Idaho	79.0
50	Hawaii	24.7		11	Utah	76.8
10	Idaho	79.0		12	Indiana	76.5
37	Illinois	52.6		13	South Dakota	76.2
12	Indiana	76.5		14	Ohio	75.9
5	Iowa	84.4		15	Missouri	75.8
19	Kansas	72.2		16	Wisconsin	74.5
6	Kentucky	84.0		17	Nebraska	73.8
36	Louisiana	53.2		18	Minnesota	72.7
3	Maine	92.9		19	Kansas	72.2
42	Maryland	46.1		20	Pennsylvania	70.9
23	Massachusetts	67.8		21	Michigan	69.8
21	Michigan	69.8		22	Oregon	69.4
18	Minnesota	72.7		23	Massachusetts	67.8
38	Mississippi	50.2		24	Tennessee	67.4
15	Missouri	75.8		25	Arkansas	67.0
7	Montana	82.0		26	Oklahoma	64.2
17	Nebraska	73.8		27	Washington	63.2
46	Nevada	41.1		28	Connecticut	59.3
4	New Hampshire	89.2		29	Colorado	59.2
41	New Jersey	47.5		30	Alabama	59.1
48	New Mexico	28.1		31	Virginia	57.6
40	New York	48.2		32	Alaska	56.9
33	North Carolina	55.1		33	North Carolina	55.1
8	North Dakota	81.9		34	South Carolina	55.0
14	Ohio	75.9		35	Delaware	53.4
26	Oklahoma	64.2		36	Louisiana	53.2
22	Oregon	69.4		37	Illinois	52.6
20	Pennsylvania	70.9		38	Mississippi	50.2
39	Rhode Island	49.8		39	Rhode Island	49.8
34	South Carolina	55.0		40	New York	48.2
13	South Dakota	76.2		41	New Jersey	47.5
24	Tennessee	67.4		42	Maryland	46.1
47	Texas	34.4		43	Florida	45.7
11	Utah	76.8		44	Georgia	43.5
1	Vermont	95.2		45	Arizona	42.4
31	Virginia	57.6		46	Nevada	41.1
27	Washington	63.2		47	Texas	34.4
2	West Virginia	94.0		48	New Mexico	28.1
16	Wisconsin	74.5		49	California	27.4
9	Wyoming	79.9		50	Hawaii	24.7
					District of Columbia	25.9

Source: CQ Press using data from U.S. Department of Health and Human Services, National Center for Health Statistics
   "National Vital Statistics Reports" (Vol. 59, No. 1, December 2010, http://www.cdc.gov/nchs/births.htm)
*Final data by state of residence. By race of mother. Does not include births to white Hispanic mothers.

Births to Black Women in 2008

National Total = 623,029 Live Births to Black Women*

ALPHA ORDER					RANK ORDER			
RANK	STATE	BIRTHS	% of USA		RANK	STATE	BIRTHS	% of USA
15	Alabama	19,913	3.2%		1	Florida	51,699	8.3%
42	Alaska	403	0.1%		2	Georgia	48,298	7.8%
28	Arizona	4,052	0.7%		3	Texas	45,951	7.4%
21	Arkansas	8,029	1.3%		4	New York	40,418	6.5%
5	California	31,975	5.1%		5	California	31,975	5.1%
33	Colorado	3,140	0.5%		6	North Carolina	31,163	5.0%
26	Connecticut	5,142	0.8%		7	Illinois	30,845	5.0%
31	Delaware	3,226	0.5%		8	Maryland	25,929	4.2%
1	Florida	51,699	8.3%		9	Louisiana	25,565	4.1%
2	Georgia	48,298	7.8%		10	Ohio	24,266	3.9%
41	Hawaii	478	0.1%		11	Virginia	23,270	3.7%
46	Idaho	154	0.0%		12	Michigan	22,449	3.6%
7	Illinois	30,845	5.0%		13	Pennsylvania	21,654	3.5%
20	Indiana	10,449	1.7%		14	South Carolina	20,624	3.3%
34	Iowa	1,782	0.3%		15	Alabama	19,913	3.2%
32	Kansas	3,156	0.5%		16	Mississippi	19,836	3.2%
25	Kentucky	5,445	0.9%		17	Tennessee	18,133	2.9%
9	Louisiana	25,565	4.1%		18	New Jersey	17,430	2.8%
43	Maine	360	0.1%		19	Missouri	12,478	2.0%
8	Maryland	25,929	4.2%		20	Indiana	10,449	1.7%
23	Massachusetts	7,201	1.2%		21	Arkansas	8,029	1.3%
12	Michigan	22,449	3.6%		22	Wisconsin	7,241	1.2%
24	Minnesota	6,675	1.1%		23	Massachusetts	7,201	1.2%
16	Mississippi	19,836	3.2%		24	Minnesota	6,675	1.1%
19	Missouri	12,478	2.0%		25	Kentucky	5,445	0.9%
49	Montana	72	0.0%		26	Connecticut	5,142	0.8%
35	Nebraska	1,753	0.3%		27	Oklahoma	4,960	0.8%
30	Nevada	3,601	0.6%		28	Arizona	4,052	0.7%
44	New Hampshire	233	0.0%		29	Washington	3,961	0.6%
18	New Jersey	17,430	2.8%		30	Nevada	3,601	0.6%
40	New Mexico	489	0.1%		31	Delaware	3,226	0.5%
4	New York	40,418	6.5%		32	Kansas	3,156	0.5%
6	North Carolina	31,163	5.0%		33	Colorado	3,140	0.5%
47	North Dakota	148	0.0%		34	Iowa	1,782	0.3%
10	Ohio	24,266	3.9%		35	Nebraska	1,753	0.3%
27	Oklahoma	4,960	0.8%		36	Oregon	1,211	0.2%
36	Oregon	1,211	0.2%		37	Rhode Island	1,009	0.2%
13	Pennsylvania	21,654	3.5%		38	West Virginia	821	0.1%
37	Rhode Island	1,009	0.2%		39	Utah	560	0.1%
14	South Carolina	20,624	3.3%		40	New Mexico	489	0.1%
45	South Dakota	215	0.0%		41	Hawaii	478	0.1%
17	Tennessee	18,133	2.9%		42	Alaska	403	0.1%
3	Texas	45,951	7.4%		43	Maine	360	0.1%
39	Utah	560	0.1%		44	New Hampshire	233	0.0%
48	Vermont	97	0.0%		45	South Dakota	215	0.0%
11	Virginia	23,270	3.7%		46	Idaho	154	0.0%
29	Washington	3,961	0.6%		47	North Dakota	148	0.0%
38	West Virginia	821	0.1%		48	Vermont	97	0.0%
22	Wisconsin	7,241	1.2%		49	Montana	72	0.0%
50	Wyoming	58	0.0%		50	Wyoming	58	0.0%
						District of Columbia	5,012	0.8%

Source: U.S. Department of Health and Human Services, National Center for Health Statistics
    "National Vital Statistics Reports" (Vol. 59, No. 1, December 2010, http://www.cdc.gov/nchs/births.htm)
*Final data by state of residence. By race of mother. Does not include births to black Hispanic mothers.

Black Births as a Percent of All Births in 2008

National Percent = 14.7% of Live Births*

ALPHA ORDER			RANK ORDER		
RANK	STATE	PERCENT	RANK	STATE	PERCENT
6	Alabama	30.9	1	Mississippi	44.1
38	Alaska	3.5	2	Louisiana	39.2
36	Arizona	4.1	3	Maryland	33.5
12	Arkansas	19.7	4	Georgia	32.9
32	California	5.8	5	South Carolina	32.7
33	Colorado	4.5	6	Alabama	30.9
20	Connecticut	12.7	7	Delaware	26.7
7	Delaware	26.7	8	North Carolina	23.8
9	Florida	22.3	9	Florida	22.3
4	Georgia	32.9	10	Virginia	21.8
40	Hawaii	2.5	11	Tennessee	21.2
49	Idaho	0.6	12	Arkansas	19.7
14	Illinois	17.4	13	Michigan	18.5
21	Indiana	11.8	14	Illinois	17.4
34	Iowa	4.4	15	Ohio	16.3
30	Kansas	7.5	16	New York	16.1
24	Kentucky	9.3	17	New Jersey	15.5
2	Louisiana	39.2	18	Missouri	15.4
39	Maine	2.6	19	Pennsylvania	14.5
3	Maryland	33.5	20	Connecticut	12.7
24	Massachusetts	9.3	21	Indiana	11.8
13	Michigan	18.5	22	Texas	11.3
26	Minnesota	9.2	23	Wisconsin	10.0
1	Mississippi	44.1	24	Kentucky	9.3
18	Missouri	15.4	24	Massachusetts	9.3
49	Montana	0.6	26	Minnesota	9.2
31	Nebraska	6.5	27	Nevada	9.1
27	Nevada	9.1	27	Oklahoma	9.1
43	New Hampshire	1.7	29	Rhode Island	8.4
17	New Jersey	15.5	30	Kansas	7.5
45	New Mexico	1.6	31	Nebraska	6.5
16	New York	16.1	32	California	5.8
8	North Carolina	23.8	33	Colorado	4.5
43	North Dakota	1.7	34	Iowa	4.4
15	Ohio	16.3	34	Washington	4.4
27	Oklahoma	9.1	36	Arizona	4.1
40	Oregon	2.5	37	West Virginia	3.8
19	Pennsylvania	14.5	38	Alaska	3.5
29	Rhode Island	8.4	39	Maine	2.6
5	South Carolina	32.7	40	Hawaii	2.5
42	South Dakota	1.8	40	Oregon	2.5
11	Tennessee	21.2	42	South Dakota	1.8
22	Texas	11.3	43	New Hampshire	1.7
47	Utah	1.0	43	North Dakota	1.7
46	Vermont	1.5	45	New Mexico	1.6
10	Virginia	21.8	46	Vermont	1.5
34	Washington	4.4	47	Utah	1.0
37	West Virginia	3.8	48	Wyoming	0.7
23	Wisconsin	10.0	49	Idaho	0.6
48	Wyoming	0.7	49	Montana	0.6
				District of Columbia	54.9

Source: CQ Press using data from U.S. Department of Health and Human Services, National Center for Health Statistics
   "National Vital Statistics Reports" (Vol. 59, No. 1, December 2010, http://www.cdc.gov/nchs/births.htm)
*Final data by state of residence. By race of mother. Does not include births to black Hispanic mothers.

Births to Hispanic Women in 2008

National Total = 1,041,239 Live Births to Hispanic Women*

ALPHA ORDER

RANK	STATE	BIRTHS	% of USA
30	Alabama	5,350	0.5%
43	Alaska	651	0.1%
5	Arizona	43,329	4.2%
32	Arkansas	4,341	0.4%
1	California	287,560	27.6%
9	Colorado	21,867	2.1%
21	Connecticut	8,674	0.8%
40	Delaware	1,837	0.2%
3	Florida	66,019	6.3%
8	Georgia	25,842	2.5%
37	Hawaii	3,062	0.3%
34	Idaho	4,055	0.4%
6	Illinois	42,765	4.1%
22	Indiana	8,519	0.8%
36	Iowa	3,324	0.3%
27	Kansas	6,784	0.7%
38	Kentucky	2,912	0.3%
35	Louisiana	3,363	0.3%
49	Maine	221	0.0%
17	Maryland	10,545	1.0%
16	Massachusetts	10,941	1.1%
20	Michigan	8,894	0.9%
29	Minnesota	5,732	0.6%
41	Mississippi	1,750	0.2%
31	Missouri	4,528	0.4%
46	Montana	432	0.0%
33	Nebraska	4,274	0.4%
13	Nevada	15,364	1.5%
44	New Hampshire	548	0.1%
7	New Jersey	29,296	2.8%
12	New Mexico	16,885	1.6%
4	New York	60,070	5.8%
10	North Carolina	21,630	2.1%
47	North Dakota	279	0.0%
26	Ohio	6,914	0.7%
24	Oklahoma	7,071	0.7%
18	Oregon	10,363	1.0%
15	Pennsylvania	13,972	1.3%
39	Rhode Island	2,607	0.3%
28	South Carolina	6,220	0.6%
45	South Dakota	462	0.0%
23	Tennessee	7,969	0.8%
2	Texas	202,980	19.5%
19	Utah	9,465	0.9%
50	Vermont	75	0.0%
14	Virginia	14,273	1.4%
11	Washington	17,353	1.7%
48	West Virginia	231	0.0%
25	Wisconsin	7,060	0.7%
42	Wyoming	1,075	0.1%

RANK ORDER

RANK	STATE	BIRTHS	% of USA
1	California	287,560	27.6%
2	Texas	202,980	19.5%
3	Florida	66,019	6.3%
4	New York	60,070	5.8%
5	Arizona	43,329	4.2%
6	Illinois	42,765	4.1%
7	New Jersey	29,296	2.8%
8	Georgia	25,842	2.5%
9	Colorado	21,867	2.1%
10	North Carolina	21,630	2.1%
11	Washington	17,353	1.7%
12	New Mexico	16,885	1.6%
13	Nevada	15,364	1.5%
14	Virginia	14,273	1.4%
15	Pennsylvania	13,972	1.3%
16	Massachusetts	10,941	1.1%
17	Maryland	10,545	1.0%
18	Oregon	10,363	1.0%
19	Utah	9,465	0.9%
20	Michigan	8,894	0.9%
21	Connecticut	8,674	0.8%
22	Indiana	8,519	0.8%
23	Tennessee	7,969	0.8%
24	Oklahoma	7,071	0.7%
25	Wisconsin	7,060	0.7%
26	Ohio	6,914	0.7%
27	Kansas	6,784	0.7%
28	South Carolina	6,220	0.6%
29	Minnesota	5,732	0.6%
30	Alabama	5,350	0.5%
31	Missouri	4,528	0.4%
32	Arkansas	4,341	0.4%
33	Nebraska	4,274	0.4%
34	Idaho	4,055	0.4%
35	Louisiana	3,363	0.3%
36	Iowa	3,324	0.3%
37	Hawaii	3,062	0.3%
38	Kentucky	2,912	0.3%
39	Rhode Island	2,607	0.3%
40	Delaware	1,837	0.2%
41	Mississippi	1,750	0.2%
42	Wyoming	1,075	0.1%
43	Alaska	651	0.1%
44	New Hampshire	548	0.1%
45	South Dakota	462	0.0%
46	Montana	432	0.0%
47	North Dakota	279	0.0%
48	West Virginia	231	0.0%
49	Maine	221	0.0%
50	Vermont	75	0.0%
	District of Columbia	1,506	0.1%

Source: U.S. Department of Health and Human Services, National Center for Health Statistics
"National Vital Statistics Reports" (Vol. 59, No. 1, December 2010, http://www.cdc.gov/nchs/births.htm)
*Final data by state of residence. By race of mother. Persons of Hispanic origin may be of any race.

Hispanic Births as a Percent of All Births in 2008

National Percent = 24.5% of Live Births*

ALPHA ORDER

RANK	STATE	PERCENT
34	Alabama	8.3
38	Alaska	5.7
4	Arizona	43.6
28	Arkansas	10.7
2	California	52.1
6	Colorado	31.2
12	Connecticut	21.5
22	Delaware	15.2
7	Florida	28.5
15	Georgia	17.6
21	Hawaii	15.7
19	Idaho	16.1
9	Illinois	24.2
31	Indiana	9.6
34	Iowa	8.3
18	Kansas	16.2
41	Kentucky	5.0
40	Louisiana	5.2
48	Maine	1.6
24	Maryland	13.6
23	Massachusetts	14.2
37	Michigan	7.3
36	Minnesota	7.9
44	Mississippi	3.9
39	Missouri	5.6
46	Montana	3.4
20	Nebraska	15.8
5	Nevada	38.9
43	New Hampshire	4.0
8	New Jersey	26.0
1	New Mexico	56.0
10	New York	24.0
17	North Carolina	16.5
47	North Dakota	3.1
42	Ohio	4.6
27	Oklahoma	12.9
13	Oregon	21.1
32	Pennsylvania	9.4
11	Rhode Island	21.6
29	South Carolina	9.9
45	South Dakota	3.8
33	Tennessee	9.3
3	Texas	50.1
16	Utah	17.0
49	Vermont	1.2
25	Virginia	13.4
14	Washington	19.2
50	West Virginia	1.1
30	Wisconsin	9.8
25	Wyoming	13.4

RANK ORDER

RANK	STATE	PERCENT
1	New Mexico	56.0
2	California	52.1
3	Texas	50.1
4	Arizona	43.6
5	Nevada	38.9
6	Colorado	31.2
7	Florida	28.5
8	New Jersey	26.0
9	Illinois	24.2
10	New York	24.0
11	Rhode Island	21.6
12	Connecticut	21.5
13	Oregon	21.1
14	Washington	19.2
15	Georgia	17.6
16	Utah	17.0
17	North Carolina	16.5
18	Kansas	16.2
19	Idaho	16.1
20	Nebraska	15.8
21	Hawaii	15.7
22	Delaware	15.2
23	Massachusetts	14.2
24	Maryland	13.6
25	Virginia	13.4
25	Wyoming	13.4
27	Oklahoma	12.9
28	Arkansas	10.7
29	South Carolina	9.9
30	Wisconsin	9.8
31	Indiana	9.6
32	Pennsylvania	9.4
33	Tennessee	9.3
34	Alabama	8.3
34	Iowa	8.3
36	Minnesota	7.9
37	Michigan	7.3
38	Alaska	5.7
39	Missouri	5.6
40	Louisiana	5.2
41	Kentucky	5.0
42	Ohio	4.6
43	New Hampshire	4.0
44	Mississippi	3.9
45	South Dakota	3.8
46	Montana	3.4
47	North Dakota	3.1
48	Maine	1.6
49	Vermont	1.2
50	West Virginia	1.1

District of Columbia   16.5

Source: CQ Press using data from U.S. Department of Health and Human Services, National Center for Health Statistics
"National Vital Statistics Reports" (Vol. 59, No. 1, December 2010, http://www.cdc.gov/nchs/births.htm)
*Final data by state of residence. By race of mother. Persons of Hispanic origin may be of any race.

Percent of Births That Are Pre-Term in 2008

National Percent = 12.3% of Births*

RANK	STATE	PERCENT
2	Alabama	15.7
44	Alaska	10.3
15	Arizona	12.9
8	Arkansas	13.5
42	California	10.5
32	Colorado	11.4
43	Connecticut	10.4
15	Delaware	12.9
6	Florida	13.8
11	Georgia	13.4
18	Hawaii	12.8
48	Idaho	9.8
19	Illinois	12.7
23	Indiana	12.4
30	Iowa	11.5
34	Kansas	11.2
5	Kentucky	14.0
3	Louisiana	15.4
44	Maine	10.3
14	Maryland	13.0
40	Massachusetts	10.8
19	Michigan	12.7
47	Minnesota	10.0
1	Mississippi	18.0
24	Missouri	12.3
30	Montana	11.5
28	Nebraska	11.8
8	Nevada	13.5
49	New Hampshire	9.6
22	New Jersey	12.5
24	New Mexico	12.3
26	New York	12.0
15	North Carolina	12.9
37	North Dakota	11.1
21	Ohio	12.6
11	Oklahoma	13.4
46	Oregon	10.1
29	Pennsylvania	11.6
34	Rhode Island	11.2
4	South Carolina	14.3
27	South Dakota	11.9
8	Tennessee	13.5
13	Texas	13.3
39	Utah	11.0
50	Vermont	9.5
33	Virginia	11.3
41	Washington	10.7
7	West Virginia	13.7
37	Wisconsin	11.1
34	Wyoming	11.2

RANK	STATE	PERCENT
1	Mississippi	18.0
2	Alabama	15.7
3	Louisiana	15.4
4	South Carolina	14.3
5	Kentucky	14.0
6	Florida	13.8
7	West Virginia	13.7
8	Arkansas	13.5
8	Nevada	13.5
8	Tennessee	13.5
11	Georgia	13.4
11	Oklahoma	13.4
13	Texas	13.3
14	Maryland	13.0
15	Arizona	12.9
15	Delaware	12.9
15	North Carolina	12.9
18	Hawaii	12.8
19	Illinois	12.7
19	Michigan	12.7
21	Ohio	12.6
22	New Jersey	12.5
23	Indiana	12.4
24	Missouri	12.3
24	New Mexico	12.3
26	New York	12.0
27	South Dakota	11.9
28	Nebraska	11.8
29	Pennsylvania	11.6
30	Iowa	11.5
30	Montana	11.5
32	Colorado	11.4
33	Virginia	11.3
34	Kansas	11.2
34	Rhode Island	11.2
34	Wyoming	11.2
37	North Dakota	11.1
37	Wisconsin	11.1
39	Utah	11.0
40	Massachusetts	10.8
41	Washington	10.7
42	California	10.5
43	Connecticut	10.4
44	Alaska	10.3
44	Maine	10.3
46	Oregon	10.1
47	Minnesota	10.0
48	Idaho	9.8
49	New Hampshire	9.6
50	Vermont	9.5

	District of Columbia	15.5

Source: CQ Press using data from U.S. Department of Health and Human Services, National Center for Health Statistics
"Vital Stats" (http://www.cdc.gov/nchs/VitalStats.htm)
*Final data by state of residence. Births before 37 weeks of gestation.

Births of Low Birthweight in 2008

National Total = 347,209 Live Births*

ALPHA ORDER

RANK	STATE	BIRTHS	% of USA
18	Alabama	6,820	2.0%
47	Alaska	680	0.2%
17	Arizona	7,030	2.0%
30	Arkansas	3,757	1.1%
1	California	37,598	10.8%
20	Colorado	6,243	1.8%
31	Connecticut	3,237	0.9%
41	Delaware	1,027	0.3%
4	Florida	20,319	5.9%
6	Georgia	13,975	4.0%
40	Hawaii	1,574	0.5%
39	Idaho	1,637	0.5%
5	Illinois	14,790	4.3%
14	Indiana	7,398	2.1%
35	Iowa	2,673	0.8%
33	Kansas	3,005	0.9%
24	Kentucky	5,360	1.5%
16	Louisiana	7,046	2.0%
44	Maine	907	0.3%
15	Maryland	7,138	2.1%
22	Massachusetts	5,951	1.7%
10	Michigan	10,378	3.0%
27	Minnesota	4,605	1.3%
25	Mississippi	5,306	1.5%
19	Missouri	6,573	1.9%
43	Montana	929	0.3%
38	Nebraska	1,901	0.5%
32	Nevada	3,175	0.9%
45	New Hampshire	890	0.3%
11	New Jersey	9,515	2.7%
36	New Mexico	2,547	0.7%
3	New York	20,508	5.9%
9	North Carolina	11,890	3.4%
49	North Dakota	610	0.2%
7	Ohio	12,797	3.7%
28	Oklahoma	4,536	1.3%
34	Oregon	2,975	0.9%
8	Pennsylvania	12,361	3.6%
42	Rhode Island	953	0.3%
21	South Carolina	6,218	1.8%
46	South Dakota	780	0.2%
13	Tennessee	7,853	2.3%
2	Texas	34,194	9.8%
29	Utah	3,785	1.1%
50	Vermont	443	0.1%
12	Virginia	8,865	2.6%
23	Washington	5,717	1.6%
37	West Virginia	2,048	0.6%
26	Wisconsin	5,068	1.5%
48	Wyoming	667	0.2%

RANK ORDER

RANK	STATE	BIRTHS	% of USA
1	California	37,598	10.8%
2	Texas	34,194	9.8%
3	New York	20,508	5.9%
4	Florida	20,319	5.9%
5	Illinois	14,790	4.3%
6	Georgia	13,975	4.0%
7	Ohio	12,797	3.7%
8	Pennsylvania	12,361	3.6%
9	North Carolina	11,890	3.4%
10	Michigan	10,378	3.0%
11	New Jersey	9,515	2.7%
12	Virginia	8,865	2.6%
13	Tennessee	7,853	2.3%
14	Indiana	7,398	2.1%
15	Maryland	7,138	2.1%
16	Louisiana	7,046	2.0%
17	Arizona	7,030	2.0%
18	Alabama	6,820	2.0%
19	Missouri	6,573	1.9%
20	Colorado	6,243	1.8%
21	South Carolina	6,218	1.8%
22	Massachusetts	5,951	1.7%
23	Washington	5,717	1.6%
24	Kentucky	5,360	1.5%
25	Mississippi	5,306	1.5%
26	Wisconsin	5,068	1.5%
27	Minnesota	4,605	1.3%
28	Oklahoma	4,536	1.3%
29	Utah	3,785	1.1%
30	Arkansas	3,757	1.1%
31	Connecticut	3,237	0.9%
32	Nevada	3,175	0.9%
33	Kansas	3,005	0.9%
34	Oregon	2,975	0.9%
35	Iowa	2,673	0.8%
36	New Mexico	2,547	0.7%
37	West Virginia	2,048	0.6%
38	Nebraska	1,901	0.5%
39	Idaho	1,637	0.5%
40	Hawaii	1,574	0.5%
41	Delaware	1,027	0.3%
42	Rhode Island	953	0.3%
43	Montana	929	0.3%
44	Maine	907	0.3%
45	New Hampshire	890	0.3%
46	South Dakota	780	0.2%
47	Alaska	680	0.2%
48	Wyoming	667	0.2%
49	North Dakota	610	0.2%
50	Vermont	443	0.1%
	District of Columbia	957	0.3%

Source: U.S. Department of Health and Human Services, National Center for Health Statistics
"National Vital Statistics Reports" (Vol. 59, No. 1, December 2010, http://www.cdc.gov/nchs/births.htm)
*Final data by state of residence. Births of less than 2,500 grams (5 pounds 8 ounces).

Births of Low Birthweight as a Percent of All Births in 2008

National Percent = 8.2% of Live Births*

ALPHA ORDER			RANK ORDER		
RANK	STATE	PERCENT	RANK	STATE	PERCENT
3	Alabama	10.6	1	Mississippi	11.8
50	Alaska	6.0	2	Louisiana	10.8
35	Arizona	7.1	3	Alabama	10.6
7	Arkansas	9.2	4	South Carolina	9.9
39	California	6.8	5	Georgia	9.6
12	Colorado	8.9	6	West Virginia	9.5
29	Connecticut	8.0	7	Arkansas	9.2
16	Delaware	8.5	7	Kentucky	9.2
13	Florida	8.8	7	Maryland	9.2
5	Georgia	9.6	7	Tennessee	9.2
27	Hawaii	8.1	11	North Carolina	9.1
44	Idaho	6.5	12	Colorado	8.9
18	Illinois	8.4	13	Florida	8.8
21	Indiana	8.3	14	Michigan	8.6
43	Iowa	6.6	14	Ohio	8.6
34	Kansas	7.2	16	Delaware	8.5
7	Kentucky	9.2	16	New Mexico	8.5
2	Louisiana	10.8	18	Illinois	8.4
42	Maine	6.7	18	New Jersey	8.4
7	Maryland	9.2	18	Texas	8.4
32	Massachusetts	7.8	21	Indiana	8.3
14	Michigan	8.6	21	Oklahoma	8.3
47	Minnesota	6.4	21	Pennsylvania	8.3
1	Mississippi	11.8	21	Virginia	8.3
27	Missouri	8.1	21	Wyoming	8.3
33	Montana	7.4	26	New York	8.2
36	Nebraska	7.0	27	Hawaii	8.1
29	Nevada	8.0	27	Missouri	8.1
44	New Hampshire	6.5	29	Connecticut	8.0
18	New Jersey	8.4	29	Nevada	8.0
16	New Mexico	8.5	31	Rhode Island	7.9
26	New York	8.2	32	Massachusetts	7.8
11	North Carolina	9.1	33	Montana	7.4
39	North Dakota	6.8	34	Kansas	7.2
14	Ohio	8.6	35	Arizona	7.1
21	Oklahoma	8.3	36	Nebraska	7.0
49	Oregon	6.1	36	Vermont	7.0
21	Pennsylvania	8.3	36	Wisconsin	7.0
31	Rhode Island	7.9	39	California	6.8
4	South Carolina	9.9	39	North Dakota	6.8
44	South Dakota	6.5	39	Utah	6.8
7	Tennessee	9.2	42	Maine	6.7
18	Texas	8.4	43	Iowa	6.6
39	Utah	6.8	44	Idaho	6.5
36	Vermont	7.0	44	New Hampshire	6.5
21	Virginia	8.3	44	South Dakota	6.5
48	Washington	6.3	47	Minnesota	6.4
6	West Virginia	9.5	48	Washington	6.3
36	Wisconsin	7.0	49	Oregon	6.1
21	Wyoming	8.3	50	Alaska	6.0
				District of Columbia	10.5

Source: U.S. Department of Health and Human Services, National Center for Health Statistics
"National Vital Statistics Reports" (Vol. 59, No. 1, December 2010, http://www.cdc.gov/nchs/births.htm)
*Final data by state of residence. Births of less than 2,500 grams (5 pounds 8 ounces).

Births of Low Birthweight to White Women
as a Percent of All Births to White Women in 2008
National Percent = 7.2% of Live Births to White Women*

ALPHA ORDER

RANK	STATE	PERCENT
5	Alabama	8.4
50	Alaska	5.0
31	Arizona	6.8
9	Arkansas	8.0
40	California	6.4
4	Colorado	8.5
36	Connecticut	6.6
28	Delaware	7.0
18	Florida	7.5
17	Georgia	7.6
40	Hawaii	6.4
45	Idaho	6.2
21	Illinois	7.3
13	Indiana	7.7
43	Iowa	6.3
31	Kansas	6.8
2	Kentucky	8.7
9	Louisiana	8.0
36	Maine	6.6
23	Maryland	7.2
26	Massachusetts	7.1
23	Michigan	7.2
49	Minnesota	5.7
3	Mississippi	8.6
23	Missouri	7.2
21	Montana	7.3
38	Nebraska	6.5
9	Nevada	8.0
40	New Hampshire	6.4
19	New Jersey	7.4
6	New Mexico	8.2
31	New York	6.8
13	North Carolina	7.7
35	North Dakota	6.7
19	Ohio	7.4
12	Oklahoma	7.8
48	Oregon	5.9
26	Pennsylvania	7.1
31	Rhode Island	6.8
13	South Carolina	7.7
45	South Dakota	6.2
7	Tennessee	8.1
13	Texas	7.7
38	Utah	6.5
28	Vermont	7.0
28	Virginia	7.0
47	Washington	6.0
1	West Virginia	9.4
43	Wisconsin	6.3
7	Wyoming	8.1

RANK ORDER

RANK	STATE	PERCENT
1	West Virginia	9.4
2	Kentucky	8.7
3	Mississippi	8.6
4	Colorado	8.5
5	Alabama	8.4
6	New Mexico	8.2
7	Tennessee	8.1
7	Wyoming	8.1
9	Arkansas	8.0
9	Louisiana	8.0
9	Nevada	8.0
12	Oklahoma	7.8
13	Indiana	7.7
13	North Carolina	7.7
13	South Carolina	7.7
13	Texas	7.7
17	Georgia	7.6
18	Florida	7.5
19	New Jersey	7.4
19	Ohio	7.4
21	Illinois	7.3
21	Montana	7.3
23	Maryland	7.2
23	Michigan	7.2
23	Missouri	7.2
26	Massachusetts	7.1
26	Pennsylvania	7.1
28	Delaware	7.0
28	Vermont	7.0
28	Virginia	7.0
31	Arizona	6.8
31	Kansas	6.8
31	New York	6.8
31	Rhode Island	6.8
35	North Dakota	6.7
36	Connecticut	6.6
36	Maine	6.6
38	Nebraska	6.5
38	Utah	6.5
40	California	6.4
40	Hawaii	6.4
40	New Hampshire	6.4
43	Iowa	6.3
43	Wisconsin	6.3
45	Idaho	6.2
45	South Dakota	6.2
47	Washington	6.0
48	Oregon	5.9
49	Minnesota	5.7
50	Alaska	5.0

	District of Columbia	6.8

Source: U.S. Department of Health and Human Services, National Center for Health Statistics
"National Vital Statistics Reports" (Vol. 59, No. 1, December 2010, http://www.cdc.gov/nchs/births.htm)
*Final data by state of residence. Births of less than 2,500 grams (5 pounds 8 ounces). Includes only non-Hispanic whites.

Births of Low Birthweight to Black Women
as a Percent of All Births to Black Women in 2008
National Percent = 13.7% of Live Births to Black Women*

ALPHA ORDER			RANK ORDER		
RANK	STATE	PERCENT	RANK	STATE	PERCENT
2	Alabama	15.8	1	Mississippi	16.1
34	Alaska	11.9	2	Alabama	15.8
36	Arizona	11.8	3	Arkansas	15.1
3	Arkansas	15.1	3	Louisiana	15.1
33	California	12.1	3	Oklahoma	15.1
7	Colorado	14.8	6	Kentucky	15.0
18	Connecticut	13.6	7	Colorado	14.8
29	Delaware	12.6	8	Michigan	14.5
19	Florida	13.5	8	Ohio	14.5
16	Georgia	13.8	8	South Carolina	14.5
41	Hawaii	10.7	8	West Virginia	14.5
NA	Idaho**	NA	12	North Carolina	14.4
16	Illinois	13.8	13	Indiana	14.1
13	Indiana	14.1	14	Texas	14.0
34	Iowa	11.9	15	Tennessee	13.9
31	Kansas	12.4	16	Georgia	13.8
6	Kentucky	15.0	16	Illinois	13.8
3	Louisiana	15.1	18	Connecticut	13.6
43	Maine	9.7	19	Florida	13.5
22	Maryland	13.1	19	Pennsylvania	13.5
37	Massachusetts	11.1	21	Missouri	13.3
8	Michigan	14.5	22	Maryland	13.1
39	Minnesota	10.8	22	Nevada	13.1
1	Mississippi	16.1	22	New Jersey	13.1
21	Missouri	13.3	25	Utah	13.0
NA	Montana**	NA	25	Virginia	13.0
30	Nebraska	12.5	25	Wisconsin	13.0
22	Nevada	13.1	28	New York	12.8
NA	New Hampshire**	NA	29	Delaware	12.6
22	New Jersey	13.1	30	Nebraska	12.5
32	New Mexico	12.3	31	Kansas	12.4
28	New York	12.8	32	New Mexico	12.3
12	North Carolina	14.4	33	California	12.1
NA	North Dakota**	NA	34	Alaska	11.9
8	Ohio	14.5	34	Iowa	11.9
3	Oklahoma	15.1	36	Arizona	11.8
39	Oregon	10.8	37	Massachusetts	11.1
19	Pennsylvania	13.5	38	Rhode Island	11.0
38	Rhode Island	11.0	39	Minnesota	10.8
8	South Carolina	14.5	39	Oregon	10.8
42	South Dakota	9.8	41	Hawaii	10.7
15	Tennessee	13.9	42	South Dakota	9.8
14	Texas	14.0	43	Maine	9.7
25	Utah	13.0	44	Washington	9.0
NA	Vermont**	NA	NA	Idaho**	NA
25	Virginia	13.0	NA	Montana**	NA
44	Washington	9.0	NA	New Hampshire**	NA
8	West Virginia	14.5	NA	North Dakota**	NA
25	Wisconsin	13.0	NA	Vermont**	NA
NA	Wyoming**	NA	NA	Wyoming**	NA

District of Columbia   13.7

Source: U.S. Department of Health and Human Services, National Center for Health Statistics
"National Vital Statistics Reports" (Vol. 59, No. 1, December 2010, http://www.cdc.gov/nchs/births.htm)
*Final data by state of residence. Births of less than 2,500 grams (5 pounds 8 ounces). Includes only non-Hispanic blacks.
**Not available. Fewer than 20 births of low birthweight to black women.

Births of Low Birthweight to Hispanic Women
as a Percent of All Births to Hispanic Women in 2008
National Percent = 7.0% of Live Births to Hispanic Women*

ALPHA ORDER

RANK	STATE	PERCENT
25	Alabama	6.9
5	Alaska	8.6
31	Arizona	6.7
36	Arkansas	6.4
41	California	6.1
6	Colorado	8.5
9	Connecticut	8.1
21	Delaware	7.0
20	Florida	7.3
28	Georgia	6.8
11	Hawaii	7.6
17	Idaho	7.4
33	Illinois	6.6
28	Indiana	6.8
21	Iowa	7.0
41	Kansas	6.1
41	Kentucky	6.1
21	Louisiana	7.0
NA	Maine**	NA
21	Maryland	7.0
7	Massachusetts	8.3
28	Michigan	6.8
45	Minnesota	6.0
35	Mississippi	6.5
41	Missouri	6.1
17	Montana	7.4
25	Nebraska	6.9
25	Nevada	6.9
15	New Hampshire	7.5
11	New Jersey	7.6
3	New Mexico	8.7
10	New York	7.9
38	North Carolina	6.2
15	North Dakota	7.5
11	Ohio	7.6
31	Oklahoma	6.7
47	Oregon	5.8
3	Pennsylvania	8.7
7	Rhode Island	8.3
36	South Carolina	6.4
2	South Dakota	8.9
38	Tennessee	6.2
11	Texas	7.6
17	Utah	7.4
NA	Vermont**	NA
33	Virginia	6.6
45	Washington	6.0
NA	West Virginia**	NA
38	Wisconsin	6.2
1	Wyoming	9.0

RANK ORDER

RANK	STATE	PERCENT
1	Wyoming	9.0
2	South Dakota	8.9
3	New Mexico	8.7
3	Pennsylvania	8.7
5	Alaska	8.6
6	Colorado	8.5
7	Massachusetts	8.3
7	Rhode Island	8.3
9	Connecticut	8.1
10	New York	7.9
11	Hawaii	7.6
11	New Jersey	7.6
11	Ohio	7.6
11	Texas	7.6
15	New Hampshire	7.5
15	North Dakota	7.5
17	Idaho	7.4
17	Montana	7.4
17	Utah	7.4
20	Florida	7.3
21	Delaware	7.0
21	Iowa	7.0
21	Louisiana	7.0
21	Maryland	7.0
25	Alabama	6.9
25	Nebraska	6.9
25	Nevada	6.9
28	Georgia	6.8
28	Indiana	6.8
28	Michigan	6.8
31	Arizona	6.7
31	Oklahoma	6.7
33	Illinois	6.6
33	Virginia	6.6
35	Mississippi	6.5
36	Arkansas	6.4
36	South Carolina	6.4
38	North Carolina	6.2
38	Tennessee	6.2
38	Wisconsin	6.2
41	California	6.1
41	Kansas	6.1
41	Kentucky	6.1
41	Missouri	6.1
45	Minnesota	6.0
45	Washington	6.0
47	Oregon	5.8
NA	Maine**	NA
NA	Vermont**	NA
NA	West Virginia**	NA
	District of Columbia	5.8

Source: U.S. Department of Health and Human Services, National Center for Health Statistics
    "National Vital Statistics Reports" (Vol. 59, No. 1, December 2010, http://www.cdc.gov/nchs/births.htm)
*Final data. Births of less than 2,500 grams (5 pounds 8 ounces). Hispanic can be of any race.
**Not available. Fewer than 20 births of low birthweight to Hispanic women.

Births to Unmarried Women in 2008

National Total = 1,726,566 Live Births*

ALPHA ORDER

ALPHA ORDER

RANK	STATE	BIRTHS	% of USA
23	Alabama	25,746	1.5%
47	Alaska	4,300	0.2%
11	Arizona	45,039	2.6%
28	Arkansas	18,158	1.1%
1	California	221,568	12.8%
30	Colorado	17,444	1.0%
34	Connecticut	14,721	0.9%
41	Delaware	5,807	0.3%
3	Florida	108,536	6.3%
6	Georgia	66,603	3.9%
39	Hawaii	7,392	0.4%
40	Idaho	6,370	0.4%
5	Illinois	71,932	4.2%
13	Indiana	38,444	2.2%
35	Iowa	14,140	0.8%
33	Kansas	15,792	0.9%
26	Kentucky	23,787	1.4%
16	Louisiana	34,576	2.0%
42	Maine	5,406	0.3%
18	Maryland	32,742	1.9%
22	Massachusetts	26,191	1.5%
10	Michigan	48,662	2.8%
25	Minnesota	24,149	1.4%
24	Mississippi	24,486	1.4%
17	Missouri	33,087	1.9%
45	Montana	4,624	0.3%
37	Nebraska	9,140	0.5%
31	Nevada	16,803	1.0%
46	New Hampshire	4,495	0.3%
12	New Jersey	39,462	2.3%
32	New Mexico	15,953	0.9%
4	New York	103,555	6.0%
9	North Carolina	55,014	3.2%
48	North Dakota	3,003	0.2%
7	Ohio	64,522	3.7%
27	Oklahoma	23,145	1.3%
29	Oregon	17,724	1.0%
8	Pennsylvania	60,950	3.5%
43	Rhode Island	5,284	0.3%
20	South Carolina	30,122	1.7%
44	South Dakota	4,634	0.3%
15	Tennessee	37,696	2.2%
2	Texas	169,318	9.8%
36	Utah	11,350	0.7%
50	Vermont	2,458	0.1%
14	Virginia	38,215	2.2%
19	Washington	30,676	1.8%
38	West Virginia	9,021	0.5%
21	Wisconsin	26,260	1.5%
49	Wyoming	2,785	0.2%

RANK ORDER

RANK	STATE	BIRTHS	% of USA
1	California	221,568	12.8%
2	Texas	169,318	9.8%
3	Florida	108,536	6.3%
4	New York	103,555	6.0%
5	Illinois	71,932	4.2%
6	Georgia	66,603	3.9%
7	Ohio	64,522	3.7%
8	Pennsylvania	60,950	3.5%
9	North Carolina	55,014	3.2%
10	Michigan	48,662	2.8%
11	Arizona	45,039	2.6%
12	New Jersey	39,462	2.3%
13	Indiana	38,444	2.2%
14	Virginia	38,215	2.2%
15	Tennessee	37,696	2.2%
16	Louisiana	34,576	2.0%
17	Missouri	33,087	1.9%
18	Maryland	32,742	1.9%
19	Washington	30,676	1.8%
20	South Carolina	30,122	1.7%
21	Wisconsin	26,260	1.5%
22	Massachusetts	26,191	1.5%
23	Alabama	25,746	1.5%
24	Mississippi	24,486	1.4%
25	Minnesota	24,149	1.4%
26	Kentucky	23,787	1.4%
27	Oklahoma	23,145	1.3%
28	Arkansas	18,158	1.1%
29	Oregon	17,724	1.0%
30	Colorado	17,444	1.0%
31	Nevada	16,803	1.0%
32	New Mexico	15,953	0.9%
33	Kansas	15,792	0.9%
34	Connecticut	14,721	0.9%
35	Iowa	14,140	0.8%
36	Utah	11,350	0.7%
37	Nebraska	9,140	0.5%
38	West Virginia	9,021	0.5%
39	Hawaii	7,392	0.4%
40	Idaho	6,370	0.4%
41	Delaware	5,807	0.3%
42	Maine	5,406	0.3%
43	Rhode Island	5,284	0.3%
44	South Dakota	4,634	0.3%
45	Montana	4,624	0.3%
46	New Hampshire	4,495	0.3%
47	Alaska	4,300	0.2%
48	North Dakota	3,003	0.2%
49	Wyoming	2,785	0.2%
50	Vermont	2,458	0.1%
	District of Columbia	5,279	0.3%

Source: U.S. Department of Health and Human Services, National Center for Health Statistics
"National Vital Statistics Reports" (Vol. 59, No. 1, December 2010, http://www.cdc.gov/nchs/births.htm)
*Final data by state of residence.

Births to Unmarried Women as a Percent of All Births in 2008

National Percent = 40.6% of Live Births*

ALPHA ORDER			RANK ORDER		
RANK	STATE	PERCENT	RANK	STATE	PERCENT
27	Alabama	39.9	1	Mississippi	54.5
33	Alaska	37.6	2	Louisiana	53.0
8	Arizona	45.3	3	New Mexico	52.9
9	Arkansas	44.6	4	Delaware	48.0
25	California	40.2	5	South Carolina	47.8
49	Colorado	24.9	6	Florida	46.9
35	Connecticut	36.4	7	Georgia	45.4
4	Delaware	48.0	8	Arizona	45.3
6	Florida	46.9	9	Arkansas	44.6
7	Georgia	45.4	10	Tennessee	44.1
31	Hawaii	37.9	11	Rhode Island	43.9
48	Idaho	25.3	12	Ohio	43.4
23	Illinois	40.7	13	Indiana	43.3
13	Indiana	43.3	14	Nevada	42.5
39	Iowa	35.2	15	Maryland	42.4
32	Kansas	37.8	16	Oklahoma	42.3
23	Kentucky	40.7	17	North Carolina	42.0
2	Louisiana	53.0	17	West Virginia	42.0
28	Maine	39.7	19	Texas	41.7
15	Maryland	42.4	20	New York	41.4
42	Massachusetts	34.0	21	Missouri	40.9
25	Michigan	40.2	22	Pennsylvania	40.8
46	Minnesota	33.3	23	Illinois	40.7
1	Mississippi	54.5	23	Kentucky	40.7
21	Missouri	40.9	25	California	40.2
34	Montana	36.7	25	Michigan	40.2
44	Nebraska	33.9	27	Alabama	39.9
14	Nevada	42.5	28	Maine	39.7
47	New Hampshire	32.9	29	Vermont	38.8
40	New Jersey	35.0	30	South Dakota	38.4
3	New Mexico	52.9	31	Hawaii	37.9
20	New York	41.4	32	Kansas	37.8
17	North Carolina	42.0	33	Alaska	37.6
45	North Dakota	33.6	34	Montana	36.7
12	Ohio	43.4	35	Connecticut	36.4
16	Oklahoma	42.3	36	Wisconsin	36.3
37	Oregon	36.1	37	Oregon	36.1
22	Pennsylvania	40.8	38	Virginia	35.8
11	Rhode Island	43.9	39	Iowa	35.2
5	South Carolina	47.8	40	New Jersey	35.0
30	South Dakota	38.4	41	Wyoming	34.6
10	Tennessee	44.1	42	Massachusetts	34.0
19	Texas	41.7	42	Washington	34.0
50	Utah	20.4	44	Nebraska	33.9
29	Vermont	38.8	45	North Dakota	33.6
38	Virginia	35.8	46	Minnesota	33.3
42	Washington	34.0	47	New Hampshire	32.9
17	West Virginia	42.0	48	Idaho	25.3
36	Wisconsin	36.3	49	Colorado	24.9
41	Wyoming	34.6	50	Utah	20.4
				District of Columbia	57.8

Source: U.S. Department of Health and Human Services, National Center for Health Statistics
"National Vital Statistics Reports" (Vol. 59, No. 1, December 2010, http://www.cdc.gov/nchs/births.htm)
*Final data by state of residence.

Births to Unmarried White Women
as a Percent of All Births to White Women in 2008
National Percent = 28.7% of Live Births*

RANK	STATE	PERCENT
41	Alabama	25.6
43	Alaska	24.3
27	Arizona	29.7
11	Arkansas	33.8
44	California	24.1
49	Colorado	17.5
46	Connecticut	22.1
9	Delaware	34.3
7	Florida	35.3
32	Georgia	26.9
39	Hawaii	25.9
47	Idaho	21.0
39	Illinois	25.9
4	Indiana	36.8
19	Iowa	31.6
20	Kansas	31.1
5	Kentucky	36.5
10	Louisiana	34.2
2	Maine	39.9
34	Maryland	26.7
37	Massachusetts	26.0
24	Michigan	30.2
37	Minnesota	26.0
18	Mississippi	31.8
13	Missouri	33.1
23	Montana	30.3
31	Nebraska	27.0
22	Nevada	30.4
13	New Hampshire	33.1
48	New Jersey	17.7
17	New Mexico	31.9
42	New York	24.6
34	North Carolina	26.7
32	North Dakota	26.9
6	Ohio	35.5
8	Oklahoma	34.4
16	Oregon	32.0
21	Pennsylvania	30.9
11	Rhode Island	33.8
25	South Carolina	30.1
29	South Dakota	27.9
15	Tennessee	32.8
34	Texas	26.7
50	Utah	13.6
3	Vermont	39.1
45	Virginia	23.9
28	Washington	28.6
1	West Virginia	40.8
29	Wisconsin	27.9
26	Wyoming	30.0

RANK	STATE	PERCENT
1	West Virginia	40.8
2	Maine	39.9
3	Vermont	39.1
4	Indiana	36.8
5	Kentucky	36.5
6	Ohio	35.5
7	Florida	35.3
8	Oklahoma	34.4
9	Delaware	34.3
10	Louisiana	34.2
11	Arkansas	33.8
11	Rhode Island	33.8
13	Missouri	33.1
13	New Hampshire	33.1
15	Tennessee	32.8
16	Oregon	32.0
17	New Mexico	31.9
18	Mississippi	31.8
19	Iowa	31.6
20	Kansas	31.1
21	Pennsylvania	30.9
22	Nevada	30.4
23	Montana	30.3
24	Michigan	30.2
25	South Carolina	30.1
26	Wyoming	30.0
27	Arizona	29.7
28	Washington	28.6
29	South Dakota	27.9
29	Wisconsin	27.9
31	Nebraska	27.0
32	Georgia	26.9
32	North Dakota	26.9
34	Maryland	26.7
34	North Carolina	26.7
34	Texas	26.7
37	Massachusetts	26.0
37	Minnesota	26.0
39	Hawaii	25.9
39	Illinois	25.9
41	Alabama	25.6
42	New York	24.6
43	Alaska	24.3
44	California	24.1
45	Virginia	23.9
46	Connecticut	22.1
47	Idaho	21.0
48	New Jersey	17.7
49	Colorado	17.5
50	Utah	13.6

District of Columbia	7.0

Source: U.S. Department of Health and Human Services, National Center for Health Statistics
"National Vital Statistics Reports" (Vol. 59, No. 1, December 2010, http://www.cdc.gov/nchs/births.htm)
*Final data by state of residence. By race of mother. Includes only non-Hispanic whites.

Births to Unmarried Black Women
as a Percent of All Births to Black Women in 2008
National Percent = 72.3% of Live Births*

ALPHA ORDER

RANK	STATE	PERCENT
18	Alabama	72.9
44	Alaska	47.1
34	Arizona	62.8
3	Arkansas	80.3
28	California	68.0
42	Colorado	49.3
24	Connecticut	69.8
19	Delaware	72.7
23	Florida	69.9
22	Georgia	70.2
50	Hawaii	29.7
47	Idaho	37.7
4	Illinois	79.8
5	Indiana	79.5
13	Iowa	77.1
17	Kansas	74.6
14	Kentucky	76.7
6	Louisiana	79.4
49	Maine	31.7
32	Maryland	64.2
37	Massachusetts	58.4
9	Michigan	78.9
35	Minnesota	60.9
2	Mississippi	80.5
7	Missouri	79.1
40	Montana	52.8
26	Nebraska	68.3
21	Nevada	71.0
46	New Hampshire	39.5
27	New Jersey	68.2
36	New Mexico	60.5
25	New York	69.5
20	North Carolina	72.4
48	North Dakota	37.2
7	Ohio	79.1
15	Oklahoma	75.7
33	Oregon	63.2
11	Pennsylvania	78.0
28	Rhode Island	68.0
11	South Carolina	78.0
41	South Dakota	52.1
10	Tennessee	78.2
31	Texas	66.5
43	Utah	47.7
45	Vermont	40.2
30	Virginia	66.8
39	Washington	54.2
16	West Virginia	75.0
1	Wisconsin	83.9
38	Wyoming	56.9

RANK ORDER

RANK	STATE	PERCENT
1	Wisconsin	83.9
2	Mississippi	80.5
3	Arkansas	80.3
4	Illinois	79.8
5	Indiana	79.5
6	Louisiana	79.4
7	Missouri	79.1
7	Ohio	79.1
9	Michigan	78.9
10	Tennessee	78.2
11	Pennsylvania	78.0
11	South Carolina	78.0
13	Iowa	77.1
14	Kentucky	76.7
15	Oklahoma	75.7
16	West Virginia	75.0
17	Kansas	74.6
18	Alabama	72.9
19	Delaware	72.7
20	North Carolina	72.4
21	Nevada	71.0
22	Georgia	70.2
23	Florida	69.9
24	Connecticut	69.8
25	New York	69.5
26	Nebraska	68.3
27	New Jersey	68.2
28	California	68.0
28	Rhode Island	68.0
30	Virginia	66.8
31	Texas	66.5
32	Maryland	64.2
33	Oregon	63.2
34	Arizona	62.8
35	Minnesota	60.9
36	New Mexico	60.5
37	Massachusetts	58.4
38	Wyoming	56.9
39	Washington	54.2
40	Montana	52.8
41	South Dakota	52.1
42	Colorado	49.3
43	Utah	47.7
44	Alaska	47.1
45	Vermont	40.2
46	New Hampshire	39.5
47	Idaho	37.7
48	North Dakota	37.2
49	Maine	31.7
50	Hawaii	29.7

	District of Columbia	79.1

Source: U.S. Department of Health and Human Services, National Center for Health Statistics
"National Vital Statistics Reports" (Vol. 59, No. 1, December 2010, http://www.cdc.gov/nchs/births.htm)
*Final data by state of residence. By race of mother. Includes only non-Hispanic blacks.

Births to Unmarried Hispanic Women
as a Percent of All Births to Hispanic Women in 2008
National Percent = 52.6% of Live Births*

ALPHA ORDER

RANK	STATE	PERCENT
50	Alabama	24.1
49	Alaska	34.9
15	Arizona	56.5
35	Arkansas	50.1
24	California	51.6
48	Colorado	36.3
6	Connecticut	64.2
5	Delaware	64.7
33	Florida	50.5
29	Georgia	50.9
38	Hawaii	49.5
47	Idaho	43.3
22	Illinois	52.1
12	Indiana	57.5
32	Iowa	50.8
19	Kansas	53.2
21	Kentucky	53.0
13	Louisiana	57.1
45	Maine	45.7
13	Maryland	57.1
2	Massachusetts	66.1
36	Michigan	49.8
11	Minnesota	57.9
9	Mississippi	59.0
25	Missouri	51.5
22	Montana	52.1
34	Nebraska	50.4
29	Nevada	50.9
42	New Hampshire	48.7
8	New Jersey	59.4
10	New Mexico	58.8
4	New York	65.7
19	North Carolina	53.2
43	North Dakota	45.9
7	Ohio	59.5
39	Oklahoma	49.0
39	Oregon	49.0
1	Pennsylvania	66.4
3	Rhode Island	65.8
36	South Carolina	49.8
25	South Dakota	51.5
18	Tennessee	53.7
39	Texas	49.0
44	Utah	45.8
16	Vermont	56.0
27	Virginia	51.4
29	Washington	50.9
46	West Virginia	45.0
17	Wisconsin	53.8
28	Wyoming	51.2

RANK ORDER

RANK	STATE	PERCENT
1	Pennsylvania	66.4
2	Massachusetts	66.1
3	Rhode Island	65.8
4	New York	65.7
5	Delaware	64.7
6	Connecticut	64.2
7	Ohio	59.5
8	New Jersey	59.4
9	Mississippi	59.0
10	New Mexico	58.8
11	Minnesota	57.9
12	Indiana	57.5
13	Louisiana	57.1
13	Maryland	57.1
15	Arizona	56.5
16	Vermont	56.0
17	Wisconsin	53.8
18	Tennessee	53.7
19	Kansas	53.2
19	North Carolina	53.2
21	Kentucky	53.0
22	Illinois	52.1
22	Montana	52.1
24	California	51.6
25	Missouri	51.5
25	South Dakota	51.5
27	Virginia	51.4
28	Wyoming	51.2
29	Georgia	50.9
29	Nevada	50.9
29	Washington	50.9
32	Iowa	50.8
33	Florida	50.5
34	Nebraska	50.4
35	Arkansas	50.1
36	Michigan	49.8
36	South Carolina	49.8
38	Hawaii	49.5
39	Oklahoma	49.0
39	Oregon	49.0
39	Texas	49.0
42	New Hampshire	48.7
43	North Dakota	45.9
44	Utah	45.8
45	Maine	45.7
46	West Virginia	45.0
47	Idaho	43.3
48	Colorado	36.3
49	Alaska	34.9
50	Alabama	24.1
	District of Columbia	72.6

Source: U.S. Department of Health and Human Services, National Center for Health Statistics
"National Vital Statistics Reports" (Vol. 59, No. 1, December 2010, http://www.cdc.gov/nchs/births.htm)
*Final data by state of residence. Hispanic can be of any race.

Births to Teenage Mothers in 2008

National Total = 434,758 Births*

ALPHA ORDER

RANK	STATE	BIRTHS	% of USA
17	Alabama	8,559	2.0%
43	Alaska	1,135	0.3%
10	Arizona	12,051	2.8%
27	Arkansas	5,940	1.4%
2	California	51,730	11.9%
24	Colorado	6,638	1.5%
36	Connecticut	2,789	0.6%
42	Delaware	1,237	0.3%
3	Florida	24,077	5.5%
6	Georgia	17,273	4.0%
40	Hawaii	1,625	0.4%
39	Idaho	2,261	0.5%
4	Illinois	17,410	4.0%
13	Indiana	9,607	2.2%
35	Iowa	3,591	0.8%
32	Kansas	4,403	1.0%
19	Kentucky	7,636	1.8%
15	Louisiana	8,817	2.0%
45	Maine	1,117	0.3%
25	Maryland	6,560	1.5%
29	Massachusetts	4,586	1.1%
11	Michigan	11,985	2.8%
28	Minnesota	4,885	1.1%
22	Mississippi	7,193	1.7%
14	Missouri	9,160	2.1%
41	Montana	1,312	0.3%
38	Nebraska	2,286	0.5%
33	Nevada	4,262	1.0%
47	New Hampshire	902	0.2%
23	New Jersey	7,008	1.6%
30	New Mexico	4,540	1.0%
5	New York	17,289	4.0%
8	North Carolina	15,136	3.5%
49	North Dakota	666	0.2%
7	Ohio	16,204	3.7%
20	Oklahoma	7,494	1.7%
31	Oregon	4,476	1.0%
9	Pennsylvania	13,724	3.2%
44	Rhode Island	1,124	0.3%
18	South Carolina	8,329	1.9%
45	South Dakota	1,117	0.3%
12	Tennessee	11,157	2.6%
1	Texas	54,284	12.5%
34	Utah	3,749	0.9%
50	Vermont	472	0.1%
16	Virginia	8,801	2.0%
21	Washington	7,386	1.7%
37	West Virginia	2,772	0.6%
26	Wisconsin	6,041	1.4%
48	Wyoming	879	0.2%

RANK ORDER

RANK	STATE	BIRTHS	% of USA
1	Texas	54,284	12.5%
2	California	51,730	11.9%
3	Florida	24,077	5.5%
4	Illinois	17,410	4.0%
5	New York	17,289	4.0%
6	Georgia	17,273	4.0%
7	Ohio	16,204	3.7%
8	North Carolina	15,136	3.5%
9	Pennsylvania	13,724	3.2%
10	Arizona	12,051	2.8%
11	Michigan	11,985	2.8%
12	Tennessee	11,157	2.6%
13	Indiana	9,607	2.2%
14	Missouri	9,160	2.1%
15	Louisiana	8,817	2.0%
16	Virginia	8,801	2.0%
17	Alabama	8,559	2.0%
18	South Carolina	8,329	1.9%
19	Kentucky	7,636	1.8%
20	Oklahoma	7,494	1.7%
21	Washington	7,386	1.7%
22	Mississippi	7,193	1.7%
23	New Jersey	7,008	1.6%
24	Colorado	6,638	1.5%
25	Maryland	6,560	1.5%
26	Wisconsin	6,041	1.4%
27	Arkansas	5,940	1.4%
28	Minnesota	4,885	1.1%
29	Massachusetts	4,586	1.1%
30	New Mexico	4,540	1.0%
31	Oregon	4,476	1.0%
32	Kansas	4,403	1.0%
33	Nevada	4,262	1.0%
34	Utah	3,749	0.9%
35	Iowa	3,591	0.8%
36	Connecticut	2,789	0.6%
37	West Virginia	2,772	0.6%
38	Nebraska	2,286	0.5%
39	Idaho	2,261	0.5%
40	Hawaii	1,625	0.4%
41	Montana	1,312	0.3%
42	Delaware	1,237	0.3%
43	Alaska	1,135	0.3%
44	Rhode Island	1,124	0.3%
45	Maine	1,117	0.3%
45	South Dakota	1,117	0.3%
47	New Hampshire	902	0.2%
48	Wyoming	879	0.2%
49	North Dakota	666	0.2%
50	Vermont	472	0.1%
	District of Columbia	1,083	0.2%

Source: U.S. Department of Health and Human Services, National Center for Health Statistics
"Vital Stats" (http://www.cdc.gov/nchs/VitalStats.htm)
*Final data. Live births to women 15 to 19 years old by state of residence of mother.

Births to Teenage Mothers as a Percent of All Births in 2008

National Percent = 10.2% of Live Births*

RANK	STATE (ALPHA ORDER)	PERCENT		RANK	STATE (RANK ORDER)	PERCENT
7	Alabama	13.3		1	Mississippi	16.0
24	Alaska	9.9		2	New Mexico	15.0
12	Arizona	12.1		3	Arkansas	14.6
3	Arkansas	14.6		4	Oklahoma	13.7
28	California	9.4		5	Louisiana	13.5
27	Colorado	9.5		6	Texas	13.4
44	Connecticut	6.9		7	Alabama	13.3
23	Delaware	10.2		8	South Carolina	13.2
21	Florida	10.4		9	Kentucky	13.1
13	Georgia	11.8		10	Tennessee	13.0
38	Hawaii	8.3		11	West Virginia	12.9
33	Idaho	9.0		12	Arizona	12.1
26	Illinois	9.8		13	Georgia	11.8
18	Indiana	10.8		14	North Carolina	11.6
34	Iowa	8.9		15	Missouri	11.3
20	Kansas	10.5		16	Ohio	10.9
9	Kentucky	13.1		16	Wyoming	10.9
5	Louisiana	13.5		18	Indiana	10.8
39	Maine	8.2		18	Nevada	10.8
35	Maryland	8.5		20	Kansas	10.5
50	Massachusetts	6.0		21	Florida	10.4
24	Michigan	9.9		21	Montana	10.4
46	Minnesota	6.7		23	Delaware	10.2
1	Mississippi	16.0		24	Alaska	9.9
15	Missouri	11.3		24	Michigan	9.9
21	Montana	10.4		26	Illinois	9.8
35	Nebraska	8.5		27	Colorado	9.5
18	Nevada	10.8		28	California	9.4
48	New Hampshire	6.6		29	Rhode Island	9.3
49	New Jersey	6.2		29	South Dakota	9.3
2	New Mexico	15.0		31	Pennsylvania	9.2
44	New York	6.9		32	Oregon	9.1
14	North Carolina	11.6		33	Idaho	9.0
42	North Dakota	7.5		34	Iowa	8.9
16	Ohio	10.9		35	Maryland	8.5
4	Oklahoma	13.7		35	Nebraska	8.5
32	Oregon	9.1		37	Wisconsin	8.4
31	Pennsylvania	9.2		38	Hawaii	8.3
29	Rhode Island	9.3		39	Maine	8.2
8	South Carolina	13.2		39	Virginia	8.2
29	South Dakota	9.3		39	Washington	8.2
10	Tennessee	13.0		42	North Dakota	7.5
6	Texas	13.4		43	Vermont	7.4
46	Utah	6.7		44	Connecticut	6.9
43	Vermont	7.4		44	New York	6.9
39	Virginia	8.2		46	Minnesota	6.7
39	Washington	8.2		46	Utah	6.7
11	West Virginia	12.9		48	New Hampshire	6.6
37	Wisconsin	8.4		49	New Jersey	6.2
16	Wyoming	10.9		50	Massachusetts	6.0

District of Columbia   11.9

Source: CQ Press using data from U.S. Department of Health and Human Services, National Center for Health Statistics
"National Vital Statistics Reports" (Vol. 59, No. 1, December 2010, http://www.cdc.gov/nchs/births.htm)
"Vital Stats" (http://www.cdc.gov/nchs/VitalStats.htm)
*Final data. Live births to women 15 to 19 years old by state of residence.

Teenage Birth Rate in 2008

National Rate = 41.5 Live Births per 1,000 Women 15 to 19 Years Old*

ALPHA ORDER

RANK	STATE	RATE
12	Alabama	53.0
17	Alaska	46.8
6	Arizona	56.2
4	Arkansas	61.8
29	California	38.4
22	Colorado	42.5
47	Connecticut	22.9
27	Delaware	40.4
21	Florida	42.8
13	Georgia	51.8
23	Hawaii	42.1
24	Idaho	41.2
30	Illinois	38.1
20	Indiana	43.7
35	Iowa	33.9
18	Kansas	45.6
7	Kentucky	55.6
9	Louisiana	54.1
44	Maine	26.1
38	Maryland	32.8
49	Massachusetts	20.1
37	Michigan	33.2
43	Minnesota	27.2
1	Mississippi	65.7
19	Missouri	45.5
26	Montana	40.7
32	Nebraska	36.5
10	Nevada	53.5
50	New Hampshire	19.8
46	New Jersey	24.5
2	New Mexico	64.1
45	New York	25.2
14	North Carolina	49.4
41	North Dakota	28.6
25	Ohio	41.0
5	Oklahoma	61.6
31	Oregon	37.2
39	Pennsylvania	31.5
42	Rhode Island	28.5
11	South Carolina	53.1
28	South Dakota	40.0
7	Tennessee	55.6
3	Texas	63.4
33	Utah	35.1
48	Vermont	21.3
36	Virginia	33.5
34	Washington	34.6
16	West Virginia	48.8
40	Wisconsin	31.3
15	Wyoming	49.2

RANK ORDER

RANK	STATE	RATE
1	Mississippi	65.7
2	New Mexico	64.1
3	Texas	63.4
4	Arkansas	61.8
5	Oklahoma	61.6
6	Arizona	56.2
7	Kentucky	55.6
7	Tennessee	55.6
9	Louisiana	54.1
10	Nevada	53.5
11	South Carolina	53.1
12	Alabama	53.0
13	Georgia	51.8
14	North Carolina	49.4
15	Wyoming	49.2
16	West Virginia	48.8
17	Alaska	46.8
18	Kansas	45.6
19	Missouri	45.5
20	Indiana	43.7
21	Florida	42.8
22	Colorado	42.5
23	Hawaii	42.1
24	Idaho	41.2
25	Ohio	41.0
26	Montana	40.7
27	Delaware	40.4
28	South Dakota	40.0
29	California	38.4
30	Illinois	38.1
31	Oregon	37.2
32	Nebraska	36.5
33	Utah	35.1
34	Washington	34.6
35	Iowa	33.9
36	Virginia	33.5
37	Michigan	33.2
38	Maryland	32.8
39	Pennsylvania	31.5
40	Wisconsin	31.3
41	North Dakota	28.6
42	Rhode Island	28.5
43	Minnesota	27.2
44	Maine	26.1
45	New York	25.2
46	New Jersey	24.5
47	Connecticut	22.9
48	Vermont	21.3
49	Massachusetts	20.1
50	New Hampshire	19.8
	District of Columbia	50.9

Source: U.S. Department of Health and Human Services, National Center for Health Statistics
"National Vital Statistics Reports" (Vol. 59, No. 1, December 2010, http://www.cdc.gov/nchs/births.htm)
*Final data by state of residence.

Percent Change in Teenage Birth Rate: 2007 to 2008

National Percent Change = 2.4% Decrease*

ALPHA ORDER				RANK ORDER		
RANK	STATE	PERCENT CHANGE		RANK	STATE	PERCENT CHANGE
24	Alabama	(2.0)		1	Montana	10.6
2	Alaska	4.7		2	Alaska	4.7
48	Arizona	(8.2)		3	Kansas	4.3
10	Arkansas	0.2		4	Oregon	3.6
36	California	(3.3)		5	West Virginia	3.0
25	Colorado	(2.1)		6	Iowa	2.1
18	Connecticut	(0.9)		7	Hawaii	1.9
14	Delaware	(0.5)		8	Nebraska	1.1
47	Florida	(5.9)		9	Kentucky	0.9
46	Georgia	(5.6)		10	Arkansas	0.2
7	Hawaii	1.9		10	Oklahoma	0.2
14	Idaho	(0.5)		12	Pennsylvania	0.0
41	Illinois	(4.8)		13	Missouri	(0.4)
36	Indiana	(3.3)		14	Delaware	(0.5)
6	Iowa	2.1		14	Idaho	(0.5)
3	Kansas	4.3		16	Washington	(0.6)
9	Kentucky	0.9		17	Ohio	(0.7)
34	Louisiana	(3.2)		18	Connecticut	(0.9)
32	Maine	(3.0)		18	South Carolina	(0.9)
40	Maryland	(4.7)		20	New Hampshire	(1.0)
50	Massachusetts	(9.0)		20	North Carolina	(1.0)
31	Michigan	(2.9)		22	Tennessee	(1.1)
42	Minnesota	(4.9)		23	Texas	(1.2)
49	Mississippi	(8.6)		24	Alabama	(2.0)
13	Missouri	(0.4)		25	Colorado	(2.1)
1	Montana	10.6		26	New York	(2.3)
8	Nebraska	1.1		27	North Dakota	(2.4)
36	Nevada	(3.3)		28	New Jersey	(2.8)
20	New Hampshire	(1.0)		28	Utah	(2.8)
28	New Jersey	(2.8)		28	Wisconsin	(2.8)
32	New Mexico	(3.0)		31	Michigan	(2.9)
26	New York	(2.3)		32	Maine	(3.0)
20	North Carolina	(1.0)		32	New Mexico	(3.0)
27	North Dakota	(2.4)		34	Louisiana	(3.2)
17	Ohio	(0.7)		34	Vermont	(3.2)
10	Oklahoma	0.2		36	California	(3.3)
4	Oregon	3.6		36	Indiana	(3.3)
12	Pennsylvania	0.0		36	Nevada	(3.3)
43	Rhode Island	(5.0)		39	Virginia	(4.6)
18	South Carolina	(0.9)		40	Maryland	(4.7)
44	South Dakota	(5.2)		41	Illinois	(4.8)
22	Tennessee	(1.1)		42	Minnesota	(4.9)
23	Texas	(1.2)		43	Rhode Island	(5.0)
28	Utah	(2.8)		44	South Dakota	(5.2)
34	Vermont	(3.2)		44	Wyoming	(5.2)
39	Virginia	(4.6)		46	Georgia	(5.6)
16	Washington	(0.6)		47	Florida	(5.9)
5	West Virginia	3.0		48	Arizona	(8.2)
28	Wisconsin	(2.8)		49	Mississippi	(8.6)
44	Wyoming	(5.2)		50	Massachusetts	(9.0)

District of Columbia   2.0

Source: CQ Press using data from U.S. Department of Health and Human Services, National Center for Health Statistics
"National Vital Statistics Reports" (Vol. 59, No. 1, December 2010, http://www.cdc.gov/nchs/births.htm)
*Final data by state of residence. Births to women 15 to 19 years old.

Births to White Teenage Mothers in 2008

National Total = 306,402 Live Births*

ALPHA ORDER

RANK	STATE	BIRTHS	% of USA
20	Alabama	4,840	1.6%
47	Alaska	492	0.2%
7	Arizona	10,063	3.3%
21	Arkansas	4,144	1.4%
2	California	44,331	14.5%
17	Colorado	5,906	1.9%
38	Connecticut	2,017	0.7%
45	Delaware	716	0.2%
3	Florida	14,816	4.8%
9	Georgia	8,594	2.8%
50	Hawaii	389	0.1%
37	Idaho	2,097	0.7%
6	Illinois	10,823	3.5%
11	Indiana	7,587	2.5%
33	Iowa	3,130	1.0%
28	Kansas	3,643	1.2%
15	Kentucky	6,499	2.1%
26	Louisiana	3,859	1.3%
40	Maine	1,055	0.3%
35	Maryland	2,907	0.9%
29	Massachusetts	3,479	1.1%
13	Michigan	7,120	2.3%
32	Minnesota	3,223	1.1%
34	Mississippi	3,106	1.0%
14	Missouri	6,631	2.2%
41	Montana	936	0.3%
39	Nebraska	1,797	0.6%
31	Nevada	3,415	1.1%
42	New Hampshire	873	0.3%
23	New Jersey	4,091	1.3%
27	New Mexico	3,704	1.2%
4	New York	11,148	3.6%
8	North Carolina	8,925	2.9%
49	North Dakota	409	0.1%
5	Ohio	10,970	3.6%
19	Oklahoma	5,168	1.7%
24	Oregon	4,002	1.3%
10	Pennsylvania	8,393	2.7%
43	Rhode Island	866	0.3%
22	South Carolina	4,118	1.3%
46	South Dakota	647	0.2%
12	Tennessee	7,339	2.4%
1	Texas	45,416	14.8%
30	Utah	3,460	1.1%
48	Vermont	454	0.1%
18	Virginia	5,221	1.7%
16	Washington	6,064	2.0%
36	West Virginia	2,634	0.9%
25	Wisconsin	3,925	1.3%
44	Wyoming	792	0.3%

RANK ORDER

RANK	STATE	BIRTHS	% of USA
1	Texas	45,416	14.8%
2	California	44,331	14.5%
3	Florida	14,816	4.8%
4	New York	11,148	3.6%
5	Ohio	10,970	3.6%
6	Illinois	10,823	3.5%
7	Arizona	10,063	3.3%
8	North Carolina	8,925	2.9%
9	Georgia	8,594	2.8%
10	Pennsylvania	8,393	2.7%
11	Indiana	7,587	2.5%
12	Tennessee	7,339	2.4%
13	Michigan	7,120	2.3%
14	Missouri	6,631	2.2%
15	Kentucky	6,499	2.1%
16	Washington	6,064	2.0%
17	Colorado	5,906	1.9%
18	Virginia	5,221	1.7%
19	Oklahoma	5,168	1.7%
20	Alabama	4,840	1.6%
21	Arkansas	4,144	1.4%
22	South Carolina	4,118	1.3%
23	New Jersey	4,091	1.3%
24	Oregon	4,002	1.3%
25	Wisconsin	3,925	1.3%
26	Louisiana	3,859	1.3%
27	New Mexico	3,704	1.2%
28	Kansas	3,643	1.2%
29	Massachusetts	3,479	1.1%
30	Utah	3,460	1.1%
31	Nevada	3,415	1.1%
32	Minnesota	3,223	1.1%
33	Iowa	3,130	1.0%
34	Mississippi	3,106	1.0%
35	Maryland	2,907	0.9%
36	West Virginia	2,634	0.9%
37	Idaho	2,097	0.7%
38	Connecticut	2,017	0.7%
39	Nebraska	1,797	0.6%
40	Maine	1,055	0.3%
41	Montana	936	0.3%
42	New Hampshire	873	0.3%
43	Rhode Island	866	0.3%
44	Wyoming	792	0.3%
45	Delaware	716	0.2%
46	South Dakota	647	0.2%
47	Alaska	492	0.2%
48	Vermont	454	0.1%
49	North Dakota	409	0.1%
50	Hawaii	389	0.1%
	District of Columbia	168	0.1%

Source: U.S. Department of Health and Human Services, National Center for Health Statistics
   "Vital Stats" (http://www.cdc.gov/nchs/VitalStats.htm)
*Final data. Live births to women 15 to 19 years old by state of residence.

White Teenage Birth Rate in 2008

National Rate = 37.3 Births per 1,000 White Teenage Women*

ALPHA ORDER

RANK	STATE	RATE
12	Alabama	46.3
33	Alaska	28.5
3	Arizona	55.7
3	Arkansas	55.7
13	California	42.9
19	Colorado	40.7
46	Connecticut	19.5
27	Delaware	32.8
24	Florida	35.0
15	Georgia	42.2
43	Hawaii	22.2
22	Idaho	38.4
29	Illinois	31.5
20	Indiana	38.8
31	Iowa	31.0
16	Kansas	41.9
7	Kentucky	52.0
18	Louisiana	41.6
38	Maine	24.9
39	Maryland	24.1
50	Massachusetts	17.7
37	Michigan	25.1
45	Minnesota	20.0
5	Mississippi	54.1
20	Missouri	38.8
29	Montana	31.5
32	Nebraska	30.8
7	Nevada	52.0
48	New Hampshire	19.0
47	New Jersey	19.3
1	New Mexico	64.7
40	New York	22.9
17	North Carolina	41.8
49	North Dakota	18.9
26	Ohio	33.0
5	Oklahoma	54.1
23	Oregon	35.4
40	Pennsylvania	22.9
36	Rhode Island	25.4
14	South Carolina	42.4
35	South Dakota	26.4
10	Tennessee	47.2
2	Texas	64.6
25	Utah	34.1
44	Vermont	20.3
34	Virginia	27.9
28	Washington	32.7
9	West Virginia	48.6
42	Wisconsin	22.6
11	Wyoming	46.9

RANK ORDER

RANK	STATE	RATE
1	New Mexico	64.7
2	Texas	64.6
3	Arizona	55.7
3	Arkansas	55.7
5	Mississippi	54.1
5	Oklahoma	54.1
7	Kentucky	52.0
7	Nevada	52.0
9	West Virginia	48.6
10	Tennessee	47.2
11	Wyoming	46.9
12	Alabama	46.3
13	California	42.9
14	South Carolina	42.4
15	Georgia	42.2
16	Kansas	41.9
17	North Carolina	41.8
18	Louisiana	41.6
19	Colorado	40.7
20	Indiana	38.8
20	Missouri	38.8
22	Idaho	38.4
23	Oregon	35.4
24	Florida	35.0
25	Utah	34.1
26	Ohio	33.0
27	Delaware	32.8
28	Washington	32.7
29	Illinois	31.5
29	Montana	31.5
31	Iowa	31.0
32	Nebraska	30.8
33	Alaska	28.5
34	Virginia	27.9
35	South Dakota	26.4
36	Rhode Island	25.4
37	Michigan	25.1
38	Maine	24.9
39	Maryland	24.1
40	New York	22.9
40	Pennsylvania	22.9
42	Wisconsin	22.6
43	Hawaii	22.2
44	Vermont	20.3
45	Minnesota	20.0
46	Connecticut	19.5
47	New Jersey	19.3
48	New Hampshire	19.0
49	North Dakota	18.9
50	Massachusetts	17.7

District of Columbia   22.7

Source: CQ Press using data from U.S. Department of Health and Human Services, National Center for Health Statistics
"Vital Stats" (http://www.cdc.gov/nchs/VitalStats.htm)
*Final data. Live births to women 15 to 19 years old by state of residence.

Births to White Teenage Mothers as a Percent of All White Births in 2008

National Percent = 9.4% of White Live Births*

ALPHA ORDER

RANK	STATE	PERCENT
10	Alabama	11.1
37	Alaska	6.9
8	Arizona	11.8
3	Arkansas	13.1
15	California	10.1
21	Colorado	9.3
45	Connecticut	6.3
25	Delaware	8.7
24	Florida	9.0
18	Georgia	9.9
41	Hawaii	6.6
25	Idaho	8.7
32	Illinois	8.0
17	Indiana	10.0
29	Iowa	8.4
18	Kansas	9.9
6	Kentucky	12.6
14	Louisiana	10.2
30	Maine	8.2
44	Maryland	6.4
47	Massachusetts	5.7
33	Michigan	7.6
48	Minnesota	5.5
5	Mississippi	12.8
15	Missouri	10.1
25	Montana	8.7
33	Nebraska	7.6
11	Nevada	10.7
39	New Hampshire	6.8
50	New Jersey	5.1
1	New Mexico	14.8
45	New York	6.3
20	North Carolina	9.5
49	North Dakota	5.4
22	Ohio	9.2
7	Oklahoma	12.3
23	Oregon	9.1
36	Pennsylvania	7.2
28	Rhode Island	8.6
13	South Carolina	10.3
40	South Dakota	6.7
9	Tennessee	11.4
2	Texas	13.4
41	Utah	6.6
35	Vermont	7.4
37	Virginia	6.9
30	Washington	8.2
4	West Virginia	12.9
43	Wisconsin	6.5
12	Wyoming	10.5

RANK ORDER

RANK	STATE	PERCENT
1	New Mexico	14.8
2	Texas	13.4
3	Arkansas	13.1
4	West Virginia	12.9
5	Mississippi	12.8
6	Kentucky	12.6
7	Oklahoma	12.3
8	Arizona	11.8
9	Tennessee	11.4
10	Alabama	11.1
11	Nevada	10.7
12	Wyoming	10.5
13	South Carolina	10.3
14	Louisiana	10.2
15	California	10.1
15	Missouri	10.1
17	Indiana	10.0
18	Georgia	9.9
18	Kansas	9.9
20	North Carolina	9.5
21	Colorado	9.3
22	Ohio	9.2
23	Oregon	9.1
24	Florida	9.0
25	Delaware	8.7
25	Idaho	8.7
25	Montana	8.7
28	Rhode Island	8.6
29	Iowa	8.4
30	Maine	8.2
30	Washington	8.2
32	Illinois	8.0
33	Michigan	7.6
33	Nebraska	7.6
35	Vermont	7.4
36	Pennsylvania	7.2
37	Alaska	6.9
37	Virginia	6.9
39	New Hampshire	6.8
40	South Dakota	6.7
41	Hawaii	6.6
41	Utah	6.6
43	Wisconsin	6.5
44	Maryland	6.4
45	Connecticut	6.3
45	New York	6.3
47	Massachusetts	5.7
48	Minnesota	5.5
49	North Dakota	5.4
50	New Jersey	5.1

District of Columbia		4.7

Source: CQ Press using data from U.S. Department of Health and Human Services, National Center for Health Statistics
   "Vital Stats" (http://www.cdc.gov/nchs/VitalStats.htm)
*Final data. Live births to women 15 to 19 years old by state of residence.

Births to Black Teenage Mothers in 2008

National Total = 112,004 Live Births*

ALPHA ORDER

RANK	STATE	BIRTHS	% of USA
15	Alabama	3,660	3.3%
41	Alaska	54	0.0%
28	Arizona	682	0.6%
21	Arkansas	1,713	1.5%
9	California	4,952	4.4%
32	Colorado	524	0.5%
27	Connecticut	748	0.7%
33	Delaware	511	0.5%
1	Florida	8,916	8.0%
2	Georgia	8,498	7.6%
42	Hawaii	50	0.0%
43	Idaho	41	0.0%
4	Illinois	6,449	5.8%
20	Indiana	1,961	1.8%
34	Iowa	375	0.3%
29	Kansas	623	0.6%
23	Kentucky	1,082	1.0%
10	Louisiana	4,838	4.3%
44	Maine	32	0.0%
16	Maryland	3,577	3.2%
25	Massachusetts	939	0.8%
11	Michigan	4,662	4.2%
26	Minnesota	898	0.8%
13	Mississippi	4,016	3.6%
19	Missouri	2,396	2.1%
48	Montana	15	0.0%
35	Nebraska	340	0.3%
30	Nevada	622	0.6%
45	New Hampshire	23	0.0%
18	New Jersey	2,832	2.5%
39	New Mexico	107	0.1%
5	New York	5,729	5.1%
6	North Carolina	5,699	5.1%
46	North Dakota	21	0.0%
7	Ohio	5,102	4.6%
24	Oklahoma	988	0.9%
36	Oregon	203	0.2%
8	Pennsylvania	5,041	4.5%
37	Rhode Island	190	0.2%
12	South Carolina	4,100	3.7%
48	South Dakota	15	0.0%
14	Tennessee	3,677	3.3%
3	Texas	8,313	7.4%
40	Utah	78	0.1%
47	Vermont	16	0.0%
17	Virginia	3,472	3.1%
31	Washington	589	0.5%
38	West Virginia	130	0.1%
22	Wisconsin	1,582	1.4%
48	Wyoming	15	0.0%

RANK ORDER

RANK	STATE	BIRTHS	% of USA
1	Florida	8,916	8.0%
2	Georgia	8,498	7.6%
3	Texas	8,313	7.4%
4	Illinois	6,449	5.8%
5	New York	5,729	5.1%
6	North Carolina	5,699	5.1%
7	Ohio	5,102	4.6%
8	Pennsylvania	5,041	4.5%
9	California	4,952	4.4%
10	Louisiana	4,838	4.3%
11	Michigan	4,662	4.2%
12	South Carolina	4,100	3.7%
13	Mississippi	4,016	3.6%
14	Tennessee	3,677	3.3%
15	Alabama	3,660	3.3%
16	Maryland	3,577	3.2%
17	Virginia	3,472	3.1%
18	New Jersey	2,832	2.5%
19	Missouri	2,396	2.1%
20	Indiana	1,961	1.8%
21	Arkansas	1,713	1.5%
22	Wisconsin	1,582	1.4%
23	Kentucky	1,082	1.0%
24	Oklahoma	988	0.9%
25	Massachusetts	939	0.8%
26	Minnesota	898	0.8%
27	Connecticut	748	0.7%
28	Arizona	682	0.6%
29	Kansas	623	0.6%
30	Nevada	622	0.6%
31	Washington	589	0.5%
32	Colorado	524	0.5%
33	Delaware	511	0.5%
34	Iowa	375	0.3%
35	Nebraska	340	0.3%
36	Oregon	203	0.2%
37	Rhode Island	190	0.2%
38	West Virginia	130	0.1%
39	New Mexico	107	0.1%
40	Utah	78	0.1%
41	Alaska	54	0.0%
42	Hawaii	50	0.0%
43	Idaho	41	0.0%
44	Maine	32	0.0%
45	New Hampshire	23	0.0%
46	North Dakota	21	0.0%
47	Vermont	16	0.0%
48	Montana	15	0.0%
48	South Dakota	15	0.0%
48	Wyoming	15	0.0%
	District of Columbia	908	0.8%

Source: U.S. Department of Health and Human Services, National Center for Health Statistics
    "Vital Stats" (http://www.cdc.gov/nchs/VitalStats.htm)
*Final data. Live births to women 15 to 19 years old by state of residence.

Black Teenage Birth Rate in 2008

National Rate = 61.5 Births per 1,000 Black Teenage Women*

ALPHA ORDER

RANK	STATE	RATE
21	Alabama	64.9
43	Alaska	35.4
27	Arizona	51.3
4	Arkansas	79.4
37	California	41.3
29	Colorado	49.8
36	Connecticut	41.5
25	Delaware	60.8
18	Florida	66.3
19	Georgia	65.1
49	Hawaii	24.6
35	Idaho	43.3
12	Illinois	71.4
13	Indiana	70.6
5	Iowa	76.7
10	Kansas	73.1
15	Kentucky	68.7
9	Louisiana	73.4
45	Maine	33.2
28	Maryland	50.6
39	Massachusetts	40.2
22	Michigan	64.4
15	Minnesota	68.7
3	Mississippi	79.7
11	Missouri	72.7
47	Montana	30.6
2	Nebraska	80.1
24	Nevada	62.1
50	New Hampshire	22.9
26	New Jersey	52.3
44	New Mexico	33.3
41	New York	38.4
23	North Carolina	63.0
30	North Dakota	49.6
6	Ohio	76.5
17	Oklahoma	68.1
33	Oregon	44.5
8	Pennsylvania	74.9
30	Rhode Island	49.6
14	South Carolina	70.3
48	South Dakota	28.1
6	Tennessee	76.5
20	Texas	65.0
46	Utah	32.7
40	Vermont	38.7
30	Virginia	49.6
34	Washington	44.4
38	West Virginia	41.2
1	Wisconsin	84.3
42	Wyoming	37.1

RANK ORDER

RANK	STATE	RATE
1	Wisconsin	84.3
2	Nebraska	80.1
3	Mississippi	79.7
4	Arkansas	79.4
5	Iowa	76.7
6	Ohio	76.5
6	Tennessee	76.5
8	Pennsylvania	74.9
9	Louisiana	73.4
10	Kansas	73.1
11	Missouri	72.7
12	Illinois	71.4
13	Indiana	70.6
14	South Carolina	70.3
15	Kentucky	68.7
15	Minnesota	68.7
17	Oklahoma	68.1
18	Florida	66.3
19	Georgia	65.1
20	Texas	65.0
21	Alabama	64.9
22	Michigan	64.4
23	North Carolina	63.0
24	Nevada	62.1
25	Delaware	60.8
26	New Jersey	52.3
27	Arizona	51.3
28	Maryland	50.6
29	Colorado	49.8
30	North Dakota	49.6
30	Rhode Island	49.6
30	Virginia	49.6
33	Oregon	44.5
34	Washington	44.4
35	Idaho	43.3
36	Connecticut	41.5
37	California	41.3
38	West Virginia	41.2
39	Massachusetts	40.2
40	Vermont	38.7
41	New York	38.4
42	Wyoming	37.1
43	Alaska	35.4
44	New Mexico	33.3
45	Maine	33.2
46	Utah	32.7
47	Montana	30.6
48	South Dakota	28.1
49	Hawaii	24.6
50	New Hampshire	22.9

District of Columbia 66.8

Source: CQ Press using data from U.S. Department of Health and Human Services, National Center for Health Statistics
"Vital Stats" (http://www.cdc.gov/nchs/VitalStats.htm)
*Final data. Live births to women 15 to 19 years old by state of residence.

Births to Black Teenage Mothers as a Percent of All Black Births in 2008

National Percent = 16.7% of Black Live Births*

ALPHA ORDER

RANK	STATE	PERCENT
20	Alabama	18.3
42	Alaska	12.4
32	Arizona	15.2
2	Arkansas	21.2
36	California	14.3
33	Colorado	15.0
39	Connecticut	13.3
29	Delaware	15.5
29	Florida	15.5
26	Georgia	15.9
48	Hawaii	8.3
4	Idaho	20.6
3	Illinois	20.7
19	Indiana	18.4
7	Iowa	19.7
17	Kansas	18.6
13	Kentucky	19.0
16	Louisiana	18.8
47	Maine	8.6
38	Maryland	13.4
46	Massachusetts	10.0
5	Michigan	20.3
40	Minnesota	12.7
6	Mississippi	20.2
13	Missouri	19.0
18	Montana	18.5
22	Nebraska	17.1
25	Nevada	16.4
49	New Hampshire	8.0
37	New Jersey	13.7
23	New Mexico	16.9
45	New York	11.5
21	North Carolina	18.1
44	North Dakota	11.6
7	Ohio	19.7
7	Oklahoma	19.7
31	Oregon	15.3
13	Pennsylvania	19.0
34	Rhode Island	14.9
12	South Carolina	19.1
50	South Dakota	6.9
11	Tennessee	19.4
24	Texas	16.8
40	Utah	12.7
28	Vermont	15.7
35	Virginia	14.7
43	Washington	12.1
27	West Virginia	15.8
1	Wisconsin	21.5
10	Wyoming	19.5

RANK ORDER

RANK	STATE	PERCENT
1	Wisconsin	21.5
2	Arkansas	21.2
3	Illinois	20.7
4	Idaho	20.6
5	Michigan	20.3
6	Mississippi	20.2
7	Iowa	19.7
7	Ohio	19.7
7	Oklahoma	19.7
10	Wyoming	19.5
11	Tennessee	19.4
12	South Carolina	19.1
13	Kentucky	19.0
13	Missouri	19.0
13	Pennsylvania	19.0
16	Louisiana	18.8
17	Kansas	18.6
18	Montana	18.5
19	Indiana	18.4
20	Alabama	18.3
21	North Carolina	18.1
22	Nebraska	17.1
23	New Mexico	16.9
24	Texas	16.8
25	Nevada	16.4
26	Georgia	15.9
27	West Virginia	15.8
28	Vermont	15.7
29	Delaware	15.5
29	Florida	15.5
31	Oregon	15.3
32	Arizona	15.2
33	Colorado	15.0
34	Rhode Island	14.9
35	Virginia	14.7
36	California	14.3
37	New Jersey	13.7
38	Maryland	13.4
39	Connecticut	13.3
40	Minnesota	12.7
40	Utah	12.7
42	Alaska	12.4
43	Washington	12.1
44	North Dakota	11.6
45	New York	11.5
46	Massachusetts	10.0
47	Maine	8.6
48	Hawaii	8.3
49	New Hampshire	8.0
50	South Dakota	6.9

	District of Columbia	17.1

Source: CQ Press using data from U.S. Department of Health and Human Services, National Center for Health Statistics
"Vital Stats" (http://www.cdc.gov/nchs/VitalStats.htm)
*Final data. Live births to women 15 to 19 years old by state of residence.

Births to Young Teenagers in 2008

National Total = 5,764 Live Births*

RANK	STATE	BIRTHS	% of USA
10	Alabama	160	2.8%
47	Alaska	5	0.1%
9	Arizona	164	2.8%
25	Arkansas	76	1.3%
2	California	625	10.8%
23	Colorado	84	1.5%
36	Connecticut	26	0.5%
38	Delaware	23	0.4%
3	Florida	356	6.2%
4	Georgia	258	4.5%
42	Hawaii	15	0.3%
41	Idaho	18	0.3%
5	Illinois	254	4.4%
16	Indiana	114	2.0%
33	Iowa	38	0.7%
31	Kansas	40	0.7%
20	Kentucky	92	1.6%
14	Louisiana	139	2.4%
45	Maine	6	0.1%
19	Maryland	98	1.7%
31	Massachusetts	40	0.7%
13	Michigan	144	2.5%
29	Minnesota	66	1.1%
15	Mississippi	132	2.3%
20	Missouri	92	1.6%
44	Montana	9	0.2%
38	Nebraska	23	0.4%
28	Nevada	67	1.2%
49	New Hampshire	4	0.1%
27	New Jersey	69	1.2%
30	New Mexico	63	1.1%
6	New York	244	4.2%
7	North Carolina	234	4.1%
47	North Dakota	5	0.1%
8	Ohio	201	3.5%
22	Oklahoma	89	1.5%
33	Oregon	38	0.7%
11	Pennsylvania	158	2.7%
40	Rhode Island	20	0.3%
17	South Carolina	108	1.9%
43	South Dakota	13	0.2%
12	Tennessee	150	2.6%
1	Texas	843	14.6%
35	Utah	32	0.6%
45	Vermont	6	0.1%
18	Virginia	105	1.8%
24	Washington	82	1.4%
36	West Virginia	26	0.5%
25	Wisconsin	76	1.3%
50	Wyoming	2	0.0%

RANK	STATE	BIRTHS	% of USA
1	Texas	843	14.6%
2	California	625	10.8%
3	Florida	356	6.2%
4	Georgia	258	4.5%
5	Illinois	254	4.4%
6	New York	244	4.2%
7	North Carolina	234	4.1%
8	Ohio	201	3.5%
9	Arizona	164	2.8%
10	Alabama	160	2.8%
11	Pennsylvania	158	2.7%
12	Tennessee	150	2.6%
13	Michigan	144	2.5%
14	Louisiana	139	2.4%
15	Mississippi	132	2.3%
16	Indiana	114	2.0%
17	South Carolina	108	1.9%
18	Virginia	105	1.8%
19	Maryland	98	1.7%
20	Kentucky	92	1.6%
20	Missouri	92	1.6%
22	Oklahoma	89	1.5%
23	Colorado	84	1.5%
24	Washington	82	1.4%
25	Arkansas	76	1.3%
25	Wisconsin	76	1.3%
27	New Jersey	69	1.2%
28	Nevada	67	1.2%
29	Minnesota	66	1.1%
30	New Mexico	63	1.1%
31	Kansas	40	0.7%
31	Massachusetts	40	0.7%
33	Iowa	38	0.7%
33	Oregon	38	0.7%
35	Utah	32	0.6%
36	Connecticut	26	0.5%
36	West Virginia	26	0.5%
38	Delaware	23	0.4%
38	Nebraska	23	0.4%
40	Rhode Island	20	0.3%
41	Idaho	18	0.3%
42	Hawaii	15	0.3%
43	South Dakota	13	0.2%
44	Montana	9	0.2%
45	Maine	6	0.1%
45	Vermont	6	0.1%
47	Alaska	5	0.1%
47	North Dakota	5	0.1%
49	New Hampshire	4	0.1%
50	Wyoming	2	0.0%
	District of Columbia	32	0.6%

Source: U.S. Department of Health and Human Services, National Center for Health Statistics
   "Vital Stats" (http://www.cdc.gov/nchs/VitalStats.htm)
*Final data. Births to 10- to 14-year-olds by state of residence.

Young Teen Birth Rate in 2008

National Rate = 0.6 Live Births per 1,000 10- to 14-Year-Old Females*

RANK	STATE	RATE		RANK	STATE	RATE
2	Alabama	1.1		1	Mississippi	1.3
NA	Alaska**	NA		2	Alabama	1.1
7	Arizona	0.8		3	New Mexico	1.0
7	Arkansas	0.8		3	Texas	1.0
19	California	0.5		5	Delaware	0.9
19	Colorado	0.5		5	Louisiana	0.9
38	Connecticut	0.2		7	Arizona	0.8
5	Delaware	0.9		7	Arkansas	0.8
15	Florida	0.7		7	Georgia	0.8
7	Georgia	0.8		7	Nevada	0.8
NA	Hawaii**	NA		7	North Carolina	0.8
NA	Idaho**	NA		7	Oklahoma	0.8
17	Illinois	0.6		7	South Carolina	0.8
19	Indiana	0.5		7	Tennessee	0.8
26	Iowa	0.4		15	Florida	0.7
26	Kansas	0.4		15	Kentucky	0.7
15	Kentucky	0.7		17	Illinois	0.6
5	Louisiana	0.9		17	Rhode Island	0.6
NA	Maine**	NA		19	California	0.5
19	Maryland	0.5		19	Colorado	0.5
38	Massachusetts	0.2		19	Indiana	0.5
26	Michigan	0.4		19	Maryland	0.5
26	Minnesota	0.4		19	Missouri	0.5
1	Mississippi	1.3		19	Ohio	0.5
19	Missouri	0.5		19	West Virginia	0.5
NA	Montana**	NA		26	Iowa	0.4
26	Nebraska	0.4		26	Kansas	0.4
7	Nevada	0.8		26	Michigan	0.4
NA	New Hampshire**	NA		26	Minnesota	0.4
38	New Jersey	0.2		26	Nebraska	0.4
3	New Mexico	1.0		26	New York	0.4
26	New York	0.4		26	Pennsylvania	0.4
7	North Carolina	0.8		26	Virginia	0.4
NA	North Dakota**	NA		26	Washington	0.4
19	Ohio	0.5		26	Wisconsin	0.4
7	Oklahoma	0.8		36	Oregon	0.3
36	Oregon	0.3		36	Utah	0.3
26	Pennsylvania	0.4		38	Connecticut	0.2
17	Rhode Island	0.6		38	Massachusetts	0.2
7	South Carolina	0.8		38	New Jersey	0.2
NA	South Dakota**	NA		NA	Alaska**	NA
7	Tennessee	0.8		NA	Hawaii**	NA
3	Texas	1.0		NA	Idaho**	NA
36	Utah	0.3		NA	Maine**	NA
NA	Vermont**	NA		NA	Montana**	NA
26	Virginia	0.4		NA	New Hampshire**	NA
26	Washington	0.4		NA	North Dakota**	NA
19	West Virginia	0.5		NA	South Dakota**	NA
26	Wisconsin	0.4		NA	Vermont**	NA
NA	Wyoming**	NA		NA	Wyoming**	NA

District of Columbia 2.3

Source: U.S. Department of Health and Human Services, National Center for Health Statistics
"National Vital Statistics Reports" (Vol. 59, No. 1, December 2010, http://www.cdc.gov/nchs/births.htm)
*Final data by state of residence.
**Insufficient data for a reliable rate.

Births to Women 35 to 54 Years Old in 2008

National Total = 602,498 Live Births*

RANK	STATE	BIRTHS	% of USA		RANK	STATE	BIRTHS	% of USA
26	Alabama	5,822	1.0%		1	California	97,256	16.1%
45	Alaska	1,375	0.2%		2	New York	49,662	8.2%
16	Arizona	12,118	2.0%		3	Texas	47,391	7.9%
36	Arkansas	3,194	0.5%		4	Florida	33,765	5.6%
1	California	97,256	16.1%		5	Illinois	27,237	4.5%
17	Colorado	10,891	1.8%		6	New Jersey	24,030	4.0%
21	Connecticut	8,723	1.4%		7	Pennsylvania	22,713	3.8%
44	Delaware	1,672	0.3%		8	Georgia	18,933	3.1%
4	Florida	33,765	5.6%		9	Massachusetts	17,701	2.9%
8	Georgia	18,933	3.1%		10	Ohio	17,436	2.9%
34	Hawaii	3,430	0.6%		11	Virginia	17,342	2.9%
39	Idaho	2,478	0.4%		12	North Carolina	16,577	2.8%
5	Illinois	27,237	4.5%		13	Michigan	16,003	2.7%
20	Indiana	9,182	1.5%		14	Maryland	14,009	2.3%
33	Iowa	4,237	0.7%		15	Washington	13,751	2.3%
32	Kansas	4,373	0.7%		16	Arizona	12,118	2.0%
28	Kentucky	5,515	0.9%		17	Colorado	10,891	1.8%
27	Louisiana	5,648	0.9%		18	Minnesota	10,445	1.7%
43	Maine	1,852	0.3%		19	Wisconsin	9,330	1.5%
14	Maryland	14,009	2.3%		20	Indiana	9,182	1.5%
9	Massachusetts	17,701	2.9%		21	Connecticut	8,723	1.4%
13	Michigan	16,003	2.7%		22	Tennessee	8,625	1.4%
18	Minnesota	10,445	1.7%		23	Missouri	8,413	1.4%
35	Mississippi	3,395	0.6%		24	Oregon	6,865	1.1%
23	Missouri	8,413	1.4%		25	South Carolina	6,712	1.1%
46	Montana	1,324	0.2%		26	Alabama	5,822	1.0%
37	Nebraska	3,055	0.5%		27	Louisiana	5,648	0.9%
29	Nevada	5,404	0.9%		28	Kentucky	5,515	0.9%
40	New Hampshire	2,346	0.4%		29	Nevada	5,404	0.9%
6	New Jersey	24,030	4.0%		30	Utah	5,213	0.9%
38	New Mexico	3,033	0.5%		31	Oklahoma	4,473	0.7%
2	New York	49,662	8.2%		32	Kansas	4,373	0.7%
12	North Carolina	16,577	2.8%		33	Iowa	4,237	0.7%
49	North Dakota	897	0.1%		34	Hawaii	3,430	0.6%
10	Ohio	17,436	2.9%		35	Mississippi	3,395	0.6%
31	Oklahoma	4,473	0.7%		36	Arkansas	3,194	0.5%
24	Oregon	6,865	1.1%		37	Nebraska	3,055	0.5%
7	Pennsylvania	22,713	3.8%		38	New Mexico	3,033	0.5%
41	Rhode Island	2,036	0.3%		39	Idaho	2,478	0.4%
25	South Carolina	6,712	1.1%		40	New Hampshire	2,346	0.4%
47	South Dakota	1,151	0.2%		41	Rhode Island	2,036	0.3%
22	Tennessee	8,625	1.4%		42	West Virginia	1,936	0.3%
3	Texas	47,391	7.9%		43	Maine	1,852	0.3%
30	Utah	5,213	0.9%		44	Delaware	1,672	0.3%
48	Vermont	981	0.2%		45	Alaska	1,375	0.2%
11	Virginia	17,342	2.9%		46	Montana	1,324	0.2%
15	Washington	13,751	2.3%		47	South Dakota	1,151	0.2%
42	West Virginia	1,936	0.3%		48	Vermont	981	0.2%
19	Wisconsin	9,330	1.5%		49	North Dakota	897	0.1%
50	Wyoming	712	0.1%		50	Wyoming	712	0.1%
					District of Columbia	1,836	0.3%

ALPHA ORDER

RANK ORDER

Source: CQ Press using data from U.S. Department of Health and Human Services, National Center for Health Statistics
   "Vital Stats" (http://www.cdc.gov/nchs/VitalStats.htm)
*Final data by state of residence.

Birth Rate for Women 35 to 54 Years Old in 2008

National Rate = 13.8 Live Births per 1,000 35- to 54-Year-Old Women*

ALPHA ORDER

RANK	STATE	RATE
47	Alabama	8.8
16	Alaska	14.2
14	Arizona	14.3
49	Arkansas	8.2
2	California	18.9
9	Colorado	15.2
7	Connecticut	16.1
20	Delaware	13.1
19	Florida	13.1
18	Georgia	13.3
1	Hawaii	19.7
24	Idaho	12.6
12	Illinois	14.8
38	Indiana	10.2
36	Iowa	10.4
27	Kansas	11.5
46	Kentucky	8.9
45	Louisiana	9.0
44	Maine	9.1
8	Maryland	15.9
4	Massachusetts	17.7
33	Michigan	10.9
17	Minnesota	13.9
48	Mississippi	8.4
40	Missouri	9.9
39	Montana	9.9
22	Nebraska	12.9
10	Nevada	15.2
29	New Hampshire	11.3
3	New Jersey	18.1
30	New Mexico	11.3
5	New York	17.1
26	North Carolina	12.3
32	North Dakota	10.9
37	Ohio	10.4
43	Oklahoma	9.2
21	Oregon	13.0
25	Pennsylvania	12.4
23	Rhode Island	12.8
34	South Carolina	10.5
31	South Dakota	11.0
42	Tennessee	9.5
15	Texas	14.2
6	Utah	16.6
35	Vermont	10.4
11	Virginia	14.9
13	Washington	14.5
50	West Virginia	7.5
28	Wisconsin	11.5
41	Wyoming	9.9

RANK ORDER

RANK	STATE	RATE
1	Hawaii	19.7
2	California	18.9
3	New Jersey	18.1
4	Massachusetts	17.7
5	New York	17.1
6	Utah	16.6
7	Connecticut	16.1
8	Maryland	15.9
9	Colorado	15.2
10	Nevada	15.2
11	Virginia	14.9
12	Illinois	14.8
13	Washington	14.5
14	Arizona	14.3
15	Texas	14.2
16	Alaska	14.2
17	Minnesota	13.9
18	Georgia	13.3
19	Florida	13.1
20	Delaware	13.1
21	Oregon	13.0
22	Nebraska	12.9
23	Rhode Island	12.8
24	Idaho	12.6
25	Pennsylvania	12.4
26	North Carolina	12.3
27	Kansas	11.5
28	Wisconsin	11.5
29	New Hampshire	11.3
30	New Mexico	11.3
31	South Dakota	11.0
32	North Dakota	10.9
33	Michigan	10.9
34	South Carolina	10.5
35	Vermont	10.4
36	Iowa	10.4
37	Ohio	10.4
38	Indiana	10.2
39	Montana	9.9
40	Missouri	9.9
41	Wyoming	9.9
42	Tennessee	9.5
43	Oklahoma	9.2
44	Maine	9.1
45	Louisiana	9.0
46	Kentucky	8.9
47	Alabama	8.8
48	Mississippi	8.4
49	Arkansas	8.2
50	West Virginia	7.5

	District of Columbia	22.1

Source: CQ Press using data from U.S. Department of Health and Human Services, National Center for Health Statistics
"Vital Stats" (http://www.cdc.gov/nchs/VitalStats.htm)
*Final data by state of residence.

Average Age of Woman at First Birth in 2006

National Average = 25.0 Years Old

ALPHA ORDER

RANK	STATE	AVERAGE AGE
45	Alabama	23.6
31	Alaska	24.3
34	Arizona	24.0
48	Arkansas	23.0
14	California	25.6
12	Colorado	25.7
2	Connecticut	27.2
20	Delaware	25.0
20	Florida	25.0
28	Georgia	24.5
12	Hawaii	25.7
42	Idaho	23.8
17	Illinois	25.4
34	Indiana	24.0
28	Iowa	24.5
32	Kansas	24.2
42	Kentucky	23.8
46	Louisiana	23.3
14	Maine	25.6
8	Maryland	26.1
1	Massachusetts	27.7
20	Michigan	25.0
10	Minnesota	25.8
50	Mississippi	22.6
33	Missouri	24.1
28	Montana	24.5
23	Nebraska	24.7
26	Nevada	24.6
5	New Hampshire	26.7
2	New Jersey	27.2
48	New Mexico	23.0
4	New York	26.8
26	North Carolina	24.6
23	North Dakota	24.7
23	Ohio	24.7
47	Oklahoma	23.1
17	Oregon	25.4
16	Pennsylvania	25.5
7	Rhode Island	26.2
34	South Carolina	24.0
34	South Dakota	24.0
34	Tennessee	24.0
39	Texas	23.9
39	Utah	23.9
6	Vermont	26.5
10	Virginia	25.8
9	Washington	25.9
39	West Virginia	23.9
19	Wisconsin	25.3
44	Wyoming	23.7

RANK ORDER

RANK	STATE	AVERAGE AGE
1	Massachusetts	27.7
2	Connecticut	27.2
2	New Jersey	27.2
4	New York	26.8
5	New Hampshire	26.7
6	Vermont	26.5
7	Rhode Island	26.2
8	Maryland	26.1
9	Washington	25.9
10	Minnesota	25.8
10	Virginia	25.8
12	Colorado	25.7
12	Hawaii	25.7
14	California	25.6
14	Maine	25.6
16	Pennsylvania	25.5
17	Illinois	25.4
17	Oregon	25.4
19	Wisconsin	25.3
20	Delaware	25.0
20	Florida	25.0
20	Michigan	25.0
23	Nebraska	24.7
23	North Dakota	24.7
23	Ohio	24.7
26	Nevada	24.6
26	North Carolina	24.6
28	Georgia	24.5
28	Iowa	24.5
28	Montana	24.5
31	Alaska	24.3
32	Kansas	24.2
33	Missouri	24.1
34	Arizona	24.0
34	Indiana	24.0
34	South Carolina	24.0
34	South Dakota	24.0
34	Tennessee	24.0
39	Texas	23.9
39	Utah	23.9
39	West Virginia	23.9
42	Idaho	23.8
42	Kentucky	23.8
44	Wyoming	23.7
45	Alabama	23.6
46	Louisiana	23.3
47	Oklahoma	23.1
48	Arkansas	23.0
48	New Mexico	23.0
50	Mississippi	22.6

	District of Columbia	26.5

Source: U.S. Department of Health and Human Services, National Center for Health Statistics
"Delayed Childbearing" (NCHS Data Brief, No. 21, August 2009, www.cdc.gov/nchs/data/databriefs/db21.pdf)

Births by Vaginal Delivery in 2008

National Total = 2,875,689 Live Births*

ALPHA ORDER					RANK ORDER			
RANK	STATE	BIRTHS	% of USA		RANK	STATE	BIRTHS	% of USA
24	Alabama	42,019	1.5%		1	California	371,899	12.9%
45	Alaska	8,856	0.3%		2	Texas	265,638	9.2%
11	Arizona	72,493	2.5%		3	New York	164,001	5.7%
33	Arkansas	26,598	0.9%		4	Florida	144,422	5.0%
1	California	371,899	12.9%		5	Illinois	122,165	4.2%
20	Colorado	51,893	1.8%		6	Ohio	103,282	3.6%
34	Connecticut	26,219	0.9%		7	Pennsylvania	103,148	3.6%
46	Delaware	8,076	0.3%		8	Georgia	98,371	3.4%
4	Florida	144,422	5.0%		9	North Carolina	90,541	3.1%
8	Georgia	98,371	3.4%		10	Michigan	82,972	2.9%
39	Hawaii	14,262	0.5%		11	Arizona	72,493	2.5%
37	Idaho	19,013	0.7%		12	Virginia	70,413	2.4%
5	Illinois	122,165	4.2%		13	New Jersey	69,091	2.4%
15	Indiana	62,119	2.2%		14	Washington	63,767	2.2%
31	Iowa	28,438	1.0%		15	Indiana	62,119	2.2%
30	Kansas	29,241	1.0%		16	Tennessee	56,641	2.0%
27	Kentucky	37,944	1.3%		17	Missouri	55,784	1.9%
26	Louisiana	40,466	1.4%		18	Wisconsin	54,051	1.9%
41	Maine	9,472	0.3%		19	Minnesota	53,302	1.9%
21	Maryland	51,706	1.8%		20	Colorado	51,893	1.8%
22	Massachusetts	50,757	1.8%		21	Maryland	51,706	1.8%
10	Michigan	82,972	2.9%		22	Massachusetts	50,757	1.8%
19	Minnesota	53,302	1.9%		23	Utah	43,395	1.5%
32	Mississippi	28,272	1.0%		24	Alabama	42,019	1.5%
17	Missouri	55,784	1.9%		25	South Carolina	41,501	1.4%
43	Montana	8,917	0.3%		26	Louisiana	40,466	1.4%
38	Nebraska	18,622	0.6%		27	Kentucky	37,944	1.3%
35	Nevada	26,192	0.9%		28	Oklahoma	36,046	1.3%
42	New Hampshire	9,318	0.3%		29	Oregon	34,907	1.2%
13	New Jersey	69,091	2.4%		30	Kansas	29,241	1.0%
36	New Mexico	23,263	0.8%		31	Iowa	28,438	1.0%
3	New York	164,001	5.7%		32	Mississippi	28,272	1.0%
9	North Carolina	90,541	3.1%		33	Arkansas	26,598	0.9%
48	North Dakota	6,426	0.2%		34	Connecticut	26,219	0.9%
6	Ohio	103,282	3.6%		35	Nevada	26,192	0.9%
28	Oklahoma	36,046	1.3%		36	New Mexico	23,263	0.8%
29	Oregon	34,907	1.2%		37	Idaho	19,013	0.7%
7	Pennsylvania	103,148	3.6%		38	Nebraska	18,622	0.6%
47	Rhode Island	8,036	0.3%		39	Hawaii	14,262	0.5%
25	South Carolina	41,501	1.4%		40	West Virginia	13,868	0.5%
44	South Dakota	8,860	0.3%		41	Maine	9,472	0.3%
16	Tennessee	56,641	2.0%		42	New Hampshire	9,318	0.3%
2	Texas	265,638	9.2%		43	Montana	8,917	0.3%
23	Utah	43,395	1.5%		44	South Dakota	8,860	0.3%
50	Vermont	4,615	0.2%		45	Alaska	8,856	0.3%
12	Virginia	70,413	2.4%		46	Delaware	8,076	0.3%
14	Washington	63,767	2.2%		47	Rhode Island	8,036	0.3%
40	West Virginia	13,868	0.5%		48	North Dakota	6,426	0.2%
18	Wisconsin	54,051	1.9%		49	Wyoming	5,868	0.2%
49	Wyoming	5,868	0.2%		50	Vermont	4,615	0.2%
						District of Columbia	6,263	0.2%

Source: CQ Press using data from U.S. Department of Health and Human Services, National Center for Health Statistics
"National Vital Statistics Reports" (Vol. 59, No. 1, December 2010, http://www.cdc.gov/nchs/births.htm)
*Estimates by state of residence.

Percent of Births by Vaginal Delivery in 2008

National Percent = 67.7% of Live Births*

ALPHA ORDER				RANK ORDER		
RANK	STATE	PERCENT		RANK	STATE	PERCENT
43	Alabama	65.1		1	Utah	78.0
2	Alaska	77.4		2	Alaska	77.4
11	Arizona	72.9		3	New Mexico	77.1
42	Arkansas	65.4		4	Idaho	75.6
29	California	67.4		5	Wisconsin	74.8
6	Colorado	74.1		6	Colorado	74.1
45	Connecticut	64.9		7	Minnesota	73.6
32	Delaware	66.8		8	South Dakota	73.4
48	Florida	62.4		9	Hawaii	73.2
30	Georgia	67.1		10	Wyoming	73.0
9	Hawaii	73.2		11	Arizona	72.9
4	Idaho	75.6		12	Vermont	72.8
23	Illinois	69.1		13	North Dakota	71.9
18	Indiana	70.0		14	Oregon	71.1
16	Iowa	70.7		15	Montana	70.8
19	Kansas	69.9		16	Iowa	70.7
44	Kentucky	65.0		17	Washington	70.6
49	Louisiana	62.0		18	Indiana	70.0
20	Maine	69.6		19	Kansas	69.9
31	Maryland	66.9		20	Maine	69.6
37	Massachusetts	65.9		21	Ohio	69.4
27	Michigan	68.5		22	North Carolina	69.2
7	Minnesota	73.6		23	Illinois	69.1
47	Mississippi	62.9		23	Pennsylvania	69.1
26	Missouri	68.9		25	Nebraska	69.0
15	Montana	70.8		26	Missouri	68.9
25	Nebraska	69.0		27	Michigan	68.5
34	Nevada	66.3		28	New Hampshire	68.1
28	New Hampshire	68.1		29	California	67.4
50	New Jersey	61.3		30	Georgia	67.1
3	New Mexico	77.1		31	Maryland	66.9
40	New York	65.5		32	Delaware	66.8
22	North Carolina	69.2		33	Rhode Island	66.7
13	North Dakota	71.9		34	Nevada	66.3
21	Ohio	69.4		35	Tennessee	66.2
38	Oklahoma	65.8		36	Virginia	66.0
14	Oregon	71.1		37	Massachusetts	65.9
23	Pennsylvania	69.1		38	Oklahoma	65.8
33	Rhode Island	66.7		38	South Carolina	65.8
38	South Carolina	65.8		40	New York	65.5
8	South Dakota	73.4		40	Texas	65.5
35	Tennessee	66.2		42	Arkansas	65.4
40	Texas	65.5		43	Alabama	65.1
1	Utah	78.0		44	Kentucky	65.0
12	Vermont	72.8		45	Connecticut	64.9
36	Virginia	66.0		46	West Virginia	64.5
17	Washington	70.6		47	Mississippi	62.9
46	West Virginia	64.5		48	Florida	62.4
5	Wisconsin	74.8		49	Louisiana	62.0
10	Wyoming	73.0		50	New Jersey	61.3

District of Columbia 68.6

Source: CQ Press using data from U.S. Department of Health and Human Services, National Center for Health Statistics "National Vital Statistics Reports" (Vol. 59, No. 1, December 2010, http://www.cdc.gov/nchs/births.htm)
*Estimates by state of residence.

Births by Cesarean Delivery in 2008

National Total = 1,372,005 Live Cesarean Births*

ALPHA ORDER

RANK	STATE	BIRTHS	% of USA
21	Alabama	22,527	1.6%
47	Alaska	2,586	0.2%
14	Arizona	26,949	2.0%
31	Arkansas	14,071	1.0%
1	California	179,880	13.1%
27	Colorado	18,138	1.3%
30	Connecticut	14,180	1.0%
43	Delaware	4,014	0.3%
3	Florida	87,023	6.3%
6	Georgia	48,232	3.5%
40	Hawaii	5,222	0.4%
39	Idaho	6,136	0.4%
5	Illinois	54,630	4.0%
15	Indiana	26,623	1.9%
35	Iowa	11,786	0.9%
33	Kansas	12,592	0.9%
23	Kentucky	20,431	1.5%
20	Louisiana	24,802	1.8%
42	Maine	4,137	0.3%
18	Maryland	25,583	1.9%
17	Massachusetts	26,265	1.9%
11	Michigan	38,155	2.8%
24	Minnesota	19,119	1.4%
28	Mississippi	16,675	1.2%
19	Missouri	25,179	1.8%
45	Montana	3,677	0.3%
36	Nebraska	8,367	0.6%
32	Nevada	13,314	1.0%
41	New Hampshire	4,365	0.3%
9	New Jersey	43,619	3.2%
38	New Mexico	6,910	0.5%
4	New York	86,382	6.3%
10	North Carolina	40,298	2.9%
48	North Dakota	2,512	0.2%
8	Ohio	45,539	3.3%
25	Oklahoma	18,735	1.4%
29	Oregon	14,189	1.0%
7	Pennsylvania	46,125	3.4%
44	Rhode Island	4,012	0.3%
22	South Carolina	21,570	1.6%
46	South Dakota	3,211	0.2%
13	Tennessee	28,919	2.1%
2	Texas	139,916	10.2%
34	Utah	12,239	0.9%
50	Vermont	1,724	0.1%
12	Virginia	36,273	2.6%
16	Washington	26,554	1.9%
37	West Virginia	7,633	0.6%
26	Wisconsin	18,210	1.3%
49	Wyoming	2,170	0.2%

RANK ORDER

RANK	STATE	BIRTHS	% of USA
1	California	179,880	13.1%
2	Texas	139,916	10.2%
3	Florida	87,023	6.3%
4	New York	86,382	6.3%
5	Illinois	54,630	4.0%
6	Georgia	48,232	3.5%
7	Pennsylvania	46,125	3.4%
8	Ohio	45,539	3.3%
9	New Jersey	43,619	3.2%
10	North Carolina	40,298	2.9%
11	Michigan	38,155	2.8%
12	Virginia	36,273	2.6%
13	Tennessee	28,919	2.1%
14	Arizona	26,949	2.0%
15	Indiana	26,623	1.9%
16	Washington	26,554	1.9%
17	Massachusetts	26,265	1.9%
18	Maryland	25,583	1.9%
19	Missouri	25,179	1.8%
20	Louisiana	24,802	1.8%
21	Alabama	22,527	1.6%
22	South Carolina	21,570	1.6%
23	Kentucky	20,431	1.5%
24	Minnesota	19,119	1.4%
25	Oklahoma	18,735	1.4%
26	Wisconsin	18,210	1.3%
27	Colorado	18,138	1.3%
28	Mississippi	16,675	1.2%
29	Oregon	14,189	1.0%
30	Connecticut	14,180	1.0%
31	Arkansas	14,071	1.0%
32	Nevada	13,314	1.0%
33	Kansas	12,592	0.9%
34	Utah	12,239	0.9%
35	Iowa	11,786	0.9%
36	Nebraska	8,367	0.6%
37	West Virginia	7,633	0.6%
38	New Mexico	6,910	0.5%
39	Idaho	6,136	0.4%
40	Hawaii	5,222	0.4%
41	New Hampshire	4,365	0.3%
42	Maine	4,137	0.3%
43	Delaware	4,014	0.3%
44	Rhode Island	4,012	0.3%
45	Montana	3,677	0.3%
46	South Dakota	3,211	0.2%
47	Alaska	2,586	0.2%
48	North Dakota	2,512	0.2%
49	Wyoming	2,170	0.2%
50	Vermont	1,724	0.1%
	District of Columbia	2,867	0.2%

Source: CQ Press using data from U.S. Department of Health and Human Services, National Center for Health Statistics
   "National Vital Statistics Reports" (Vol. 59, No. 1, December 2010, http://www.cdc.gov/nchs/births.htm)
*Estimates by state of residence.

Percent of Births by Cesarean Delivery in 2008

National Percent = 32.3% of Live Births*

ALPHA ORDER

RANK	STATE	PERCENT
8	Alabama	34.9
49	Alaska	22.6
40	Arizona	27.1
9	Arkansas	34.6
22	California	32.6
45	Colorado	25.9
6	Connecticut	35.1
19	Delaware	33.2
3	Florida	37.6
21	Georgia	32.9
42	Hawaii	26.8
47	Idaho	24.4
27	Illinois	30.9
33	Indiana	30.0
35	Iowa	29.3
32	Kansas	30.1
7	Kentucky	35.0
2	Louisiana	38.0
31	Maine	30.4
20	Maryland	33.1
14	Massachusetts	34.1
24	Michigan	31.5
44	Minnesota	26.4
4	Mississippi	37.1
25	Missouri	31.1
36	Montana	29.2
26	Nebraska	31.0
17	Nevada	33.7
23	New Hampshire	31.9
1	New Jersey	38.7
48	New Mexico	22.9
10	New York	34.5
29	North Carolina	30.8
38	North Dakota	28.1
30	Ohio	30.6
12	Oklahoma	34.2
37	Oregon	28.9
27	Pennsylvania	30.9
18	Rhode Island	33.3
12	South Carolina	34.2
43	South Dakota	26.6
16	Tennessee	33.8
10	Texas	34.5
50	Utah	22.0
39	Vermont	27.2
15	Virginia	34.0
34	Washington	29.4
5	West Virginia	35.5
46	Wisconsin	25.2
41	Wyoming	27.0

RANK ORDER

RANK	STATE	PERCENT
1	New Jersey	38.7
2	Louisiana	38.0
3	Florida	37.6
4	Mississippi	37.1
5	West Virginia	35.5
6	Connecticut	35.1
7	Kentucky	35.0
8	Alabama	34.9
9	Arkansas	34.6
10	New York	34.5
10	Texas	34.5
12	Oklahoma	34.2
12	South Carolina	34.2
14	Massachusetts	34.1
15	Virginia	34.0
16	Tennessee	33.8
17	Nevada	33.7
18	Rhode Island	33.3
19	Delaware	33.2
20	Maryland	33.1
21	Georgia	32.9
22	California	32.6
23	New Hampshire	31.9
24	Michigan	31.5
25	Missouri	31.1
26	Nebraska	31.0
27	Illinois	30.9
27	Pennsylvania	30.9
29	North Carolina	30.8
30	Ohio	30.6
31	Maine	30.4
32	Kansas	30.1
33	Indiana	30.0
34	Washington	29.4
35	Iowa	29.3
36	Montana	29.2
37	Oregon	28.9
38	North Dakota	28.1
39	Vermont	27.2
40	Arizona	27.1
41	Wyoming	27.0
42	Hawaii	26.8
43	South Dakota	26.6
44	Minnesota	26.4
45	Colorado	25.9
46	Wisconsin	25.2
47	Idaho	24.4
48	New Mexico	22.9
49	Alaska	22.6
50	Utah	22.0

District of Columbia	31.4

Source: U.S. Department of Health and Human Services, National Center for Health Statistics
"National Vital Statistics Reports" (Vol. 59, No. 1, December 2010, http://www.cdc.gov/nchs/births.htm)
*Preliminary data by state of residence.

Percent Change in Rate of Cesarean Births: 2005 to 2008

National Percent Change = 6.6% Increase*

<table>
<tr><td colspan="3">ALPHA ORDER</td><td colspan="3">RANK ORDER</td></tr>
<tr><th>RANK</th><th>STATE</th><th>PERCENT CHANGE</th><th>RANK</th><th>STATE</th><th>PERCENT CHANGE</th></tr>
<tr><td>7</td><td>Alabama</td><td>9.7</td><td>1</td><td>New Hampshire</td><td>13.9</td></tr>
<tr><td>47</td><td>Alaska</td><td>3.2</td><td>2</td><td>Montana</td><td>13.2</td></tr>
<tr><td>7</td><td>Arizona</td><td>9.7</td><td>3</td><td>Delaware</td><td>10.7</td></tr>
<tr><td>5</td><td>Arkansas</td><td>9.8</td><td>4</td><td>Rhode Island</td><td>9.9</td></tr>
<tr><td>29</td><td>California</td><td>6.2</td><td>5</td><td>Arkansas</td><td>9.8</td></tr>
<tr><td>35</td><td>Colorado</td><td>5.3</td><td>5</td><td>Wyoming</td><td>9.8</td></tr>
<tr><td>16</td><td>Connecticut</td><td>8.3</td><td>7</td><td>Alabama</td><td>9.7</td></tr>
<tr><td>3</td><td>Delaware</td><td>10.7</td><td>7</td><td>Arizona</td><td>9.7</td></tr>
<tr><td>20</td><td>Florida</td><td>7.7</td><td>7</td><td>Iowa</td><td>9.7</td></tr>
<tr><td>19</td><td>Georgia</td><td>7.9</td><td>10</td><td>New York</td><td>9.5</td></tr>
<tr><td>39</td><td>Hawaii</td><td>4.7</td><td>11</td><td>Michigan</td><td>9.4</td></tr>
<tr><td>18</td><td>Idaho</td><td>8.0</td><td>12</td><td>Ohio</td><td>8.9</td></tr>
<tr><td>22</td><td>Illinois</td><td>7.3</td><td>13</td><td>Nevada</td><td>8.7</td></tr>
<tr><td>25</td><td>Indiana</td><td>6.4</td><td>13</td><td>Tennessee</td><td>8.7</td></tr>
<tr><td>7</td><td>Iowa</td><td>9.7</td><td>15</td><td>Nebraska</td><td>8.4</td></tr>
<tr><td>44</td><td>Kansas</td><td>4.2</td><td>16</td><td>Connecticut</td><td>8.3</td></tr>
<tr><td>47</td><td>Kentucky</td><td>3.2</td><td>16</td><td>Virginia</td><td>8.3</td></tr>
<tr><td>46</td><td>Louisiana</td><td>3.3</td><td>18</td><td>Idaho</td><td>8.0</td></tr>
<tr><td>21</td><td>Maine</td><td>7.4</td><td>19</td><td>Georgia</td><td>7.9</td></tr>
<tr><td>25</td><td>Maryland</td><td>6.4</td><td>20</td><td>Florida</td><td>7.7</td></tr>
<tr><td>31</td><td>Massachusetts</td><td>5.9</td><td>21</td><td>Maine</td><td>7.4</td></tr>
<tr><td>11</td><td>Michigan</td><td>9.4</td><td>22</td><td>Illinois</td><td>7.3</td></tr>
<tr><td>43</td><td>Minnesota</td><td>4.3</td><td>23</td><td>Pennsylvania</td><td>6.9</td></tr>
<tr><td>34</td><td>Mississippi</td><td>5.7</td><td>24</td><td>New Jersey</td><td>6.6</td></tr>
<tr><td>39</td><td>Missouri</td><td>4.7</td><td>25</td><td>Indiana</td><td>6.4</td></tr>
<tr><td>2</td><td>Montana</td><td>13.2</td><td>25</td><td>Maryland</td><td>6.4</td></tr>
<tr><td>15</td><td>Nebraska</td><td>8.4</td><td>25</td><td>North Dakota</td><td>6.4</td></tr>
<tr><td>13</td><td>Nevada</td><td>8.7</td><td>28</td><td>Wisconsin</td><td>6.3</td></tr>
<tr><td>1</td><td>New Hampshire</td><td>13.9</td><td>29</td><td>California</td><td>6.2</td></tr>
<tr><td>24</td><td>New Jersey</td><td>6.6</td><td>30</td><td>South Dakota</td><td>6.0</td></tr>
<tr><td>47</td><td>New Mexico</td><td>3.2</td><td>31</td><td>Massachusetts</td><td>5.9</td></tr>
<tr><td>10</td><td>New York</td><td>9.5</td><td>32</td><td>Texas</td><td>5.8</td></tr>
<tr><td>37</td><td>North Carolina</td><td>5.1</td><td>32</td><td>Washington</td><td>5.8</td></tr>
<tr><td>25</td><td>North Dakota</td><td>6.4</td><td>34</td><td>Mississippi</td><td>5.7</td></tr>
<tr><td>12</td><td>Ohio</td><td>8.9</td><td>35</td><td>Colorado</td><td>5.3</td></tr>
<tr><td>36</td><td>Oklahoma</td><td>5.2</td><td>36</td><td>Oklahoma</td><td>5.2</td></tr>
<tr><td>39</td><td>Oregon</td><td>4.7</td><td>37</td><td>North Carolina</td><td>5.1</td></tr>
<tr><td>23</td><td>Pennsylvania</td><td>6.9</td><td>38</td><td>Vermont</td><td>5.0</td></tr>
<tr><td>4</td><td>Rhode Island</td><td>9.9</td><td>39</td><td>Hawaii</td><td>4.7</td></tr>
<tr><td>42</td><td>South Carolina</td><td>4.6</td><td>39</td><td>Missouri</td><td>4.7</td></tr>
<tr><td>30</td><td>South Dakota</td><td>6.0</td><td>39</td><td>Oregon</td><td>4.7</td></tr>
<tr><td>13</td><td>Tennessee</td><td>8.7</td><td>42</td><td>South Carolina</td><td>4.6</td></tr>
<tr><td>32</td><td>Texas</td><td>5.8</td><td>43</td><td>Minnesota</td><td>4.3</td></tr>
<tr><td>50</td><td>Utah</td><td>1.9</td><td>44</td><td>Kansas</td><td>4.2</td></tr>
<tr><td>38</td><td>Vermont</td><td>5.0</td><td>45</td><td>West Virginia</td><td>3.8</td></tr>
<tr><td>16</td><td>Virginia</td><td>8.3</td><td>46</td><td>Louisiana</td><td>3.3</td></tr>
<tr><td>32</td><td>Washington</td><td>5.8</td><td>47</td><td>Alaska</td><td>3.2</td></tr>
<tr><td>45</td><td>West Virginia</td><td>3.8</td><td>47</td><td>Kentucky</td><td>3.2</td></tr>
<tr><td>28</td><td>Wisconsin</td><td>6.3</td><td>47</td><td>New Mexico</td><td>3.2</td></tr>
<tr><td>5</td><td>Wyoming</td><td>9.8</td><td>50</td><td>Utah</td><td>1.9</td></tr>
<tr><td></td><td></td><td></td><td></td><td>District of Columbia</td><td>3.0</td></tr>
</table>

Source: CQ Press using data from U.S. Department of Health and Human Services, National Center for Health Statistics
   "National Vital Statistics Reports" (Vol. 59, No. 1, December 2010, http://www.cdc.gov/nchs/births.htm)
*Estimates by state of residence.

Percent of Women Beginning Prenatal Care in First Trimester in 2008

National Percent = 71.0% of Women*

<table>
<tr><td colspan="3">ALPHA ORDER</td><td colspan="3">RANK ORDER</td></tr>
<tr><td>RANK</td><td>STATE</td><td>PERCENT</td><td>RANK</td><td>STATE</td><td>PERCENT</td></tr>
<tr><td>NA</td><td>Alabama**</td><td>NA</td><td>1</td><td>Vermont</td><td>82.6</td></tr>
<tr><td>NA</td><td>Alaska**</td><td>NA</td><td>2</td><td>New Hampshire</td><td>82.1</td></tr>
<tr><td>NA</td><td>Arizona**</td><td>NA</td><td>3</td><td>California</td><td>80.2</td></tr>
<tr><td>NA</td><td>Arkansas**</td><td>NA</td><td>4</td><td>Michigan</td><td>77.2</td></tr>
<tr><td>3</td><td>California</td><td>80.2</td><td>5</td><td>Nebraska</td><td>73.9</td></tr>
<tr><td>22</td><td>Colorado</td><td>68.1</td><td>6</td><td>Montana</td><td>73.4</td></tr>
<tr><td>NA</td><td>Conncoticut**</td><td>NA</td><td>7</td><td>Kansas</td><td>73.3</td></tr>
<tr><td>13</td><td>Delaware</td><td>71.1</td><td>8</td><td>Georgia</td><td>72.6</td></tr>
<tr><td>18</td><td>Florida</td><td>69.7</td><td>9</td><td>Iowa</td><td>72.5</td></tr>
<tr><td>8</td><td>Georgia</td><td>72.6</td><td>10</td><td>New York</td><td>72.4</td></tr>
<tr><td>NA</td><td>Hawaii**</td><td>NA</td><td>10</td><td>North Dakota</td><td>72.4</td></tr>
<tr><td>19</td><td>Idaho</td><td>69.3</td><td>12</td><td>Kentucky</td><td>72.2</td></tr>
<tr><td>NA</td><td>Illinois**</td><td>NA</td><td>13</td><td>Delaware</td><td>71.1</td></tr>
<tr><td>24</td><td>Indiana</td><td>67.4</td><td>13</td><td>Oregon</td><td>71.1</td></tr>
<tr><td>9</td><td>Iowa</td><td>72.5</td><td>15</td><td>Pennsylvania</td><td>70.8</td></tr>
<tr><td>7</td><td>Kansas</td><td>73.3</td><td>16</td><td>Ohio</td><td>70.6</td></tr>
<tr><td>12</td><td>Kentucky</td><td>72.2</td><td>17</td><td>Wyoming</td><td>70.1</td></tr>
<tr><td>NA</td><td>Louisiana**</td><td>NA</td><td>18</td><td>Florida</td><td>69.7</td></tr>
<tr><td>NA</td><td>Maine**</td><td>NA</td><td>19</td><td>Idaho</td><td>69.3</td></tr>
<tr><td>NA</td><td>Maryland**</td><td>NA</td><td>19</td><td>South Dakota</td><td>69.3</td></tr>
<tr><td>NA</td><td>Massachusetts**</td><td>NA</td><td>21</td><td>Washington</td><td>68.5</td></tr>
<tr><td>4</td><td>Michigan</td><td>77.2</td><td>22</td><td>Colorado</td><td>68.1</td></tr>
<tr><td>NA</td><td>Minnesota**</td><td>NA</td><td>23</td><td>Tennessee</td><td>67.8</td></tr>
<tr><td>NA</td><td>Mississippi**</td><td>NA</td><td>24</td><td>Indiana</td><td>67.4</td></tr>
<tr><td>NA</td><td>Missouri**</td><td>NA</td><td>25</td><td>South Carolina</td><td>66.5</td></tr>
<tr><td>6</td><td>Montana</td><td>73.4</td><td>26</td><td>New Mexico</td><td>62.2</td></tr>
<tr><td>5</td><td>Nebraska</td><td>73.9</td><td>27</td><td>Texas</td><td>59.3</td></tr>
<tr><td>NA</td><td>Nevada**</td><td>NA</td><td>NA</td><td>Alabama**</td><td>NA</td></tr>
<tr><td>2</td><td>New Hampshire</td><td>82.1</td><td>NA</td><td>Alaska**</td><td>NA</td></tr>
<tr><td>NA</td><td>New Jersey**</td><td>NA</td><td>NA</td><td>Arizona**</td><td>NA</td></tr>
<tr><td>26</td><td>New Mexico</td><td>62.2</td><td>NA</td><td>Arkansas**</td><td>NA</td></tr>
<tr><td>10</td><td>New York</td><td>72.4</td><td>NA</td><td>Connecticut**</td><td>NA</td></tr>
<tr><td>NA</td><td>North Carolina**</td><td>NA</td><td>NA</td><td>Hawaii**</td><td>NA</td></tr>
<tr><td>10</td><td>North Dakota</td><td>72.4</td><td>NA</td><td>Illinois**</td><td>NA</td></tr>
<tr><td>16</td><td>Ohio</td><td>70.6</td><td>NA</td><td>Louisiana**</td><td>NA</td></tr>
<tr><td>NA</td><td>Oklahoma**</td><td>NA</td><td>NA</td><td>Maine**</td><td>NA</td></tr>
<tr><td>13</td><td>Oregon</td><td>71.1</td><td>NA</td><td>Maryland**</td><td>NA</td></tr>
<tr><td>15</td><td>Pennsylvania</td><td>70.8</td><td>NA</td><td>Massachusetts**</td><td>NA</td></tr>
<tr><td>NA</td><td>Rhode Island**</td><td>NA</td><td>NA</td><td>Minnesota**</td><td>NA</td></tr>
<tr><td>25</td><td>South Carolina</td><td>66.5</td><td>NA</td><td>Mississippi**</td><td>NA</td></tr>
<tr><td>19</td><td>South Dakota</td><td>69.3</td><td>NA</td><td>Missouri**</td><td>NA</td></tr>
<tr><td>23</td><td>Tennessee</td><td>67.8</td><td>NA</td><td>Nevada**</td><td>NA</td></tr>
<tr><td>27</td><td>Texas</td><td>59.3</td><td>NA</td><td>New Jersey**</td><td>NA</td></tr>
<tr><td>NA</td><td>Utah**</td><td>NA</td><td>NA</td><td>North Carolina**</td><td>NA</td></tr>
<tr><td>1</td><td>Vermont</td><td>82.6</td><td>NA</td><td>Oklahoma**</td><td>NA</td></tr>
<tr><td>NA</td><td>Virginia**</td><td>NA</td><td>NA</td><td>Rhode Island**</td><td>NA</td></tr>
<tr><td>21</td><td>Washington</td><td>68.5</td><td>NA</td><td>Utah**</td><td>NA</td></tr>
<tr><td>NA</td><td>West Virginia**</td><td>NA</td><td>NA</td><td>Virginia**</td><td>NA</td></tr>
<tr><td>NA</td><td>Wisconsin**</td><td>NA</td><td>NA</td><td>West Virginia**</td><td>NA</td></tr>
<tr><td>17</td><td>Wyoming</td><td>70.1</td><td>NA</td><td>Wisconsin**</td><td>NA</td></tr>
<tr><td></td><td></td><td></td><td></td><td>District of Columbia**</td><td>NA</td></tr>
</table>

Source: CQ Press using data from U.S. Department of Health and Human Services, National Center for Health Statistics
    "Vital Stats" (http://www.cdc.gov/nchs/VitalStats.htm)
*Final data by state of residence. National figure is for reporting states only.
**Not available.

Percent of White Women Beginning Prenatal Care in First Trimester in 2008

National Percent = 76.6% of White Women*

ALPHA ORDER

RANK	STATE	PERCENT
NA	Alabama**	NA
NA	Alaska**	NA
NA	Arizona**	NA
NA	Arkansas**	NA
1	California	85.2
13	Colorado	75.7
NA	Connecticut**	NA
7	Delaware	79.3
14	Florida	75.4
6	Georgia	80.3
NA	Hawaii**	NA
24	Idaho	72.6
NA	Illinois**	NA
26	Indiana	71.5
16	Iowa	75.3
8	Kansas	78.5
19	Kentucky	74.4
NA	Louisiana**	NA
NA	Maine**	NA
NA	Maryland**	NA
NA	Massachusetts**	NA
4	Michigan	80.8
NA	Minnesota**	NA
NA	Mississippi**	NA
NA	Missouri**	NA
10	Montana	77.2
9	Nebraska	78.3
NA	Nevada**	NA
3	New Hampshire	83.1
NA	New Jersey**	NA
25	New Mexico	71.8
5	New York	80.5
NA	North Carolina**	NA
11	North Dakota	76.9
21	Ohio	74.1
NA	Oklahoma**	NA
14	Oregon	75.4
12	Pennsylvania	76.4
NA	Rhode Island**	NA
20	South Carolina	74.2
17	South Dakota	75.2
18	Tennessee	74.7
27	Texas	70.3
NA	Utah**	NA
2	Vermont	83.2
NA	Virginia**	NA
23	Washington	73.1
NA	West Virginia**	NA
NA	Wisconsin**	NA
22	Wyoming	73.7

RANK ORDER

RANK	STATE	PERCENT
1	California	85.2
2	Vermont	83.2
3	New Hampshire	83.1
4	Michigan	80.8
5	New York	80.5
6	Georgia	80.3
7	Delaware	79.3
8	Kansas	78.5
9	Nebraska	78.3
10	Montana	77.2
11	North Dakota	76.9
12	Pennsylvania	76.4
13	Colorado	75.7
14	Florida	75.4
14	Oregon	75.4
16	Iowa	75.3
17	South Dakota	75.2
18	Tennessee	74.7
19	Kentucky	74.4
20	South Carolina	74.2
21	Ohio	74.1
22	Wyoming	73.7
23	Washington	73.1
24	Idaho	72.6
25	New Mexico	71.8
26	Indiana	71.5
27	Texas	70.3
NA	Alabama**	NA
NA	Alaska**	NA
NA	Arizona**	NA
NA	Arkansas**	NA
NA	Connecticut**	NA
NA	Hawaii**	NA
NA	Illinois**	NA
NA	Louisiana**	NA
NA	Maine**	NA
NA	Maryland**	NA
NA	Massachusetts**	NA
NA	Minnesota**	NA
NA	Mississippi**	NA
NA	Missouri**	NA
NA	Nevada**	NA
NA	New Jersey**	NA
NA	North Carolina**	NA
NA	Oklahoma**	NA
NA	Rhode Island**	NA
NA	Utah**	NA
NA	Virginia**	NA
NA	West Virginia**	NA
NA	Wisconsin**	NA
NA	District of Columbia**	NA

Source: CQ Press using data from U.S. Department of Health and Human Services, National Center for Health Statistics
"Vital Stats" (http://www.cdc.gov/nchs/VitalStats.htm)
*Final data by state of residence. National figure is for reporting states only. Includes only non-Hispanic whites.
**Not available.

Percent of Black Women Beginning Prenatal Care in First Trimester in 2008

National Percent = 60.3% of Black Women*

ALPHA ORDER

RANK	STATE	PERCENT
NA	Alabama**	NA
NA	Alaska**	NA
NA	Arizona**	NA
NA	Arkansas**	NA
1	California	75.5
25	Colorado	52.5
NA	Connecticut**	NA
3	Delaware	67.3
12	Florida	60.1
4	Georgia	66.2
NA	Hawaii**	NA
23	Idaho	53.9
NA	Illinois**	NA
24	Indiana	53.7
21	Iowa	55.3
8	Kansas	61.6
6	Kentucky	63.4
NA	Louisiana**	NA
NA	Maine**	NA
NA	Maryland**	NA
NA	Massachusetts**	NA
5	Michigan	65.4
NA	Minnesota**	NA
NA	Mississippi**	NA
NA	Missouri**	NA
2	Montana	73.1
13	Nebraska	59.8
NA	Nevada**	NA
7	New Hampshire	61.7
NA	New Jersey**	NA
9	New Mexico	61.4
10	New York	61.0
NA	North Carolina**	NA
18	North Dakota	56.6
18	Ohio	56.6
NA	Oklahoma**	NA
14	Oregon	58.8
22	Pennsylvania	54.3
NA	Rhode Island**	NA
11	South Carolina	60.3
27	South Dakota	42.9
20	Tennessee	55.5
26	Texas	51.9
NA	Utah**	NA
16	Vermont	57.3
NA	Virginia**	NA
15	Washington	58.2
NA	West Virginia**	NA
NA	Wisconsin**	NA
17	Wyoming	56.9

RANK ORDER

RANK	STATE	PERCENT
1	California	75.5
2	Montana	73.1
3	Delaware	67.3
4	Georgia	66.2
5	Michigan	65.4
6	Kentucky	63.4
7	New Hampshire	61.7
8	Kansas	61.6
9	New Mexico	61.4
10	New York	61.0
11	South Carolina	60.3
12	Florida	60.1
13	Nebraska	59.8
14	Oregon	58.8
15	Washington	58.2
16	Vermont	57.3
17	Wyoming	56.9
18	North Dakota	56.6
18	Ohio	56.6
20	Tennessee	55.5
21	Iowa	55.3
22	Pennsylvania	54.3
23	Idaho	53.9
24	Indiana	53.7
25	Colorado	52.5
26	Texas	51.9
27	South Dakota	42.9
NA	Alabama**	NA
NA	Alaska**	NA
NA	Arizona**	NA
NA	Arkansas**	NA
NA	Connecticut**	NA
NA	Hawaii**	NA
NA	Illinois**	NA
NA	Louisiana**	NA
NA	Maine**	NA
NA	Maryland**	NA
NA	Massachusetts**	NA
NA	Minnesota**	NA
NA	Mississippi**	NA
NA	Missouri**	NA
NA	Nevada**	NA
NA	New Jersey**	NA
NA	North Carolina**	NA
NA	Oklahoma**	NA
NA	Rhode Island**	NA
NA	Utah**	NA
NA	Virginia**	NA
NA	West Virginia**	NA
NA	Wisconsin**	NA
	District of Columbia**	NA

Source: CQ Press using data from U.S. Department of Health and Human Services, National Center for Health Statistics
"Vital Stats" (http://www.cdc.gov/nchs/VitalStats.htm)
*Final data by state of residence. National figure is for reporting states only. Includes only non-Hispanic blacks.
**Not available.

Percent of Hispanic Women Beginning Prenatal Care in First Trimester in 2008

National Percent = 64.7% of Hispanic Women*

ALPHA ORDER

RANK ORDER

RANK	STATE	PERCENT		RANK	STATE	PERCENT
NA	Alabama**	NA		1	California	77.3
NA	Alaska**	NA		2	New Hampshire	72.2
NA	Arizona**	NA		3	Vermont	69.3
NA	Arkansas**	NA		4	Michigan	68.5
1	California	77.3		5	Florida	67.5
15	Colorado	56.0		6	Montana	67.0
NA	Connecticut**	NA		7	New York	64.3
25	Delaware	48.9		8	Georgia	63.0
5	Florida	67.5		9	New Mexico	61.3
8	Georgia	63.0		10	North Dakota	60.5
NA	Hawaii**	NA		11	Nebraska	59.9
18	Idaho	55.7		12	Oregon	59.4
NA	Illinois**	NA		13	Washington	58.1
23	Indiana	52.2		14	Ohio	56.9
19	Iowa	55.5		15	Colorado	56.0
17	Kansas	55.9		15	Pennsylvania	56.0
21	Kentucky	53.4		17	Kansas	55.9
NA	Louisiana**	NA		18	Idaho	55.7
NA	Maine**	NA		19	Iowa	55.5
NA	Maryland**	NA		20	Wyoming	55.2
NA	Massachusetts**	NA		21	Kentucky	53.4
4	Michigan	68.5		22	Texas	52.5
NA	Minnesota**	NA		23	Indiana	52.2
NA	Mississippi**	NA		24	South Dakota	51.8
NA	Missouri**	NA		25	Delaware	48.9
6	Montana	67.0		26	South Carolina	45.7
11	Nebraska	59.9		27	Tennessee	44.4
NA	Nevada**	NA		NA	Alabama**	NA
2	New Hampshire	72.2		NA	Alaska**	NA
NA	New Jersey**	NA		NA	Arizona**	NA
9	New Mexico	61.3		NA	Arkansas**	NA
7	New York	64.3		NA	Connecticut**	NA
NA	North Carolina**	NA		NA	Hawaii**	NA
10	North Dakota	60.5		NA	Illinois**	NA
14	Ohio	56.9		NA	Louisiana**	NA
NA	Oklahoma**	NA		NA	Maine**	NA
12	Oregon	59.4		NA	Maryland**	NA
15	Pennsylvania	56.0		NA	Massachusetts**	NA
NA	Rhode Island**	NA		NA	Minnesota**	NA
26	South Carolina	45.7		NA	Mississippi**	NA
24	South Dakota	51.8		NA	Missouri**	NA
27	Tennessee	44.4		NA	Nevada**	NA
22	Texas	52.5		NA	New Jersey**	NA
NA	Utah**	NA		NA	North Carolina**	NA
3	Vermont	69.3		NA	Oklahoma**	NA
NA	Virginia**	NA		NA	Rhode Island**	NA
13	Washington	58.1		NA	Utah**	NA
NA	West Virginia**	NA		NA	Virginia**	NA
NA	Wisconsin**	NA		NA	West Virginia**	NA
20	Wyoming	55.2		NA	Wisconsin**	NA
					District of Columbia**	NA

Source: CQ Press using data from U.S. Department of Health and Human Services, National Center for Health Statistics
"Vital Stats" (http://www.cdc.gov/nchs/VitalStats.htm)

*Final data by state of residence. National figure is for reporting states only. Persons of Hispanic origin may be of any race.

**Not available.

Percent of Women Receiving Late or No Prenatal Care in 2008

National Percent = 7.0% of Women*

ALPHA ORDER				RANK ORDER		
RANK	STATE	PERCENT		RANK	STATE	PERCENT
NA	Alabama**	NA		1	Texas	12.4
NA	Alaska**	NA		2	New Mexico	10.8
NA	Arizona**	NA		3	Delaware	9.5
NA	Arkansas**	NA		4	Tennessee	8.7
25	California	3.6		5	Colorado	7.9
5	Colorado	7.9		6	South Carolina	7.8
NA	Connecticut**	NA		7	Georgia	7.7
3	Delaware	9.5		8	Wyoming	7.6
9	Florida	7.3		9	Florida	7.3
7	Georgia	7.7		10	Ohio	7.2
NA	Hawaii**	NA		10	Washington	7.2
17	Idaho	6.0		12	Indiana	7.1
NA	Illinois**	NA		13	Pennsylvania	7.0
12	Indiana	7.1		14	North Dakota	6.6
23	Iowa	4.5		15	New York	6.3
20	Kansas	5.3		16	South Dakota	6.2
17	Kentucky	6.0		17	Idaho	6.0
NA	Louisiana**	NA		17	Kentucky	6.0
NA	Maine**	NA		19	Oregon	5.5
NA	Maryland**	NA		20	Kansas	5.3
NA	Massachusetts**	NA		20	Montana	5.3
22	Michigan	4.6		22	Michigan	4.6
NA	Minnesota**	NA		23	Iowa	4.5
NA	Mississippi**	NA		24	Nebraska	4.4
NA	Missouri**	NA		25	California	3.6
20	Montana	5.3		25	New Hampshire	3.6
24	Nebraska	4.4		27	Vermont	2.8
NA	Nevada**	NA		NA	Alabama**	NA
25	New Hampshire	3.6		NA	Alaska**	NA
NA	New Jersey**	NA		NA	Arizona**	NA
2	New Mexico	10.8		NA	Arkansas**	NA
15	New York	6.3		NA	Connecticut**	NA
NA	North Carolina**	NA		NA	Hawaii**	NA
14	North Dakota	6.6		NA	Illinois**	NA
10	Ohio	7.2		NA	Louisiana**	NA
NA	Oklahoma**	NA		NA	Maine**	NA
19	Oregon	5.5		NA	Maryland**	NA
13	Pennsylvania	7.0		NA	Massachusetts**	NA
NA	Rhode Island**	NA		NA	Minnesota**	NA
6	South Carolina	7.8		NA	Mississippi**	NA
16	South Dakota	6.2		NA	Missouri**	NA
4	Tennessee	8.7		NA	Nevada**	NA
1	Texas	12.4		NA	New Jersey**	NA
NA	Utah**	NA		NA	North Carolina**	NA
27	Vermont	2.8		NA	Oklahoma**	NA
NA	Virginia**	NA		NA	Rhode Island**	NA
10	Washington	7.2		NA	Utah**	NA
NA	West Virginia**	NA		NA	Virginia**	NA
NA	Wisconsin**	NA		NA	West Virginia**	NA
8	Wyoming	7.6		NA	Wisconsin**	NA
				NA	District of Columbia**	NA

Source: CQ Press using data from U.S. Department of Health and Human Services, National Center for Health Statistics
  "Vital Stats" (http://www.cdc.gov/nchs/VitalStats.htm)
*Final data by state of residence. "Late" means care begun in third trimester. National figure is for reporting states only.
**Not available.

Percent of White Women Receiving Late or No Prenatal Care in 2008

National Percent = 4.8% of White Women*

ALPHA ORDER

RANK	STATE	PERCENT
NA	Alabama**	NA
NA	Alaska**	NA
NA	Arizona**	NA
NA	Arkansas**	NA
27	California	2.5
7	Colorado	5.5
NA	Connecticut**	NA
4	Delaware	6.5
10	Florida	5.3
17	Georgia	4.2
NA	Hawaii**	NA
14	Idaho	4.8
NA	Illinois**	NA
7	Indiana	5.5
21	Iowa	3.6
19	Kansas	3.7
10	Kentucky	5.3
NA	Louisiana**	NA
NA	Maine**	NA
NA	Maryland**	NA
NA	Massachusetts**	NA
21	Michigan	3.6
NA	Minnesota**	NA
NA	Mississippi**	NA
NA	Missouri**	NA
19	Montana	3.7
23	Nebraska	3.4
NA	Nevada**	NA
24	New Hampshire	3.3
NA	New Jersey**	NA
2	New Mexico	6.7
24	New York	3.3
NA	North Carolina**	NA
15	North Dakota	4.6
5	Ohio	5.7
NA	Oklahoma**	NA
15	Oregon	4.6
12	Pennsylvania	5.1
NA	Rhode Island**	NA
12	South Carolina	5.1
18	South Dakota	4.0
9	Tennessee	5.4
1	Texas	8.0
NA	Utah**	NA
26	Vermont	2.6
NA	Virginia**	NA
6	Washington	5.6
NA	West Virginia**	NA
NA	Wisconsin**	NA
3	Wyoming	6.6

RANK ORDER

RANK	STATE	PERCENT
1	Texas	8.0
2	New Mexico	6.7
3	Wyoming	6.6
4	Delaware	6.5
5	Ohio	5.7
6	Washington	5.6
7	Colorado	5.5
7	Indiana	5.5
9	Tennessee	5.4
10	Florida	5.3
10	Kentucky	5.3
12	Pennsylvania	5.1
12	South Carolina	5.1
14	Idaho	4.8
15	North Dakota	4.6
15	Oregon	4.6
17	Georgia	4.2
18	South Dakota	4.0
19	Kansas	3.7
19	Montana	3.7
21	Iowa	3.6
21	Michigan	3.6
23	Nebraska	3.4
24	New Hampshire	3.3
24	New York	3.3
26	Vermont	2.6
27	California	2.5
NA	Alabama**	NA
NA	Alaska**	NA
NA	Arizona**	NA
NA	Arkansas**	NA
NA	Connecticut**	NA
NA	Hawaii**	NA
NA	Illinois**	NA
NA	Louisiana**	NA
NA	Maine**	NA
NA	Maryland**	NA
NA	Massachusetts**	NA
NA	Minnesota**	NA
NA	Mississippi**	NA
NA	Missouri**	NA
NA	Nevada**	NA
NA	New Jersey**	NA
NA	North Carolina**	NA
NA	Oklahoma**	NA
NA	Rhode Island**	NA
NA	Utah**	NA
NA	Virginia**	NA
NA	West Virginia**	NA
NA	Wisconsin**	NA
	District of Columbia**	NA

Source: CQ Press using data from U.S. Department of Health and Human Services, National Center for Health Statistics
"Vital Stats" (http://www.cdc.gov/nchs/VitalStats.htm)
*Final data by state of residence. "Late" means care begun in third trimester. National figure is for reporting states only.
Includes only non-Hispanic whites.
**Not available.

Percent of Black Women Receiving Late or No Prenatal Care in 2008

National Percent = 11.3% of Black Women*

ALPHA ORDER			RANK ORDER		
RANK	STATE	PERCENT	RANK	STATE	PERCENT
NA	Alabama**	NA	1	Texas	16.2
NA	Alaska**	NA	2	Colorado	14.5
NA	Arizona**	NA	3	Tennessee	14.3
NA	Arkansas**	NA	4	Pennsylvania	13.9
27	California	4.8	5	Indiana	13.4
2	Colorado	14.5	6	Ohio	12.9
NA	Connecticut**	NA	7	Wyoming	12.1
9	Delaware	11.7	8	New Mexico	11.9
14	Florida	10.5	9	Delaware	11.7
15	Georgia	9.8	10	New York	11.4
NA	Hawaii**	NA	11	Iowa	11.3
16	Idaho	9.7	11	Washington	11.3
NA	Illinois**	NA	13	South Dakota	10.8
5	Indiana	13.4	14	Florida	10.5
11	Iowa	11.3	15	Georgia	9.8
21	Kansas	8.4	16	Idaho	9.7
20	Kentucky	8.7	17	South Carolina	9.4
NA	Louisiana**	NA	18	Oregon	9.2
NA	Maine**	NA	19	North Dakota	9.0
NA	Maryland**	NA	20	Kentucky	8.7
NA	Massachusetts**	NA	21	Kansas	8.4
22	Michigan	8.3	22	Michigan	8.3
NA	Minnesota**	NA	22	Vermont	8.3
NA	Mississippi**	NA	24	Nebraska	8.1
NA	Missouri**	NA	25	Montana	7.5
25	Montana	7.5	25	New Hampshire	7.5
24	Nebraska	8.1	27	California	4.8
NA	Nevada**	NA	NA	Alabama**	NA
25	New Hampshire	7.5	NA	Alaska**	NA
NA	New Jersey**	NA	NA	Arizona**	NA
8	New Mexico	11.9	NA	Arkansas**	NA
10	New York	11.4	NA	Connecticut**	NA
NA	North Carolina**	NA	NA	Hawaii**	NA
19	North Dakota	9.0	NA	Illinois**	NA
6	Ohio	12.9	NA	Louisiana**	NA
NA	Oklahoma**	NA	NA	Maine**	NA
18	Oregon	9.2	NA	Maryland**	NA
4	Pennsylvania	13.9	NA	Massachusetts**	NA
NA	Rhode Island**	NA	NA	Minnesota**	NA
17	South Carolina	9.4	NA	Mississippi**	NA
13	South Dakota	10.8	NA	Missouri**	NA
3	Tennessee	14.3	NA	Nevada**	NA
1	Texas	16.2	NA	New Jersey**	NA
NA	Utah**	NA	NA	North Carolina**	NA
22	Vermont	8.3	NA	Oklahoma**	NA
NA	Virginia**	NA	NA	Rhode Island**	NA
11	Washington	11.3	NA	Utah**	NA
NA	West Virginia**	NA	NA	Virginia**	NA
NA	Wisconsin**	NA	NA	West Virginia**	NA
7	Wyoming	12.1	NA	Wisconsin**	NA
				District of Columbia**	NA

Source: CQ Press using data from U.S. Department of Health and Human Services, National Center for Health Statistics
   "Vital Stats" (http://www.cdc.gov/nchs/VitalStats.htm)
*Final data by state of residence. "Late" means care begun in third trimester. National figure is for reporting states only.
Includes only non-Hispanic blacks.
**Not available.

Percent of Hispanic Women Receiving Late or No Prenatal Care in 2008

National Percent = 9.2% of Hispanic Women*

ALPHA ORDER			RANK ORDER		
RANK	**STATE**	**PERCENT**	**RANK**	**STATE**	**PERCENT**
NA	Alabama**	NA	1	Tennessee	20.5
NA	Alaska**	NA	2	South Carolina	16.5
NA	Arizona**	NA	3	Delaware	15.7
NA	Arkansas**	NA	4	Texas	14.9
27	California	4.2	5	Georgia	13.7
11	Colorado	11.4	6	South Dakota	13.2
NA	Connecticut**	NA	7	Ohio	12.7
3	Delaware	15.7	8	Kentucky	11.9
20	Florida	7.9	9	Wyoming	11.8
5	Georgia	13.7	10	New Mexico	11.6
NA	Hawaii**	NA	11	Colorado	11.4
13	Idaho	10.4	12	Indiana	11.1
NA	Illinois**	NA	13	Idaho	10.4
12	Indiana	11.1	13	Kansas	10.4
18	Iowa	8.5	13	Washington	10.4
13	Kansas	10.4	16	North Dakota	10.2
8	Kentucky	11.9	16	Pennsylvania	10.2
NA	Louisiana**	NA	18	Iowa	8.5
NA	Maine**	NA	18	New York	8.5
NA	Maryland**	NA	20	Florida	7.9
NA	Massachusetts**	NA	21	Nebraska	7.5
23	Michigan	6.6	22	Oregon	7.4
NA	Minnesota**	NA	23	Michigan	6.6
NA	Mississippi**	NA	24	Montana	6.3
NA	Missouri**	NA	25	New Hampshire	5.5
24	Montana	6.3	26	Vermont	5.3
21	Nebraska	7.5	27	California	4.2
NA	Nevada**	NA	NA	Alabama**	NA
25	New Hampshire	5.5	NA	Alaska**	NA
NA	New Jersey**	NA	NA	Arizona**	NA
10	New Mexico	11.6	NA	Arkansas**	NA
18	New York	8.5	NA	Connecticut**	NA
NA	North Carolina**	NA	NA	Hawaii**	NA
16	North Dakota	10.2	NA	Illinois**	NA
7	Ohio	12.7	NA	Louisiana**	NA
NA	Oklahoma**	NA	NA	Maine**	NA
22	Oregon	7.4	NA	Maryland**	NA
16	Pennsylvania	10.2	NA	Massachusetts**	NA
NA	Rhode Island**	NA	NA	Minnesota**	NA
2	South Carolina	16.5	NA	Mississippi**	NA
6	South Dakota	13.2	NA	Missouri**	NA
1	Tennessee	20.5	NA	Nevada**	NA
4	Texas	14.9	NA	New Jersey**	NA
NA	Utah**	NA	NA	North Carolina**	NA
26	Vermont	5.3	NA	Oklahoma**	NA
NA	Virginia**	NA	NA	Rhode Island**	NA
13	Washington	10.4	NA	Utah**	NA
NA	West Virginia**	NA	NA	Virginia**	NA
NA	Wisconsin**	NA	NA	West Virginia**	NA
9	Wyoming	11.8	NA	Wisconsin**	NA
				District of Columbia**	NA

Source: CQ Press using data from U.S. Department of Health and Human Services, National Center for Health Statistics
 "Vital Stats" (http://www.cdc.gov/nchs/VitalStats.htm)
*Final data by state of residence. "Late" means care begun in third trimester. National figure is for reporting states only.
Persons of Hispanic origin may be of any race.
**Not available.

Assisted Reproductive Technology Procedures in 2006

National Total = 136,181 Procedures*

ALPHA ORDER			
RANK	STATE	PROCEDURES	% of USA
30	Alabama	868	0.6%
47	Alaska	189	0.1%
17	Arizona	2,313	1.7%
40	Arkansas	415	0.3%
1	California	18,886	13.9%
21	Colorado	1,706	1.3%
12	Connecticut	3,341	2.5%
41	Delaware	301	0.2%
6	Florida	6,389	4.7%
14	Georgia	2,991	2.2%
37	Hawaii	570	0.4%
38	Idaho	506	0.4%
3	Illinois	9,594	7.0%
19	Indiana	1,844	1.4%
28	Iowa	899	0.7%
34	Kansas	704	0.5%
27	Kentucky	948	0.7%
29	Louisiana	891	0.7%
44	Maine	221	0.2%
8	Maryland	4,677	3.4%
5	Massachusetts	8,305	6.1%
13	Michigan	3,264	2.4%
18	Minnesota	2,008	1.5%
39	Mississippi	438	0.3%
20	Missouri	1,842	1.4%
49	Montana	176	0.1%
36	Nebraska	582	0.4%
23	Nevada	1,254	0.9%
32	New Hampshire	796	0.6%
4	New Jersey	9,237	6.8%
42	New Mexico	288	0.2%
2	New York	17,687	13.0%
15	North Carolina	2,608	1.9%
45	North Dakota	216	0.2%
11	Ohio	3,344	2.5%
35	Oklahoma	627	0.5%
24	Oregon	1,148	0.8%
9	Pennsylvania	4,611	3.4%
33	Rhode Island	760	0.6%
26	South Carolina	990	0.7%
46	South Dakota	197	0.1%
25	Tennessee	1,090	0.8%
7	Texas	6,181	4.5%
31	Utah	831	0.6%
48	Vermont	180	0.1%
10	Virginia	4,367	3.2%
16	Washington	2,382	1.7%
43	West Virginia	261	0.2%
22	Wisconsin	1,483	1.1%
50	Wyoming	63	0.0%

RANK ORDER			
RANK	STATE	PROCEDURES	% of USA
1	California	18,886	13.9%
2	New York	17,687	13.0%
3	Illinois	9,594	7.0%
4	New Jersey	9,237	6.8%
5	Massachusetts	8,305	6.1%
6	Florida	6,389	4.7%
7	Texas	6,181	4.5%
8	Maryland	4,677	3.4%
9	Pennsylvania	4,611	3.4%
10	Virginia	4,367	3.2%
11	Ohio	3,344	2.5%
12	Connecticut	3,341	2.5%
13	Michigan	3,264	2.4%
14	Georgia	2,991	2.2%
15	North Carolina	2,608	1.9%
16	Washington	2,382	1.7%
17	Arizona	2,313	1.7%
18	Minnesota	2,008	1.5%
19	Indiana	1,844	1.4%
20	Missouri	1,842	1.4%
21	Colorado	1,706	1.3%
22	Wisconsin	1,483	1.1%
23	Nevada	1,254	0.9%
24	Oregon	1,148	0.8%
25	Tennessee	1,090	0.8%
26	South Carolina	990	0.7%
27	Kentucky	948	0.7%
28	Iowa	899	0.7%
29	Louisiana	891	0.7%
30	Alabama	868	0.6%
31	Utah	831	0.6%
32	New Hampshire	796	0.6%
33	Rhode Island	760	0.6%
34	Kansas	704	0.5%
35	Oklahoma	627	0.5%
36	Nebraska	582	0.4%
37	Hawaii	570	0.4%
38	Idaho	506	0.4%
39	Mississippi	438	0.3%
40	Arkansas	415	0.3%
41	Delaware	301	0.2%
42	New Mexico	288	0.2%
43	West Virginia	261	0.2%
44	Maine	221	0.2%
45	North Dakota	216	0.2%
46	South Dakota	197	0.1%
47	Alaska	189	0.1%
48	Vermont	180	0.1%
49	Montana	176	0.1%
50	Wyoming	63	0.0%
	District of Columbia	712	0.5%

Source: U.S. Department of Health and Human Services, Centers for Disease Control and Prevention
"Assisted Reproductive Technology, 2006" (MMWR, Vol. 58, No. SS-5, 06/12/09, http://www.cdc.gov/mmwr/mmwr_ss.html)
*By patient's residence. Does not include 2,002 procedures for patients with residences outside the U.S. Assisted reproductive technology (ART) includes treatments in which both eggs and sperm are handled in the laboratory. In 2006, 72% of ART treatments were freshly fertilized embryos using the patient's eggs, 16% were thawed embryos using the patient's eggs, 8% were freshly fertilized embryos from donor eggs, and 4% were thawed embryos from donor eggs.

Infants Born from Assisted Reproductive Technology Procedures in 2006

National Total = 53,768 Live Births*

ALPHA ORDER

RANK	STATE	BIRTHS	% of USA
30	Alabama	369	0.7%
49	Alaska	73	0.1%
19	Arizona	890	1.7%
38	Arkansas	203	0.4%
1	California	7,288	13.6%
17	Colorado	1,025	1.9%
14	Connecticut	1,303	2.4%
42	Delaware	138	0.3%
7	Florida	2,505	4.7%
13	Georgia	1,317	2.4%
39	Hawaii	198	0.4%
37	Idaho	232	0.4%
4	Illinois	3,297	6.1%
21	Indiana	630	1.2%
27	Iowa	437	0.8%
34	Kansas	295	0.5%
28	Kentucky	425	0.8%
31	Louisiana	343	0.6%
43	Maine	128	0.2%
8	Maryland	1,798	3.3%
6	Massachusetts	2,965	5.5%
11	Michigan	1,390	2.6%
18	Minnesota	947	1.8%
40	Mississippi	178	0.3%
20	Missouri	795	1.5%
44	Montana	109	0.2%
36	Nebraska	243	0.5%
22	Nevada	563	1.0%
33	New Hampshire	304	0.6%
3	New Jersey	3,622	6.7%
41	New Mexico	163	0.3%
2	New York	5,802	10.8%
15	North Carolina	1,179	2.2%
46	North Dakota	91	0.2%
12	Ohio	1,373	2.6%
32	Oklahoma	321	0.6%
23	Oregon	558	1.0%
10	Pennsylvania	1,643	3.1%
35	Rhode Island	272	0.5%
26	South Carolina	516	1.0%
47	South Dakota	85	0.2%
25	Tennessee	519	1.0%
5	Texas	2,996	5.6%
29	Utah	416	0.8%
48	Vermont	76	0.1%
9	Virginia	1,675	3.1%
16	Washington	1,082	2.0%
45	West Virginia	107	0.2%
24	Wisconsin	557	1.0%
50	Wyoming	39	0.1%

RANK ORDER

RANK	STATE	BIRTHS	% of USA
1	California	7,288	13.6%
2	New York	5,802	10.8%
3	New Jersey	3,622	6.7%
4	Illinois	3,297	6.1%
5	Texas	2,996	5.6%
6	Massachusetts	2,965	5.5%
7	Florida	2,505	4.7%
8	Maryland	1,798	3.3%
9	Virginia	1,675	3.1%
10	Pennsylvania	1,643	3.1%
11	Michigan	1,390	2.6%
12	Ohio	1,373	2.6%
13	Georgia	1,317	2.4%
14	Connecticut	1,303	2.4%
15	North Carolina	1,179	2.2%
16	Washington	1,082	2.0%
17	Colorado	1,025	1.9%
18	Minnesota	947	1.8%
19	Arizona	890	1.7%
20	Missouri	795	1.5%
21	Indiana	630	1.2%
22	Nevada	563	1.0%
23	Oregon	558	1.0%
24	Wisconsin	557	1.0%
25	Tennessee	519	1.0%
26	South Carolina	516	1.0%
27	Iowa	437	0.8%
28	Kentucky	425	0.8%
29	Utah	416	0.8%
30	Alabama	369	0.7%
31	Louisiana	343	0.6%
32	Oklahoma	321	0.6%
33	New Hampshire	304	0.6%
34	Kansas	295	0.5%
35	Rhode Island	272	0.5%
36	Nebraska	243	0.5%
37	Idaho	232	0.4%
38	Arkansas	203	0.4%
39	Hawaii	198	0.4%
40	Mississippi	178	0.3%
41	New Mexico	163	0.3%
42	Delaware	138	0.3%
43	Maine	128	0.2%
44	Montana	109	0.2%
45	West Virginia	107	0.2%
46	North Dakota	91	0.2%
47	South Dakota	85	0.2%
48	Vermont	76	0.1%
49	Alaska	73	0.1%
50	Wyoming	39	0.1%
	District of Columbia	288	0.5%

Source: U.S. Department of Health and Human Services, Centers for Disease Control and Prevention
   "Assisted Reproductive Technology, 2006" (MMWR, Vol. 58, No. SS-5, 06/12/09, http://www.cdc.gov/mmwr/mmwr_ss.html)
*By patient's residence. Does not include the 879 births for patients with residences outside the U.S. Assisted reproductive
technology (ART) includes treatments in which both eggs and sperm are handled in the laboratory. In 2006, 72% of ART
treatments were freshly fertilized embryos using the patient's eggs, 16% were thawed embryos using the patient's eggs, 8% were
freshly fertilized embryos from donor eggs, and 4% were thawed embryos from donor eggs.

Percent of Assisted Reproductive Technology Procedures That Resulted in Live Births in 2006
National Percent = 29.9%*

ALPHA ORDER

RANK	STATE	PERCENT
24	Alabama	32.3
40	Alaska	29.1
38	Arizona	29.2
17	Arkansas	34.0
41	California	28.9
2	Colorado	44.3
32	Connecticut	30.6
13	Delaware	35.2
36	Florida	29.4
19	Georgia	33.1
49	Hawaii	25.4
15	Idaho	34.4
47	Illinois	26.3
48	Indiana	25.5
8	Iowa	38.0
21	Kansas	32.7
19	Kentucky	33.1
46	Louisiana	27.6
5	Maine	38.9
34	Maryland	29.7
43	Massachusetts	28.3
28	Michigan	31.5
10	Minnesota	36.4
29	Mississippi	31.1
26	Missouri	32.0
1	Montana	46.0
30	Nebraska	30.9
21	Nevada	32.7
35	New Hampshire	29.6
38	New Jersey	29.2
4	New Mexico	39.6
49	New York	25.4
16	North Carolina	34.1
33	North Dakota	30.1
31	Ohio	30.8
6	Oklahoma	38.8
14	Oregon	35.1
44	Pennsylvania	27.8
44	Rhode Island	27.8
7	South Carolina	38.4
23	South Dakota	32.5
12	Tennessee	35.4
11	Texas	35.5
9	Utah	37.2
25	Vermont	32.2
36	Virginia	29.4
17	Washington	34.0
27	West Virginia	31.8
41	Wisconsin	28.9
3	Wyoming	41.3

RANK ORDER

RANK	STATE	PERCENT
1	Montana	46.0
2	Colorado	44.3
3	Wyoming	41.3
4	New Mexico	39.6
5	Maine	38.9
6	Oklahoma	38.8
7	South Carolina	38.4
8	Iowa	38.0
9	Utah	37.2
10	Minnesota	36.4
11	Texas	35.5
12	Tennessee	35.4
13	Delaware	35.2
14	Oregon	35.1
15	Idaho	34.4
16	North Carolina	34.1
17	Arkansas	34.0
17	Washington	34.0
19	Georgia	33.1
19	Kentucky	33.1
21	Kansas	32.7
21	Nevada	32.7
23	South Dakota	32.5
24	Alabama	32.3
25	Vermont	32.2
26	Missouri	32.0
27	West Virginia	31.8
28	Michigan	31.5
29	Mississippi	31.1
30	Nebraska	30.9
31	Ohio	30.8
32	Connecticut	30.6
33	North Dakota	30.1
34	Maryland	29.7
35	New Hampshire	29.6
36	Florida	29.4
36	Virginia	29.4
38	Arizona	29.2
38	New Jersey	29.2
40	Alaska	29.1
41	California	28.9
41	Wisconsin	28.9
43	Massachusetts	28.3
44	Pennsylvania	27.8
44	Rhode Island	27.8
46	Louisiana	27.6
47	Illinois	26.3
48	Indiana	25.5
49	Hawaii	25.4
49	New York	25.4

| | District of Columbia | 31.2 |

Source: CQ Press using data from U.S. Department of Health and Human Services, Centers for Disease Control and Prevention
"Assisted Reproductive Technology, 2006" (MMWR, Vol. 58, No. SS-5, 06/12/09, http://www.cdc.gov/mmwr/mmwr_ss.html)
*By patient's residence. Assisted reproductive technology (ART) includes treatments in which both eggs and sperm are handled in the laboratory. In 2006, 72% of ART treatments were freshly fertilized embryos using the patient's eggs, 16% were thawed embryos using the patient's eggs, 8% were freshly fertilized embryos from donor eggs, and 4% were thawed embryos from donor eggs.

Percent of Total Live Births Resulting from Assisted Reproductive Technology Procedures in 2006
National Percent = 1.3% of Live Births*

ALPHA ORDER

RANK	STATE	PERCENT
42	Alabama	0.6
36	Alaska	0.7
26	Arizona	0.9
45	Arkansas	0.5
12	California	1.3
10	Colorado	1.4
2	Connecticut	3.1
14	Delaware	1.2
17	Florida	1.1
26	Georgia	0.9
23	Hawaii	1.0
23	Idaho	1.0
8	Illinois	1.8
36	Indiana	0.7
17	Iowa	1.1
36	Kansas	0.7
36	Kentucky	0.7
45	Louisiana	0.5
26	Maine	0.9
4	Maryland	2.3
1	Massachusetts	3.8
17	Michigan	1.1
12	Minnesota	1.3
50	Mississippi	0.4
23	Missouri	1.0
26	Montana	0.9
26	Nebraska	0.9
10	Nevada	1.4
7	New Hampshire	2.1
2	New Jersey	3.1
45	New Mexico	0.5
4	New York	2.3
26	North Carolina	0.9
17	North Dakota	1.1
26	Ohio	0.9
42	Oklahoma	0.6
17	Oregon	1.1
17	Pennsylvania	1.1
6	Rhode Island	2.2
33	South Carolina	0.8
36	South Dakota	0.7
42	Tennessee	0.6
36	Texas	0.7
33	Utah	0.8
14	Vermont	1.2
9	Virginia	1.6
14	Washington	1.2
45	West Virginia	0.5
33	Wisconsin	0.8
45	Wyoming	0.5

RANK ORDER

RANK	STATE	PERCENT
1	Massachusetts	3.8
2	Connecticut	3.1
2	New Jersey	3.1
4	Maryland	2.3
4	New York	2.3
6	Rhode Island	2.2
7	New Hampshire	2.1
8	Illinois	1.8
9	Virginia	1.6
10	Colorado	1.4
10	Nevada	1.4
12	California	1.3
12	Minnesota	1.3
14	Delaware	1.2
14	Vermont	1.2
14	Washington	1.2
17	Florida	1.1
17	Iowa	1.1
17	Michigan	1.1
17	North Dakota	1.1
17	Oregon	1.1
17	Pennsylvania	1.1
23	Hawaii	1.0
23	Idaho	1.0
23	Missouri	1.0
26	Arizona	0.9
26	Georgia	0.9
26	Maine	0.9
26	Montana	0.9
26	Nebraska	0.9
26	North Carolina	0.9
26	Ohio	0.9
33	South Carolina	0.8
33	Utah	0.8
33	Wisconsin	0.8
36	Alaska	0.7
36	Indiana	0.7
36	Kansas	0.7
36	Kentucky	0.7
36	South Dakota	0.7
36	Texas	0.7
42	Alabama	0.6
42	Oklahoma	0.6
42	Tennessee	0.6
45	Arkansas	0.5
45	Louisiana	0.5
45	New Mexico	0.5
45	West Virginia	0.5
45	Wyoming	0.5
50	Mississippi	0.4

District of Columbia 3.4

Source: CQ Press using data from U.S. Department of Health and Human Services, Centers for Disease Control and Prevention "Assisted Reproductive Technology, 2006" (MMWR, Vol. 58, No. SS-5, 06/12/09, http://www.cdc.gov/mmwr/mmwr_ss.html) "National Vital Statistics Reports" (Vol. 57, No. 7, January 7, 2009, http://www.cdc.gov/nchs/births.htm)

*By patient's residence. Does not include births or procedures to patients with residences outside the U.S. Assisted reproductive technology (ART) includes treatments in which both eggs and sperm are handled in the laboratory (that is, in vitro fertilization and related procedures).

Percent of Assisted Reproductive Technology Procedure Infants Born in Multiple Birth Deliveries in 2006
National Percent = 47.5% of Assisted Reproductive Technology Births*

ALPHA ORDER

RANK	STATE	PERCENT
31	Alabama	47.2
27	Alaska	47.9
35	Arizona	46.2
3	Arkansas	59.1
23	California	48.8
13	Colorado	51.2
49	Connecticut	42.3
38	Delaware	45.7
22	Florida	48.9
24	Georgia	48.5
9	Hawaii	52.5
28	Idaho	47.8
39	Illinois	45.6
26	Indiana	48.1
47	Iowa	42.8
48	Kansas	42.7
14	Kentucky	50.6
7	Louisiana	53.4
2	Maine	61.7
42	Maryland	44.2
50	Massachusetts	40.9
17	Michigan	50.4
37	Minnesota	45.9
33	Mississippi	46.6
19	Missouri	49.7
16	Montana	50.5
14	Nebraska	50.6
8	Nevada	52.6
43	New Hampshire	44.1
18	New Jersey	50.0
4	New Mexico	57.1
41	New York	44.3
28	North Carolina	47.8
5	North Dakota	54.9
25	Ohio	48.3
30	Oklahoma	47.7
6	Oregon	54.5
46	Pennsylvania	43.5
45	Rhode Island	43.8
12	South Carolina	51.7
32	South Dakota	47.1
21	Tennessee	49.1
11	Texas	51.9
10	Utah	52.2
36	Vermont	46.1
34	Virginia	46.4
20	Washington	49.4
44	West Virginia	43.9
40	Wisconsin	45.4
1	Wyoming	64.1

RANK ORDER

RANK	STATE	PERCENT
1	Wyoming	64.1
2	Maine	61.7
3	Arkansas	59.1
4	New Mexico	57.1
5	North Dakota	54.9
6	Oregon	54.5
7	Louisiana	53.4
8	Nevada	52.6
9	Hawaii	52.5
10	Utah	52.2
11	Texas	51.9
12	South Carolina	51.7
13	Colorado	51.2
14	Kentucky	50.6
14	Nebraska	50.6
16	Montana	50.5
17	Michigan	50.4
18	New Jersey	50.0
19	Missouri	49.7
20	Washington	49.4
21	Tennessee	49.1
22	Florida	48.9
23	California	48.8
24	Georgia	48.5
25	Ohio	48.3
26	Indiana	48.1
27	Alaska	47.9
28	Idaho	47.8
28	North Carolina	47.8
30	Oklahoma	47.7
31	Alabama	47.2
32	South Dakota	47.1
33	Mississippi	46.6
34	Virginia	46.4
35	Arizona	46.2
36	Vermont	46.1
37	Minnesota	45.9
38	Delaware	45.7
39	Illinois	45.6
40	Wisconsin	45.4
41	New York	44.3
42	Maryland	44.2
43	New Hampshire	44.1
44	West Virginia	43.9
45	Rhode Island	43.8
46	Pennsylvania	43.5
47	Iowa	42.8
48	Kansas	42.7
49	Connecticut	42.3
50	Massachusetts	40.9
	District of Columbia	45.1

Source: U.S. Department of Health and Human Services, Centers for Disease Control and Prevention
  "Assisted Reproductive Technology, 2006" (MMWR, Vol. 58, No. SS-5, 06/12/09, http://www.cdc.gov/mmwr/mmwr_ss.html)
*By patient's residence. Includes births and procedures to patients with residences outside the U.S. Assisted reproductive
technology (ART) includes treatments in which both eggs and sperm are handled in the laboratory (that is, in vitro fertilization and
related procedures).

Pregnancy Rate in 2006

National Rate = 71.1 Births and Abortions per 1,000 Women 15 to 49 Years Old*

ALPHA ORDER

RANK	STATE	RATE
29	Alabama	66.9
11	Alaska	75.3
7	Arizona	77.6
22	Arkansas	69.0
NA	California**	NA
24	Colorado	68.8
32	Connecticut	65.8
4	Delaware	79.9
5	Florida	79.8
12	Georgia	75.0
9	Hawaii	76.9
14	Idaho	73.2
16	Illinois	71.4
35	Indiana	64.8
28	Iowa	67.9
6	Kansas	78.9
44	Kentucky	60.3
NA	Louisiana**	NA
47	Maine	53.6
42	Maryland	60.7
40	Massachusetts	62.4
41	Michigan	62.1
21	Minnesota	69.1
26	Mississippi	68.6
39	Missouri	62.5
30	Montana	66.7
18	Nebraska	70.7
2	Nevada	87.2
NA	New Hampshire**	NA
23	New Jersey	68.9
10	New Mexico	76.7
8	New York	77.4
13	North Carolina	74.5
33	North Dakota	65.7
31	Ohio	65.9
15	Oklahoma	71.7
24	Oregon	68.8
38	Pennsylvania	63.0
36	Rhode Island	64.5
34	South Carolina	65.4
20	South Dakota	69.4
27	Tennessee	68.5
3	Texas	82.2
1	Utah	87.6
46	Vermont	53.8
19	Virginia	70.1
17	Washington	71.2
45	West Virginia	54.6
43	Wisconsin	60.6
37	Wyoming	63.3

RANK ORDER

RANK	STATE	RATE
1	Utah	87.6
2	Nevada	87.2
3	Texas	82.2
4	Delaware	79.9
5	Florida	79.8
6	Kansas	78.9
7	Arizona	77.6
8	New York	77.4
9	Hawaii	76.9
10	New Mexico	76.7
11	Alaska	75.3
12	Georgia	75.0
13	North Carolina	74.5
14	Idaho	73.2
15	Oklahoma	71.7
16	Illinois	71.4
17	Washington	71.2
18	Nebraska	70.7
19	Virginia	70.1
20	South Dakota	69.4
21	Minnesota	69.1
22	Arkansas	69.0
23	New Jersey	68.9
24	Colorado	68.8
24	Oregon	68.8
26	Mississippi	68.6
27	Tennessee	68.5
28	Iowa	67.9
29	Alabama	66.9
30	Montana	66.7
31	Ohio	65.9
32	Connecticut	65.8
33	North Dakota	65.7
34	South Carolina	65.4
35	Indiana	64.8
36	Rhode Island	64.5
37	Wyoming	63.3
38	Pennsylvania	63.0
39	Missouri	62.5
40	Massachusetts	62.4
41	Michigan	62.1
42	Maryland	60.7
43	Wisconsin	60.6
44	Kentucky	60.3
45	West Virginia	54.6
46	Vermont	53.8
47	Maine	53.6
NA	California**	NA
NA	Louisiana**	NA
NA	New Hampshire**	NA

District of Columbia 67.3

Source: CQ Press using data from U.S. Department of Health and Human Services, Centers for Disease Control and Prevention
    "Abortion Surveillance-United States, 2006" (MMWR, Vol. 58, No. SS-8, 11/27/09, http://www.cdc.gov/mmwr/mmwr_ss.html)
*The sum of live births and legal induced abortions per 1,000 women 15 to 49 years old. Births by state of residence, abortions
by state of occurrence. Miscarriages are not included in these rates. National rate includes only states reporting abortions and
births.
**Not available.

Teenage Pregnancy Rate in 2006

National Rate = 57.7 Births and Abortions per 1,000 Women 15 to 19 Years Old*

ALPHA ORDER

RANK ORDER

RANK	STATE	RATE		RANK	STATE	RATE
11	Alabama	67.3		1	New Mexico	82.2
18	Alaska	58.5		2	Nevada	81.4
6	Arizona	72.2		3	Texas	76.6
5	Arkansas	72.3		4	Mississippi	73.0
NA	California**	NA		5	Arkansas	72.3
19	Colorado	57.0		6	Arizona	72.2
31	Connecticut	46.2		7	Georgia	69.3
12	Delaware	63.2		7	Tennessee	69.3
NA	Florida**	NA		9	Oklahoma	69.2
7	Georgia	69.3		10	North Carolina	68.4
13	Hawaii	62.6		11	Alabama	67.3
35	Idaho	44.5		12	Delaware	63.2
NA	Illinois**	NA		13	Hawaii	62.6
25	Indiana	51.7		14	Kansas	62.2
34	Iowa	44.7		15	South Carolina	61.7
14	Kansas	62.2		16	Kentucky	59.7
16	Kentucky	59.7		17	New York	59.6
NA	Louisiana**	NA		18	Alaska	58.5
42	Maine	37.0		19	Colorado	57.0
NA	Maryland**	NA		20	Ohio	55.1
41	Massachusetts	38.3		20	Washington	55.1
30	Michigan	46.9		22	Oregon	53.1
38	Minnesota	39.8		23	Missouri	52.1
4	Mississippi	73.0		23	Montana	52.1
23	Missouri	52.1		25	Indiana	51.7
23	Montana	52.1		26	West Virginia	51.4
37	Nebraska	40.9		27	Rhode Island	50.3
2	Nevada	81.4		28	Virginia	50.2
NA	New Hampshire**	NA		29	Wyoming	47.6
33	New Jersey	44.8		30	Michigan	46.9
1	New Mexico	82.2		31	Connecticut	46.2
17	New York	59.6		32	Pennsylvania	45.8
10	North Carolina	68.4		33	New Jersey	44.8
43	North Dakota	35.9		34	Iowa	44.7
20	Ohio	55.1		35	Idaho	44.5
9	Oklahoma	69.2		36	South Dakota	44.1
22	Oregon	53.1		37	Nebraska	40.9
32	Pennsylvania	45.8		38	Minnesota	39.8
27	Rhode Island	50.3		39	Utah	39.6
15	South Carolina	61.7		40	Wisconsin	39.4
36	South Dakota	44.1		41	Massachusetts	38.3
7	Tennessee	69.3		42	Maine	37.0
3	Texas	76.6		43	North Dakota	35.9
39	Utah	39.6		44	Vermont	34.0
44	Vermont	34.0		NA	California**	NA
28	Virginia	50.2		NA	Florida**	NA
20	Washington	55.1		NA	Illinois**	NA
26	West Virginia	51.4		NA	Louisiana**	NA
40	Wisconsin	39.4		NA	Maryland**	NA
29	Wyoming	47.6		NA	New Hampshire**	NA

District of Columbia 71.5

Source: CQ Press using data from U.S. Department of Health and Human Services, Centers for Disease Control and Prevention
"Abortion Surveillance-United States, 2006" (MMWR, Vol. 58, No. SS-8, 11/27/09, http://www.cdc.gov/mmwr/mmwr_ss.html)
*The sum of live births and legal induced abortions per 1,000 women 15 to 19 years old. Births by state of residence, abortions by state of occurrence. Miscarriages are not included in these rates. National rate includes only states reporting abortions and births.
**Not available.

Reported Legal Abortions in 2006

Reporting States' Total = 846,181 Abortions*

ALPHA ORDER

RANK	STATE	ABORTIONS	% of USA
18	Alabama	11,654	1.4%
42	Alaska	1,923	0.2%
22	Arizona	10,836	1.3%
31	Arkansas	4,988	0.6%
NA	California**	NA	NA
21	Colorado	11,048	1.3%
15	Connecticut	14,112	1.7%
33	Delaware	4,804	0.6%
2	Florida	95,586	11.3%
9	Georgia	30,550	3.6%
34	Hawaii	3,990	0.5%
45	Idaho	1,249	0.1%
4	Illinois	46,467	5.5%
23	Indiana	10,614	1.3%
29	Iowa	6,722	0.8%
20	Kansas	11,173	1.3%
35	Kentucky	3,912	0.5%
NA	Louisiana**	NA	NA
39	Maine	2,670	0.3%
25	Maryland	9,530	1.1%
13	Massachusetts	24,246	2.9%
11	Michigan	25,636	3.0%
16	Minnesota	14,065	1.7%
37	Mississippi	2,949	0.3%
26	Missouri	7,556	0.9%
40	Montana	2,119	0.3%
38	Nebraska	2,927	0.3%
19	Nevada	11,471	1.4%
NA	New Hampshire**	NA	NA
8	New Jersey	30,986	3.7%
30	New Mexico	6,087	0.7%
1	New York	127,437	15.1%
6	North Carolina	35,088	4.1%
44	North Dakota	1,298	0.2%
7	Ohio	32,936	3.9%
27	Oklahoma	7,088	0.8%
17	Oregon	11,732	1.4%
5	Pennsylvania	36,731	4.3%
32	Rhode Island	4,828	0.6%
28	South Carolina	7,005	0.8%
46	South Dakota	748	0.1%
14	Tennessee	17,883	2.1%
3	Texas	81,883	9.7%
36	Utah	3,753	0.4%
43	Vermont	1,610	0.2%
10	Virginia	27,349	3.2%
12	Washington	24,627	2.9%
41	West Virginia	2,036	0.2%
24	Wisconsin	9,580	1.1%
47	Wyoming	7	0.0%

RANK ORDER

RANK	STATE	ABORTIONS	% of USA
1	New York	127,437	15.1%
2	Florida	95,586	11.3%
3	Texas	81,883	9.7%
4	Illinois	46,467	5.5%
5	Pennsylvania	36,731	4.3%
6	North Carolina	35,088	4.1%
7	Ohio	32,936	3.9%
8	New Jersey	30,986	3.7%
9	Georgia	30,550	3.6%
10	Virginia	27,349	3.2%
11	Michigan	25,636	3.0%
12	Washington	24,627	2.9%
13	Massachusetts	24,246	2.9%
14	Tennessee	17,883	2.1%
15	Connecticut	14,112	1.7%
16	Minnesota	14,065	1.7%
17	Oregon	11,732	1.4%
18	Alabama	11,654	1.4%
19	Nevada	11,471	1.4%
20	Kansas	11,173	1.3%
21	Colorado	11,048	1.3%
22	Arizona	10,836	1.3%
23	Indiana	10,614	1.3%
24	Wisconsin	9,580	1.1%
25	Maryland	9,530	1.1%
26	Missouri	7,556	0.9%
27	Oklahoma	7,088	0.8%
28	South Carolina	7,005	0.8%
29	Iowa	6,722	0.8%
30	New Mexico	6,087	0.7%
31	Arkansas	4,988	0.6%
32	Rhode Island	4,828	0.6%
33	Delaware	4,804	0.6%
34	Hawaii	3,990	0.5%
35	Kentucky	3,912	0.5%
36	Utah	3,753	0.4%
37	Mississippi	2,949	0.3%
38	Nebraska	2,927	0.3%
39	Maine	2,670	0.3%
40	Montana	2,119	0.3%
41	West Virginia	2,036	0.2%
42	Alaska	1,923	0.2%
43	Vermont	1,610	0.2%
44	North Dakota	1,298	0.2%
45	Idaho	1,249	0.1%
46	South Dakota	748	0.1%
47	Wyoming	7	0.0%
NA	California**	NA	NA
NA	Louisiana**	NA	NA
NA	New Hampshire**	NA	NA
	District of Columbia	2,692	0.3%

Source: U.S. Department of Health and Human Services, Centers for Disease Control and Prevention
"Abortion Surveillance-United States, 2006" (MMWR, Vol. 58, No. SS-8, 11/27/09, http://www.cdc.gov/mmwr/mmwr_ss.html)
*By state of occurrence. Total is for reporting states only.
**Not reported.

Percent Change in Reported Legal Abortions: 2002 to 2006

National Percent Change = 0.1% Increase*

ALPHA ORDER

RANK	STATE	PERCENT CHANGE
30	Alabama	(4.9)
NA	Alaska**	NA
20	Arizona	1.5
34	Arkansas	(6.2)
NA	California**	NA
2	Colorado	42.4
16	Connecticut	4.8
12	Delaware	6.9
10	Florida	8.7
39	Georgia	(10.4)
19	Hawaii	1.8
1	Idaho	50.7
25	Illinois	(1.0)
28	Indiana	(3.0)
11	Iowa	7.7
31	Kansas	(5.0)
7	Kentucky	11.7
NA	Louisiana**	NA
5	Maine	15.3
45	Maryland	(29.9)
29	Massachusetts	(4.0)
41	Michigan	(12.3)
24	Minnesota	(0.9)
43	Mississippi	(18.2)
35	Missouri	(7.9)
32	Montana	(5.7)
44	Nebraska	(22.5)
6	Nevada	15.2
NA	New Hampshire**	NA
32	New Jersey	(5.7)
3	New Mexico	20.1
22	New York	(0.4)
4	North Carolina	20.0
13	North Dakota	6.5
36	Ohio	(8.1)
9	Oklahoma	9.0
40	Oregon	(10.9)
17	Pennsylvania	4.4
42	Rhode Island	(13.0)
15	South Carolina	5.2
38	South Dakota	(9.4)
21	Tennessee	0.4
18	Texas	2.4
13	Utah	6.5
26	Vermont	(1.5)
8	Virginia	9.4
27	Washington	(2.1)
23	West Virginia	(0.6)
37	Wisconsin	(8.7)
46	Wyoming	(30.0)

RANK ORDER

RANK	STATE	PERCENT CHANGE
1	Idaho	50.7
2	Colorado	42.4
3	New Mexico	20.1
4	North Carolina	20.0
5	Maine	15.3
6	Nevada	15.2
7	Kentucky	11.7
8	Virginia	9.4
9	Oklahoma	9.0
10	Florida	8.7
11	Iowa	7.7
12	Delaware	6.9
13	North Dakota	6.5
13	Utah	6.5
15	South Carolina	5.2
16	Connecticut	4.8
17	Pennsylvania	4.4
18	Texas	2.4
19	Hawaii	1.8
20	Arizona	1.5
21	Tennessee	0.4
22	New York	(0.4)
23	West Virginia	(0.6)
24	Minnesota	(0.9)
25	Illinois	(1.0)
26	Vermont	(1.5)
27	Washington	(2.1)
28	Indiana	(3.0)
29	Massachusetts	(4.0)
30	Alabama	(4.9)
31	Kansas	(5.0)
32	Montana	(5.7)
32	New Jersey	(5.7)
34	Arkansas	(6.2)
35	Missouri	(7.9)
36	Ohio	(8.1)
37	Wisconsin	(8.7)
38	South Dakota	(9.4)
39	Georgia	(10.4)
40	Oregon	(10.9)
41	Michigan	(12.3)
42	Rhode Island	(13.0)
43	Mississippi	(18.2)
44	Nebraska	(22.5)
45	Maryland	(29.9)
46	Wyoming	(30.0)
NA	Alaska**	NA
NA	California**	NA
NA	Louisiana**	NA
NA	New Hampshire**	NA

District of Columbia (51.2)

Source: CQ Press using data from U.S. Department of Health and Human Services, Centers for Disease Control and Prevention
"Abortion Surveillance-United States, 2006" (MMWR, Vol. 58, No. SS-8, 11/27/09, http://www.cdc.gov/mmwr/mmwr_ss.html)
"Abortion Surveillance-United States, 2002" (MMWR, Vol. 54, No. SS-7, 11/25/05)
*By state of occurrence. National percent change is only for states reporting in both years.
**Not reported.

Reported Legal Abortions per 1,000 Live Births in 2006

Reporting States' Ratio = 233 Abortions per 1,000 Live Births*

ALPHA ORDER				RANK ORDER		
RANK	STATE	RATIO		RANK	STATE	RATIO
26	Alabama	184		1	New York	510
27	Alaska	175		2	Florida	404
39	Arizona	106		3	Delaware	401
35	Arkansas	122		4	Rhode Island	390
NA	California**	NA		5	Connecticut	337
30	Colorado	156		6	Massachusetts	312
5	Connecticut	337		7	Nevada	287
3	Delaware	401		8	Washington	283
2	Florida	404		9	North Carolina	274
20	Georgia	206		10	Kansas	273
19	Hawaii	210		11	New Jersey	269
46	Idaho	52		12	Illinois	257
12	Illinois	257		13	Virginia	254
36	Indiana	120		14	Vermont	247
29	Iowa	166		15	Pennsylvania	246
10	Kansas	273		16	Oregon	241
43	Kentucky	67		17	Ohio	219
NA	Louisiana**	NA		18	Tennessee	212
25	Maine	189		19	Hawaii	210
34	Maryland	123		20	Georgia	206
6	Massachusetts	312		21	Texas	205
23	Michigan	201		22	New Mexico	203
24	Minnesota	191		23	Michigan	201
44	Mississippi	64		24	Minnesota	191
41	Missouri	93		25	Maine	189
28	Montana	169		26	Alabama	184
38	Nebraska	110		27	Alaska	175
7	Nevada	287		28	Montana	169
NA	New Hampshire**	NA		29	Iowa	166
11	New Jersey	269		30	Colorado	156
22	New Mexico	203		31	North Dakota	151
1	New York	510		32	Wisconsin	132
9	North Carolina	274		33	Oklahoma	131
31	North Dakota	151		34	Maryland	123
17	Ohio	219		35	Arkansas	122
33	Oklahoma	131		36	Indiana	120
16	Oregon	241		37	South Carolina	113
15	Pennsylvania	246		38	Nebraska	110
4	Rhode Island	390		39	Arizona	106
37	South Carolina	113		40	West Virginia	97
45	South Dakota	63		41	Missouri	93
18	Tennessee	212		42	Utah	70
21	Texas	205		43	Kentucky	67
42	Utah	70		44	Mississippi	64
14	Vermont	247		45	South Dakota	63
13	Virginia	254		46	Idaho	52
8	Washington	283		47	Wyoming	1
40	West Virginia	97		NA	California**	NA
32	Wisconsin	132		NA	Louisiana**	NA
47	Wyoming	1		NA	New Hampshire**	NA

District of Columbia   316

Source: U.S. Department of Health and Human Services, Centers for Disease Control and Prevention
"Abortion Surveillance-United States, 2006" (MMWR, Vol. 58, No. SS-8, 11/27/09, http://www.cdc.gov/mmwr/mmwr_ss.html)
*By state of occurrence. National figure is for reporting states only.
**Not reported.

Reported Legal Abortions per 1,000 Women 15 to 44 Years Old in 2006

Reporting States' Rate = 15.9 Abortions per 1,000 Women 15 to 44 Years Old*

ALPHA ORDER				RANK ORDER		
RANK	STATE	RATE		RANK	STATE	RATE
25	Alabama	12.4		1	New York	31.1
22	Alaska	13.4		2	Florida	27.3
34	Arizona	8.7		3	Delaware	27.1
33	Arkansas	8.8		4	Nevada	22.7
NA	California**	NA		5	Rhode Island	21.5
29	Colorado	11.0		6	Kansas	20.1
7	Connecticut	20.0		7	Connecticut	20.0
3	Delaware	27.1		8	North Carolina	18.9
2	Florida	27.3		9	Washington	18.6
18	Georgia	15.0		10	Massachusetts	17.7
16	Hawaii	15.7		11	New Jersey	17.5
46	Idaho	4.2		12	Illinois	17.3
12	Illinois	17.3		13	Virginia	16.8
37	Indiana	8.2		14	Texas	16.3
28	Iowa	11.5		15	Oregon	15.9
6	Kansas	20.1		16	Hawaii	15.7
45	Kentucky	4.5		17	New Mexico	15.3
NA	Louisiana**	NA		18	Georgia	15.0
30	Maine	10.4		18	Pennsylvania	15.0
38	Maryland	7.9		20	Ohio	14.2
10	Massachusetts	17.7		20	Tennessee	14.2
25	Michigan	12.4		22	Alaska	13.4
23	Minnesota	13.2		23	Minnesota	13.2
43	Mississippi	4.9		24	Vermont	13.0
41	Missouri	6.3		25	Alabama	12.4
27	Montana	11.7		25	Michigan	12.4
36	Nebraska	8.3		27	Montana	11.7
4	Nevada	22.7		28	Iowa	11.5
NA	New Hampshire**	NA		29	Colorado	11.0
11	New Jersey	17.5		30	Maine	10.4
17	New Mexico	15.3		31	North Dakota	10.2
1	New York	31.1		32	Oklahoma	9.8
8	North Carolina	18.9		33	Arkansas	8.8
31	North Dakota	10.2		34	Arizona	8.7
20	Ohio	14.2		35	Wisconsin	8.5
32	Oklahoma	9.8		36	Nebraska	8.3
15	Oregon	15.9		37	Indiana	8.2
18	Pennsylvania	15.0		38	Maryland	7.9
5	Rhode Island	21.5		39	South Carolina	7.8
39	South Carolina	7.8		40	Utah	6.5
43	South Dakota	4.9		41	Missouri	6.3
20	Tennessee	14.2		42	West Virginia	5.8
14	Texas	16.3		43	Mississippi	4.9
40	Utah	6.5		43	South Dakota	4.9
24	Vermont	13.0		45	Kentucky	4.5
13	Virginia	16.8		46	Idaho	4.2
9	Washington	18.6		47	Wyoming	0.1
42	West Virginia	5.8		NA	California**	NA
35	Wisconsin	8.5		NA	Louisiana**	NA
47	Wyoming	0.1		NA	New Hampshire**	NA
				District of Columbia		18.4

Source: U.S. Department of Health and Human Services, Centers for Disease Control and Prevention
   "Abortion Surveillance-United States, 2006" (MMWR, Vol. 58, No. SS-8, 11/27/09, http://www.cdc.gov/mmwr/mmwr_ss.html)
*By state of occurrence. National figure is for reporting states only.
**Not reported.

Percent of Legal Abortions Obtained by Out-of-State Residents in 2006

Reporting States' Percent = 8.4% of Abortions*

ALPHA ORDER				RANK ORDER		
RANK	STATE	PERCENT		RANK	STATE	PERCENT
6	Alabama	18.7		1	Kansas	48.2
41	Alaska	0.6		2	North Dakota	40.1
34	Arizona	3.4		3	Delaware	28.2
11	Arkansas	14.0		4	Rhode Island	23.6
NA	California**	NA		5	Tennessee	22.2
42	Colorado	0.4		6	Alabama	18.7
36	Connecticut	3.0		7	North Carolina	17.4
3	Delaware	28.2		8	Iowa	16.7
NA	Florida**	NA		9	South Dakota	15.4
14	Georgia	10.7		10	Maryland	14.3
43	Hawaii	0.3		11	Arkansas	14.0
38	Idaho	2.7		12	Oregon	12.5
18	Illinois	8.7		13	Nebraska	12.4
31	Indiana	4.0		14	Georgia	10.7
8	Iowa	16.7		15	West Virginia	10.3
1	Kansas	48.2		16	Vermont	9.6
NA	Kentucky**	NA		17	Montana	8.9
NA	Louisiana**	NA		18	Illinois	8.7
35	Maine	3.2		19	Utah	8.2
10	Maryland	14.3		20	Minnesota	7.9
30	Massachusetts	4.1		21	Missouri	7.5
37	Michigan	2.8		22	Ohio	6.0
20	Minnesota	7.9		23	Nevada	5.7
39	Mississippi	2.5		24	New Mexico	5.3
21	Missouri	7.5		24	Virginia	5.3
17	Montana	8.9		26	New Jersey	5.2
13	Nebraska	12.4		27	Washington	4.8
23	Nevada	5.7		28	Pennsylvania	4.2
NA	New Hampshire**	NA		28	South Carolina	4.2
26	New Jersey	5.2		30	Massachusetts	4.1
24	New Mexico	5.3		31	Indiana	4.0
NA	New York**	NA		32	Texas	3.6
7	North Carolina	17.4		33	Oklahoma	3.5
2	North Dakota	40.1		34	Arizona	3.4
22	Ohio	6.0		35	Maine	3.2
33	Oklahoma	3.5		36	Connecticut	3.0
12	Oregon	12.5		37	Michigan	2.8
28	Pennsylvania	4.2		38	Idaho	2.7
4	Rhode Island	23.6		39	Mississippi	2.5
28	South Carolina	4.2		40	Wisconsin	2.4
9	South Dakota	15.4		41	Alaska	0.6
5	Tennessee	22.2		42	Colorado	0.4
32	Texas	3.6		43	Hawaii	0.3
19	Utah	8.2		44	Wyoming	0.0
16	Vermont	9.6		NA	California**	NA
24	Virginia	5.3		NA	Florida**	NA
27	Washington	4.8		NA	Kentucky**	NA
15	West Virginia	10.3		NA	Louisiana**	NA
40	Wisconsin	2.4		NA	New Hampshire**	NA
44	Wyoming	0.0		NA	New York**	NA

District of Columbia 54.3

Source: U.S. Department of Health and Human Services, Centers for Disease Control and Prevention
    "Abortion Surveillance-United States, 2006" (MMWR, Vol. 58, No. SS-8, 11/27/09, http://www.cdc.gov/mmwr/mmwr_ss.html)
*By state of occurrence. National figure is for reporting states only.
**Not reported.

Percent of Reported Legal Abortions That Were First-Time Abortions: 2006

Reporting States' Percent = 54.1% of Abortions*

ALPHA ORDER				RANK ORDER		
RANK	STATE	PERCENT		RANK	STATE	PERCENT
7	Alabama	65.3		1	Idaho	78.1
17	Alaska	59.6		2	South Dakota	70.5
15	Arizona	61.0		3	North Dakota	68.8
13	Arkansas	62.4		4	Utah	66.4
NA	California**	NA		5	New Jersey	66.1
9	Colorado	64.0		6	Maine	65.8
NA	Connecticut**	NA		7	Alabama	65.3
20	Delaware	59.3		8	Iowa	65.0
NA	Florida**	NA		9	Colorado	64.0
16	Georgia	60.4		10	Nebraska	63.9
34	Hawaii	50.8		11	Oklahoma	63.4
1	Idaho	78.1		12	Mississippi	62.9
NA	Illinois**	NA		13	Arkansas	62.4
26	Indiana	56.4		14	Kansas	61.7
8	Iowa	65.0		15	Arizona	61.0
14	Kansas	61.7		16	Georgia	60.4
21	Kentucky	58.8		17	Alaska	59.6
NA	Louisiana**	NA		18	Vermont	59.5
6	Maine	65.8		18	West Virginia	59.5
40	Maryland	21.6		20	Delaware	59.3
36	Massachusetts	48.1		21	Kentucky	58.8
32	Michigan	51.5		22	Minnesota	58.5
22	Minnesota	58.5		23	Texas	58.0
12	Mississippi	62.9		24	Missouri	57.8
24	Missouri	57.8		25	South Carolina	57.0
39	Montana	32.2		26	Indiana	56.4
10	Nebraska	63.9		26	Virginia	56.4
35	Nevada	50.7		28	Oregon	56.1
NA	New Hampshire**	NA		29	Pennsylvania	55.3
5	New Jersey	66.1		30	Washington	53.3
NA	New Mexico**	NA		31	Tennessee	52.2
38	New York	45.1		32	Michigan	51.5
NA	North Carolina**	NA		33	Rhode Island	51.3
3	North Dakota	68.8		34	Hawaii	50.8
36	Ohio	48.1		35	Nevada	50.7
11	Oklahoma	63.4		36	Massachusetts	48.1
28	Oregon	56.1		36	Ohio	48.1
29	Pennsylvania	55.3		38	New York	45.1
33	Rhode Island	51.3		39	Montana	32.2
25	South Carolina	57.0		40	Maryland	21.6
2	South Dakota	70.5		NA	California**	NA
31	Tennessee	52.2		NA	Connecticut**	NA
23	Texas	58.0		NA	Florida**	NA
4	Utah	66.4		NA	Illinois**	NA
18	Vermont	59.5		NA	Louisiana**	NA
26	Virginia	56.4		NA	New Hampshire**	NA
30	Washington	53.3		NA	New Mexico**	NA
18	West Virginia	59.5		NA	North Carolina**	NA
NA	Wisconsin**	NA		NA	Wisconsin**	NA
NA	Wyoming**	NA		NA	Wyoming**	NA
				District of Columbia**		NA

Source: U.S. Department of Health and Human Services, Centers for Disease Control and Prevention
"Abortion Surveillance-United States, 2006" (MMWR, Vol. 58, No. SS-8, 11/27/09, http://www.cdc.gov/mmwr/mmwr_ss.html)
*By state of occurrence. National figure is for reporting states only. Percent of abortions to women who had no previous abortions.
**Not reported.

Percent of Reported Legal Abortions Obtained by White Women in 2006

Reporting States' Percent = 55.8% of Abortions*

ALPHA ORDER				RANK ORDER		
RANK	STATE	PERCENT		RANK	STATE	PERCENT
31	Alabama	42.3		1	Vermont	94.7
21	Alaska	57.8		2	Idaho	90.7
NA	Arizona**	NA		3	Maine	90.0
19	Arkansas	61.7		4	West Virginia	85.1
NA	California**	NA		5	Oregon	84.2
14	Colorado	67.2		6	South Dakota	84.0
NA	Connecticut**	NA		7	North Dakota	81.7
25	Delaware	53.8		8	Montana	80.2
NA	Florida**	NA		9	Iowa	79.3
33	Georgia	37.9		10	Oklahoma	72.0
35	Hawaii	24.1		11	Texas	70.6
2	Idaho	90.7		12	Wisconsin	69.1
NA	Illinois**	NA		13	Kansas	68.2
17	Indiana	64.1		14	Colorado	67.2
9	Iowa	79.3		15	Kentucky	66.6
13	Kansas	68.2		16	Rhode Island	64.6
15	Kentucky	66.6		17	Indiana	64.1
NA	Louisiana**	NA		18	Minnesota	62.9
3	Maine	90.0		19	Arkansas	61.7
37	Maryland	20.5		20	South Carolina	58.9
27	Massachusetts	50.1		21	Alaska	57.8
26	Michigan	53.5		22	Ohio	56.8
18	Minnesota	62.9		23	Pennsylvania	55.9
36	Mississippi	22.6		24	Missouri	54.8
24	Missouri	54.8		25	Delaware	53.8
8	Montana	80.2		26	Michigan	53.5
NA	Nebraska**	NA		27	Massachusetts	50.1
NA	Nevada**	NA		28	Tennessee	49.0
NA	New Hampshire**	NA		29	New York**	47.0
34	New Jersey	31.8		30	Virginia	44.5
NA	New Mexico**	NA		31	Alabama	42.3
29	New York**	47.0		32	North Carolina	41.1
32	North Carolina	41.1		33	Georgia	37.9
7	North Dakota	81.7		34	New Jersey	31.8
22	Ohio	56.8		35	Hawaii	24.1
10	Oklahoma	72.0		36	Mississippi	22.6
5	Oregon	84.2		37	Maryland	20.5
23	Pennsylvania	55.9		NA	Arizona**	NA
16	Rhode Island	64.6		NA	California**	NA
20	South Carolina	58.9		NA	Connecticut**	NA
6	South Dakota	84.0		NA	Florida**	NA
28	Tennessee	49.0		NA	Illinois**	NA
11	Texas	70.6		NA	Louisiana**	NA
NA	Utah**	NA		NA	Nebraska**	NA
1	Vermont	94.7		NA	Nevada**	NA
30	Virginia	44.5		NA	New Hampshire**	NA
NA	Washington**	NA		NA	New Mexico**	NA
4	West Virginia	85.1		NA	Utah**	NA
12	Wisconsin	69.1		NA	Washington**	NA
NA	Wyoming**	NA		NA	Wyoming**	NA

District of Columbia	21.0

Source: U.S. Department of Health and Human Services, Centers for Disease Control and Prevention
   "Abortion Surveillance-United States, 2006" (MMWR, Vol. 58, No. SS-8, 11/27/09, http://www.cdc.gov/mmwr/mmwr_ss.html)
*By state of occurrence. Includes those of Hispanic ethnicity. National percent is for reporting states only.
**Not reported. New York's number is for New York City only.

Percent of Reported Legal Abortions Obtained by Black Women in 2006

Reporting States' Percent = 36.4% of Abortions*

ALPHA ORDER			RANK ORDER		
RANK	STATE	PERCENT	RANK	STATE	PERCENT
4	Alabama	56.0	1	Mississippi	76.3
28	Alaska	7.3	2	Maryland	67.4
NA	Arizona**	NA	3	Georgia	57.4
16	Arkansas	30.6	4	Alabama	56.0
NA	California**	NA	5	Tennessee	46.0
29	Colorado	6.2	6	North Carolina	45.4
NA	Connecticut**	NA	7	New Jersey	44.6
9	Delaware	41.5	8	Virginia	41.8
NA	Florida**	NA	9	Delaware	41.5
3	Georgia	57.4	10	New York**	40.9
32	Hawaii	3.6	11	Missouri	40.1
35	Idaho	1.1	12	Michigan	39.5
NA	Illinois**	NA	13	Pennsylvania	38.9
17	Indiana	28.7	14	South Carolina	38.5
27	Iowa	9.9	15	Ohio	35.5
22	Kansas	21.5	16	Arkansas	30.6
20	Kentucky	21.7	17	Indiana	28.7
NA	Louisiana**	NA	18	Wisconsin	24.3
34	Maine	1.9	19	Texas	23.2
2	Maryland	67.4	20	Kentucky	21.7
23	Massachusetts	19.2	20	Minnesota	21.7
12	Michigan	39.5	22	Kansas	21.5
20	Minnesota	21.7	23	Massachusetts	19.2
1	Mississippi	76.3	24	Oklahoma	18.8
11	Missouri	40.1	25	Rhode Island	15.2
36	Montana	0.7	26	West Virginia	11.2
NA	Nebraska**	NA	27	Iowa	9.9
NA	Nevada**	NA	28	Alaska	7.3
NA	New Hampshire**	NA	29	Colorado	6.2
7	New Jersey	44.6	30	Oregon	5.7
NA	New Mexico**	NA	31	North Dakota	3.7
10	New York**	40.9	32	Hawaii	3.6
6	North Carolina	45.4	33	Vermont	2.2
31	North Dakota	3.7	34	Maine	1.9
15	Ohio	35.5	35	Idaho	1.1
24	Oklahoma	18.8	36	Montana	0.7
30	Oregon	5.7	37	South Dakota	0.0
13	Pennsylvania	38.9	NA	Arizona**	NA
25	Rhode Island	15.2	NA	California**	NA
14	South Carolina	38.5	NA	Connecticut**	NA
37	South Dakota	0.0	NA	Florida**	NA
5	Tennessee	46.0	NA	Illinois**	NA
19	Texas	23.2	NA	Louisiana**	NA
NA	Utah**	NA	NA	Nebraska**	NA
33	Vermont	2.2	NA	Nevada**	NA
8	Virginia	41.8	NA	New Hampshire**	NA
NA	Washington**	NA	NA	New Mexico**	NA
26	West Virginia	11.2	NA	Utah**	NA
18	Wisconsin	24.3	NA	Washington**	NA
NA	Wyoming**	NA	NA	Wyoming**	NA
				District of Columbia	52.5

Source: U.S. Department of Health and Human Services, Centers for Disease Control and Prevention
   "Abortion Surveillance-United States, 2006" (MMWR, Vol. 58, No. SS-8, 11/27/09, http://www.cdc.gov/mmwr/mmwr_ss.html)
*By state of occurrence. National percent is for reporting states only.
**Not reported. New York's number is for New York City only.

Percent of Reported Legal Abortions Obtained by Hispanic Women in 2006

Reporting States' Percent = 20.1%*

ALPHA ORDER			RANK ORDER		
RANK	STATE	PERCENT	RANK	STATE	PERCENT
NA	Alabama**	NA	1	New Mexico	50.9
NA	Alaska**	NA	2	Arizona	37.9
2	Arizona	37.9	3	Texas	36.7
19	Arkansas	5.0	4	New York	27.1
NA	California**	NA	5	New Jersey	26.9
7	Colorado	22.3	6	Utah	24.0
NA	Connecticut**	NA	7	Colorado	22.3
9	Delaware	11.2	8	Oregon	11.4
NA	Florida**	NA	9	Delaware	11.2
16	Georgia	5.7	10	Idaho	10.9
14	Hawaii	6.6	11	Kansas	10.5
10	Idaho	10.9	12	Wisconsin	9.1
NA	Illinois**	NA	13	Indiana	7.5
13	Indiana	7.5	14	Hawaii	6.6
NA	Iowa**	NA	15	Pennsylvania	6.0
11	Kansas	10.5	16	Georgia	5.7
NA	Kentucky**	NA	16	Minnesota	5.7
NA	Louisiana**	NA	18	South Dakota	5.2
23	Maine	2.3	19	Arkansas	5.0
NA	Maryland**	NA	20	Tennessee	4.3
NA	Massachusetts**	NA	21	Ohio	3.6
NA	Michigan**	NA	22	Missouri	3.1
16	Minnesota	5.7	23	Maine	2.3
25	Mississippi	1.2	24	Vermont	2.2
22	Missouri	3.1	25	Mississippi	1.2
NA	Montana**	NA	NA	Alabama**	NA
NA	Nebraska**	NA	NA	Alaska**	NA
NA	Nevada**	NA	NA	California**	NA
NA	New Hampshire**	NA	NA	Connecticut**	NA
5	New Jersey	26.9	NA	Florida**	NA
1	New Mexico	50.9	NA	Illinois**	NA
4	New York	27.1	NA	Iowa**	NA
NA	North Carolina**	NA	NA	Kentucky**	NA
NA	North Dakota**	NA	NA	Louisiana**	NA
21	Ohio	3.6	NA	Maryland**	NA
NA	Oklahoma**	NA	NA	Massachusetts**	NA
8	Oregon	11.4	NA	Michigan**	NA
15	Pennsylvania	6.0	NA	Montana**	NA
NA	Rhode Island**	NA	NA	Nebraska**	NA
NA	South Carolina**	NA	NA	Nevada**	NA
18	South Dakota	5.2	NA	New Hampshire**	NA
20	Tennessee	4.3	NA	North Carolina**	NA
3	Texas	36.7	NA	North Dakota**	NA
6	Utah	24.0	NA	Oklahoma**	NA
24	Vermont	2.2	NA	Rhode Island**	NA
NA	Virginia**	NA	NA	South Carolina**	NA
NA	Washington**	NA	NA	Virginia**	NA
NA	West Virginia**	NA	NA	Washington**	NA
12	Wisconsin	9.1	NA	West Virginia**	NA
NA	Wyoming**	NA	NA	Wyoming**	NA

District of Columbia   13.7

Source: U.S. Department of Health and Human Services, Centers for Disease Control and Prevention
   "Abortion Surveillance-United States, 2006" (MMWR, Vol. 58, No. SS-8, 11/27/09, http://www.cdc.gov/mmwr/mmwr_ss.html)
*By state of occurrence. National percent is for reporting states only. Hispanic can be of any race.
**Not reported.

Percent of Reported Legal Abortions Obtained by Married Women in 2006

Reporting States' Percent = 16.5% of Abortions*

ALPHA ORDER

RANK	STATE	PERCENT
38	Alabama	11.6
12	Alaska	17.6
16	Arizona	16.9
NA	Arkansas**	NA
NA	California**	NA
11	Colorado	17.7
NA	Connecticut**	NA
39	Delaware	11.4
NA	Florida**	NA
15	Georgia	17.0
34	Hawaii	13.7
3	Idaho	20.5
23	Illinois	15.3
20	Indiana	16.1
16	Iowa	16.9
NA	Kansas**	NA
25	Kentucky	15.1
NA	Louisiana**	NA
29	Maine	14.5
9	Maryland	17.9
33	Massachusetts	13.8
37	Michigan	12.6
19	Minnesota	16.4
NA	Mississippi**	NA
10	Missouri	17.8
27	Montana	14.8
NA	Nebraska**	NA
5	Nevada	19.6
NA	New Hampshire**	NA
35	New Jersey	13.6
30	New Mexico	14.4
32	New York**	14.1
4	North Carolina	20.3
35	North Dakota	13.6
26	Ohio	15.0
2	Oklahoma	20.8
6	Oregon	19.4
28	Pennsylvania	14.6
16	Rhode Island	16.9
20	South Carolina	16.1
24	South Dakota	15.2
22	Tennessee	15.5
7	Texas	18.4
1	Utah	23.8
14	Vermont	17.2
8	Virginia	18.0
NA	Washington**	NA
12	West Virginia	17.6
31	Wisconsin	14.3
NA	Wyoming**	NA

RANK ORDER

RANK	STATE	PERCENT
1	Utah	23.8
2	Oklahoma	20.8
3	Idaho	20.5
4	North Carolina	20.3
5	Nevada	19.6
6	Oregon	19.4
7	Texas	18.4
8	Virginia	18.0
9	Maryland	17.9
10	Missouri	17.8
11	Colorado	17.7
12	Alaska	17.6
12	West Virginia	17.6
14	Vermont	17.2
15	Georgia	17.0
16	Arizona	16.9
16	Iowa	16.9
16	Rhode Island	16.9
19	Minnesota	16.4
20	Indiana	16.1
20	South Carolina	16.1
22	Tennessee	15.5
23	Illinois	15.3
24	South Dakota	15.2
25	Kentucky	15.1
26	Ohio	15.0
27	Montana	14.8
28	Pennsylvania	14.6
29	Maine	14.5
30	New Mexico	14.4
31	Wisconsin	14.3
32	New York**	14.1
33	Massachusetts	13.8
34	Hawaii	13.7
35	New Jersey	13.6
35	North Dakota	13.6
37	Michigan	12.6
38	Alabama	11.6
39	Delaware	11.4
NA	Arkansas**	NA
NA	California**	NA
NA	Connecticut**	NA
NA	Florida**	NA
NA	Kansas**	NA
NA	Louisiana**	NA
NA	Mississippi**	NA
NA	Nebraska**	NA
NA	New Hampshire**	NA
NA	Washington**	NA
NA	Wyoming**	NA

District of Columbia   10.0

Source: U.S. Department of Health and Human Services, Centers for Disease Control and Prevention
"Abortion Surveillance-United States, 2006" (MMWR, Vol. 58, No. SS-8, 11/27/09, http://www.cdc.gov/mmwr/mmwr_ss.html)
*By state of occurrence. National percent is for reporting states only.
**Not reported. New York's number is for New York City only.

Percent of Reported Legal Abortions Obtained by Unmarried Women in 2006

Reporting States' Percent = 83.5% of Abortions*

ALPHA ORDER

RANK	STATE	PERCENT
2	Alabama	87.8
28	Alaska	79.7
15	Arizona	83.1
NA	Arkansas**	NA
NA	California**	NA
32	Colorado	79.1
NA	Connecticut**	NA
4	Delaware	86.6
NA	Florida**	NA
35	Georgia	77.4
6	Hawaii	86.0
29	Idaho	79.5
16	Illinois	82.8
21	Indiana	81.7
18	Iowa	82.7
19	Kansas	82.6
10	Kentucky	84.9
NA	Louisiana**	NA
20	Maine	81.9
32	Maryland	79.1
34	Massachusetts	77.7
3	Michigan	86.7
16	Minnesota	82.8
1	Mississippi	92.0
25	Missouri	80.7
39	Montana	73.7
NA	Nebraska**	NA
37	Nevada	74.5
NA	New Hampshire**	NA
5	New Jersey	86.4
14	New Mexico	83.2
13	New York**	83.6
38	North Carolina	74.4
6	North Dakota	86.0
22	Ohio	81.4
31	Oklahoma	79.2
36	Oregon	77.3
9	Pennsylvania	85.4
29	Rhode Island	79.5
12	South Carolina	83.7
11	South Dakota	84.8
22	Tennessee	81.4
26	Texas	80.6
41	Utah	64.1
26	Vermont	80.6
40	Virginia	71.5
NA	Washington**	NA
24	West Virginia	81.0
8	Wisconsin	85.5
NA	Wyoming**	NA

RANK ORDER

RANK	STATE	PERCENT
1	Mississippi	92.0
2	Alabama	87.8
3	Michigan	86.7
4	Delaware	86.6
5	New Jersey	86.4
6	Hawaii	86.0
6	North Dakota	86.0
8	Wisconsin	85.5
9	Pennsylvania	85.4
10	Kentucky	84.9
11	South Dakota	84.8
12	South Carolina	83.7
13	New York**	83.6
14	New Mexico	83.2
15	Arizona	83.1
16	Illinois	82.8
16	Minnesota	82.8
18	Iowa	82.7
19	Kansas	82.6
20	Maine	81.9
21	Indiana	81.7
22	Ohio	81.4
22	Tennessee	81.4
24	West Virginia	81.0
25	Missouri	80.7
26	Texas	80.6
26	Vermont	80.6
28	Alaska	79.7
29	Idaho	79.5
29	Rhode Island	79.5
31	Oklahoma	79.2
32	Colorado	79.1
32	Maryland	79.1
34	Massachusetts	77.7
35	Georgia	77.4
36	Oregon	77.3
37	Nevada	74.5
38	North Carolina	74.4
39	Montana	73.7
40	Virginia	71.5
41	Utah	64.1
NA	Arkansas**	NA
NA	California**	NA
NA	Connecticut**	NA
NA	Florida**	NA
NA	Louisiana**	NA
NA	Nebraska**	NA
NA	New Hampshire**	NA
NA	Washington**	NA
NA	Wyoming**	NA

| | District of Columbia | 89.6 |

Source: U.S. Department of Health and Human Services, Centers for Disease Control and Prevention
   "Abortion Surveillance-United States, 2006" (MMWR, Vol. 58, No. SS-8, 11/27/09, http://www.cdc.gov/mmwr/mmwr_ss.html)
*By state of occurrence. National percent is for reporting states only.
**Not reported. New York's number is for New York City only.

Reported Legal Abortions Obtained by Teenagers in 2006

Reporting States' Total = 116,613 Abortions Obtained by Teenagers*

ALPHA ORDER				RANK ORDER			
RANK	STATE	ABORTIONS	% of USA	RANK	STATE	ABORTIONS	% of USA
14	Alabama	2,180	1.9%	1	New York	23,286	20.0%
38	Alaska	369	0.3%	2	Texas	10,530	9.0%
18	Arizona	1,967	1.7%	3	Pennsylvania	6,415	5.5%
28	Arkansas	956	0.8%	4	Ohio	5,895	5.1%
NA	California**	NA	NA	5	New Jersey	5,592	4.8%
17	Colorado	1,994	1.7%	6	North Carolina	5,430	4.7%
13	Connecticut	2,733	2.3%	7	Michigan	4,694	4.0%
32	Delaware	632	0.5%	8	Georgia	4,520	3.9%
NA	Florida**	NA	NA	9	Washington	4,515	3.9%
8	Georgia	4,520	3.9%	10	Massachusetts	4,019	3.4%
30	Hawaii	824	0.7%	11	Virginia	3,981	3.4%
41	Idaho	265	0.2%	12	Tennessee	2,881	2.5%
NA	Illinois**	NA	NA	13	Connecticut	2,733	2.3%
21	Indiana	1,700	1.5%	14	Alabama	2,180	1.9%
25	Iowa	1,222	1.0%	15	Minnesota	2,141	1.8%
19	Kansas	1,950	1.7%	16	Oregon	2,053	1.8%
31	Kentucky	662	0.6%	17	Colorado	1,994	1.7%
NA	Louisiana**	NA	NA	18	Arizona	1,967	1.7%
34	Maine	483	0.4%	19	Kansas	1,950	1.7%
NA	Maryland**	NA	NA	20	Nevada	1,833	1.6%
10	Massachusetts	4,019	3.4%	21	Indiana	1,700	1.5%
7	Michigan	4,694	4.0%	22	Wisconsin	1,662	1.4%
15	Minnesota	2,141	1.8%	23	South Carolina	1,294	1.1%
35	Mississippi	467	0.4%	24	Missouri	1,278	1.1%
24	Missouri	1,278	1.1%	25	Iowa	1,222	1.0%
37	Montana	413	0.4%	26	New Mexico	1,208	1.0%
36	Nebraska	460	0.4%	27	Oklahoma	1,148	1.0%
20	Nevada	1,833	1.6%	28	Arkansas	956	0.8%
NA	New Hampshire**	NA	NA	29	Rhode Island	865	0.7%
5	New Jersey	5,592	4.8%	30	Hawaii	824	0.7%
26	New Mexico	1,208	1.0%	31	Kentucky	662	0.6%
1	New York	23,286	20.0%	32	Delaware	632	0.5%
6	North Carolina	5,430	4.7%	33	Utah	628	0.5%
42	North Dakota	229	0.2%	34	Maine	483	0.4%
4	Ohio	5,895	5.1%	35	Mississippi	467	0.4%
27	Oklahoma	1,148	1.0%	36	Nebraska	460	0.4%
16	Oregon	2,053	1.8%	37	Montana	413	0.4%
3	Pennsylvania	6,415	5.5%	38	Alaska	369	0.3%
29	Rhode Island	865	0.7%	39	West Virginia	320	0.3%
23	South Carolina	1,294	1.1%	40	Vermont	300	0.3%
43	South Dakota	124	0.1%	41	Idaho	265	0.2%
12	Tennessee	2,881	2.5%	42	North Dakota	229	0.2%
2	Texas	10,530	9.0%	43	South Dakota	124	0.1%
33	Utah	628	0.5%	44	Wyoming	1	0.0%
40	Vermont	300	0.3%	NA	California**	NA	NA
11	Virginia	3,981	3.4%	NA	Florida**	NA	NA
9	Washington	4,515	3.9%	NA	Illinois**	NA	NA
39	West Virginia	320	0.3%	NA	Louisiana**	NA	NA
22	Wisconsin	1,662	1.4%	NA	Maryland**	NA	NA
44	Wyoming	1	0.0%	NA	New Hampshire**	NA	NA
					District of Columbia	494	0.4%

Source: U.S. Department of Health and Human Services, Centers for Disease Control and Prevention
   "Abortion Surveillance-United States, 2006" (MMWR, Vol. 58, No. SS-8, 11/27/09, http://www.cdc.gov/mmwr/mmwr_ss.html)
*19 years old and younger by state of occurrence. National total is for reporting states only.
**Not reported.

Percent of Reported Legal Abortions Obtained by Teenagers in 2006

Reporting States' Percent = 16.8% of Abortions*

ALPHA ORDER				RANK ORDER		
RANK	STATE	PERCENT		RANK	STATE	PERCENT
8	Alabama	18.7		1	Idaho	21.2
6	Alaska	19.2		2	Hawaii	20.7
14	Arizona	18.2		3	New Mexico	19.8
6	Arkansas	19.2		4	Montana	19.5
NA	California**	NA		5	Connecticut	19.4
17	Colorado	18.0		6	Alaska	19.2
5	Connecticut	19.4		6	Arkansas	19.2
43	Delaware	13.2		8	Alabama	18.7
NA	Florida**	NA		9	Vermont	18.6
40	Georgia	14.8		10	South Carolina	18.5
2	Hawaii	20.7		11	Michigan	18.3
1	Idaho	21.2		11	New York	18.3
NA	Illinois**	NA		11	Washington	18.3
33	Indiana	16.0		14	Arizona	18.2
14	Iowa	18.2		14	Iowa	18.2
22	Kansas	17.5		16	Maine	18.1
26	Kentucky	16.9		17	Colorado	18.0
NA	Louisiana**	NA		17	New Jersey	18.0
16	Maine	18.1		19	Ohio	17.9
NA	Maryland**	NA		19	Rhode Island	17.9
29	Massachusetts	16.6		21	North Dakota	17.6
11	Michigan	18.3		22	Kansas	17.5
39	Minnesota	15.2		22	Oregon	17.5
35	Mississippi	15.8		22	Pennsylvania	17.5
26	Missouri	16.9		25	Wisconsin	17.3
4	Montana	19.5		26	Kentucky	16.9
36	Nebraska	15.7		26	Missouri	16.9
33	Nevada	16.0		28	Utah	16.7
NA	New Hampshire**	NA		29	Massachusetts	16.6
17	New Jersey	18.0		29	South Dakota	16.6
3	New Mexico	19.8		31	Oklahoma	16.2
11	New York	18.3		32	Tennessee	16.1
38	North Carolina	15.5		33	Indiana	16.0
21	North Dakota	17.6		33	Nevada	16.0
19	Ohio	17.9		35	Mississippi	15.8
31	Oklahoma	16.2		36	Nebraska	15.7
22	Oregon	17.5		36	West Virginia	15.7
22	Pennsylvania	17.5		38	North Carolina	15.5
19	Rhode Island	17.9		39	Minnesota	15.2
10	South Carolina	18.5		40	Georgia	14.8
29	South Dakota	16.6		41	Virginia	14.6
32	Tennessee	16.1		42	Wyoming	14.3
44	Texas	12.9		43	Delaware	13.2
28	Utah	16.7		44	Texas	12.9
9	Vermont	18.6		NA	California**	NA
41	Virginia	14.6		NA	Florida**	NA
11	Washington	18.3		NA	Illinois**	NA
36	West Virginia	15.7		NA	Louisiana**	NA
25	Wisconsin	17.3		NA	Maryland**	NA
42	Wyoming	14.3		NA	New Hampshire**	NA

District of Columbia 18.4

Source: CQ Press using data from U.S. Department of Health and Human Services, Centers for Disease Control and Prevention "Abortion Surveillance-United States, 2006" (MMWR, Vol. 58, No. SS-8, 11/27/09, http://www.cdc.gov/mmwr/mmwr_ss.html)
*19 years old and younger by state of occurrence. National percent is for reporting states only.
**Not reported.

Reported Legal Abortions Obtained by Teenagers 17 Years and Younger in 2006

Reporting States' Total = 44,322 Abortions*

ALPHA ORDER

RANK	STATE	ABORTIONS	% of USA
14	Alabama	842	1.9%
38	Alaska	128	0.3%
19	Arizona	705	1.6%
27	Arkansas	401	0.9%
NA	California**	NA	NA
20	Colorado	701	1.6%
12	Connecticut	1,147	2.6%
30	Delaware	264	0.6%
NA	Florida**	NA	NA
9	Georgia	1,687	3.8%
29	Hawaii	386	0.9%
39	Idaho	121	0.3%
NA	Illinois**	NA	NA
22	Indiana	595	1.3%
25	Iowa	463	1.0%
17	Kansas	758	1.7%
32	Kentucky	255	0.6%
NA	Louisiana**	NA	NA
34	Maine	189	0.4%
NA	Maryland**	NA	NA
10	Massachusetts	1,372	3.1%
7	Michigan	1,772	4.0%
16	Minnesota	793	1.8%
37	Mississippi	158	0.4%
26	Missouri	448	1.0%
36	Montana	161	0.4%
35	Nebraska	162	0.4%
18	Nevada	748	1.7%
NA	New Hampshire**	NA	NA
5	New Jersey	2,198	5.0%
24	New Mexico	502	1.1%
1	New York	9,953	22.5%
6	North Carolina	1,969	4.4%
42	North Dakota	64	0.1%
3	Ohio	2,380	5.4%
28	Oklahoma	400	0.9%
15	Oregon	829	1.9%
4	Pennsylvania	2,278	5.1%
31	Rhode Island	261	0.6%
23	South Carolina	549	1.2%
43	South Dakota	44	0.1%
13	Tennessee	1,002	2.3%
2	Texas	3,434	7.7%
33	Utah	197	0.4%
41	Vermont	103	0.2%
11	Virginia	1,249	2.8%
8	Washington	1,716	3.9%
40	West Virginia	108	0.2%
21	Wisconsin	596	1.3%
NA	Wyoming**	NA	NA

RANK ORDER

RANK	STATE	ABORTIONS	% of USA
1	New York	9,953	22.5%
2	Texas	3,434	7.7%
3	Ohio	2,380	5.4%
4	Pennsylvania	2,278	5.1%
5	New Jersey	2,198	5.0%
6	North Carolina	1,969	4.4%
7	Michigan	1,772	4.0%
8	Washington	1,716	3.9%
9	Georgia	1,687	3.8%
10	Massachusetts	1,372	3.1%
11	Virginia	1,249	2.8%
12	Connecticut	1,147	2.6%
13	Tennessee	1,002	2.3%
14	Alabama	842	1.9%
15	Oregon	829	1.9%
16	Minnesota	793	1.8%
17	Kansas	758	1.7%
18	Nevada	748	1.7%
19	Arizona	705	1.6%
20	Colorado	701	1.6%
21	Wisconsin	596	1.3%
22	Indiana	595	1.3%
23	South Carolina	549	1.2%
24	New Mexico	502	1.1%
25	Iowa	463	1.0%
26	Missouri	448	1.0%
27	Arkansas	401	0.9%
28	Oklahoma	400	0.9%
29	Hawaii	386	0.9%
30	Delaware	264	0.6%
31	Rhode Island	261	0.6%
32	Kentucky	255	0.6%
33	Utah	197	0.4%
34	Maine	189	0.4%
35	Nebraska	162	0.4%
36	Montana	161	0.4%
37	Mississippi	158	0.4%
38	Alaska	128	0.3%
39	Idaho	121	0.3%
40	West Virginia	108	0.2%
41	Vermont	103	0.2%
42	North Dakota	64	0.1%
43	South Dakota	44	0.1%
NA	California**	NA	NA
NA	Florida**	NA	NA
NA	Illinois**	NA	NA
NA	Louisiana**	NA	NA
NA	Maryland**	NA	NA
NA	New Hampshire**	NA	NA
NA	Wyoming**	NA	NA
	District of Columbia	241	0.5%

Source: U.S. Department of Health and Human Services, Centers for Disease Control and Prevention
   "Abortion Surveillance-United States, 2006" (MMWR, Vol. 58, No. SS-8, 11/27/09, http://www.cdc.gov/mmwr/mmwr_ss.html)
*By state of occurrence. National total is for reporting states only.
**Not reported.

Percent of Reported Legal Abortions Obtained
by Teenagers 17 Years and Younger in 2006
Reporting States' Percent = 6.4% of Abortions*

ALPHA ORDER

RANK	STATE	PERCENT
9	Alabama	7.2
18	Alaska	6.7
19	Arizona	6.5
5	Arkansas	8.0
NA	California**	NA
23	Colorado	6.3
4	Connecticut	8.1
34	Delaware	5.5
NA	Florida**	NA
34	Georgia	5.5
1	Hawaii	9.7
1	Idaho	9.7
NA	Illinois**	NA
29	Indiana	5.6
15	Iowa	6.9
17	Kansas	6.8
19	Kentucky	6.5
NA	Louisiana**	NA
11	Maine	7.1
NA	Maryland**	NA
28	Massachusetts	5.7
15	Michigan	6.9
29	Minnesota	5.6
37	Mississippi	5.4
26	Missouri	5.9
8	Montana	7.6
34	Nebraska	5.5
19	Nevada	6.5
NA	New Hampshire**	NA
11	New Jersey	7.1
3	New Mexico	8.2
6	New York	7.8
29	North Carolina	5.6
41	North Dakota	4.9
9	Ohio	7.2
29	Oklahoma	5.6
11	Oregon	7.1
24	Pennsylvania	6.2
37	Rhode Island	5.4
6	South Carolina	7.8
26	South Dakota	5.9
29	Tennessee	5.6
43	Texas	4.2
40	Utah	5.2
22	Vermont	6.4
42	Virginia	4.6
14	Washington	7.0
39	West Virginia	5.3
24	Wisconsin	6.2
NA	Wyoming**	NA

RANK ORDER

RANK	STATE	PERCENT
1	Hawaii	9.7
1	Idaho	9.7
3	New Mexico	8.2
4	Connecticut	8.1
5	Arkansas	8.0
6	New York	7.8
6	South Carolina	7.8
8	Montana	7.6
9	Alabama	7.2
9	Ohio	7.2
11	Maine	7.1
11	New Jersey	7.1
11	Oregon	7.1
14	Washington	7.0
15	Iowa	6.9
15	Michigan	6.9
17	Kansas	6.8
18	Alaska	6.7
19	Arizona	6.5
19	Kentucky	6.5
19	Nevada	6.5
22	Vermont	6.4
23	Colorado	6.3
24	Pennsylvania	6.2
24	Wisconsin	6.2
26	Missouri	5.9
26	South Dakota	5.9
28	Massachusetts	5.7
29	Indiana	5.6
29	Minnesota	5.6
29	North Carolina	5.6
29	Oklahoma	5.6
29	Tennessee	5.6
34	Delaware	5.5
34	Georgia	5.5
34	Nebraska	5.5
37	Mississippi	5.4
37	Rhode Island	5.4
39	West Virginia	5.3
40	Utah	5.2
41	North Dakota	4.9
42	Virginia	4.6
43	Texas	4.2
NA	California**	NA
NA	Florida**	NA
NA	Illinois**	NA
NA	Louisiana**	NA
NA	Maryland**	NA
NA	New Hampshire**	NA
NA	Wyoming**	NA

District of Columbia   9.0

Source: CQ Press using data from U.S. Department of Health and Human Services, Centers for Disease Control and Prevention
    "Abortion Surveillance-United States, 2006" (MMWR, Vol. 58, No. SS-8, 11/27/09, http://www.cdc.gov/mmwr/mmwr_ss.html)
*By state of occurrence. National percent is for reporting states only.
**Not reported.

Percent of Teenage Abortions Obtained
by Teenagers 17 Years and Younger in 2006
Reporting States' Percent = 38.0% of Teenage Abortions*

ALPHA ORDER

RANK	STATE	PERCENT
16	Alabama	38.6
34	Alaska	34.7
25	Arizona	35.8
6	Arkansas	41.9
NA	California**	NA
28	Colorado	35.2
5	Connecticut	42.0
7	Delaware	41.8
NA	Florida**	NA
21	Georgia	37.3
1	Hawaii	46.8
2	Idaho	45.7
NA	Illinois**	NA
31	Indiana	35.0
19	Iowa	37.9
15	Kansas	38.9
17	Kentucky	38.5
NA	Louisiana**	NA
13	Maine	39.1
NA	Maryland**	NA
36	Massachusetts	34.1
20	Michigan	37.8
22	Minnesota	37.0
37	Mississippi	33.8
30	Missouri	35.1
14	Montana	39.0
28	Nebraska	35.2
9	Nevada	40.8
NA	New Hampshire**	NA
12	New Jersey	39.3
8	New Mexico	41.6
3	New York	42.7
23	North Carolina	36.3
43	North Dakota	27.9
10	Ohio	40.4
32	Oklahoma	34.8
10	Oregon	40.4
26	Pennsylvania	35.5
42	Rhode Island	30.2
4	South Carolina	42.4
26	South Dakota	35.5
32	Tennessee	34.8
39	Texas	32.6
40	Utah	31.4
35	Vermont	34.3
40	Virginia	31.4
18	Washington	38.0
37	West Virginia	33.8
24	Wisconsin	35.9
NA	Wyoming**	NA

RANK ORDER

RANK	STATE	PERCENT
1	Hawaii	46.8
2	Idaho	45.7
3	New York	42.7
4	South Carolina	42.4
5	Connecticut	42.0
6	Arkansas	41.9
7	Delaware	41.8
8	New Mexico	41.6
9	Nevada	40.8
10	Ohio	40.4
10	Oregon	40.4
12	New Jersey	39.3
13	Maine	39.1
14	Montana	39.0
15	Kansas	38.9
16	Alabama	38.6
17	Kentucky	38.5
18	Washington	38.0
19	Iowa	37.9
20	Michigan	37.8
21	Georgia	37.3
22	Minnesota	37.0
23	North Carolina	36.3
24	Wisconsin	35.9
25	Arizona	35.8
26	Pennsylvania	35.5
26	South Dakota	35.5
28	Colorado	35.2
28	Nebraska	35.2
30	Missouri	35.1
31	Indiana	35.0
32	Oklahoma	34.8
32	Tennessee	34.8
34	Alaska	34.7
35	Vermont	34.3
36	Massachusetts	34.1
37	Mississippi	33.8
37	West Virginia	33.8
39	Texas	32.6
40	Utah	31.4
40	Virginia	31.4
42	Rhode Island	30.2
43	North Dakota	27.9
NA	California**	NA
NA	Florida**	NA
NA	Illinois**	NA
NA	Louisiana**	NA
NA	Maryland**	NA
NA	New Hampshire**	NA
NA	Wyoming**	NA

| | District of Columbia | 48.8 |

Source: CQ Press using data from U.S. Department of Health and Human Services, Centers for Disease Control and Prevention "Abortion Surveillance-United States, 2006" (MMWR, Vol. 58, No. SS-8, 11/27/09, http://www.cdc.gov/mmwr/mmwr_ss.html)

*By state of occurrence. National percent is for reporting states only.

**Not reported.

Reported Legal Abortions Performed at 12 Weeks or Fewer of Gestation in 2006

Reporting States' Total = 574,497 Abortions*

ALPHA ORDER

RANK	STATE	ABORTIONS	% of USA
15	Alabama	10,138	1.8%
35	Alaska	1,808	0.3%
16	Arizona	9,766	1.7%
27	Arkansas	4,264	0.7%
NA	California**	NA	NA
17	Colorado	9,751	1.7%
13	Connecticut	12,332	2.1%
32	Delaware	3,109	0.5%
NA	Florida**	NA	NA
6	Georgia	26,373	4.6%
29	Hawaii	3,429	0.6%
39	Idaho	1,197	0.2%
NA	Illinois**	NA	NA
20	Indiana	8,967	1.6%
25	Iowa	6,280	1.1%
18	Kansas	9,584	1.7%
30	Kentucky	3,248	0.6%
NA	Louisiana**	NA	NA
33	Maine	2,547	0.4%
NA	Maryland**	NA	NA
NA	Massachusetts**	NA	NA
9	Michigan	23,055	4.0%
12	Minnesota	12,462	2.2%
NA	Mississippi**	NA	NA
23	Missouri	6,838	1.2%
34	Montana	1,855	0.3%
NA	Nebraska**	NA	NA
19	Nevada	9,076	1.6%
NA	New Hampshire**	NA	NA
8	New Jersey	24,502	4.3%
26	New Mexico	5,162	0.9%
1	New York	105,653	18.4%
5	North Carolina	27,417	4.8%
38	North Dakota	1,215	0.2%
4	Ohio	27,817	4.8%
24	Oklahoma	6,357	1.1%
14	Oregon	10,202	1.8%
3	Pennsylvania	32,346	5.6%
28	Rhode Island	4,069	0.7%
22	South Carolina	6,906	1.2%
40	South Dakota	705	0.1%
11	Tennessee	16,904	2.9%
2	Texas	75,032	13.1%
31	Utah	3,219	0.6%
37	Vermont	1,511	0.3%
7	Virginia	26,077	4.5%
10	Washington	21,468	3.7%
36	West Virginia	1,793	0.3%
21	Wisconsin	7,821	1.4%
41	Wyoming	0	0.0%

RANK ORDER

RANK	STATE	ABORTIONS	% of USA
1	New York	105,653	18.4%
2	Texas	75,032	13.1%
3	Pennsylvania	32,346	5.6%
4	Ohio	27,817	4.8%
5	North Carolina	27,417	4.8%
6	Georgia	26,373	4.6%
7	Virginia	26,077	4.5%
8	New Jersey	24,502	4.3%
9	Michigan	23,055	4.0%
10	Washington	21,468	3.7%
11	Tennessee	16,904	2.9%
12	Minnesota	12,462	2.2%
13	Connecticut	12,332	2.1%
14	Oregon	10,202	1.8%
15	Alabama	10,138	1.8%
16	Arizona	9,766	1.7%
17	Colorado	9,751	1.7%
18	Kansas	9,584	1.7%
19	Nevada	9,076	1.6%
20	Indiana	8,967	1.6%
21	Wisconsin	7,821	1.4%
22	South Carolina	6,906	1.2%
23	Missouri	6,838	1.2%
24	Oklahoma	6,357	1.1%
25	Iowa	6,280	1.1%
26	New Mexico	5,162	0.9%
27	Arkansas	4,264	0.7%
28	Rhode Island	4,069	0.7%
29	Hawaii	3,429	0.6%
30	Kentucky	3,248	0.6%
31	Utah	3,219	0.6%
32	Delaware	3,109	0.5%
33	Maine	2,547	0.4%
34	Montana	1,855	0.3%
35	Alaska	1,808	0.3%
36	West Virginia	1,793	0.3%
37	Vermont	1,511	0.3%
38	North Dakota	1,215	0.2%
39	Idaho	1,197	0.2%
40	South Dakota	705	0.1%
41	Wyoming	0	0.0%
NA	California**	NA	NA
NA	Florida**	NA	NA
NA	Illinois**	NA	NA
NA	Louisiana**	NA	NA
NA	Maryland**	NA	NA
NA	Massachusetts**	NA	NA
NA	Mississippi**	NA	NA
NA	Nebraska**	NA	NA
NA	New Hampshire**	NA	NA

District of Columbia 2,242 0.4%

Source: CQ Press using data from U.S. Department of Health and Human Services, Centers for Disease Control and Prevention
   "Abortion Surveillance-United States, 2006" (MMWR, Vol. 58, No. SS-8, 11/27/09, http://www.cdc.gov/mmwr/mmwr_ss.html)
*By state of occurrence. National total is for reporting states only.
**Not reported.

Percent of Reported Legal Abortions Performed
at 12 Weeks or Fewer of Gestation in 2006
Reporting States' Percent = 86.5% of Abortions*

ALPHA ORDER

RANK	STATE	PERCENT
23	Alabama	87.0
7	Alaska	94.0
13	Arizona	90.1
29	Arkansas	85.5
NA	California**	NA
17	Colorado	88.3
21	Connecticut	87.4
40	Delaware	64.7
NA	Florida**	NA
25	Georgia	86.3
26	Hawaii	85.9
2	Idaho	95.8
NA	Illinois**	NA
31	Indiana	84.5
10	Iowa	93.4
27	Kansas	85.8
34	Kentucky	83.0
NA	Louisiana**	NA
3	Maine	95.4
NA	Maryland**	NA
NA	Massachusetts**	NA
14	Michigan	89.9
16	Minnesota	88.6
NA	Mississippi**	NA
12	Missouri	90.5
20	Montana	87.5
NA	Nebraska**	NA
37	Nevada	79.1
NA	New Hampshire**	NA
37	New Jersey	79.1
30	New Mexico	84.8
35	New York	82.9
39	North Carolina	78.1
9	North Dakota	93.6
31	Ohio	84.5
15	Oklahoma	89.7
23	Oregon	87.0
18	Pennsylvania	88.1
33	Rhode Island	84.3
1	South Carolina	98.6
6	South Dakota	94.3
5	Tennessee	94.5
11	Texas	91.6
27	Utah	85.8
8	Vermont	93.9
4	Virginia	95.3
22	Washington	87.2
18	West Virginia	88.1
36	Wisconsin	81.6
41	Wyoming	0.0

RANK ORDER

RANK	STATE	PERCENT
1	South Carolina	98.6
2	Idaho	95.8
3	Maine	95.4
4	Virginia	95.3
5	Tennessee	94.5
6	South Dakota	94.3
7	Alaska	94.0
8	Vermont	93.9
9	North Dakota	93.6
10	Iowa	93.4
11	Texas	91.6
12	Missouri	90.5
13	Arizona	90.1
14	Michigan	89.9
15	Oklahoma	89.7
16	Minnesota	88.6
17	Colorado	88.3
18	Pennsylvania	88.1
18	West Virginia	88.1
20	Montana	87.5
21	Connecticut	87.4
22	Washington	87.2
23	Alabama	87.0
23	Oregon	87.0
25	Georgia	86.3
26	Hawaii	85.9
27	Kansas	85.8
27	Utah	85.8
29	Arkansas	85.5
30	New Mexico	84.8
31	Indiana	84.5
31	Ohio	84.5
33	Rhode Island	84.3
34	Kentucky	83.0
35	New York	82.9
36	Wisconsin	81.6
37	Nevada	79.1
37	New Jersey	79.1
39	North Carolina	78.1
40	Delaware	64.7
41	Wyoming	0.0
NA	California**	NA
NA	Florida**	NA
NA	Illinois**	NA
NA	Louisiana**	NA
NA	Maryland**	NA
NA	Massachusetts**	NA
NA	Mississippi**	NA
NA	Nebraska**	NA
NA	New Hampshire**	NA

District of Columbia 83.3

Source: CQ Press using data from U.S. Department of Health and Human Services, Centers for Disease Control and Prevention
    "Abortion Surveillance-United States, 2006" (MMWR, Vol. 58, No. SS-8, 11/27/09, http://www.cdc.gov/mmwr/mmwr_ss.html)
*By state of occurrence. National percent is for reporting states only.
**Not reported.

Reported Legal Abortions Performed at or after 21 Weeks of Gestation in 2006

Reporting States' Total = 8,360 Abortions*

<table>
<tr><td colspan="4">ALPHA ORDER</td><td colspan="4">RANK ORDER</td></tr>
<tr><th>RANK</th><th>STATE</th><th>ABORTIONS</th><th>% of USA</th><th>RANK</th><th>STATE</th><th>ABORTIONS</th><th>% of USA</th></tr>
<tr><td>21</td><td>Alabama</td><td>26</td><td>0.3%</td><td>1</td><td>New York</td><td>2,974</td><td>35.6%</td></tr>
<tr><td>23</td><td>Alaska</td><td>15</td><td>0.2%</td><td>2</td><td>New Jersey</td><td>931</td><td>11.1%</td></tr>
<tr><td>13</td><td>Arizona</td><td>95</td><td>1.1%</td><td>3</td><td>Georgia</td><td>900</td><td>10.8%</td></tr>
<tr><td>33</td><td>Arkansas</td><td>0</td><td>0.0%</td><td>4</td><td>Texas</td><td>551</td><td>6.6%</td></tr>
<tr><td>NA</td><td>California**</td><td>NA</td><td>NA</td><td>5</td><td>Ohio</td><td>510</td><td>6.1%</td></tr>
<tr><td>8</td><td>Colorado</td><td>258</td><td>3.1%</td><td>6</td><td>Washington</td><td>431</td><td>5.2%</td></tr>
<tr><td>22</td><td>Connecticut</td><td>17</td><td>0.2%</td><td>7</td><td>Kansas</td><td>418</td><td>5.0%</td></tr>
<tr><td>23</td><td>Delaware</td><td>15</td><td>0.2%</td><td>8</td><td>Colorado</td><td>258</td><td>3.1%</td></tr>
<tr><td>NA</td><td>Florida**</td><td>NA</td><td>NA</td><td>9</td><td>Pennsylvania</td><td>247</td><td>3.0%</td></tr>
<tr><td>3</td><td>Georgia</td><td>900</td><td>10.8%</td><td>10</td><td>Oregon</td><td>230</td><td>2.8%</td></tr>
<tr><td>20</td><td>Hawaii</td><td>28</td><td>0.3%</td><td>11</td><td>Wisconsin</td><td>192</td><td>2.3%</td></tr>
<tr><td>33</td><td>Idaho</td><td>0</td><td>0.0%</td><td>12</td><td>New Mexico</td><td>114</td><td>1.4%</td></tr>
<tr><td>NA</td><td>Illinois**</td><td>NA</td><td>NA</td><td>13</td><td>Arizona</td><td>95</td><td>1.1%</td></tr>
<tr><td>33</td><td>Indiana</td><td>0</td><td>0.0%</td><td>14</td><td>Michigan</td><td>88</td><td>1.1%</td></tr>
<tr><td>28</td><td>Iowa</td><td>9</td><td>0.1%</td><td>15</td><td>Minnesota</td><td>53</td><td>0.6%</td></tr>
<tr><td>7</td><td>Kansas</td><td>418</td><td>5.0%</td><td>16</td><td>Kentucky</td><td>51</td><td>0.6%</td></tr>
<tr><td>16</td><td>Kentucky</td><td>51</td><td>0.6%</td><td>17</td><td>Nevada</td><td>48</td><td>0.6%</td></tr>
<tr><td>NA</td><td>Louisiana**</td><td>NA</td><td>NA</td><td>18</td><td>Missouri</td><td>46</td><td>0.6%</td></tr>
<tr><td>28</td><td>Maine</td><td>9</td><td>0.1%</td><td>19</td><td>Virginia</td><td>45</td><td>0.5%</td></tr>
<tr><td>NA</td><td>Maryland**</td><td>NA</td><td>NA</td><td>20</td><td>Hawaii</td><td>28</td><td>0.3%</td></tr>
<tr><td>NA</td><td>Massachusetts**</td><td>NA</td><td>NA</td><td>21</td><td>Alabama</td><td>26</td><td>0.3%</td></tr>
<tr><td>14</td><td>Michigan</td><td>88</td><td>1.1%</td><td>22</td><td>Connecticut</td><td>17</td><td>0.2%</td></tr>
<tr><td>15</td><td>Minnesota</td><td>53</td><td>0.6%</td><td>23</td><td>Alaska</td><td>15</td><td>0.2%</td></tr>
<tr><td>NA</td><td>Mississippi**</td><td>NA</td><td>NA</td><td>23</td><td>Delaware</td><td>15</td><td>0.2%</td></tr>
<tr><td>18</td><td>Missouri</td><td>46</td><td>0.6%</td><td>23</td><td>Tennessee</td><td>15</td><td>0.2%</td></tr>
<tr><td>33</td><td>Montana</td><td>0</td><td>0.0%</td><td>26</td><td>South Carolina</td><td>13</td><td>0.2%</td></tr>
<tr><td>NA</td><td>Nebraska**</td><td>NA</td><td>NA</td><td>26</td><td>Utah</td><td>13</td><td>0.2%</td></tr>
<tr><td>17</td><td>Nevada</td><td>48</td><td>0.6%</td><td>28</td><td>Iowa</td><td>9</td><td>0.1%</td></tr>
<tr><td>NA</td><td>New Hampshire**</td><td>NA</td><td>NA</td><td>28</td><td>Maine</td><td>9</td><td>0.1%</td></tr>
<tr><td>2</td><td>New Jersey</td><td>931</td><td>11.1%</td><td>30</td><td>South Dakota</td><td>7</td><td>0.1%</td></tr>
<tr><td>12</td><td>New Mexico</td><td>114</td><td>1.4%</td><td>31</td><td>West Virginia</td><td>6</td><td>0.1%</td></tr>
<tr><td>1</td><td>New York</td><td>2,974</td><td>35.6%</td><td>32</td><td>Vermont</td><td>5</td><td>0.1%</td></tr>
<tr><td>33</td><td>North Carolina</td><td>0</td><td>0.0%</td><td>33</td><td>Arkansas</td><td>0</td><td>0.0%</td></tr>
<tr><td>33</td><td>North Dakota</td><td>0</td><td>0.0%</td><td>33</td><td>Idaho</td><td>0</td><td>0.0%</td></tr>
<tr><td>5</td><td>Ohio</td><td>510</td><td>6.1%</td><td>33</td><td>Indiana</td><td>0</td><td>0.0%</td></tr>
<tr><td>33</td><td>Oklahoma</td><td>0</td><td>0.0%</td><td>33</td><td>Montana</td><td>0</td><td>0.0%</td></tr>
<tr><td>10</td><td>Oregon</td><td>230</td><td>2.8%</td><td>33</td><td>North Carolina</td><td>0</td><td>0.0%</td></tr>
<tr><td>9</td><td>Pennsylvania</td><td>247</td><td>3.0%</td><td>33</td><td>North Dakota</td><td>0</td><td>0.0%</td></tr>
<tr><td>33</td><td>Rhode Island</td><td>0</td><td>0.0%</td><td>33</td><td>Oklahoma</td><td>0</td><td>0.0%</td></tr>
<tr><td>26</td><td>South Carolina</td><td>13</td><td>0.2%</td><td>33</td><td>Rhode Island</td><td>0</td><td>0.0%</td></tr>
<tr><td>30</td><td>South Dakota</td><td>7</td><td>0.1%</td><td>33</td><td>Wyoming</td><td>0</td><td>0.0%</td></tr>
<tr><td>23</td><td>Tennessee</td><td>15</td><td>0.2%</td><td>NA</td><td>California**</td><td>NA</td><td>NA</td></tr>
<tr><td>4</td><td>Texas</td><td>551</td><td>6.6%</td><td>NA</td><td>Florida**</td><td>NA</td><td>NA</td></tr>
<tr><td>26</td><td>Utah</td><td>13</td><td>0.2%</td><td>NA</td><td>Illinois**</td><td>NA</td><td>NA</td></tr>
<tr><td>32</td><td>Vermont</td><td>5</td><td>0.1%</td><td>NA</td><td>Louisiana**</td><td>NA</td><td>NA</td></tr>
<tr><td>19</td><td>Virginia</td><td>45</td><td>0.5%</td><td>NA</td><td>Maryland**</td><td>NA</td><td>NA</td></tr>
<tr><td>6</td><td>Washington</td><td>431</td><td>5.2%</td><td>NA</td><td>Massachusetts**</td><td>NA</td><td>NA</td></tr>
<tr><td>31</td><td>West Virginia</td><td>6</td><td>0.1%</td><td>NA</td><td>Mississippi**</td><td>NA</td><td>NA</td></tr>
<tr><td>11</td><td>Wisconsin</td><td>192</td><td>2.3%</td><td>NA</td><td>Nebraska**</td><td>NA</td><td>NA</td></tr>
<tr><td>33</td><td>Wyoming</td><td>0</td><td>0.0%</td><td>NA</td><td>New Hampshire**</td><td>NA</td><td>NA</td></tr>
<tr><td></td><td></td><td></td><td></td><td></td><td>District of Columbia</td><td>0</td><td>0.0%</td></tr>
</table>

Source: U.S. Department of Health and Human Services, Centers for Disease Control and Prevention
   "Abortion Surveillance-United States, 2006" (MMWR, Vol. 58, No. SS-8, 11/27/09, http://www.cdc.gov/mmwr/mmwr_ss.html)
*By state of occurrence. National total is for reporting states only.
**Not reported.

Percent of Reported Legal Abortions Performed at or after
21 Weeks of Gestation in 2006
Reporting States' Percent = 1.3% of Abortions*

RANK	STATE	PERCENT
27	Alabama	0.2
14	Alaska	0.8
12	Arizona	0.9
33	Arkansas	0.0
NA	California**	NA
4	Colorado	2.3
30	Connecticut	0.1
19	Delaware	0.4
NA	Florida**	NA
3	Georgia	2.9
15	Hawaii	0.7
33	Idaho	0.0
NA	Illinois**	NA
33	Indiana	0.0
30	Iowa	0.1
1	Kansas	3.7
11	Kentucky	1.3
NA	Louisiana**	NA
22	Maine	0.3
NA	Maryland**	NA
NA	Massachusetts**	NA
22	Michigan	0.3
19	Minnesota	0.4
NA	Mississippi**	NA
18	Missouri	0.6
33	Montana	0.0
NA	Nebraska**	NA
19	Nevada	0.4
NA	New Hampshire**	NA
2	New Jersey	3.0
8	New Mexico	1.9
4	New York	2.3
33	North Carolina	0.0
33	North Dakota	0.0
10	Ohio	1.5
33	Oklahoma	0.0
7	Oregon	2.0
15	Pennsylvania	0.7
33	Rhode Island	0.0
27	South Carolina	0.2
12	South Dakota	0.9
30	Tennessee	0.1
15	Texas	0.7
22	Utah	0.3
22	Vermont	0.3
27	Virginia	0.2
9	Washington	1.8
22	West Virginia	0.3
6	Wisconsin	2.1
33	Wyoming	0.0

RANK	STATE	PERCENT
1	Kansas	3.7
2	New Jersey	3.0
3	Georgia	2.9
4	Colorado	2.3
4	New York	2.3
6	Wisconsin	2.1
7	Oregon	2.0
8	New Mexico	1.9
9	Washington	1.8
10	Ohio	1.5
11	Kentucky	1.3
12	Arizona	0.9
12	South Dakota	0.9
14	Alaska	0.8
15	Hawaii	0.7
15	Pennsylvania	0.7
15	Texas	0.7
18	Missouri	0.6
19	Delaware	0.4
19	Minnesota	0.4
19	Nevada	0.4
22	Maine	0.3
22	Michigan	0.3
22	Utah	0.3
22	Vermont	0.3
22	West Virginia	0.3
27	Alabama	0.2
27	South Carolina	0.2
27	Virginia	0.2
30	Connecticut	0.1
30	Iowa	0.1
30	Tennessee	0.1
33	Arkansas	0.0
33	Idaho	0.0
33	Indiana	0.0
33	Montana	0.0
33	North Carolina	0.0
33	North Dakota	0.0
33	Oklahoma	0.0
33	Rhode Island	0.0
33	Wyoming	0.0
NA	California**	NA
NA	Florida**	NA
NA	Illinois**	NA
NA	Louisiana**	NA
NA	Maryland**	NA
NA	Massachusetts**	NA
NA	Mississippi**	NA
NA	Nebraska**	NA
NA	New Hampshire**	NA

	District of Columbia	0.0

Source: U.S. Department of Health and Human Services, Centers for Disease Control and Prevention
"Abortion Surveillance-United States, 2006" (MMWR, Vol. 58, No. SS-8, 11/27/09, http://www.cdc.gov/mmwr/mmwr_ss.html)
*By state of occurrence. National percent is for reporting states only.
**Not reported.

II. Deaths

Deaths in 2009 90
Death Rate in 2009 91
Deaths in 2008 92
Death Rate in 2008 93
Age-Adjusted Death Rate in 2008 94
Percent Change in Death Rate: 1999 to 2008 95
Deaths in 2007 96
Death Rate in 2007 97
Age-Adjusted Death Rate in 2007 98
Infant Deaths in 2007 99
Infant Mortality Rate in 2007 100
White Infant Mortality Rate in 2007. 101
Black Infant Mortality Rate in 2007 102
Neonatal Deaths in 2007. 103
Neonatal Death Rate in 2007 104
White Neonatal Death Rate in 2007 105
Black Neonatal Death Rate in 2007 106
Estimated Deaths by Cancer in 2010 107
Estimated Death Rate by Cancer in 2010 108
Age-Adjusted Death Rate by Cancer for Males in 2006 . . 109
Age-Adjusted Death Rate by Cancer for Females
    in 2006 110
Estimated Deaths by Brain Cancer in 2010 111
Estimated Death Rate by Brain Cancer in 2010 112
Estimated Deaths by Female Breast Cancer in 2010 113
Age-Adjusted Death Rate by Female Breast Cancer
    in 2006 114
Estimated Deaths by Colon and Rectum Cancer in 2010. . 115
Estimated Death Rate by Colon and Rectum Cancer
    in 2010 116
Estimated Deaths by Leukemia in 2010 117
Estimated Death Rate by Leukemia in 2010. 118
Estimated Deaths by Liver Cancer in 2010 119
Estimated Death Rate by Liver Cancer in 2010 120
Estimated Deaths by Lung Cancer in 2010. 121
Estimated Death Rate by Lung Cancer in 2010 122
Estimated Deaths by Non-Hodgkin's Lymphoma
    in 2010 123
Estimated Death Rate by Non-Hodgkin's Lymphoma
    in 2010 124

Estimated Deaths by Ovarian Cancer in 2010 125
Estimated Death Rate by Ovarian Cancer in 2010 126
Estimated Deaths by Pancreatic Cancer in 2010 127
Estimated Death Rate by Pancreatic Cancer in 2010 128
Estimated Deaths by Prostate Cancer in 2010 129
Age-Adjusted Death Rate by Prostate Cancer in 2006. . . . 130
Deaths by AIDS in 2007. 131
Death Rate by AIDS in 2007 132
Age-Adjusted Death Rate by AIDS in 2007. 133
Deaths by Alzheimer's Disease in 2007 134
Death Rate by Alzheimer's Disease in 2007 135
Age-Adjusted Death Rate by Alzheimer's Disease
    in 2007 136
Deaths by Cerebrovascular Diseases in 2007 137
Death Rate by Cerebrovascular Diseases in 2007 138
Age-Adjusted Death Rate by Cerebrovascular Diseases
    in 2007 139
Deaths by Chronic Liver Disease and Cirrhosis in 2007 . . 140
Death Rate by Chronic Liver Disease and Cirrhosis
    in 2007 141
Age-Adjusted Death Rate by Chronic Liver Disease and
    Cirrhosis in 2007 142
Deaths by Chronic Lower Respiratory Diseases in 2007 . . 143
Death Rate by Chronic Lower Respiratory Diseases
    in 2007 144
Age-Adjusted Death Rate by Chronic Lower Respiratory
    Diseases in 2007. 145
Deaths by Diabetes Mellitus in 2007 146
Death Rate by Diabetes Mellitus in 2007 147
Age-Adjusted Death Rate by Diabetes Mellitus in 2007 . . 148
Deaths by Diseases of the Heart in 2007 149
Death Rate by Diseases of the Heart in 2007 150
Age-Adjusted Death Rate by Diseases of the Heart
    in 2007 151
Deaths by Malignant Neoplasms in 2007 152
Death Rate by Malignant Neoplasms in 2007 153
Age-Adjusted Death Rate by Malignant Neoplasms
    in 2007 154
Deaths by Nephritis and Other Kidney Diseases
    in 2007 155

Death Rate by Nephritis and Other Kidney Diseases
in 2007 156
Age-Adjusted Death Rate by Nephritis and Other Kidney
Diseases in 2007. 157
Deaths by Influenza and Pneumonia in 2007 158
Death Rate by Influenza and Pneumonia in 2007. 159
Age-Adjusted Death Rate by Influenza and Pneumonia
in 2007 160
Deaths by Injury in 2007. 161
Death Rate by Injury in 2007 162
Age-Adjusted Death Rate by Injury in 2007 163
Deaths by Accidents in 2007 164
Death Rate by Accidents in 2007 165
Age-Adjusted Death Rate by Accidents in 2007 166
Deaths by Motor Vehicle Accidents in 2007 167
Death Rate by Motor Vehicle Accidents in 2007. 168
Age-Adjusted Death Rate by Motor Vehicle Accidents
in 2007 169
Deaths by Firearm Injury in 2007. 170

Death Rate by Firearm Injury in 2007 171
Age-Adjusted Death Rate by Firearm Injury in 2007. 172
Deaths by Homicide in 2007. 173
Death Rate by Homicide in 2007 174
Age-Adjusted Death Rate by Homicide in 2007 175
Deaths by Suicide in 2007 176
Death Rate by Suicide in 2007 177
Age-Adjusted Death Rate by Suicide in 2007 178
Alcohol-Induced Deaths in 2007 179
Death Rate by Alcohol-Induced Deaths in 2007 180
Age-Adjusted Death Rate by Alcohol-Induced Deaths
in 2007 181
Drug-Induced Deaths in 2007. 182
Death Rate by Drug-Induced Deaths in 2007. 183
Age-Adjusted Death Rate by Drug-Induced Deaths
in 2007 184
Occupational Fatalities in 2009 185
Occupational Fatality Rate in 2009. 186

Deaths in 2009

National Total = 2,425,580 Deaths*

ALPHA ORDER

RANK	STATE	DEATHS	% of USA
18	Alabama	47,366	2.0%
50	Alaska	3,610	0.1%
19	Arizona	45,464	1.9%
29	Arkansas	28,810	1.2%
1	California	232,409	9.6%
28	Colorado	31,162	1.3%
30	Connecticut	28,446	1.2%
45	Delaware	7,650	0.3%
2	Florida	169,959	7.0%
11	Georgia	67,402	2.8%
42	Hawaii	9,727	0.4%
40	Idaho	11,124	0.5%
7	Illinois	100,431	4.1%
14	Indiana	56,088	2.3%
32	Iowa	27,563	1.1%
33	Kansas	23,690	1.0%
22	Kentucky	40,230	1.7%
23	Louisiana	39,217	1.6%
39	Maine	12,579	0.5%
21	Maryland	43,448	1.8%
16	Massachusetts	51,912	2.1%
8	Michigan	85,546	3.5%
25	Minnesota	37,767	1.6%
31	Mississippi	28,081	1.2%
15	Missouri	54,601	2.3%
44	Montana	8,721	0.4%
37	Nebraska	14,900	0.6%
35	Nevada	19,680	0.8%
41	New Hampshire	10,157	0.4%
10	New Jersey	68,339	2.8%
36	New Mexico	15,200	0.6%
4	New York	145,952	6.0%
9	North Carolina	77,164	3.2%
47	North Dakota	6,022	0.2%
6	Ohio	107,268	4.4%
26	Oklahoma	35,447	1.5%
27	Oregon	31,538	1.3%
5	Pennsylvania	124,724	5.1%
43	Rhode Island	9,410	0.4%
24	South Carolina	38,435	1.6%
46	South Dakota	6,948	0.3%
13	Tennessee	58,067	2.4%
3	Texas	162,289	6.7%
38	Utah	14,205	0.6%
48	Vermont	4,981	0.2%
12	Virginia	58,418	2.4%
17	Washington	47,973	2.0%
34	West Virginia	21,291	0.9%
20	Wisconsin	45,121	1.9%
49	Wyoming	4,200	0.2%

RANK ORDER

RANK	STATE	DEATHS	% of USA
1	California	232,409	9.6%
2	Florida	169,959	7.0%
3	Texas	162,289	6.7%
4	New York	145,952	6.0%
5	Pennsylvania	124,724	5.1%
6	Ohio	107,268	4.4%
7	Illinois	100,431	4.1%
8	Michigan	85,546	3.5%
9	North Carolina	77,164	3.2%
10	New Jersey	68,339	2.8%
11	Georgia	67,402	2.8%
12	Virginia	58,418	2.4%
13	Tennessee	58,067	2.4%
14	Indiana	56,088	2.3%
15	Missouri	54,601	2.3%
16	Massachusetts	51,912	2.1%
17	Washington	47,973	2.0%
18	Alabama	47,366	2.0%
19	Arizona	45,464	1.9%
20	Wisconsin	45,121	1.9%
21	Maryland	43,448	1.8%
22	Kentucky	40,230	1.7%
23	Louisiana	39,217	1.6%
24	South Carolina	38,435	1.6%
25	Minnesota	37,767	1.6%
26	Oklahoma	35,447	1.5%
27	Oregon	31,538	1.3%
28	Colorado	31,162	1.3%
29	Arkansas	28,810	1.2%
30	Connecticut	28,446	1.2%
31	Mississippi	28,081	1.2%
32	Iowa	27,563	1.1%
33	Kansas	23,690	1.0%
34	West Virginia	21,291	0.9%
35	Nevada	19,680	0.8%
36	New Mexico	15,200	0.6%
37	Nebraska	14,900	0.6%
38	Utah	14,205	0.6%
39	Maine	12,579	0.5%
40	Idaho	11,124	0.5%
41	New Hampshire	10,157	0.4%
42	Hawaii	9,727	0.4%
43	Rhode Island	9,410	0.4%
44	Montana	8,721	0.4%
45	Delaware	7,650	0.3%
46	South Dakota	6,948	0.3%
47	North Dakota	6,022	0.2%
48	Vermont	4,981	0.2%
49	Wyoming	4,200	0.2%
50	Alaska	3,610	0.1%
	District of Columbia	4,848	0.2%

Source: U.S. Department of Health and Human Services, National Center for Health Statistics
"National Vital Statistics Reports" (Vol. 58, No. 25, August 27, 2010, http://www.cdc.gov/nchs/deaths.htm)
*Provisional data for 12 months ending with December by state of residence.

Death Rate in 2009

National Rate = 790.1 Deaths per 100,000 Population*

ALPHA ORDER

RANK	STATE	RATE
2	Alabama	1,005.9
49	Alaska	516.8
44	Arizona	689.3
3	Arkansas	997.1
47	California	628.8
48	Colorado	620.2
27	Conncotiout	808.5
19	Delaware	864.3
12	Florida	916.8
45	Georgia	685.7
37	Hawaii	751.0
42	Idaho	719.6
32	Illinois	777.9
17	Indiana	873.2
13	Iowa	916.4
23	Kansas	840.4
8	Kentucky	932.5
18	Louisiana	873.0
6	Maine	954.2
35	Maryland	762.3
30	Massachusetts	787.3
20	Michigan	858.1
43	Minnesota	717.2
7	Mississippi	951.3
14	Missouri	911.9
15	Montana	894.5
24	Nebraska	829.3
39	Nevada	744.6
34	New Hampshire	766.8
31	New Jersey	784.8
36	New Mexico	756.3
38	New York	746.9
26	North Carolina	822.6
9	North Dakota	931.0
10	Ohio	929.3
5	Oklahoma	961.4
25	Oregon	824.4
4	Pennsylvania	989.5
16	Rhode Island	893.5
22	South Carolina	842.6
21	South Dakota	855.3
11	Tennessee	922.2
46	Texas	654.9
50	Utah	510.1
28	Vermont	801.1
40	Virginia	741.1
41	Washington	719.9
1	West Virginia	1,170.0
29	Wisconsin	797.9
33	Wyoming	771.7

RANK ORDER

RANK	STATE	RATE
1	West Virginia	1,170.0
2	Alabama	1,005.9
3	Arkansas	997.1
4	Pennsylvania	989.5
5	Oklahoma	961.4
6	Maine	954.2
7	Mississippi	951.3
8	Kentucky	932.5
9	North Dakota	931.0
10	Ohio	929.3
11	Tennessee	922.2
12	Florida	916.8
13	Iowa	916.4
14	Missouri	911.9
15	Montana	894.5
16	Rhode Island	893.5
17	Indiana	873.2
18	Louisiana	873.0
19	Delaware	864.3
20	Michigan	858.1
21	South Dakota	855.3
22	South Carolina	842.6
23	Kansas	840.4
24	Nebraska	829.3
25	Oregon	824.4
26	North Carolina	822.6
27	Connecticut	808.5
28	Vermont	801.1
29	Wisconsin	797.9
30	Massachusetts	787.3
31	New Jersey	784.8
32	Illinois	777.9
33	Wyoming	771.7
34	New Hampshire	766.8
35	Maryland	762.3
36	New Mexico	756.3
37	Hawaii	751.0
38	New York	746.9
39	Nevada	744.6
40	Virginia	741.1
41	Washington	719.9
42	Idaho	719.6
43	Minnesota	717.2
44	Arizona	689.3
45	Georgia	685.7
46	Texas	654.9
47	California	628.8
48	Colorado	620.2
49	Alaska	516.8
50	Utah	510.1

District of Columbia	808.5

Source: CQ Press using data from U.S. Department of Health and Human Services, National Center for Health Statistics
  "National Vital Statistics Reports" (Vol. 58, No. 25, August 27, 2010, http://www.cdc.gov/nchs/deaths.htm)
*Provisional data for 12 months ending with December by state of residence. Not age-adjusted.

Deaths in 2008

National Total = 2,473,018 Deaths*

ALPHA ORDER

RANK	STATE	DEATHS	% of USA
18	Alabama	47,712	1.9%
50	Alaska	3,483	0.1%
20	Arizona	45,610	1.8%
29	Arkansas	29,310	1.2%
1	California	234,229	9.5%
28	Colorado	31,256	1.3%
31	Connecticut	28,797	1.2%
45	Delaware	7,623	0.3%
2	Florida	170,668	6.9%
11	Georgia	69,942	2.8%
43	Hawaii	9,475	0.4%
40	Idaho	10,942	0.4%
7	Illinois	103,615	4.2%
14	Indiana	56,743	2.3%
32	Iowa	28,533	1.2%
33	Kansas	24,969	1.0%
22	Kentucky	41,280	1.7%
23	Louisiana	41,217	1.7%
39	Maine	12,531	0.5%
21	Maryland	43,885	1.8%
16	Massachusetts	53,521	2.2%
8	Michigan	88,418	3.6%
25	Minnesota	38,487	1.6%
30	Mississippi	28,980	1.2%
15	Missouri	56,566	2.3%
44	Montana	8,903	0.4%
37	Nebraska	15,455	0.6%
35	Nevada	20,790	0.8%
41	New Hampshire	10,268	0.4%
10	New Jersey	69,993	2.8%
36	New Mexico	15,996	0.6%
4	New York	148,660	6.0%
9	North Carolina	77,277	3.1%
47	North Dakota	5,870	0.2%
6	Ohio	109,749	4.4%
26	Oklahoma	37,061	1.5%
27	Oregon	31,939	1.3%
5	Pennsylvania	127,450	5.2%
42	Rhode Island	9,740	0.4%
24	South Carolina	40,305	1.6%
46	South Dakota	7,080	0.3%
13	Tennessee	58,882	2.4%
3	Texas	165,197	6.7%
38	Utah	13,991	0.6%
48	Vermont	5,213	0.2%
12	Virginia	59,093	2.4%
17	Washington	48,603	2.0%
34	West Virginia	21,549	0.9%
19	Wisconsin	46,799	1.9%
49	Wyoming	4,222	0.2%

RANK ORDER

RANK	STATE	DEATHS	% of USA
1	California	234,229	9.5%
2	Florida	170,668	6.9%
3	Texas	165,197	6.7%
4	New York	148,660	6.0%
5	Pennsylvania	127,450	5.2%
6	Ohio	109,749	4.4%
7	Illinois	103,615	4.2%
8	Michigan	88,418	3.6%
9	North Carolina	77,277	3.1%
10	New Jersey	69,993	2.8%
11	Georgia	69,942	2.8%
12	Virginia	59,093	2.4%
13	Tennessee	58,882	2.4%
14	Indiana	56,743	2.3%
15	Missouri	56,566	2.3%
16	Massachusetts	53,521	2.2%
17	Washington	48,603	2.0%
18	Alabama	47,712	1.9%
19	Wisconsin	46,799	1.9%
20	Arizona	45,610	1.8%
21	Maryland	43,885	1.8%
22	Kentucky	41,280	1.7%
23	Louisiana	41,217	1.7%
24	South Carolina	40,305	1.6%
25	Minnesota	38,487	1.6%
26	Oklahoma	37,061	1.5%
27	Oregon	31,939	1.3%
28	Colorado	31,256	1.3%
29	Arkansas	29,310	1.2%
30	Mississippi	28,980	1.2%
31	Connecticut	28,797	1.2%
32	Iowa	28,533	1.2%
33	Kansas	24,969	1.0%
34	West Virginia	21,549	0.9%
35	Nevada	20,790	0.8%
36	New Mexico	15,996	0.6%
37	Nebraska	15,455	0.6%
38	Utah	13,991	0.6%
39	Maine	12,531	0.5%
40	Idaho	10,942	0.4%
41	New Hampshire	10,268	0.4%
42	Rhode Island	9,740	0.4%
43	Hawaii	9,475	0.4%
44	Montana	8,903	0.4%
45	Delaware	7,623	0.3%
46	South Dakota	7,080	0.3%
47	North Dakota	5,870	0.2%
48	Vermont	5,213	0.2%
49	Wyoming	4,222	0.2%
50	Alaska	3,483	0.1%
	District of Columbia	5,139	0.2%

Source: U.S. Department of Health and Human Services, National Center for Health Statistics
    "National Vital Statistics Reports" (Vol. 59, No. 2, December 9, 2010, http://www.cdc.gov/nchs/deaths.htm)
*Preliminary data by state of residence.

Death Rate in 2008

National Rate = 813.3 Deaths per 100,000 Population*

<table>
<tr><th colspan="3">ALPHA ORDER</th><th colspan="3">RANK ORDER</th></tr>
<tr><th>RANK</th><th>STATE</th><th>RATE</th><th>RANK</th><th>STATE</th><th>RATE</th></tr>
<tr><td>4</td><td>Alabama</td><td>1,023.4</td><td>1</td><td>West Virginia</td><td>1,187.6</td></tr>
<tr><td>50</td><td>Alaska</td><td>507.5</td><td>2</td><td>Arkansas</td><td>1,026.5</td></tr>
<tr><td>45</td><td>Arizona</td><td>701.7</td><td>3</td><td>Pennsylvania</td><td>1,023.8</td></tr>
<tr><td>2</td><td>Arkansas</td><td>1,026.5</td><td>4</td><td>Alabama</td><td>1,023.4</td></tr>
<tr><td>47</td><td>California</td><td>637.2</td><td>5</td><td>Oklahoma</td><td>1,017.5</td></tr>
<tr><td>48</td><td>Colorado</td><td>632.8</td><td>6</td><td>Kentucky</td><td>966.9</td></tr>
<tr><td>30</td><td>Connecticut</td><td>822.5</td><td>7</td><td>Missouri</td><td>956.9</td></tr>
<tr><td>23</td><td>Delaware</td><td>873.1</td><td>8</td><td>Mississippi</td><td>956.2</td></tr>
<tr><td>14</td><td>Florida</td><td>931.2</td><td>9</td><td>Ohio</td><td>955.5</td></tr>
<tr><td>43</td><td>Georgia</td><td>722.1</td><td>10</td><td>Maine</td><td>951.9</td></tr>
<tr><td>42</td><td>Hawaii</td><td>735.5</td><td>11</td><td>Iowa</td><td>950.3</td></tr>
<tr><td>44</td><td>Idaho</td><td>718.1</td><td>12</td><td>Tennessee</td><td>947.4</td></tr>
<tr><td>33</td><td>Illinois</td><td>803.1</td><td>13</td><td>Louisiana</td><td>934.5</td></tr>
<tr><td>20</td><td>Indiana</td><td>889.8</td><td>14</td><td>Florida</td><td>931.2</td></tr>
<tr><td>11</td><td>Iowa</td><td>950.3</td><td>15</td><td>Rhode Island</td><td>926.9</td></tr>
<tr><td>19</td><td>Kansas</td><td>891.1</td><td>16</td><td>Montana</td><td>920.3</td></tr>
<tr><td>6</td><td>Kentucky</td><td>966.9</td><td>17</td><td>North Dakota</td><td>915.1</td></tr>
<tr><td>13</td><td>Louisiana</td><td>934.5</td><td>18</td><td>South Carolina</td><td>899.7</td></tr>
<tr><td>10</td><td>Maine</td><td>951.9</td><td>19</td><td>Kansas</td><td>891.1</td></tr>
<tr><td>37</td><td>Maryland</td><td>779.0</td><td>20</td><td>Indiana</td><td>889.8</td></tr>
<tr><td>29</td><td>Massachusetts</td><td>823.7</td><td>21</td><td>Michigan</td><td>883.9</td></tr>
<tr><td>21</td><td>Michigan</td><td>883.9</td><td>22</td><td>South Dakota</td><td>880.4</td></tr>
<tr><td>41</td><td>Minnesota</td><td>737.2</td><td>23</td><td>Delaware</td><td>873.1</td></tr>
<tr><td>8</td><td>Mississippi</td><td>956.2</td><td>24</td><td>Nebraska</td><td>866.6</td></tr>
<tr><td>7</td><td>Missouri</td><td>956.9</td><td>25</td><td>Oregon</td><td>842.7</td></tr>
<tr><td>16</td><td>Montana</td><td>920.3</td><td>26</td><td>Vermont</td><td>839.1</td></tr>
<tr><td>24</td><td>Nebraska</td><td>866.6</td><td>27</td><td>North Carolina</td><td>837.9</td></tr>
<tr><td>34</td><td>Nevada</td><td>799.6</td><td>28</td><td>Wisconsin</td><td>831.5</td></tr>
<tr><td>36</td><td>New Hampshire</td><td>780.4</td><td>29</td><td>Massachusetts</td><td>823.7</td></tr>
<tr><td>31</td><td>New Jersey</td><td>806.1</td><td>30</td><td>Connecticut</td><td>822.5</td></tr>
<tr><td>32</td><td>New Mexico</td><td>805.1</td><td>31</td><td>New Jersey</td><td>806.1</td></tr>
<tr><td>38</td><td>New York</td><td>762.7</td><td>32</td><td>New Mexico</td><td>805.1</td></tr>
<tr><td>27</td><td>North Carolina</td><td>837.9</td><td>33</td><td>Illinois</td><td>803.1</td></tr>
<tr><td>17</td><td>North Dakota</td><td>915.1</td><td>34</td><td>Nevada</td><td>799.6</td></tr>
<tr><td>9</td><td>Ohio</td><td>955.5</td><td>35</td><td>Wyoming</td><td>792.6</td></tr>
<tr><td>5</td><td>Oklahoma</td><td>1,017.5</td><td>36</td><td>New Hampshire</td><td>780.4</td></tr>
<tr><td>25</td><td>Oregon</td><td>842.7</td><td>37</td><td>Maryland</td><td>779.0</td></tr>
<tr><td>3</td><td>Pennsylvania</td><td>1,023.8</td><td>38</td><td>New York</td><td>762.7</td></tr>
<tr><td>15</td><td>Rhode Island</td><td>926.9</td><td>39</td><td>Virginia</td><td>760.6</td></tr>
<tr><td>18</td><td>South Carolina</td><td>899.7</td><td>40</td><td>Washington</td><td>742.1</td></tr>
<tr><td>22</td><td>South Dakota</td><td>880.4</td><td>41</td><td>Minnesota</td><td>737.2</td></tr>
<tr><td>12</td><td>Tennessee</td><td>947.4</td><td>42</td><td>Hawaii</td><td>735.5</td></tr>
<tr><td>46</td><td>Texas</td><td>679.1</td><td>43</td><td>Georgia</td><td>722.1</td></tr>
<tr><td>49</td><td>Utah</td><td>511.3</td><td>44</td><td>Idaho</td><td>718.1</td></tr>
<tr><td>26</td><td>Vermont</td><td>839.1</td><td>45</td><td>Arizona</td><td>701.7</td></tr>
<tr><td>39</td><td>Virginia</td><td>760.6</td><td>46</td><td>Texas</td><td>679.1</td></tr>
<tr><td>40</td><td>Washington</td><td>742.1</td><td>47</td><td>California</td><td>637.2</td></tr>
<tr><td>1</td><td>West Virginia</td><td>1,187.6</td><td>48</td><td>Colorado</td><td>632.8</td></tr>
<tr><td>28</td><td>Wisconsin</td><td>831.5</td><td>49</td><td>Utah</td><td>511.3</td></tr>
<tr><td>35</td><td>Wyoming</td><td>792.6</td><td>50</td><td>Alaska</td><td>507.5</td></tr>
<tr><td></td><td></td><td></td><td></td><td>District of Columbia</td><td>868.3</td></tr>
</table>

Source: U.S. Department of Health and Human Services, National Center for Health Statistics
   "National Vital Statistics Reports" (Vol. 59, No. 2, December 9, 2010, http://www.cdc.gov/nchs/deaths.htm)
*Preliminary data by state of residence. Not age-adjusted.

Age-Adjusted Death Rate in 2008

National Rate = 758.7 Deaths per 100,000 Population*

ALPHA ORDER				RANK ORDER		
RANK	STATE	RATE		RANK	STATE	RATE
4	Alabama	930.3		1	West Virginia	958.1
32	Alaska	739.6		2	Mississippi	950.0
49	Arizona	650.6		3	Oklahoma	932.2
7	Arkansas	899.2		4	Alabama	930.3
47	California	658.8		5	Louisiana	922.0
40	Colorado	708.6		6	Kentucky	901.2
43	Connecticut	691.4		7	Arkansas	899.2
20	Delaware	780.8		8	Tennessee	889.7
44	Florida	679.0		9	Nevada	868.2
13	Georgia	835.4		10	Missouri	847.0
50	Hawaii	589.0		11	Ohio	844.0
36	Idaho	721.7		12	South Carolina	839.7
23	Illinois	772.0		13	Georgia	835.4
14	Indiana	835.1		14	Indiana	835.1
30	Iowa	744.0		15	North Carolina	825.6
19	Kansas	784.7		16	Michigan	811.7
6	Kentucky	901.2		17	Pennsylvania	796.5
5	Louisiana	922.0		18	Montana	785.9
25	Maine	764.1		19	Kansas	784.7
24	Maryland	771.6		20	Delaware	780.8
42	Massachusetts	705.9		21	Texas	777.3
16	Michigan	811.7		22	Wyoming	772.5
46	Minnesota	675.2		23	Illinois	772.0
2	Mississippi	950.0		24	Maryland	771.6
10	Missouri	847.0		25	Maine	764.1
18	Montana	785.9		26	Virginia	762.6
31	Nebraska	741.1		27	New Mexico	758.2
9	Nevada	868.2		28	Rhode Island	749.6
39	New Hampshire	712.5		29	Oregon	747.9
37	New Jersey	716.8		30	Iowa	744.0
27	New Mexico	758.2		31	Nebraska	741.1
45	New York	675.8		32	Alaska	739.6
15	North Carolina	825.6		33	Wisconsin	729.7
38	North Dakota	713.0		34	Washington	723.3
11	Ohio	844.0		35	Vermont	722.2
3	Oklahoma	932.2		36	Idaho	721.7
29	Oregon	747.9		37	New Jersey	716.8
17	Pennsylvania	796.5		38	North Dakota	713.0
28	Rhode Island	749.6		39	New Hampshire	712.5
12	South Carolina	839.7		40	Colorado	708.6
41	South Dakota	708.4		41	South Dakota	708.4
8	Tennessee	889.7		42	Massachusetts	705.9
21	Texas	777.3		43	Connecticut	691.4
48	Utah	656.9		44	Florida	679.0
35	Vermont	722.2		45	New York	675.8
26	Virginia	762.6		46	Minnesota	675.2
34	Washington	723.3		47	California	658.8
1	West Virginia	958.1		48	Utah	656.9
33	Wisconsin	729.7		49	Arizona	650.6
22	Wyoming	772.5		50	Hawaii	589.0
				District of Columbia		849.9

Source: U.S. Department of Health and Human Services, National Center for Health Statistics
"National Vital Statistics Reports" (Vol. 59, No. 2, December 9, 2010, http://www.cdc.gov/nchs/deaths.htm)
*Preliminary data by state of residence. Age-adjusted rates eliminate the distorting effects of the aging of the population. Rates based on the year 2000 standard population.

Percent Change in Death Rate: 1999 to 2008

National Percent Change = 7.3% Decrease*

ALPHA ORDER

RANK	STATE	PERCENT CHANGE
7	Alabama	(0.2)
1	Alaska	16.1
50	Arizona	(16.3)
31	Arkansas	(6.2)
39	California	(7.9)
25	Colorado	(5.3)
41	Connccticut	(8.3)
11	Delaware	(1.3)
49	Florida	(13.8)
44	Georgia	(9.3)
2	Hawaii	5.4
31	Idaho	(6.2)
46	Illinois	(10.2)
22	Indiana	(4.4)
20	Iowa	(4.0)
18	Kansas	(3.4)
14	Kentucky	(2.6)
9	Louisiana	(0.9)
16	Maine	(2.7)
34	Maryland	(6.5)
43	Massachusetts	(8.9)
6	Michigan	(0.1)
42	Minnesota	(8.6)
30	Mississippi	(6.1)
33	Missouri	(6.4)
5	Montana	0.0
37	Nebraska	(7.3)
21	Nevada	(4.1)
13	New Hampshire	(1.7)
47	New Jersey	(11.3)
3	New Mexico	2.4
48	New York	(13.2)
39	North Carolina	(7.9)
23	North Dakota	(5.0)
9	Ohio	(0.9)
12	Oklahoma	(1.5)
23	Oregon	(5.0)
28	Pennsylvania	(5.7)
26	Rhode Island	(5.4)
17	South Carolina	(3.0)
36	South Dakota	(7.2)
18	Tennessee	(3.4)
37	Texas	(7.3)
45	Utah	(9.7)
7	Vermont	(0.2)
27	Virginia	(5.5)
14	Washington	(2.6)
4	West Virginia	1.9
34	Wisconsin	(6.5)
29	Wyoming	(6.0)

RANK ORDER

RANK	STATE	PERCENT CHANGE
1	Alaska	16.1
2	Hawaii	5.4
3	New Mexico	2.4
4	West Virginia	1.9
5	Montana	0.0
6	Michigan	(0.1)
7	Alabama	(0.2)
7	Vermont	(0.2)
9	Louisiana	(0.9)
9	Ohio	(0.9)
11	Delaware	(1.3)
12	Oklahoma	(1.5)
13	New Hampshire	(1.7)
14	Kentucky	(2.6)
14	Washington	(2.6)
16	Maine	(2.7)
17	South Carolina	(3.0)
18	Kansas	(3.4)
18	Tennessee	(3.4)
20	Iowa	(4.0)
21	Nevada	(4.1)
22	Indiana	(4.4)
23	North Dakota	(5.0)
23	Oregon	(5.0)
25	Colorado	(5.3)
26	Rhode Island	(5.4)
27	Virginia	(5.5)
28	Pennsylvania	(5.7)
29	Wyoming	(6.0)
30	Mississippi	(6.1)
31	Arkansas	(6.2)
31	Idaho	(6.2)
33	Missouri	(6.4)
34	Maryland	(6.5)
34	Wisconsin	(6.5)
36	South Dakota	(7.2)
37	Nebraska	(7.3)
37	Texas	(7.3)
39	California	(7.9)
39	North Carolina	(7.9)
41	Connecticut	(8.3)
42	Minnesota	(8.6)
43	Massachusetts	(8.9)
44	Georgia	(9.3)
45	Utah	(9.7)
46	Illinois	(10.2)
47	New Jersey	(11.3)
48	New York	(13.2)
49	Florida	(13.8)
50	Arizona	(16.3)

District of Columbia (25.8)

Source: CQ Press using data from U.S. Department of Health and Human Services, National Center for Health Statistics
"National Vital Statistics Reports" (Vol. 59, No. 2, December 9, 2010, http://www.cdc.gov/nchs/deaths.htm)
"National Vital Statistics Reports" (Vol. 49, No. 8, September 21, 2001, www.cdc.gov/nchs/data/nvsr/nvsr49/nvs49_08.pdf)
*By state of residence. Not age-adjusted.

Deaths in 2007

National Total = 2,423,712 Deaths*

ALPHA ORDER

RANK	STATE	DEATHS	% of USA
18	Alabama	46,696	1.9%
50	Alaska	3,463	0.1%
20	Arizona	45,554	1.9%
31	Arkansas	28,191	1.2%
1	California	233,720	9.6%
28	Colorado	29,993	1.2%
29	Connecticut	28,651	1.2%
45	Delaware	7,327	0.3%
2	Florida	168,096	6.9%
11	Georgia	68,331	2.8%
43	Hawaii	9,495	0.4%
40	Idaho	10,822	0.4%
7	Illinois	100,503	4.1%
15	Indiana	54,000	2.2%
32	Iowa	27,221	1.1%
33	Kansas	24,491	1.0%
22	Kentucky	40,090	1.7%
23	Louisiana	39,966	1.6%
39	Maine	12,493	0.5%
21	Maryland	43,757	1.8%
16	Massachusetts	52,917	2.2%
8	Michigan	86,721	3.6%
25	Minnesota	37,138	1.5%
30	Mississippi	28,255	1.2%
14	Missouri	54,166	2.2%
44	Montana	8,624	0.4%
37	Nebraska	15,263	0.6%
35	Nevada	18,687	0.8%
41	New Hampshire	10,303	0.4%
10	New Jersey	69,662	2.9%
36	New Mexico	15,482	0.6%
4	New York	147,680	6.1%
9	North Carolina	76,046	3.1%
47	North Dakota	5,561	0.2%
6	Ohio	106,534	4.4%
26	Oklahoma	36,032	1.5%
27	Oregon	31,403	1.3%
5	Pennsylvania	125,104	5.2%
42	Rhode Island	9,723	0.4%
24	South Carolina	39,439	1.6%
46	South Dakota	6,826	0.3%
13	Tennessee	57,087	2.4%
3	Texas	160,548	6.6%
38	Utah	14,143	0.6%
48	Vermont	5,179	0.2%
12	Virginia	58,225	2.4%
17	Washington	47,323	2.0%
34	West Virginia	21,086	0.9%
19	Wisconsin	46,241	1.9%
49	Wyoming	4,266	0.2%

RANK ORDER

RANK	STATE	DEATHS	% of USA
1	California	233,720	9.6%
2	Florida	168,096	6.9%
3	Texas	160,548	6.6%
4	New York	147,680	6.1%
5	Pennsylvania	125,104	5.2%
6	Ohio	106,534	4.4%
7	Illinois	100,503	4.1%
8	Michigan	86,721	3.6%
9	North Carolina	76,046	3.1%
10	New Jersey	69,662	2.9%
11	Georgia	68,331	2.8%
12	Virginia	58,225	2.4%
13	Tennessee	57,087	2.4%
14	Missouri	54,166	2.2%
15	Indiana	54,000	2.2%
16	Massachusetts	52,917	2.2%
17	Washington	47,323	2.0%
18	Alabama	46,696	1.9%
19	Wisconsin	46,241	1.9%
20	Arizona	45,554	1.9%
21	Maryland	43,757	1.8%
22	Kentucky	40,090	1.7%
23	Louisiana	39,966	1.6%
24	South Carolina	39,439	1.6%
25	Minnesota	37,138	1.5%
26	Oklahoma	36,032	1.5%
27	Oregon	31,403	1.3%
28	Colorado	29,993	1.2%
29	Connecticut	28,651	1.2%
30	Mississippi	28,255	1.2%
31	Arkansas	28,191	1.2%
32	Iowa	27,221	1.1%
33	Kansas	24,491	1.0%
34	West Virginia	21,086	0.9%
35	Nevada	18,687	0.8%
36	New Mexico	15,482	0.6%
37	Nebraska	15,263	0.6%
38	Utah	14,143	0.6%
39	Maine	12,493	0.5%
40	Idaho	10,822	0.4%
41	New Hampshire	10,303	0.4%
42	Rhode Island	9,723	0.4%
43	Hawaii	9,495	0.4%
44	Montana	8,624	0.4%
45	Delaware	7,327	0.3%
46	South Dakota	6,826	0.3%
47	North Dakota	5,561	0.2%
48	Vermont	5,179	0.2%
49	Wyoming	4,266	0.2%
50	Alaska	3,463	0.1%
	District of Columbia	5,188	0.2%

Source: U.S. Department of Health and Human Services, National Center for Health Statistics
"National Vital Statistics Reports" (Vol. 58, No. 19, May 20, 2010, http://www.cdc.gov/nchs/deaths.htm)
*Final data by state of residence.

Death Rate in 2007

National Rate = 803.6 Deaths per 100,000 Population*

ALPHA ORDER			RANK ORDER		
RANK	STATE	RATE	RANK	STATE	RATE
2	Alabama	1,009.0	1	West Virginia	1,163.7
50	Alaska	506.7	2	Alabama	1,009.0
43	Arizona	718.7	3	Pennsylvania	1,006.2
5	Arkansas	994.5	4	Oklahoma	996.1
47	California	639.4	5	Arkansas	994.5
48	Colorado	616.9	6	Mississippi	968.0
30	Connecticut	818.1	7	Maine	948.4
24	Delaware	847.3	8	Kentucky	945.2
13	Florida	921.0	9	Louisiana	930.9
44	Georgia	715.9	10	Ohio	929.1
39	Hawaii	739.8	11	Tennessee	927.2
42	Idaho	721.8	12	Missouri	921.4
35	Illinois	782.0	13	Florida	921.0
23	Indiana	851.0	14	Rhode Island	919.1
15	Iowa	911.0	15	Iowa	911.0
18	Kansas	882.2	16	Montana	900.3
8	Kentucky	945.2	17	South Carolina	894.8
9	Louisiana	930.9	18	Kansas	882.2
7	Maine	948.4	19	North Dakota	869.3
36	Maryland	778.8	20	Michigan	861.0
29	Massachusetts	820.4	21	Nebraska	860.1
20	Michigan	861.0	22	South Dakota	857.3
45	Minnesota	714.5	23	Indiana	851.0
6	Mississippi	968.0	24	Delaware	847.3
12	Missouri	921.4	25	North Carolina	839.3
16	Montana	900.3	26	Oregon	838.0
21	Nebraska	860.1	27	Vermont	833.6
41	Nevada	728.4	28	Wisconsin	825.5
34	New Hampshire	783.0	29	Massachusetts	820.4
32	New Jersey	802.0	30	Connecticut	818.1
33	New Mexico	785.9	31	Wyoming	815.9
37	New York	765.3	32	New Jersey	802.0
25	North Carolina	839.3	33	New Mexico	785.9
19	North Dakota	869.3	34	New Hampshire	783.0
10	Ohio	929.1	35	Illinois	782.0
4	Oklahoma	996.1	36	Maryland	778.8
26	Oregon	838.0	37	New York	765.3
3	Pennsylvania	1,006.2	38	Virginia	755.0
14	Rhode Island	919.1	39	Hawaii	739.8
17	South Carolina	894.8	40	Washington	731.6
22	South Dakota	857.3	41	Nevada	728.4
11	Tennessee	927.2	42	Idaho	721.8
46	Texas	671.6	43	Arizona	718.7
49	Utah	534.6	44	Georgia	715.9
27	Vermont	833.6	45	Minnesota	714.5
38	Virginia	755.0	46	Texas	671.6
40	Washington	731.6	47	California	639.4
1	West Virginia	1,163.7	48	Colorado	616.9
28	Wisconsin	825.5	49	Utah	534.6
31	Wyoming	815.9	50	Alaska	506.7
				District of Columbia	881.9

Source: U.S. Department of Health and Human Services, National Center for Health Statistics
"National Vital Statistics Reports" (Vol. 58, No. 19, May 20, 2010, http://www.cdc.gov/nchs/deaths.htm)
*Final data by state of residence. Not age-adjusted.

Age-Adjusted Death Rate in 2007

National Rate = 760.2 Deaths per 100,000 Population*

ALPHA ORDER			RANK ORDER		
RANK	STATE	RATE	RANK	STATE	RATE
3	Alabama	930.7	1	West Virginia	951.7
28	Alaska	755.1	2	Mississippi	943.0
46	Arizona	682.1	3	Alabama	930.7
8	Arkansas	882.8	4	Louisiana	926.4
48	California	674.2	5	Oklahoma	920.4
40	Colorado	700.8	6	Kentucky	896.9
42	Connecticut	694.1	7	Tennessee	885.2
22	Delaware	773.6	8	Arkansas	882.8
45	Florida	685.9	9	South Carolina	849.7
10	Georgia	839.8	10	Georgia	839.8
50	Hawaii	607.4	11	North Carolina	834.4
32	Idaho	734.6	12	Ohio	830.8
26	Illinois	759.8	13	Missouri	826.7
14	Indiana	809.9	14	Indiana	809.9
38	Iowa	718.6	15	Michigan	806.1
19	Kansas	783.0	16	Nevada	803.5
6	Kentucky	896.9	17	Wyoming	802.0
4	Louisiana	926.4	18	Pennsylvania	790.1
22	Maine	773.6	19	Kansas	783.0
20	Maryland	782.7	20	Maryland	782.7
39	Massachusetts	707.5	21	Texas	777.7
15	Michigan	806.1	22	Delaware	773.6
49	Minnesota	661.5	22	Maine	773.6
2	Mississippi	943.0	24	Montana	772.7
13	Missouri	826.7	25	Virginia	770.6
24	Montana	772.7	26	Illinois	759.8
31	Nebraska	743.7	27	New Mexico	755.9
16	Nevada	803.5	28	Alaska	755.1
35	New Hampshire	727.0	29	Oregon	753.9
36	New Jersey	724.2	30	Rhode Island	750.0
27	New Mexico	755.9	31	Nebraska	743.7
44	New York	686.4	32	Idaho	734.6
11	North Carolina	834.4	33	Wisconsin	732.3
47	North Dakota	679.5	34	Vermont	729.3
12	Ohio	830.8	35	New Hampshire	727.0
5	Oklahoma	920.4	36	New Jersey	724.2
29	Oregon	753.9	37	Washington	722.2
18	Pennsylvania	790.1	38	Iowa	718.6
30	Rhode Island	750.0	39	Massachusetts	707.5
9	South Carolina	849.7	40	Colorado	700.8
43	South Dakota	693.5	41	Utah	694.2
7	Tennessee	885.2	42	Connecticut	694.1
21	Texas	777.7	43	South Dakota	693.5
41	Utah	694.2	44	New York	686.4
34	Vermont	729.3	45	Florida	685.9
25	Virginia	770.6	46	Arizona	682.1
37	Washington	722.2	47	North Dakota	679.5
1	West Virginia	951.7	48	California	674.2
33	Wisconsin	732.3	49	Minnesota	661.5
17	Wyoming	802.0	50	Hawaii	607.4
				District of Columbia	866.9

Source: U.S. Department of Health and Human Services, National Center for Health Statistics
    "National Vital Statistics Reports" (Vol. 58, No. 19, May 20, 2010, http://www.cdc.gov/nchs/deaths.htm)
*Final data by state of residence. Age-adjusted rates eliminate the distorting effects of the aging of the population. Rates based
on the year 2000 standard population.

Infant Deaths in 2007

National Total = 29,138 Infant Deaths*

ALPHA ORDER

RANK	STATE	DEATHS	% of USA
15	Alabama	641	2.2%
47	Alaska	72	0.2%
13	Arizona	711	2.4%
30	Arkansas	317	1.1%
1	California	2,944	10.1%
24	Colorado	433	1.5%
33	Connecticut	276	0.9%
41	Delaware	91	0.3%
3	Florida	1,685	5.8%
6	Georgia	1,206	4.1%
40	Hawaii	124	0.4%
38	Idaho	169	0.6%
5	Illinois	1,217	4.2%
14	Indiana	681	2.3%
35	Iowa	225	0.8%
29	Kansas	333	1.1%
27	Kentucky	397	1.4%
18	Louisiana	608	2.1%
43	Maine	89	0.3%
16	Maryland	625	2.1%
28	Massachusetts	384	1.3%
10	Michigan	995	3.4%
26	Minnesota	409	1.4%
23	Mississippi	467	1.6%
17	Missouri	613	2.1%
44	Montana	79	0.3%
37	Nebraska	182	0.6%
34	Nevada	262	0.9%
46	New Hampshire	76	0.3%
19	New Jersey	601	2.1%
36	New Mexico	192	0.7%
4	New York	1,412	4.8%
9	North Carolina	1,112	3.8%
48	North Dakota	66	0.2%
7	Ohio	1,160	4.0%
22	Oklahoma	469	1.6%
31	Oregon	284	1.0%
8	Pennsylvania	1,139	3.9%
41	Rhode Island	91	0.3%
20	South Carolina	539	1.8%
44	South Dakota	79	0.3%
12	Tennessee	721	2.5%
2	Texas	2,564	8.8%
32	Utah	280	1.0%
50	Vermont	33	0.1%
11	Virginia	848	2.9%
25	Washington	429	1.5%
39	West Virginia	164	0.6%
21	Wisconsin	470	1.6%
49	Wyoming	58	0.2%

RANK ORDER

RANK	STATE	DEATHS	% of USA
1	California	2,944	10.1%
2	Texas	2,564	8.8%
3	Florida	1,685	5.8%
4	New York	1,412	4.8%
5	Illinois	1,217	4.2%
6	Georgia	1,206	4.1%
7	Ohio	1,160	4.0%
8	Pennsylvania	1,139	3.9%
9	North Carolina	1,112	3.8%
10	Michigan	995	3.4%
11	Virginia	848	2.9%
12	Tennessee	721	2.5%
13	Arizona	711	2.4%
14	Indiana	681	2.3%
15	Alabama	641	2.2%
16	Maryland	625	2.1%
17	Missouri	613	2.1%
18	Louisiana	608	2.1%
19	New Jersey	601	2.1%
20	South Carolina	539	1.8%
21	Wisconsin	470	1.6%
22	Oklahoma	469	1.6%
23	Mississippi	467	1.6%
24	Colorado	433	1.5%
25	Washington	429	1.5%
26	Minnesota	409	1.4%
27	Kentucky	397	1.4%
28	Massachusetts	384	1.3%
29	Kansas	333	1.1%
30	Arkansas	317	1.1%
31	Oregon	284	1.0%
32	Utah	280	1.0%
33	Connecticut	276	0.9%
34	Nevada	262	0.9%
35	Iowa	225	0.8%
36	New Mexico	192	0.7%
37	Nebraska	182	0.6%
38	Idaho	169	0.6%
39	West Virginia	164	0.6%
40	Hawaii	124	0.4%
41	Delaware	91	0.3%
41	Rhode Island	91	0.3%
43	Maine	89	0.3%
44	Montana	79	0.3%
44	South Dakota	79	0.3%
46	New Hampshire	76	0.3%
47	Alaska	72	0.2%
48	North Dakota	66	0.2%
49	Wyoming	58	0.2%
50	Vermont	33	0.1%
	District of Columbia	116	0.4%

Source: U.S. Department of Health and Human Services, National Center for Health Statistics
"National Vital Statistics Reports" (Vol. 58, No. 19, May 20, 2010, http://www.cdc.gov/nchs/deaths.htm)
*Final data. Deaths of infants under 1 year old by state of residence.

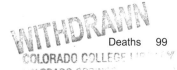

Infant Mortality Rate in 2007

National Rate = 6.8 Infant Deaths per 1,000 Live Births*

ALPHA ORDER

RANK	STATE	RATE
2	Alabama	9.9
30	Alaska	6.5
24	Arizona	6.9
13	Arkansas	7.7
45	California	5.2
39	Colorado	6.1
29	Connecticut	6.6
17	Delaware	7.5
23	Florida	7.1
8	Georgia	8.0
30	Hawaii	6.5
25	Idaho	6.8
27	Illinois	6.7
15	Indiana	7.6
43	Iowa	5.5
10	Kansas	7.9
27	Kentucky	6.7
3	Louisiana	9.2
36	Maine	6.3
8	Maryland	8.0
49	Massachusetts	4.9
10	Michigan	7.9
41	Minnesota	5.6
1	Mississippi	10.0
17	Missouri	7.5
33	Montana	6.4
25	Nebraska	6.8
33	Nevada	6.4
44	New Hampshire	5.4
45	New Jersey	5.2
36	New Mexico	6.3
41	New York	5.6
5	North Carolina	8.5
17	North Dakota	7.5
13	Ohio	7.7
5	Oklahoma	8.5
40	Oregon	5.8
15	Pennsylvania	7.6
21	Rhode Island	7.4
4	South Carolina	8.6
33	South Dakota	6.4
7	Tennessee	8.3
36	Texas	6.3
47	Utah	5.1
47	Vermont	5.1
12	Virginia	7.8
50	Washington	4.8
17	West Virginia	7.5
30	Wisconsin	6.5
21	Wyoming	7.4

RANK ORDER

RANK	STATE	RATE
1	Mississippi	10.0
2	Alabama	9.9
3	Louisiana	9.2
4	South Carolina	8.6
5	North Carolina	8.5
5	Oklahoma	8.5
7	Tennessee	8.3
8	Georgia	8.0
8	Maryland	8.0
10	Kansas	7.9
10	Michigan	7.9
12	Virginia	7.8
13	Arkansas	7.7
13	Ohio	7.7
15	Indiana	7.6
15	Pennsylvania	7.6
17	Delaware	7.5
17	Missouri	7.5
17	North Dakota	7.5
17	West Virginia	7.5
21	Rhode Island	7.4
21	Wyoming	7.4
23	Florida	7.1
24	Arizona	6.9
25	Idaho	6.8
25	Nebraska	6.8
27	Illinois	6.7
27	Kentucky	6.7
29	Connecticut	6.6
30	Alaska	6.5
30	Hawaii	6.5
30	Wisconsin	6.5
33	Montana	6.4
33	Nevada	6.4
33	South Dakota	6.4
36	Maine	6.3
36	New Mexico	6.3
36	Texas	6.3
39	Colorado	6.1
40	Oregon	5.8
41	Minnesota	5.6
41	New York	5.6
43	Iowa	5.5
44	New Hampshire	5.4
45	California	5.2
45	New Jersey	5.2
47	Utah	5.1
47	Vermont	5.1
49	Massachusetts	4.9
50	Washington	4.8
	District of Columbia	13.1

Source: U.S. Department of Health and Human Services, National Center for Health Statistics
   "National Vital Statistics Reports" (Vol. 58, No. 19, May 20, 2010, http://www.cdc.gov/nchs/deaths.htm)
*Final data. Deaths of infants under 1 year old by state of residence.

White Infant Mortality Rate in 2007

National Rate = 5.6 White Infant Deaths per 1,000 White Live Births*

ALPHA ORDER

RANK	STATE	RATE
1	Alabama	8.0
40	Alaska	5.2
8	Arizona	6.6
11	Arkansas	6.5
44	California	4.9
27	Colorado	5.9
27	Connecticut	5.9
17	Delaware	6.1
36	Florida	5.5
34	Georgia	5.6
17	Hawaii	6.1
8	Idaho	6.6
40	Illinois	5.2
8	Indiana	6.6
38	Iowa	5.3
3	Kansas	7.0
23	Kentucky	6.0
17	Louisiana	6.1
15	Maine	6.3
45	Maryland	4.8
48	Massachusetts	4.5
17	Michigan	6.1
47	Minnesota	4.7
6	Mississippi	6.7
27	Missouri	5.9
27	Montana	5.9
17	Nebraska	6.1
23	Nevada	6.0
38	New Hampshire	5.3
50	New Jersey	4.1
23	New Mexico	6.0
42	New York	5.0
13	North Carolina	6.4
5	North Dakota	6.8
15	Ohio	6.3
2	Oklahoma	7.3
32	Oregon	5.7
17	Pennsylvania	6.1
11	Rhode Island	6.5
23	South Carolina	6.0
34	South Dakota	5.6
13	Tennessee	6.4
32	Texas	5.7
42	Utah	5.0
45	Vermont	4.8
31	Virginia	5.8
49	Washington	4.3
3	West Virginia	7.0
37	Wisconsin	5.4
6	Wyoming	6.7

RANK ORDER

RANK	STATE	RATE
1	Alabama	8.0
2	Oklahoma	7.3
3	Kansas	7.0
3	West Virginia	7.0
5	North Dakota	6.8
6	Mississippi	6.7
6	Wyoming	6.7
8	Arizona	6.6
8	Idaho	6.6
8	Indiana	6.6
11	Arkansas	6.5
11	Rhode Island	6.5
13	North Carolina	6.4
13	Tennessee	6.4
15	Maine	6.3
15	Ohio	6.3
17	Delaware	6.1
17	Hawaii	6.1
17	Louisiana	6.1
17	Michigan	6.1
17	Nebraska	6.1
17	Pennsylvania	6.1
23	Kentucky	6.0
23	Nevada	6.0
23	New Mexico	6.0
23	South Carolina	6.0
27	Colorado	5.9
27	Connecticut	5.9
27	Missouri	5.9
27	Montana	5.9
31	Virginia	5.8
32	Oregon	5.7
32	Texas	5.7
34	Georgia	5.6
34	South Dakota	5.6
36	Florida	5.5
37	Wisconsin	5.4
38	Iowa	5.3
38	New Hampshire	5.3
40	Alaska	5.2
40	Illinois	5.2
42	New York	5.0
42	Utah	5.0
44	California	4.9
45	Maryland	4.8
45	Vermont	4.8
47	Minnesota	4.7
48	Massachusetts	4.5
49	Washington	4.3
50	New Jersey	4.1

| | District of Columbia | 8.5 |

Source: U.S. Department of Health and Human Services, National Center for Health Statistics
"National Vital Statistics Reports" (Vol. 58, No. 19, May 20, 2010, http://www.cdc.gov/nchs/deaths.htm)
*Final data. Deaths of infants under 1 year old, exclusive of fetal deaths. Based on race of the mother.

Black Infant Mortality Rate in 2007

National Rate = 13.2 Black Infant Deaths per 1,000 Black Live Births*

ALPHA ORDER				RANK ORDER		
RANK	STATE	RATE		RANK	STATE	RATE
14	Alabama	14.4		1	Kansas	19.0
NA	Alaska**	NA		2	Oklahoma	18.0
12	Arizona	15.0		3	Missouri	16.5
21	Arkansas	13.2		4	Michigan	16.4
25	California	12.4		5	Indiana	16.0
21	Colorado	13.2		5	Rhode Island	16.0
28	Connecticut	12.1		7	Tennessee	15.7
29	Delaware	11.8		8	Virginia	15.4
27	Florida	12.2		9	Wisconsin	15.2
23	Georgia	12.8		10	North Carolina	15.1
NA	Hawaii**	NA		10	Pennsylvania	15.1
NA	Idaho**	NA		12	Arizona	15.0
15	Illinois	14.2		13	Ohio	14.8
5	Indiana	16.0		14	Alabama	14.4
31	Iowa	11.6		15	Illinois	14.2
1	Kansas	19.0		16	Louisiana	14.1
24	Kentucky	12.7		17	Nebraska	14.0
16	Louisiana	14.1		18	Mississippi	13.9
NA	Maine**	NA		19	South Carolina	13.7
20	Maryland	13.6		20	Maryland	13.6
35	Massachusetts	8.8		21	Arkansas	13.2
4	Michigan	16.4		21	Colorado	13.2
30	Minnesota	11.7		23	Georgia	12.8
18	Mississippi	13.9		24	Kentucky	12.7
3	Missouri	16.5		25	California	12.4
NA	Montana**	NA		25	Nevada	12.4
17	Nebraska	14.0		27	Florida	12.2
25	Nevada	12.4		28	Connecticut	12.1
NA	New Hampshire**	NA		29	Delaware	11.8
33	New Jersey	11.0		30	Minnesota	11.7
NA	New Mexico**	NA		31	Iowa	11.6
35	New York	8.8		32	Texas	11.5
10	North Carolina	15.1		33	New Jersey	11.0
NA	North Dakota**	NA		34	Washington	10.3
13	Ohio	14.8		35	Massachusetts	8.8
2	Oklahoma	18.0		35	New York	8.8
NA	Oregon**	NA		NA	Alaska**	NA
10	Pennsylvania	15.1		NA	Hawaii**	NA
5	Rhode Island	16.0		NA	Idaho**	NA
19	South Carolina	13.7		NA	Maine**	NA
NA	South Dakota**	NA		NA	Montana**	NA
7	Tennessee	15.7		NA	New Hampshire**	NA
32	Texas	11.5		NA	New Mexico**	NA
NA	Utah**	NA		NA	North Dakota**	NA
NA	Vermont**	NA		NA	Oregon**	NA
8	Virginia	15.4		NA	South Dakota**	NA
34	Washington	10.3		NA	Utah**	NA
NA	West Virginia**	NA		NA	Vermont**	NA
9	Wisconsin	15.2		NA	West Virginia**	NA
NA	Wyoming**	NA		NA	Wyoming**	NA
					District of Columbia	16.6

Source: U.S. Department of Health and Human Services, National Center for Health Statistics
"National Vital Statistics Reports" (Vol. 58, No. 19, May 20, 2010, http://www.cdc.gov/nchs/deaths.htm)
*Final data. Deaths of infants under 1 year old, exclusive of fetal deaths. Based on race of the mother.
**With fewer than 20 deaths, the rate would be considered statistically unreliable.

Neonatal Deaths in 2007

National Total = 19,058 Deaths*

ALPHA ORDER

RANK	STATE	DEATHS	% of USA
17	Alabama	406	2.1%
48	Alaska	35	0.2%
12	Arizona	488	2.6%
33	Arkansas	179	0.9%
1	California	2,009	10.5%
21	Colorado	295	1.5%
29	Connecticut	211	1.1%
42	Delaware	65	0.3%
3	Florida	1,058	5.6%
7	Georgia	766	4.0%
40	Hawaii	81	0.4%
38	Idaho	113	0.6%
5	Illinois	865	4.5%
15	Indiana	430	2.3%
35	Iowa	135	0.7%
30	Kansas	210	1.1%
28	Kentucky	241	1.3%
20	Louisiana	355	1.9%
43	Maine	63	0.3%
13	Maryland	453	2.4%
25	Massachusetts	267	1.4%
10	Michigan	696	3.7%
23	Minnesota	280	1.5%
24	Mississippi	274	1.4%
16	Missouri	409	2.1%
46	Montana	45	0.2%
36	Nebraska	131	0.7%
34	Nevada	166	0.9%
45	New Hampshire	46	0.2%
18	New Jersey	399	2.1%
37	New Mexico	119	0.6%
4	New York	937	4.9%
9	North Carolina	747	3.9%
47	North Dakota	43	0.2%
6	Ohio	781	4.1%
26	Oklahoma	263	1.4%
31	Oregon	195	1.0%
8	Pennsylvania	751	3.9%
41	Rhode Island	67	0.4%
19	South Carolina	356	1.9%
44	South Dakota	51	0.3%
14	Tennessee	450	2.4%
2	Texas	1,572	8.2%
32	Utah	187	1.0%
50	Vermont	20	0.1%
11	Virginia	583	3.1%
27	Washington	254	1.3%
39	West Virginia	103	0.5%
22	Wisconsin	293	1.5%
49	Wyoming	29	0.2%

RANK ORDER

RANK	STATE	DEATHS	% of USA
1	California	2,009	10.5%
2	Texas	1,572	8.2%
3	Florida	1,058	5.6%
4	New York	937	4.9%
5	Illinois	865	4.5%
6	Ohio	781	4.1%
7	Georgia	766	4.0%
8	Pennsylvania	751	3.9%
9	North Carolina	747	3.9%
10	Michigan	696	3.7%
11	Virginia	583	3.1%
12	Arizona	488	2.6%
13	Maryland	453	2.4%
14	Tennessee	450	2.4%
15	Indiana	430	2.3%
16	Missouri	409	2.1%
17	Alabama	406	2.1%
18	New Jersey	399	2.1%
19	South Carolina	356	1.9%
20	Louisiana	355	1.9%
21	Colorado	295	1.5%
22	Wisconsin	293	1.5%
23	Minnesota	280	1.5%
24	Mississippi	274	1.4%
25	Massachusetts	267	1.4%
26	Oklahoma	263	1.4%
27	Washington	254	1.3%
28	Kentucky	241	1.3%
29	Connecticut	211	1.1%
30	Kansas	210	1.1%
31	Oregon	195	1.0%
32	Utah	187	1.0%
33	Arkansas	179	0.9%
34	Nevada	166	0.9%
35	Iowa	135	0.7%
36	Nebraska	131	0.7%
37	New Mexico	119	0.6%
38	Idaho	113	0.6%
39	West Virginia	103	0.5%
40	Hawaii	81	0.4%
41	Rhode Island	67	0.4%
42	Delaware	65	0.3%
43	Maine	63	0.3%
44	South Dakota	51	0.3%
45	New Hampshire	46	0.2%
46	Montana	45	0.2%
47	North Dakota	43	0.2%
48	Alaska	35	0.2%
49	Wyoming	29	0.2%
50	Vermont	20	0.1%
	District of Columbia	86	0.5%

Source: U.S. Department of Health and Human Services, National Center for Health Statistics
    "National Vital Statistics Reports" (Vol. 58, No. 19, May 20, 2010, http://www.cdc.gov/nchs/deaths.htm)
*Final data. Deaths of infants under 28 days old, exclusive of fetal deaths.

Neonatal Death Rate in 2007

National Rate = 4.4 Deaths per 1,000 Live Births*

ALPHA ORDER

RANK	STATE	RATE
1	Alabama	6.3
48	Alaska	3.2
23	Arizona	4.7
28	Arkansas	4.3
41	California	3.6
29	Colorado	4.2
13	Connecticut	5.1
10	Delaware	5.3
27	Florida	4.4
13	Georgia	5.1
29	Hawaii	4.2
25	Idaho	4.5
20	Illinois	4.8
20	Indiana	4.8
46	Iowa	3.3
15	Kansas	5.0
32	Kentucky	4.1
7	Louisiana	5.4
25	Maine	4.5
3	Maryland	5.8
43	Massachusetts	3.4
6	Michigan	5.6
38	Minnesota	3.8
2	Mississippi	5.9
15	Missouri	5.0
41	Montana	3.6
18	Nebraska	4.9
33	Nevada	4.0
46	New Hampshire	3.3
43	New Jersey	3.4
36	New Mexico	3.9
39	New York	3.7
4	North Carolina	5.7
18	North Dakota	4.9
11	Ohio	5.2
20	Oklahoma	4.8
33	Oregon	4.0
15	Pennsylvania	5.0
7	Rhode Island	5.4
4	South Carolina	5.7
29	South Dakota	4.2
11	Tennessee	5.2
36	Texas	3.9
43	Utah	3.4
49	Vermont	3.1
7	Virginia	5.4
50	Washington	2.9
23	West Virginia	4.7
33	Wisconsin	4.0
39	Wyoming	3.7

RANK ORDER

RANK	STATE	RATE
1	Alabama	6.3
2	Mississippi	5.9
3	Maryland	5.8
4	North Carolina	5.7
4	South Carolina	5.7
6	Michigan	5.6
7	Louisiana	5.4
7	Rhode Island	5.4
7	Virginia	5.4
10	Delaware	5.3
11	Ohio	5.2
11	Tennessee	5.2
13	Connecticut	5.1
13	Georgia	5.1
15	Kansas	5.0
15	Missouri	5.0
15	Pennsylvania	5.0
18	Nebraska	4.9
18	North Dakota	4.9
20	Illinois	4.8
20	Indiana	4.8
20	Oklahoma	4.8
23	Arizona	4.7
23	West Virginia	4.7
25	Idaho	4.5
25	Maine	4.5
27	Florida	4.4
28	Arkansas	4.3
29	Colorado	4.2
29	Hawaii	4.2
29	South Dakota	4.2
32	Kentucky	4.1
33	Nevada	4.0
33	Oregon	4.0
33	Wisconsin	4.0
36	New Mexico	3.9
36	Texas	3.9
38	Minnesota	3.8
39	New York	3.7
39	Wyoming	3.7
41	California	3.6
41	Montana	3.6
43	Massachusetts	3.4
43	New Jersey	3.4
43	Utah	3.4
46	Iowa	3.3
46	New Hampshire	3.3
48	Alaska	3.2
49	Vermont	3.1
50	Washington	2.9
	District of Columbia	9.7

Source: U.S. Department of Health and Human Services, National Center for Health Statistics
"National Vital Statistics Reports" (Vol. 58, No. 19, May 20, 2010, http://www.cdc.gov/nchs/deaths.htm)
*Final data. Deaths of infants under 28 days old, exclusive of fetal deaths.

White Neonatal Death Rate in 2007

National Rate = 3.7 White Neonatal Deaths per 1,000 White Live Births*

ALPHA ORDER				RANK ORDER		
RANK	STATE	RATE		RANK	STATE	RATE
2	Alabama	4.9		1	North Dakota	5.1
47	Alaska	3.0		2	Alabama	4.9
4	Arizona	4.6		3	Rhode Island	4.8
38	Arkansas	3.4		4	Arizona	4.6
41	California	3.3		5	Connecticut	4.5
18	Colorado	4.0		5	Idaho	4.5
5	Connecticut	4.5		5	Kansas	4.5
11	Delaware	4.3		5	Maine	4.5
34	Florida	3.5		9	Michigan	4.4
31	Georgia	3.6		9	Nebraska	4.4
31	Hawaii	3.6		11	Delaware	4.3
5	Idaho	4.5		11	West Virginia	4.3
24	Illinois	3.8		13	North Carolina	4.2
16	Indiana	4.1		13	Ohio	4.2
41	Iowa	3.3		13	Oklahoma	4.2
5	Kansas	4.5		16	Indiana	4.1
29	Kentucky	3.7		16	Pennsylvania	4.1
34	Louisiana	3.5		18	Colorado	4.0
5	Maine	4.5		18	South Dakota	4.0
34	Maryland	3.5		20	New Mexico	3.9
46	Massachusetts	3.1		20	Oregon	3.9
9	Michigan	4.4		20	South Carolina	3.9
41	Minnesota	3.3		20	Tennessee	3.9
24	Mississippi	3.8		24	Illinois	3.8
24	Missouri	3.8		24	Mississippi	3.8
34	Montana	3.5		24	Missouri	3.8
9	Nebraska	4.4		24	Nevada	3.8
24	Nevada	3.8		24	Virginia	3.8
41	New Hampshire	3.3		29	Kentucky	3.7
48	New Jersey	2.9		29	Wyoming	3.7
20	New Mexico	3.9		31	Georgia	3.6
41	New York	3.3		31	Hawaii	3.6
13	North Carolina	4.2		31	Wisconsin	3.6
1	North Dakota	5.1		34	Florida	3.5
13	Ohio	4.2		34	Louisiana	3.5
13	Oklahoma	4.2		34	Maryland	3.5
20	Oregon	3.9		34	Montana	3.5
16	Pennsylvania	4.1		38	Arkansas	3.4
3	Rhode Island	4.8		38	Texas	3.4
20	South Carolina	3.9		38	Utah	3.4
18	South Dakota	4.0		41	California	3.3
20	Tennessee	3.9		41	Iowa	3.3
38	Texas	3.4		41	Minnesota	3.3
38	Utah	3.4		41	New Hampshire	3.3
NA	Vermont**	NA		41	New York	3.3
24	Virginia	3.8		46	Massachusetts	3.1
49	Washington	2.6		47	Alaska	3.0
11	West Virginia	4.3		48	New Jersey	2.9
31	Wisconsin	3.6		49	Washington	2.6
29	Wyoming	3.7		NA	Vermont**	NA
					District of Columbia	5.9

Source: U.S. Department of Health and Human Services, National Center for Health Statistics
   "National Vital Statistics Reports" (Vol. 58, No. 19, May 20, 2010, http://www.cdc.gov/nchs/deaths.htm)
*Final data. Deaths of infants under 28 days old, exclusive of fetal deaths. Based on race of the mother.
**With fewer than 20 deaths, the rate would be considered statistically unreliable.

Black Neonatal Death Rate in 2007

National Rate = 8.7 Black Neonatal Deaths per 1,000 Black Live Births*

<table>
<tr><td colspan="3">ALPHA ORDER</td><td colspan="3">RANK ORDER</td></tr>
<tr><td>RANK</td><td>STATE</td><td>RATE</td><td>RANK</td><td>STATE</td><td>RATE</td></tr>
<tr><td>13</td><td>Alabama</td><td>9.5</td><td>1</td><td>Missouri</td><td>11.7</td></tr>
<tr><td>NA</td><td>Alaska**</td><td>NA</td><td>2</td><td>Kansas</td><td>11.6</td></tr>
<tr><td>11</td><td>Arizona</td><td>10.1</td><td>3</td><td>Virginia</td><td>11.3</td></tr>
<tr><td>19</td><td>Arkansas</td><td>8.6</td><td>4</td><td>Michigan</td><td>11.1</td></tr>
<tr><td>25</td><td>California</td><td>8.0</td><td>5</td><td>Oklahoma</td><td>10.8</td></tr>
<tr><td>23</td><td>Colorado</td><td>8.2</td><td>6</td><td>Nebraska</td><td>10.5</td></tr>
<tr><td>16</td><td>Connecticut</td><td>9.4</td><td>7</td><td>Indiana</td><td>10.4</td></tr>
<tr><td>18</td><td>Delaware</td><td>8.8</td><td>8</td><td>North Carolina</td><td>10.3</td></tr>
<tr><td>28</td><td>Florida</td><td>7.5</td><td>9</td><td>Ohio</td><td>10.2</td></tr>
<tr><td>26</td><td>Georgia</td><td>7.9</td><td>9</td><td>Tennessee</td><td>10.2</td></tr>
<tr><td>NA</td><td>Hawaii**</td><td>NA</td><td>11</td><td>Arizona</td><td>10.1</td></tr>
<tr><td>NA</td><td>Idaho**</td><td>NA</td><td>12</td><td>Maryland</td><td>9.7</td></tr>
<tr><td>13</td><td>Illinois</td><td>9.5</td><td>13</td><td>Alabama</td><td>9.5</td></tr>
<tr><td>7</td><td>Indiana</td><td>10.4</td><td>13</td><td>Illinois</td><td>9.5</td></tr>
<tr><td>NA</td><td>Iowa**</td><td>NA</td><td>13</td><td>Pennsylvania</td><td>9.5</td></tr>
<tr><td>2</td><td>Kansas</td><td>11.6</td><td>16</td><td>Connecticut</td><td>9.4</td></tr>
<tr><td>27</td><td>Kentucky</td><td>7.6</td><td>17</td><td>South Carolina</td><td>9.1</td></tr>
<tr><td>20</td><td>Louisiana</td><td>8.4</td><td>18</td><td>Delaware</td><td>8.8</td></tr>
<tr><td>NA</td><td>Maine**</td><td>NA</td><td>19</td><td>Arkansas</td><td>8.6</td></tr>
<tr><td>12</td><td>Maryland</td><td>9.7</td><td>20</td><td>Louisiana</td><td>8.4</td></tr>
<tr><td>32</td><td>Massachusetts</td><td>6.1</td><td>20</td><td>Mississippi</td><td>8.4</td></tr>
<tr><td>4</td><td>Michigan</td><td>11.1</td><td>22</td><td>Wisconsin</td><td>8.3</td></tr>
<tr><td>30</td><td>Minnesota</td><td>7.1</td><td>23</td><td>Colorado</td><td>8.2</td></tr>
<tr><td>20</td><td>Mississippi</td><td>8.4</td><td>23</td><td>Nevada</td><td>8.2</td></tr>
<tr><td>1</td><td>Missouri</td><td>11.7</td><td>25</td><td>California</td><td>8.0</td></tr>
<tr><td>NA</td><td>Montana**</td><td>NA</td><td>26</td><td>Georgia</td><td>7.9</td></tr>
<tr><td>6</td><td>Nebraska</td><td>10.5</td><td>27</td><td>Kentucky</td><td>7.6</td></tr>
<tr><td>23</td><td>Nevada</td><td>8.2</td><td>28</td><td>Florida</td><td>7.5</td></tr>
<tr><td>NA</td><td>New Hampshire**</td><td>NA</td><td>29</td><td>Texas</td><td>7.4</td></tr>
<tr><td>31</td><td>New Jersey</td><td>6.9</td><td>30</td><td>Minnesota</td><td>7.1</td></tr>
<tr><td>NA</td><td>New Mexico**</td><td>NA</td><td>31</td><td>New Jersey</td><td>6.9</td></tr>
<tr><td>33</td><td>New York</td><td>6.0</td><td>32</td><td>Massachusetts</td><td>6.1</td></tr>
<tr><td>8</td><td>North Carolina</td><td>10.3</td><td>33</td><td>New York</td><td>6.0</td></tr>
<tr><td>NA</td><td>North Dakota**</td><td>NA</td><td>34</td><td>Washington</td><td>5.6</td></tr>
<tr><td>9</td><td>Ohio</td><td>10.2</td><td>NA</td><td>Alaska**</td><td>NA</td></tr>
<tr><td>5</td><td>Oklahoma</td><td>10.8</td><td>NA</td><td>Hawaii**</td><td>NA</td></tr>
<tr><td>NA</td><td>Oregon**</td><td>NA</td><td>NA</td><td>Idaho**</td><td>NA</td></tr>
<tr><td>13</td><td>Pennsylvania</td><td>9.5</td><td>NA</td><td>Iowa**</td><td>NA</td></tr>
<tr><td>NA</td><td>Rhode Island**</td><td>NA</td><td>NA</td><td>Maine**</td><td>NA</td></tr>
<tr><td>17</td><td>South Carolina</td><td>9.1</td><td>NA</td><td>Montana**</td><td>NA</td></tr>
<tr><td>NA</td><td>South Dakota**</td><td>NA</td><td>NA</td><td>New Hampshire**</td><td>NA</td></tr>
<tr><td>9</td><td>Tennessee</td><td>10.2</td><td>NA</td><td>New Mexico**</td><td>NA</td></tr>
<tr><td>29</td><td>Texas</td><td>7.4</td><td>NA</td><td>North Dakota**</td><td>NA</td></tr>
<tr><td>NA</td><td>Utah**</td><td>NA</td><td>NA</td><td>Oregon**</td><td>NA</td></tr>
<tr><td>NA</td><td>Vermont**</td><td>NA</td><td>NA</td><td>Rhode Island**</td><td>NA</td></tr>
<tr><td>3</td><td>Virginia</td><td>11.3</td><td>NA</td><td>South Dakota**</td><td>NA</td></tr>
<tr><td>34</td><td>Washington</td><td>5.6</td><td>NA</td><td>Utah**</td><td>NA</td></tr>
<tr><td>NA</td><td>West Virginia**</td><td>NA</td><td>NA</td><td>Vermont**</td><td>NA</td></tr>
<tr><td>22</td><td>Wisconsin</td><td>8.3</td><td>NA</td><td>West Virginia**</td><td>NA</td></tr>
<tr><td>NA</td><td>Wyoming**</td><td>NA</td><td>NA</td><td>Wyoming**</td><td>NA</td></tr>
<tr><td></td><td></td><td></td><td></td><td>District of Columbia</td><td>12.6</td></tr>
</table>

Source: U.S. Department of Health and Human Services, National Center for Health Statistics
"National Vital Statistics Reports" (Vol. 58, No. 19, May 20, 2010, http://www.cdc.gov/nchs/deaths.htm)
*Final data. Deaths of infants under 28 days old, exclusive of fetal deaths. Based on race of the mother.
**With fewer than 20 deaths, the rate would be considered statistically unreliable.

Estimated Deaths by Cancer in 2010

National Estimated Total = 569,490 Deaths

ALPHA ORDER

RANK	STATE	DEATHS	% of USA
21	Alabama	10,150	1.8%
50	Alaska	880	0.2%
19	Arizona	10,630	1.9%
30	Arkansas	6,460	1.1%
1	California	55,710	9.8%
28	Colorado	6,880	1.2%
29	Connecticut	6,850	1.2%
45	Delaware	1,900	0.3%
2	Florida	40,880	7.2%
11	Georgia	15,570	2.7%
42	Hawaii	2,330	0.4%
41	Idaho	2,530	0.4%
7	Illinois	23,360	4.1%
15	Indiana	12,900	2.3%
31	Iowa	6,370	1.1%
33	Kansas	5,370	0.9%
22	Kentucky	9,670	1.7%
25	Louisiana	8,480	1.5%
38	Maine	3,170	0.6%
20	Maryland	10,250	1.8%
14	Massachusetts	12,990	2.3%
8	Michigan	20,740	3.6%
23	Minnesota	9,200	1.6%
32	Mississippi	6,060	1.1%
16	Missouri	12,620	2.2%
44	Montana	1,980	0.3%
36	Nebraska	3,500	0.6%
35	Nevada	4,640	0.8%
40	New Hampshire	2,660	0.5%
10	New Jersey	16,520	2.9%
37	New Mexico	3,400	0.6%
4	New York	34,540	6.1%
9	North Carolina	19,100	3.4%
47	North Dakota	1,280	0.2%
6	Ohio	24,980	4.4%
26	Oklahoma	7,660	1.3%
27	Oregon	7,510	1.3%
5	Pennsylvania	28,690	5.0%
43	Rhode Island	2,170	0.4%
24	South Carolina	9,180	1.6%
46	South Dakota	1,670	0.3%
13	Tennessee	13,600	2.4%
3	Texas	36,540	6.4%
39	Utah	2,820	0.5%
47	Vermont	1,280	0.2%
12	Virginia	14,230	2.5%
17	Washington	11,640	2.0%
34	West Virginia	4,670	0.8%
18	Wisconsin	11,310	2.0%
49	Wyoming	1,000	0.2%

RANK ORDER

RANK	STATE	DEATHS	% of USA
1	California	55,710	9.8%
2	Florida	40,880	7.2%
3	Texas	36,540	6.4%
4	New York	34,540	6.1%
5	Pennsylvania	28,690	5.0%
6	Ohio	24,980	4.4%
7	Illinois	23,360	4.1%
8	Michigan	20,740	3.6%
9	North Carolina	19,100	3.4%
10	New Jersey	16,520	2.9%
11	Georgia	15,570	2.7%
12	Virginia	14,230	2.5%
13	Tennessee	13,600	2.4%
14	Massachusetts	12,990	2.3%
15	Indiana	12,900	2.3%
16	Missouri	12,620	2.2%
17	Washington	11,640	2.0%
18	Wisconsin	11,310	2.0%
19	Arizona	10,630	1.9%
20	Maryland	10,250	1.8%
21	Alabama	10,150	1.8%
22	Kentucky	9,670	1.7%
23	Minnesota	9,200	1.6%
24	South Carolina	9,180	1.6%
25	Louisiana	8,480	1.5%
26	Oklahoma	7,660	1.3%
27	Oregon	7,510	1.3%
28	Colorado	6,880	1.2%
29	Connecticut	6,850	1.2%
30	Arkansas	6,460	1.1%
31	Iowa	6,370	1.1%
32	Mississippi	6,060	1.1%
33	Kansas	5,370	0.9%
34	West Virginia	4,670	0.8%
35	Nevada	4,640	0.8%
36	Nebraska	3,500	0.6%
37	New Mexico	3,400	0.6%
38	Maine	3,170	0.6%
39	Utah	2,820	0.5%
40	New Hampshire	2,660	0.5%
41	Idaho	2,530	0.4%
42	Hawaii	2,330	0.4%
43	Rhode Island	2,170	0.4%
44	Montana	1,980	0.3%
45	Delaware	1,900	0.3%
46	South Dakota	1,670	0.3%
47	North Dakota	1,280	0.2%
47	Vermont	1,280	0.2%
49	Wyoming	1,000	0.2%
50	Alaska	880	0.2%
	District of Columbia	960	0.2%

Estimated Death Rate by Cancer in 2010

National Estimated Rate = 185.5 Deaths per 100,000 Population*

ALPHA ORDER

RANK	STATE	RATE
9	Alabama	215.6
49	Alaska	126.0
44	Arizona	161.2
5	Arkansas	223.6
46	California	150.7
48	Colorado	136.9
29	Connecticut	194.7
10	Delaware	214.7
6	Florida	220.5
45	Georgia	158.4
36	Hawaii	179.9
43	Idaho	163.7
34	Illinois	180.9
22	Indiana	200.8
11	Iowa	211.8
30	Kansas	190.5
4	Kentucky	224.1
32	Louisiana	188.8
2	Maine	240.5
37	Maryland	179.8
26	Massachusetts	197.0
13	Michigan	208.0
40	Minnesota	174.7
18	Mississippi	205.3
12	Missouri	210.8
20	Montana	203.1
28	Nebraska	194.8
39	Nevada	175.6
22	New Hampshire	200.8
31	New Jersey	189.7
42	New Mexico	169.2
38	New York	176.8
19	North Carolina	203.6
25	North Dakota	197.9
7	Ohio	216.4
14	Oklahoma	207.8
27	Oregon	196.3
3	Pennsylvania	227.6
15	Rhode Island	206.0
21	South Carolina	201.3
17	South Dakota	205.6
8	Tennessee	216.0
47	Texas	147.4
50	Utah	101.3
16	Vermont	205.9
35	Virginia	180.5
40	Washington	174.7
1	West Virginia	256.6
24	Wisconsin	200.0
33	Wyoming	183.7

RANK ORDER

RANK	STATE	RATE
1	West Virginia	256.6
2	Maine	240.5
3	Pennsylvania	227.6
4	Kentucky	224.1
5	Arkansas	223.6
6	Florida	220.5
7	Ohio	216.4
8	Tennessee	216.0
9	Alabama	215.6
10	Delaware	214.7
11	Iowa	211.8
12	Missouri	210.8
13	Michigan	208.0
14	Oklahoma	207.8
15	Rhode Island	206.0
16	Vermont	205.9
17	South Dakota	205.6
18	Mississippi	205.3
19	North Carolina	203.6
20	Montana	203.1
21	South Carolina	201.3
22	Indiana	200.8
22	New Hampshire	200.8
24	Wisconsin	200.0
25	North Dakota	197.9
26	Massachusetts	197.0
27	Oregon	196.3
28	Nebraska	194.8
29	Connecticut	194.7
30	Kansas	190.5
31	New Jersey	189.7
32	Louisiana	188.8
33	Wyoming	183.7
34	Illinois	180.9
35	Virginia	180.5
36	Hawaii	179.9
37	Maryland	179.8
38	New York	176.8
39	Nevada	175.6
40	Minnesota	174.7
40	Washington	174.7
42	New Mexico	169.2
43	Idaho	163.7
44	Arizona	161.2
45	Georgia	158.4
46	California	150.7
47	Texas	147.4
48	Colorado	136.9
49	Alaska	126.0
50	Utah	101.3
	District of Columbia	160.1

Source: CQ Press using data from American Cancer Society
"Cancer Facts & Figures 2010" (Copyright 2010, American Cancer Society, http://www.cancer.org/docroot/stt/stt_0.asp)
*Rates calculated using 2009 Census resident population estimates. Not age-adjusted.

Age-Adjusted Death Rate by Cancer for Males in 2006

National Rate = 229.9 Deaths per 100,000 Male Population*

ALPHA ORDER

RANK	STATE	RATE
5	Alabama	267.7
36	Alaska	217.0
47	Arizona	196.9
7	Arkansas	261.6
45	California	202.2
48	Colorado	196.0
30	Connecticut	223.4
15	Delaware	246.0
39	Florida	215.2
16	Georgia	245.9
49	Hawaii	186.2
44	Idaho	205.5
19	Illinois	240.5
9	Indiana	253.0
25	Iowa	229.1
27	Kansas	227.1
1	Kentucky	280.7
3	Louisiana	278.6
11	Maine	251.3
21	Maryland	236.8
23	Massachusetts	235.4
22	Michigan	236.2
38	Minnesota	215.4
2	Mississippi	280.1
12	Missouri	249.4
40	Montana	214.9
34	Nebraska	220.5
31	Nevada	223.3
24	New Hampshire	233.2
28	New Jersey	226.7
46	New Mexico	199.2
42	New York	211.7
13	North Carolina	248.3
41	North Dakota	214.1
10	Ohio	251.9
14	Oklahoma	247.6
32	Oregon	223.2
17	Pennsylvania	243.2
20	Rhode Island	240.4
8	South Carolina	256.2
33	South Dakota	221.8
4	Tennessee	268.0
26	Texas	227.3
50	Utah	167.0
37	Vermont	216.2
18	Virginia	241.4
35	Washington	217.3
6	West Virginia	263.1
29	Wisconsin	226.3
43	Wyoming	206.7

RANK ORDER

RANK	STATE	RATE
1	Kentucky	280.7
2	Mississippi	280.1
3	Louisiana	278.6
4	Tennessee	268.0
5	Alabama	267.7
6	West Virginia	263.1
7	Arkansas	261.6
8	South Carolina	256.2
9	Indiana	253.0
10	Ohio	251.9
11	Maine	251.3
12	Missouri	249.4
13	North Carolina	248.3
14	Oklahoma	247.6
15	Delaware	246.0
16	Georgia	245.9
17	Pennsylvania	243.2
18	Virginia	241.4
19	Illinois	240.5
20	Rhode Island	240.4
21	Maryland	236.8
22	Michigan	236.2
23	Massachusetts	235.4
24	New Hampshire	233.2
25	Iowa	229.1
26	Texas	227.3
27	Kansas	227.1
28	New Jersey	226.7
29	Wisconsin	226.3
30	Connecticut	223.4
31	Nevada	223.3
32	Oregon	223.2
33	South Dakota	221.8
34	Nebraska	220.5
35	Washington	217.3
36	Alaska	217.0
37	Vermont	216.2
38	Minnesota	215.4
39	Florida	215.2
40	Montana	214.9
41	North Dakota	214.1
42	New York	211.7
43	Wyoming	206.7
44	Idaho	205.5
45	California	202.2
46	New Mexico	199.2
47	Arizona	196.9
48	Colorado	196.0
49	Hawaii	186.2
50	Utah	167.0
	District of Columbia	270.2

Source: American Cancer Society
"Cancer Facts & Figures 2010" (Copyright 2010, American Cancer Society, http://www.cancer.org/docroot/stt/stt_0.asp)
*For 2002 to 2006. Age-adjusted to the 2000 U.S. standard population.

Age-Adjusted Death Rate by Cancer for Females in 2006

National Rate = 157.8 Deaths per 100,000 Female Population*

ALPHA ORDER

RANK	STATE	RATE
22	Alabama	161.5
32	Alaska	155.2
48	Arizona	138.4
17	Arkansas	165.2
44	California	147.6
46	Colorado	142.3
29	Connecticut	156.8
13	Delaware	165.8
43	Florida	147.9
33	Georgia	155.1
49	Hawaii	122.4
45	Idaho	146.2
15	Illinois	165.3
6	Indiana	170.1
35	Iowa	154.6
31	Kansas	156.5
1	Kentucky	178.7
3	Louisiana	175.8
4	Maine	172.4
15	Maryland	165.3
20	Massachusetts	163.5
18	Michigan	164.9
38	Minnesota	151.7
12	Mississippi	166.0
9	Missouri	167.1
25	Montana	160.0
40	Nebraska	149.7
8	Nevada	168.2
21	New Hampshire	163.1
11	New Jersey	166.2
47	New Mexico	140.2
37	New York	153.9
27	North Carolina	158.9
41	North Dakota	149.3
5	Ohio	170.2
19	Oklahoma	163.7
14	Oregon	165.5
10	Pennsylvania	166.3
23	Rhode Island	161.2
28	South Carolina	158.3
42	South Dakota	148.1
7	Tennessee	169.5
39	Texas	150.3
50	Utah	118.7
33	Vermont	155.1
26	Virginia	159.9
24	Washington	160.2
2	West Virginia	175.9
30	Wisconsin	156.6
36	Wyoming	154.4

RANK ORDER

RANK	STATE	RATE
1	Kentucky	178.7
2	West Virginia	175.9
3	Louisiana	175.8
4	Maine	172.4
5	Ohio	170.2
6	Indiana	170.1
7	Tennessee	169.5
8	Nevada	168.2
9	Missouri	167.1
10	Pennsylvania	166.3
11	New Jersey	166.2
12	Mississippi	166.0
13	Delaware	165.8
14	Oregon	165.5
15	Illinois	165.3
15	Maryland	165.3
17	Arkansas	165.2
18	Michigan	164.9
19	Oklahoma	163.7
20	Massachusetts	163.5
21	New Hampshire	163.1
22	Alabama	161.5
23	Rhode Island	161.2
24	Washington	160.2
25	Montana	160.0
26	Virginia	159.9
27	North Carolina	158.9
28	South Carolina	158.3
29	Connecticut	156.8
30	Wisconsin	156.6
31	Kansas	156.5
32	Alaska	155.2
33	Georgia	155.1
33	Vermont	155.1
35	Iowa	154.6
36	Wyoming	154.4
37	New York	153.9
38	Minnesota	151.7
39	Texas	150.3
40	Nebraska	149.7
41	North Dakota	149.3
42	South Dakota	148.1
43	Florida	147.9
44	California	147.6
45	Idaho	146.2
46	Colorado	142.3
47	New Mexico	140.2
48	Arizona	138.4
49	Hawaii	122.4
50	Utah	118.7
	District of Columbia	164.3

Source: American Cancer Society
"Cancer Facts & Figures 2010" (Copyright 2010, American Cancer Society, http://www.cancer.org/docroot/stt/stt_0.asp)
*For 2002 to 2006. Age-adjusted to the 2000 U.S. standard population.

Estimated Deaths by Brain Cancer in 2010

National Estimated Total = 13,140 Deaths

ALPHA ORDER

RANK	STATE	DEATHS	% of USA
21	Alabama	210	1.6%
NA	Alaska*	NA	NA
16	Arizona	280	2.1%
30	Arkansas	150	1.1%
1	California	1,490	11.3%
21	Colorado	210	1.6%
30	Connecticut	150	1.1%
NA	Delaware*	NA	NA
3	Florida	800	6.1%
11	Georgia	340	2.6%
NA	Hawaii*	NA	NA
38	Idaho	80	0.6%
8	Illinois	470	3.6%
11	Indiana	340	2.6%
28	Iowa	170	1.3%
32	Kansas	140	1.1%
27	Kentucky	180	1.4%
21	Louisiana	210	1.6%
38	Maine	80	0.6%
21	Maryland	210	1.6%
16	Massachusetts	280	2.1%
7	Michigan	500	3.8%
20	Minnesota	240	1.8%
33	Mississippi	130	1.0%
16	Missouri	280	2.1%
42	Montana	60	0.5%
37	Nebraska	90	0.7%
34	Nevada	120	0.9%
41	New Hampshire	70	0.5%
11	New Jersey	340	2.6%
38	New Mexico	80	0.6%
3	New York	800	6.1%
10	North Carolina	350	2.7%
NA	North Dakota*	NA	NA
6	Ohio	540	4.1%
28	Oklahoma	170	1.3%
21	Oregon	210	1.6%
5	Pennsylvania	550	4.2%
43	Rhode Island	50	0.4%
26	South Carolina	200	1.5%
NA	South Dakota*	NA	NA
11	Tennessee	340	2.6%
2	Texas	840	6.4%
35	Utah	100	0.8%
NA	Vermont*	NA	NA
15	Virginia	300	2.3%
9	Washington	370	2.8%
35	West Virginia	100	0.8%
19	Wisconsin	270	2.1%
NA	Wyoming*	NA	NA

RANK ORDER

RANK	STATE	DEATHS	% of USA
1	California	1,490	11.3%
2	Texas	840	6.4%
3	Florida	800	6.1%
3	New York	800	6.1%
5	Pennsylvania	550	4.2%
6	Ohio	540	4.1%
7	Michigan	500	3.8%
8	Illinois	470	3.6%
9	Washington	370	2.8%
10	North Carolina	350	2.7%
11	Georgia	340	2.6%
11	Indiana	340	2.6%
11	New Jersey	340	2.6%
11	Tennessee	340	2.6%
15	Virginia	300	2.3%
16	Arizona	280	2.1%
16	Massachusetts	280	2.1%
16	Missouri	280	2.1%
19	Wisconsin	270	2.1%
20	Minnesota	240	1.8%
21	Alabama	210	1.6%
21	Colorado	210	1.6%
21	Louisiana	210	1.6%
21	Maryland	210	1.6%
21	Oregon	210	1.6%
26	South Carolina	200	1.5%
27	Kentucky	180	1.4%
28	Iowa	170	1.3%
28	Oklahoma	170	1.3%
30	Arkansas	150	1.1%
30	Connecticut	150	1.1%
32	Kansas	140	1.1%
33	Mississippi	130	1.0%
34	Nevada	120	0.9%
35	Utah	100	0.8%
35	West Virginia	100	0.8%
37	Nebraska	90	0.7%
38	Idaho	80	0.6%
38	Maine	80	0.6%
38	New Mexico	80	0.6%
41	New Hampshire	70	0.5%
42	Montana	60	0.5%
43	Rhode Island	50	0.4%
NA	Alaska*	NA	NA
NA	Delaware*	NA	NA
NA	Hawaii*	NA	NA
NA	North Dakota*	NA	NA
NA	South Dakota*	NA	NA
NA	Vermont*	NA	NA
NA	Wyoming*	NA	NA
	District of Columbia	80	0.6%

Source: American Cancer Society
"Cancer Facts & Figures 2010" (Copyright 2010, American Cancer Society, http://www.cancer.org/docroot/stt/stt_0.asp)
*Fewer than 50 deaths.

Estimated Death Rate by Brain Cancer in 2010

National Estimated Rate = 4.3 Deaths per 100,000 Population*

ALPHA ORDER			RANK ORDER		
RANK	STATE	RATE	RANK	STATE	RATE
22	Alabama	4.5	1	Montana	6.2
NA	Alaska**	NA	2	Maine	6.1
29	Arizona	4.2	3	Iowa	5.7
10	Arkansas	5.2	4	Washington	5.6
34	California	4.0	5	Oregon	5.5
29	Colorado	4.2	5	West Virginia	5.5
27	Connecticut	4.3	7	Tennessee	5.4
NA	Delaware**	NA	8	Indiana	5.3
27	Florida	4.3	8	New Hampshire	5.3
42	Georgia	3.5	10	Arkansas	5.2
NA	Hawaii**	NA	10	Idaho	5.2
10	Idaho	5.2	12	Kansas	5.0
40	Illinois	3.6	12	Michigan	5.0
8	Indiana	5.3	12	Nebraska	5.0
3	Iowa	5.7	15	Wisconsin	4.8
12	Kansas	5.0	16	Louisiana	4.7
29	Kentucky	4.2	16	Missouri	4.7
16	Louisiana	4.7	16	Ohio	4.7
2	Maine	6.1	16	Rhode Island	4.7
38	Maryland	3.7	20	Minnesota	4.6
29	Massachusetts	4.2	20	Oklahoma	4.6
12	Michigan	5.0	22	Alabama	4.5
20	Minnesota	4.6	22	Nevada	4.5
24	Mississippi	4.4	24	Mississippi	4.4
16	Missouri	4.7	24	Pennsylvania	4.4
1	Montana	6.2	24	South Carolina	4.4
12	Nebraska	5.0	27	Connecticut	4.3
22	Nevada	4.5	27	Florida	4.3
8	New Hampshire	5.3	29	Arizona	4.2
36	New Jersey	3.9	29	Colorado	4.2
34	New Mexico	4.0	29	Kentucky	4.2
33	New York	4.1	29	Massachusetts	4.2
38	North Carolina	3.7	33	New York	4.1
NA	North Dakota**	NA	34	California	4.0
16	Ohio	4.7	34	New Mexico	4.0
20	Oklahoma	4.6	36	New Jersey	3.9
5	Oregon	5.5	37	Virginia	3.8
24	Pennsylvania	4.4	38	Maryland	3.7
16	Rhode Island	4.7	38	North Carolina	3.7
24	South Carolina	4.4	40	Illinois	3.6
NA	South Dakota**	NA	40	Utah	3.6
7	Tennessee	5.4	42	Georgia	3.5
43	Texas	3.4	43	Texas	3.4
40	Utah	3.6	NA	Alaska**	NA
NA	Vermont**	NA	NA	Delaware**	NA
37	Virginia	3.8	NA	Hawaii**	NA
4	Washington	5.6	NA	North Dakota**	NA
5	West Virginia	5.5	NA	South Dakota**	NA
15	Wisconsin	4.8	NA	Vermont**	NA
NA	Wyoming**	NA	NA	Wyoming**	NA
				District of Columbia	13.3

Source: CQ Press using data from American Cancer Society
    "Cancer Facts & Figures 2010" (Copyright 2010, American Cancer Society, http://www.cancer.org/docroot/stt/stt_0.asp)
*Rates calculated using 2009 Census resident population estimates. Not age-adjusted.
**Fewer than 50 deaths.

Estimated Deaths by Female Breast Cancer in 2010

National Estimated Total = 39,840 Deaths

ALPHA ORDER				RANK ORDER			
RANK	STATE	DEATHS	% of USA	RANK	STATE	DEATHS	% of USA
20	Alabama	690	1.7%	1	California	4,230	10.6%
49	Alaska	70	0.2%	2	Texas	2,780	7.0%
19	Arizona	740	1.9%	3	Florida	2,650	6.7%
30	Arkansas	430	1.1%	4	New York	2,490	6.3%
1	California	4,230	10.6%	5	Pennsylvania	1,980	5.0%
27	Colorado	500	1.3%	6	Illinois	1,790	4.5%
28	Connecticut	490	1.2%	7	Ohio	1,730	4.3%
44	Delaware	120	0.3%	8	New Jersey	1,430	3.6%
3	Florida	2,650	6.7%	9	North Carolina	1,340	3.4%
12	Georgia	1,100	2.8%	10	Michigan	1,320	3.3%
42	Hawaii	140	0.4%	11	Virginia	1,120	2.8%
41	Idaho	160	0.4%	12	Georgia	1,100	2.8%
6	Illinois	1,790	4.5%	13	Tennessee	890	2.2%
14	Indiana	860	2.2%	14	Indiana	860	2.2%
32	Iowa	380	1.0%	14	Missouri	860	2.2%
33	Kansas	370	0.9%	16	Maryland	800	2.0%
25	Kentucky	580	1.5%	17	Washington	790	2.0%
23	Louisiana	620	1.6%	18	Massachusetts	780	2.0%
40	Maine	170	0.4%	19	Arizona	740	1.9%
16	Maryland	800	2.0%	20	Alabama	690	1.7%
18	Massachusetts	780	2.0%	20	Wisconsin	690	1.7%
10	Michigan	1,320	3.3%	22	South Carolina	640	1.6%
24	Minnesota	610	1.5%	23	Louisiana	620	1.6%
31	Mississippi	400	1.0%	24	Minnesota	610	1.5%
14	Missouri	860	2.2%	25	Kentucky	580	1.5%
45	Montana	110	0.3%	26	Oklahoma	520	1.3%
38	Nebraska	210	0.5%	27	Colorado	500	1.3%
34	Nevada	330	0.8%	28	Connecticut	490	1.2%
39	New Hampshire	190	0.5%	28	Oregon	490	1.2%
8	New Jersey	1,430	3.6%	30	Arkansas	430	1.1%
37	New Mexico	230	0.6%	31	Mississippi	400	1.0%
4	New York	2,490	6.3%	32	Iowa	380	1.0%
9	North Carolina	1,340	3.4%	33	Kansas	370	0.9%
48	North Dakota	80	0.2%	34	Nevada	330	0.8%
7	Ohio	1,730	4.3%	35	West Virginia	270	0.7%
26	Oklahoma	520	1.3%	36	Utah	250	0.6%
28	Oregon	490	1.2%	37	New Mexico	230	0.6%
5	Pennsylvania	1,980	5.0%	38	Nebraska	210	0.5%
43	Rhode Island	130	0.3%	39	New Hampshire	190	0.5%
22	South Carolina	640	1.6%	40	Maine	170	0.4%
46	South Dakota	100	0.3%	41	Idaho	160	0.4%
13	Tennessee	890	2.2%	42	Hawaii	140	0.4%
2	Texas	2,780	7.0%	43	Rhode Island	130	0.3%
36	Utah	250	0.6%	44	Delaware	120	0.3%
47	Vermont	90	0.2%	45	Montana	110	0.3%
11	Virginia	1,120	2.8%	46	South Dakota	100	0.3%
17	Washington	790	2.0%	47	Vermont	90	0.2%
35	West Virginia	270	0.7%	48	North Dakota	80	0.2%
20	Wisconsin	690	1.7%	49	Alaska	70	0.2%
50	Wyoming	60	0.2%	50	Wyoming	60	0.2%
					District of Columbia	80	0.2%

Source: American Cancer Society
"Cancer Facts & Figures 2010" (Copyright 2010, American Cancer Society, http://www.cancer.org/docroot/stt/stt_0.asp)

Age-Adjusted Death Rate by Female Breast Cancer in 2006

National Rate = 24.5 Deaths per 100,000 Female Population*

ALPHA ORDER

RANK	STATE	RATE
11	Alabama	25.1
49	Alaska	21.7
48	Arizona	21.8
24	Arkansas	24.3
34	California	23.2
45	Colorado	22.2
21	Connecticut	24.4
26	Delaware	24.0
42	Florida	22.6
20	Georgia	24.5
50	Hawaii	17.7
44	Idaho	22.3
10	Illinois	25.7
16	Indiana	24.8
38	Iowa	22.9
19	Kansas	24.6
16	Kentucky	24.8
1	Louisiana	28.9
29	Maine	23.4
4	Maryland	26.8
25	Massachusetts	24.2
11	Michigan	25.1
45	Minnesota	22.2
5	Mississippi	26.4
7	Missouri	26.3
35	Montana	23.1
38	Nebraska	22.9
21	Nevada	24.4
32	New Hampshire	23.3
2	New Jersey	27.4
43	New Mexico	22.5
18	New York	24.7
11	North Carolina	25.1
37	North Dakota	23.0
3	Ohio	27.1
11	Oklahoma	25.1
27	Oregon	23.9
5	Pennsylvania	26.4
35	Rhode Island	23.1
15	South Carolina	25.0
38	South Dakota	22.9
9	Tennessee	25.9
29	Texas	23.4
28	Utah	23.8
38	Vermont	22.9
8	Virginia	26.0
32	Washington	23.3
21	West Virginia	24.4
29	Wisconsin	23.4
47	Wyoming	22.0

RANK ORDER

RANK	STATE	RATE
1	Louisiana	28.9
2	New Jersey	27.4
3	Ohio	27.1
4	Maryland	26.8
5	Mississippi	26.4
5	Pennsylvania	26.4
7	Missouri	26.3
8	Virginia	26.0
9	Tennessee	25.9
10	Illinois	25.7
11	Alabama	25.1
11	Michigan	25.1
11	North Carolina	25.1
11	Oklahoma	25.1
15	South Carolina	25.0
16	Indiana	24.8
16	Kentucky	24.8
18	New York	24.7
19	Kansas	24.6
20	Georgia	24.5
21	Connecticut	24.4
21	Nevada	24.4
21	West Virginia	24.4
24	Arkansas	24.3
25	Massachusetts	24.2
26	Delaware	24.0
27	Oregon	23.9
28	Utah	23.8
29	Maine	23.4
29	Texas	23.4
29	Wisconsin	23.4
32	New Hampshire	23.3
32	Washington	23.3
34	California	23.2
35	Montana	23.1
35	Rhode Island	23.1
37	North Dakota	23.0
38	Iowa	22.9
38	Nebraska	22.9
38	South Dakota	22.9
38	Vermont	22.9
42	Florida	22.6
43	New Mexico	22.5
44	Idaho	22.3
45	Colorado	22.2
45	Minnesota	22.2
47	Wyoming	22.0
48	Arizona	21.8
49	Alaska	21.7
50	Hawaii	17.7

	District of Columbia	28.9

Source: American Cancer Society
"Cancer Facts & Figures 2010" (Copyright 2010, American Cancer Society, http://www.cancer.org/docroot/stt/stt_0.asp)
*For 2002 to 2006. Age-adjusted to the 2000 U.S. standard population.

Estimated Deaths by Colon and Rectum Cancer in 2010

National Estimated Total = 51,370 Deaths

ALPHA ORDER

RANK	STATE	DEATHS	% of USA
19	Alabama	950	1.8%
50	Alaska	80	0.2%
17	Arizona	1,020	2.0%
31	Arkansas	600	1.2%
1	California	4,970	9.7%
28	Colorado	660	1.3%
32	Connecticut	540	1.1%
44	Delaware	160	0.3%
2	Florida	3,540	6.9%
11	Georgia	1,430	2.8%
40	Hawaii	220	0.4%
40	Idaho	220	0.4%
6	Illinois	2,310	4.5%
14	Indiana	1,130	2.2%
30	Iowa	620	1.2%
33	Kansas	530	1.0%
23	Kentucky	880	1.7%
21	Louisiana	920	1.8%
38	Maine	270	0.5%
19	Maryland	950	1.8%
16	Massachusetts	1,050	2.0%
8	Michigan	1,740	3.4%
24	Minnesota	780	1.5%
29	Mississippi	630	1.2%
15	Missouri	1,120	2.2%
43	Montana	170	0.3%
36	Nebraska	360	0.7%
33	Nevada	530	1.0%
42	New Hampshire	210	0.4%
9	New Jersey	1,600	3.1%
37	New Mexico	340	0.7%
4	New York	3,120	6.1%
10	North Carolina	1,520	3.0%
47	North Dakota	120	0.2%
7	Ohio	2,280	4.4%
26	Oklahoma	700	1.4%
27	Oregon	690	1.3%
5	Pennsylvania	2,610	5.1%
46	Rhode Island	150	0.3%
25	South Carolina	770	1.5%
44	South Dakota	160	0.3%
13	Tennessee	1,190	2.3%
3	Texas	3,340	6.5%
39	Utah	250	0.5%
47	Vermont	120	0.2%
12	Virginia	1,300	2.5%
18	Washington	980	1.9%
35	West Virginia	440	0.9%
22	Wisconsin	900	1.8%
49	Wyoming	110	0.2%

RANK ORDER

RANK	STATE	DEATHS	% of USA
1	California	4,970	9.7%
2	Florida	3,540	6.9%
3	Texas	3,340	6.5%
4	New York	3,120	6.1%
5	Pennsylvania	2,610	5.1%
6	Illinois	2,310	4.5%
7	Ohio	2,280	4.4%
8	Michigan	1,740	3.4%
9	New Jersey	1,600	3.1%
10	North Carolina	1,520	3.0%
11	Georgia	1,430	2.8%
12	Virginia	1,300	2.5%
13	Tennessee	1,190	2.3%
14	Indiana	1,130	2.2%
15	Missouri	1,120	2.2%
16	Massachusetts	1,050	2.0%
17	Arizona	1,020	2.0%
18	Washington	980	1.9%
19	Alabama	950	1.8%
19	Maryland	950	1.8%
21	Louisiana	920	1.8%
22	Wisconsin	900	1.8%
23	Kentucky	880	1.7%
24	Minnesota	780	1.5%
25	South Carolina	770	1.5%
26	Oklahoma	700	1.4%
27	Oregon	690	1.3%
28	Colorado	660	1.3%
29	Mississippi	630	1.2%
30	Iowa	620	1.2%
31	Arkansas	600	1.2%
32	Connecticut	540	1.1%
33	Kansas	530	1.0%
33	Nevada	530	1.0%
35	West Virginia	440	0.9%
36	Nebraska	360	0.7%
37	New Mexico	340	0.7%
38	Maine	270	0.5%
39	Utah	250	0.5%
40	Hawaii	220	0.4%
40	Idaho	220	0.4%
42	New Hampshire	210	0.4%
43	Montana	170	0.3%
44	Delaware	160	0.3%
44	South Dakota	160	0.3%
46	Rhode Island	150	0.3%
47	North Dakota	120	0.2%
47	Vermont	120	0.2%
49	Wyoming	110	0.2%
50	Alaska	80	0.2%
	District of Columbia**	NA	NA

Source: American Cancer Society
   "Cancer Facts & Figures 2010" (Copyright 2010, American Cancer Society, http://www.cancer.org/docroot/stt/stt_0.asp)

Estimated Death Rate by Colon and Rectum Cancer in 2010

National Estimated Rate = 16.7 Deaths per 100,000 Population*

ALPHA ORDER				RANK ORDER		
RANK	STATE	RATE		RANK	STATE	RATE
9	Alabama	20.2		1	West Virginia	24.2
49	Alaska	11.5		2	Mississippi	21.3
39	Arizona	15.5		3	Arkansas	20.8
3	Arkansas	20.8		4	Pennsylvania	20.7
47	California	13.4		5	Iowa	20.6
48	Colorado	13.1		6	Louisiana	20.5
40	Connecticut	15.3		6	Maine	20.5
23	Delaware	18.1		8	Kentucky	20.4
16	Florida	19.1		9	Alabama	20.2
43	Georgia	14.5		9	Wyoming	20.2
29	Hawaii	17.0		11	Nevada	20.1
44	Idaho	14.2		12	Nebraska	20.0
25	Illinois	17.9		13	Ohio	19.8
26	Indiana	17.6		14	South Dakota	19.7
5	Iowa	20.6		15	Vermont	19.3
19	Kansas	18.8		16	Florida	19.1
8	Kentucky	20.4		17	Oklahoma	19.0
6	Louisiana	20.5		18	Tennessee	18.9
6	Maine	20.5		19	Kansas	18.8
32	Maryland	16.7		20	Missouri	18.7
36	Massachusetts	15.9		21	North Dakota	18.6
27	Michigan	17.5		22	New Jersey	18.4
41	Minnesota	14.8		23	Delaware	18.1
2	Mississippi	21.3		24	Oregon	18.0
20	Missouri	18.7		25	Illinois	17.9
28	Montana	17.4		26	Indiana	17.6
12	Nebraska	20.0		27	Michigan	17.5
11	Nevada	20.1		28	Montana	17.4
36	New Hampshire	15.9		29	Hawaii	17.0
22	New Jersey	18.4		30	New Mexico	16.9
30	New Mexico	16.9		30	South Carolina	16.9
35	New York	16.0		32	Maryland	16.7
34	North Carolina	16.2		33	Virginia	16.5
21	North Dakota	18.6		34	North Carolina	16.2
13	Ohio	19.8		35	New York	16.0
17	Oklahoma	19.0		36	Massachusetts	15.9
24	Oregon	18.0		36	New Hampshire	15.9
4	Pennsylvania	20.7		36	Wisconsin	15.9
44	Rhode Island	14.2		39	Arizona	15.5
30	South Carolina	16.9		40	Connecticut	15.3
14	South Dakota	19.7		41	Minnesota	14.8
18	Tennessee	18.9		42	Washington	14.7
46	Texas	13.5		43	Georgia	14.5
50	Utah	9.0		44	Idaho	14.2
15	Vermont	19.3		44	Rhode Island	14.2
33	Virginia	16.5		46	Texas	13.5
42	Washington	14.7		47	California	13.4
1	West Virginia	24.2		48	Colorado	13.1
36	Wisconsin	15.9		49	Alaska	11.5
9	Wyoming	20.2		50	Utah	9.0
					District of Columbia**	NA

Source: CQ Press using data from American Cancer Society
"Cancer Facts & Figures 2010" (Copyright 2010, American Cancer Society, http://www.cancer.org/docroot/stt/stt_0.asp)
*Rates calculated using 2009 Census resident population estimates. Not age-adjusted.

Estimated Deaths by Leukemia in 2010

National Estimated Total = 21,840 Deaths

ALPHA ORDER

RANK	STATE	DEATHS	% of USA
22	Alabama	350	1.6%
NA	Alaska*	NA	NA
19	Arizona	420	1.9%
31	Arkansas	240	1.1%
1	California	2,220	10.2%
29	Colorado	270	1.2%
32	Connecticut	230	1.1%
45	Delaware	70	0.3%
2	Florida	1,560	7.1%
11	Georgia	560	2.6%
44	Hawaii	80	0.4%
37	Idaho	120	0.5%
7	Illinois	900	4.1%
13	Indiana	520	2.4%
26	Iowa	300	1.4%
30	Kansas	260	1.2%
24	Kentucky	320	1.5%
25	Louisiana	310	1.4%
39	Maine	110	0.5%
20	Maryland	390	1.8%
18	Massachusetts	470	2.2%
8	Michigan	810	3.7%
20	Minnesota	390	1.8%
32	Mississippi	230	1.1%
12	Missouri	540	2.5%
41	Montana	90	0.4%
35	Nebraska	140	0.6%
39	Nevada	110	0.5%
41	New Hampshire	90	0.4%
10	New Jersey	600	2.7%
37	New Mexico	120	0.5%
4	New York	1,380	6.3%
9	North Carolina	650	3.0%
47	North Dakota	60	0.3%
6	Ohio	930	4.3%
27	Oklahoma	290	1.3%
28	Oregon	280	1.3%
5	Pennsylvania	1,100	5.0%
41	Rhode Island	90	0.4%
23	South Carolina	330	1.5%
45	South Dakota	70	0.3%
15	Tennessee	490	2.2%
3	Texas	1,410	6.5%
35	Utah	140	0.6%
48	Vermont	50	0.2%
14	Virginia	510	2.3%
17	Washington	480	2.2%
34	West Virginia	150	0.7%
15	Wisconsin	490	2.2%
NA	Wyoming*	NA	NA

RANK ORDER

RANK	STATE	DEATHS	% of USA
1	California	2,220	10.2%
2	Florida	1,560	7.1%
3	Texas	1,410	6.5%
4	New York	1,380	6.3%
5	Pennsylvania	1,100	5.0%
6	Ohio	930	4.3%
7	Illinois	900	4.1%
8	Michigan	810	3.7%
9	North Carolina	650	3.0%
10	New Jersey	600	2.7%
11	Georgia	560	2.6%
12	Missouri	540	2.5%
13	Indiana	520	2.4%
14	Virginia	510	2.3%
15	Tennessee	490	2.2%
15	Wisconsin	490	2.2%
17	Washington	480	2.2%
18	Massachusetts	470	2.2%
19	Arizona	420	1.9%
20	Maryland	390	1.8%
20	Minnesota	390	1.8%
22	Alabama	350	1.6%
23	South Carolina	330	1.5%
24	Kentucky	320	1.5%
25	Louisiana	310	1.4%
26	Iowa	300	1.4%
27	Oklahoma	290	1.3%
28	Oregon	280	1.3%
29	Colorado	270	1.2%
30	Kansas	260	1.2%
31	Arkansas	240	1.1%
32	Connecticut	230	1.1%
32	Mississippi	230	1.1%
34	West Virginia	150	0.7%
35	Nebraska	140	0.6%
35	Utah	140	0.6%
37	Idaho	120	0.5%
37	New Mexico	120	0.5%
39	Maine	110	0.5%
39	Nevada	110	0.5%
41	Montana	90	0.4%
41	New Hampshire	90	0.4%
41	Rhode Island	90	0.4%
44	Hawaii	80	0.4%
45	Delaware	70	0.3%
45	South Dakota	70	0.3%
47	North Dakota	60	0.3%
48	Vermont	50	0.2%
NA	Alaska*	NA	NA
NA	Wyoming*	NA	NA
	District of Columbia*	NA	NA

Source: American Cancer Society
   "Cancer Facts & Figures 2010" (Copyright 2010, American Cancer Society, http://www.cancer.org/docroot/stt/stt_0.asp)
*Fewer than 50 deaths.

Estimated Death Rate by Leukemia in 2010

National Estimated Rate = 7.1 Deaths per 100,000 Population*

ALPHA ORDER

RANK	STATE	RATE
24	Alabama	7.4
NA	Alaska**	NA
40	Arizona	6.4
11	Arkansas	8.3
42	California	6.0
46	Colorado	5.4
38	Connecticut	6.5
18	Delaware	7.9
10	Florida	8.4
44	Georgia	5.7
41	Hawaii	6.2
20	Idaho	7.8
32	Illinois	7.0
14	Indiana	8.1
1	Iowa	10.0
3	Kansas	9.2
24	Kentucky	7.4
33	Louisiana	6.9
11	Maine	8.3
36	Maryland	6.8
30	Massachusetts	7.1
14	Michigan	8.1
24	Minnesota	7.4
20	Mississippi	7.8
5	Missouri	9.0
3	Montana	9.2
20	Nebraska	7.8
48	Nevada	4.2
36	New Hampshire	6.8
33	New Jersey	6.9
42	New Mexico	6.0
30	New York	7.1
33	North Carolina	6.9
2	North Dakota	9.3
14	Ohio	8.1
18	Oklahoma	7.9
27	Oregon	7.3
6	Pennsylvania	8.7
9	Rhode Island	8.5
28	South Carolina	7.2
8	South Dakota	8.6
20	Tennessee	7.8
44	Texas	5.7
47	Utah	5.0
17	Vermont	8.0
38	Virginia	6.5
28	Washington	7.2
13	West Virginia	8.2
6	Wisconsin	8.7
NA	Wyoming**	NA

RANK ORDER

RANK	STATE	RATE
1	Iowa	10.0
2	North Dakota	9.3
3	Kansas	9.2
3	Montana	9.2
5	Missouri	9.0
6	Pennsylvania	8.7
6	Wisconsin	8.7
8	South Dakota	8.6
9	Rhode Island	8.5
10	Florida	8.4
11	Arkansas	8.3
11	Maine	8.3
13	West Virginia	8.2
14	Indiana	8.1
14	Michigan	8.1
14	Ohio	8.1
17	Vermont	8.0
18	Delaware	7.9
18	Oklahoma	7.9
20	Idaho	7.8
20	Mississippi	7.8
20	Nebraska	7.8
20	Tennessee	7.8
24	Alabama	7.4
24	Kentucky	7.4
24	Minnesota	7.4
27	Oregon	7.3
28	South Carolina	7.2
28	Washington	7.2
30	Massachusetts	7.1
30	New York	7.1
32	Illinois	7.0
33	Louisiana	6.9
33	New Jersey	6.9
33	North Carolina	6.9
36	Maryland	6.8
36	New Hampshire	6.8
38	Connecticut	6.5
38	Virginia	6.5
40	Arizona	6.4
41	Hawaii	6.2
42	California	6.0
42	New Mexico	6.0
44	Georgia	5.7
44	Texas	5.7
46	Colorado	5.4
47	Utah	5.0
48	Nevada	4.2
NA	Alaska**	NA
NA	Wyoming**	NA
	District of Columbia**	NA

Source: CQ Press using data from American Cancer Society
"Cancer Facts & Figures 2010" (Copyright 2010, American Cancer Society, http://www.cancer.org/docroot/stt/stt_0.asp)
*Rates calculated using 2009 Census resident population estimates. Not age-adjusted.
**Fewer than 50 deaths.

Estimated Deaths by Liver Cancer in 2010

National Estimated Total = 18,910 Deaths

ALPHA ORDER					RANK ORDER			
RANK	STATE	DEATHS	% of USA		RANK	STATE	DEATHS	% of USA
22	Alabama	310	1.6%		1	California	2,600	13.7%
NA	Alaska*	NA	NA		2	Texas	1,660	8.8%
15	Arizona	380	2.0%		3	Florida	1,360	7.2%
29	Arkansas	200	1.1%		4	New York	1,270	6.7%
1	California	2,600	13.7%		5	Pennsylvania	840	4.4%
26	Colorado	230	1.2%		6	Illinois	700	3.7%
29	Connecticut	200	1.1%		7	Ohio	680	3.6%
44	Delaware	50	0.3%		8	Michigan	600	3.2%
3	Florida	1,360	7.2%		9	North Carolina	500	2.6%
13	Georgia	430	2.3%		10	New Jersey	470	2.5%
36	Hawaii	120	0.6%		11	Massachusetts	440	2.3%
42	Idaho	70	0.4%		11	Washington	440	2.3%
6	Illinois	700	3.7%		13	Georgia	430	2.3%
19	Indiana	340	1.8%		14	Virginia	410	2.2%
33	Iowa	160	0.8%		15	Arizona	380	2.0%
35	Kansas	140	0.7%		15	Missouri	380	2.0%
25	Kentucky	250	1.3%		15	Tennessee	380	2.0%
19	Louisiana	340	1.8%		18	Maryland	360	1.9%
38	Maine	80	0.4%		19	Indiana	340	1.8%
18	Maryland	360	1.9%		19	Louisiana	340	1.8%
11	Massachusetts	440	2.3%		21	Wisconsin	330	1.7%
8	Michigan	600	3.2%		22	Alabama	310	1.6%
23	Minnesota	280	1.5%		23	Minnesota	280	1.5%
31	Mississippi	190	1.0%		24	South Carolina	270	1.4%
15	Missouri	380	2.0%		25	Kentucky	250	1.3%
44	Montana	50	0.3%		26	Colorado	230	1.2%
38	Nebraska	80	0.4%		26	Oregon	230	1.2%
32	Nevada	180	1.0%		28	Oklahoma	220	1.2%
38	New Hampshire	80	0.4%		29	Arkansas	200	1.1%
10	New Jersey	470	2.5%		29	Connecticut	200	1.1%
34	New Mexico	150	0.8%		31	Mississippi	190	1.0%
4	New York	1,270	6.7%		32	Nevada	180	1.0%
9	North Carolina	500	2.6%		33	Iowa	160	0.8%
NA	North Dakota*	NA	NA		34	New Mexico	150	0.8%
7	Ohio	680	3.6%		35	Kansas	140	0.7%
28	Oklahoma	220	1.2%		36	Hawaii	120	0.6%
26	Oregon	230	1.2%		36	West Virginia	120	0.6%
5	Pennsylvania	840	4.4%		38	Maine	80	0.4%
42	Rhode Island	70	0.4%		38	Nebraska	80	0.4%
24	South Carolina	270	1.4%		38	New Hampshire	80	0.4%
NA	South Dakota*	NA	NA		38	Utah	80	0.4%
15	Tennessee	380	2.0%		42	Idaho	70	0.4%
2	Texas	1,660	8.8%		42	Rhode Island	70	0.4%
38	Utah	80	0.4%		44	Delaware	50	0.3%
NA	Vermont*	NA	NA		44	Montana	50	0.3%
14	Virginia	410	2.2%		NA	Alaska*	NA	NA
11	Washington	440	2.3%		NA	North Dakota*	NA	NA
36	West Virginia	120	0.6%		NA	South Dakota*	NA	NA
21	Wisconsin	330	1.7%		NA	Vermont*	NA	NA
NA	Wyoming*	NA	NA		NA	Wyoming*	NA	NA
					District of Columbia*		NA	NA

Source: American Cancer Society
"Cancer Facts & Figures 2010" (Copyright 2010, American Cancer Society, http://www.cancer.org/docroot/stt/stt_0.asp)
*Fewer than 50 deaths.

Estimated Death Rate by Liver Cancer in 2010

National Estimated Rate = 6.2 Deaths per 100,000 Population*

ALPHA ORDER

RANK	STATE	RATE
11	Alabama	6.6
NA	Alaska**	NA
27	Arizona	5.8
6	Arkansas	6.9
5	California	7.0
41	Colorado	4.6
30	Connecticut	5.7
31	Delaware	5.6
4	Florida	7.3
44	Georgia	4.4
1	Hawaii	9.3
42	Idaho	4.5
32	Illinois	5.4
34	Indiana	5.3
34	Iowa	5.3
40	Kansas	5.0
27	Kentucky	5.8
2	Louisiana	7.6
19	Maine	6.1
17	Maryland	6.3
8	Massachusetts	6.7
20	Michigan	6.0
34	Minnesota	5.3
16	Mississippi	6.4
17	Missouri	6.3
39	Montana	5.1
42	Nebraska	4.5
7	Nevada	6.8
20	New Hampshire	6.0
32	New Jersey	5.4
3	New Mexico	7.5
15	New York	6.5
34	North Carolina	5.3
NA	North Dakota**	NA
25	Ohio	5.9
20	Oklahoma	6.0
20	Oregon	6.0
8	Pennsylvania	6.7
11	Rhode Island	6.6
25	South Carolina	5.9
NA	South Dakota**	NA
20	Tennessee	6.0
8	Texas	6.7
45	Utah	2.9
NA	Vermont**	NA
38	Virginia	5.2
11	Washington	6.6
11	West Virginia	6.6
27	Wisconsin	5.8
NA	Wyoming**	NA

RANK ORDER

RANK	STATE	RATE
1	Hawaii	9.3
2	Louisiana	7.6
3	New Mexico	7.5
4	Florida	7.3
5	California	7.0
6	Arkansas	6.9
7	Nevada	6.8
8	Massachusetts	6.7
8	Pennsylvania	6.7
8	Texas	6.7
11	Alabama	6.6
11	Rhode Island	6.6
11	Washington	6.6
11	West Virginia	6.6
15	New York	6.5
16	Mississippi	6.4
17	Maryland	6.3
17	Missouri	6.3
19	Maine	6.1
20	Michigan	6.0
20	New Hampshire	6.0
20	Oklahoma	6.0
20	Oregon	6.0
20	Tennessee	6.0
25	Ohio	5.9
25	South Carolina	5.9
27	Arizona	5.8
27	Kentucky	5.8
27	Wisconsin	5.8
30	Connecticut	5.7
31	Delaware	5.6
32	Illinois	5.4
32	New Jersey	5.4
34	Indiana	5.3
34	Iowa	5.3
34	Minnesota	5.3
34	North Carolina	5.3
38	Virginia	5.2
39	Montana	5.1
40	Kansas	5.0
41	Colorado	4.6
42	Idaho	4.5
42	Nebraska	4.5
44	Georgia	4.4
45	Utah	2.9
NA	Alaska**	NA
NA	North Dakota**	NA
NA	South Dakota**	NA
NA	Vermont**	NA
NA	Wyoming**	NA
	District of Columbia**	NA

Source: CQ Press using data from American Cancer Society
"Cancer Facts & Figures 2010" (Copyright 2010, American Cancer Society, http://www.cancer.org/docroot/stt/stt_0.asp)
*Rates calculated using 2009 Census resident population estimates. Not age-adjusted.
**Fewer than 50 deaths.

Estimated Deaths by Lung Cancer in 2010

National Estimated Total = 157,300 Deaths

ALPHA ORDER

RANK	STATE	DEATHS	% of USA
18	Alabama	3,190	2.0%
50	Alaska	250	0.2%
23	Arizona	2,670	1.7%
29	Arkansas	1,900	1.2%
1	California	12,630	8.0%
32	Colorado	1,670	1.1%
31	Connecticut	1,760	1.1%
42	Delaware	580	0.4%
2	Florida	11,620	7.4%
10	Georgia	4,620	2.9%
44	Hawaii	570	0.4%
40	Idaho	640	0.4%
7	Illinois	6,490	4.1%
14	Indiana	4,000	2.5%
30	Iowa	1,770	1.1%
33	Kansas	1,590	1.0%
17	Kentucky	3,410	2.2%
24	Louisiana	2,550	1.6%
36	Maine	960	0.6%
22	Maryland	2,760	1.8%
16	Massachusetts	3,530	2.2%
8	Michigan	5,830	3.7%
25	Minnesota	2,450	1.6%
28	Mississippi	2,010	1.3%
15	Missouri	3,950	2.5%
42	Montana	580	0.4%
37	Nebraska	900	0.6%
35	Nevada	1,300	0.8%
39	New Hampshire	750	0.5%
12	New Jersey	4,220	2.7%
38	New Mexico	780	0.5%
4	New York	8,720	5.5%
9	North Carolina	5,650	3.6%
48	North Dakota	320	0.2%
6	Ohio	7,260	4.6%
26	Oklahoma	2,390	1.5%
27	Oregon	2,100	1.3%
5	Pennsylvania	7,960	5.1%
41	Rhode Island	600	0.4%
21	South Carolina	2,870	1.8%
46	South Dakota	450	0.3%
11	Tennessee	4,520	2.9%
3	Texas	9,600	6.1%
45	Utah	480	0.3%
47	Vermont	370	0.2%
13	Virginia	4,050	2.6%
19	Washington	3,110	2.0%
34	West Virginia	1,480	0.9%
20	Wisconsin	2,940	1.9%
49	Wyoming	260	0.2%

RANK ORDER

RANK	STATE	DEATHS	% of USA
1	California	12,630	8.0%
2	Florida	11,620	7.4%
3	Texas	9,600	6.1%
4	New York	8,720	5.5%
5	Pennsylvania	7,960	5.1%
6	Ohio	7,260	4.6%
7	Illinois	6,490	4.1%
8	Michigan	5,830	3.7%
9	North Carolina	5,650	3.6%
10	Georgia	4,620	2.9%
11	Tennessee	4,520	2.9%
12	New Jersey	4,220	2.7%
13	Virginia	4,050	2.6%
14	Indiana	4,000	2.5%
15	Missouri	3,950	2.5%
16	Massachusetts	3,530	2.2%
17	Kentucky	3,410	2.2%
18	Alabama	3,190	2.0%
19	Washington	3,110	2.0%
20	Wisconsin	2,940	1.9%
21	South Carolina	2,870	1.8%
22	Maryland	2,760	1.8%
23	Arizona	2,670	1.7%
24	Louisiana	2,550	1.6%
25	Minnesota	2,450	1.6%
26	Oklahoma	2,390	1.5%
27	Oregon	2,100	1.3%
28	Mississippi	2,010	1.3%
29	Arkansas	1,900	1.2%
30	Iowa	1,770	1.1%
31	Connecticut	1,760	1.1%
32	Colorado	1,670	1.1%
33	Kansas	1,590	1.0%
34	West Virginia	1,480	0.9%
35	Nevada	1,300	0.8%
36	Maine	960	0.6%
37	Nebraska	900	0.6%
38	New Mexico	780	0.5%
39	New Hampshire	750	0.5%
40	Idaho	640	0.4%
41	Rhode Island	600	0.4%
42	Delaware	580	0.4%
42	Montana	580	0.4%
44	Hawaii	570	0.4%
45	Utah	480	0.3%
46	South Dakota	450	0.3%
47	Vermont	370	0.2%
48	North Dakota	320	0.2%
49	Wyoming	260	0.2%
50	Alaska	250	0.2%
	District of Columbia	230	0.1%

Source: American Cancer Society
"Cancer Facts & Figures 2010" (Copyright 2010, American Cancer Society, http://www.cancer.org/docroot/stt/stt_0.asp)

Estimated Death Rate by Lung Cancer in 2010

National Estimated Rate = 51.2 Deaths per 100,000 Population*

ALPHA ORDER

RANK	STATE	RATE
6	Alabama	67.7
47	Alaska	35.8
44	Arizona	40.5
8	Arkansas	65.8
48	California	34.2
49	Colorado	33.2
32	Connecticut	50.0
9	Delaware	65.5
14	Florida	62.7
38	Georgia	47.0
42	Hawaii	44.0
43	Idaho	41.4
30	Illinois	50.3
15	Indiana	62.3
19	Iowa	58.8
24	Kansas	56.4
2	Kentucky	79.0
22	Louisiana	56.8
3	Maine	72.8
36	Maryland	48.4
27	Massachusetts	53.5
20	Michigan	58.5
40	Minnesota	46.5
5	Mississippi	68.1
7	Missouri	66.0
17	Montana	59.5
31	Nebraska	50.1
34	Nevada	49.2
23	New Hampshire	56.6
35	New Jersey	48.5
45	New Mexico	38.8
41	New York	44.6
16	North Carolina	60.2
33	North Dakota	49.5
12	Ohio	62.9
10	Oklahoma	64.8
26	Oregon	54.9
11	Pennsylvania	63.2
21	Rhode Island	57.0
12	South Carolina	62.9
25	South Dakota	55.4
4	Tennessee	71.8
46	Texas	38.7
50	Utah	17.2
17	Vermont	59.5
29	Virginia	51.4
39	Washington	46.7
1	West Virginia	81.3
28	Wisconsin	52.0
37	Wyoming	47.8

RANK ORDER

RANK	STATE	RATE
1	West Virginia	81.3
2	Kentucky	79.0
3	Maine	72.8
4	Tennessee	71.8
5	Mississippi	68.1
6	Alabama	67.7
7	Missouri	66.0
8	Arkansas	65.8
9	Delaware	65.5
10	Oklahoma	64.8
11	Pennsylvania	63.2
12	Ohio	62.9
12	South Carolina	62.9
14	Florida	62.7
15	Indiana	62.3
16	North Carolina	60.2
17	Montana	59.5
17	Vermont	59.5
19	Iowa	58.8
20	Michigan	58.5
21	Rhode Island	57.0
22	Louisiana	56.8
23	New Hampshire	56.6
24	Kansas	56.4
25	South Dakota	55.4
26	Oregon	54.9
27	Massachusetts	53.5
28	Wisconsin	52.0
29	Virginia	51.4
30	Illinois	50.3
31	Nebraska	50.1
32	Connecticut	50.0
33	North Dakota	49.5
34	Nevada	49.2
35	New Jersey	48.5
36	Maryland	48.4
37	Wyoming	47.8
38	Georgia	47.0
39	Washington	46.7
40	Minnesota	46.5
41	New York	44.6
42	Hawaii	44.0
43	Idaho	41.4
44	Arizona	40.5
45	New Mexico	38.8
46	Texas	38.7
47	Alaska	35.8
48	California	34.2
49	Colorado	33.2
50	Utah	17.2
	District of Columbia	38.4

Source: CQ Press using data from American Cancer Society
 "Cancer Facts & Figures 2010" (Copyright 2010, American Cancer Society, http://www.cancer.org/docroot/stt/stt_0.asp)
*Rates calculated using 2009 Census resident population estimates. Not age-adjusted.

Estimated Deaths by Non-Hodgkin's Lymphoma in 2010

National Estimated Total = 20,210 Deaths

ALPHA ORDER

RANK	STATE	DEATHS	% of USA
21	Alabama	320	1.6%
NA	Alaska*	NA	NA
19	Arizona	360	1.8%
31	Arkansas	200	1.0%
1	California	2,110	10.4%
27	Colorado	280	1.4%
30	Connecticut	230	1.1%
44	Delaware	60	0.3%
2	Florida	1,480	7.3%
11	Georgia	500	2.5%
39	Hawaii	90	0.4%
39	Idaho	90	0.4%
7	Illinois	740	3.7%
15	Indiana	440	2.2%
26	Iowa	290	1.4%
31	Kansas	200	1.0%
22	Kentucky	310	1.5%
27	Louisiana	280	1.4%
39	Maine	90	0.4%
22	Maryland	310	1.5%
18	Massachusetts	400	2.0%
8	Michigan	700	3.5%
20	Minnesota	330	1.6%
33	Mississippi	190	0.9%
13	Missouri	450	2.2%
42	Montana	80	0.4%
35	Nebraska	150	0.7%
35	Nevada	150	0.7%
43	New Hampshire	70	0.3%
9	New Jersey	640	3.2%
37	New Mexico	120	0.6%
2	New York	1,480	7.3%
10	North Carolina	570	2.8%
NA	North Dakota*	NA	NA
6	Ohio	840	4.2%
27	Oklahoma	280	1.4%
22	Oregon	310	1.5%
5	Pennsylvania	1,100	5.4%
44	Rhode Island	60	0.3%
25	South Carolina	300	1.5%
44	South Dakota	60	0.3%
12	Tennessee	470	2.3%
4	Texas	1,280	6.3%
38	Utah	100	0.5%
NA	Vermont*	NA	NA
13	Virginia	450	2.2%
15	Washington	440	2.2%
33	West Virginia	190	0.9%
17	Wisconsin	410	2.0%
47	Wyoming	50	0.2%

RANK ORDER

RANK	STATE	DEATHS	% of USA
1	California	2,110	10.4%
2	Florida	1,480	7.3%
2	New York	1,480	7.3%
4	Texas	1,280	6.3%
5	Pennsylvania	1,100	5.4%
6	Ohio	840	4.2%
7	Illinois	740	3.7%
8	Michigan	700	3.5%
9	New Jersey	640	3.2%
10	North Carolina	570	2.8%
11	Georgia	500	2.5%
12	Tennessee	470	2.3%
13	Missouri	450	2.2%
13	Virginia	450	2.2%
15	Indiana	440	2.2%
15	Washington	440	2.2%
17	Wisconsin	410	2.0%
18	Massachusetts	400	2.0%
19	Arizona	360	1.8%
20	Minnesota	330	1.6%
21	Alabama	320	1.6%
22	Kentucky	310	1.5%
22	Maryland	310	1.5%
22	Oregon	310	1.5%
25	South Carolina	300	1.5%
26	Iowa	290	1.4%
27	Colorado	280	1.4%
27	Louisiana	280	1.4%
27	Oklahoma	280	1.4%
30	Connecticut	230	1.1%
31	Arkansas	200	1.0%
31	Kansas	200	1.0%
33	Mississippi	190	0.9%
33	West Virginia	190	0.9%
35	Nebraska	150	0.7%
35	Nevada	150	0.7%
37	New Mexico	120	0.6%
38	Utah	100	0.5%
39	Hawaii	90	0.4%
39	Idaho	90	0.4%
39	Maine	90	0.4%
42	Montana	80	0.4%
43	New Hampshire	70	0.3%
44	Delaware	60	0.3%
44	Rhode Island	60	0.3%
44	South Dakota	60	0.3%
47	Wyoming	50	0.2%
NA	Alaska*	NA	NA
NA	North Dakota*	NA	NA
NA	Vermont*	NA	NA
	District of Columbia*	NA	NA

Source: American Cancer Society
"Cancer Facts & Figures 2010" (Copyright 2010, American Cancer Society, http://www.cancer.org/docroot/stt/stt_0.asp)
*Fewer than 50 deaths.

Estimated Death Rate by Non-Hodgkin's Lymphoma in 2010

National Estimated Rate = 6.6 Deaths per 100,000 Population*

ALPHA ORDER				RANK ORDER		
RANK	STATE	RATE		RANK	STATE	RATE
23	Alabama	6.8		1	West Virginia	10.4
NA	Alaska**	NA		2	Iowa	9.6
42	Arizona	5.5		3	Wyoming	9.2
20	Arkansas	6.9		4	Pennsylvania	8.7
36	California	5.7		5	Nebraska	8.3
41	Colorado	5.6		6	Montana	8.2
28	Connecticut	6.5		7	Oregon	8.1
23	Delaware	6.8		8	Florida	8.0
8	Florida	8.0		9	New York	7.6
46	Georgia	5.1		9	Oklahoma	7.6
20	Hawaii	6.9		11	Missouri	7.5
35	Idaho	5.8		11	Tennessee	7.5
36	Illinois	5.7		13	South Dakota	7.4
20	Indiana	6.9		14	New Jersey	7.3
2	Iowa	9.6		14	Ohio	7.3
18	Kansas	7.1		14	Wisconsin	7.3
17	Kentucky	7.2		17	Kentucky	7.2
31	Louisiana	6.2		18	Kansas	7.1
23	Maine	6.8		19	Michigan	7.0
43	Maryland	5.4		20	Arkansas	6.9
32	Massachusetts	6.1		20	Hawaii	6.9
19	Michigan	7.0		20	Indiana	6.9
30	Minnesota	6.3		23	Alabama	6.8
29	Mississippi	6.4		23	Delaware	6.8
11	Missouri	7.5		23	Maine	6.8
6	Montana	8.2		26	South Carolina	6.6
5	Nebraska	8.3		26	Washington	6.6
36	Nevada	5.7		28	Connecticut	6.5
44	New Hampshire	5.3		29	Mississippi	6.4
14	New Jersey	7.3		30	Minnesota	6.3
34	New Mexico	6.0		31	Louisiana	6.2
9	New York	7.6		32	Massachusetts	6.1
32	North Carolina	6.1		32	North Carolina	6.1
NA	North Dakota**	NA		34	New Mexico	6.0
14	Ohio	7.3		35	Idaho	5.8
9	Oklahoma	7.6		36	California	5.7
7	Oregon	8.1		36	Illinois	5.7
4	Pennsylvania	8.7		36	Nevada	5.7
36	Rhode Island	5.7		36	Rhode Island	5.7
26	South Carolina	6.6		36	Virginia	5.7
13	South Dakota	7.4		41	Colorado	5.6
11	Tennessee	7.5		42	Arizona	5.5
45	Texas	5.2		43	Maryland	5.4
47	Utah	3.6		44	New Hampshire	5.3
NA	Vermont**	NA		45	Texas	5.2
36	Virginia	5.7		46	Georgia	5.1
26	Washington	6.6		47	Utah	3.6
1	West Virginia	10.4		NA	Alaska**	NA
14	Wisconsin	7.3		NA	North Dakota**	NA
3	Wyoming	9.2		NA	Vermont**	NA
				District of Columbia**		NA

Source: CQ Press using data from American Cancer Society
   "Cancer Facts & Figures 2010" (Copyright 2010, American Cancer Society, http://www.cancer.org/docroot/stt/stt_0.asp)
*Rates calculated using 2009 Census resident population estimates. Not age-adjusted.
**Fewer than 50 deaths.

Estimated Deaths by Ovarian Cancer in 2010

National Estimated Total = 13,850 Deaths

ALPHA ORDER

RANK ORDER

RANK	STATE	DEATHS	% of USA		RANK	STATE	DEATHS	% of USA
18	Alabama	260	1.9%		1	California	1,500	10.8%
NA	Alaska*	NA	NA		2	Florida	930	6.7%
16	Arizona	290	2.1%		3	New York	910	6.6%
31	Arkansas	140	1.0%		4	Texas	840	6.1%
1	California	1,500	10.8%		5	Pennsylvania	730	5.3%
24	Colorado	210	1.5%		6	Illinois	570	4.1%
28	Connecticut	180	1.3%		7	Ohio	540	3.9%
NA	Delaware*	NA	NA		8	Michigan	500	3.6%
2	Florida	930	6.7%		9	New Jersey	430	3.1%
10	Georgia	390	2.8%		10	Georgia	390	2.8%
43	Hawaii	50	0.4%		10	North Carolina	390	2.8%
40	Idaho	60	0.4%		12	Virginia	370	2.7%
6	Illinois	570	4.1%		13	Massachusetts	330	2.4%
15	Indiana	300	2.2%		13	Washington	330	2.4%
29	Iowa	170	1.2%		15	Indiana	300	2.2%
31	Kansas	140	1.0%		16	Arizona	290	2.1%
26	Kentucky	200	1.4%		16	Wisconsin	290	2.1%
26	Louisiana	200	1.4%		18	Alabama	260	1.9%
39	Maine	70	0.5%		19	Maryland	250	1.8%
19	Maryland	250	1.8%		19	Missouri	250	1.8%
13	Massachusetts	330	2.4%		19	Tennessee	250	1.8%
8	Michigan	500	3.6%		22	Minnesota	220	1.6%
22	Minnesota	220	1.6%		22	South Carolina	220	1.6%
33	Mississippi	130	0.9%		24	Colorado	210	1.5%
19	Missouri	250	1.8%		24	Oregon	210	1.5%
43	Montana	50	0.4%		26	Kentucky	200	1.4%
36	Nebraska	80	0.6%		26	Louisiana	200	1.4%
34	Nevada	110	0.8%		28	Connecticut	180	1.3%
40	New Hampshire	60	0.4%		29	Iowa	170	1.2%
9	New Jersey	430	3.1%		30	Oklahoma	160	1.2%
36	New Mexico	80	0.6%		31	Arkansas	140	1.0%
3	New York	910	6.6%		31	Kansas	140	1.0%
10	North Carolina	390	2.8%		33	Mississippi	130	0.9%
NA	North Dakota*	NA	NA		34	Nevada	110	0.8%
7	Ohio	540	3.9%		34	West Virginia	110	0.8%
30	Oklahoma	160	1.2%		36	Nebraska	80	0.6%
24	Oregon	210	1.5%		36	New Mexico	80	0.6%
5	Pennsylvania	730	5.3%		36	Utah	80	0.6%
40	Rhode Island	60	0.4%		39	Maine	70	0.5%
22	South Carolina	220	1.6%		40	Idaho	60	0.4%
43	South Dakota	50	0.4%		40	New Hampshire	60	0.4%
19	Tennessee	250	1.8%		40	Rhode Island	60	0.4%
4	Texas	840	6.1%		43	Hawaii	50	0.4%
36	Utah	80	0.6%		43	Montana	50	0.4%
NA	Vermont*	NA	NA		43	South Dakota	50	0.4%
12	Virginia	370	2.7%		NA	Alaska*	NA	NA
13	Washington	330	2.4%		NA	Delaware*	NA	NA
34	West Virginia	110	0.8%		NA	North Dakota*	NA	NA
16	Wisconsin	290	2.1%		NA	Vermont*	NA	NA
NA	Wyoming*	NA	NA		NA	Wyoming*	NA	NA
					District of Columbia*	NA	NA	

Source: American Cancer Society
   "Cancer Facts & Figures 2010" (Copyright 2010, American Cancer Society, http://www.cancer.org/docroot/stt/stt_0.asp)
*Fewer than 50 deaths.

Estimated Death Rate by Ovarian Cancer in 2010

National Estimated Rate = 8.9 Deaths per 100,000 Female Population*

ALPHA ORDER

RANK	STATE	RATE
7	Alabama	10.7
NA	Alaska**	NA
26	Arizona	8.8
18	Arkansas	9.5
37	California	8.1
34	Colorado	8.4
11	Connecticut	10.0
NA	Delaware**	NA
12	Florida	9.9
40	Georgia	7.8
40	Hawaii	7.8
40	Idaho	7.8
28	Illinois	8.7
20	Indiana	9.2
4	Iowa	11.2
12	Kansas	9.9
22	Kentucky	9.1
28	Louisiana	8.7
8	Maine	10.4
31	Maryland	8.5
16	Massachusetts	9.7
12	Michigan	9.9
35	Minnesota	8.3
31	Mississippi	8.5
36	Missouri	8.2
9	Montana	10.3
26	Nebraska	8.8
31	Nevada	8.5
25	New Hampshire	8.9
16	New Jersey	9.7
39	New Mexico	7.9
22	New York	9.1
37	North Carolina	8.1
NA	North Dakota**	NA
22	Ohio	9.1
30	Oklahoma	8.6
6	Oregon	10.9
3	Pennsylvania	11.3
5	Rhode Island	11.1
19	South Carolina	9.4
1	South Dakota	12.3
43	Tennessee	7.7
44	Texas	6.8
45	Utah	5.8
NA	Vermont**	NA
20	Virginia	9.2
12	Washington	9.9
2	West Virginia	11.9
10	Wisconsin	10.2
NA	Wyoming**	NA

RANK ORDER

RANK	STATE	RATE
1	South Dakota	12.3
2	West Virginia	11.9
3	Pennsylvania	11.3
4	Iowa	11.2
5	Rhode Island	11.1
6	Oregon	10.9
7	Alabama	10.7
8	Maine	10.4
9	Montana	10.3
10	Wisconsin	10.2
11	Connecticut	10.0
12	Florida	9.9
12	Kansas	9.9
12	Michigan	9.9
12	Washington	9.9
16	Massachusetts	9.7
16	New Jersey	9.7
18	Arkansas	9.5
19	South Carolina	9.4
20	Indiana	9.2
20	Virginia	9.2
22	Kentucky	9.1
22	New York	9.1
22	Ohio	9.1
25	New Hampshire	8.9
26	Arizona	8.8
26	Nebraska	8.8
28	Illinois	8.7
28	Louisiana	8.7
30	Oklahoma	8.6
31	Maryland	8.5
31	Mississippi	8.5
31	Nevada	8.5
34	Colorado	8.4
35	Minnesota	8.3
36	Missouri	8.2
37	California	8.1
37	North Carolina	8.1
39	New Mexico	7.9
40	Georgia	7.8
40	Hawaii	7.8
40	Idaho	7.8
43	Tennessee	7.7
44	Texas	6.8
45	Utah	5.8
NA	Alaska**	NA
NA	Delaware**	NA
NA	North Dakota**	NA
NA	Vermont**	NA
NA	Wyoming**	NA
	District of Columbia**	NA

Source: CQ Press using data from American Cancer Society
   "Cancer Facts & Figures 2010" (Copyright 2010, American Cancer Society, http://www.cancer.org/docroot/stt/stt_0.asp)
*Rates calculated using 2009 Census female population estimates. Not age-adjusted.
**Fewer than 50 deaths.

Estimated Deaths by Pancreatic Cancer in 2010

National Estimated Total = 36,800 Deaths

ALPHA ORDER

RANK	STATE	DEATHS	% of USA
22	Alabama	590	1.6%
50	Alaska	60	0.2%
18	Arizona	740	2.0%
29	Arkansas	430	1.2%
1	California	3,900	10.6%
28	Colorado	460	1.3%
24	Connecticut	540	1.5%
43	Delaware	120	0.3%
2	Florida	2,560	7.0%
11	Georgia	940	2.6%
42	Hawaii	180	0.5%
40	Idaho	190	0.5%
6	Illinois	1,580	4.3%
14	Indiana	790	2.1%
31	Iowa	380	1.0%
33	Kansas	330	0.9%
24	Kentucky	540	1.5%
24	Louisiana	540	1.5%
37	Maine	200	0.5%
20	Maryland	710	1.9%
13	Massachusetts	920	2.5%
8	Michigan	1,330	3.6%
21	Minnesota	600	1.6%
32	Mississippi	360	1.0%
14	Missouri	790	2.1%
43	Montana	120	0.3%
37	Nebraska	200	0.5%
34	Nevada	300	0.8%
40	New Hampshire	190	0.5%
10	New Jersey	1,130	3.1%
35	New Mexico	230	0.6%
3	New York	2,440	6.6%
9	North Carolina	1,160	3.2%
47	North Dakota	90	0.2%
7	Ohio	1,530	4.2%
30	Oklahoma	400	1.1%
27	Oregon	490	1.3%
5	Pennsylvania	2,010	5.5%
43	Rhode Island	120	0.3%
23	South Carolina	560	1.5%
46	South Dakota	100	0.3%
17	Tennessee	750	2.0%
4	Texas	2,200	6.0%
37	Utah	200	0.5%
48	Vermont	80	0.2%
12	Virginia	930	2.5%
16	Washington	760	2.1%
36	West Virginia	220	0.6%
19	Wisconsin	720	2.0%
49	Wyoming	70	0.2%

RANK ORDER

RANK	STATE	DEATHS	% of USA
1	California	3,900	10.6%
2	Florida	2,560	7.0%
3	New York	2,440	6.6%
4	Texas	2,200	6.0%
5	Pennsylvania	2,010	5.5%
6	Illinois	1,580	4.3%
7	Ohio	1,530	4.2%
8	Michigan	1,330	3.6%
9	North Carolina	1,160	3.2%
10	New Jersey	1,130	3.1%
11	Georgia	940	2.6%
12	Virginia	930	2.5%
13	Massachusetts	920	2.5%
14	Indiana	790	2.1%
14	Missouri	790	2.1%
16	Washington	760	2.1%
17	Tennessee	750	2.0%
18	Arizona	740	2.0%
19	Wisconsin	720	2.0%
20	Maryland	710	1.9%
21	Minnesota	600	1.6%
22	Alabama	590	1.6%
23	South Carolina	560	1.5%
24	Connecticut	540	1.5%
24	Kentucky	540	1.5%
24	Louisiana	540	1.5%
27	Oregon	490	1.3%
28	Colorado	460	1.3%
29	Arkansas	430	1.2%
30	Oklahoma	400	1.1%
31	Iowa	380	1.0%
32	Mississippi	360	1.0%
33	Kansas	330	0.9%
34	Nevada	300	0.8%
35	New Mexico	230	0.6%
36	West Virginia	220	0.6%
37	Maine	200	0.5%
37	Nebraska	200	0.5%
37	Utah	200	0.5%
40	Idaho	190	0.5%
40	New Hampshire	190	0.5%
42	Hawaii	180	0.5%
43	Delaware	120	0.3%
43	Montana	120	0.3%
43	Rhode Island	120	0.3%
46	South Dakota	100	0.3%
47	North Dakota	90	0.2%
48	Vermont	80	0.2%
49	Wyoming	70	0.2%
50	Alaska	60	0.2%
	District of Columbia	70	0.2%

Source: American Cancer Society
"Cancer Facts & Figures 2010" (Copyright 2010, American Cancer Society, http://www.cancer.org/docroot/stt/stt_0.asp)

Estimated Death Rate by Pancreatic Cancer in 2010

National Estimated Rate = 12.0 Deaths per 100,000 Population*

ALPHA ORDER

RANK	STATE	RATE
20	Alabama	12.5
49	Alaska	8.6
42	Arizona	11.2
4	Arkansas	14.9
45	California	10.6
47	Colorado	9.2
2	Connecticut	15.3
10	Delaware	13.6
9	Florida	13.8
46	Georgia	9.6
7	Hawaii	13.9
25	Idaho	12.3
30	Illinois	12.2
25	Indiana	12.3
19	Iowa	12.6
36	Kansas	11.7
20	Kentucky	12.5
33	Louisiana	12.0
3	Maine	15.2
20	Maryland	12.5
6	Massachusetts	14.0
11	Michigan	13.3
37	Minnesota	11.4
30	Mississippi	12.2
13	Missouri	13.2
25	Montana	12.3
43	Nebraska	11.1
37	Nevada	11.4
5	New Hampshire	14.3
14	New Jersey	13.0
37	New Mexico	11.4
20	New York	12.5
24	North Carolina	12.4
7	North Dakota	13.9
11	Ohio	13.3
44	Oklahoma	10.8
17	Oregon	12.8
1	Pennsylvania	15.9
37	Rhode Island	11.4
25	South Carolina	12.3
25	South Dakota	12.3
34	Tennessee	11.9
48	Texas	8.9
50	Utah	7.2
15	Vermont	12.9
35	Virginia	11.8
37	Washington	11.4
32	West Virginia	12.1
18	Wisconsin	12.7
15	Wyoming	12.9

RANK ORDER

RANK	STATE	RATE
1	Pennsylvania	15.9
2	Connecticut	15.3
3	Maine	15.2
4	Arkansas	14.9
5	New Hampshire	14.3
6	Massachusetts	14.0
7	Hawaii	13.9
7	North Dakota	13.9
9	Florida	13.8
10	Delaware	13.6
11	Michigan	13.3
11	Ohio	13.3
13	Missouri	13.2
14	New Jersey	13.0
15	Vermont	12.9
15	Wyoming	12.9
17	Oregon	12.8
18	Wisconsin	12.7
19	Iowa	12.6
20	Alabama	12.5
20	Kentucky	12.5
20	Maryland	12.5
20	New York	12.5
24	North Carolina	12.4
25	Idaho	12.3
25	Indiana	12.3
25	Montana	12.3
25	South Carolina	12.3
25	South Dakota	12.3
30	Illinois	12.2
30	Mississippi	12.2
32	West Virginia	12.1
33	Louisiana	12.0
34	Tennessee	11.9
35	Virginia	11.8
36	Kansas	11.7
37	Minnesota	11.4
37	Nevada	11.4
37	New Mexico	11.4
37	Rhode Island	11.4
37	Washington	11.4
42	Arizona	11.2
43	Nebraska	11.1
44	Oklahoma	10.8
45	California	10.6
46	Georgia	9.6
47	Colorado	9.2
48	Texas	8.9
49	Alaska	8.6
50	Utah	7.2

District of Columbia	11.7

Source: CQ Press using data from American Cancer Society
   "Cancer Facts & Figures 2010" (Copyright 2010, American Cancer Society, http://www.cancer.org/docroot/stt/stt_0.asp)
*Rates calculated using 2009 Census resident population estimates. Not age-adjusted.

Estimated Deaths by Prostate Cancer in 2010

National Estimated Total = 32,050 Deaths

ALPHA ORDER

RANK	STATE	DEATHS	% of USA
19	Alabama	600	1.9%
NA	Alaska*	NA	NA
16	Arizona	650	2.0%
24	Arkansas	460	1.4%
1	California	3,710	11.6%
29	Colorado	390	1.2%
28	Connecticut	410	1.3%
44	Delaware	100	0.3%
2	Florida	2,590	8.1%
11	Georgia	930	2.9%
43	Hawaii	120	0.4%
38	Idaho	180	0.6%
7	Illinois	1,420	4.4%
18	Indiana	620	1.9%
30	Iowa	370	1.2%
33	Kansas	300	0.9%
23	Kentucky	470	1.5%
25	Louisiana	440	1.4%
39	Maine	150	0.5%
16	Maryland	650	2.0%
19	Massachusetts	600	1.9%
8	Michigan	1,010	3.2%
25	Minnesota	440	1.4%
31	Mississippi	330	1.0%
13	Missouri	710	2.2%
41	Montana	130	0.4%
35	Nebraska	240	0.7%
34	Nevada	270	0.8%
40	New Hampshire	140	0.4%
10	New Jersey	940	2.9%
35	New Mexico	240	0.7%
4	New York	1,690	5.3%
9	North Carolina	980	3.1%
47	North Dakota	70	0.2%
6	Ohio	1,440	4.5%
32	Oklahoma	320	1.0%
27	Oregon	430	1.3%
5	Pennsylvania	1,660	5.2%
46	Rhode Island	80	0.2%
22	South Carolina	490	1.5%
44	South Dakota	100	0.3%
15	Tennessee	690	2.2%
3	Texas	1,820	5.7%
37	Utah	200	0.6%
48	Vermont	50	0.2%
13	Virginia	710	2.2%
12	Washington	770	2.4%
41	West Virginia	130	0.4%
19	Wisconsin	600	1.9%
NA	Wyoming*	NA	NA

RANK ORDER

RANK	STATE	DEATHS	% of USA
1	California	3,710	11.6%
2	Florida	2,590	8.1%
3	Texas	1,820	5.7%
4	New York	1,690	5.3%
5	Pennsylvania	1,660	5.2%
6	Ohio	1,440	4.5%
7	Illinois	1,420	4.4%
8	Michigan	1,010	3.2%
9	North Carolina	980	3.1%
10	New Jersey	940	2.9%
11	Georgia	930	2.9%
12	Washington	770	2.4%
13	Missouri	710	2.2%
13	Virginia	710	2.2%
15	Tennessee	690	2.2%
16	Arizona	650	2.0%
16	Maryland	650	2.0%
18	Indiana	620	1.9%
19	Alabama	600	1.9%
19	Massachusetts	600	1.9%
19	Wisconsin	600	1.9%
22	South Carolina	490	1.5%
23	Kentucky	470	1.5%
24	Arkansas	460	1.4%
25	Louisiana	440	1.4%
25	Minnesota	440	1.4%
27	Oregon	430	1.3%
28	Connecticut	410	1.3%
29	Colorado	390	1.2%
30	Iowa	370	1.2%
31	Mississippi	330	1.0%
32	Oklahoma	320	1.0%
33	Kansas	300	0.9%
34	Nevada	270	0.8%
35	Nebraska	240	0.7%
35	New Mexico	240	0.7%
37	Utah	200	0.6%
38	Idaho	180	0.6%
39	Maine	150	0.5%
40	New Hampshire	140	0.4%
41	Montana	130	0.4%
41	West Virginia	130	0.4%
43	Hawaii	120	0.4%
44	Delaware	100	0.3%
44	South Dakota	100	0.3%
46	Rhode Island	80	0.2%
47	North Dakota	70	0.2%
48	Vermont	50	0.2%
NA	Alaska*	NA	NA
NA	Wyoming*	NA	NA
	District of Columbia	70	0.2%

Source: American Cancer Society
"Cancer Facts & Figures 2010" (Copyright 2010, American Cancer Society, http://www.cancer.org/docroot/stt/stt_0.asp)
*Fewer than 50 deaths.

Age-Adjusted Death Rate by Prostate Cancer in 2006

National Rate = 25.6 Deaths per 100,000 Male Population*

ALPHA ORDER

RANK	STATE	RATE
2	Alabama	31.2
41	Alaska	24.2
48	Arizona	22.1
14	Arkansas	27.5
41	California	24.2
32	Colorado	25.5
23	Connecticut	26.6
20	Delaware	26.8
49	Florida	21.3
5	Georgia	29.7
50	Hawaii	17.4
11	Idaho	28.2
17	Illinois	27.0
29	Indiana	26.0
22	Iowa	26.7
47	Kansas	23.5
23	Kentucky	26.6
4	Louisiana	30.4
26	Maine	26.2
8	Maryland	28.4
32	Massachusetts	25.5
36	Michigan	24.8
20	Minnesota	26.8
1	Mississippi	34.2
45	Missouri	24.0
8	Montana	28.4
38	Nebraska	24.5
35	Nevada	25.4
16	New Hampshire	27.2
38	New Jersey	24.5
25	New Mexico	26.3
37	New York	24.6
6	North Carolina	28.9
12	North Dakota	27.9
17	Ohio	27.0
43	Oklahoma	24.1
19	Oregon	26.9
29	Pennsylvania	26.0
32	Rhode Island	25.5
3	South Carolina	30.6
15	South Dakota	27.4
10	Tennessee	28.3
40	Texas	24.3
29	Utah	26.0
26	Vermont	26.2
6	Virginia	28.9
28	Washington	26.1
46	West Virginia	23.9
13	Wisconsin	27.8
43	Wyoming	24.1

RANK ORDER

RANK	STATE	RATE
1	Mississippi	34.2
2	Alabama	31.2
3	South Carolina	30.6
4	Louisiana	30.4
5	Georgia	29.7
6	North Carolina	28.9
6	Virginia	28.9
8	Maryland	28.4
8	Montana	28.4
10	Tennessee	28.3
11	Idaho	28.2
12	North Dakota	27.9
13	Wisconsin	27.8
14	Arkansas	27.5
15	South Dakota	27.4
16	New Hampshire	27.2
17	Illinois	27.0
17	Ohio	27.0
19	Oregon	26.9
20	Delaware	26.8
20	Minnesota	26.8
22	Iowa	26.7
23	Connecticut	26.6
23	Kentucky	26.6
25	New Mexico	26.3
26	Maine	26.2
26	Vermont	26.2
28	Washington	26.1
29	Indiana	26.0
29	Pennsylvania	26.0
29	Utah	26.0
32	Colorado	25.5
32	Massachusetts	25.5
32	Rhode Island	25.5
35	Nevada	25.4
36	Michigan	24.8
37	New York	24.6
38	Nebraska	24.5
38	New Jersey	24.5
40	Texas	24.3
41	Alaska	24.2
41	California	24.2
43	Oklahoma	24.1
43	Wyoming	24.1
45	Missouri	24.0
46	West Virginia	23.9
47	Kansas	23.5
48	Arizona	22.1
49	Florida	21.3
50	Hawaii	17.4

District of Columbia   43.3

Source: American Cancer Society
"Cancer Facts & Figures 2010" (Copyright 2010, American Cancer Society, http://www.cancer.org/docroot/stt/stt_0.asp)
*For 2002 to 2006. Age-adjusted to the 2000 U.S. standard population.

Deaths by AIDS in 2007

National Total = 11,295 Deaths*

ALPHA ORDER

RANK	STATE	DEATHS	% of USA
17	Alabama	183	1.6%
44	Alaska	7	0.1%
22	Arizona	109	1.0%
25	Arkansas	91	0.8%
3	California	1,101	9.7%
27	Colorado	82	0.7%
20	Connecticut	140	1.2%
29	Delaware	55	0.5%
1	Florida	1,530	13.5%
5	Georgia	689	6.1%
40	Hawaii	21	0.2%
45	Idaho	6	0.1%
12	Illinois	303	2.7%
24	Indiana	97	0.9%
41	Iowa	18	0.2%
38	Kansas	22	0.2%
29	Kentucky	55	0.5%
10	Louisiana	344	3.0%
42	Maine	13	0.1%
7	Maryland	436	3.9%
19	Massachusetts	143	1.3%
16	Michigan	187	1.7%
32	Minnesota	49	0.4%
18	Mississippi	163	1.4%
21	Missouri	128	1.1%
46	Montana	5	0.0%
35	Nebraska	28	0.2%
28	Nevada	80	0.7%
43	New Hampshire	10	0.1%
6	New Jersey	495	4.4%
34	New Mexico	35	0.3%
2	New York	1,342	11.9%
8	North Carolina	384	3.4%
48	North Dakota	3	0.0%
15	Ohio	207	1.8%
25	Oklahoma	91	0.8%
31	Oregon	54	0.5%
9	Pennsylvania	378	3.3%
36	Rhode Island	24	0.2%
11	South Carolina	315	2.8%
46	South Dakota	5	0.0%
13	Tennessee	252	2.2%
4	Texas	988	8.7%
37	Utah	23	0.2%
49	Vermont	2	0.0%
14	Virginia	230	2.0%
23	Washington	107	0.9%
38	West Virginia	22	0.2%
32	Wisconsin	49	0.4%
50	Wyoming	0	0.0%

RANK ORDER

RANK	STATE	DEATHS	% of USA
1	Florida	1,530	13.5%
2	New York	1,342	11.9%
3	California	1,101	9.7%
4	Texas	988	8.7%
5	Georgia	689	6.1%
6	New Jersey	495	4.4%
7	Maryland	436	3.9%
8	North Carolina	384	3.4%
9	Pennsylvania	378	3.3%
10	Louisiana	344	3.0%
11	South Carolina	315	2.8%
12	Illinois	303	2.7%
13	Tennessee	252	2.2%
14	Virginia	230	2.0%
15	Ohio	207	1.8%
16	Michigan	187	1.7%
17	Alabama	183	1.6%
18	Mississippi	163	1.4%
19	Massachusetts	143	1.3%
20	Connecticut	140	1.2%
21	Missouri	128	1.1%
22	Arizona	109	1.0%
23	Washington	107	0.9%
24	Indiana	97	0.9%
25	Arkansas	91	0.8%
25	Oklahoma	91	0.8%
27	Colorado	82	0.7%
28	Nevada	80	0.7%
29	Delaware	55	0.5%
29	Kentucky	55	0.5%
31	Oregon	54	0.5%
32	Minnesota	49	0.4%
32	Wisconsin	49	0.4%
34	New Mexico	35	0.3%
35	Nebraska	28	0.2%
36	Rhode Island	24	0.2%
37	Utah	23	0.2%
38	Kansas	22	0.2%
38	West Virginia	22	0.2%
40	Hawaii	21	0.2%
41	Iowa	18	0.2%
42	Maine	13	0.1%
43	New Hampshire	10	0.1%
44	Alaska	7	0.1%
45	Idaho	6	0.1%
46	Montana	5	0.0%
46	South Dakota	5	0.0%
48	North Dakota	3	0.0%
49	Vermont	2	0.0%
50	Wyoming	0	0.0%
	District of Columbia	194	1.7%

Source: U.S. Department of Health and Human Services, National Center for Health Statistics
"National Vital Statistics Reports" (Vol. 58, No. 19, May 20, 2010, http://www.cdc.gov/nchs/deaths.htm)
*Final data by state of residence. AIDS is Acquired Immunodeficiency Syndrome. It is a specific group of diseases or
conditions which are indicative of severe immunosuppression related to infection with the Human Immunodeficiency Virus (HIV).

Death Rate by AIDS in 2007

National Rate = 3.7 Deaths per 100,000 Population*

ALPHA ORDER

RANK	STATE	RATE
13	Alabama	4.0
NA	Alaska**	NA
28	Arizona	1.7
15	Arkansas	3.2
17	California	3.0
28	Colorado	1.7
13	Connecticut	4.0
7	Delaware	6.4
1	Florida	8.4
4	Georgia	7.2
31	Hawaii	1.6
NA	Idaho**	NA
21	Illinois	2.4
33	Indiana	1.5
NA	Iowa**	NA
40	Kansas	0.8
35	Kentucky	1.3
2	Louisiana	8.0
NA	Maine**	NA
3	Maryland	7.8
23	Massachusetts	2.2
25	Michigan	1.9
37	Minnesota	0.9
9	Mississippi	5.6
23	Missouri	2.2
NA	Montana**	NA
31	Nebraska	1.6
16	Nevada	3.1
NA	New Hampshire**	NA
8	New Jersey	5.7
26	New Mexico	1.8
6	New York	7.0
10	North Carolina	4.2
NA	North Dakota**	NA
26	Ohio	1.8
20	Oklahoma	2.5
34	Oregon	1.4
17	Pennsylvania	3.0
22	Rhode Island	2.3
5	South Carolina	7.1
NA	South Dakota**	NA
11	Tennessee	4.1
11	Texas	4.1
37	Utah	0.9
NA	Vermont**	NA
17	Virginia	3.0
28	Washington	1.7
36	West Virginia	1.2
37	Wisconsin	0.9
NA	Wyoming**	NA

RANK ORDER

RANK	STATE	RATE
1	Florida	8.4
2	Louisiana	8.0
3	Maryland	7.8
4	Georgia	7.2
5	South Carolina	7.1
6	New York	7.0
7	Delaware	6.4
8	New Jersey	5.7
9	Mississippi	5.6
10	North Carolina	4.2
11	Tennessee	4.1
11	Texas	4.1
13	Alabama	4.0
13	Connecticut	4.0
15	Arkansas	3.2
16	Nevada	3.1
17	California	3.0
17	Pennsylvania	3.0
17	Virginia	3.0
20	Oklahoma	2.5
21	Illinois	2.4
22	Rhode Island	2.3
23	Massachusetts	2.2
23	Missouri	2.2
25	Michigan	1.9
26	New Mexico	1.8
26	Ohio	1.8
28	Arizona	1.7
28	Colorado	1.7
28	Washington	1.7
31	Hawaii	1.6
31	Nebraska	1.6
33	Indiana	1.5
34	Oregon	1.4
35	Kentucky	1.3
36	West Virginia	1.2
37	Minnesota	0.9
37	Utah	0.9
37	Wisconsin	0.9
40	Kansas	0.8
NA	Alaska**	NA
NA	Idaho**	NA
NA	Iowa**	NA
NA	Maine**	NA
NA	Montana**	NA
NA	New Hampshire**	NA
NA	North Dakota**	NA
NA	South Dakota**	NA
NA	Vermont**	NA
NA	Wyoming**	NA

District of Columbia   33.0

Source: U.S. Department of Health and Human Services, National Center for Health Statistics
"National Vital Statistics Reports" (Vol. 58, No. 19, May 20, 2010, http://www.cdc.gov/nchs/deaths.htm)
*Final data by state of residence. AIDS is Acquired Immunodeficiency Syndrome. It is a specific group of diseases or conditions which are indicative of severe immunosuppression related to infection with the Human Immunodeficiency Virus (HIV). Not age-adjusted.
**Insufficient data to determine a reliable rate.

Age-Adjusted Death Rate by AIDS in 2007

National Rate = 3.7 Deaths per 100,000 Population*

ALPHA ORDER				RANK ORDER		
RANK	STATE	RATE		RANK	STATE	RATE
13	Alabama	4.0		1	Florida	8.3
NA	Alaska**	NA		1	Louisiana	8.3
26	Arizona	1.8		3	Maryland	7.4
15	Arkansas	3.2		4	Georgia	7.1
17	California	3.0		4	South Carolina	7.1
30	Colorado	1.6		6	New York	6.6
14	Connecticut	3.6		7	Delaware	6.2
7	Delaware	6.2		8	Mississippi	5.9
1	Florida	8.3		9	New Jersey	5.3
4	Georgia	7.1		10	Texas	4.3
30	Hawaii	1.6		11	North Carolina	4.1
NA	Idaho**	NA		11	Tennessee	4.1
21	Illinois	2.3		13	Alabama	4.0
33	Indiana	1.5		14	Connecticut	3.6
NA	Iowa**	NA		15	Arkansas	3.2
40	Kansas	0.8		16	Nevada	3.1
35	Kentucky	1.3		17	California	3.0
1	Louisiana	8.3		18	Pennsylvania	2.9
NA	Maine**	NA		19	Virginia	2.8
3	Maryland	7.4		20	Oklahoma	2.7
24	Massachusetts	2.0		21	Illinois	2.3
26	Michigan	1.8		22	Missouri	2.2
38	Minnesota	0.9		22	Rhode Island	2.2
8	Mississippi	5.9		24	Massachusetts	2.0
22	Missouri	2.2		25	New Mexico	1.9
NA	Montana**	NA		26	Arizona	1.8
29	Nebraska	1.7		26	Michigan	1.8
16	Nevada	3.1		26	Ohio	1.8
NA	New Hampshire**	NA		29	Nebraska	1.7
9	New Jersey	5.3		30	Colorado	1.6
25	New Mexico	1.9		30	Hawaii	1.6
6	New York	6.6		30	Washington	1.6
11	North Carolina	4.1		33	Indiana	1.5
NA	North Dakota**	NA		34	Oregon	1.4
26	Ohio	1.8		35	Kentucky	1.3
20	Oklahoma	2.7		36	West Virginia	1.2
34	Oregon	1.4		37	Utah	1.0
18	Pennsylvania	2.9		38	Minnesota	0.9
22	Rhode Island	2.2		38	Wisconsin	0.9
4	South Carolina	7.1		40	Kansas	0.8
NA	South Dakota**	NA		NA	Alaska**	NA
11	Tennessee	4.1		NA	Idaho**	NA
10	Texas	4.3		NA	Iowa**	NA
37	Utah	1.0		NA	Maine**	NA
NA	Vermont**	NA		NA	Montana**	NA
19	Virginia	2.8		NA	New Hampshire**	NA
30	Washington	1.6		NA	North Dakota**	NA
36	West Virginia	1.2		NA	South Dakota**	NA
38	Wisconsin	0.9		NA	Vermont**	NA
NA	Wyoming**	NA		NA	Wyoming**	NA

District of Columbia   32.8

Source: U.S. Department of Health and Human Services, National Center for Health Statistics
    "National Vital Statistics Reports" (Vol. 58, No. 19, May 20, 2010, http://www.cdc.gov/nchs/deaths.htm)
*Final data by state of residence. AIDS is Acquired Immunodeficiency Syndrome. It is a specific group of diseases or
conditions which are indicative of severe immunosuppression related to infection with the Human Immunodeficiency Virus (HIV).
Age-adjusted rates based on the year 2000 standard population.
**Insufficient data to determine a reliable rate.

Deaths by Alzheimer's Disease in 2007

National Total = 74,632 Deaths*

ALPHA ORDER					RANK ORDER			
RANK	STATE		DEATHS	% of USA	RANK	STATE	DEATHS	% of USA
20	Alabama		1,517	2.0%	1	California	8,497	11.4%
50	Alaska		65	0.1%	2	Texas	4,814	6.5%
11	Arizona		2,051	2.7%	3	Florida	4,644	6.2%
31	Arkansas		824	1.1%	4	Ohio	3,671	4.9%
1	California		8,497	11.4%	5	Pennsylvania	3,505	4.7%
27	Colorado		1,109	1.5%	6	Illinois	2,734	3.7%
33	Connecticut		764	1.0%	7	Washington	2,689	3.6%
48	Delaware		201	0.3%	8	North Carolina	2,460	3.3%
3	Florida		4,644	6.2%	9	Michigan	2,432	3.3%
13	Georgia		1,849	2.5%	10	Tennessee	2,276	3.0%
46	Hawaii		247	0.3%	11	Arizona	2,051	2.7%
38	Idaho		416	0.6%	12	New York	1,999	2.7%
6	Illinois		2,734	3.7%	13	Georgia	1,849	2.5%
18	Indiana		1,663	2.2%	14	New Jersey	1,823	2.4%
23	Iowa		1,202	1.6%	15	Virginia	1,703	2.3%
30	Kansas		860	1.2%	16	Massachusetts	1,695	2.3%
25	Kentucky		1,198	1.6%	17	Missouri	1,681	2.3%
22	Louisiana		1,324	1.8%	18	Indiana	1,663	2.2%
36	Maine		470	0.6%	19	Wisconsin	1,658	2.2%
29	Maryland		881	1.2%	20	Alabama	1,517	2.0%
16	Massachusetts		1,695	2.3%	21	South Carolina	1,396	1.9%
9	Michigan		2,432	3.3%	22	Louisiana	1,324	1.8%
26	Minnesota		1,179	1.6%	23	Iowa	1,202	1.6%
32	Mississippi		797	1.1%	24	Oregon	1,200	1.6%
17	Missouri		1,681	2.3%	25	Kentucky	1,198	1.6%
44	Montana		260	0.3%	26	Minnesota	1,179	1.6%
35	Nebraska		512	0.7%	27	Colorado	1,109	1.5%
45	Nevada		248	0.3%	28	Oklahoma	927	1.2%
37	New Hampshire		418	0.6%	29	Maryland	881	1.2%
14	New Jersey		1,823	2.4%	30	Kansas	860	1.2%
43	New Mexico		322	0.4%	31	Arkansas	824	1.1%
12	New York		1,999	2.7%	32	Mississippi	797	1.1%
8	North Carolina		2,460	3.3%	33	Connecticut	764	1.0%
39	North Dakota		395	0.5%	34	West Virginia	534	0.7%
4	Ohio		3,671	4.9%	35	Nebraska	512	0.7%
28	Oklahoma		927	1.2%	36	Maine	470	0.6%
24	Oregon		1,200	1.6%	37	New Hampshire	418	0.6%
5	Pennsylvania		3,505	4.7%	38	Idaho	416	0.6%
42	Rhode Island		328	0.4%	39	North Dakota	395	0.5%
21	South Carolina		1,396	1.9%	40	Utah	393	0.5%
41	South Dakota		346	0.5%	41	South Dakota	346	0.5%
10	Tennessee		2,276	3.0%	42	Rhode Island	328	0.4%
2	Texas		4,814	6.5%	43	New Mexico	322	0.4%
40	Utah		393	0.5%	44	Montana	260	0.3%
47	Vermont		205	0.3%	45	Nevada	248	0.3%
15	Virginia		1,703	2.3%	46	Hawaii	247	0.3%
7	Washington		2,689	3.6%	47	Vermont	205	0.3%
34	West Virginia		534	0.7%	48	Delaware	201	0.3%
19	Wisconsin		1,658	2.2%	49	Wyoming	110	0.1%
49	Wyoming		110	0.1%	50	Alaska	65	0.1%
						District of Columbia	140	0.2%

Source: U.S. Department of Health and Human Services, National Center for Health Statistics
"National Vital Statistics Reports" (Vol. 58, No. 19, May 20, 2010, http://www.cdc.gov/nchs/deaths.htm)
*Final data by state of residence. A degenerative disease of the brain cells producing loss of memory and general intellectual impairment. It usually affects people over age 65. As the disease progresses, a variety of symptoms may become apparent, including confusion, irritability, and restlessness, as well as disorientation and impaired judgment and concentration.

Death Rate by Alzheimer's Disease in 2007

National Rate = 24.7 Deaths per 100,000 Population*

ALPHA ORDER			RANK ORDER		
RANK	**STATE**	**RATE**	**RANK**	**STATE**	**RATE**
8	Alabama	32.8	1	North Dakota	61.7
50	Alaska	9.5	2	South Dakota	43.5
9	Arizona	32.4	3	Washington	41.6
19	Arkansas	29.1	4	Iowa	40.2
33	California	23.2	5	Tennessee	37.0
35	Colorado	22.8	6	Maine	35.7
38	Connecticut	21.8	7	Vermont	33.0
33	Delaware	23.2	8	Alabama	32.8
31	Florida	25.4	9	Arizona	32.4
43	Georgia	19.4	10	Ohio	32.0
44	Hawaii	19.2	10	Oregon	32.0
24	Idaho	27.7	12	New Hampshire	31.8
39	Illinois	21.3	13	South Carolina	31.7
29	Indiana	26.2	14	Kansas	31.0
4	Iowa	40.2	14	Rhode Island	31.0
14	Kansas	31.0	16	Louisiana	30.8
22	Kentucky	28.2	17	Wisconsin	29.6
16	Louisiana	30.8	18	West Virginia	29.5
6	Maine	35.7	19	Arkansas	29.1
46	Maryland	15.7	20	Nebraska	28.9
28	Massachusetts	26.3	21	Missouri	28.6
32	Michigan	24.1	22	Kentucky	28.2
36	Minnesota	22.7	22	Pennsylvania	28.2
25	Mississippi	27.3	24	Idaho	27.7
21	Missouri	28.6	25	Mississippi	27.3
26	Montana	27.1	26	Montana	27.1
20	Nebraska	28.9	26	North Carolina	27.1
49	Nevada	9.7	28	Massachusetts	26.3
12	New Hampshire	31.8	29	Indiana	26.2
40	New Jersey	21.0	30	Oklahoma	25.6
45	New Mexico	16.3	31	Florida	25.4
48	New York	10.4	32	Michigan	24.1
26	North Carolina	27.1	33	California	23.2
1	North Dakota	61.7	33	Delaware	23.2
10	Ohio	32.0	35	Colorado	22.8
30	Oklahoma	25.6	36	Minnesota	22.7
10	Oregon	32.0	37	Virginia	22.1
22	Pennsylvania	28.2	38	Connecticut	21.8
14	Rhode Island	31.0	39	Illinois	21.3
13	South Carolina	31.7	40	New Jersey	21.0
2	South Dakota	43.5	40	Wyoming	21.0
5	Tennessee	37.0	42	Texas	20.1
42	Texas	20.1	43	Georgia	19.4
47	Utah	14.9	44	Hawaii	19.2
7	Vermont	33.0	45	New Mexico	16.3
37	Virginia	22.1	46	Maryland	15.7
3	Washington	41.6	47	Utah	14.9
18	West Virginia	29.5	48	New York	10.4
17	Wisconsin	29.6	49	Nevada	9.7
40	Wyoming	21.0	50	Alaska	9.5
				District of Columbia	23.8

Source: U.S. Department of Health and Human Services, National Center for Health Statistics
   "National Vital Statistics Reports" (Vol. 58, No. 19, May 20, 2010, http://www.cdc.gov/nchs/deaths.htm)
*Final data by state of residence. A degenerative disease of the brain cells producing loss of memory and general intellectual impairment. It usually affects people over age 65. As the disease progresses, a variety of symptoms may become apparent, including confusion, irritability, and restlessness, as well as disorientation and impaired judgment and concentration. Not age-adjusted.

Age-Adjusted Death Rate by Alzheimer's Disease in 2007

National Rate = 22.7 Deaths per 100,000 Population*

RANK	STATE	RATE
7	Alabama	30.1
38	Alaska	20.8
8	Arizona	29.6
23	Arkansas	24.6
24	California	24.3
14	Colorado	27.8
44	Connecticut	16.9
36	Delaware	20.9
45	Florida	16.2
20	Georgia	25.3
48	Hawaii	14.1
11	Idaho	28.2
40	Illinois	19.9
27	Indiana	24.2
12	Iowa	27.9
21	Kansas	25.2
18	Kentucky	27.1
4	Louisiana	31.3
12	Maine	27.9
46	Maryland	16.0
36	Massachusetts	20.9
33	Michigan	22.1
42	Minnesota	19.6
19	Mississippi	26.5
24	Missouri	24.3
33	Montana	22.1
31	Nebraska	22.9
49	Nevada	12.3
9	New Hampshire	28.9
43	New Jersey	18.0
47	New Mexico	15.5
50	New York	8.8
15	North Carolina	27.7
2	North Dakota	40.4
17	Ohio	27.4
30	Oklahoma	23.0
16	Oregon	27.6
41	Pennsylvania	19.8
32	Rhode Island	22.2
5	South Carolina	30.9
6	South Dakota	30.2
3	Tennessee	35.9
22	Texas	24.7
39	Utah	20.5
10	Vermont	28.4
28	Virginia	23.4
1	Washington	40.7
29	West Virginia	23.1
24	Wisconsin	24.3
35	Wyoming	21.0

RANK	STATE	RATE
1	Washington	40.7
2	North Dakota	40.4
3	Tennessee	35.9
4	Louisiana	31.3
5	South Carolina	30.9
6	South Dakota	30.2
7	Alabama	30.1
8	Arizona	29.6
9	New Hampshire	28.9
10	Vermont	28.4
11	Idaho	28.2
12	Iowa	27.9
12	Maine	27.9
14	Colorado	27.8
15	North Carolina	27.7
16	Oregon	27.6
17	Ohio	27.4
18	Kentucky	27.1
19	Mississippi	26.5
20	Georgia	25.3
21	Kansas	25.2
22	Texas	24.7
23	Arkansas	24.6
24	California	24.3
24	Missouri	24.3
24	Wisconsin	24.3
27	Indiana	24.2
28	Virginia	23.4
29	West Virginia	23.1
30	Oklahoma	23.0
31	Nebraska	22.9
32	Rhode Island	22.2
33	Michigan	22.1
33	Montana	22.1
35	Wyoming	21.0
36	Delaware	20.9
36	Massachusetts	20.9
38	Alaska	20.8
39	Utah	20.5
40	Illinois	19.9
41	Pennsylvania	19.8
42	Minnesota	19.6
43	New Jersey	18.0
44	Connecticut	16.9
45	Florida	16.2
46	Maryland	16.0
47	New Mexico	15.5
48	Hawaii	14.1
49	Nevada	12.3
50	New York	8.8
	District of Columbia	21.8

Source: U.S. Department of Health and Human Services, National Center for Health Statistics
   "National Vital Statistics Reports" (Vol. 58, No. 19, May 20, 2010, http://www.cdc.gov/nchs/deaths.htm)
*Final data by state of residence. A degenerative disease of the brain cells producing loss of memory and general intellectual impairment. It usually affects people over age 65. As the disease progresses, a variety of symptoms may become apparent, including confusion, irritability, and restlessness, as well as disorientation and impaired judgment and concentration. Age-adjusted rates based on the year 2000 standard population.

Deaths by Cerebrovascular Diseases in 2007

National Total = 135,952 Deaths*

ALPHA ORDER

RANK	STATE	DEATHS	% of USA
17	Alabama	2,747	2.0%
50	Alaska	157	0.1%
22	Arizona	2,207	1.6%
27	Arkansas	1,873	1.4%
1	California	14,557	10.7%
30	Colorado	1,600	1.2%
33	Connecticut	1,463	1.1%
46	Delaware	374	0.3%
3	Florida	8,781	6.5%
10	Georgia	3,894	2.9%
40	Hawaii	643	0.5%
41	Idaho	640	0.5%
7	Illinois	5,864	4.3%
15	Indiana	3,083	2.3%
29	Iowa	1,686	1.2%
32	Kansas	1,498	1.1%
25	Kentucky	2,144	1.6%
24	Louisiana	2,147	1.6%
39	Maine	664	0.5%
21	Maryland	2,364	1.7%
16	Massachusetts	2,832	2.1%
8	Michigan	4,798	3.5%
23	Minnesota	2,193	1.6%
31	Mississippi	1,589	1.2%
14	Missouri	3,229	2.4%
44	Montana	443	0.3%
35	Nebraska	921	0.7%
36	Nevada	850	0.6%
42	New Hampshire	489	0.4%
11	New Jersey	3,492	2.6%
37	New Mexico	804	0.6%
5	New York	6,160	4.5%
9	North Carolina	4,530	3.3%
47	North Dakota	330	0.2%
6	Ohio	5,905	4.3%
26	Oklahoma	2,126	1.6%
28	Oregon	1,835	1.3%
4	Pennsylvania	7,152	5.3%
43	Rhode Island	457	0.3%
20	South Carolina	2,466	1.8%
45	South Dakota	410	0.3%
12	Tennessee	3,450	2.5%
2	Texas	9,796	7.2%
38	Utah	755	0.6%
48	Vermont	269	0.2%
13	Virginia	3,313	2.4%
19	Washington	2,692	2.0%
34	West Virginia	1,113	0.8%
18	Wisconsin	2,738	2.0%
49	Wyoming	209	0.2%

RANK ORDER

RANK	STATE	DEATHS	% of USA
1	California	14,557	10.7%
2	Texas	9,796	7.2%
3	Florida	8,781	6.5%
4	Pennsylvania	7,152	5.3%
5	New York	6,160	4.5%
6	Ohio	5,905	4.3%
7	Illinois	5,864	4.3%
8	Michigan	4,798	3.5%
9	North Carolina	4,530	3.3%
10	Georgia	3,894	2.9%
11	New Jersey	3,492	2.6%
12	Tennessee	3,450	2.5%
13	Virginia	3,313	2.4%
14	Missouri	3,229	2.4%
15	Indiana	3,083	2.3%
16	Massachusetts	2,832	2.1%
17	Alabama	2,747	2.0%
18	Wisconsin	2,738	2.0%
19	Washington	2,692	2.0%
20	South Carolina	2,466	1.8%
21	Maryland	2,364	1.7%
22	Arizona	2,207	1.6%
23	Minnesota	2,193	1.6%
24	Louisiana	2,147	1.6%
25	Kentucky	2,144	1.6%
26	Oklahoma	2,126	1.6%
27	Arkansas	1,873	1.4%
28	Oregon	1,835	1.3%
29	Iowa	1,686	1.2%
30	Colorado	1,600	1.2%
31	Mississippi	1,589	1.2%
32	Kansas	1,498	1.1%
33	Connecticut	1,463	1.1%
34	West Virginia	1,113	0.8%
35	Nebraska	921	0.7%
36	Nevada	850	0.6%
37	New Mexico	804	0.6%
38	Utah	755	0.6%
39	Maine	664	0.5%
40	Hawaii	643	0.5%
41	Idaho	640	0.5%
42	New Hampshire	489	0.4%
43	Rhode Island	457	0.3%
44	Montana	443	0.3%
45	South Dakota	410	0.3%
46	Delaware	374	0.3%
47	North Dakota	330	0.2%
48	Vermont	269	0.2%
49	Wyoming	209	0.2%
50	Alaska	157	0.1%
	District of Columbia	220	0.2%

Source: U.S. Department of Health and Human Services, National Center for Health Statistics
"National Vital Statistics Reports" (Vol. 58, No. 19, May 20, 2010, http://www.cdc.gov/nchs/deaths.htm)
*Final data by state of residence. Cerebrovascular diseases include stroke and other disorders of the blood vessels of the brain.

Death Rate by Cerebrovascular Diseases in 2007

National Rate = 45.1 Deaths per 100,000 Population*

ALPHA ORDER

RANK	STATE	RATE
3	Alabama	59.4
50	Alaska	23.0
45	Arizona	34.8
1	Arkansas	66.1
43	California	39.8
47	Colorado	32.9
36	Connecticut	41.8
30	Delaware	43.2
24	Florida	48.1
39	Georgia	40.8
18	Hawaii	50.1
33	Idaho	42.7
27	Illinois	45.6
23	Indiana	48.6
6	Iowa	56.4
11	Kansas	54.0
16	Kentucky	50.5
19	Louisiana	50.0
17	Maine	50.4
35	Maryland	42.1
28	Massachusetts	43.9
25	Michigan	47.6
34	Minnesota	42.2
10	Mississippi	54.4
9	Missouri	54.9
26	Montana	46.2
12	Nebraska	51.9
46	Nevada	33.1
44	New Hampshire	37.2
41	New Jersey	40.2
39	New Mexico	40.8
48	New York	31.9
19	North Carolina	50.0
13	North Dakota	51.6
14	Ohio	51.5
4	Oklahoma	58.8
21	Oregon	49.0
5	Pennsylvania	57.5
30	Rhode Island	43.2
8	South Carolina	55.9
14	South Dakota	51.5
7	Tennessee	56.0
38	Texas	41.0
49	Utah	28.5
29	Vermont	43.3
32	Virginia	43.0
37	Washington	41.6
2	West Virginia	61.4
22	Wisconsin	48.9
42	Wyoming	40.0

RANK ORDER

RANK	STATE	RATE
1	Arkansas	66.1
2	West Virginia	61.4
3	Alabama	59.4
4	Oklahoma	58.8
5	Pennsylvania	57.5
6	Iowa	56.4
7	Tennessee	56.0
8	South Carolina	55.9
9	Missouri	54.9
10	Mississippi	54.4
11	Kansas	54.0
12	Nebraska	51.9
13	North Dakota	51.6
14	Ohio	51.5
14	South Dakota	51.5
16	Kentucky	50.5
17	Maine	50.4
18	Hawaii	50.1
19	Louisiana	50.0
19	North Carolina	50.0
21	Oregon	49.0
22	Wisconsin	48.9
23	Indiana	48.6
24	Florida	48.1
25	Michigan	47.6
26	Montana	46.2
27	Illinois	45.6
28	Massachusetts	43.9
29	Vermont	43.3
30	Delaware	43.2
30	Rhode Island	43.2
32	Virginia	43.0
33	Idaho	42.7
34	Minnesota	42.2
35	Maryland	42.1
36	Connecticut	41.8
37	Washington	41.6
38	Texas	41.0
39	Georgia	40.8
39	New Mexico	40.8
41	New Jersey	40.2
42	Wyoming	40.0
43	California	39.8
44	New Hampshire	37.2
45	Arizona	34.8
46	Nevada	33.1
47	Colorado	32.9
48	New York	31.9
49	Utah	28.5
50	Alaska	23.0

District of Columbia	37.4

Source: U.S. Department of Health and Human Services, National Center for Health Statistics
"National Vital Statistics Reports" (Vol. 58, No. 19, May 20, 2010, http://www.cdc.gov/nchs/deaths.htm)
*Final data by state of residence. Cerebrovascular diseases include stroke and other disorders of the blood vessels of the brain.
Not age-adjusted.

Age-Adjusted Death Rate by Cerebrovascular Diseases in 2007

National Rate = 42.2 Deaths per 100,000 Population*

ALPHA ORDER

RANK	STATE	RATE
2	Alabama	54.5
18	Alaska	44.3
49	Arizona	32.7
1	Arkansas	57.4
27	California	42.2
35	Colorado	39.0
46	Connecticut	34.2
33	Delaware	39.4
47	Florida	33.6
9	Georgia	49.7
31	Hawaii	39.6
22	Idaho	43.2
20	Illinois	43.9
15	Indiana	45.7
28	Iowa	42.1
14	Kansas	46.0
13	Kentucky	48.1
8	Louisiana	50.1
30	Maine	40.3
25	Maryland	42.7
43	Massachusetts	36.5
18	Michigan	44.3
40	Minnesota	38.1
6	Mississippi	53.0
12	Missouri	48.2
38	Montana	38.5
23	Nebraska	43.1
39	Nevada	38.3
45	New Hampshire	34.3
44	New Jersey	35.8
34	New Mexico	39.2
50	New York	28.2
7	North Carolina	50.3
42	North Dakota	37.3
16	Ohio	45.3
4	Oklahoma	53.8
21	Oregon	43.6
24	Pennsylvania	42.9
48	Rhode Island	33.5
5	South Carolina	53.4
37	South Dakota	38.7
3	Tennessee	53.9
10	Texas	49.0
36	Utah	38.9
41	Vermont	37.6
17	Virginia	44.5
29	Washington	41.4
11	West Virginia	48.9
26	Wisconsin	42.3
32	Wyoming	39.5

RANK ORDER

RANK	STATE	RATE
1	Arkansas	57.4
2	Alabama	54.5
3	Tennessee	53.9
4	Oklahoma	53.8
5	South Carolina	53.4
6	Mississippi	53.0
7	North Carolina	50.3
8	Louisiana	50.1
9	Georgia	49.7
10	Texas	49.0
11	West Virginia	48.9
12	Missouri	48.2
13	Kentucky	48.1
14	Kansas	46.0
15	Indiana	45.7
16	Ohio	45.3
17	Virginia	44.5
18	Alaska	44.3
18	Michigan	44.3
20	Illinois	43.9
21	Oregon	43.6
22	Idaho	43.2
23	Nebraska	43.1
24	Pennsylvania	42.9
25	Maryland	42.7
26	Wisconsin	42.3
27	California	42.2
28	Iowa	42.1
29	Washington	41.4
30	Maine	40.3
31	Hawaii	39.6
32	Wyoming	39.5
33	Delaware	39.4
34	New Mexico	39.2
35	Colorado	39.0
36	Utah	38.9
37	South Dakota	38.7
38	Montana	38.5
39	Nevada	38.3
40	Minnesota	38.1
41	Vermont	37.6
42	North Dakota	37.3
43	Massachusetts	36.5
44	New Jersey	35.8
45	New Hampshire	34.3
46	Connecticut	34.2
47	Florida	33.6
48	Rhode Island	33.5
49	Arizona	32.7
50	New York	28.2
	District of Columbia	36.9

Source: U.S. Department of Health and Human Services, National Center for Health Statistics
    "National Vital Statistics Reports" (Vol. 58, No. 19, May 20, 2010, http://www.cdc.gov/nchs/deaths.htm)
*Final data by state of residence. Cerebrovascular diseases include stroke and other disorders of the blood vessels of the brain.
Age-adjusted rates based on the year 2000 standard population.

Deaths by Chronic Liver Disease and Cirrhosis in 2007

National Total = 29,165 Deaths*

ALPHA ORDER

RANK	STATE	DEATHS	% of USA
19	Alabama	505	1.7%
47	Alaska	70	0.2%
10	Arizona	752	2.6%
32	Arkansas	271	0.9%
1	California	4,065	13.9%
17	Colorado	542	1.9%
30	Connecticut	288	1.0%
47	Delaware	70	0.2%
3	Florida	2,260	7.7%
11	Georgia	686	2.4%
44	Hawaii	112	0.4%
37	Idaho	156	0.5%
7	Illinois	1,035	3.5%
21	Indiana	489	1.7%
35	Iowa	239	0.8%
36	Kansas	230	0.8%
26	Kentucky	390	1.3%
29	Louisiana	357	1.2%
37	Maine	156	0.5%
24	Maryland	447	1.5%
16	Massachusetts	609	2.1%
8	Michigan	1,008	3.5%
27	Minnesota	379	1.3%
34	Mississippi	263	0.9%
25	Missouri	433	1.5%
40	Montana	138	0.5%
42	Nebraska	116	0.4%
33	Nevada	268	0.9%
42	New Hampshire	116	0.4%
13	New Jersey	646	2.2%
28	New Mexico	372	1.3%
4	New York	1,308	4.5%
9	North Carolina	888	3.0%
50	North Dakota	43	0.1%
5	Ohio	1,152	3.9%
19	Oklahoma	505	1.7%
23	Oregon	466	1.6%
6	Pennsylvania	1,084	3.7%
41	Rhode Island	119	0.4%
18	South Carolina	512	1.8%
45	South Dakota	95	0.3%
14	Tennessee	629	2.2%
2	Texas	2,535	8.7%
39	Utah	142	0.5%
49	Vermont	54	0.2%
15	Virginia	613	2.1%
12	Washington	661	2.3%
31	West Virginia	273	0.9%
22	Wisconsin	487	1.7%
46	Wyoming	86	0.3%

RANK ORDER

RANK	STATE	DEATHS	% of USA
1	California	4,065	13.9%
2	Texas	2,535	8.7%
3	Florida	2,260	7.7%
4	New York	1,308	4.5%
5	Ohio	1,152	3.9%
6	Pennsylvania	1,084	3.7%
7	Illinois	1,035	3.5%
8	Michigan	1,008	3.5%
9	North Carolina	888	3.0%
10	Arizona	752	2.6%
11	Georgia	686	2.4%
12	Washington	661	2.3%
13	New Jersey	646	2.2%
14	Tennessee	629	2.2%
15	Virginia	613	2.1%
16	Massachusetts	609	2.1%
17	Colorado	542	1.9%
18	South Carolina	512	1.8%
19	Alabama	505	1.7%
19	Oklahoma	505	1.7%
21	Indiana	489	1.7%
22	Wisconsin	487	1.7%
23	Oregon	466	1.6%
24	Maryland	447	1.5%
25	Missouri	433	1.5%
26	Kentucky	390	1.3%
27	Minnesota	379	1.3%
28	New Mexico	372	1.3%
29	Louisiana	357	1.2%
30	Connecticut	288	1.0%
31	West Virginia	273	0.9%
32	Arkansas	271	0.9%
33	Nevada	268	0.9%
34	Mississippi	263	0.9%
35	Iowa	239	0.8%
36	Kansas	230	0.8%
37	Idaho	156	0.5%
37	Maine	156	0.5%
39	Utah	142	0.5%
40	Montana	138	0.5%
41	Rhode Island	119	0.4%
42	Nebraska	116	0.4%
42	New Hampshire	116	0.4%
44	Hawaii	112	0.4%
45	South Dakota	95	0.3%
46	Wyoming	86	0.3%
47	Alaska	70	0.2%
47	Delaware	70	0.2%
49	Vermont	54	0.2%
50	North Dakota	43	0.1%
	District of Columbia	45	0.2%

Source: U.S. Department of Health and Human Services, National Center for Health Statistics
"National Vital Statistics Reports" (Vol. 58, No. 19, May 20, 2010, http://www.cdc.gov/nchs/deaths.htm)
*Final data by state of residence. Cirrhosis of the liver is characterized by the replacement of normal tissue with fibrous tissue and the loss of functional liver cells. It can result from alcohol abuse, nutritional deprivation, or infection especially by the hepatitis virus.

Death Rate by Chronic Liver Disease and Cirrhosis in 2007

National Rate = 9.7 Deaths per 100,000 Population*

ALPHA ORDER				RANK ORDER		
RANK	STATE	RATE		RANK	STATE	RATE
15	Alabama	10.9		1	New Mexico	18.9
19	Alaska	10.2		2	Wyoming	16.4
8	Arizona	11.9		3	West Virginia	15.1
25	Arkansas	9.6		4	Montana	14.4
13	California	11.1		5	Oklahoma	14.0
13	Colorado	11.1		6	Florida	12.4
36	Connecticut	8.2		6	Oregon	12.4
37	Delaware	8.1		8	Arizona	11.9
6	Florida	12.4		8	South Dakota	11.9
46	Georgia	7.2		10	Maine	11.8
30	Hawaii	8.7		11	South Carolina	11.6
17	Idaho	10.4		12	Rhode Island	11.2
37	Illinois	8.1		13	California	11.1
42	Indiana	7.7		13	Colorado	11.1
39	Iowa	8.0		15	Alabama	10.9
34	Kansas	8.3		16	Texas	10.6
27	Kentucky	9.2		17	Idaho	10.4
34	Louisiana	8.3		17	Nevada	10.4
10	Maine	11.8		19	Alaska	10.2
39	Maryland	8.0		19	Tennessee	10.2
26	Massachusetts	9.4		19	Washington	10.2
22	Michigan	10.0		22	Michigan	10.0
45	Minnesota	7.3		22	Ohio	10.0
28	Mississippi	9.0		24	North Carolina	9.8
43	Missouri	7.4		25	Arkansas	9.6
4	Montana	14.4		26	Massachusetts	9.4
49	Nebraska	6.5		27	Kentucky	9.2
17	Nevada	10.4		28	Mississippi	9.0
29	New Hampshire	8.8		29	New Hampshire	8.8
43	New Jersey	7.4		30	Hawaii	8.7
1	New Mexico	18.9		30	Pennsylvania	8.7
47	New York	6.8		30	Vermont	8.7
24	North Carolina	9.8		30	Wisconsin	8.7
48	North Dakota	6.7		34	Kansas	8.3
22	Ohio	10.0		34	Louisiana	8.3
5	Oklahoma	14.0		36	Connecticut	8.2
6	Oregon	12.4		37	Delaware	8.1
30	Pennsylvania	8.7		37	Illinois	8.1
12	Rhode Island	11.2		39	Iowa	8.0
11	South Carolina	11.6		39	Maryland	8.0
8	South Dakota	11.9		41	Virginia	7.9
19	Tennessee	10.2		42	Indiana	7.7
16	Texas	10.6		43	Missouri	7.4
50	Utah	5.4		43	New Jersey	7.4
30	Vermont	8.7		45	Minnesota	7.3
41	Virginia	7.9		46	Georgia	7.2
19	Washington	10.2		47	New York	6.8
3	West Virginia	15.1		48	North Dakota	6.7
30	Wisconsin	8.7		49	Nebraska	6.5
2	Wyoming	16.4		50	Utah	5.4
					District of Columbia	7.6

Source: U.S. Department of Health and Human Services, National Center for Health Statistics
   "National Vital Statistics Reports" (Vol. 58, No. 19, May 20, 2010, http://www.cdc.gov/nchs/deaths.htm)
*Final data by state of residence. Cirrhosis of the liver is characterized by the replacement of normal tissue with fibrous tissue and the loss of functional liver cells. It can result from alcohol abuse, nutritional deprivation, or infection especially by the hepatitis virus. Not age-adjusted.

Age-Adjusted Death Rate by Chronic Liver Disease and Cirrhosis in 2007

National Rate = 9.1 Deaths per 100,000 Population*

ALPHA ORDER

RANK	STATE	RATE
17	Alabama	9.9
7	Alaska	11.4
6	Arizona	11.7
26	Arkansas	8.6
9	California	11.3
12	Colorado	11.0
40	Connecticut	7.3
36	Delaware	7.5
14	Florida	10.4
35	Georgia	7.6
34	Hawaii	7.7
15	Idaho	10.2
30	Illinois	7.9
40	Indiana	7.3
42	Iowa	7.2
32	Kansas	7.8
27	Kentucky	8.5
29	Louisiana	8.0
19	Maine	9.6
38	Maryland	7.4
28	Massachusetts	8.4
23	Michigan	9.1
44	Minnesota	6.9
25	Mississippi	8.8
45	Missouri	6.7
4	Montana	12.6
48	Nebraska	6.3
16	Nevada	10.0
32	New Hampshire	7.8
45	New Jersey	6.7
1	New Mexico	18.4
50	New York	6.2
21	North Carolina	9.2
48	North Dakota	6.3
23	Ohio	9.1
3	Oklahoma	13.2
11	Oregon	11.1
38	Pennsylvania	7.4
17	Rhode Island	9.9
13	South Carolina	10.5
9	South Dakota	11.3
21	Tennessee	9.2
7	Texas	11.4
47	Utah	6.5
43	Vermont	7.0
36	Virginia	7.5
20	Washington	9.5
5	West Virginia	12.5
30	Wisconsin	7.9
2	Wyoming	15.5

RANK ORDER

RANK	STATE	RATE
1	New Mexico	18.4
2	Wyoming	15.5
3	Oklahoma	13.2
4	Montana	12.6
5	West Virginia	12.5
6	Arizona	11.7
7	Alaska	11.4
7	Texas	11.4
9	California	11.3
9	South Dakota	11.3
11	Oregon	11.1
12	Colorado	11.0
13	South Carolina	10.5
14	Florida	10.4
15	Idaho	10.2
16	Nevada	10.0
17	Alabama	9.9
17	Rhode Island	9.9
19	Maine	9.6
20	Washington	9.5
21	North Carolina	9.2
21	Tennessee	9.2
23	Michigan	9.1
23	Ohio	9.1
25	Mississippi	8.8
26	Arkansas	8.6
27	Kentucky	8.5
28	Massachusetts	8.4
29	Louisiana	8.0
30	Illinois	7.9
30	Wisconsin	7.9
32	Kansas	7.8
32	New Hampshire	7.8
34	Hawaii	7.7
35	Georgia	7.6
36	Delaware	7.5
36	Virginia	7.5
38	Maryland	7.4
38	Pennsylvania	7.4
40	Connecticut	7.3
40	Indiana	7.3
42	Iowa	7.2
43	Vermont	7.0
44	Minnesota	6.9
45	Missouri	6.7
45	New Jersey	6.7
47	Utah	6.5
48	Nebraska	6.3
48	North Dakota	6.3
50	New York	6.2

District of Columbia	7.5

Source: U.S. Department of Health and Human Services, National Center for Health Statistics
"National Vital Statistics Reports" (Vol. 58, No. 19, May 20, 2010, http://www.cdc.gov/nchs/deaths.htm)
*Final data by state of residence. Cirrhosis of the liver is characterized by the replacement of normal tissue with fibrous tissue and the loss of functional liver cells. It can result from alcohol abuse, nutritional deprivation, or infection especially by the hepatitis virus. Age-adjusted rates based on the year 2000 standard population.

Deaths by Chronic Lower Respiratory Diseases in 2007

National Total = 127,924 Deaths*

ALPHA ORDER				RANK ORDER			
RANK	STATE	DEATHS	% of USA	RANK	STATE	DEATHS	% of USA
19	Alabama	2,530	2.0%	1	California	12,532	9.8%
50	Alaska	175	0.1%	2	Florida	9,357	7.3%
16	Arizona	2,686	2.1%	3	Texas	8,107	6.3%
30	Arkansas	1,656	1.3%	4	New York	6,561	5.1%
1	California	12,532	9.8%	5	Ohio	6,454	5.0%
24	Colorado	2,002	1.6%	6	Pennsylvania	6,077	4.8%
33	Connecticut	1,353	1.1%	7	Illinois	4,742	3.7%
45	Delaware	379	0.3%	8	Michigan	4,624	3.6%
2	Florida	9,357	7.3%	9	North Carolina	4,231	3.3%
10	Georgia	3,384	2.6%	10	Georgia	3,384	2.6%
47	Hawaii	299	0.2%	11	Indiana	3,227	2.5%
39	Idaho	666	0.5%	12	Tennessee	3,167	2.5%
7	Illinois	4,742	3.7%	13	Missouri	3,081	2.4%
11	Indiana	3,227	2.5%	14	New Jersey	2,991	2.3%
29	Iowa	1,660	1.3%	15	Virginia	2,770	2.2%
31	Kansas	1,476	1.2%	16	Arizona	2,686	2.1%
18	Kentucky	2,629	2.1%	17	Washington	2,684	2.1%
28	Louisiana	1,685	1.3%	18	Kentucky	2,629	2.1%
38	Maine	728	0.6%	19	Alabama	2,530	2.0%
25	Maryland	1,901	1.5%	20	Wisconsin	2,399	1.9%
22	Massachusetts	2,332	1.8%	21	Oklahoma	2,386	1.9%
8	Michigan	4,624	3.6%	22	Massachusetts	2,332	1.8%
27	Minnesota	1,758	1.4%	23	South Carolina	2,036	1.6%
32	Mississippi	1,408	1.1%	24	Colorado	2,002	1.6%
13	Missouri	3,081	2.4%	25	Maryland	1,901	1.5%
42	Montana	604	0.5%	26	Oregon	1,892	1.5%
36	Nebraska	919	0.7%	27	Minnesota	1,758	1.4%
35	Nevada	1,050	0.8%	28	Louisiana	1,685	1.3%
41	New Hampshire	611	0.5%	29	Iowa	1,660	1.3%
14	New Jersey	2,991	2.3%	30	Arkansas	1,656	1.3%
37	New Mexico	884	0.7%	31	Kansas	1,476	1.2%
4	New York	6,561	5.1%	32	Mississippi	1,408	1.1%
9	North Carolina	4,231	3.3%	33	Connecticut	1,353	1.1%
49	North Dakota	265	0.2%	34	West Virginia	1,331	1.0%
5	Ohio	6,454	5.0%	35	Nevada	1,050	0.8%
21	Oklahoma	2,386	1.9%	36	Nebraska	919	0.7%
26	Oregon	1,892	1.5%	37	New Mexico	884	0.7%
6	Pennsylvania	6,077	4.8%	38	Maine	728	0.6%
44	Rhode Island	421	0.3%	39	Idaho	666	0.5%
23	South Carolina	2,036	1.6%	40	Utah	617	0.5%
43	South Dakota	457	0.4%	41	New Hampshire	611	0.5%
12	Tennessee	3,167	2.5%	42	Montana	604	0.5%
3	Texas	8,107	6.3%	43	South Dakota	457	0.4%
40	Utah	617	0.5%	44	Rhode Island	421	0.3%
46	Vermont	316	0.2%	45	Delaware	379	0.3%
15	Virginia	2,770	2.2%	46	Vermont	316	0.2%
17	Washington	2,684	2.1%	47	Hawaii	299	0.2%
34	West Virginia	1,331	1.0%	48	Wyoming	295	0.2%
20	Wisconsin	2,399	1.9%	49	North Dakota	265	0.2%
48	Wyoming	295	0.2%	50	Alaska	175	0.1%
					District of Columbia	129	0.1%

Source: U.S. Department of Health and Human Services, National Center for Health Statistics
"National Vital Statistics Reports" (Vol. 58, No. 19, May 20, 2010, http://www.cdc.gov/nchs/deaths.htm)
*Final data by state of residence. Chronic lower respiratory diseases are diseases of the lungs including bronchitis, emphysema, and asthma. Includes allied conditions.

Death Rate by Chronic Lower Respiratory Diseases in 2007

National Rate = 42.4 Deaths per 100,000 Population*

ALPHA ORDER

RANK	STATE	RATE
11	Alabama	54.7
48	Alaska	25.6
30	Arizona	42.4
5	Arkansas	58.4
43	California	34.3
33	Colorado	41.2
37	Connecticut	38.6
28	Delaware	43.8
16	Florida	51.3
41	Georgia	35.5
49	Hawaii	23.3
27	Idaho	44.4
38	Illinois	36.9
17	Indiana	50.9
9	Iowa	55.6
12	Kansas	53.2
4	Kentucky	62.0
36	Louisiana	39.2
10	Maine	55.3
46	Maryland	33.8
39	Massachusetts	36.2
25	Michigan	45.9
46	Minnesota	33.8
21	Mississippi	48.2
13	Missouri	52.4
3	Montana	63.1
14	Nebraska	51.8
34	Nevada	40.9
23	New Hampshire	46.4
42	New Jersey	34.4
26	New Mexico	44.9
44	New York	34.0
22	North Carolina	46.7
32	North Dakota	41.4
8	Ohio	56.3
2	Oklahoma	66.0
19	Oregon	50.5
20	Pennsylvania	48.9
35	Rhode Island	39.8
24	South Carolina	46.2
6	South Dakota	57.4
15	Tennessee	51.4
45	Texas	33.9
49	Utah	23.3
17	Vermont	50.9
40	Virginia	35.9
31	Washington	41.5
1	West Virginia	73.5
29	Wisconsin	42.8
7	Wyoming	56.4

RANK ORDER

RANK	STATE	RATE
1	West Virginia	73.5
2	Oklahoma	66.0
3	Montana	63.1
4	Kentucky	62.0
5	Arkansas	58.4
6	South Dakota	57.4
7	Wyoming	56.4
8	Ohio	56.3
9	Iowa	55.6
10	Maine	55.3
11	Alabama	54.7
12	Kansas	53.2
13	Missouri	52.4
14	Nebraska	51.8
15	Tennessee	51.4
16	Florida	51.3
17	Indiana	50.9
17	Vermont	50.9
19	Oregon	50.5
20	Pennsylvania	48.9
21	Mississippi	48.2
22	North Carolina	46.7
23	New Hampshire	46.4
24	South Carolina	46.2
25	Michigan	45.9
26	New Mexico	44.9
27	Idaho	44.4
28	Delaware	43.8
29	Wisconsin	42.8
30	Arizona	42.4
31	Washington	41.5
32	North Dakota	41.4
33	Colorado	41.2
34	Nevada	40.9
35	Rhode Island	39.8
36	Louisiana	39.2
37	Connecticut	38.6
38	Illinois	36.9
39	Massachusetts	36.2
40	Virginia	35.9
41	Georgia	35.5
42	New Jersey	34.4
43	California	34.3
44	New York	34.0
45	Texas	33.9
46	Maryland	33.8
46	Minnesota	33.8
48	Alaska	25.6
49	Hawaii	23.3
49	Utah	23.3

District of Columbia	21.9

Source: U.S. Department of Health and Human Services, National Center for Health Statistics
   "National Vital Statistics Reports" (Vol. 58, No. 19, May 20, 2010, http://www.cdc.gov/nchs/deaths.htm)
*Final data by state of residence. Chronic lower respiratory diseases are diseases of the lungs including bronchitis, emphysema, and asthma. Includes allied conditions. Not age-adjusted.

Age-Adjusted Death Rate by Chronic Lower Respiratory Diseases in 2007

National Rate = 40.8 Deaths per 100,000 Population*

ALPHA ORDER

RANK	STATE	RATE
8	Alabama	50.2
23	Alaska	44.4
32	Arizona	40.2
6	Arkansas	51.7
38	California	37.4
11	Colorado	49.1
42	Connecticut	33.1
33	Delaware	40.1
39	Florida	36.7
26	Georgia	43.8
50	Hawaii	19.3
17	Idaho	46.6
39	Illinois	36.7
9	Indiana	49.2
22	Iowa	44.7
12	Kansas	48.8
2	Kentucky	59.0
34	Louisiana	39.7
21	Maine	44.8
41	Maryland	35.1
47	Massachusetts	31.6
27	Michigan	43.6
44	Minnesota	32.8
13	Mississippi	47.5
15	Missouri	47.4
5	Montana	55.0
19	Nebraska	45.8
13	Nevada	47.5
24	New Hampshire	44.0
48	New Jersey	31.3
27	New Mexico	43.6
49	New York	30.8
31	North Carolina	41.1
43	North Dakota	32.9
7	Ohio	50.7
1	Oklahoma	61.2
18	Oregon	46.3
36	Pennsylvania	38.1
45	Rhode Island	32.7
24	South Carolina	44.0
16	South Dakota	47.0
9	Tennessee	49.2
30	Texas	41.2
46	Utah	31.9
20	Vermont	44.9
37	Virginia	37.7
29	Washington	42.4
3	West Virginia	58.6
35	Wisconsin	38.7
4	Wyoming	56.5

RANK ORDER

RANK	STATE	RATE
1	Oklahoma	61.2
2	Kentucky	59.0
3	West Virginia	58.6
4	Wyoming	56.5
5	Montana	55.0
6	Arkansas	51.7
7	Ohio	50.7
8	Alabama	50.2
9	Indiana	49.2
9	Tennessee	49.2
11	Colorado	49.1
12	Kansas	48.8
13	Mississippi	47.5
13	Nevada	47.5
15	Missouri	47.4
16	South Dakota	47.0
17	Idaho	46.6
18	Oregon	46.3
19	Nebraska	45.8
20	Vermont	44.9
21	Maine	44.8
22	Iowa	44.7
23	Alaska	44.4
24	New Hampshire	44.0
24	South Carolina	44.0
26	Georgia	43.8
27	Michigan	43.6
27	New Mexico	43.6
29	Washington	42.4
30	Texas	41.2
31	North Carolina	41.1
32	Arizona	40.2
33	Delaware	40.1
34	Louisiana	39.7
35	Wisconsin	38.7
36	Pennsylvania	38.1
37	Virginia	37.7
38	California	37.4
39	Florida	36.7
39	Illinois	36.7
41	Maryland	35.1
42	Connecticut	33.1
43	North Dakota	32.9
44	Minnesota	32.8
45	Rhode Island	32.7
46	Utah	31.9
47	Massachusetts	31.6
48	New Jersey	31.3
49	New York	30.8
50	Hawaii	19.3
	District of Columbia	22.4

Source: U.S. Department of Health and Human Services, National Center for Health Statistics
   "National Vital Statistics Reports" (Vol. 58, No. 19, May 20, 2010, http://www.cdc.gov/nchs/deaths.htm)
*Final data by state of residence. Chronic lower respiratory diseases are diseases of the lungs including bronchitis, emphysema, and asthma. Includes allied conditions. Age-adjusted rates based on the year 2000 standard population.

Deaths by Diabetes Mellitus in 2007

National Total = 71,382 Deaths*

ALPHA ORDER					RANK ORDER			
RANK	STATE	DEATHS	% of USA		RANK	STATE	DEATHS	% of USA
18	Alabama	1,313	1.8%		1	California	7,413	10.4%
50	Alaska	105	0.1%		2	Florida	5,110	7.2%
22	Arizona	1,159	1.6%		3	Texas	5,109	7.2%
28	Arkansas	838	1.2%		4	Ohio	3,722	5.2%
1	California	7,413	10.4%		5	New York	3,715	5.2%
31	Colorado	710	1.0%		6	Pennsylvania	3,442	4.8%
35	Connecticut	646	0.9%		7	Illinois	2,851	4.0%
47	Delaware	223	0.3%		8	Michigan	2,826	4.0%
2	Florida	5,110	7.2%		9	New Jersey	2,329	3.3%
12	Georgia	1,604	2.2%		10	North Carolina	2,156	3.0%
41	Hawaii	291	0.4%		11	Tennessee	1,700	2.4%
39	Idaho	331	0.5%		12	Georgia	1,604	2.2%
7	Illinois	2,851	4.0%		13	Indiana	1,564	2.2%
13	Indiana	1,564	2.2%		14	Washington	1,508	2.1%
30	Iowa	767	1.1%		15	Virginia	1,507	2.1%
32	Kansas	702	1.0%		16	Missouri	1,444	2.0%
26	Kentucky	1,091	1.5%		17	Louisiana	1,437	2.0%
17	Louisiana	1,437	2.0%		18	Alabama	1,313	1.8%
38	Maine	355	0.5%		19	Maryland	1,301	1.8%
19	Maryland	1,301	1.8%		20	South Carolina	1,231	1.7%
21	Massachusetts	1,222	1.7%		21	Massachusetts	1,222	1.7%
8	Michigan	2,826	4.0%		22	Arizona	1,159	1.6%
27	Minnesota	1,084	1.5%		23	Oklahoma	1,148	1.6%
34	Mississippi	654	0.9%		24	Wisconsin	1,136	1.6%
16	Missouri	1,444	2.0%		25	Oregon	1,113	1.6%
43	Montana	258	0.4%		26	Kentucky	1,091	1.5%
37	Nebraska	472	0.7%		27	Minnesota	1,084	1.5%
40	Nevada	312	0.4%		28	Arkansas	838	1.2%
42	New Hampshire	280	0.4%		29	West Virginia	800	1.1%
9	New Jersey	2,329	3.3%		30	Iowa	767	1.1%
33	New Mexico	673	0.9%		31	Colorado	710	1.0%
5	New York	3,715	5.2%		32	Kansas	702	1.0%
10	North Carolina	2,156	3.0%		33	New Mexico	673	0.9%
46	North Dakota	226	0.3%		34	Mississippi	654	0.9%
4	Ohio	3,722	5.2%		35	Connecticut	646	0.9%
23	Oklahoma	1,148	1.6%		36	Utah	548	0.8%
25	Oregon	1,113	1.6%		37	Nebraska	472	0.7%
6	Pennsylvania	3,442	4.8%		38	Maine	355	0.5%
44	Rhode Island	248	0.3%		39	Idaho	331	0.5%
20	South Carolina	1,231	1.7%		40	Nevada	312	0.4%
45	South Dakota	247	0.3%		41	Hawaii	291	0.4%
11	Tennessee	1,700	2.4%		42	New Hampshire	280	0.4%
3	Texas	5,109	7.2%		43	Montana	258	0.4%
36	Utah	548	0.8%		44	Rhode Island	248	0.3%
48	Vermont	170	0.2%		45	South Dakota	247	0.3%
15	Virginia	1,507	2.1%		46	North Dakota	226	0.3%
14	Washington	1,508	2.1%		47	Delaware	223	0.3%
29	West Virginia	800	1.1%		48	Vermont	170	0.2%
24	Wisconsin	1,136	1.6%		49	Wyoming	139	0.2%
49	Wyoming	139	0.2%		50	Alaska	105	0.1%
						District of Columbia	152	0.2%

Source: U.S. Department of Health and Human Services, National Center for Health Statistics
"National Vital Statistics Reports" (Vol. 58, No. 19, May 20, 2010, http://www.cdc.gov/nchs/deaths.htm)
*Final data by state of residence. A severe, chronic form of diabetes caused by insufficient production of insulin and resulting in abnormal metabolism of carbohydrates, fats, and proteins. The disease, which typically appears in childhood or adolescence, is characterized by increased sugar levels in the blood and urine, excessive thirst, and frequent urination.

Death Rate by Diabetes Mellitus in 2007

National Rate = 23.7 Deaths per 100,000 Population*

ALPHA ORDER

RANK	STATE	RATE
10	Alabama	28.4
48	Alaska	15.4
46	Arizona	18.3
9	Arkansas	29.6
40	California	20.3
49	Colorado	14.6
45	Connecticut	18.4
22	Delaware	25.8
12	Florida	28.0
47	Georgia	16.8
32	Hawaii	22.7
35	Idaho	22.1
34	Illinois	22.2
26	Indiana	24.6
23	Iowa	25.7
25	Kansas	25.3
23	Kentucky	25.7
4	Louisiana	33.5
17	Maine	27.0
31	Maryland	23.2
44	Massachusetts	18.9
11	Michigan	28.1
38	Minnesota	20.9
33	Mississippi	22.4
26	Missouri	24.6
18	Montana	26.9
20	Nebraska	26.6
50	Nevada	12.2
37	New Hampshire	21.3
19	New Jersey	26.8
3	New Mexico	34.2
43	New York	19.3
28	North Carolina	23.8
2	North Dakota	35.3
5	Ohio	32.5
6	Oklahoma	31.7
8	Oregon	29.7
14	Pennsylvania	27.7
29	Rhode Island	23.4
13	South Carolina	27.9
7	South Dakota	31.0
15	Tennessee	27.6
36	Texas	21.4
39	Utah	20.7
16	Vermont	27.4
42	Virginia	19.5
30	Washington	23.3
1	West Virginia	44.1
40	Wisconsin	20.3
20	Wyoming	26.6

RANK ORDER

RANK	STATE	RATE
1	West Virginia	44.1
2	North Dakota	35.3
3	New Mexico	34.2
4	Louisiana	33.5
5	Ohio	32.5
6	Oklahoma	31.7
7	South Dakota	31.0
8	Oregon	29.7
9	Arkansas	29.6
10	Alabama	28.4
11	Michigan	28.1
12	Florida	28.0
13	South Carolina	27.9
14	Pennsylvania	27.7
15	Tennessee	27.6
16	Vermont	27.4
17	Maine	27.0
18	Montana	26.9
19	New Jersey	26.8
20	Nebraska	26.6
20	Wyoming	26.6
22	Delaware	25.8
23	Iowa	25.7
23	Kentucky	25.7
25	Kansas	25.3
26	Indiana	24.6
26	Missouri	24.6
28	North Carolina	23.8
29	Rhode Island	23.4
30	Washington	23.3
31	Maryland	23.2
32	Hawaii	22.7
33	Mississippi	22.4
34	Illinois	22.2
35	Idaho	22.1
36	Texas	21.4
37	New Hampshire	21.3
38	Minnesota	20.9
39	Utah	20.7
40	California	20.3
40	Wisconsin	20.3
42	Virginia	19.5
43	New York	19.3
44	Massachusetts	18.9
45	Connecticut	18.4
46	Arizona	18.3
47	Georgia	16.8
48	Alaska	15.4
49	Colorado	14.6
50	Nevada	12.2
	District of Columbia	25.8

Source: U.S. Department of Health and Human Services, National Center for Health Statistics
   "National Vital Statistics Reports" (Vol. 58, No. 19, May 20, 2010, http://www.cdc.gov/nchs/deaths.htm)
*Final data by state of residence. A severe, chronic form of diabetes caused by insufficient production of insulin and resulting in abnormal metabolism of carbohydrates, fats, and proteins. The disease, which typically appears in childhood or adolescence, is characterized by increased sugar levels in the blood and urine, excessive thirst, and frequent urination. Not age-adjusted.

Age-Adjusted Death Rate by Diabetes Mellitus in 2007

National Rate = 22.5 Deaths per 100,000 Population*

ALPHA ORDER

RANK	STATE	RATE
14	Alabama	26.0
20	Alaska	23.4
46	Arizona	17.4
9	Arkansas	26.5
33	California	21.8
47	Colorado	16.7
49	Connecticut	15.8
20	Delaware	23.4
36	Florida	21.1
41	Georgia	19.5
43	Hawaii	18.5
29	Idaho	22.7
33	Illinois	21.8
20	Indiana	23.4
37	Iowa	20.5
28	Kansas	22.8
19	Kentucky	24.1
2	Louisiana	33.3
32	Maine	21.9
20	Maryland	23.4
48	Massachusetts	16.6
10	Michigan	26.3
40	Minnesota	19.6
33	Mississippi	21.8
30	Missouri	22.3
27	Montana	23.1
25	Nebraska	23.3
50	Nevada	12.9
38	New Hampshire	20.1
17	New Jersey	24.4
3	New Mexico	32.7
45	New York	17.5
20	North Carolina	23.4
6	North Dakota	28.3
5	Ohio	29.1
4	Oklahoma	29.3
8	Oregon	27.0
31	Pennsylvania	22.0
42	Rhode Island	19.2
11	South Carolina	26.2
15	South Dakota	25.6
11	Tennessee	26.2
16	Texas	24.9
7	Utah	27.6
17	Vermont	24.4
39	Virginia	19.7
26	Washington	23.2
1	West Virginia	35.5
44	Wisconsin	18.3
11	Wyoming	26.2

RANK ORDER

RANK	STATE	RATE
1	West Virginia	35.5
2	Louisiana	33.3
3	New Mexico	32.7
4	Oklahoma	29.3
5	Ohio	29.1
6	North Dakota	28.3
7	Utah	27.6
8	Oregon	27.0
9	Arkansas	26.5
10	Michigan	26.3
11	South Carolina	26.2
11	Tennessee	26.2
11	Wyoming	26.2
14	Alabama	26.0
15	South Dakota	25.6
16	Texas	24.9
17	New Jersey	24.4
17	Vermont	24.4
19	Kentucky	24.1
20	Alaska	23.4
20	Delaware	23.4
20	Indiana	23.4
20	Maryland	23.4
20	North Carolina	23.4
25	Nebraska	23.3
26	Washington	23.2
27	Montana	23.1
28	Kansas	22.8
29	Idaho	22.7
30	Missouri	22.3
31	Pennsylvania	22.0
32	Maine	21.9
33	California	21.8
33	Illinois	21.8
33	Mississippi	21.8
36	Florida	21.1
37	Iowa	20.5
38	New Hampshire	20.1
39	Virginia	19.7
40	Minnesota	19.6
41	Georgia	19.5
42	Rhode Island	19.2
43	Hawaii	18.5
44	Wisconsin	18.3
45	New York	17.5
46	Arizona	17.4
47	Colorado	16.7
48	Massachusetts	16.6
49	Connecticut	15.8
50	Nevada	12.9
	District of Columbia	25.2

Source: U.S. Department of Health and Human Services, National Center for Health Statistics
 "National Vital Statistics Reports" (Vol. 58, No. 19, May 20, 2010, http://www.cdc.gov/nchs/deaths.htm)
*Final data by state of residence. A severe, chronic form of diabetes caused by insufficient production of insulin and resulting in abnormal metabolism of carbohydrates, fats, and proteins. The disease, which typically appears in childhood or adolescence, is characterized by increased sugar levels in the blood and urine, excessive thirst, and frequent urination. Age-adjusted rates based on the year 2000 standard population.

Deaths by Diseases of the Heart in 2007

National Total = 616,067 Deaths*

ALPHA ORDER

ALPHA ORDER

RANK	STATE	DEATHS	% of USA
17	Alabama	11,926	1.9%
50	Alaska	613	0.1%
21	Arizona	10,302	1.7%
29	Arkansas	7,214	1.2%
1	California	61,690	10.0%
32	Colorado	6,106	1.0%
28	Connecticut	7,289	1.2%
44	Delaware	1,914	0.3%
3	Florida	42,254	6.9%
11	Georgia	16,184	2.6%
43	Hawaii	2,227	0.4%
42	Idaho	2,433	0.4%
7	Illinois	25,813	4.2%
15	Indiana	13,682	2.2%
30	Iowa	6,880	1.1%
33	Kansas	5,749	0.9%
23	Kentucky	9,916	1.6%
22	Louisiana	9,947	1.6%
39	Maine	2,852	0.5%
18	Maryland	11,314	1.8%
16	Massachusetts	12,710	2.1%
8	Michigan	24,149	3.9%
27	Minnesota	7,477	1.2%
26	Mississippi	8,037	1.3%
12	Missouri	14,338	2.3%
45	Montana	1,870	0.3%
36	Nebraska	3,520	0.6%
35	Nevada	4,591	0.7%
41	New Hampshire	2,511	0.4%
9	New Jersey	18,831	3.1%
37	New Mexico	3,305	0.5%
2	New York	49,528	8.0%
10	North Carolina	17,395	2.8%
47	North Dakota	1,414	0.2%
6	Ohio	26,757	4.3%
24	Oklahoma	9,602	1.6%
31	Oregon	6,655	1.1%
5	Pennsylvania	32,862	5.3%
40	Rhode Island	2,751	0.4%
25	South Carolina	8,992	1.5%
46	South Dakota	1,633	0.3%
13	Tennessee	14,280	2.3%
4	Texas	38,912	6.3%
38	Utah	2,980	0.5%
48	Vermont	1,166	0.2%
14	Virginia	13,750	2.2%
20	Washington	11,037	1.8%
34	West Virginia	5,208	0.8%
19	Wisconsin	11,110	1.8%
49	Wyoming	957	0.2%

RANK ORDER

RANK	STATE	DEATHS	% of USA
1	California	61,690	10.0%
2	New York	49,528	8.0%
3	Florida	42,254	6.9%
4	Texas	38,912	6.3%
5	Pennsylvania	32,862	5.3%
6	Ohio	26,757	4.3%
7	Illinois	25,813	4.2%
8	Michigan	24,149	3.9%
9	New Jersey	18,831	3.1%
10	North Carolina	17,395	2.8%
11	Georgia	16,184	2.6%
12	Missouri	14,338	2.3%
13	Tennessee	14,280	2.3%
14	Virginia	13,750	2.2%
15	Indiana	13,682	2.2%
16	Massachusetts	12,710	2.1%
17	Alabama	11,926	1.9%
18	Maryland	11,314	1.8%
19	Wisconsin	11,110	1.8%
20	Washington	11,037	1.8%
21	Arizona	10,302	1.7%
22	Louisiana	9,947	1.6%
23	Kentucky	9,916	1.6%
24	Oklahoma	9,602	1.6%
25	South Carolina	8,992	1.5%
26	Mississippi	8,037	1.3%
27	Minnesota	7,477	1.2%
28	Connecticut	7,289	1.2%
29	Arkansas	7,214	1.2%
30	Iowa	6,880	1.1%
31	Oregon	6,655	1.1%
32	Colorado	6,106	1.0%
33	Kansas	5,749	0.9%
34	West Virginia	5,208	0.8%
35	Nevada	4,591	0.7%
36	Nebraska	3,520	0.6%
37	New Mexico	3,305	0.5%
38	Utah	2,980	0.5%
39	Maine	2,852	0.5%
40	Rhode Island	2,751	0.4%
41	New Hampshire	2,511	0.4%
42	Idaho	2,433	0.4%
43	Hawaii	2,227	0.4%
44	Delaware	1,914	0.3%
45	Montana	1,870	0.3%
46	South Dakota	1,633	0.3%
47	North Dakota	1,414	0.2%
48	Vermont	1,166	0.2%
49	Wyoming	957	0.2%
50	Alaska	613	0.1%
	District of Columbia	1,434	0.2%

Source: U.S. Department of Health and Human Services, National Center for Health Statistics
"National Vital Statistics Reports" (Vol. 58, No. 19, May 20, 2010, http://www.cdc.gov/nchs/deaths.htm)
*Final data by state of residence.

Death Rate by Diseases of the Heart in 2007

National Rate = 204.3 Deaths per 100,000 Population*

ALPHA ORDER				RANK ORDER		
RANK	STATE	RATE		RANK	STATE	RATE
6	Alabama	257.7		1	West Virginia	287.4
50	Alaska	89.7		2	Mississippi	275.4
45	Arizona	162.5		3	Oklahoma	265.4
8	Arkansas	254.5		4	Pennsylvania	264.3
42	California	168.8		5	Rhode Island	260.1
48	Colorado	125.6		6	Alabama	257.7
22	Connecticut	208.1		7	New York	256.7
17	Delaware	221.3		8	Arkansas	254.5
15	Florida	231.5		9	Missouri	243.9
41	Georgia	169.6		10	Michigan	239.8
39	Hawaii	173.5		11	Kentucky	233.8
46	Idaho	162.3		12	Ohio	233.3
27	Illinois	200.8		13	Tennessee	231.9
21	Indiana	215.6		14	Louisiana	231.7
16	Iowa	230.3		15	Florida	231.5
23	Kansas	207.1		16	Iowa	230.3
11	Kentucky	233.8		17	Delaware	221.3
14	Louisiana	231.7		18	North Dakota	221.0
20	Maine	216.5		19	New Jersey	216.8
26	Maryland	201.4		20	Maine	216.5
30	Massachusetts	197.1		21	Indiana	215.6
10	Michigan	239.8		22	Connecticut	208.1
47	Minnesota	143.9		23	Kansas	207.1
2	Mississippi	275.4		24	South Dakota	205.1
9	Missouri	243.9		25	South Carolina	204.0
31	Montana	195.2		26	Maryland	201.4
28	Nebraska	198.4		27	Illinois	200.8
36	Nevada	179.0		28	Nebraska	198.4
33	New Hampshire	190.8		29	Wisconsin	198.3
19	New Jersey	216.8		30	Massachusetts	197.1
43	New Mexico	167.8		31	Montana	195.2
7	New York	256.7		32	North Carolina	192.0
32	North Carolina	192.0		33	New Hampshire	190.8
18	North Dakota	221.0		34	Vermont	187.7
12	Ohio	233.3		35	Wyoming	183.0
3	Oklahoma	265.4		36	Nevada	179.0
38	Oregon	177.6		37	Virginia	178.3
4	Pennsylvania	264.3		38	Oregon	177.6
5	Rhode Island	260.1		39	Hawaii	173.5
25	South Carolina	204.0		40	Washington	170.6
24	South Dakota	205.1		41	Georgia	169.6
13	Tennessee	231.9		42	California	168.8
44	Texas	162.8		43	New Mexico	167.8
49	Utah	112.7		44	Texas	162.8
34	Vermont	187.7		45	Arizona	162.5
37	Virginia	178.3		46	Idaho	162.3
40	Washington	170.6		47	Minnesota	143.9
1	West Virginia	287.4		48	Colorado	125.6
29	Wisconsin	198.3		49	Utah	112.7
35	Wyoming	183.0		50	Alaska	89.7
					District of Columbia	243.8

Source: U.S. Department of Health and Human Services, National Center for Health Statistics
    "National Vital Statistics Reports" (Vol. 58, No. 19, May 20, 2010, http://www.cdc.gov/nchs/deaths.htm)
*Final data by state of residence. Not age-adjusted.

Age-Adjusted Death Rate by Diseases of the Heart in 2007

National Rate = 190.9 Deaths per 100,000 Population*

ALPHA ORDER

RANK	STATE	RATE
3	Alabama	235.5
47	Alaska	147.9
45	Arizona	152.5
7	Arkansas	221.8
28	California	177.9
48	Colorado	145.3
33	Connecticut	171.0
17	Delaware	200.2
40	Florida	162.4
14	Georgia	203.0
49	Hawaii	140.2
37	Idaho	164.1
21	Illinois	192.8
14	Indiana	203.0
30	Iowa	174.8
26	Kansas	178.7
9	Kentucky	220.9
4	Louisiana	230.0
31	Maine	172.9
16	Maryland	202.4
35	Massachusetts	165.5
8	Michigan	221.5
50	Minnesota	129.8
1	Mississippi	266.5
11	Missouri	214.4
39	Montana	163.1
36	Nebraska	165.3
18	Nevada	200.0
29	New Hampshire	174.9
22	New Jersey	191.9
42	New Mexico	159.2
6	New York	225.1
24	North Carolina	191.0
37	North Dakota	164.1
12	Ohio	204.8
2	Oklahoma	241.6
44	Oregon	156.9
19	Pennsylvania	199.4
13	Rhode Island	203.6
20	South Carolina	192.9
43	South Dakota	159.1
10	Tennessee	220.6
22	Texas	191.9
46	Utah	152.1
41	Vermont	161.2
25	Virginia	182.7
34	Washington	167.2
5	West Virginia	229.4
32	Wisconsin	171.9
27	Wyoming	178.3

RANK ORDER

RANK	STATE	RATE
1	Mississippi	266.5
2	Oklahoma	241.6
3	Alabama	235.5
4	Louisiana	230.0
5	West Virginia	229.4
6	New York	225.1
7	Arkansas	221.8
8	Michigan	221.5
9	Kentucky	220.9
10	Tennessee	220.6
11	Missouri	214.4
12	Ohio	204.8
13	Rhode Island	203.6
14	Georgia	203.0
14	Indiana	203.0
16	Maryland	202.4
17	Delaware	200.2
18	Nevada	200.0
19	Pennsylvania	199.4
20	South Carolina	192.9
21	Illinois	192.8
22	New Jersey	191.9
22	Texas	191.9
24	North Carolina	191.0
25	Virginia	182.7
26	Kansas	178.7
27	Wyoming	178.3
28	California	177.9
29	New Hampshire	174.9
30	Iowa	174.8
31	Maine	172.9
32	Wisconsin	171.9
33	Connecticut	171.0
34	Washington	167.2
35	Massachusetts	165.5
36	Nebraska	165.3
37	Idaho	164.1
37	North Dakota	164.1
39	Montana	163.1
40	Florida	162.4
41	Vermont	161.2
42	New Mexico	159.2
43	South Dakota	159.1
44	Oregon	156.9
45	Arizona	152.5
46	Utah	152.1
47	Alaska	147.9
48	Colorado	145.3
49	Hawaii	140.2
50	Minnesota	129.8

	District of Columbia	239.4

Source: U.S. Department of Health and Human Services, National Center for Health Statistics
"National Vital Statistics Reports" (Vol. 58, No. 19, May 20, 2010, http://www.cdc.gov/nchs/deaths.htm)
*Final data by state of residence. Age-adjusted rates based on the year 2000 standard population.

Deaths by Malignant Neoplasms in 2007

National Total = 562,875 Deaths*

ALPHA ORDER

RANK ORDER

RANK	STATE	DEATHS	% of USA		RANK	STATE	DEATHS	% of USA
21	Alabama	10,025	1.8%		1	California	55,011	9.8%
50	Alaska	839	0.1%		2	Florida	40,088	7.1%
20	Arizona	10,134	1.8%		3	New York	35,485	6.3%
30	Arkansas	6,388	1.1%		4	Texas	35,074	6.2%
1	California	55,011	9.8%		5	Pennsylvania	29,014	5.2%
29	Colorado	6,617	1.2%		6	Ohio	25,230	4.5%
28	Connecticut	6,827	1.2%		7	Illinois	24,115	4.3%
45	Delaware	1,853	0.3%		8	Michigan	20,087	3.6%
2	Florida	40,088	7.1%		9	North Carolina	17,478	3.1%
11	Georgia	14,983	2.7%		10	New Jersey	17,096	3.0%
42	Hawaii	2,214	0.4%		11	Georgia	14,983	2.7%
41	Idaho	2,405	0.4%		12	Virginia	14,009	2.5%
7	Illinois	24,115	4.3%		13	Tennessee	13,161	2.3%
15	Indiana	12,778	2.3%		14	Massachusetts	13,003	2.3%
31	Iowa	6,376	1.1%		15	Indiana	12,778	2.3%
33	Kansas	5,406	1.0%		16	Missouri	12,380	2.2%
22	Kentucky	9,692	1.7%		17	Washington	11,568	2.1%
25	Louisiana	8,736	1.6%		18	Wisconsin	10,963	1.9%
38	Maine	3,112	0.6%		19	Maryland	10,179	1.8%
19	Maryland	10,179	1.8%		20	Arizona	10,134	1.8%
14	Massachusetts	13,003	2.3%		21	Alabama	10,025	1.8%
8	Michigan	20,087	3.6%		22	Kentucky	9,692	1.7%
23	Minnesota	9,176	1.6%		23	Minnesota	9,176	1.6%
32	Mississippi	6,002	1.1%		24	South Carolina	8,867	1.6%
16	Missouri	12,380	2.2%		25	Louisiana	8,736	1.6%
44	Montana	1,921	0.3%		26	Oklahoma	7,727	1.4%
36	Nebraska	3,479	0.6%		27	Oregon	7,393	1.3%
35	Nevada	4,331	0.8%		28	Connecticut	6,827	1.2%
39	New Hampshire	2,609	0.5%		29	Colorado	6,617	1.2%
10	New Jersey	17,096	3.0%		30	Arkansas	6,388	1.1%
37	New Mexico	3,238	0.6%		31	Iowa	6,376	1.1%
3	New York	35,485	6.3%		32	Mississippi	6,002	1.1%
9	North Carolina	17,478	3.1%		33	Kansas	5,406	1.0%
48	North Dakota	1,264	0.2%		34	West Virginia	4,690	0.8%
6	Ohio	25,230	4.5%		35	Nevada	4,331	0.8%
26	Oklahoma	7,727	1.4%		36	Nebraska	3,479	0.6%
27	Oregon	7,393	1.3%		37	New Mexico	3,238	0.6%
5	Pennsylvania	29,014	5.2%		38	Maine	3,112	0.6%
43	Rhode Island	2,213	0.4%		39	New Hampshire	2,609	0.5%
24	South Carolina	8,867	1.6%		40	Utah	2,572	0.5%
46	South Dakota	1,612	0.3%		41	Idaho	2,405	0.4%
13	Tennessee	13,161	2.3%		42	Hawaii	2,214	0.4%
4	Texas	35,074	6.2%		43	Rhode Island	2,213	0.4%
40	Utah	2,572	0.5%		44	Montana	1,921	0.3%
47	Vermont	1,346	0.2%		45	Delaware	1,853	0.3%
12	Virginia	14,009	2.5%		46	South Dakota	1,612	0.3%
17	Washington	11,568	2.1%		47	Vermont	1,346	0.2%
34	West Virginia	4,690	0.8%		48	North Dakota	1,264	0.2%
18	Wisconsin	10,963	1.9%		49	Wyoming	940	0.2%
49	Wyoming	940	0.2%		50	Alaska	839	0.1%
					District of Columbia	1,169	0.2%	

Source: U.S. Department of Health and Human Services, National Center for Health Statistics
   "National Vital Statistics Reports" (Vol. 58, No. 19, May 20, 2010, http://www.cdc.gov/nchs/deaths.htm)
*Final data by state of residence. Neoplasms are abnormal tissue, tumors. Includes many cancers.

Death Rate by Malignant Neoplasms in 2007

National Rate = 186.6 Deaths per 100,000 Population*

ALPHA ORDER			RANK ORDER		
RANK	STATE	RATE	RANK	STATE	RATE
9	Alabama	216.6	1	West Virginia	258.8
49	Alaska	122.8	2	Maine	236.3
44	Arizona	159.9	3	Pennsylvania	233.4
5	Arkansas	225.3	4	Kentucky	228.5
46	California	150.5	5	Arkansas	225.3
48	Colorado	136.1	6	Ohio	220.0
30	Connecticut	194.9	7	Florida	219.6
10	Delaware	214.3	8	Vermont	216.7
7	Florida	219.6	9	Alabama	216.6
45	Georgia	157.0	10	Delaware	214.3
40	Hawaii	172.5	11	Tennessee	213.8
43	Idaho	160.4	12	Oklahoma	213.6
33	Illinois	187.6	13	Iowa	213.4
20	Indiana	201.4	14	Missouri	210.6
13	Iowa	213.4	15	Rhode Island	209.2
31	Kansas	194.7	16	Mississippi	205.6
4	Kentucky	228.5	17	Louisiana	203.5
17	Louisiana	203.5	18	South Dakota	202.5
2	Maine	236.3	19	Massachusetts	201.6
36	Maryland	181.2	20	Indiana	201.4
19	Massachusetts	201.6	21	South Carolina	201.2
23	Michigan	199.4	22	Montana	200.6
39	Minnesota	176.5	23	Michigan	199.4
16	Mississippi	205.6	24	New Hampshire	198.3
14	Missouri	210.6	25	North Dakota	197.6
22	Montana	200.6	26	Oregon	197.3
28	Nebraska	196.0	27	New Jersey	196.8
41	Nevada	168.8	28	Nebraska	196.0
24	New Hampshire	198.3	29	Wisconsin	195.7
27	New Jersey	196.8	30	Connecticut	194.9
42	New Mexico	164.4	31	Kansas	194.7
34	New York	183.9	32	North Carolina	192.9
32	North Carolina	192.9	33	Illinois	187.6
25	North Dakota	197.6	34	New York	183.9
6	Ohio	220.0	35	Virginia	181.6
12	Oklahoma	213.6	36	Maryland	181.2
26	Oregon	197.3	37	Wyoming	179.8
3	Pennsylvania	233.4	38	Washington	178.8
15	Rhode Island	209.2	39	Minnesota	176.5
21	South Carolina	201.2	40	Hawaii	172.5
18	South Dakota	202.5	41	Nevada	168.8
11	Tennessee	213.8	42	New Mexico	164.4
47	Texas	146.7	43	Idaho	160.4
50	Utah	97.2	44	Arizona	159.9
8	Vermont	216.7	45	Georgia	157.0
35	Virginia	181.6	46	California	150.5
38	Washington	178.8	47	Texas	146.7
1	West Virginia	258.8	48	Colorado	136.1
29	Wisconsin	195.7	49	Alaska	122.8
37	Wyoming	179.8	50	Utah	97.2
				District of Columbia	198.7

Source: U.S. Department of Health and Human Services, National Center for Health Statistics
    "National Vital Statistics Reports" (Vol. 58, No. 19, May 20, 2010, http://www.cdc.gov/nchs/deaths.htm)
*Final data by state of residence. Neoplasms are abnormal tissue, tumors. Includes many cancers. Not age-adjusted.

Age-Adjusted Death Rate by Malignant Neoplasms in 2007

National Rate = 178.4 Deaths per 100,000 Population*

<table>
<tr><td colspan="3">ALPHA ORDER</td><td colspan="3">RANK ORDER</td></tr>
<tr><td>RANK</td><td>STATE</td><td>RATE</td><td>RANK</td><td>STATE</td><td>RATE</td></tr>
<tr><td>9</td><td>Alabama</td><td>197.3</td><td>1</td><td>Kentucky</td><td>213.5</td></tr>
<tr><td>27</td><td>Alaska</td><td>179.9</td><td>2</td><td>West Virginia</td><td>207.6</td></tr>
<tr><td>48</td><td>Arizona</td><td>152.8</td><td>3</td><td>Arkansas</td><td>200.4</td></tr>
<tr><td>3</td><td>Arkansas</td><td>200.4</td><td>3</td><td>Mississippi</td><td>200.4</td></tr>
<tr><td>45</td><td>California</td><td>161.7</td><td>5</td><td>Louisiana</td><td>200.3</td></tr>
<tr><td>47</td><td>Colorado</td><td>153.7</td><td>5</td><td>Tennessee</td><td>200.3</td></tr>
<tr><td>38</td><td>Connecticut</td><td>170.7</td><td>7</td><td>Oklahoma</td><td>198.2</td></tr>
<tr><td>10</td><td>Delaware</td><td>193.9</td><td>8</td><td>Ohio</td><td>197.9</td></tr>
<tr><td>42</td><td>Florida</td><td>166.6</td><td>9</td><td>Alabama</td><td>197.3</td></tr>
<tr><td>22</td><td>Georgia</td><td>181.8</td><td>10</td><td>Delaware</td><td>193.9</td></tr>
<tr><td>49</td><td>Hawaii</td><td>146.2</td><td>11</td><td>Indiana</td><td>193.2</td></tr>
<tr><td>43</td><td>Idaho</td><td>165.6</td><td>12</td><td>Maine</td><td>191.9</td></tr>
<tr><td>19</td><td>Illinois</td><td>185.9</td><td>13</td><td>Missouri</td><td>191.6</td></tr>
<tr><td>11</td><td>Indiana</td><td>193.2</td><td>14</td><td>North Carolina</td><td>189.0</td></tr>
<tr><td>32</td><td>Iowa</td><td>177.7</td><td>15</td><td>Vermont</td><td>188.5</td></tr>
<tr><td>26</td><td>Kansas</td><td>180.0</td><td>16</td><td>Pennsylvania</td><td>188.2</td></tr>
<tr><td>1</td><td>Kentucky</td><td>213.5</td><td>17</td><td>Michigan</td><td>187.3</td></tr>
<tr><td>5</td><td>Louisiana</td><td>200.3</td><td>18</td><td>South Carolina</td><td>186.7</td></tr>
<tr><td>12</td><td>Maine</td><td>191.9</td><td>19</td><td>Illinois</td><td>185.9</td></tr>
<tr><td>23</td><td>Maryland</td><td>180.7</td><td>20</td><td>New Hampshire</td><td>184.5</td></tr>
<tr><td>28</td><td>Massachusetts</td><td>179.8</td><td>21</td><td>Virginia</td><td>182.7</td></tr>
<tr><td>17</td><td>Michigan</td><td>187.3</td><td>22</td><td>Georgia</td><td>181.8</td></tr>
<tr><td>40</td><td>Minnesota</td><td>169.7</td><td>23</td><td>Maryland</td><td>180.7</td></tr>
<tr><td>3</td><td>Mississippi</td><td>200.4</td><td>24</td><td>New Jersey</td><td>180.4</td></tr>
<tr><td>13</td><td>Missouri</td><td>191.6</td><td>25</td><td>Nevada</td><td>180.2</td></tr>
<tr><td>36</td><td>Montana</td><td>172.1</td><td>26</td><td>Kansas</td><td>180.0</td></tr>
<tr><td>34</td><td>Nebraska</td><td>177.3</td><td>27</td><td>Alaska</td><td>179.9</td></tr>
<tr><td>25</td><td>Nevada</td><td>180.2</td><td>28</td><td>Massachusetts</td><td>179.8</td></tr>
<tr><td>20</td><td>New Hampshire</td><td>184.5</td><td>29</td><td>Rhode Island</td><td>179.6</td></tr>
<tr><td>24</td><td>New Jersey</td><td>180.4</td><td>30</td><td>Oregon</td><td>179.3</td></tr>
<tr><td>46</td><td>New Mexico</td><td>157.3</td><td>31</td><td>Wisconsin</td><td>177.9</td></tr>
<tr><td>41</td><td>New York</td><td>168.0</td><td>32</td><td>Iowa</td><td>177.7</td></tr>
<tr><td>14</td><td>North Carolina</td><td>189.0</td><td>32</td><td>Washington</td><td>177.7</td></tr>
<tr><td>44</td><td>North Dakota</td><td>165.3</td><td>34</td><td>Nebraska</td><td>177.3</td></tr>
<tr><td>8</td><td>Ohio</td><td>197.9</td><td>35</td><td>Wyoming</td><td>174.4</td></tr>
<tr><td>7</td><td>Oklahoma</td><td>198.2</td><td>36</td><td>Montana</td><td>172.1</td></tr>
<tr><td>30</td><td>Oregon</td><td>179.3</td><td>37</td><td>South Dakota</td><td>171.3</td></tr>
<tr><td>16</td><td>Pennsylvania</td><td>188.2</td><td>38</td><td>Connecticut</td><td>170.7</td></tr>
<tr><td>29</td><td>Rhode Island</td><td>179.6</td><td>39</td><td>Texas</td><td>170.3</td></tr>
<tr><td>18</td><td>South Carolina</td><td>186.7</td><td>40</td><td>Minnesota</td><td>169.7</td></tr>
<tr><td>37</td><td>South Dakota</td><td>171.3</td><td>41</td><td>New York</td><td>168.0</td></tr>
<tr><td>5</td><td>Tennessee</td><td>200.3</td><td>42</td><td>Florida</td><td>166.6</td></tr>
<tr><td>39</td><td>Texas</td><td>170.3</td><td>43</td><td>Idaho</td><td>165.6</td></tr>
<tr><td>50</td><td>Utah</td><td>128.8</td><td>44</td><td>North Dakota</td><td>165.3</td></tr>
<tr><td>15</td><td>Vermont</td><td>188.5</td><td>45</td><td>California</td><td>161.7</td></tr>
<tr><td>21</td><td>Virginia</td><td>182.7</td><td>46</td><td>New Mexico</td><td>157.3</td></tr>
<tr><td>32</td><td>Washington</td><td>177.7</td><td>47</td><td>Colorado</td><td>153.7</td></tr>
<tr><td>2</td><td>West Virginia</td><td>207.6</td><td>48</td><td>Arizona</td><td>152.8</td></tr>
<tr><td>31</td><td>Wisconsin</td><td>177.9</td><td>49</td><td>Hawaii</td><td>146.2</td></tr>
<tr><td>35</td><td>Wyoming</td><td>174.4</td><td>50</td><td>Utah</td><td>128.8</td></tr>
<tr><td></td><td></td><td></td><td></td><td>District of Columbia</td><td>199.1</td></tr>
</table>

Source: U.S. Department of Health and Human Services, National Center for Health Statistics
"National Vital Statistics Reports" (Vol. 58, No. 19, May 20, 2010, http://www.cdc.gov/nchs/deaths.htm)
*Final data by state of residence. Neoplasms are abnormal tissue, tumors. Includes many cancers. Age-adjusted rates based on the year 2000 standard population.

Deaths by Nephritis and Other Kidney Diseases in 2007

National Total = 46,448 Deaths*

ALPHA ORDER

RANK	STATE	DEATHS	% of USA
17	Alabama	1,051	2.3%
50	Alaska	40	0.1%
29	Arizona	528	1.1%
25	Arkansas	666	1.4%
4	California	2,835	6.1%
32	Colorado	444	1.0%
27	Connecticut	566	1.2%
42	Delaware	163	0.4%
3	Florida	2,923	6.3%
10	Georgia	1,689	3.6%
40	Hawaii	176	0.4%
44	Idaho	134	0.3%
5	Illinois	2,536	5.5%
14	Indiana	1,293	2.8%
35	Iowa	272	0.6%
28	Kansas	554	1.2%
19	Kentucky	994	2.1%
16	Louisiana	1,152	2.5%
36	Maine	269	0.6%
23	Maryland	731	1.6%
13	Massachusetts	1,361	2.9%
11	Michigan	1,610	3.5%
22	Minnesota	780	1.7%
24	Mississippi	697	1.5%
15	Missouri	1,184	2.5%
45	Montana	110	0.2%
36	Nebraska	269	0.6%
31	Nevada	461	1.0%
43	New Hampshire	149	0.3%
9	New Jersey	1,690	3.6%
38	New Mexico	252	0.5%
6	New York	2,387	5.1%
8	North Carolina	1,723	3.7%
48	North Dakota	56	0.1%
7	Ohio	1,747	3.8%
26	Oklahoma	623	1.3%
34	Oregon	426	0.9%
2	Pennsylvania	2,965	6.4%
41	Rhode Island	167	0.4%
21	South Carolina	806	1.7%
46	South Dakota	77	0.2%
20	Tennessee	831	1.8%
1	Texas	3,291	7.1%
39	Utah	220	0.5%
49	Vermont	54	0.1%
12	Virginia	1,439	3.1%
33	Washington	440	0.9%
30	West Virginia	480	1.0%
18	Wisconsin	1,002	2.2%
47	Wyoming	68	0.1%

RANK ORDER

RANK	STATE	DEATHS	% of USA
1	Texas	3,291	7.1%
2	Pennsylvania	2,965	6.4%
3	Florida	2,923	6.3%
4	California	2,835	6.1%
5	Illinois	2,536	5.5%
6	New York	2,387	5.1%
7	Ohio	1,747	3.8%
8	North Carolina	1,723	3.7%
9	New Jersey	1,690	3.6%
10	Georgia	1,689	3.6%
11	Michigan	1,610	3.5%
12	Virginia	1,439	3.1%
13	Massachusetts	1,361	2.9%
14	Indiana	1,293	2.8%
15	Missouri	1,184	2.5%
16	Louisiana	1,152	2.5%
17	Alabama	1,051	2.3%
18	Wisconsin	1,002	2.2%
19	Kentucky	994	2.1%
20	Tennessee	831	1.8%
21	South Carolina	806	1.7%
22	Minnesota	780	1.7%
23	Maryland	731	1.6%
24	Mississippi	697	1.5%
25	Arkansas	666	1.4%
26	Oklahoma	623	1.3%
27	Connecticut	566	1.2%
28	Kansas	554	1.2%
29	Arizona	528	1.1%
30	West Virginia	480	1.0%
31	Nevada	461	1.0%
32	Colorado	444	1.0%
33	Washington	440	0.9%
34	Oregon	426	0.9%
35	Iowa	272	0.6%
36	Maine	269	0.6%
36	Nebraska	269	0.6%
38	New Mexico	252	0.5%
39	Utah	220	0.5%
40	Hawaii	176	0.4%
41	Rhode Island	167	0.4%
42	Delaware	163	0.4%
43	New Hampshire	149	0.3%
44	Idaho	134	0.3%
45	Montana	110	0.2%
46	South Dakota	77	0.2%
47	Wyoming	68	0.1%
48	North Dakota	56	0.1%
49	Vermont	54	0.1%
50	Alaska	40	0.1%
	District of Columbia	67	0.1%

Source: U.S. Department of Health and Human Services, National Center for Health Statistics
    "National Vital Statistics Reports" (Vol. 58, No. 19, May 20, 2010, http://www.cdc.gov/nchs/deaths.htm)
*Final data by state of residence. Includes nephrotic syndrome and nephrosis.

Death Rate by Nephritis and Other Kidney Diseases in 2007

National Rate = 15.4 Deaths per 100,000 Population*

<table>
<tr><td colspan="3">ALPHA ORDER</td><td colspan="3">RANK ORDER</td></tr>
<tr><td>RANK</td><td>STATE</td><td>RATE</td><td>RANK</td><td>STATE</td><td>RATE</td></tr>
<tr><td>7</td><td>Alabama</td><td>22.7</td><td>1</td><td>Louisiana</td><td>26.8</td></tr>
<tr><td>50</td><td>Alaska</td><td>5.9</td><td>2</td><td>West Virginia</td><td>26.5</td></tr>
<tr><td>46</td><td>Arizona</td><td>8.3</td><td>3</td><td>Mississippi</td><td>23.9</td></tr>
<tr><td>5</td><td>Arkansas</td><td>23.5</td><td>4</td><td>Pennsylvania</td><td>23.8</td></tr>
<tr><td>48</td><td>California</td><td>7.8</td><td>5</td><td>Arkansas</td><td>23.5</td></tr>
<tr><td>41</td><td>Colorado</td><td>9.1</td><td>6</td><td>Kentucky</td><td>23.4</td></tr>
<tr><td>23</td><td>Connecticut</td><td>16.2</td><td>7</td><td>Alabama</td><td>22.7</td></tr>
<tr><td>16</td><td>Delaware</td><td>18.8</td><td>8</td><td>Massachusetts</td><td>21.1</td></tr>
<tr><td>24</td><td>Florida</td><td>16.0</td><td>9</td><td>Indiana</td><td>20.4</td></tr>
<tr><td>21</td><td>Georgia</td><td>17.7</td><td>9</td><td>Maine</td><td>20.4</td></tr>
<tr><td>31</td><td>Hawaii</td><td>13.7</td><td>11</td><td>Missouri</td><td>20.1</td></tr>
<tr><td>43</td><td>Idaho</td><td>8.9</td><td>12</td><td>Kansas</td><td>20.0</td></tr>
<tr><td>13</td><td>Illinois</td><td>19.7</td><td>13</td><td>Illinois</td><td>19.7</td></tr>
<tr><td>9</td><td>Indiana</td><td>20.4</td><td>14</td><td>New Jersey</td><td>19.5</td></tr>
<tr><td>41</td><td>Iowa</td><td>9.1</td><td>15</td><td>North Carolina</td><td>19.0</td></tr>
<tr><td>12</td><td>Kansas</td><td>20.0</td><td>16</td><td>Delaware</td><td>18.8</td></tr>
<tr><td>6</td><td>Kentucky</td><td>23.4</td><td>17</td><td>Virginia</td><td>18.7</td></tr>
<tr><td>1</td><td>Louisiana</td><td>26.8</td><td>18</td><td>South Carolina</td><td>18.3</td></tr>
<tr><td>9</td><td>Maine</td><td>20.4</td><td>19</td><td>Nevada</td><td>18.0</td></tr>
<tr><td>33</td><td>Maryland</td><td>13.0</td><td>20</td><td>Wisconsin</td><td>17.9</td></tr>
<tr><td>8</td><td>Massachusetts</td><td>21.1</td><td>21</td><td>Georgia</td><td>17.7</td></tr>
<tr><td>24</td><td>Michigan</td><td>16.0</td><td>22</td><td>Oklahoma</td><td>17.2</td></tr>
<tr><td>29</td><td>Minnesota</td><td>15.0</td><td>23</td><td>Connecticut</td><td>16.2</td></tr>
<tr><td>3</td><td>Mississippi</td><td>23.9</td><td>24</td><td>Florida</td><td>16.0</td></tr>
<tr><td>11</td><td>Missouri</td><td>20.1</td><td>24</td><td>Michigan</td><td>16.0</td></tr>
<tr><td>37</td><td>Montana</td><td>11.5</td><td>26</td><td>Rhode Island</td><td>15.8</td></tr>
<tr><td>27</td><td>Nebraska</td><td>15.2</td><td>27</td><td>Nebraska</td><td>15.2</td></tr>
<tr><td>19</td><td>Nevada</td><td>18.0</td><td>27</td><td>Ohio</td><td>15.2</td></tr>
<tr><td>39</td><td>New Hampshire</td><td>11.3</td><td>29</td><td>Minnesota</td><td>15.0</td></tr>
<tr><td>14</td><td>New Jersey</td><td>19.5</td><td>30</td><td>Texas</td><td>13.8</td></tr>
<tr><td>35</td><td>New Mexico</td><td>12.8</td><td>31</td><td>Hawaii</td><td>13.7</td></tr>
<tr><td>36</td><td>New York</td><td>12.4</td><td>32</td><td>Tennessee</td><td>13.5</td></tr>
<tr><td>15</td><td>North Carolina</td><td>19.0</td><td>33</td><td>Maryland</td><td>13.0</td></tr>
<tr><td>44</td><td>North Dakota</td><td>8.8</td><td>33</td><td>Wyoming</td><td>13.0</td></tr>
<tr><td>27</td><td>Ohio</td><td>15.2</td><td>35</td><td>New Mexico</td><td>12.8</td></tr>
<tr><td>22</td><td>Oklahoma</td><td>17.2</td><td>36</td><td>New York</td><td>12.4</td></tr>
<tr><td>38</td><td>Oregon</td><td>11.4</td><td>37</td><td>Montana</td><td>11.5</td></tr>
<tr><td>4</td><td>Pennsylvania</td><td>23.8</td><td>38</td><td>Oregon</td><td>11.4</td></tr>
<tr><td>26</td><td>Rhode Island</td><td>15.8</td><td>39</td><td>New Hampshire</td><td>11.3</td></tr>
<tr><td>18</td><td>South Carolina</td><td>18.3</td><td>40</td><td>South Dakota</td><td>9.7</td></tr>
<tr><td>40</td><td>South Dakota</td><td>9.7</td><td>41</td><td>Colorado</td><td>9.1</td></tr>
<tr><td>32</td><td>Tennessee</td><td>13.5</td><td>41</td><td>Iowa</td><td>9.1</td></tr>
<tr><td>30</td><td>Texas</td><td>13.8</td><td>43</td><td>Idaho</td><td>8.9</td></tr>
<tr><td>46</td><td>Utah</td><td>8.3</td><td>44</td><td>North Dakota</td><td>8.8</td></tr>
<tr><td>45</td><td>Vermont</td><td>8.7</td><td>45</td><td>Vermont</td><td>8.7</td></tr>
<tr><td>17</td><td>Virginia</td><td>18.7</td><td>46</td><td>Arizona</td><td>8.3</td></tr>
<tr><td>49</td><td>Washington</td><td>6.8</td><td>46</td><td>Utah</td><td>8.3</td></tr>
<tr><td>2</td><td>West Virginia</td><td>26.5</td><td>48</td><td>California</td><td>7.8</td></tr>
<tr><td>20</td><td>Wisconsin</td><td>17.9</td><td>49</td><td>Washington</td><td>6.8</td></tr>
<tr><td>33</td><td>Wyoming</td><td>13.0</td><td>50</td><td>Alaska</td><td>5.9</td></tr>
<tr><td></td><td></td><td></td><td></td><td>District of Columbia</td><td>11.4</td></tr>
</table>

Source: U.S. Department of Health and Human Services, National Center for Health Statistics
   "National Vital Statistics Reports" (Vol. 58, No. 19, May 20, 2010, http://www.cdc.gov/nchs/deaths.htm)
*Final data by state of residence. Includes nephrotic syndrome and nephrosis. Not age-adjusted.

Age-Adjusted Death Rate by Nephritis and Other Kidney Diseases in 2007

National Rate = 14.5 Deaths per 100,000 Population*

ALPHA ORDER

RANK	STATE	RATE
6	Alabama	20.7
40	Alaska	10.5
45	Arizona	7.9
7	Arkansas	20.6
44	California	8.3
38	Colorado	10.8
27	Connecticut	13.4
19	Delaware	17.0
34	Florida	11.4
4	Georgia	21.5
36	Hawaii	11.1
43	Idaho	9.1
11	Illinois	19.2
9	Indiana	19.3
48	Iowa	6.8
16	Kansas	17.5
3	Kentucky	22.4
1	Louisiana	26.9
20	Maine	16.5
28	Maryland	13.1
14	Massachusetts	17.9
24	Michigan	14.9
25	Minnesota	13.7
2	Mississippi	23.4
15	Missouri	17.8
42	Montana	9.7
32	Nebraska	12.6
7	Nevada	20.6
39	New Hampshire	10.7
17	New Jersey	17.4
33	New Mexico	12.3
37	New York	11.0
12	North Carolina	19.0
50	North Dakota	6.2
26	Ohio	13.5
22	Oklahoma	15.7
41	Oregon	10.2
13	Pennsylvania	18.2
31	Rhode Island	12.7
18	South Carolina	17.3
47	South Dakota	7.4
30	Tennessee	13.0
21	Texas	16.3
34	Utah	11.4
46	Vermont	7.5
9	Virginia	19.3
49	Washington	6.7
5	West Virginia	21.1
23	Wisconsin	15.6
28	Wyoming	13.1

RANK ORDER

RANK	STATE	RATE
1	Louisiana	26.9
2	Mississippi	23.4
3	Kentucky	22.4
4	Georgia	21.5
5	West Virginia	21.1
6	Alabama	20.7
7	Arkansas	20.6
7	Nevada	20.6
9	Indiana	19.3
9	Virginia	19.3
11	Illinois	19.2
12	North Carolina	19.0
13	Pennsylvania	18.2
14	Massachusetts	17.9
15	Missouri	17.8
16	Kansas	17.5
17	New Jersey	17.4
18	South Carolina	17.3
19	Delaware	17.0
20	Maine	16.5
21	Texas	16.3
22	Oklahoma	15.7
23	Wisconsin	15.6
24	Michigan	14.9
25	Minnesota	13.7
26	Ohio	13.5
27	Connecticut	13.4
28	Maryland	13.1
28	Wyoming	13.1
30	Tennessee	13.0
31	Rhode Island	12.7
32	Nebraska	12.6
33	New Mexico	12.3
34	Florida	11.4
34	Utah	11.4
36	Hawaii	11.1
37	New York	11.0
38	Colorado	10.8
39	New Hampshire	10.7
40	Alaska	10.5
41	Oregon	10.2
42	Montana	9.7
43	Idaho	9.1
44	California	8.3
45	Arizona	7.9
46	Vermont	7.5
47	South Dakota	7.4
48	Iowa	6.8
49	Washington	6.7
50	North Dakota	6.2
	District of Columbia	11.2

Source: U.S. Department of Health and Human Services, National Center for Health Statistics
    "National Vital Statistics Reports" (Vol. 58, No. 19, May 20, 2010, http://www.cdc.gov/nchs/deaths.htm)
*Final data by state of residence. Includes nephrotic syndrome and nephrosis. Age-adjusted rates based on the year 2000 standard population.

Deaths by Influenza and Pneumonia in 2007

National Total = 52,717 Deaths*

RANK	STATE	DEATHS	% of USA
20	Alabama	898	1.7%
50	Alaska	48	0.1%
19	Arizona	905	1.7%
27	Arkansas	734	1.4%
1	California	6,546	12.4%
31	Colorado	592	1.1%
24	Connecticut	776	1.5%
47	Delaware	117	0.2%
6	Florida	2,246	4.3%
12	Georgia	1,407	2.7%
43	Hawaii	199	0.4%
40	Idaho	228	0.4%
5	Illinois	2,550	4.8%
16	Indiana	1,098	2.1%
25	Iowa	749	1.4%
29	Kansas	665	1.3%
21	Kentucky	897	1.7%
22	Louisiana	870	1.7%
39	Maine	236	0.4%
18	Maryland	994	1.9%
10	Massachusetts	1,538	2.9%
9	Michigan	1,637	3.1%
30	Minnesota	603	1.1%
32	Mississippi	554	1.1%
14	Missouri	1,289	2.4%
45	Montana	183	0.3%
36	Nebraska	331	0.6%
34	Nevada	408	0.8%
42	New Hampshire	207	0.4%
13	New Jersey	1,343	2.5%
38	New Mexico	298	0.6%
2	New York	4,431	8.4%
8	North Carolina	1,645	3.1%
46	North Dakota	133	0.3%
7	Ohio	1,743	3.3%
23	Oklahoma	801	1.5%
33	Oregon	477	0.9%
4	Pennsylvania	2,555	4.8%
41	Rhode Island	224	0.4%
28	South Carolina	723	1.4%
44	South Dakota	189	0.4%
11	Tennessee	1,438	2.7%
3	Texas	3,230	6.1%
37	Utah	313	0.6%
49	Vermont	70	0.1%
15	Virginia	1,231	2.3%
26	Washington	743	1.4%
34	West Virginia	408	0.8%
17	Wisconsin	1,022	1.9%
48	Wyoming	113	0.2%

RANK ORDER

RANK	STATE	DEATHS	% of USA
1	California	6,546	12.4%
2	New York	4,431	8.4%
3	Texas	3,230	6.1%
4	Pennsylvania	2,555	4.8%
5	Illinois	2,550	4.8%
6	Florida	2,246	4.3%
7	Ohio	1,743	3.3%
8	North Carolina	1,645	3.1%
9	Michigan	1,637	3.1%
10	Massachusetts	1,538	2.9%
11	Tennessee	1,438	2.7%
12	Georgia	1,407	2.7%
13	New Jersey	1,343	2.5%
14	Missouri	1,289	2.4%
15	Virginia	1,231	2.3%
16	Indiana	1,098	2.1%
17	Wisconsin	1,022	1.9%
18	Maryland	994	1.9%
19	Arizona	905	1.7%
20	Alabama	898	1.7%
21	Kentucky	897	1.7%
22	Louisiana	870	1.7%
23	Oklahoma	801	1.5%
24	Connecticut	776	1.5%
25	Iowa	749	1.4%
26	Washington	743	1.4%
27	Arkansas	734	1.4%
28	South Carolina	723	1.4%
29	Kansas	665	1.3%
30	Minnesota	603	1.1%
31	Colorado	592	1.1%
32	Mississippi	554	1.1%
33	Oregon	477	0.9%
34	Nevada	408	0.8%
34	West Virginia	408	0.8%
36	Nebraska	331	0.6%
37	Utah	313	0.6%
38	New Mexico	298	0.6%
39	Maine	236	0.4%
40	Idaho	228	0.4%
41	Rhode Island	224	0.4%
42	New Hampshire	207	0.4%
43	Hawaii	199	0.4%
44	South Dakota	189	0.4%
45	Montana	183	0.3%
46	North Dakota	133	0.3%
47	Delaware	117	0.2%
48	Wyoming	113	0.2%
49	Vermont	70	0.1%
50	Alaska	48	0.1%
	District of Columbia	82	0.2%

Source: U.S. Department of Health and Human Services, National Center for Health Statistics
    "National Vital Statistics Reports" (Vol. 58, No. 19, May 20, 2010, http://www.cdc.gov/nchs/deaths.htm)
*Final data by state of residence.

Death Rate by Influenza and Pneumonia in 2007

National Rate = 17.5 Deaths per 100,000 Population*

ALPHA ORDER

RANK	STATE	RATE
19	Alabama	19.4
50	Alaska	7.0
40	Arizona	14.3
1	Arkansas	25.9
25	California	17.9
45	Colorado	12.2
9	Connecticut	22.2
41	Delaware	13.5
44	Florida	12.3
39	Georgia	14.7
34	Hawaii	15.5
36	Idaho	15.2
18	Illinois	19.8
28	Indiana	17.3
2	Iowa	25.1
3	Kansas	24.0
14	Kentucky	21.1
17	Louisiana	20.3
25	Maine	17.9
27	Maryland	17.7
4	Massachusetts	23.8
30	Michigan	16.3
47	Minnesota	11.6
21	Mississippi	19.0
11	Missouri	21.9
20	Montana	19.1
22	Nebraska	18.7
32	Nevada	15.9
33	New Hampshire	15.7
34	New Jersey	15.5
38	New Mexico	15.1
7	New York	23.0
23	North Carolina	18.2
15	North Dakota	20.8
36	Ohio	15.2
10	Oklahoma	22.1
43	Oregon	12.7
16	Pennsylvania	20.6
13	Rhode Island	21.2
29	South Carolina	16.4
5	South Dakota	23.7
6	Tennessee	23.4
41	Texas	13.5
46	Utah	11.8
49	Vermont	11.3
31	Virginia	16.0
48	Washington	11.5
8	West Virginia	22.5
23	Wisconsin	18.2
12	Wyoming	21.6

RANK ORDER

RANK	STATE	RATE
1	Arkansas	25.9
2	Iowa	25.1
3	Kansas	24.0
4	Massachusetts	23.8
5	South Dakota	23.7
6	Tennessee	23.4
7	New York	23.0
8	West Virginia	22.5
9	Connecticut	22.2
10	Oklahoma	22.1
11	Missouri	21.9
12	Wyoming	21.6
13	Rhode Island	21.2
14	Kentucky	21.1
15	North Dakota	20.8
16	Pennsylvania	20.6
17	Louisiana	20.3
18	Illinois	19.8
19	Alabama	19.4
20	Montana	19.1
21	Mississippi	19.0
22	Nebraska	18.7
23	North Carolina	18.2
23	Wisconsin	18.2
25	California	17.9
25	Maine	17.9
27	Maryland	17.7
28	Indiana	17.3
29	South Carolina	16.4
30	Michigan	16.3
31	Virginia	16.0
32	Nevada	15.9
33	New Hampshire	15.7
34	Hawaii	15.5
34	New Jersey	15.5
36	Idaho	15.2
36	Ohio	15.2
38	New Mexico	15.1
39	Georgia	14.7
40	Arizona	14.3
41	Delaware	13.5
41	Texas	13.5
43	Oregon	12.7
44	Florida	12.3
45	Colorado	12.2
46	Utah	11.8
47	Minnesota	11.6
48	Washington	11.5
49	Vermont	11.3
50	Alaska	7.0
	District of Columbia	13.9

Source: U.S. Department of Health and Human Services, National Center for Health Statistics
"National Vital Statistics Reports" (Vol. 58, No. 19, May 20, 2010, http://www.cdc.gov/nchs/deaths.htm)
*Final data by state of residence. Not age-adjusted.

Age-Adjusted Death Rate by Influenza and Pneumonia in 2007

National Rate = 16.2 Deaths per 100,000 Population*

ALPHA ORDER

RANK	STATE	RATE
20	Alabama	17.8
43	Alaska	12.9
41	Arizona	13.5
2	Arkansas	22.3
10	California	18.9
38	Colorado	14.3
22	Connecticut	17.6
44	Delaware	12.2
50	Florida	8.6
15	Georgia	18.3
45	Hawaii	11.6
32	Idaho	15.1
12	Illinois	18.8
24	Indiana	16.1
17	Iowa	18.0
8	Kansas	19.9
5	Kentucky	20.1
4	Louisiana	20.3
39	Maine	14.1
18	Maryland	17.9
9	Massachusetts	19.5
34	Michigan	15.0
48	Minnesota	10.2
15	Mississippi	18.3
10	Missouri	18.9
28	Montana	15.8
32	Nebraska	15.1
13	Nevada	18.4
37	New Hampshire	14.5
40	New Jersey	13.7
35	New Mexico	14.6
7	New York	20.0
13	North Carolina	18.4
35	North Dakota	14.6
42	Ohio	13.3
5	Oklahoma	20.1
46	Oregon	11.1
31	Pennsylvania	15.2
24	Rhode Island	16.1
28	South Carolina	15.8
18	South Dakota	17.9
1	Tennessee	22.5
24	Texas	16.1
27	Utah	16.0
49	Vermont	9.8
23	Virginia	16.6
46	Washington	11.1
20	West Virginia	17.8
30	Wisconsin	15.5
3	Wyoming	20.9

RANK ORDER

RANK	STATE	RATE
1	Tennessee	22.5
2	Arkansas	22.3
3	Wyoming	20.9
4	Louisiana	20.3
5	Kentucky	20.1
5	Oklahoma	20.1
7	New York	20.0
8	Kansas	19.9
9	Massachusetts	19.5
10	California	18.9
10	Missouri	18.9
12	Illinois	18.8
13	Nevada	18.4
13	North Carolina	18.4
15	Georgia	18.3
15	Mississippi	18.3
17	Iowa	18.0
18	Maryland	17.9
18	South Dakota	17.9
20	Alabama	17.8
20	West Virginia	17.8
22	Connecticut	17.6
23	Virginia	16.6
24	Indiana	16.1
24	Rhode Island	16.1
24	Texas	16.1
27	Utah	16.0
28	Montana	15.8
28	South Carolina	15.8
30	Wisconsin	15.5
31	Pennsylvania	15.2
32	Idaho	15.1
32	Nebraska	15.1
34	Michigan	15.0
35	New Mexico	14.6
35	North Dakota	14.6
37	New Hampshire	14.5
38	Colorado	14.3
39	Maine	14.1
40	New Jersey	13.7
41	Arizona	13.5
42	Ohio	13.3
43	Alaska	12.9
44	Delaware	12.2
45	Hawaii	11.6
46	Oregon	11.1
46	Washington	11.1
48	Minnesota	10.2
49	Vermont	9.8
50	Florida	8.6

	District of Columbia	13.2

Source: U.S. Department of Health and Human Services, National Center for Health Statistics
"National Vital Statistics Reports" (Vol. 58, No. 19, May 20, 2010, http://www.cdc.gov/nchs/deaths.htm)
*Final data by state of residence. Age-adjusted rates based on the year 2000 standard population.

Deaths by Injury in 2007

National Total = 182,598 Deaths*

ALPHA ORDER

ALPHA ORDER

RANK	STATE	DEATHS	% of USA
18	Alabama	3,696	2.0%
44	Alaska	570	0.3%
11	Arizona	4,847	2.7%
30	Arkansas	2,204	1.2%
1	California	18,041	9.9%
24	Colorado	3,172	1.7%
34	Connecticut	1,766	1.0%
47	Delaware	471	0.3%
3	Florida	13,183	7.2%
9	Georgia	5,890	3.2%
43	Hawaii	693	0.4%
39	Idaho	940	0.5%
7	Illinois	6,430	3.5%
15	Indiana	3,878	2.1%
36	Iowa	1,663	0.9%
33	Kansas	1,768	1.0%
23	Kentucky	3,332	1.8%
17	Louisiana	3,770	2.1%
41	Maine	818	0.4%
21	Maryland	3,366	1.8%
26	Massachusetts	2,965	1.6%
10	Michigan	5,883	3.2%
27	Minnesota	2,833	1.6%
28	Mississippi	2,534	1.4%
14	Missouri	4,280	2.3%
40	Montana	865	0.5%
38	Nebraska	961	0.5%
32	Nevada	1,913	1.0%
42	New Hampshire	706	0.4%
20	New Jersey	3,483	1.9%
31	New Mexico	1,956	1.1%
5	New York	7,708	4.2%
8	North Carolina	6,225	3.4%
50	North Dakota	397	0.2%
6	Ohio	6,956	3.8%
25	Oklahoma	3,010	1.6%
29	Oregon	2,440	1.3%
4	Pennsylvania	7,970	4.4%
45	Rhode Island	550	0.3%
22	South Carolina	3,333	1.8%
46	South Dakota	492	0.3%
12	Tennessee	4,746	2.6%
2	Texas	13,576	7.4%
37	Utah	1,612	0.9%
49	Vermont	411	0.2%
13	Virginia	4,306	2.4%
16	Washington	3,827	2.1%
35	West Virginia	1,688	0.9%
19	Wisconsin	3,634	2.0%
48	Wyoming	428	0.2%

RANK ORDER

RANK	STATE	DEATHS	% of USA
1	California	18,041	9.9%
2	Texas	13,576	7.4%
3	Florida	13,183	7.2%
4	Pennsylvania	7,970	4.4%
5	New York	7,708	4.2%
6	Ohio	6,956	3.8%
7	Illinois	6,430	3.5%
8	North Carolina	6,225	3.4%
9	Georgia	5,890	3.2%
10	Michigan	5,883	3.2%
11	Arizona	4,847	2.7%
12	Tennessee	4,746	2.6%
13	Virginia	4,306	2.4%
14	Missouri	4,280	2.3%
15	Indiana	3,878	2.1%
16	Washington	3,827	2.1%
17	Louisiana	3,770	2.1%
18	Alabama	3,696	2.0%
19	Wisconsin	3,634	2.0%
20	New Jersey	3,483	1.9%
21	Maryland	3,366	1.8%
22	South Carolina	3,333	1.8%
23	Kentucky	3,332	1.8%
24	Colorado	3,172	1.7%
25	Oklahoma	3,010	1.6%
26	Massachusetts	2,965	1.6%
27	Minnesota	2,833	1.6%
28	Mississippi	2,534	1.4%
29	Oregon	2,440	1.3%
30	Arkansas	2,204	1.2%
31	New Mexico	1,956	1.1%
32	Nevada	1,913	1.0%
33	Kansas	1,768	1.0%
34	Connecticut	1,766	1.0%
35	West Virginia	1,688	0.9%
36	Iowa	1,663	0.9%
37	Utah	1,612	0.9%
38	Nebraska	961	0.5%
39	Idaho	940	0.5%
40	Montana	865	0.5%
41	Maine	818	0.4%
42	New Hampshire	706	0.4%
43	Hawaii	693	0.4%
44	Alaska	570	0.3%
45	Rhode Island	550	0.3%
46	South Dakota	492	0.3%
47	Delaware	471	0.3%
48	Wyoming	428	0.2%
49	Vermont	411	0.2%
50	North Dakota	397	0.2%
	District of Columbia	412	0.2%

Source: U.S. Department of Health and Human Services, National Center for Health Statistics
   (http://wonder.cdc.gov)
*By state of residence. Injury as used here includes accidents (including motor vehicle), suicides, homicides, and "other"
undetermined.

Death Rate by Injury in 2007

National Rate = 60.6 Deaths per 100,000 Population*

ALPHA ORDER

RANK	STATE	RATE
9	Alabama	79.9
6	Alaska	83.7
13	Arizona	76.3
11	Arkansas	77.9
47	California	49.6
20	Colorado	65.5
45	Connecticut	50.6
40	Delaware	54.6
17	Florida	72.4
28	Georgia	61.8
41	Hawaii	54.3
25	Idaho	62.8
46	Illinois	50.1
30	Indiana	61.2
38	Iowa	55.7
24	Kansas	63.7
10	Kentucky	78.7
5	Louisiana	86.2
26	Maine	62.2
33	Maryland	59.9
48	Massachusetts	45.8
35	Michigan	58.5
39	Minnesota	54.7
4	Mississippi	86.8
16	Missouri	72.8
3	Montana	90.4
41	Nebraska	54.3
15	Nevada	74.9
43	New Hampshire	53.8
49	New Jersey	40.3
1	New Mexico	99.6
50	New York	39.7
18	North Carolina	68.8
26	North Dakota	62.2
31	Ohio	60.6
7	Oklahoma	83.4
21	Oregon	65.3
23	Pennsylvania	64.2
44	Rhode Island	52.2
14	South Carolina	75.7
28	South Dakota	61.8
12	Tennessee	77.2
36	Texas	56.9
32	Utah	60.4
19	Vermont	66.2
37	Virginia	55.9
34	Washington	59.3
2	West Virginia	93.3
22	Wisconsin	64.9
8	Wyoming	81.8

RANK ORDER

RANK	STATE	RATE
1	New Mexico	99.6
2	West Virginia	93.3
3	Montana	90.4
4	Mississippi	86.8
5	Louisiana	86.2
6	Alaska	83.7
7	Oklahoma	83.4
8	Wyoming	81.8
9	Alabama	79.9
10	Kentucky	78.7
11	Arkansas	77.9
12	Tennessee	77.2
13	Arizona	76.3
14	South Carolina	75.7
15	Nevada	74.9
16	Missouri	72.8
17	Florida	72.4
18	North Carolina	68.8
19	Vermont	66.2
20	Colorado	65.5
21	Oregon	65.3
22	Wisconsin	64.9
23	Pennsylvania	64.2
24	Kansas	63.7
25	Idaho	62.8
26	Maine	62.2
26	North Dakota	62.2
28	Georgia	61.8
28	South Dakota	61.8
30	Indiana	61.2
31	Ohio	60.6
32	Utah	60.4
33	Maryland	59.9
34	Washington	59.3
35	Michigan	58.5
36	Texas	56.9
37	Virginia	55.9
38	Iowa	55.7
39	Minnesota	54.7
40	Delaware	54.6
41	Hawaii	54.3
41	Nebraska	54.3
43	New Hampshire	53.8
44	Rhode Island	52.2
45	Connecticut	50.6
46	Illinois	50.1
47	California	49.6
48	Massachusetts	45.8
49	New Jersey	40.3
50	New York	39.7
	District of Columbia	70.1

Source: U.S. Department of Health and Human Services, National Center for Health Statistics
(http://wonder.cdc.gov)

*By state of residence. Injury as used here includes accidents (including motor vehicle), suicides, homicides, and "other" undetermined. Not age-adjusted.

Age-Adjusted Death Rate by Injury in 2007

National Rate = 59.3 Deaths per 100,000 Population*

<table>
<tr><td colspan="3">ALPHA ORDER</td><td colspan="3">RANK ORDER</td></tr>
<tr><th>RANK</th><th>STATE</th><th>RATE</th><th>RANK</th><th>STATE</th><th>RATE</th></tr>
<tr><td>9</td><td>Alabama</td><td>78.7</td><td>1</td><td>New Mexico</td><td>99.0</td></tr>
<tr><td>3</td><td>Alaska</td><td>87.3</td><td>2</td><td>West Virginia</td><td>90.1</td></tr>
<tr><td>14</td><td>Arizona</td><td>75.8</td><td>3</td><td>Alaska</td><td>87.3</td></tr>
<tr><td>11</td><td>Arkansas</td><td>76.9</td><td>4</td><td>Mississippi</td><td>86.9</td></tr>
<tr><td>44</td><td>California</td><td>49.5</td><td>5</td><td>Louisiana</td><td>86.5</td></tr>
<tr><td>19</td><td>Colorado</td><td>66.8</td><td>6</td><td>Montana</td><td>85.5</td></tr>
<tr><td>46</td><td>Connecticut</td><td>47.6</td><td>7</td><td>Oklahoma</td><td>82.5</td></tr>
<tr><td>38</td><td>Delaware</td><td>53.5</td><td>8</td><td>Wyoming</td><td>82.2</td></tr>
<tr><td>17</td><td>Florida</td><td>68.5</td><td>9</td><td>Alabama</td><td>78.7</td></tr>
<tr><td>21</td><td>Georgia</td><td>64.1</td><td>10</td><td>Kentucky</td><td>77.6</td></tr>
<tr><td>43</td><td>Hawaii</td><td>50.5</td><td>11</td><td>Arkansas</td><td>76.9</td></tr>
<tr><td>22</td><td>Idaho</td><td>63.4</td><td>12</td><td>Tennessee</td><td>76.0</td></tr>
<tr><td>45</td><td>Illinois</td><td>49.4</td><td>13</td><td>Nevada</td><td>75.9</td></tr>
<tr><td>27</td><td>Indiana</td><td>60.4</td><td>14</td><td>Arizona</td><td>75.8</td></tr>
<tr><td>42</td><td>Iowa</td><td>51.1</td><td>15</td><td>South Carolina</td><td>74.7</td></tr>
<tr><td>26</td><td>Kansas</td><td>61.3</td><td>16</td><td>Missouri</td><td>70.4</td></tr>
<tr><td>10</td><td>Kentucky</td><td>77.6</td><td>17</td><td>Florida</td><td>68.5</td></tr>
<tr><td>5</td><td>Louisiana</td><td>86.5</td><td>17</td><td>North Carolina</td><td>68.5</td></tr>
<tr><td>32</td><td>Maine</td><td>58.6</td><td>19</td><td>Colorado</td><td>66.8</td></tr>
<tr><td>29</td><td>Maryland</td><td>59.4</td><td>20</td><td>Utah</td><td>65.9</td></tr>
<tr><td>48</td><td>Massachusetts</td><td>43.1</td><td>21</td><td>Georgia</td><td>64.1</td></tr>
<tr><td>36</td><td>Michigan</td><td>57.1</td><td>22</td><td>Idaho</td><td>63.4</td></tr>
<tr><td>40</td><td>Minnesota</td><td>52.0</td><td>23</td><td>Oregon</td><td>62.1</td></tr>
<tr><td>4</td><td>Mississippi</td><td>86.9</td><td>24</td><td>Vermont</td><td>61.8</td></tr>
<tr><td>16</td><td>Missouri</td><td>70.4</td><td>25</td><td>Wisconsin</td><td>61.7</td></tr>
<tr><td>6</td><td>Montana</td><td>85.5</td><td>26</td><td>Kansas</td><td>61.3</td></tr>
<tr><td>39</td><td>Nebraska</td><td>52.2</td><td>27</td><td>Indiana</td><td>60.4</td></tr>
<tr><td>13</td><td>Nevada</td><td>75.9</td><td>28</td><td>Pennsylvania</td><td>60.1</td></tr>
<tr><td>41</td><td>New Hampshire</td><td>51.3</td><td>29</td><td>Maryland</td><td>59.4</td></tr>
<tr><td>49</td><td>New Jersey</td><td>39.1</td><td>30</td><td>Texas</td><td>59.2</td></tr>
<tr><td>1</td><td>New Mexico</td><td>99.0</td><td>31</td><td>Ohio</td><td>58.7</td></tr>
<tr><td>50</td><td>New York</td><td>38.0</td><td>32</td><td>Maine</td><td>58.6</td></tr>
<tr><td>17</td><td>North Carolina</td><td>68.5</td><td>33</td><td>Washington</td><td>58.0</td></tr>
<tr><td>34</td><td>North Dakota</td><td>57.5</td><td>34</td><td>North Dakota</td><td>57.5</td></tr>
<tr><td>31</td><td>Ohio</td><td>58.7</td><td>35</td><td>South Dakota</td><td>57.2</td></tr>
<tr><td>7</td><td>Oklahoma</td><td>82.5</td><td>36</td><td>Michigan</td><td>57.1</td></tr>
<tr><td>23</td><td>Oregon</td><td>62.1</td><td>37</td><td>Virginia</td><td>55.6</td></tr>
<tr><td>28</td><td>Pennsylvania</td><td>60.1</td><td>38</td><td>Delaware</td><td>53.5</td></tr>
<tr><td>47</td><td>Rhode Island</td><td>47.0</td><td>39</td><td>Nebraska</td><td>52.2</td></tr>
<tr><td>15</td><td>South Carolina</td><td>74.7</td><td>40</td><td>Minnesota</td><td>52.0</td></tr>
<tr><td>35</td><td>South Dakota</td><td>57.2</td><td>41</td><td>New Hampshire</td><td>51.3</td></tr>
<tr><td>12</td><td>Tennessee</td><td>76.0</td><td>42</td><td>Iowa</td><td>51.1</td></tr>
<tr><td>30</td><td>Texas</td><td>59.2</td><td>43</td><td>Hawaii</td><td>50.5</td></tr>
<tr><td>20</td><td>Utah</td><td>65.9</td><td>44</td><td>California</td><td>49.5</td></tr>
<tr><td>24</td><td>Vermont</td><td>61.8</td><td>45</td><td>Illinois</td><td>49.4</td></tr>
<tr><td>37</td><td>Virginia</td><td>55.6</td><td>46</td><td>Connecticut</td><td>47.6</td></tr>
<tr><td>33</td><td>Washington</td><td>58.0</td><td>47</td><td>Rhode Island</td><td>47.0</td></tr>
<tr><td>2</td><td>West Virginia</td><td>90.1</td><td>48</td><td>Massachusetts</td><td>43.1</td></tr>
<tr><td>25</td><td>Wisconsin</td><td>61.7</td><td>49</td><td>New Jersey</td><td>39.1</td></tr>
<tr><td>8</td><td>Wyoming</td><td>82.2</td><td>50</td><td>New York</td><td>38.0</td></tr>
<tr><td></td><td></td><td></td><td></td><td>District of Columbia</td><td>66.0</td></tr>
</table>

Source: U.S. Department of Health and Human Services, National Center for Health Statistics
(http://wonder.cdc.gov)

*By state of residence. Injury as used here includes accidents (including motor vehicle), suicides, homicides, and "other" undetermined. Age-adjusted rates based on the year 2000 standard population.

Deaths by Accidents in 2007

National Total = 123,706 Deaths*

ALPHA ORDER

RANK	STATE	DEATHS	% of USA
17	Alabama	2,542	2.1%
46	Alaska	354	0.3%
12	Arizona	3,161	2.6%
30	Arkansas	1,391	1.1%
1	California	11,614	9.4%
26	Colorado	2,056	1.7%
31	Connecticut	1,343	1.1%
47	Delaware	309	0.2%
3	Florida	9,113	7.4%
9	Georgia	4,012	3.2%
43	Hawaii	470	0.4%
39	Idaho	641	0.5%
8	Illinois	4,367	3.5%
18	Indiana	2,499	2.0%
33	Iowa	1,252	1.0%
36	Kansas	1,205	1.0%
21	Kentucky	2,372	1.9%
19	Louisiana	2,466	2.0%
41	Maine	584	0.5%
29	Maryland	1,480	1.2%
24	Massachusetts	2,139	1.7%
10	Michigan	3,764	3.0%
25	Minnesota	2,066	1.7%
27	Mississippi	1,808	1.5%
13	Missouri	2,975	2.4%
40	Montana	614	0.5%
38	Nebraska	674	0.5%
35	Nevada	1,212	1.0%
42	New Hampshire	527	0.4%
20	New Jersey	2,425	2.0%
32	New Mexico	1,329	1.1%
5	New York	5,160	4.2%
7	North Carolina	4,389	3.5%
50	North Dakota	279	0.2%
6	Ohio	4,922	4.0%
23	Oklahoma	2,149	1.7%
28	Oregon	1,646	1.3%
4	Pennsylvania	5,568	4.5%
44	Rhode Island	416	0.3%
22	South Carolina	2,364	1.9%
45	South Dakota	366	0.3%
11	Tennessee	3,257	2.6%
2	Texas	9,392	7.6%
37	Utah	811	0.7%
48	Vermont	303	0.2%
14	Virginia	2,931	2.4%
15	Washington	2,637	2.1%
34	West Virginia	1,241	1.0%
16	Wisconsin	2,619	2.1%
49	Wyoming	299	0.2%

RANK ORDER

RANK	STATE	DEATHS	% of USA
1	California	11,614	9.4%
2	Texas	9,392	7.6%
3	Florida	9,113	7.4%
4	Pennsylvania	5,568	4.5%
5	New York	5,160	4.2%
6	Ohio	4,922	4.0%
7	North Carolina	4,389	3.5%
8	Illinois	4,367	3.5%
9	Georgia	4,012	3.2%
10	Michigan	3,764	3.0%
11	Tennessee	3,257	2.6%
12	Arizona	3,161	2.6%
13	Missouri	2,975	2.4%
14	Virginia	2,931	2.4%
15	Washington	2,637	2.1%
16	Wisconsin	2,619	2.1%
17	Alabama	2,542	2.1%
18	Indiana	2,499	2.0%
19	Louisiana	2,466	2.0%
20	New Jersey	2,425	2.0%
21	Kentucky	2,372	1.9%
22	South Carolina	2,364	1.9%
23	Oklahoma	2,149	1.7%
24	Massachusetts	2,139	1.7%
25	Minnesota	2,066	1.7%
26	Colorado	2,056	1.7%
27	Mississippi	1,808	1.5%
28	Oregon	1,646	1.3%
29	Maryland	1,480	1.2%
30	Arkansas	1,391	1.1%
31	Connecticut	1,343	1.1%
32	New Mexico	1,329	1.1%
33	Iowa	1,252	1.0%
34	West Virginia	1,241	1.0%
35	Nevada	1,212	1.0%
36	Kansas	1,205	1.0%
37	Utah	811	0.7%
38	Nebraska	674	0.5%
39	Idaho	641	0.5%
40	Montana	614	0.5%
41	Maine	584	0.5%
42	New Hampshire	527	0.4%
43	Hawaii	470	0.4%
44	Rhode Island	416	0.3%
45	South Dakota	366	0.3%
46	Alaska	354	0.3%
47	Delaware	309	0.2%
48	Vermont	303	0.2%
49	Wyoming	299	0.2%
50	North Dakota	279	0.2%
	District of Columbia	193	0.2%

Source: U.S. Department of Health and Human Services, National Center for Health Statistics
"National Vital Statistics Reports" (Vol. 58, No. 19, May 20, 2010, http://www.cdc.gov/nchs/deaths.htm)
*Final data by state of residence. Includes motor vehicle deaths, poisoning, falls, drowning, and other accidents.

Death Rate by Accidents in 2007

National Rate = 41.0 Deaths per 100,000 Population*

ALPHA ORDER			RANK ORDER		
RANK	STATE	RATE	RANK	STATE	RATE
9	Alabama	54.9	1	West Virginia	68.5
12	Alaska	51.8	2	New Mexico	67.5
14	Arizona	49.9	3	Montana	64.1
16	Arkansas	49.1	4	Mississippi	61.9
46	California	31.8	5	Oklahoma	59.4
29	Colorado	42.3	6	Louisiana	57.4
38	Connecticut	38.3	7	Wyoming	57.2
43	Delaware	35.7	8	Kentucky	55.9
14	Florida	49.9	9	Alabama	54.9
30	Georgia	42.0	10	South Carolina	53.6
42	Hawaii	36.6	11	Tennessee	52.9
28	Idaho	42.8	12	Alaska	51.8
44	Illinois	34.0	13	Missouri	50.6
35	Indiana	39.4	14	Arizona	49.9
31	Iowa	41.9	14	Florida	49.9
26	Kansas	43.4	16	Arkansas	49.1
8	Kentucky	55.9	17	Vermont	48.8
6	Louisiana	57.4	18	North Carolina	48.4
23	Maine	44.3	19	Nevada	47.2
50	Maryland	26.3	20	Wisconsin	46.8
45	Massachusetts	33.2	21	South Dakota	46.0
41	Michigan	37.4	22	Pennsylvania	44.8
34	Minnesota	39.7	23	Maine	44.3
4	Mississippi	61.9	24	Oregon	43.9
13	Missouri	50.6	25	North Dakota	43.6
3	Montana	64.1	26	Kansas	43.4
39	Nebraska	38.0	27	Ohio	42.9
19	Nevada	47.2	28	Idaho	42.8
33	New Hampshire	40.1	29	Colorado	42.3
48	New Jersey	27.9	30	Georgia	42.0
2	New Mexico	67.5	31	Iowa	41.9
49	New York	26.7	32	Washington	40.8
18	North Carolina	48.4	33	New Hampshire	40.1
25	North Dakota	43.6	34	Minnesota	39.7
27	Ohio	42.9	35	Indiana	39.4
5	Oklahoma	59.4	36	Rhode Island	39.3
24	Oregon	43.9	36	Texas	39.3
22	Pennsylvania	44.8	38	Connecticut	38.3
36	Rhode Island	39.3	39	Nebraska	38.0
10	South Carolina	53.6	39	Virginia	38.0
21	South Dakota	46.0	41	Michigan	37.4
11	Tennessee	52.9	42	Hawaii	36.6
36	Texas	39.3	43	Delaware	35.7
47	Utah	30.7	44	Illinois	34.0
17	Vermont	48.8	45	Massachusetts	33.2
39	Virginia	38.0	46	California	31.8
32	Washington	40.8	47	Utah	30.7
1	West Virginia	68.5	48	New Jersey	27.9
20	Wisconsin	46.8	49	New York	26.7
7	Wyoming	57.2	50	Maryland	26.3
				District of Columbia	32.8

Source: U.S. Department of Health and Human Services, National Center for Health Statistics
"National Vital Statistics Reports" (Vol. 58, No. 19, May 20, 2010, http://www.cdc.gov/nchs/deaths.htm)
*Final data by state of residence. Includes motor vehicle deaths, poisoning, falls, drowning, and other accidents. Not age-adjusted.

Age-Adjusted Death Rate by Accidents in 2007

National Rate = 40.0 Deaths per 100,000 Population*

ALPHA ORDER

RANK	STATE	RATE
10	Alabama	53.9
8	Alaska	55.3
13	Arizona	49.4
17	Arkansas	47.6
46	California	31.9
20	Colorado	44.2
39	Connecticut	35.8
41	Delaware	34.8
18	Florida	46.5
20	Georgia	44.2
45	Hawaii	33.3
23	Idaho	43.1
44	Illinois	33.4
33	Indiana	38.7
37	Iowa	37.3
28	Kansas	41.2
9	Kentucky	55.1
6	Louisiana	57.6
25	Maine	41.5
49	Maryland	26.2
47	Massachusetts	30.8
38	Michigan	36.1
36	Minnesota	37.4
3	Mississippi	61.9
14	Missouri	48.4
4	Montana	60.2
40	Nebraska	35.7
14	Nevada	48.4
34	New Hampshire	38.5
48	New Jersey	26.8
1	New Mexico	66.7
50	New York	25.3
16	North Carolina	48.3
32	North Dakota	39.3
29	Ohio	41.1
5	Oklahoma	58.4
25	Oregon	41.5
30	Pennsylvania	40.9
42	Rhode Island	34.6
11	South Carolina	53.0
24	South Dakota	41.8
12	Tennessee	52.1
27	Texas	41.4
43	Utah	34.4
19	Vermont	44.7
35	Virginia	38.1
31	Washington	39.8
2	West Virginia	65.9
22	Wisconsin	43.8
7	Wyoming	57.0

RANK ORDER

RANK	STATE	RATE
1	New Mexico	66.7
2	West Virginia	65.9
3	Mississippi	61.9
4	Montana	60.2
5	Oklahoma	58.4
6	Louisiana	57.6
7	Wyoming	57.0
8	Alaska	55.3
9	Kentucky	55.1
10	Alabama	53.9
11	South Carolina	53.0
12	Tennessee	52.1
13	Arizona	49.4
14	Missouri	48.4
14	Nevada	48.4
16	North Carolina	48.3
17	Arkansas	47.6
18	Florida	46.5
19	Vermont	44.7
20	Colorado	44.2
20	Georgia	44.2
22	Wisconsin	43.8
23	Idaho	43.1
24	South Dakota	41.8
25	Maine	41.5
25	Oregon	41.5
27	Texas	41.4
28	Kansas	41.2
29	Ohio	41.1
30	Pennsylvania	40.9
31	Washington	39.8
32	North Dakota	39.3
33	Indiana	38.7
34	New Hampshire	38.5
35	Virginia	38.1
36	Minnesota	37.4
37	Iowa	37.3
38	Michigan	36.1
39	Connecticut	35.8
40	Nebraska	35.7
41	Delaware	34.8
42	Rhode Island	34.6
43	Utah	34.4
44	Illinois	33.4
45	Hawaii	33.3
46	California	31.9
47	Massachusetts	30.8
48	New Jersey	26.8
49	Maryland	26.2
50	New York	25.3

	District of Columbia	32.4

Source: U.S. Department of Health and Human Services, National Center for Health Statistics
   "National Vital Statistics Reports" (Vol. 58, No. 19, May 20, 2010, http://www.cdc.gov/nchs/deaths.htm)
*Final data by state of residence. Includes motor vehicle deaths, poisoning, falls, drowning, and other accidents. Age-adjusted rates based on the year 2000 standard population.

Deaths by Motor Vehicle Accidents in 2007

National Total = 43,945 Deaths*

ALPHA ORDER

RANK	STATE	DEATHS	% of USA
12	Alabama	1,212	2.8%
48	Alaska	107	0.2%
13	Arizona	1,104	2.5%
24	Arkansas	675	1.5%
1	California	4,306	9.8%
28	Colorado	593	1.3%
37	Connocticut	309	0.7%
46	Delaware	118	0.3%
3	Florida	3,329	7.6%
5	Georgia	1,745	4.0%
44	Hawaii	136	0.3%
39	Idaho	273	0.6%
9	Illinois	1,375	3.1%
18	Indiana	942	2.1%
30	Iowa	459	1.0%
32	Kansas	447	1.0%
20	Kentucky	853	1.9%
17	Louisiana	1,036	2.4%
41	Maine	198	0.5%
24	Maryland	675	1.5%
31	Massachusetts	450	1.0%
11	Michigan	1,229	2.8%
27	Minnesota	618	1.4%
19	Mississippi	914	2.1%
16	Missouri	1,054	2.4%
40	Montana	268	0.6%
38	Nebraska	284	0.6%
34	Nevada	407	0.9%
43	New Hampshire	138	0.3%
23	New Jersey	719	1.6%
35	New Mexico	379	0.9%
7	New York	1,478	3.4%
4	North Carolina	1,818	4.1%
47	North Dakota	115	0.3%
8	Ohio	1,399	3.2%
22	Oklahoma	743	1.7%
29	Oregon	490	1.1%
6	Pennsylvania	1,604	3.7%
49	Rhode Island	85	0.2%
15	South Carolina	1,062	2.4%
42	South Dakota	149	0.3%
10	Tennessee	1,303	3.0%
2	Texas	3,800	8.6%
36	Utah	320	0.7%
50	Vermont	71	0.2%
14	Virginia	1,081	2.5%
26	Washington	649	1.5%
33	West Virginia	429	1.0%
21	Wisconsin	809	1.8%
45	Wyoming	134	0.3%

RANK ORDER

RANK	STATE	DEATHS	% of USA
1	California	4,306	9.8%
2	Texas	3,800	8.6%
3	Florida	3,329	7.6%
4	North Carolina	1,818	4.1%
5	Georgia	1,745	4.0%
6	Pennsylvania	1,604	3.7%
7	New York	1,478	3.4%
8	Ohio	1,399	3.2%
9	Illinois	1,375	3.1%
10	Tennessee	1,303	3.0%
11	Michigan	1,229	2.8%
12	Alabama	1,212	2.8%
13	Arizona	1,104	2.5%
14	Virginia	1,081	2.5%
15	South Carolina	1,062	2.4%
16	Missouri	1,054	2.4%
17	Louisiana	1,036	2.4%
18	Indiana	942	2.1%
19	Mississippi	914	2.1%
20	Kentucky	853	1.9%
21	Wisconsin	809	1.8%
22	Oklahoma	743	1.7%
23	New Jersey	719	1.6%
24	Arkansas	675	1.5%
24	Maryland	675	1.5%
26	Washington	649	1.5%
27	Minnesota	618	1.4%
28	Colorado	593	1.3%
29	Oregon	490	1.1%
30	Iowa	459	1.0%
31	Massachusetts	450	1.0%
32	Kansas	447	1.0%
33	West Virginia	429	1.0%
34	Nevada	407	0.9%
35	New Mexico	379	0.9%
36	Utah	320	0.7%
37	Connecticut	309	0.7%
38	Nebraska	284	0.6%
39	Idaho	273	0.6%
40	Montana	268	0.6%
41	Maine	198	0.5%
42	South Dakota	149	0.3%
43	New Hampshire	138	0.3%
44	Hawaii	136	0.3%
45	Wyoming	134	0.3%
46	Delaware	118	0.3%
47	North Dakota	115	0.3%
48	Alaska	107	0.2%
49	Rhode Island	85	0.2%
50	Vermont	71	0.2%
	District of Columbia	54	0.1%

Source: U.S. Department of Health and Human Services, National Center for Health Statistics
"National Vital Statistics Reports" (Vol. 58, No. 19, May 20, 2010, http://www.cdc.gov/nchs/deaths.htm)
*Final data by state of residence. These numbers are compiled from death certificates by the Centers for Disease Control and Prevention. They may differ from motor vehicle deaths collected by the U.S. Department of Transportation from other sources.

Death Rate by Motor Vehicle Accidents in 2007

National Rate = 14.6 Deaths per 100,000 Population*

ALPHA ORDER				RANK ORDER		
RANK	STATE	RATE		RANK	STATE	RATE
3	Alabama	26.2		1	Mississippi	31.3
25	Alaska	15.7		2	Montana	28.0
20	Arizona	17.4		3	Alabama	26.2
7	Arkansas	23.8		4	Wyoming	25.6
40	California	11.8		5	Louisiana	24.1
34	Colorado	12.2		5	South Carolina	24.1
46	Connecticut	8.8		7	Arkansas	23.8
31	Delaware	13.6		8	West Virginia	23.7
16	Florida	18.2		9	Tennessee	21.2
15	Georgia	18.3		10	Oklahoma	20.5
43	Hawaii	10.6		11	Kentucky	20.1
16	Idaho	18.2		11	North Carolina	20.1
42	Illinois	10.7		13	New Mexico	19.2
28	Indiana	14.8		14	South Dakota	18.7
26	Iowa	15.4		15	Georgia	18.3
21	Kansas	16.1		16	Florida	18.2
11	Kentucky	20.1		16	Idaho	18.2
5	Louisiana	24.1		18	North Dakota	18.0
27	Maine	15.0		19	Missouri	17.9
38	Maryland	12.0		20	Arizona	17.4
50	Massachusetts	7.0		21	Kansas	16.1
34	Michigan	12.2		22	Nebraska	16.0
39	Minnesota	11.9		23	Nevada	15.9
1	Mississippi	31.3		23	Texas	15.9
19	Missouri	17.9		25	Alaska	15.7
2	Montana	28.0		26	Iowa	15.4
22	Nebraska	16.0		27	Maine	15.0
23	Nevada	15.9		28	Indiana	14.8
44	New Hampshire	10.5		29	Wisconsin	14.4
47	New Jersey	8.3		30	Virginia	14.0
13	New Mexico	19.2		31	Delaware	13.6
49	New York	7.7		32	Oregon	13.1
11	North Carolina	20.1		33	Pennsylvania	12.9
18	North Dakota	18.0		34	Colorado	12.2
34	Ohio	12.2		34	Michigan	12.2
10	Oklahoma	20.5		34	Ohio	12.2
32	Oregon	13.1		37	Utah	12.1
33	Pennsylvania	12.9		38	Maryland	12.0
48	Rhode Island	8.0		39	Minnesota	11.9
5	South Carolina	24.1		40	California	11.8
14	South Dakota	18.7		41	Vermont	11.4
9	Tennessee	21.2		42	Illinois	10.7
23	Texas	15.9		43	Hawaii	10.6
37	Utah	12.1		44	New Hampshire	10.5
41	Vermont	11.4		45	Washington	10.0
30	Virginia	14.0		46	Connecticut	8.8
45	Washington	10.0		47	New Jersey	8.3
8	West Virginia	23.7		48	Rhode Island	8.0
29	Wisconsin	14.4		49	New York	7.7
4	Wyoming	25.6		50	Massachusetts	7.0
				District of Columbia		9.2

Source: U.S. Department of Health and Human Services, National Center for Health Statistics
"National Vital Statistics Reports" (Vol. 58, No. 19, May 20, 2010, http://www.cdc.gov/nchs/deaths.htm)
*Final data by state of residence. These numbers are compiled from death certificates by the Centers for Disease Control and Prevention. They may differ from motor vehicle deaths collected by the U.S. Department of Transportation from other sources. Not age-adjusted.

Age-Adjusted Death Rate by Motor Vehicle Accidents in 2007

National Rate = 14.4 Deaths per 100,000 Population*

ALPHA ORDER				RANK ORDER		
RANK	STATE	RATE		RANK	STATE	RATE
3	Alabama	25.9		1	Mississippi	31.6
25	Alaska	15.2		2	Montana	27.6
18	Arizona	17.6		3	Alabama	25.9
7	Arkansas	23.7		4	Wyoming	25.3
39	California	11.7		5	South Carolina	24.2
35	Colorado	12.3		6	Louisiana	24.0
46	Connecticut	8.7		7	Arkansas	23.7
31	Delaware	13.6		8	West Virginia	23.6
17	Florida	18.1		9	Tennessee	21.0
14	Georgia	18.5		10	Oklahoma	20.4
43	Hawaii	10.3		11	Kentucky	20.0
14	Idaho	18.5		11	North Carolina	20.0
42	Illinois	10.6		13	New Mexico	19.2
27	Indiana	14.8		14	Georgia	18.5
26	Iowa	15.0		14	Idaho	18.5
23	Kansas	15.9		16	South Dakota	18.3
11	Kentucky	20.0		17	Florida	18.1
6	Louisiana	24.0		18	Arizona	17.6
28	Maine	14.7		18	Missouri	17.6
37	Maryland	12.0		20	North Dakota	17.5
50	Massachusetts	6.7		21	Texas	16.2
37	Michigan	12.0		22	Nevada	16.0
39	Minnesota	11.7		23	Kansas	15.9
1	Mississippi	31.6		24	Nebraska	15.7
18	Missouri	17.6		25	Alaska	15.2
2	Montana	27.6		26	Iowa	15.0
24	Nebraska	15.7		27	Indiana	14.8
22	Nevada	16.0		28	Maine	14.7
43	New Hampshire	10.3		29	Wisconsin	14.2
47	New Jersey	8.2		30	Virginia	13.9
13	New Mexico	19.2		31	Delaware	13.6
49	New York	7.4		32	Oregon	13.0
11	North Carolina	20.0		33	Pennsylvania	12.5
20	North Dakota	17.5		34	Utah	12.4
36	Ohio	12.1		35	Colorado	12.3
10	Oklahoma	20.4		36	Ohio	12.1
32	Oregon	13.0		37	Maryland	12.0
33	Pennsylvania	12.5		37	Michigan	12.0
48	Rhode Island	7.6		39	California	11.7
5	South Carolina	24.2		39	Minnesota	11.7
16	South Dakota	18.3		41	Vermont	10.9
9	Tennessee	21.0		42	Illinois	10.6
21	Texas	16.2		43	Hawaii	10.3
34	Utah	12.4		43	New Hampshire	10.3
41	Vermont	10.9		45	Washington	9.9
30	Virginia	13.9		46	Connecticut	8.7
45	Washington	9.9		47	New Jersey	8.2
8	West Virginia	23.6		48	Rhode Island	7.6
29	Wisconsin	14.2		49	New York	7.4
4	Wyoming	25.3		50	Massachusetts	6.7
					District of Columbia	8.9

Source: U.S. Department of Health and Human Services, National Center for Health Statistics
  "National Vital Statistics Reports" (Vol. 58, No. 19, May 20, 2010, http://www.cdc.gov/nchs/deaths.htm)
*Final data by state of residence. These numbers are compiled from death certificates by the Centers for Disease Control and Prevention. They may differ from motor vehicle deaths collected by the U.S. Department of Transportation from other sources. Age-adjusted rates based on the year 2000 standard population.

Deaths by Firearm Injury in 2007

National Total = 31,224 Deaths*

RANK	STATE	DEATHS	% of USA
15	Alabama	812	2.6%
41	Alaska	120	0.4%
11	Arizona	951	3.0%
27	Arkansas	426	1.4%
1	California	3,268	10.5%
23	Colorado	505	1.6%
38	Connecticut	149	0.5%
43	Delaware	79	0.3%
3	Florida	2,272	7.3%
5	Georgia	1,244	4.0%
50	Hawaii	36	0.1%
36	Idaho	187	0.6%
9	Illinois	1,032	3.3%
18	Indiana	670	2.1%
37	Iowa	157	0.5%
32	Kansas	292	0.9%
19	Kentucky	612	2.0%
13	Louisiana	869	2.8%
42	Maine	107	0.3%
17	Maryland	678	2.2%
35	Massachusetts	235	0.8%
8	Michigan	1,095	3.5%
30	Minnesota	344	1.1%
22	Mississippi	535	1.7%
16	Missouri	759	2.4%
40	Montana	139	0.4%
39	Nebraska	142	0.5%
28	Nevada	414	1.3%
44	New Hampshire	78	0.2%
26	New Jersey	446	1.4%
31	New Mexico	295	0.9%
10	New York	985	3.2%
6	North Carolina	1,116	3.6%
46	North Dakota	57	0.2%
7	Ohio	1,105	3.5%
25	Oklahoma	482	1.5%
29	Oregon	387	1.2%
4	Pennsylvania	1,325	4.2%
49	Rhode Island	37	0.1%
20	South Carolina	592	1.9%
47	South Dakota	52	0.2%
12	Tennessee	924	3.0%
2	Texas	2,561	8.2%
34	Utah	253	0.8%
47	Vermont	52	0.2%
14	Virginia	825	2.6%
21	Washington	548	1.8%
33	West Virginia	267	0.9%
24	Wisconsin	488	1.6%
45	Wyoming	76	0.2%

RANK	STATE	DEATHS	% of USA
1	California	3,268	10.5%
2	Texas	2,561	8.2%
3	Florida	2,272	7.3%
4	Pennsylvania	1,325	4.2%
5	Georgia	1,244	4.0%
6	North Carolina	1,116	3.6%
7	Ohio	1,105	3.5%
8	Michigan	1,095	3.5%
9	Illinois	1,032	3.3%
10	New York	985	3.2%
11	Arizona	951	3.0%
12	Tennessee	924	3.0%
13	Louisiana	869	2.8%
14	Virginia	825	2.6%
15	Alabama	812	2.6%
16	Missouri	759	2.4%
17	Maryland	678	2.2%
18	Indiana	670	2.1%
19	Kentucky	612	2.0%
20	South Carolina	592	1.9%
21	Washington	548	1.8%
22	Mississippi	535	1.7%
23	Colorado	505	1.6%
24	Wisconsin	488	1.6%
25	Oklahoma	482	1.5%
26	New Jersey	446	1.4%
27	Arkansas	426	1.4%
28	Nevada	414	1.3%
29	Oregon	387	1.2%
30	Minnesota	344	1.1%
31	New Mexico	295	0.9%
32	Kansas	292	0.9%
33	West Virginia	267	0.9%
34	Utah	253	0.8%
35	Massachusetts	235	0.8%
36	Idaho	187	0.6%
37	Iowa	157	0.5%
38	Connecticut	149	0.5%
39	Nebraska	142	0.5%
40	Montana	139	0.4%
41	Alaska	120	0.4%
42	Maine	107	0.3%
43	Delaware	79	0.3%
44	New Hampshire	78	0.2%
45	Wyoming	76	0.2%
46	North Dakota	57	0.2%
47	South Dakota	52	0.2%
47	Vermont	52	0.2%
49	Rhode Island	37	0.1%
50	Hawaii	36	0.1%
	District of Columbia	144	0.5%

Source: U.S. Department of Health and Human Services, National Center for Health Statistics
"National Vital Statistics Reports" (Vol. 58, No. 19, May 20, 2010, http://www.cdc.gov/nchs/deaths.htm)
*Final data by state of residence.

Death Rate by Firearm Injury in 2007

National Rate = 10.4 Deaths per 100,000 Population*

ALPHA ORDER

RANK	STATE	RATE
4	Alabama	17.5
3	Alaska	17.6
6	Arizona	15.0
6	Arkansas	15.0
33	California	8.9
28	Colorado	10.4
47	Connecticut	4.3
32	Delaware	9.1
19	Florida	12.4
16	Georgia	13.0
50	Hawaii	2.8
18	Idaho	12.5
39	Illinois	8.0
26	Indiana	10.6
44	Iowa	5.3
27	Kansas	10.5
13	Kentucky	14.4
1	Louisiana	20.2
38	Maine	8.1
21	Maryland	12.1
48	Massachusetts	3.6
22	Michigan	10.9
41	Minnesota	6.6
2	Mississippi	18.3
17	Missouri	12.9
11	Montana	14.5
39	Nebraska	8.0
5	Nevada	16.1
43	New Hampshire	5.9
45	New Jersey	5.1
6	New Mexico	15.0
45	New York	5.1
20	North Carolina	12.3
33	North Dakota	8.9
30	Ohio	9.6
15	Oklahoma	13.3
29	Oregon	10.3
23	Pennsylvania	10.7
49	Rhode Island	3.5
14	South Carolina	13.4
42	South Dakota	6.5
6	Tennessee	15.0
23	Texas	10.7
30	Utah	9.6
37	Vermont	8.4
23	Virginia	10.7
36	Washington	8.5
10	West Virginia	14.7
35	Wisconsin	8.7
11	Wyoming	14.5

RANK ORDER

RANK	STATE	RATE
1	Louisiana	20.2
2	Mississippi	18.3
3	Alaska	17.6
4	Alabama	17.5
5	Nevada	16.1
6	Arizona	15.0
6	Arkansas	15.0
6	New Mexico	15.0
6	Tennessee	15.0
10	West Virginia	14.7
11	Montana	14.5
11	Wyoming	14.5
13	Kentucky	14.4
14	South Carolina	13.4
15	Oklahoma	13.3
16	Georgia	13.0
17	Missouri	12.9
18	Idaho	12.5
19	Florida	12.4
20	North Carolina	12.3
21	Maryland	12.1
22	Michigan	10.9
23	Pennsylvania	10.7
23	Texas	10.7
23	Virginia	10.7
26	Indiana	10.6
27	Kansas	10.5
28	Colorado	10.4
29	Oregon	10.3
30	Ohio	9.6
30	Utah	9.6
32	Delaware	9.1
33	California	8.9
33	North Dakota	8.9
35	Wisconsin	8.7
36	Washington	8.5
37	Vermont	8.4
38	Maine	8.1
39	Illinois	8.0
39	Nebraska	8.0
41	Minnesota	6.6
42	South Dakota	6.5
43	New Hampshire	5.9
44	Iowa	5.3
45	New Jersey	5.1
45	New York	5.1
47	Connecticut	4.3
48	Massachusetts	3.6
49	Rhode Island	3.5
50	Hawaii	2.8
	District of Columbia	24.5

Source: U.S. Department of Health and Human Services, National Center for Health Statistics
"National Vital Statistics Reports" (Vol. 58, No. 19, May 20, 2010, http://www.cdc.gov/nchs/deaths.htm)
*Final data by state of residence. Not age-adjusted.

Age-Adjusted Death Rate by Firearm Injury in 2007

National Rate = 10.2 Deaths per 100,000 Population*

ALPHA ORDER

RANK	STATE	RATE
4	Alabama	17.5
3	Alaska	17.8
7	Arizona	15.1
6	Arkansas	15.2
33	California	8.8
28	Colorado	10.3
47	Connecticut	4.2
32	Delaware	9.0
20	Florida	12.2
15	Georgia	13.2
50	Hawaii	2.6
18	Idaho	12.7
38	Illinois	7.9
24	Indiana	10.6
45	Iowa	5.0
28	Kansas	10.3
11	Kentucky	14.2
1	Louisiana	20.2
40	Maine	7.6
21	Maryland	12.1
48	Massachusetts	3.6
23	Michigan	10.8
41	Minnesota	6.5
2	Mississippi	18.5
17	Missouri	12.8
13	Montana	13.7
38	Nebraska	7.9
5	Nevada	16.3
43	New Hampshire	5.5
44	New Jersey	5.2
8	New Mexico	15.0
45	New York	5.0
19	North Carolina	12.3
34	North Dakota	8.6
31	Ohio	9.6
15	Oklahoma	13.2
30	Oregon	9.8
24	Pennsylvania	10.6
49	Rhode Island	3.4
14	South Carolina	13.3
42	South Dakota	6.1
10	Tennessee	14.8
22	Texas	10.9
27	Utah	10.4
37	Vermont	8.1
26	Virginia	10.5
36	Washington	8.3
11	West Virginia	14.2
34	Wisconsin	8.6
8	Wyoming	15.0

RANK ORDER

RANK	STATE	RATE
1	Louisiana	20.2
2	Mississippi	18.5
3	Alaska	17.8
4	Alabama	17.5
5	Nevada	16.3
6	Arkansas	15.2
7	Arizona	15.1
8	New Mexico	15.0
8	Wyoming	15.0
10	Tennessee	14.8
11	Kentucky	14.2
11	West Virginia	14.2
13	Montana	13.7
14	South Carolina	13.3
15	Georgia	13.2
15	Oklahoma	13.2
17	Missouri	12.8
18	Idaho	12.7
19	North Carolina	12.3
20	Florida	12.2
21	Maryland	12.1
22	Texas	10.9
23	Michigan	10.8
24	Indiana	10.6
24	Pennsylvania	10.6
26	Virginia	10.5
27	Utah	10.4
28	Colorado	10.3
28	Kansas	10.3
30	Oregon	9.8
31	Ohio	9.6
32	Delaware	9.0
33	California	8.8
34	North Dakota	8.6
34	Wisconsin	8.6
36	Washington	8.3
37	Vermont	8.1
38	Illinois	7.9
38	Nebraska	7.9
40	Maine	7.6
41	Minnesota	6.5
42	South Dakota	6.1
43	New Hampshire	5.5
44	New Jersey	5.2
45	Iowa	5.0
45	New York	5.0
47	Connecticut	4.2
48	Massachusetts	3.6
49	Rhode Island	3.4
50	Hawaii	2.6

| | District of Columbia | 21.7 |

Source: U.S. Department of Health and Human Services, National Center for Health Statistics
"National Vital Statistics Reports" (Vol. 58, No. 19, May 20, 2010, http://www.cdc.gov/nchs/deaths.htm)
*Final data by state of residence. Age-adjusted rates based on the year 2000 standard population.

Deaths by Homicide in 2007

National Total = 18,361 Homicides*

ALPHA ORDER

RANK	STATE	DEATHS	% of USA
14	Alabama	480	2.6%
39	Alaska	50	0.3%
13	Arizona	528	2.9%
23	Arkansas	243	1.3%
1	California	2,376	12.9%
29	Colorado	173	0.9%
33	Connecticut	106	0.6%
40	Delaware	48	0.3%
3	Florida	1,324	7.2%
6	Georgia	771	4.2%
43	Hawaii	24	0.1%
40	Idaho	48	0.3%
4	Illinois	863	4.7%
20	Indiana	374	2.0%
38	Iowa	51	0.3%
32	Kansas	115	0.6%
24	Kentucky	213	1.2%
11	Louisiana	627	3.4%
42	Maine	26	0.1%
12	Maryland	573	3.1%
27	Massachusetts	188	1.0%
8	Michigan	704	3.8%
31	Minnesota	120	0.7%
21	Mississippi	286	1.6%
18	Missouri	384	2.1%
43	Montana	24	0.1%
36	Nebraska	71	0.4%
27	Nevada	188	1.0%
48	New Hampshire	14	0.1%
17	New Jersey	403	2.2%
30	New Mexico	160	0.9%
5	New York	840	4.6%
9	North Carolina	674	3.7%
48	North Dakota	14	0.1%
10	Ohio	639	3.5%
22	Oklahoma	251	1.4%
35	Oregon	81	0.4%
7	Pennsylvania	750	4.1%
43	Rhode Island	24	0.1%
19	South Carolina	382	2.1%
47	South Dakota	15	0.1%
15	Tennessee	475	2.6%
2	Texas	1,495	8.1%
37	Utah	68	0.4%
50	Vermont	13	0.1%
16	Virginia	420	2.3%
26	Washington	201	1.1%
34	West Virginia	86	0.5%
25	Wisconsin	202	1.1%
46	Wyoming	17	0.1%

RANK ORDER

RANK	STATE	DEATHS	% of USA
1	California	2,376	12.9%
2	Texas	1,495	8.1%
3	Florida	1,324	7.2%
4	Illinois	863	4.7%
5	New York	840	4.6%
6	Georgia	771	4.2%
7	Pennsylvania	750	4.1%
8	Michigan	704	3.8%
9	North Carolina	674	3.7%
10	Ohio	639	3.5%
11	Louisiana	627	3.4%
12	Maryland	573	3.1%
13	Arizona	528	2.9%
14	Alabama	480	2.6%
15	Tennessee	475	2.6%
16	Virginia	420	2.3%
17	New Jersey	403	2.2%
18	Missouri	384	2.1%
19	South Carolina	382	2.1%
20	Indiana	374	2.0%
21	Mississippi	286	1.6%
22	Oklahoma	251	1.4%
23	Arkansas	243	1.3%
24	Kentucky	213	1.2%
25	Wisconsin	202	1.1%
26	Washington	201	1.1%
27	Massachusetts	188	1.0%
27	Nevada	188	1.0%
29	Colorado	173	0.9%
30	New Mexico	160	0.9%
31	Minnesota	120	0.7%
32	Kansas	115	0.6%
33	Connecticut	106	0.6%
34	West Virginia	86	0.5%
35	Oregon	81	0.4%
36	Nebraska	71	0.4%
37	Utah	68	0.4%
38	Iowa	51	0.3%
39	Alaska	50	0.3%
40	Delaware	48	0.3%
40	Idaho	48	0.3%
42	Maine	26	0.1%
43	Hawaii	24	0.1%
43	Montana	24	0.1%
43	Rhode Island	24	0.1%
46	Wyoming	17	0.1%
47	South Dakota	15	0.1%
48	New Hampshire	14	0.1%
48	North Dakota	14	0.1%
50	Vermont	13	0.1%
	District of Columbia	159	0.9%

Source: U.S. Department of Health and Human Services, National Center for Health Statistics
  "National Vital Statistics Reports" (Vol. 58, No. 19, May 20, 2010, http://www.cdc.gov/nchs/deaths.htm)
*Final data by state of residence. Includes legal intervention. Homicide data shown here are collected by the Centers for Disease Control and Prevention based on death certificates and differ from murder data collected by the F.B.I. from other sources.

Death Rate by Homicide in 2007

National Rate = 6.1 Deaths per 100,000 Population*

ALPHA ORDER

RANK	STATE	RATE
2	Alabama	10.4
12	Alaska	7.3
7	Arizona	8.3
6	Arkansas	8.6
18	California	6.5
32	Colorado	3.6
36	Connecticut	3.0
23	Delaware	5.6
12	Florida	7.3
8	Georgia	8.1
44	Hawaii	1.9
34	Idaho	3.2
17	Illinois	6.7
22	Indiana	5.9
45	Iowa	1.7
30	Kansas	4.1
26	Kentucky	5.0
1	Louisiana	14.6
43	Maine	2.0
3	Maryland	10.2
37	Massachusetts	2.9
15	Michigan	7.0
40	Minnesota	2.3
4	Mississippi	9.8
18	Missouri	6.5
39	Montana	2.5
31	Nebraska	4.0
12	Nevada	7.3
NA	New Hampshire**	NA
28	New Jersey	4.6
8	New Mexico	8.1
29	New York	4.4
11	North Carolina	7.4
NA	North Dakota**	NA
23	Ohio	5.6
16	Oklahoma	6.9
42	Oregon	2.2
21	Pennsylvania	6.0
40	Rhode Island	2.3
5	South Carolina	8.7
NA	South Dakota**	NA
10	Tennessee	7.7
20	Texas	6.3
38	Utah	2.6
NA	Vermont**	NA
25	Virginia	5.4
35	Washington	3.1
27	West Virginia	4.7
32	Wisconsin	3.6
NA	Wyoming**	NA

RANK ORDER

RANK	STATE	RATE
1	Louisiana	14.6
2	Alabama	10.4
3	Maryland	10.2
4	Mississippi	9.8
5	South Carolina	8.7
6	Arkansas	8.6
7	Arizona	8.3
8	Georgia	8.1
8	New Mexico	8.1
10	Tennessee	7.7
11	North Carolina	7.4
12	Alaska	7.3
12	Florida	7.3
12	Nevada	7.3
15	Michigan	7.0
16	Oklahoma	6.9
17	Illinois	6.7
18	California	6.5
18	Missouri	6.5
20	Texas	6.3
21	Pennsylvania	6.0
22	Indiana	5.9
23	Delaware	5.6
23	Ohio	5.6
25	Virginia	5.4
26	Kentucky	5.0
27	West Virginia	4.7
28	New Jersey	4.6
29	New York	4.4
30	Kansas	4.1
31	Nebraska	4.0
32	Colorado	3.6
32	Wisconsin	3.6
34	Idaho	3.2
35	Washington	3.1
36	Connecticut	3.0
37	Massachusetts	2.9
38	Utah	2.6
39	Montana	2.5
40	Minnesota	2.3
40	Rhode Island	2.3
42	Oregon	2.2
43	Maine	2.0
44	Hawaii	1.9
45	Iowa	1.7
NA	New Hampshire**	NA
NA	North Dakota**	NA
NA	South Dakota**	NA
NA	Vermont**	NA
NA	Wyoming**	NA

District of Columbia   27.0

Source: U.S. Department of Health and Human Services, National Center for Health Statistics
   "National Vital Statistics Reports" (Vol. 58, No. 19, May 20, 2010, http://www.cdc.gov/nchs/deaths.htm)
*Final data by state of residence. Includes legal intervention. Homicide data shown here are collected by the Centers for Disease Control and Prevention based on death certificates and differ from murder data collected by the F.B.I. from other sources. Not age-adjusted.
**Insufficient data to determine a reliable rate.

Age-Adjusted Death Rate by Homicide in 2007

National Rate = 6.1 Deaths per 100,000 Population*

ALPHA ORDER				RANK ORDER		
RANK	STATE	RATE		RANK	STATE	RATE
2	Alabama	10.5		1	Louisiana	14.6
14	Alaska	7.1		2	Alabama	10.5
7	Arizona	8.3		3	Maryland	10.4
5	Arkansas	8.8		4	Mississippi	10.0
19	California	6.3		5	Arkansas	8.8
33	Colorado	3.4		6	South Carolina	8.7
35	Connecticut	3.1		7	Arizona	8.3
23	Delaware	5.7		8	New Mexico	8.2
11	Florida	7.6		9	Georgia	8.0
9	Georgia	8.0		10	Tennessee	7.8
44	Hawaii	1.8		11	Florida	7.6
34	Idaho	3.2		12	North Carolina	7.5
17	Illinois	6.6		13	Nevada	7.4
22	Indiana	5.9		14	Alaska	7.1
44	Iowa	1.8		14	Michigan	7.1
30	Kansas	4.2		16	Oklahoma	6.9
26	Kentucky	5.0		17	Illinois	6.6
1	Louisiana	14.6		17	Missouri	6.6
43	Maine	2.0		19	California	6.3
3	Maryland	10.4		19	Pennsylvania	6.3
37	Massachusetts	3.0		21	Texas	6.2
14	Michigan	7.1		22	Indiana	5.9
40	Minnesota	2.3		23	Delaware	5.7
4	Mississippi	10.0		23	Ohio	5.7
17	Missouri	6.6		25	Virginia	5.4
38	Montana	2.5		26	Kentucky	5.0
31	Nebraska	4.1		27	West Virginia	4.9
13	Nevada	7.4		28	New Jersey	4.8
NA	New Hampshire**	NA		29	New York	4.4
28	New Jersey	4.8		30	Kansas	4.2
8	New Mexico	8.2		31	Nebraska	4.1
29	New York	4.4		32	Wisconsin	3.6
12	North Carolina	7.5		33	Colorado	3.4
NA	North Dakota**	NA		34	Idaho	3.2
23	Ohio	5.7		35	Connecticut	3.1
16	Oklahoma	6.9		35	Washington	3.1
42	Oregon	2.1		37	Massachusetts	3.0
19	Pennsylvania	6.3		38	Montana	2.5
41	Rhode Island	2.2		39	Utah	2.4
6	South Carolina	8.7		40	Minnesota	2.3
NA	South Dakota**	NA		41	Rhode Island	2.2
10	Tennessee	7.8		42	Oregon	2.1
21	Texas	6.2		43	Maine	2.0
39	Utah	2.4		44	Hawaii	1.8
NA	Vermont**	NA		44	Iowa	1.8
25	Virginia	5.4		NA	New Hampshire**	NA
35	Washington	3.1		NA	North Dakota**	NA
27	West Virginia	4.9		NA	South Dakota**	NA
32	Wisconsin	3.6		NA	Vermont**	NA
NA	Wyoming**	NA		NA	Wyoming**	NA
					District of Columbia	23.8

Source: U.S. Department of Health and Human Services, National Center for Health Statistics
"National Vital Statistics Reports" (Vol. 58, No. 19, May 20, 2010, http://www.cdc.gov/nchs/deaths.htm)
*Final data by state of residence. Includes legal intervention. Homicide data shown here are collected by the Centers for Disease Control and Prevention based on death certificates and differ from murder data collected by the F.B.I. from other sources. Age-adjusted rates based on the year 2000 standard population.
**Insufficient data to determine a reliable rate.

Deaths by Suicide in 2007

National Total = 34,598 Suicides*

ALPHA ORDER

ALPHA ORDER

RANK	STATE	DEATHS	% of USA
22	Alabama	592	1.7%
43	Alaska	149	0.4%
10	Arizona	1,016	2.9%
30	Arkansas	402	1.2%
1	California	3,602	10.4%
15	Colorado	811	2.3%
37	Connecticut	271	0.8%
48	Delaware	95	0.3%
2	Florida	2,587	7.5%
11	Georgia	997	2.9%
44	Hawaii	133	0.4%
38	Idaho	223	0.6%
8	Illinois	1,108	3.2%
17	Indiana	790	2.3%
35	Iowa	322	0.9%
33	Kansas	382	1.1%
19	Kentucky	649	1.9%
26	Louisiana	522	1.5%
40	Maine	191	0.6%
27	Maryland	518	1.5%
28	Massachusetts	516	1.5%
7	Michigan	1,131	3.3%
23	Minnesota	572	1.7%
32	Mississippi	396	1.1%
16	Missouri	808	2.3%
39	Montana	196	0.6%
41	Nebraska	181	0.5%
29	Nevada	471	1.4%
42	New Hampshire	158	0.5%
20	New Jersey	596	1.7%
31	New Mexico	401	1.2%
5	New York	1,396	4.0%
9	North Carolina	1,077	3.1%
48	North Dakota	95	0.3%
6	Ohio	1,295	3.7%
24	Oklahoma	531	1.5%
21	Oregon	594	1.7%
4	Pennsylvania	1,441	4.2%
47	Rhode Island	96	0.3%
25	South Carolina	530	1.5%
45	South Dakota	102	0.3%
14	Tennessee	844	2.4%
3	Texas	2,433	7.0%
34	Utah	378	1.1%
50	Vermont	89	0.3%
12	Virginia	880	2.5%
13	Washington	865	2.5%
36	West Virginia	300	0.9%
18	Wisconsin	729	2.1%
46	Wyoming	101	0.3%

RANK ORDER

RANK	STATE	DEATHS	% of USA
1	California	3,602	10.4%
2	Florida	2,587	7.5%
3	Texas	2,433	7.0%
4	Pennsylvania	1,441	4.2%
5	New York	1,396	4.0%
6	Ohio	1,295	3.7%
7	Michigan	1,131	3.3%
8	Illinois	1,108	3.2%
9	North Carolina	1,077	3.1%
10	Arizona	1,016	2.9%
11	Georgia	997	2.9%
12	Virginia	880	2.5%
13	Washington	865	2.5%
14	Tennessee	844	2.4%
15	Colorado	811	2.3%
16	Missouri	808	2.3%
17	Indiana	790	2.3%
18	Wisconsin	729	2.1%
19	Kentucky	649	1.9%
20	New Jersey	596	1.7%
21	Oregon	594	1.7%
22	Alabama	592	1.7%
23	Minnesota	572	1.7%
24	Oklahoma	531	1.5%
25	South Carolina	530	1.5%
26	Louisiana	522	1.5%
27	Maryland	518	1.5%
28	Massachusetts	516	1.5%
29	Nevada	471	1.4%
30	Arkansas	402	1.2%
31	New Mexico	401	1.2%
32	Mississippi	396	1.1%
33	Kansas	382	1.1%
34	Utah	378	1.1%
35	Iowa	322	0.9%
36	West Virginia	300	0.9%
37	Connecticut	271	0.8%
38	Idaho	223	0.6%
39	Montana	196	0.6%
40	Maine	191	0.6%
41	Nebraska	181	0.5%
42	New Hampshire	158	0.5%
43	Alaska	149	0.4%
44	Hawaii	133	0.4%
45	South Dakota	102	0.3%
46	Wyoming	101	0.3%
47	Rhode Island	96	0.3%
48	Delaware	95	0.3%
48	North Dakota	95	0.3%
50	Vermont	89	0.3%
	District of Columbia	36	0.1%

Source: U.S. Department of Health and Human Services, National Center for Health Statistics
"National Vital Statistics Reports" (Vol. 58, No. 19, May 20, 2010, http://www.cdc.gov/nchs/deaths.htm)
*Final data by state of residence.

Death Rate by Suicide in 2007

National Rate = 11.5 Deaths per 100,000 Population*

RANK	STATE	RATE		RANK	STATE	RATE
25	Alabama	12.8		1	Alaska	21.8
1	Alaska	21.8		2	Montana	20.5
8	Arizona	16.0		3	New Mexico	20.4
17	Arkansas	14.2		4	Wyoming	19.3
43	California	9.9		5	Nevada	18.4
6	Colorado	16.7		6	Colorado	16.7
48	Connecticut	7.7		7	West Virginia	16.6
36	Delaware	11.0		8	Arizona	16.0
17	Florida	14.2		9	Oregon	15.9
39	Georgia	10.4		10	Kentucky	15.3
39	Hawaii	10.4		11	Idaho	14.9
11	Idaho	14.9		11	North Dakota	14.9
46	Illinois	8.6		13	Oklahoma	14.7
27	Indiana	12.5		14	Maine	14.5
38	Iowa	10.8		15	Utah	14.3
19	Kansas	13.8		15	Vermont	14.3
10	Kentucky	15.3		17	Arkansas	14.2
28	Louisiana	12.2		17	Florida	14.2
14	Maine	14.5		19	Kansas	13.8
44	Maryland	9.2		20	Missouri	13.7
47	Massachusetts	8.0		20	Tennessee	13.7
35	Michigan	11.2		22	Mississippi	13.6
36	Minnesota	11.0		23	Washington	13.4
22	Mississippi	13.6		24	Wisconsin	13.0
20	Missouri	13.7		25	Alabama	12.8
2	Montana	20.5		25	South Dakota	12.8
41	Nebraska	10.2		27	Indiana	12.5
5	Nevada	18.4		28	Louisiana	12.2
29	New Hampshire	12.0		29	New Hampshire	12.0
50	New Jersey	6.9		29	South Carolina	12.0
3	New Mexico	20.4		31	North Carolina	11.9
49	New York	7.2		32	Pennsylvania	11.6
31	North Carolina	11.9		33	Virginia	11.4
11	North Dakota	14.9		34	Ohio	11.3
34	Ohio	11.3		35	Michigan	11.2
13	Oklahoma	14.7		36	Delaware	11.0
9	Oregon	15.9		36	Minnesota	11.0
32	Pennsylvania	11.6		38	Iowa	10.8
45	Rhode Island	9.1		39	Georgia	10.4
29	South Carolina	12.0		39	Hawaii	10.4
25	South Dakota	12.8		41	Nebraska	10.2
20	Tennessee	13.7		41	Texas	10.2
41	Texas	10.2		43	California	9.9
15	Utah	14.3		44	Maryland	9.2
15	Vermont	14.3		45	Rhode Island	9.1
33	Virginia	11.4		46	Illinois	8.6
23	Washington	13.4		47	Massachusetts	8.0
7	West Virginia	16.6		48	Connecticut	7.7
24	Wisconsin	13.0		49	New York	7.2
4	Wyoming	19.3		50	New Jersey	6.9
					District of Columbia	6.1

Source: U.S. Department of Health and Human Services, National Center for Health Statistics
   "National Vital Statistics Reports" (Vol. 58, No. 19, May 20, 2010, http://www.cdc.gov/nchs/deaths.htm)
*Final data by state of residence. Not age-adjusted.

Age-Adjusted Death Rate by Suicide in 2007

National Rate = 11.3 Deaths per 100,000 Population*

ALPHA ORDER

RANK	STATE	RATE
25	Alabama	12.5
1	Alaska	22.1
7	Arizona	16.1
15	Arkansas	14.3
42	California	9.8
6	Colorado	16.4
48	Connecticut	7.4
37	Delaware	10.7
21	Florida	13.3
37	Georgia	10.7
43	Hawaii	9.7
11	Idaho	15.1
46	Illinois	8.5
27	Indiana	12.4
39	Iowa	10.6
18	Kansas	13.7
11	Kentucky	15.1
28	Louisiana	12.2
18	Maine	13.7
44	Maryland	9.0
47	Massachusetts	7.6
34	Michigan	11.0
36	Minnesota	10.8
16	Mississippi	13.8
20	Missouri	13.5
4	Montana	19.4
41	Nebraska	10.2
5	Nevada	18.3
33	New Hampshire	11.1
50	New Jersey	6.7
2	New Mexico	20.4
49	New York	7.0
29	North Carolina	11.7
14	North Dakota	14.4
34	Ohio	11.0
13	Oklahoma	14.7
10	Oregon	15.2
31	Pennsylvania	11.2
45	Rhode Island	8.7
29	South Carolina	11.7
25	South Dakota	12.5
21	Tennessee	13.3
40	Texas	10.4
9	Utah	15.4
16	Vermont	13.8
31	Virginia	11.2
23	Washington	13.0
8	West Virginia	15.9
24	Wisconsin	12.7
3	Wyoming	19.7

RANK ORDER

RANK	STATE	RATE
1	Alaska	22.1
2	New Mexico	20.4
3	Wyoming	19.7
4	Montana	19.4
5	Nevada	18.3
6	Colorado	16.4
7	Arizona	16.1
8	West Virginia	15.9
9	Utah	15.4
10	Oregon	15.2
11	Idaho	15.1
11	Kentucky	15.1
13	Oklahoma	14.7
14	North Dakota	14.4
15	Arkansas	14.3
16	Mississippi	13.8
16	Vermont	13.8
18	Kansas	13.7
18	Maine	13.7
20	Missouri	13.5
21	Florida	13.3
21	Tennessee	13.3
23	Washington	13.0
24	Wisconsin	12.7
25	Alabama	12.5
25	South Dakota	12.5
27	Indiana	12.4
28	Louisiana	12.2
29	North Carolina	11.7
29	South Carolina	11.7
31	Pennsylvania	11.2
31	Virginia	11.2
33	New Hampshire	11.1
34	Michigan	11.0
34	Ohio	11.0
36	Minnesota	10.8
37	Delaware	10.7
37	Georgia	10.7
39	Iowa	10.6
40	Texas	10.4
41	Nebraska	10.2
42	California	9.8
43	Hawaii	9.7
44	Maryland	9.0
45	Rhode Island	8.7
46	Illinois	8.5
47	Massachusetts	7.6
48	Connecticut	7.4
49	New York	7.0
50	New Jersey	6.7

District of Columbia	5.8

Source: U.S. Department of Health and Human Services, National Center for Health Statistics
  "National Vital Statistics Reports" (Vol. 58, No. 19, May 20, 2010, http://www.cdc.gov/nchs/deaths.htm)
*Final data by state of residence. Age-adjusted rates based on the year 2000 standard population.

Alcohol-Induced Deaths in 2007

National Total = 23,199 Deaths*

ALPHA ORDER

RANK	STATE	DEATHS	% of USA
28	Alabama	254	1.1%
38	Alaska	144	0.6%
6	Arizona	747	3.2%
34	Arkansas	173	0.7%
1	California	4,027	17.4%
11	Colorado	610	2.6%
30	Connecticut	214	0.9%
49	Delaware	57	0.2%
2	Florida	1,770	7.6%
14	Georgia	505	2.2%
46	Hawaii	82	0.4%
37	Idaho	152	0.7%
10	Illinois	630	2.7%
26	Indiana	315	1.4%
31	Iowa	212	0.9%
32	Kansas	211	0.9%
27	Kentucky	283	1.2%
33	Louisiana	202	0.9%
41	Maine	133	0.6%
23	Maryland	338	1.5%
18	Massachusetts	440	1.9%
8	Michigan	713	3.1%
24	Minnesota	333	1.4%
36	Mississippi	160	0.7%
25	Missouri	324	1.4%
40	Montana	143	0.6%
43	Nebraska	103	0.4%
29	Nevada	253	1.1%
42	New Hampshire	120	0.5%
19	New Jersey	414	1.8%
21	New Mexico	404	1.7%
4	New York	1,167	5.0%
9	North Carolina	676	2.9%
49	North Dakota	57	0.2%
5	Ohio	780	3.4%
20	Oklahoma	412	1.8%
13	Oregon	543	2.3%
12	Pennsylvania	548	2.4%
44	Rhode Island	93	0.4%
22	South Carolina	363	1.6%
47	South Dakota	81	0.3%
16	Tennessee	481	2.1%
3	Texas	1,360	5.9%
38	Utah	144	0.6%
48	Vermont	63	0.3%
17	Virginia	445	1.9%
7	Washington	718	3.1%
35	West Virginia	165	0.7%
15	Wisconsin	489	2.1%
45	Wyoming	88	0.4%

RANK ORDER

RANK	STATE	DEATHS	% of USA
1	California	4,027	17.4%
2	Florida	1,770	7.6%
3	Texas	1,360	5.9%
4	New York	1,167	5.0%
5	Ohio	780	3.4%
6	Arizona	747	3.2%
7	Washington	718	3.1%
8	Michigan	713	3.1%
9	North Carolina	676	2.9%
10	Illinois	630	2.7%
11	Colorado	610	2.6%
12	Pennsylvania	548	2.4%
13	Oregon	543	2.3%
14	Georgia	505	2.2%
15	Wisconsin	489	2.1%
16	Tennessee	481	2.1%
17	Virginia	445	1.9%
18	Massachusetts	440	1.9%
19	New Jersey	414	1.8%
20	Oklahoma	412	1.8%
21	New Mexico	404	1.7%
22	South Carolina	363	1.6%
23	Maryland	338	1.5%
24	Minnesota	333	1.4%
25	Missouri	324	1.4%
26	Indiana	315	1.4%
27	Kentucky	283	1.2%
28	Alabama	254	1.1%
29	Nevada	253	1.1%
30	Connecticut	214	0.9%
31	Iowa	212	0.9%
32	Kansas	211	0.9%
33	Louisiana	202	0.9%
34	Arkansas	173	0.7%
35	West Virginia	165	0.7%
36	Mississippi	160	0.7%
37	Idaho	152	0.7%
38	Alaska	144	0.6%
38	Utah	144	0.6%
40	Montana	143	0.6%
41	Maine	133	0.6%
42	New Hampshire	120	0.5%
43	Nebraska	103	0.4%
44	Rhode Island	93	0.4%
45	Wyoming	88	0.4%
46	Hawaii	82	0.4%
47	South Dakota	81	0.3%
48	Vermont	63	0.3%
49	Delaware	57	0.2%
49	North Dakota	57	0.2%
	District of Columbia	60	0.3%

Source: U.S. Department of Health and Human Services, National Center for Health Statistics
"National Vital Statistics Reports" (Vol. 58, No. 19, May 20, 2010, http://www.cdc.gov/nchs/deaths.htm)
*Final data by state of residence. Includes excessive blood level of alcohol, accidental poisoning by alcohol and the following alcohol-related causes: psychoses, dependence syndrome, polyneuropathy, cardiomyopathy, gastritis, chronic liver disease, and cirrhosis. Excludes accidents, homicides, and other causes indirectly related to alcohol use.

Death Rate by Alcohol-Induced Deaths in 2007

National Rate = 7.7 Deaths per 100,000 Population*

ALPHA ORDER

RANK	STATE	RATE
41	Alabama	5.5
1	Alaska	21.1
7	Arizona	11.8
34	Arkansas	6.1
10	California	11.0
6	Colorado	12.5
34	Connecticut	6.1
31	Delaware	6.6
16	Florida	9.7
45	Georgia	5.3
32	Hawaii	6.4
12	Idaho	10.1
47	Illinois	4.9
46	Indiana	5.0
26	Iowa	7.1
24	Kansas	7.6
30	Kentucky	6.7
49	Louisiana	4.7
12	Maine	10.1
36	Maryland	6.0
28	Massachusetts	6.8
26	Michigan	7.1
32	Minnesota	6.4
41	Mississippi	5.5
41	Missouri	5.5
4	Montana	14.9
38	Nebraska	5.8
15	Nevada	9.9
17	New Hampshire	9.1
48	New Jersey	4.8
2	New Mexico	20.5
36	New York	6.0
25	North Carolina	7.5
19	North Dakota	8.9
28	Ohio	6.8
8	Oklahoma	11.4
5	Oregon	14.5
50	Pennsylvania	4.4
20	Rhode Island	8.8
22	South Carolina	8.2
11	South Dakota	10.2
23	Tennessee	7.8
40	Texas	5.7
44	Utah	5.4
12	Vermont	10.1
38	Virginia	5.8
9	Washington	11.1
17	West Virginia	9.1
21	Wisconsin	8.7
3	Wyoming	16.8

RANK ORDER

RANK	STATE	RATE
1	Alaska	21.1
2	New Mexico	20.5
3	Wyoming	16.8
4	Montana	14.9
5	Oregon	14.5
6	Colorado	12.5
7	Arizona	11.8
8	Oklahoma	11.4
9	Washington	11.1
10	California	11.0
11	South Dakota	10.2
12	Idaho	10.1
12	Maine	10.1
12	Vermont	10.1
15	Nevada	9.9
16	Florida	9.7
17	New Hampshire	9.1
17	West Virginia	9.1
19	North Dakota	8.9
20	Rhode Island	8.8
21	Wisconsin	8.7
22	South Carolina	8.2
23	Tennessee	7.8
24	Kansas	7.6
25	North Carolina	7.5
26	Iowa	7.1
26	Michigan	7.1
28	Massachusetts	6.8
28	Ohio	6.8
30	Kentucky	6.7
31	Delaware	6.6
32	Hawaii	6.4
32	Minnesota	6.4
34	Arkansas	6.1
34	Connecticut	6.1
36	Maryland	6.0
36	New York	6.0
38	Nebraska	5.8
38	Virginia	5.8
40	Texas	5.7
41	Alabama	5.5
41	Mississippi	5.5
41	Missouri	5.5
44	Utah	5.4
45	Georgia	5.3
46	Indiana	5.0
47	Illinois	4.9
48	New Jersey	4.8
49	Louisiana	4.7
50	Pennsylvania	4.4

District of Columbia	10.2

Source: U.S. Department of Health and Human Services, National Center for Health Statistics
   "National Vital Statistics Reports" (Vol. 58, No. 19, May 20, 2010, http://www.cdc.gov/nchs/deaths.htm)
*Final data by state of residence. Includes excessive blood level of alcohol, accidental poisoning by alcohol and the following alcohol-related causes: psychoses, dependence syndrome, polyneuropathy, cardiomyopathy, gastritis, chronic liver disease, and cirrhosis. Excludes accidents, homicides, and other causes indirectly related to alcohol use. Not age-adjusted.

Age-Adjusted Death Rate by Alcohol-Induced Deaths in 2007

National Rate = 7.3 Deaths per 100,000 Population*

ALPHA ORDER

RANK	STATE	RATE
45	Alabama	5.0
1	Alaska	20.6
6	Arizona	11.9
37	Arkansas	5.6
8	California	11.1
6	Colorado	11.9
38	Connecticut	5.5
31	Delaware	6.1
14	Florida	8.6
42	Georgia	5.3
35	Hawaii	5.8
11	Idaho	10.0
46	Illinois	4.7
46	Indiana	4.7
26	Iowa	6.5
23	Kansas	7.2
29	Kentucky	6.2
48	Louisiana	4.5
16	Maine	8.1
38	Maryland	5.5
31	Massachusetts	6.1
27	Michigan	6.4
33	Minnesota	6.0
41	Mississippi	5.4
44	Missouri	5.2
4	Montana	13.1
36	Nebraska	5.7
13	Nevada	9.4
18	New Hampshire	8.0
49	New Jersey	4.3
2	New Mexico	20.1
38	New York	5.5
25	North Carolina	7.0
14	North Dakota	8.6
29	Ohio	6.2
9	Oklahoma	11.0
5	Oregon	13.0
50	Pennsylvania	3.9
19	Rhode Island	7.9
22	South Carolina	7.6
12	South Dakota	9.8
24	Tennessee	7.1
33	Texas	6.0
27	Utah	6.4
16	Vermont	8.1
42	Virginia	5.3
10	Washington	10.3
19	West Virginia	7.9
19	Wisconsin	7.9
3	Wyoming	15.6

RANK ORDER

RANK	STATE	RATE
1	Alaska	20.6
2	New Mexico	20.1
3	Wyoming	15.6
4	Montana	13.1
5	Oregon	13.0
6	Arizona	11.9
6	Colorado	11.9
8	California	11.1
9	Oklahoma	11.0
10	Washington	10.3
11	Idaho	10.0
12	South Dakota	9.8
13	Nevada	9.4
14	Florida	8.6
14	North Dakota	8.6
16	Maine	8.1
16	Vermont	8.1
18	New Hampshire	8.0
19	Rhode Island	7.9
19	West Virginia	7.9
19	Wisconsin	7.9
22	South Carolina	7.6
23	Kansas	7.2
24	Tennessee	7.1
25	North Carolina	7.0
26	Iowa	6.5
27	Michigan	6.4
27	Utah	6.4
29	Kentucky	6.2
29	Ohio	6.2
31	Delaware	6.1
31	Massachusetts	6.1
33	Minnesota	6.0
33	Texas	6.0
35	Hawaii	5.8
36	Nebraska	5.7
37	Arkansas	5.6
38	Connecticut	5.5
38	Maryland	5.5
38	New York	5.5
41	Mississippi	5.4
42	Georgia	5.3
42	Virginia	5.3
44	Missouri	5.2
45	Alabama	5.0
46	Illinois	4.7
46	Indiana	4.7
48	Louisiana	4.5
49	New Jersey	4.3
50	Pennsylvania	3.9
	District of Columbia	9.6

Source: U.S. Department of Health and Human Services, National Center for Health Statistics
"National Vital Statistics Reports" (Vol. 58, No. 19, May 20, 2010, http://www.cdc.gov/nchs/deaths.htm)
*Final data by state of residence. Includes excessive blood level of alcohol, accidental poisoning by alcohol and the following alcohol-related causes: psychoses, dependence syndrome, polyneuropathy, cardiomyopathy, gastritis, chronic liver disease, and cirrhosis. Excludes accidents, homicides, and other causes indirectly related to alcohol use. Age-adjusted rates based on the year 2000 standard population.

Drug-Induced Deaths in 2007

National Total = 38,371 Deaths*

ALPHA ORDER

RANK	STATE	DEATHS	% of USA
27	Alabama	554	1.4%
46	Alaska	75	0.2%
13	Arizona	981	2.6%
35	Arkansas	326	0.8%
1	California	4,178	10.9%
19	Colorado	747	1.9%
31	Connecticut	444	1.2%
44	Delaware	102	0.3%
2	Florida	2,936	7.7%
14	Georgia	973	2.5%
40	Hawaii	142	0.4%
42	Idaho	133	0.3%
8	Illinois	1,239	3.2%
16	Indiana	827	2.2%
37	Iowa	211	0.5%
36	Kansas	294	0.8%
21	Kentucky	722	1.9%
15	Louisiana	862	2.2%
39	Maine	161	0.4%
17	Maryland	807	2.1%
11	Massachusetts	1,003	2.6%
7	Michigan	1,542	4.0%
33	Minnesota	359	0.9%
34	Mississippi	334	0.9%
20	Missouri	730	1.9%
43	Montana	132	0.3%
45	Nebraska	92	0.2%
29	Nevada	515	1.3%
38	New Hampshire	187	0.5%
18	New Jersey	797	2.1%
30	New Mexico	471	1.2%
4	New York	1,909	5.0%
9	North Carolina	1,125	2.9%
49	North Dakota	37	0.1%
6	Ohio	1,691	4.4%
23	Oklahoma	687	1.8%
26	Oregon	564	1.5%
5	Pennsylvania	1,812	4.7%
40	Rhode Island	142	0.4%
25	South Carolina	584	1.5%
50	South Dakota	34	0.1%
10	Tennessee	1,035	2.7%
3	Texas	2,343	6.1%
28	Utah	546	1.4%
47	Vermont	68	0.2%
22	Virginia	713	1.9%
11	Washington	1,003	2.6%
32	West Virginia	405	1.1%
24	Wisconsin	639	1.7%
47	Wyoming	68	0.2%

RANK ORDER

RANK	STATE	DEATHS	% of USA
1	California	4,178	10.9%
2	Florida	2,936	7.7%
3	Texas	2,343	6.1%
4	New York	1,909	5.0%
5	Pennsylvania	1,812	4.7%
6	Ohio	1,691	4.4%
7	Michigan	1,542	4.0%
8	Illinois	1,239	3.2%
9	North Carolina	1,125	2.9%
10	Tennessee	1,035	2.7%
11	Massachusetts	1,003	2.6%
11	Washington	1,003	2.6%
13	Arizona	981	2.6%
14	Georgia	973	2.5%
15	Louisiana	862	2.2%
16	Indiana	827	2.2%
17	Maryland	807	2.1%
18	New Jersey	797	2.1%
19	Colorado	747	1.9%
20	Missouri	730	1.9%
21	Kentucky	722	1.9%
22	Virginia	713	1.9%
23	Oklahoma	687	1.8%
24	Wisconsin	639	1.7%
25	South Carolina	584	1.5%
26	Oregon	564	1.5%
27	Alabama	554	1.4%
28	Utah	546	1.4%
29	Nevada	515	1.3%
30	New Mexico	471	1.2%
31	Connecticut	444	1.2%
32	West Virginia	405	1.1%
33	Minnesota	359	0.9%
34	Mississippi	334	0.9%
35	Arkansas	326	0.8%
36	Kansas	294	0.8%
37	Iowa	211	0.5%
38	New Hampshire	187	0.5%
39	Maine	161	0.4%
40	Hawaii	142	0.4%
40	Rhode Island	142	0.4%
42	Idaho	133	0.3%
43	Montana	132	0.3%
44	Delaware	102	0.3%
45	Nebraska	92	0.2%
46	Alaska	75	0.2%
47	Vermont	68	0.2%
47	Wyoming	68	0.2%
49	North Dakota	37	0.1%
50	South Dakota	34	0.1%
	District of Columbia	90	0.2%

Source: U.S. Department of Health and Human Services, National Center for Health Statistics
"National Vital Statistics Reports" (Vol. 58, No. 19, May 20, 2010, http://www.cdc.gov/nchs/deaths.htm)
*Final data by state of residence. Includes drug psychoses, drug dependence, nondependent use excluding alcohol and tobacco, accidental poisoning or suicide by drugs, medicaments, and biologicals. Excludes accidents, homicides, and other causes indirectly related to drug use.

Death Rate by Drug-Induced Deaths in 2007

National Rate = 12.7 Deaths per 100,000 Population*

ALPHA ORDER

RANK	STATE	RATE
29	Alabama	12.0
36	Alaska	11.0
11	Arizona	15.5
31	Arkansas	11.5
32	California	11.4
13	Colorado	15.4
25	Connecticut	12.7
30	Delaware	11.8
9	Florida	16.1
39	Georgia	10.2
35	Hawaii	11.1
45	Idaho	8.9
42	Illinois	9.6
23	Indiana	13.0
46	Iowa	7.1
38	Kansas	10.6
7	Kentucky	17.0
4	Louisiana	20.1
28	Maine	12.2
18	Maryland	14.4
10	Massachusetts	15.6
14	Michigan	15.3
47	Minnesota	6.9
32	Mississippi	11.4
26	Missouri	12.4
20	Montana	13.8
49	Nebraska	5.2
4	Nevada	20.1
19	New Hampshire	14.2
43	New Jersey	9.2
1	New Mexico	23.9
40	New York	9.9
26	North Carolina	12.4
48	North Dakota	5.8
16	Ohio	14.7
6	Oklahoma	19.0
15	Oregon	15.1
17	Pennsylvania	14.6
21	Rhode Island	13.4
22	South Carolina	13.2
50	South Dakota	4.3
8	Tennessee	16.8
41	Texas	9.8
3	Utah	20.6
37	Vermont	10.9
43	Virginia	9.2
11	Washington	15.5
2	West Virginia	22.4
32	Wisconsin	11.4
23	Wyoming	13.0

RANK ORDER

RANK	STATE	RATE
1	New Mexico	23.9
2	West Virginia	22.4
3	Utah	20.6
4	Louisiana	20.1
4	Nevada	20.1
6	Oklahoma	19.0
7	Kentucky	17.0
8	Tennessee	16.8
9	Florida	16.1
10	Massachusetts	15.6
11	Arizona	15.5
11	Washington	15.5
13	Colorado	15.4
14	Michigan	15.3
15	Oregon	15.1
16	Ohio	14.7
17	Pennsylvania	14.6
18	Maryland	14.4
19	New Hampshire	14.2
20	Montana	13.8
21	Rhode Island	13.4
22	South Carolina	13.2
23	Indiana	13.0
23	Wyoming	13.0
25	Connecticut	12.7
26	Missouri	12.4
26	North Carolina	12.4
28	Maine	12.2
29	Alabama	12.0
30	Delaware	11.8
31	Arkansas	11.5
32	California	11.4
32	Mississippi	11.4
32	Wisconsin	11.4
35	Hawaii	11.1
36	Alaska	11.0
37	Vermont	10.9
38	Kansas	10.6
39	Georgia	10.2
40	New York	9.9
41	Texas	9.8
42	Illinois	9.6
43	New Jersey	9.2
43	Virginia	9.2
45	Idaho	8.9
46	Iowa	7.1
47	Minnesota	6.9
48	North Dakota	5.8
49	Nebraska	5.2
50	South Dakota	4.3

	District of Columbia	15.3

Source: U.S. Department of Health and Human Services, National Center for Health Statistics
   "National Vital Statistics Reports" (Vol. 58, No. 19, May 20, 2010, http://www.cdc.gov/nchs/deaths.htm)
*Final data by state of residence. Includes drug psychoses, drug dependence, nondependent use excluding alcohol and tobacco, accidental poisoning or suicide by drugs, medicaments, and biologicals. Excludes accidents, homicides, and other causes indirectly related to drug use. Not age-adjusted.

Age-Adjusted Death Rate by Drug-Induced Deaths in 2007

National Rate = 12.6 Deaths per 100,000 Population*

ALPHA ORDER

RANK	STATE	RATE
29	Alabama	12.1
38	Alaska	10.3
10	Arizona	15.9
31	Arkansas	11.8
33	California	11.3
14	Colorado	14.7
25	Connecticut	12.6
29	Delaware	12.1
9	Florida	16.3
39	Georgia	10.0
36	Hawaii	10.8
43	Idaho	9.1
41	Illinois	9.6
22	Indiana	13.1
46	Iowa	7.1
36	Kansas	10.8
7	Kentucky	16.9
4	Louisiana	20.5
26	Maine	12.4
18	Maryland	14.0
11	Massachusetts	15.1
12	Michigan	15.0
47	Minnesota	6.7
32	Mississippi	11.7
26	Missouri	12.4
20	Montana	13.4
49	Nebraska	5.4
5	Nevada	19.8
19	New Hampshire	13.8
43	New Jersey	9.1
1	New Mexico	24.1
41	New York	9.6
28	North Carolina	12.3
48	North Dakota	5.5
14	Ohio	14.7
6	Oklahoma	19.5
16	Oregon	14.5
16	Pennsylvania	14.5
24	Rhode Island	13.0
22	South Carolina	13.1
50	South Dakota	4.3
8	Tennessee	16.6
40	Texas	9.9
3	Utah	22.4
35	Vermont	11.1
43	Virginia	9.1
13	Washington	14.8
2	West Virginia	22.9
33	Wisconsin	11.3
21	Wyoming	13.3

RANK ORDER

RANK	STATE	RATE
1	New Mexico	24.1
2	West Virginia	22.9
3	Utah	22.4
4	Louisiana	20.5
5	Nevada	19.8
6	Oklahoma	19.5
7	Kentucky	16.9
8	Tennessee	16.6
9	Florida	16.3
10	Arizona	15.9
11	Massachusetts	15.1
12	Michigan	15.0
13	Washington	14.8
14	Colorado	14.7
14	Ohio	14.7
16	Oregon	14.5
16	Pennsylvania	14.5
18	Maryland	14.0
19	New Hampshire	13.8
20	Montana	13.4
21	Wyoming	13.3
22	Indiana	13.1
22	South Carolina	13.1
24	Rhode Island	13.0
25	Connecticut	12.6
26	Maine	12.4
26	Missouri	12.4
28	North Carolina	12.3
29	Alabama	12.1
29	Delaware	12.1
31	Arkansas	11.8
32	Mississippi	11.7
33	California	11.3
33	Wisconsin	11.3
35	Vermont	11.1
36	Hawaii	10.8
36	Kansas	10.8
38	Alaska	10.3
39	Georgia	10.0
40	Texas	9.9
41	Illinois	9.6
41	New York	9.6
43	Idaho	9.1
43	New Jersey	9.1
43	Virginia	9.1
46	Iowa	7.1
47	Minnesota	6.7
48	North Dakota	5.5
49	Nebraska	5.4
50	South Dakota	4.3

District of Columbia	15.1

Source: U.S. Department of Health and Human Services, National Center for Health Statistics
"National Vital Statistics Reports" (Vol. 58, No. 19, May 20, 2010, http://www.cdc.gov/nchs/deaths.htm)
*Final data by state of residence. Includes drug psychoses, drug dependence, nondependent use excluding alcohol and tobacco, accidental poisoning or suicide by drugs, medicaments, and biologicals. Excludes accidents, homicides, and other causes indirectly related to drug use. Age-adjusted rates based on the year 2000 standard population.

Occupational Fatalities in 2009

National Total = 4,340 Deaths*

ALPHA ORDER

RANK	STATE	DEATHS	% of USA
26	Alabama	70	1.6%
44	Alaska	17	0.4%
33	Arizona	50	1.2%
23	Arkansas	75	1.7%
2	California	301	6.9%
19	Colorado	80	1.8%
38	Connecticut	34	0.8%
48	Delaware	7	0.2%
3	Florida	243	5.6%
16	Georgia	96	2.2%
46	Hawaii	13	0.3%
39	Idaho	26	0.6%
6	Illinois	158	3.6%
11	Indiana	123	2.8%
20	Iowa	78	1.8%
22	Kansas	76	1.8%
15	Kentucky	97	2.2%
8	Louisiana	138	3.2%
45	Maine	16	0.4%
28	Maryland	65	1.5%
31	Massachusetts	59	1.4%
18	Michigan	93	2.1%
30	Minnesota	60	1.4%
29	Mississippi	64	1.5%
7	Missouri	142	3.3%
33	Montana	50	1.2%
32	Nebraska	57	1.3%
41	Nevada	24	0.6%
50	New Hampshire	6	0.1%
14	New Jersey	99	2.3%
36	New Mexico	42	1.0%
4	New York	184	4.2%
10	North Carolina	125	2.9%
40	North Dakota	25	0.6%
9	Ohio	132	3.0%
21	Oklahoma	77	1.8%
27	Oregon	66	1.5%
5	Pennsylvania	166	3.8%
48	Rhode Island	7	0.2%
25	South Carolina	73	1.7%
41	South Dakota	24	0.6%
13	Tennessee	105	2.4%
1	Texas	480	11.1%
35	Utah	48	1.1%
47	Vermont	12	0.3%
12	Virginia	118	2.7%
23	Washington	75	1.7%
37	West Virginia	41	0.9%
17	Wisconsin	94	2.2%
43	Wyoming	19	0.4%

RANK ORDER

RANK	STATE	DEATHS	% of USA
1	Texas	480	11.1%
2	California	301	6.9%
3	Florida	243	5.6%
4	New York	184	4.2%
5	Pennsylvania	166	3.8%
6	Illinois	158	3.6%
7	Missouri	142	3.3%
8	Louisiana	138	3.2%
9	Ohio	132	3.0%
10	North Carolina	125	2.9%
11	Indiana	123	2.8%
12	Virginia	118	2.7%
13	Tennessee	105	2.4%
14	New Jersey	99	2.3%
15	Kentucky	97	2.2%
16	Georgia	96	2.2%
17	Wisconsin	94	2.2%
18	Michigan	93	2.1%
19	Colorado	80	1.8%
20	Iowa	78	1.8%
21	Oklahoma	77	1.8%
22	Kansas	76	1.8%
23	Arkansas	75	1.7%
23	Washington	75	1.7%
25	South Carolina	73	1.7%
26	Alabama	70	1.6%
27	Oregon	66	1.5%
28	Maryland	65	1.5%
29	Mississippi	64	1.5%
30	Minnesota	60	1.4%
31	Massachusetts	59	1.4%
32	Nebraska	57	1.3%
33	Arizona	50	1.2%
33	Montana	50	1.2%
35	Utah	48	1.1%
36	New Mexico	42	1.0%
37	West Virginia	41	0.9%
38	Connecticut	34	0.8%
39	Idaho	26	0.6%
40	North Dakota	25	0.6%
41	Nevada	24	0.6%
41	South Dakota	24	0.6%
43	Wyoming	19	0.4%
44	Alaska	17	0.4%
45	Maine	16	0.4%
46	Hawaii	13	0.3%
47	Vermont	12	0.3%
48	Delaware	7	0.2%
48	Rhode Island	7	0.2%
50	New Hampshire	6	0.1%
	District of Columbia	10	0.2%

Source: U.S. Department of Labor, Bureau of Labor Statistics
    "National Census of Fatal Occupational Injuries in 2009" (press release, August 19, 2010, http://www.bls.gov/iif/home.htm)
*Preliminary data.

Occupational Fatality Rate in 2009

National Rate = 3.1 Deaths per 100,000 Workers*

ALPHA ORDER

RANK	STATE	RATE
21	Alabama	3.8
13	Alaska	5.2
47	Arizona	1.8
6	Arkansas	5.9
45	California	1.9
27	Colorado	3.3
43	Connecticut	2.0
47	Delaware	1.8
30	Florida	3.0
38	Georgia	2.3
40	Hawaii	2.2
21	Idaho	3.8
32	Illinois	2.7
17	Indiana	4.4
14	Iowa	5.0
10	Kansas	5.4
11	Kentucky	5.3
2	Louisiana	7.3
33	Maine	2.5
35	Maryland	2.4
45	Massachusetts	1.9
38	Michigan	2.3
40	Minnesota	2.2
9	Mississippi	5.5
11	Missouri	5.3
1	Montana	10.8
5	Nebraska	6.1
43	Nevada	2.0
50	New Hampshire	0.9
35	New Jersey	2.4
15	New Mexico	4.8
42	New York	2.1
28	North Carolina	3.1
3	North Dakota	7.2
33	Ohio	2.5
16	Oklahoma	4.7
21	Oregon	3.8
31	Pennsylvania	2.9
49	Rhode Island	1.4
19	South Carolina	3.9
7	South Dakota	5.7
19	Tennessee	3.9
18	Texas	4.3
21	Utah	3.8
25	Vermont	3.6
28	Virginia	3.1
35	Washington	2.4
7	West Virginia	5.7
26	Wisconsin	3.4
4	Wyoming	7.0

RANK ORDER

RANK	STATE	RATE
1	Montana	10.8
2	Louisiana	7.3
3	North Dakota	7.2
4	Wyoming	7.0
5	Nebraska	6.1
6	Arkansas	5.9
7	South Dakota	5.7
7	West Virginia	5.7
9	Mississippi	5.5
10	Kansas	5.4
11	Kentucky	5.3
11	Missouri	5.3
13	Alaska	5.2
14	Iowa	5.0
15	New Mexico	4.8
16	Oklahoma	4.7
17	Indiana	4.4
18	Texas	4.3
19	South Carolina	3.9
19	Tennessee	3.9
21	Alabama	3.8
21	Idaho	3.8
21	Oregon	3.8
21	Utah	3.8
25	Vermont	3.6
26	Wisconsin	3.4
27	Colorado	3.3
28	North Carolina	3.1
28	Virginia	3.1
30	Florida	3.0
31	Pennsylvania	2.9
32	Illinois	2.7
33	Maine	2.5
33	Ohio	2.5
35	Maryland	2.4
35	New Jersey	2.4
35	Washington	2.4
38	Georgia	2.3
38	Michigan	2.3
40	Hawaii	2.2
40	Minnesota	2.2
42	New York	2.1
43	Connecticut	2.0
43	Nevada	2.0
45	California	1.9
45	Massachusetts	1.9
47	Arizona	1.8
47	Delaware	1.8
49	Rhode Island	1.4
50	New Hampshire	0.9
	District of Columbia	3.4

Source: CQ Press using data from U.S. Department of Labor, Bureau of Labor Statistics
"National Census of Fatal Occupational Injuries in 2009" (press release, August 19, 2010, http://www.bls.gov/iif/home.htm)
*Preliminary data. Rates based on employed civilian labor force.

III. Facilities

Community Hospitals in 2009 189
Rate of Community Hospitals in 2009 190
Community Hospitals per 1,000 Square Miles in 2009 . . . 191
Community Hospitals in Urban Areas in 2009. 192
Percent of Community Hospitals in Urban Areas
    in 2009 193
Community Hospitals in Rural Areas in 2009 194
Percent of Community Hospitals in Rural Areas in 2009. . 195
Nongovernment, Not-for-Profit Hospitals in 2009. 196
Investor-Owned, For-Profit Hospitals in 2009 197
State and Local Government-Owned Hospitals in 2009. . . 198
Beds in Community Hospitals in 2009. 199
Rate of Beds in Community Hospitals in 2009 200
Average Number of Beds per Community Hospital
    in 2009 201
Admissions to Community Hospitals in 2009 202
Inpatient Days in Community Hospitals in 2009 203
Average Daily Census in Community Hospitals in 2009. . 204
Average Stay in Community Hospitals in 2009 205
Occupancy Rate in Community Hospitals in 2009. 206
Outpatient Visits to Community Hospitals in 2009 207
Emergency Outpatient Visits to Community Hospitals
    in 2009 208
Medicare and Medicaid Certified Facilities in 2011. 209
Medicare and Medicaid Certified Hospitals in 2011 210
Beds in Medicare and Medicaid Certified Hospitals
    in 2011 211
Medicare and Medicaid Certified Children's Hospitals
    in 2011 212
Beds in Medicare and Medicaid Certified Children's
    Hospitals in 2011 213

Medicare and Medicaid Certified Rehabilitation
    Hospitals in 2011 214
Beds in Medicare and Medicaid Certified Rehabilitation
    Hospitals in 2011 215
Medicare and Medicaid Certified Psychiatric Hospitals
    in 2011 216
Beds in Medicare and Medicaid Certified Psychiatric
    Hospitals in 2011 217
Medicare and Medicaid Certified Outpatient Surgery
    Centers in 2011 218
Medicare and Medicaid Certified Community Mental
    Health Centers in 2011. 219
Medicare and Medicaid Certified Outpatient Physical
    Therapy Facilities in 2011 220
Medicare and Medicaid Certified Rural Health Clinics
    in 2011 221
Medicare and Medicaid Certified Home Health Agencies
    in 2011 222
Medicare and Medicaid Certified Hospices in 2011. 223
Hospice Patients in Residential Facilities in 2011 224
Medicare and Medicaid Certified Nursing Care Facilities
    in 2011 225
Beds in Medicare and Medicaid Certified Nursing Care
    Facilities in 2011 226
Rate of Beds in Medicare and Medicaid Certified
    Nursing Care Facilities in 2011 227
Nursing Home Occupancy Rate in 2009 228
Nursing Home Resident Rate in 2009 229
Nursing Home Population in 2009 230
Health Care Establishments in 2008. 231

Community Hospitals in 2009

National Total = 5,008 Hospitals*

ALPHA ORDER

RANK	STATE	HOSPITALS	% of USA
20	Alabama	108	2.2%
47	Alaska	22	0.4%
30	Arizona	72	1.4%
26	Arkansas	86	1.7%
2	California	343	6.8%
27	Colorado	81	1.6%
42	Connecticut	35	0.7%
50	Delaware	7	0.1%
3	Florida	210	4.2%
9	Georgia	152	3.0%
45	Hawaii	25	0.5%
38	Idaho	41	0.8%
5	Illinois	189	3.8%
16	Indiana	123	2.5%
17	Iowa	118	2.4%
11	Kansas	133	2.7%
21	Kentucky	104	2.1%
13	Louisiana	128	2.6%
40	Maine	37	0.7%
35	Maryland	49	1.0%
28	Massachusetts	78	1.6%
8	Michigan	158	3.2%
12	Minnesota	132	2.6%
22	Mississippi	97	1.9%
15	Missouri	125	2.5%
36	Montana	48	1.0%
24	Nebraska	87	1.7%
42	Nevada	35	0.7%
44	New Hampshire	28	0.6%
29	New Jersey	74	1.5%
40	New Mexico	37	0.7%
5	New York	189	3.8%
19	North Carolina	115	2.3%
38	North Dakota	41	0.8%
7	Ohio	183	3.7%
18	Oklahoma	116	2.3%
32	Oregon	58	1.2%
4	Pennsylvania	194	3.9%
49	Rhode Island	11	0.2%
31	South Carolina	70	1.4%
34	South Dakota	53	1.1%
10	Tennessee	137	2.7%
1	Texas	428	8.5%
37	Utah	44	0.9%
48	Vermont	14	0.3%
23	Virginia	90	1.8%
24	Washington	87	1.7%
33	West Virginia	56	1.1%
14	Wisconsin	126	2.5%
46	Wyoming	24	0.5%

RANK ORDER

RANK	STATE	HOSPITALS	% of USA
1	Texas	428	8.5%
2	California	343	6.8%
3	Florida	210	4.2%
4	Pennsylvania	194	3.9%
5	Illinois	189	3.8%
5	New York	189	3.8%
7	Ohio	183	3.7%
8	Michigan	158	3.2%
9	Georgia	152	3.0%
10	Tennessee	137	2.7%
11	Kansas	133	2.7%
12	Minnesota	132	2.6%
13	Louisiana	128	2.6%
14	Wisconsin	126	2.5%
15	Missouri	125	2.5%
16	Indiana	123	2.5%
17	Iowa	118	2.4%
18	Oklahoma	116	2.3%
19	North Carolina	115	2.3%
20	Alabama	108	2.2%
21	Kentucky	104	2.1%
22	Mississippi	97	1.9%
23	Virginia	90	1.8%
24	Nebraska	87	1.7%
24	Washington	87	1.7%
26	Arkansas	86	1.7%
27	Colorado	81	1.6%
28	Massachusetts	78	1.6%
29	New Jersey	74	1.5%
30	Arizona	72	1.4%
31	South Carolina	70	1.4%
32	Oregon	58	1.2%
33	West Virginia	56	1.1%
34	South Dakota	53	1.1%
35	Maryland	49	1.0%
36	Montana	48	1.0%
37	Utah	44	0.9%
38	Idaho	41	0.8%
38	North Dakota	41	0.8%
40	Maine	37	0.7%
40	New Mexico	37	0.7%
42	Connecticut	35	0.7%
42	Nevada	35	0.7%
44	New Hampshire	28	0.6%
45	Hawaii	25	0.5%
46	Wyoming	24	0.5%
47	Alaska	22	0.4%
48	Vermont	14	0.3%
49	Rhode Island	11	0.2%
50	Delaware	7	0.1%
	District of Columbia	10	0.2%

Source: American Hospital Association (Chicago, IL)
    "Hospital Statistics" (2011 edition)
*Community hospitals are all nonfederal, short-term general, and special hospitals whose facilities and services are available to the public.

Rate of Community Hospitals in 2009

National Rate = 1.6 Community Hospitals per 100,000 Population*

ALPHA ORDER				RANK ORDER		
RANK	STATE	RATE		RANK	STATE	RATE
18	Alabama	2.3		1	South Dakota	6.5
9	Alaska	3.1		2	North Dakota	6.3
41	Arizona	1.1		3	Montana	4.9
12	Arkansas	3.0		4	Nebraska	4.8
47	California	0.9		5	Kansas	4.7
28	Colorado	1.6		6	Wyoming	4.4
44	Connecticut	1.0		7	Iowa	3.9
49	Delaware	0.8		8	Mississippi	3.3
41	Florida	1.1		9	Alaska	3.1
32	Georgia	1.5		9	Oklahoma	3.1
24	Hawaii	1.9		9	West Virginia	3.1
15	Idaho	2.7		12	Arkansas	3.0
32	Illinois	1.5		13	Louisiana	2.8
24	Indiana	1.9		13	Maine	2.8
7	Iowa	3.9		15	Idaho	2.7
5	Kansas	4.7		16	Minnesota	2.5
17	Kentucky	2.4		17	Kentucky	2.4
13	Louisiana	2.8		18	Alabama	2.3
13	Maine	2.8		18	Vermont	2.3
47	Maryland	0.9		20	Tennessee	2.2
39	Massachusetts	1.2		20	Wisconsin	2.2
28	Michigan	1.6		22	Missouri	2.1
16	Minnesota	2.5		22	New Hampshire	2.1
8	Mississippi	3.3		24	Hawaii	1.9
22	Missouri	2.1		24	Indiana	1.9
3	Montana	4.9		26	New Mexico	1.8
4	Nebraska	4.8		27	Texas	1.7
37	Nevada	1.3		28	Colorado	1.6
22	New Hampshire	2.1		28	Michigan	1.6
49	New Jersey	0.8		28	Ohio	1.6
26	New Mexico	1.8		28	Utah	1.6
44	New York	1.0		32	Georgia	1.5
39	North Carolina	1.2		32	Illinois	1.5
2	North Dakota	6.3		32	Oregon	1.5
28	Ohio	1.6		32	Pennsylvania	1.5
9	Oklahoma	3.1		32	South Carolina	1.5
32	Oregon	1.5		37	Nevada	1.3
32	Pennsylvania	1.5		37	Washington	1.3
44	Rhode Island	1.0		39	Massachusetts	1.2
32	South Carolina	1.5		39	North Carolina	1.2
1	South Dakota	6.5		41	Arizona	1.1
20	Tennessee	2.2		41	Florida	1.1
27	Texas	1.7		41	Virginia	1.1
28	Utah	1.6		44	Connecticut	1.0
18	Vermont	2.3		44	New York	1.0
41	Virginia	1.1		44	Rhode Island	1.0
37	Washington	1.3		47	California	0.9
9	West Virginia	3.1		47	Maryland	0.9
20	Wisconsin	2.2		49	Delaware	0.8
6	Wyoming	4.4		49	New Jersey	0.8
					District of Columbia	1.7

Source: CQ Press using data from American Hospital Association (Chicago, IL)
"Hospital Statistics" (2011 edition)
*Community hospitals are all nonfederal, short-term general, and special hospitals whose facilities and services are available to the public.

Community Hospitals per 1,000 Square Miles in 2009

National Rate = 1.3 Community Hospitals*

ALPHA ORDER

RANK	STATE	RATE
21	Alabama	2.1
50	Alaska**	0.0
41	Arizona	0.6
30	Arkansas	1.6
21	California	2.1
39	Colorado	0.8
4	Connecticut	6.3
14	Delaware	2.8
12	Florida	3.2
15	Georgia	2.6
18	Hawaii	2.3
44	Idaho	0.5
10	Illinois	3.3
9	Indiana	3.4
21	Iowa	2.1
30	Kansas	1.6
15	Kentucky	2.6
17	Louisiana	2.5
38	Maine	1.0
7	Maryland	3.9
2	Massachusetts	7.4
30	Michigan	1.6
34	Minnesota	1.5
26	Mississippi	2.0
28	Missouri	1.8
46	Montana	0.3
37	Nebraska	1.1
46	Nevada	0.3
13	New Hampshire	3.0
1	New Jersey	8.5
46	New Mexico	0.3
8	New York	3.5
21	North Carolina	2.1
41	North Dakota	0.6
6	Ohio	4.1
29	Oklahoma	1.7
41	Oregon	0.6
5	Pennsylvania	4.2
3	Rhode Island	7.1
20	South Carolina	2.2
40	South Dakota	0.7
10	Tennessee	3.3
30	Texas	1.6
44	Utah	0.5
34	Vermont	1.5
21	Virginia	2.1
36	Washington	1.2
18	West Virginia	2.3
27	Wisconsin	1.9
49	Wyoming	0.2

RANK ORDER

RANK	STATE	RATE
1	New Jersey	8.5
2	Massachusetts	7.4
3	Rhode Island	7.1
4	Connecticut	6.3
5	Pennsylvania	4.2
6	Ohio	4.1
7	Maryland	3.9
8	New York	3.5
9	Indiana	3.4
10	Illinois	3.3
10	Tennessee	3.3
12	Florida	3.2
13	New Hampshire	3.0
14	Delaware	2.8
15	Georgia	2.6
15	Kentucky	2.6
17	Louisiana	2.5
18	Hawaii	2.3
18	West Virginia	2.3
20	South Carolina	2.2
21	Alabama	2.1
21	California	2.1
21	Iowa	2.1
21	North Carolina	2.1
21	Virginia	2.1
26	Mississippi	2.0
27	Wisconsin	1.9
28	Missouri	1.8
29	Oklahoma	1.7
30	Arkansas	1.6
30	Kansas	1.6
30	Michigan	1.6
30	Texas	1.6
34	Minnesota	1.5
34	Vermont	1.5
36	Washington	1.2
37	Nebraska	1.1
38	Maine	1.0
39	Colorado	0.8
40	South Dakota	0.7
41	Arizona	0.6
41	North Dakota	0.6
41	Oregon	0.6
44	Idaho	0.5
44	Utah	0.5
46	Montana	0.3
46	Nevada	0.3
46	New Mexico	0.3
49	Wyoming	0.2
50	Alaska**	0.0

District of Columbia***   NA

Source: CQ Press using data from American Hospital Association (Chicago, IL)
"Hospital Statistics" (2011 edition)
*Based on land and water area figures. Community hospitals are nonfederal, short-term general, and other special hospitals
whose facilities and services are available to the public.
**Alaska has 22 community hospitals for its 664,988 square miles.
***The District of Columbia has 10 community hospitals for its 68 square miles.

Community Hospitals in Urban Areas in 2009

National Total = 3,011 Hospitals*

<table>
<tr><th colspan="4">ALPHA ORDER</th><th colspan="4">RANK ORDER</th></tr>
<tr><th>RANK</th><th>STATE</th><th>HOSPITALS</th><th>% of USA</th><th>RANK</th><th>STATE</th><th>HOSPITALS</th><th>% of USA</th></tr>
<tr><td>17</td><td>Alabama</td><td>60</td><td>2.0%</td><td>1</td><td>California</td><td>313</td><td>10.4%</td></tr>
<tr><td>47</td><td>Alaska</td><td>5</td><td>0.2%</td><td>2</td><td>Texas</td><td>277</td><td>9.2%</td></tr>
<tr><td>19</td><td>Arizona</td><td>58</td><td>1.9%</td><td>3</td><td>Florida</td><td>181</td><td>6.0%</td></tr>
<tr><td>28</td><td>Arkansas</td><td>37</td><td>1.2%</td><td>4</td><td>New York</td><td>150</td><td>5.0%</td></tr>
<tr><td>1</td><td>California</td><td>313</td><td>10.4%</td><td>5</td><td>Pennsylvania</td><td>145</td><td>4.8%</td></tr>
<tr><td>25</td><td>Colorado</td><td>43</td><td>1.4%</td><td>6</td><td>Ohio</td><td>128</td><td>4.3%</td></tr>
<tr><td>31</td><td>Connecticut</td><td>30</td><td>1.0%</td><td>7</td><td>Illinois</td><td>125</td><td>4.2%</td></tr>
<tr><td>47</td><td>Delaware</td><td>5</td><td>0.2%</td><td>8</td><td>Michigan</td><td>99</td><td>3.3%</td></tr>
<tr><td>3</td><td>Florida</td><td>181</td><td>6.0%</td><td>9</td><td>Georgia</td><td>87</td><td>2.9%</td></tr>
<tr><td>9</td><td>Georgia</td><td>87</td><td>2.9%</td><td>10</td><td>Indiana</td><td>83</td><td>2.8%</td></tr>
<tr><td>41</td><td>Hawaii</td><td>13</td><td>0.4%</td><td>11</td><td>Tennessee</td><td>81</td><td>2.7%</td></tr>
<tr><td>38</td><td>Idaho</td><td>15</td><td>0.5%</td><td>12</td><td>Louisiana</td><td>77</td><td>2.6%</td></tr>
<tr><td>7</td><td>Illinois</td><td>125</td><td>4.2%</td><td>13</td><td>Massachusetts</td><td>76</td><td>2.5%</td></tr>
<tr><td>10</td><td>Indiana</td><td>83</td><td>2.8%</td><td>14</td><td>New Jersey</td><td>74</td><td>2.5%</td></tr>
<tr><td>29</td><td>Iowa</td><td>34</td><td>1.1%</td><td>15</td><td>Missouri</td><td>72</td><td>2.4%</td></tr>
<tr><td>30</td><td>Kansas</td><td>33</td><td>1.1%</td><td>16</td><td>Wisconsin</td><td>69</td><td>2.3%</td></tr>
<tr><td>27</td><td>Kentucky</td><td>42</td><td>1.4%</td><td>17</td><td>Alabama</td><td>60</td><td>2.0%</td></tr>
<tr><td>12</td><td>Louisiana</td><td>77</td><td>2.6%</td><td>17</td><td>Virginia</td><td>60</td><td>2.0%</td></tr>
<tr><td>38</td><td>Maine</td><td>15</td><td>0.5%</td><td>19</td><td>Arizona</td><td>58</td><td>1.9%</td></tr>
<tr><td>25</td><td>Maryland</td><td>43</td><td>1.4%</td><td>19</td><td>North Carolina</td><td>58</td><td>1.9%</td></tr>
<tr><td>13</td><td>Massachusetts</td><td>76</td><td>2.5%</td><td>21</td><td>Washington</td><td>53</td><td>1.8%</td></tr>
<tr><td>8</td><td>Michigan</td><td>99</td><td>3.3%</td><td>22</td><td>Minnesota</td><td>50</td><td>1.7%</td></tr>
<tr><td>22</td><td>Minnesota</td><td>50</td><td>1.7%</td><td>23</td><td>Oklahoma</td><td>49</td><td>1.6%</td></tr>
<tr><td>33</td><td>Mississippi</td><td>28</td><td>0.9%</td><td>24</td><td>South Carolina</td><td>45</td><td>1.5%</td></tr>
<tr><td>15</td><td>Missouri</td><td>72</td><td>2.4%</td><td>25</td><td>Colorado</td><td>43</td><td>1.4%</td></tr>
<tr><td>46</td><td>Montana</td><td>6</td><td>0.2%</td><td>25</td><td>Maryland</td><td>43</td><td>1.4%</td></tr>
<tr><td>37</td><td>Nebraska</td><td>16</td><td>0.5%</td><td>27</td><td>Kentucky</td><td>42</td><td>1.4%</td></tr>
<tr><td>36</td><td>Nevada</td><td>24</td><td>0.8%</td><td>28</td><td>Arkansas</td><td>37</td><td>1.2%</td></tr>
<tr><td>42</td><td>New Hampshire</td><td>11</td><td>0.4%</td><td>29</td><td>Iowa</td><td>34</td><td>1.1%</td></tr>
<tr><td>14</td><td>New Jersey</td><td>74</td><td>2.5%</td><td>30</td><td>Kansas</td><td>33</td><td>1.1%</td></tr>
<tr><td>38</td><td>New Mexico</td><td>15</td><td>0.5%</td><td>31</td><td>Connecticut</td><td>30</td><td>1.0%</td></tr>
<tr><td>4</td><td>New York</td><td>150</td><td>5.0%</td><td>32</td><td>Oregon</td><td>29</td><td>1.0%</td></tr>
<tr><td>19</td><td>North Carolina</td><td>58</td><td>1.9%</td><td>33</td><td>Mississippi</td><td>28</td><td>0.9%</td></tr>
<tr><td>45</td><td>North Dakota</td><td>8</td><td>0.3%</td><td>34</td><td>West Virginia</td><td>27</td><td>0.9%</td></tr>
<tr><td>6</td><td>Ohio</td><td>128</td><td>4.3%</td><td>35</td><td>Utah</td><td>26</td><td>0.9%</td></tr>
<tr><td>23</td><td>Oklahoma</td><td>49</td><td>1.6%</td><td>36</td><td>Nevada</td><td>24</td><td>0.8%</td></tr>
<tr><td>32</td><td>Oregon</td><td>29</td><td>1.0%</td><td>37</td><td>Nebraska</td><td>16</td><td>0.5%</td></tr>
<tr><td>5</td><td>Pennsylvania</td><td>145</td><td>4.8%</td><td>38</td><td>Idaho</td><td>15</td><td>0.5%</td></tr>
<tr><td>42</td><td>Rhode Island</td><td>11</td><td>0.4%</td><td>38</td><td>Maine</td><td>15</td><td>0.5%</td></tr>
<tr><td>24</td><td>South Carolina</td><td>45</td><td>1.5%</td><td>38</td><td>New Mexico</td><td>15</td><td>0.5%</td></tr>
<tr><td>42</td><td>South Dakota</td><td>11</td><td>0.4%</td><td>41</td><td>Hawaii</td><td>13</td><td>0.4%</td></tr>
<tr><td>11</td><td>Tennessee</td><td>81</td><td>2.7%</td><td>42</td><td>New Hampshire</td><td>11</td><td>0.4%</td></tr>
<tr><td>2</td><td>Texas</td><td>277</td><td>9.2%</td><td>42</td><td>Rhode Island</td><td>11</td><td>0.4%</td></tr>
<tr><td>35</td><td>Utah</td><td>26</td><td>0.9%</td><td>42</td><td>South Dakota</td><td>11</td><td>0.4%</td></tr>
<tr><td>49</td><td>Vermont</td><td>2</td><td>0.1%</td><td>45</td><td>North Dakota</td><td>8</td><td>0.3%</td></tr>
<tr><td>17</td><td>Virginia</td><td>60</td><td>2.0%</td><td>46</td><td>Montana</td><td>6</td><td>0.2%</td></tr>
<tr><td>21</td><td>Washington</td><td>53</td><td>1.8%</td><td>47</td><td>Alaska</td><td>5</td><td>0.2%</td></tr>
<tr><td>34</td><td>West Virginia</td><td>27</td><td>0.9%</td><td>47</td><td>Delaware</td><td>5</td><td>0.2%</td></tr>
<tr><td>16</td><td>Wisconsin</td><td>69</td><td>2.3%</td><td>49</td><td>Vermont</td><td>2</td><td>0.1%</td></tr>
<tr><td>49</td><td>Wyoming</td><td>2</td><td>0.1%</td><td>49</td><td>Wyoming</td><td>2</td><td>0.1%</td></tr>
<tr><td></td><td></td><td></td><td></td><td></td><td>District of Columbia</td><td>10</td><td>0.3%</td></tr>
</table>

Source: American Hospital Association (Chicago, IL)
   "Hospital Statistics" (2011 edition)
*Community hospitals are all nonfederal, short-term general, and special hospitals whose facilities and services are available to the public. Urban is defined as any area inside a metropolitan statistical area as defined by the U.S. Office of Management and Budget.

Percent of Community Hospitals in Urban Areas in 2009

National Percent = 60.1% of Community Hospitals*

ALPHA ORDER

RANK	STATE	PERCENT
26	Alabama	55.6
44	Alaska	22.7
8	Arizona	80.6
33	Arkansas	43.0
4	California	91.3
28	Colorado	53.1
7	Connecticut	85.7
11	Delaware	71.4
6	Florida	86.2
25	Georgia	57.2
29	Hawaii	52.0
40	Idaho	36.6
16	Illinois	66.1
14	Indiana	67.5
42	Iowa	28.8
43	Kansas	24.8
37	Kentucky	40.4
21	Louisiana	60.2
35	Maine	40.5
5	Maryland	87.8
3	Massachusetts	97.4
19	Michigan	62.7
39	Minnesota	37.9
41	Mississippi	28.9
24	Missouri	57.6
49	Montana	12.5
47	Nebraska	18.4
13	Nevada	68.6
38	New Hampshire	39.3
1	New Jersey	100.0
35	New Mexico	40.5
9	New York	79.4
30	North Carolina	50.4
46	North Dakota	19.5
12	Ohio	69.9
34	Oklahoma	42.2
31	Oregon	50.0
10	Pennsylvania	74.7
1	Rhode Island	100.0
18	South Carolina	64.3
45	South Dakota	20.8
22	Tennessee	59.1
17	Texas	64.7
22	Utah	59.1
48	Vermont	14.3
15	Virginia	66.7
20	Washington	60.9
32	West Virginia	48.2
27	Wisconsin	54.8
50	Wyoming	8.3

RANK ORDER

RANK	STATE	PERCENT
1	New Jersey	100.0
1	Rhode Island	100.0
3	Massachusetts	97.4
4	California	91.3
5	Maryland	87.8
6	Florida	86.2
7	Connecticut	85.7
8	Arizona	80.6
9	New York	79.4
10	Pennsylvania	74.7
11	Delaware	71.4
12	Ohio	69.9
13	Nevada	68.6
14	Indiana	67.5
15	Virginia	66.7
16	Illinois	66.1
17	Texas	64.7
18	South Carolina	64.3
19	Michigan	62.7
20	Washington	60.9
21	Louisiana	60.2
22	Tennessee	59.1
22	Utah	59.1
24	Missouri	57.6
25	Georgia	57.2
26	Alabama	55.6
27	Wisconsin	54.8
28	Colorado	53.1
29	Hawaii	52.0
30	North Carolina	50.4
31	Oregon	50.0
32	West Virginia	48.2
33	Arkansas	43.0
34	Oklahoma	42.2
35	Maine	40.5
35	New Mexico	40.5
37	Kentucky	40.4
38	New Hampshire	39.3
39	Minnesota	37.9
40	Idaho	36.6
41	Mississippi	28.9
42	Iowa	28.8
43	Kansas	24.8
44	Alaska	22.7
45	South Dakota	20.8
46	North Dakota	19.5
47	Nebraska	18.4
48	Vermont	14.3
49	Montana	12.5
50	Wyoming	8.3
	District of Columbia	100.0

Source: CQ Press using data from American Hospital Association (Chicago, IL)
"Hospital Statistics" (2011 edition)
*Community hospitals are all nonfederal, short-term general, and special hospitals whose facilities and services are available to the public. Urban is defined as any area inside a metropolitan statistical area as defined by the U.S. Office of Management and Budget.

Community Hospitals in Rural Areas in 2009

National Total = 1,997 Hospitals*

ALPHA ORDER

RANK	STATE	HOSPITALS	% of USA
20	Alabama	48	2.4%
39	Alaska	17	0.9%
41	Arizona	14	0.7%
18	Arkansas	49	2.5%
28	California	30	1.5%
25	Colorado	38	1.9%
46	Connecticut	5	0.3%
47	Delaware	2	0.1%
30	Florida	29	1.5%
8	Georgia	65	3.3%
42	Hawaii	12	0.6%
33	Idaho	26	1.3%
9	Illinois	64	3.2%
23	Indiana	40	2.0%
3	Iowa	84	4.2%
2	Kansas	100	5.0%
10	Kentucky	62	3.1%
17	Louisiana	51	2.6%
35	Maine	22	1.1%
45	Maryland	6	0.3%
47	Massachusetts	2	0.1%
11	Michigan	59	3.0%
4	Minnesota	82	4.1%
6	Mississippi	69	3.5%
16	Missouri	53	2.7%
21	Montana	42	2.1%
5	Nebraska	71	3.6%
44	Nevada	11	0.6%
39	New Hampshire	17	0.9%
49	New Jersey	0	0.0%
35	New Mexico	22	1.1%
24	New York	39	2.0%
12	North Carolina	57	2.9%
27	North Dakota	33	1.7%
15	Ohio	55	2.8%
7	Oklahoma	67	3.4%
30	Oregon	29	1.5%
18	Pennsylvania	49	2.5%
49	Rhode Island	0	0.0%
34	South Carolina	25	1.3%
21	South Dakota	42	2.1%
14	Tennessee	56	2.8%
1	Texas	151	7.6%
38	Utah	18	0.9%
42	Vermont	12	0.6%
28	Virginia	30	1.5%
26	Washington	34	1.7%
30	West Virginia	29	1.5%
12	Wisconsin	57	2.9%
35	Wyoming	22	1.1%

RANK ORDER

RANK	STATE	HOSPITALS	% of USA
1	Texas	151	7.6%
2	Kansas	100	5.0%
3	Iowa	84	4.2%
4	Minnesota	82	4.1%
5	Nebraska	71	3.6%
6	Mississippi	69	3.5%
7	Oklahoma	67	3.4%
8	Georgia	65	3.3%
9	Illinois	64	3.2%
10	Kentucky	62	3.1%
11	Michigan	59	3.0%
12	North Carolina	57	2.9%
12	Wisconsin	57	2.9%
14	Tennessee	56	2.8%
15	Ohio	55	2.8%
16	Missouri	53	2.7%
17	Louisiana	51	2.6%
18	Arkansas	49	2.5%
18	Pennsylvania	49	2.5%
20	Alabama	48	2.4%
21	Montana	42	2.1%
21	South Dakota	42	2.1%
23	Indiana	40	2.0%
24	New York	39	2.0%
25	Colorado	38	1.9%
26	Washington	34	1.7%
27	North Dakota	33	1.7%
28	California	30	1.5%
28	Virginia	30	1.5%
30	Florida	29	1.5%
30	Oregon	29	1.5%
30	West Virginia	29	1.5%
33	Idaho	26	1.3%
34	South Carolina	25	1.3%
35	Maine	22	1.1%
35	New Mexico	22	1.1%
35	Wyoming	22	1.1%
38	Utah	18	0.9%
39	Alaska	17	0.9%
39	New Hampshire	17	0.9%
41	Arizona	14	0.7%
42	Hawaii	12	0.6%
42	Vermont	12	0.6%
44	Nevada	11	0.6%
45	Maryland	6	0.3%
46	Connecticut	5	0.3%
47	Delaware	2	0.1%
47	Massachusetts	2	0.1%
49	New Jersey	0	0.0%
49	Rhode Island	0	0.0%
	District of Columbia	0	0.0%

Source: American Hospital Association (Chicago, IL)
    "Hospital Statistics" (2011 edition)
*Community hospitals are all nonfederal, short-term general, and special hospitals whose facilities and services are available to the public. Rural is defined as any area outside a metropolitan statistical area as defined by the U.S. Office of Management and Budget.

Percent of Community Hospitals in Rural Areas in 2009

National Percent = 39.9% of Community Hospitals*

ALPHA ORDER

RANK	STATE	PERCENT
25	Alabama	44.4
7	Alaska	77.3
43	Arizona	19.4
18	Arkansas	57.0
47	California	8.7
23	Colorado	46.9
44	Connecticut	14.3
40	Delaware	28.6
45	Florida	13.8
26	Georgia	42.8
22	Hawaii	48.0
11	Idaho	63.4
35	Illinois	33.9
37	Indiana	32.5
9	Iowa	71.2
8	Kansas	75.2
14	Kentucky	59.6
30	Louisiana	39.8
15	Maine	59.5
46	Maryland	12.2
48	Massachusetts	2.6
32	Michigan	37.3
12	Minnesota	62.1
10	Mississippi	71.1
27	Missouri	42.4
2	Montana	87.5
4	Nebraska	81.6
38	Nevada	31.4
13	New Hampshire	60.7
49	New Jersey	0.0
15	New Mexico	59.5
42	New York	20.6
21	North Carolina	49.6
5	North Dakota	80.5
39	Ohio	30.1
17	Oklahoma	57.8
20	Oregon	50.0
41	Pennsylvania	25.3
49	Rhode Island	0.0
33	South Carolina	35.7
6	South Dakota	79.2
28	Tennessee	40.9
34	Texas	35.3
28	Utah	40.9
3	Vermont	85.7
36	Virginia	33.3
31	Washington	39.1
19	West Virginia	51.8
24	Wisconsin	45.2
1	Wyoming	91.7

RANK ORDER

RANK	STATE	PERCENT
1	Wyoming	91.7
2	Montana	87.5
3	Vermont	85.7
4	Nebraska	81.6
5	North Dakota	80.5
6	South Dakota	79.2
7	Alaska	77.3
8	Kansas	75.2
9	Iowa	71.2
10	Mississippi	71.1
11	Idaho	63.4
12	Minnesota	62.1
13	New Hampshire	60.7
14	Kentucky	59.6
15	Maine	59.5
15	New Mexico	59.5
17	Oklahoma	57.8
18	Arkansas	57.0
19	West Virginia	51.8
20	Oregon	50.0
21	North Carolina	49.6
22	Hawaii	48.0
23	Colorado	46.9
24	Wisconsin	45.2
25	Alabama	44.4
26	Georgia	42.8
27	Missouri	42.4
28	Tennessee	40.9
28	Utah	40.9
30	Louisiana	39.8
31	Washington	39.1
32	Michigan	37.3
33	South Carolina	35.7
34	Texas	35.3
35	Illinois	33.9
36	Virginia	33.3
37	Indiana	32.5
38	Nevada	31.4
39	Ohio	30.1
40	Delaware	28.6
41	Pennsylvania	25.3
42	New York	20.6
43	Arizona	19.4
44	Connecticut	14.3
45	Florida	13.8
46	Maryland	12.2
47	California	8.7
48	Massachusetts	2.6
49	New Jersey	0.0
49	Rhode Island	0.0
	District of Columbia	0.0

Source: CQ Press using data from American Hospital Association (Chicago, IL)
    "Hospital Statistics" (2011 edition)
*Community hospitals are all nonfederal, short-term general, and special hospitals whose facilities and services are available to the public. Rural is defined as any area outside a metropolitan statistical area as defined by the U.S. Office of Management and Budget.

Nongovernment, Not-for-Profit Hospitals in 2009

National Total = 2,918 Hospitals*

ALPHA ORDER					RANK ORDER			
RANK	STATE	HOSPITALS	% of USA		RANK	STATE	HOSPITALS	% of USA
38	Alabama	26	0.9%		1	California	202	6.9%
44	Alaska	14	0.5%		2	New York	164	5.6%
27	Arizona	43	1.5%		3	Pennsylvania	153	5.2%
24	Arkansas	45	1.5%		4	Illinois	147	5.0%
1	California	202	6.9%		4	Texas	147	5.0%
31	Colorado	37	1.3%		6	Ohio	138	4.7%
35	Connecticut	33	1.1%		7	Michigan	126	4.3%
49	Delaware	6	0.2%		8	Wisconsin	118	4.0%
10	Florida	82	2.8%		9	Minnesota	93	3.2%
18	Georgia	63	2.2%		10	Florida	82	2.8%
42	Hawaii	18	0.6%		11	North Carolina	74	2.5%
43	Idaho	16	0.5%		12	Kentucky	73	2.5%
4	Illinois	147	5.0%		13	Massachusetts	68	2.3%
15	Indiana	64	2.2%		14	Virginia	66	2.3%
20	Iowa	58	2.0%		15	Indiana	64	2.2%
21	Kansas	54	1.9%		15	Missouri	64	2.2%
12	Kentucky	73	2.5%		15	New Jersey	64	2.2%
33	Louisiana	35	1.2%		18	Georgia	63	2.2%
34	Maine	34	1.2%		19	Tennessee	59	2.0%
22	Maryland	47	1.6%		20	Iowa	58	2.0%
13	Massachusetts	68	2.3%		21	Kansas	54	1.9%
7	Michigan	126	4.3%		22	Maryland	47	1.6%
9	Minnesota	93	3.2%		23	South Dakota	46	1.6%
37	Mississippi	28	1.0%		24	Arkansas	45	1.5%
15	Missouri	64	2.2%		24	Nebraska	45	1.5%
29	Montana	40	1.4%		26	Oregon	44	1.5%
24	Nebraska	45	1.5%		27	Arizona	43	1.5%
47	Nevada	13	0.4%		28	Washington	41	1.4%
40	New Hampshire	24	0.8%		29	Montana	40	1.4%
15	New Jersey	64	2.2%		30	North Dakota	39	1.3%
44	New Mexico	14	0.5%		31	Colorado	37	1.3%
2	New York	164	5.6%		32	Oklahoma	36	1.2%
11	North Carolina	74	2.5%		33	Louisiana	35	1.2%
30	North Dakota	39	1.3%		34	Maine	34	1.2%
6	Ohio	138	4.7%		35	Connecticut	33	1.1%
32	Oklahoma	36	1.2%		36	West Virginia	32	1.1%
26	Oregon	44	1.5%		37	Mississippi	28	1.0%
3	Pennsylvania	153	5.2%		38	Alabama	26	0.9%
48	Rhode Island	11	0.4%		39	South Carolina	25	0.9%
39	South Carolina	25	0.9%		40	New Hampshire	24	0.8%
23	South Dakota	46	1.6%		41	Utah	23	0.8%
19	Tennessee	59	2.0%		42	Hawaii	18	0.6%
4	Texas	147	5.0%		43	Idaho	16	0.5%
41	Utah	23	0.8%		44	Alaska	14	0.5%
44	Vermont	14	0.5%		44	New Mexico	14	0.5%
14	Virginia	66	2.3%		44	Vermont	14	0.5%
28	Washington	41	1.4%		47	Nevada	13	0.4%
36	West Virginia	32	1.1%		48	Rhode Island	11	0.4%
8	Wisconsin	118	4.0%		49	Delaware	6	0.2%
50	Wyoming	5	0.2%		50	Wyoming	5	0.2%
						District of Columbia	7	0.2%

Source: American Hospital Association (Chicago, IL)
   "Hospital Statistics" (2011 edition)
*Nongovernment, not-for-profit hospitals are a subset of community hospitals. Community hospitals are all nonfederal, short-term general, and other special hospitals whose facilities and services are available to the public.

Investor-Owned, For-Profit Hospitals in 2009

National Total = 998 Hospitals*

ALPHA ORDER				RANK ORDER			
RANK	STATE	HOSPITALS	% of USA	RANK	STATE	HOSPITALS	% of USA
5	Alabama	40	4.0%	1	Texas	165	16.5%
36	Alaska	2	0.2%	2	Florida	103	10.3%
16	Arizona	22	2.2%	3	California	72	7.2%
11	Arkansas	26	2.6%	4	Tennessee	56	5.6%
3	California	72	7.2%	5	Alabama	40	4.0%
21	Colorado	16	1.6%	6	Louisiana	39	3.9%
41	Conncctiout	1	0.1%	6	Pennsylvania	39	3.9%
41	Delaware	1	0.1%	8	Georgia	36	3.6%
2	Florida	103	10.3%	9	Oklahoma	35	3.5%
8	Georgia	36	3.6%	10	Mississippi	29	2.9%
47	Hawaii	0	0.0%	11	Arkansas	26	2.6%
31	Idaho	5	0.5%	11	Missouri	26	2.6%
21	Illinois	16	1.6%	13	Indiana	25	2.5%
13	Indiana	25	2.5%	13	South Carolina	25	2.5%
41	Iowa	1	0.1%	15	Ohio	23	2.3%
19	Kansas	17	1.7%	16	Arizona	22	2.2%
17	Kentucky	20	2.0%	17	Kentucky	20	2.0%
6	Louisiana	39	3.9%	17	Virginia	20	2.0%
41	Maine	1	0.1%	19	Kansas	17	1.7%
36	Maryland	2	0.2%	19	Michigan	17	1.7%
28	Massachusetts	8	0.8%	21	Colorado	16	1.6%
19	Michigan	17	1.7%	21	Illinois	16	1.6%
41	Minnesota	1	0.1%	21	Nevada	16	1.6%
10	Mississippi	29	2.9%	21	New Mexico	16	1.6%
11	Missouri	26	2.6%	25	Utah	15	1.5%
41	Montana	1	0.1%	26	West Virginia	14	1.4%
36	Nebraska	2	0.2%	27	North Carolina	9	0.9%
21	Nevada	16	1.6%	28	Massachusetts	8	0.8%
33	New Hampshire	4	0.4%	29	New Jersey	7	0.7%
29	New Jersey	7	0.7%	30	Wisconsin	6	0.6%
21	New Mexico	16	1.6%	31	Idaho	5	0.5%
47	New York	0	0.0%	31	Washington	5	0.5%
27	North Carolina	9	0.9%	33	New Hampshire	4	0.4%
36	North Dakota	2	0.2%	33	South Dakota	4	0.4%
15	Ohio	23	2.3%	35	Wyoming	3	0.3%
9	Oklahoma	35	3.5%	36	Alaska	2	0.2%
36	Oregon	2	0.2%	36	Maryland	2	0.2%
6	Pennsylvania	39	3.9%	36	Nebraska	2	0.2%
47	Rhode Island	0	0.0%	36	North Dakota	2	0.2%
13	South Carolina	25	2.5%	36	Oregon	2	0.2%
33	South Dakota	4	0.4%	41	Connecticut	1	0.1%
4	Tennessee	56	5.6%	41	Delaware	1	0.1%
1	Texas	165	16.5%	41	Iowa	1	0.1%
25	Utah	15	1.5%	41	Maine	1	0.1%
47	Vermont	0	0.0%	41	Minnesota	1	0.1%
17	Virginia	20	2.0%	41	Montana	1	0.1%
31	Washington	5	0.5%	47	Hawaii	0	0.0%
26	West Virginia	14	1.4%	47	New York	0	0.0%
30	Wisconsin	6	0.6%	47	Rhode Island	0	0.0%
35	Wyoming	3	0.3%	47	Vermont	0	0.0%
					District of Columbia	3	0.3%

Source: American Hospital Association (Chicago, IL)
"Hospital Statistics" (2011 edition)
*Investor-owned, for-profit hospitals are a subset of community hospitals. Community hospitals are all nonfederal, short-term general, and other special hospitals whose facilities and services are available to the public.

State and Local Government-Owned Hospitals in 2009

National Total = 1,092 Hospitals*

ALPHA ORDER

RANK	STATE	HOSPITALS	% of USA
8	Alabama	42	3.8%
34	Alaska	6	0.5%
30	Arizona	7	0.6%
25	Arkansas	15	1.4%
2	California	69	6.3%
16	Colorado	28	2.6%
44	Connecticut	1	0.1%
45	Delaware	0	0.0%
18	Florida	25	2.3%
6	Georgia	53	4.9%
30	Hawaii	7	0.6%
22	Idaho	20	1.8%
17	Illinois	26	2.4%
14	Indiana	34	3.1%
4	Iowa	59	5.4%
3	Kansas	62	5.7%
28	Kentucky	11	1.0%
5	Louisiana	54	4.9%
40	Maine	2	0.2%
45	Maryland	0	0.0%
40	Massachusetts	2	0.2%
25	Michigan	15	1.4%
12	Minnesota	38	3.5%
10	Mississippi	40	3.7%
13	Missouri	35	3.2%
30	Montana	7	0.6%
10	Nebraska	40	3.7%
34	Nevada	6	0.5%
45	New Hampshire	0	0.0%
38	New Jersey	3	0.3%
30	New Mexico	7	0.6%
18	New York	25	2.3%
15	North Carolina	32	2.9%
45	North Dakota	0	0.0%
20	Ohio	22	2.0%
7	Oklahoma	45	4.1%
27	Oregon	12	1.1%
40	Pennsylvania	2	0.2%
45	Rhode Island	0	0.0%
22	South Carolina	20	1.8%
38	South Dakota	3	0.3%
20	Tennessee	22	2.0%
1	Texas	116	10.6%
34	Utah	6	0.5%
45	Vermont	0	0.0%
37	Virginia	4	0.4%
9	Washington	41	3.8%
29	West Virginia	10	0.9%
40	Wisconsin	2	0.2%
24	Wyoming	16	1.5%

RANK ORDER

RANK	STATE	HOSPITALS	% of USA
1	Texas	116	10.6%
2	California	69	6.3%
3	Kansas	62	5.7%
4	Iowa	59	5.4%
5	Louisiana	54	4.9%
6	Georgia	53	4.9%
7	Oklahoma	45	4.1%
8	Alabama	42	3.8%
9	Washington	41	3.8%
10	Mississippi	40	3.7%
10	Nebraska	40	3.7%
12	Minnesota	38	3.5%
13	Missouri	35	3.2%
14	Indiana	34	3.1%
15	North Carolina	32	2.9%
16	Colorado	28	2.6%
17	Illinois	26	2.4%
18	Florida	25	2.3%
18	New York	25	2.3%
20	Ohio	22	2.0%
20	Tennessee	22	2.0%
22	Idaho	20	1.8%
22	South Carolina	20	1.8%
24	Wyoming	16	1.5%
25	Arkansas	15	1.4%
25	Michigan	15	1.4%
27	Oregon	12	1.1%
28	Kentucky	11	1.0%
29	West Virginia	10	0.9%
30	Arizona	7	0.6%
30	Hawaii	7	0.6%
30	Montana	7	0.6%
30	New Mexico	7	0.6%
34	Alaska	6	0.5%
34	Nevada	6	0.5%
34	Utah	6	0.5%
37	Virginia	4	0.4%
38	New Jersey	3	0.3%
38	South Dakota	3	0.3%
40	Maine	2	0.2%
40	Massachusetts	2	0.2%
40	Pennsylvania	2	0.2%
40	Wisconsin	2	0.2%
44	Connecticut	1	0.1%
45	Delaware	0	0.0%
45	Maryland	0	0.0%
45	New Hampshire	0	0.0%
45	North Dakota	0	0.0%
45	Rhode Island	0	0.0%
45	Vermont	0	0.0%
	District of Columbia	0	0.0%

Source: American Hospital Association (Chicago, IL)
"Hospital Statistics" (2011 edition)
*State and local government-owned hospitals are a subset of community hospitals. Community hospitals are all nonfederal, short-term general, and other special hospitals whose facilities and services are available to the public.

Beds in Community Hospitals in 2009

National Total = 805,593 Beds*

ALPHA ORDER				RANK ORDER			
RANK	STATE	BEDS	% of USA	RANK	STATE	BEDS	% of USA
19	Alabama	15,290	1.9%	1	California	68,745	8.5%
49	Alaska	1,532	0.2%	2	Texas	62,069	7.7%
22	Arizona	13,455	1.7%	3	New York	60,400	7.5%
31	Arkansas	9,565	1.2%	4	Florida	53,293	6.6%
1	California	68,745	8.5%	5	Pennsylvania	39,212	4.9%
28	Colorado	10,364	1.3%	6	Ohio	33,994	4.2%
32	Connecticut	7,935	1.0%	7	Illinois	33,856	4.2%
47	Delaware	2,125	0.3%	8	Michigan	25,863	3.2%
4	Florida	53,293	6.6%	9	Georgia	25,419	3.2%
9	Georgia	25,419	3.2%	10	North Carolina	22,830	2.8%
44	Hawaii	2,966	0.4%	11	New Jersey	21,054	2.6%
42	Idaho	3,382	0.4%	12	Tennessee	20,959	2.6%
7	Illinois	33,856	4.2%	13	Missouri	19,101	2.4%
15	Indiana	17,298	2.1%	14	Virginia	17,538	2.2%
29	Iowa	10,276	1.3%	15	Indiana	17,298	2.1%
30	Kansas	10,127	1.3%	16	Louisiana	15,857	2.0%
20	Kentucky	14,124	1.8%	17	Minnesota	15,589	1.9%
16	Louisiana	15,857	2.0%	18	Massachusetts	15,483	1.9%
41	Maine	3,583	0.4%	19	Alabama	15,290	1.9%
25	Maryland	11,887	1.5%	20	Kentucky	14,124	1.8%
18	Massachusetts	15,483	1.9%	21	Wisconsin	13,637	1.7%
8	Michigan	25,863	3.2%	22	Arizona	13,455	1.7%
17	Minnesota	15,589	1.9%	23	Mississippi	12,879	1.6%
23	Mississippi	12,879	1.6%	24	South Carolina	12,483	1.5%
13	Missouri	19,101	2.4%	25	Maryland	11,887	1.5%
40	Montana	3,820	0.5%	26	Washington	11,322	1.4%
33	Nebraska	7,442	0.9%	27	Oklahoma	11,316	1.4%
36	Nevada	5,119	0.6%	28	Colorado	10,364	1.3%
45	New Hampshire	2,863	0.4%	29	Iowa	10,276	1.3%
11	New Jersey	21,054	2.6%	30	Kansas	10,127	1.3%
39	New Mexico	3,913	0.5%	31	Arkansas	9,565	1.2%
3	New York	60,400	7.5%	32	Connecticut	7,935	1.0%
10	North Carolina	22,830	2.8%	33	Nebraska	7,442	0.9%
43	North Dakota	3,362	0.4%	34	West Virginia	7,408	0.9%
6	Ohio	33,994	4.2%	35	Oregon	6,481	0.8%
27	Oklahoma	11,316	1.4%	36	Nevada	5,119	0.6%
35	Oregon	6,481	0.8%	37	Utah	4,973	0.6%
5	Pennsylvania	39,212	4.9%	38	South Dakota	4,142	0.5%
46	Rhode Island	2,512	0.3%	39	New Mexico	3,913	0.5%
24	South Carolina	12,483	1.5%	40	Montana	3,820	0.5%
38	South Dakota	4,142	0.5%	41	Maine	3,583	0.4%
12	Tennessee	20,959	2.6%	42	Idaho	3,382	0.4%
2	Texas	62,069	7.7%	43	North Dakota	3,362	0.4%
37	Utah	4,973	0.6%	44	Hawaii	2,966	0.4%
50	Vermont	1,296	0.2%	45	New Hampshire	2,863	0.4%
14	Virginia	17,538	2.2%	46	Rhode Island	2,512	0.3%
26	Washington	11,322	1.4%	47	Delaware	2,125	0.3%
34	West Virginia	7,408	0.9%	48	Wyoming	2,002	0.2%
21	Wisconsin	13,637	1.7%	49	Alaska	1,532	0.2%
48	Wyoming	2,002	0.2%	50	Vermont	1,296	0.2%
					District of Columbia	3,452	0.4%

Source: American Hospital Association (Chicago, IL)
"Hospital Statistics" (2011 edition)
*All nonfederal, short-term general, and other special hospitals whose facilities and services are available to the public. Includes beds in hospital and nursing home units.

Rate of Beds in Community Hospitals in 2009

National Rate = 262 Beds per 100,000 Population*

RANK	STATE	RATE		RANK	STATE	RATE
14	Alabama	325		1	North Dakota	520
38	Alaska	219		2	South Dakota	510
44	Arizona	204		3	Mississippi	436
12	Arkansas	331		4	Nebraska	414
47	California	186		5	West Virginia	407
43	Colorado	206		6	Montana	392
36	Connecticut	226		7	Wyoming	368
32	Delaware	240		8	Kansas	359
21	Florida	287		9	Louisiana	353
26	Georgia	259		10	Iowa	342
35	Hawaii	229		11	Tennessee	333
38	Idaho	219		12	Arkansas	331
25	Illinois	262		13	Kentucky	327
24	Indiana	269		14	Alabama	325
10	Iowa	342		15	Missouri	319
8	Kansas	359		16	Pennsylvania	311
13	Kentucky	327		17	New York	309
9	Louisiana	353		18	Oklahoma	307
23	Maine	272		19	Minnesota	296
41	Maryland	209		20	Ohio	295
34	Massachusetts	235		21	Florida	287
26	Michigan	259		22	South Carolina	274
19	Minnesota	296		23	Maine	272
3	Mississippi	436		24	Indiana	269
15	Missouri	319		25	Illinois	262
6	Montana	392		26	Georgia	259
4	Nebraska	414		26	Michigan	259
46	Nevada	194		28	Texas	250
40	New Hampshire	216		29	North Carolina	243
30	New Jersey	242		30	New Jersey	242
45	New Mexico	195		31	Wisconsin	241
17	New York	309		32	Delaware	240
29	North Carolina	243		33	Rhode Island	239
1	North Dakota	520		34	Massachusetts	235
20	Ohio	295		35	Hawaii	229
18	Oklahoma	307		36	Connecticut	226
50	Oregon	169		37	Virginia	222
16	Pennsylvania	311		38	Alaska	219
33	Rhode Island	239		38	Idaho	219
22	South Carolina	274		40	New Hampshire	216
2	South Dakota	510		41	Maryland	209
11	Tennessee	333		42	Vermont	208
28	Texas	250		43	Colorado	206
48	Utah	179		44	Arizona	204
42	Vermont	208		45	New Mexico	195
37	Virginia	222		46	Nevada	194
49	Washington	170		47	California	186
5	West Virginia	407		48	Utah	179
31	Wisconsin	241		49	Washington	170
7	Wyoming	368		50	Oregon	169

ALPHA ORDER / RANK ORDER

District of Columbia 576

Source: CQ Press using data from American Hospital Association (Chicago, IL)
"Hospital Statistics" (2011 edition)
*All nonfederal, short-term general, and other special hospitals whose facilities and services are available to the public. Includes beds in hospital and nursing home units.

Average Number of Beds per Community Hospital in 2009

National Average = 161 Beds per Community Hospital*

ALPHA ORDER

RANK	STATE	AVERAGE
23	Alabama	142
50	Alaska	70
13	Arizona	187
35	Arkansas	111
9	California	200
29	Colorado	128
7	Connecticut	227
2	Delaware	304
4	Florida	254
17	Georgia	167
31	Hawaii	119
45	Idaho	82
15	Illinois	179
24	Indiana	141
42	Iowa	87
49	Kansas	76
25	Kentucky	136
30	Louisiana	124
40	Maine	97
5	Maryland	243
10	Massachusetts	199
18	Michigan	164
32	Minnesota	118
26	Mississippi	133
19	Missouri	153
47	Montana	80
43	Nebraska	86
21	Nevada	146
38	New Hampshire	102
3	New Jersey	285
37	New Mexico	106
1	New York	320
10	North Carolina	199
45	North Dakota	82
14	Ohio	186
39	Oklahoma	98
34	Oregon	112
8	Pennsylvania	202
6	Rhode Island	228
16	South Carolina	178
48	South Dakota	78
19	Tennessee	153
22	Texas	145
33	Utah	113
41	Vermont	93
12	Virginia	195
28	Washington	130
27	West Virginia	132
36	Wisconsin	108
44	Wyoming	83

RANK ORDER

RANK	STATE	AVERAGE
1	New York	320
2	Delaware	304
3	New Jersey	285
4	Florida	254
5	Maryland	243
6	Rhode Island	228
7	Connecticut	227
8	Pennsylvania	202
9	California	200
10	Massachusetts	199
10	North Carolina	199
12	Virginia	195
13	Arizona	187
14	Ohio	186
15	Illinois	179
16	South Carolina	178
17	Georgia	167
18	Michigan	164
19	Missouri	153
19	Tennessee	153
21	Nevada	146
22	Texas	145
23	Alabama	142
24	Indiana	141
25	Kentucky	136
26	Mississippi	133
27	West Virginia	132
28	Washington	130
29	Colorado	128
30	Louisiana	124
31	Hawaii	119
32	Minnesota	118
33	Utah	113
34	Oregon	112
35	Arkansas	111
36	Wisconsin	108
37	New Mexico	106
38	New Hampshire	102
39	Oklahoma	98
40	Maine	97
41	Vermont	93
42	Iowa	87
43	Nebraska	86
44	Wyoming	83
45	Idaho	82
45	North Dakota	82
47	Montana	80
48	South Dakota	78
49	Kansas	76
50	Alaska	70

| | District of Columbia | 345 |

Source: CQ Press using data from American Hospital Association (Chicago, IL)
"Hospital Statistics" (2011 edition)
*All nonfederal, short-term general, and other special hospitals whose facilities and services are available to the public. Includes beds in hospital and nursing home units.

Admissions to Community Hospitals in 2009

National Total = 35,527,377 Admissions*

ALPHA ORDER

RANK	STATE	ADMISSIONS	% of USA
19	Alabama	665,788	1.9%
48	Alaska	57,227	0.2%
18	Arizona	705,371	2.0%
30	Arkansas	380,478	1.1%
1	California	3,433,319	9.7%
26	Colorado	445,291	1.3%
29	Connecticut	407,710	1.1%
45	Delaware	102,153	0.3%
4	Florida	2,452,546	6.9%
11	Georgia	956,870	2.7%
43	Hawaii	111,706	0.3%
40	Idaho	129,645	0.4%
6	Illinois	1,557,816	4.4%
17	Indiana	713,456	2.0%
31	Iowa	354,534	1.0%
33	Kansas	315,820	0.9%
23	Kentucky	597,224	1.7%
20	Louisiana	639,450	1.8%
39	Maine	150,199	0.4%
16	Maryland	715,496	2.0%
14	Massachusetts	819,625	2.3%
8	Michigan	1,219,893	3.4%
21	Minnesota	623,504	1.8%
28	Mississippi	412,912	1.2%
13	Missouri	825,090	2.3%
46	Montana	101,327	0.3%
37	Nebraska	209,750	0.6%
35	Nevada	245,866	0.7%
42	New Hampshire	122,959	0.3%
9	New Jersey	1,094,810	3.1%
38	New Mexico	183,116	0.5%
3	New York	2,533,577	7.1%
10	North Carolina	1,034,112	2.9%
47	North Dakota	92,593	0.3%
7	Ohio	1,531,076	4.3%
27	Oklahoma	442,394	1.2%
32	Oregon	323,733	0.9%
5	Pennsylvania	1,841,550	5.2%
41	Rhode Island	126,761	0.4%
25	South Carolina	528,204	1.5%
44	South Dakota	102,335	0.3%
12	Tennessee	859,191	2.4%
2	Texas	2,621,436	7.4%
36	Utah	226,239	0.6%
50	Vermont	50,922	0.1%
15	Virginia	793,145	2.2%
24	Washington	588,889	1.7%
34	West Virginia	280,252	0.8%
22	Wisconsin	609,329	1.7%
49	Wyoming	52,232	0.1%

RANK ORDER

RANK	STATE	ADMISSIONS	% of USA
1	California	3,433,319	9.7%
2	Texas	2,621,436	7.4%
3	New York	2,533,577	7.1%
4	Florida	2,452,546	6.9%
5	Pennsylvania	1,841,550	5.2%
6	Illinois	1,557,816	4.4%
7	Ohio	1,531,076	4.3%
8	Michigan	1,219,893	3.4%
9	New Jersey	1,094,810	3.1%
10	North Carolina	1,034,112	2.9%
11	Georgia	956,870	2.7%
12	Tennessee	859,191	2.4%
13	Missouri	825,090	2.3%
14	Massachusetts	819,625	2.3%
15	Virginia	793,145	2.2%
16	Maryland	715,496	2.0%
17	Indiana	713,456	2.0%
18	Arizona	705,371	2.0%
19	Alabama	665,788	1.9%
20	Louisiana	639,450	1.8%
21	Minnesota	623,504	1.8%
22	Wisconsin	609,329	1.7%
23	Kentucky	597,224	1.7%
24	Washington	588,889	1.7%
25	South Carolina	528,204	1.5%
26	Colorado	445,291	1.3%
27	Oklahoma	442,394	1.2%
28	Mississippi	412,912	1.2%
29	Connecticut	407,710	1.1%
30	Arkansas	380,478	1.1%
31	Iowa	354,534	1.0%
32	Oregon	323,733	0.9%
33	Kansas	315,820	0.9%
34	West Virginia	280,252	0.8%
35	Nevada	245,866	0.7%
36	Utah	226,239	0.6%
37	Nebraska	209,750	0.6%
38	New Mexico	183,116	0.5%
39	Maine	150,199	0.4%
40	Idaho	129,645	0.4%
41	Rhode Island	126,761	0.4%
42	New Hampshire	122,959	0.3%
43	Hawaii	111,706	0.3%
44	South Dakota	102,335	0.3%
45	Delaware	102,153	0.3%
46	Montana	101,327	0.3%
47	North Dakota	92,593	0.3%
48	Alaska	57,227	0.2%
49	Wyoming	52,232	0.1%
50	Vermont	50,922	0.1%
	District of Columbia	138,456	0.4%

Source: American Hospital Association (Chicago, IL)
   "Hospital Statistics" (2011 edition)
*Admissions to all nonfederal, short-term general, and other special hospitals whose facilities and services are available to the public. Includes admissions to hospital and nursing home units.

Inpatient Days in Community Hospitals in 2009

National Total = 192,656,804 Inpatient Days*

ALPHA ORDER					RANK ORDER			
RANK	STATE	DAYS	% of USA		RANK	STATE	DAYS	% of USA
19	Alabama	3,459,946	1.8%		1	California	17,582,055	9.1%
49	Alaska	338,547	0.2%		2	New York	17,474,823	9.1%
21	Arizona	3,203,551	1.7%		3	Texas	13,590,044	7.1%
32	Arkansas	1,957,556	1.0%		4	Florida	12,261,161	6.4%
1	California	17,582,055	9.1%		5	Pennsylvania	9,865,210	5.1%
29	Colorado	2,237,893	1.2%		6	Illinois	7,769,059	4.0%
28	Connecticut	2,345,878	1.2%		7	Ohio	7,744,235	4.0%
47	Delaware	597,993	0.3%		8	Michigan	6,332,816	3.3%
4	Florida	12,261,161	6.4%		9	Georgia	6,059,475	3.1%
9	Georgia	6,059,475	3.1%		10	North Carolina	5,788,671	3.0%
42	Hawaii	772,508	0.4%		11	New Jersey	5,565,763	2.9%
46	Idaho	627,077	0.3%		12	Tennessee	4,799,858	2.5%
6	Illinois	7,769,059	4.0%		13	Virginia	4,375,451	2.3%
17	Indiana	3,687,549	1.9%		14	Missouri	4,256,929	2.2%
30	Iowa	2,185,446	1.1%		15	Massachusetts	4,187,076	2.2%
31	Kansas	2,014,165	1.0%		16	Minnesota	3,726,573	1.9%
23	Kentucky	3,113,326	1.6%		17	Indiana	3,687,549	1.9%
18	Louisiana	3,517,185	1.8%		18	Louisiana	3,517,185	1.8%
41	Maine	822,849	0.4%		19	Alabama	3,459,946	1.8%
20	Maryland	3,252,959	1.7%		20	Maryland	3,252,959	1.7%
15	Massachusetts	4,187,076	2.2%		21	Arizona	3,203,551	1.7%
8	Michigan	6,332,816	3.3%		22	Wisconsin	3,125,349	1.6%
16	Minnesota	3,726,573	1.9%		23	Kentucky	3,113,326	1.6%
26	Mississippi	2,600,075	1.3%		24	South Carolina	2,960,134	1.5%
14	Missouri	4,256,929	2.2%		25	Washington	2,660,901	1.4%
39	Montana	869,897	0.5%		26	Mississippi	2,600,075	1.3%
34	Nebraska	1,552,206	0.8%		27	Oklahoma	2,401,771	1.2%
36	Nevada	1,311,084	0.7%		28	Connecticut	2,345,878	1.2%
44	New Hampshire	655,015	0.3%		29	Colorado	2,237,893	1.2%
11	New Jersey	5,565,763	2.9%		30	Iowa	2,185,446	1.1%
40	New Mexico	844,787	0.4%		31	Kansas	2,014,165	1.0%
2	New York	17,474,823	9.1%		32	Arkansas	1,957,556	1.0%
10	North Carolina	5,788,671	3.0%		33	West Virginia	1,648,197	0.9%
43	North Dakota	751,653	0.4%		34	Nebraska	1,552,206	0.8%
7	Ohio	7,744,235	4.0%		35	Oregon	1,437,561	0.7%
27	Oklahoma	2,401,771	1.2%		36	Nevada	1,311,084	0.7%
35	Oregon	1,437,561	0.7%		37	South Dakota	1,005,265	0.5%
5	Pennsylvania	9,865,210	5.1%		38	Utah	1,003,710	0.5%
45	Rhode Island	654,695	0.3%		39	Montana	869,897	0.5%
24	South Carolina	2,960,134	1.5%		40	New Mexico	844,787	0.4%
37	South Dakota	1,005,265	0.5%		41	Maine	822,849	0.4%
12	Tennessee	4,799,858	2.5%		42	Hawaii	772,508	0.4%
3	Texas	13,590,044	7.1%		43	North Dakota	751,653	0.4%
38	Utah	1,003,710	0.5%		44	New Hampshire	655,015	0.3%
50	Vermont	321,741	0.2%		45	Rhode Island	654,695	0.3%
13	Virginia	4,375,451	2.3%		46	Idaho	627,077	0.3%
25	Washington	2,660,901	1.4%		47	Delaware	597,993	0.3%
33	West Virginia	1,648,197	0.9%		48	Wyoming	411,717	0.2%
22	Wisconsin	3,125,349	1.6%		49	Alaska	338,547	0.2%
48	Wyoming	411,717	0.2%		50	Vermont	321,741	0.2%
						District of Columbia	927,419	0.5%

Source: American Hospital Association (Chicago, IL)
"Hospital Statistics" (2011 edition)
*Inpatient days in all nonfederal, short-term general, and other special hospitals whose facilities and services are available to the public. Includes days in hospital and nursing home units.

Average Daily Census in Community Hospitals in 2009

National Average = 527,827 Inpatients*

ALPHA ORDER					RANK ORDER			

<table>
<tr><th>RANK</th><th>STATE</th><th>INPATIENTS</th><th>% of USA</th><th></th><th>RANK</th><th>STATE</th><th>INPATIENTS</th><th>% of USA</th></tr>
<tr><td>19</td><td>Alabama</td><td>9,479</td><td>1.8%</td><td></td><td>1</td><td>California</td><td>48,170</td><td>9.1%</td></tr>
<tr><td>49</td><td>Alaska</td><td>928</td><td>0.2%</td><td></td><td>2</td><td>New York</td><td>47,876</td><td>9.1%</td></tr>
<tr><td>21</td><td>Arizona</td><td>8,777</td><td>1.7%</td><td></td><td>3</td><td>Texas</td><td>37,233</td><td>7.1%</td></tr>
<tr><td>32</td><td>Arkansas</td><td>5,363</td><td>1.0%</td><td></td><td>4</td><td>Florida</td><td>33,592</td><td>6.4%</td></tr>
<tr><td>1</td><td>California</td><td>48,170</td><td>9.1%</td><td></td><td>5</td><td>Pennsylvania</td><td>27,028</td><td>5.1%</td></tr>
<tr><td>29</td><td>Colorado</td><td>6,131</td><td>1.2%</td><td></td><td>6</td><td>Illinois</td><td>21,285</td><td>4.0%</td></tr>
<tr><td>28</td><td>Connecticut</td><td>6,427</td><td>1.2%</td><td></td><td>7</td><td>Ohio</td><td>21,217</td><td>4.0%</td></tr>
<tr><td>47</td><td>Delaware</td><td>1,638</td><td>0.3%</td><td></td><td>8</td><td>Michigan</td><td>17,350</td><td>3.3%</td></tr>
<tr><td>4</td><td>Florida</td><td>33,592</td><td>6.4%</td><td></td><td>9</td><td>Georgia</td><td>16,601</td><td>3.1%</td></tr>
<tr><td>9</td><td>Georgia</td><td>16,601</td><td>3.1%</td><td></td><td>10</td><td>North Carolina</td><td>15,859</td><td>3.0%</td></tr>
<tr><td>42</td><td>Hawaii</td><td>2,116</td><td>0.4%</td><td></td><td>11</td><td>New Jersey</td><td>15,249</td><td>2.9%</td></tr>
<tr><td>46</td><td>Idaho</td><td>1,718</td><td>0.3%</td><td></td><td>12</td><td>Tennessee</td><td>13,150</td><td>2.5%</td></tr>
<tr><td>6</td><td>Illinois</td><td>21,285</td><td>4.0%</td><td></td><td>13</td><td>Virginia</td><td>11,988</td><td>2.3%</td></tr>
<tr><td>17</td><td>Indiana</td><td>10,103</td><td>1.9%</td><td></td><td>14</td><td>Missouri</td><td>11,663</td><td>2.2%</td></tr>
<tr><td>30</td><td>Iowa</td><td>5,988</td><td>1.1%</td><td></td><td>15</td><td>Massachusetts</td><td>11,471</td><td>2.2%</td></tr>
<tr><td>31</td><td>Kansas</td><td>5,518</td><td>1.0%</td><td></td><td>16</td><td>Minnesota</td><td>10,210</td><td>1.9%</td></tr>
<tr><td>23</td><td>Kentucky</td><td>8,530</td><td>1.6%</td><td></td><td>17</td><td>Indiana</td><td>10,103</td><td>1.9%</td></tr>
<tr><td>18</td><td>Louisiana</td><td>9,636</td><td>1.8%</td><td></td><td>18</td><td>Louisiana</td><td>9,636</td><td>1.8%</td></tr>
<tr><td>41</td><td>Maine</td><td>2,254</td><td>0.4%</td><td></td><td>19</td><td>Alabama</td><td>9,479</td><td>1.8%</td></tr>
<tr><td>20</td><td>Maryland</td><td>8,912</td><td>1.7%</td><td></td><td>20</td><td>Maryland</td><td>8,912</td><td>1.7%</td></tr>
<tr><td>15</td><td>Massachusetts</td><td>11,471</td><td>2.2%</td><td></td><td>21</td><td>Arizona</td><td>8,777</td><td>1.7%</td></tr>
<tr><td>8</td><td>Michigan</td><td>17,350</td><td>3.3%</td><td></td><td>22</td><td>Wisconsin</td><td>8,563</td><td>1.6%</td></tr>
<tr><td>16</td><td>Minnesota</td><td>10,210</td><td>1.9%</td><td></td><td>23</td><td>Kentucky</td><td>8,530</td><td>1.6%</td></tr>
<tr><td>26</td><td>Mississippi</td><td>7,123</td><td>1.3%</td><td></td><td>24</td><td>South Carolina</td><td>8,110</td><td>1.5%</td></tr>
<tr><td>14</td><td>Missouri</td><td>11,663</td><td>2.2%</td><td></td><td>25</td><td>Washington</td><td>7,290</td><td>1.4%</td></tr>
<tr><td>39</td><td>Montana</td><td>2,383</td><td>0.5%</td><td></td><td>26</td><td>Mississippi</td><td>7,123</td><td>1.3%</td></tr>
<tr><td>34</td><td>Nebraska</td><td>4,253</td><td>0.8%</td><td></td><td>27</td><td>Oklahoma</td><td>6,580</td><td>1.2%</td></tr>
<tr><td>36</td><td>Nevada</td><td>3,592</td><td>0.7%</td><td></td><td>28</td><td>Connecticut</td><td>6,427</td><td>1.2%</td></tr>
<tr><td>44</td><td>New Hampshire</td><td>1,795</td><td>0.3%</td><td></td><td>29</td><td>Colorado</td><td>6,131</td><td>1.2%</td></tr>
<tr><td>11</td><td>New Jersey</td><td>15,249</td><td>2.9%</td><td></td><td>30</td><td>Iowa</td><td>5,988</td><td>1.1%</td></tr>
<tr><td>40</td><td>New Mexico</td><td>2,314</td><td>0.4%</td><td></td><td>31</td><td>Kansas</td><td>5,518</td><td>1.0%</td></tr>
<tr><td>2</td><td>New York</td><td>47,876</td><td>9.1%</td><td></td><td>32</td><td>Arkansas</td><td>5,363</td><td>1.0%</td></tr>
<tr><td>10</td><td>North Carolina</td><td>15,859</td><td>3.0%</td><td></td><td>33</td><td>West Virginia</td><td>4,516</td><td>0.9%</td></tr>
<tr><td>43</td><td>North Dakota</td><td>2,059</td><td>0.4%</td><td></td><td>34</td><td>Nebraska</td><td>4,253</td><td>0.8%</td></tr>
<tr><td>7</td><td>Ohio</td><td>21,217</td><td>4.0%</td><td></td><td>35</td><td>Oregon</td><td>3,939</td><td>0.7%</td></tr>
<tr><td>27</td><td>Oklahoma</td><td>6,580</td><td>1.2%</td><td></td><td>36</td><td>Nevada</td><td>3,592</td><td>0.7%</td></tr>
<tr><td>35</td><td>Oregon</td><td>3,939</td><td>0.7%</td><td></td><td>37</td><td>South Dakota</td><td>2,754</td><td>0.5%</td></tr>
<tr><td>5</td><td>Pennsylvania</td><td>27,028</td><td>5.1%</td><td></td><td>38</td><td>Utah</td><td>2,750</td><td>0.5%</td></tr>
<tr><td>45</td><td>Rhode Island</td><td>1,794</td><td>0.3%</td><td></td><td>39</td><td>Montana</td><td>2,383</td><td>0.5%</td></tr>
<tr><td>24</td><td>South Carolina</td><td>8,110</td><td>1.5%</td><td></td><td>40</td><td>New Mexico</td><td>2,314</td><td>0.4%</td></tr>
<tr><td>37</td><td>South Dakota</td><td>2,754</td><td>0.5%</td><td></td><td>41</td><td>Maine</td><td>2,254</td><td>0.4%</td></tr>
<tr><td>12</td><td>Tennessee</td><td>13,150</td><td>2.5%</td><td></td><td>42</td><td>Hawaii</td><td>2,116</td><td>0.4%</td></tr>
<tr><td>3</td><td>Texas</td><td>37,233</td><td>7.1%</td><td></td><td>43</td><td>North Dakota</td><td>2,059</td><td>0.4%</td></tr>
<tr><td>38</td><td>Utah</td><td>2,750</td><td>0.5%</td><td></td><td>44</td><td>New Hampshire</td><td>1,795</td><td>0.3%</td></tr>
<tr><td>50</td><td>Vermont</td><td>881</td><td>0.2%</td><td></td><td>45</td><td>Rhode Island</td><td>1,794</td><td>0.3%</td></tr>
<tr><td>13</td><td>Virginia</td><td>11,988</td><td>2.3%</td><td></td><td>46</td><td>Idaho</td><td>1,718</td><td>0.3%</td></tr>
<tr><td>25</td><td>Washington</td><td>7,290</td><td>1.4%</td><td></td><td>47</td><td>Delaware</td><td>1,638</td><td>0.3%</td></tr>
<tr><td>33</td><td>West Virginia</td><td>4,516</td><td>0.9%</td><td></td><td>48</td><td>Wyoming</td><td>1,128</td><td>0.2%</td></tr>
<tr><td>22</td><td>Wisconsin</td><td>8,563</td><td>1.6%</td><td></td><td>49</td><td>Alaska</td><td>928</td><td>0.2%</td></tr>
<tr><td>48</td><td>Wyoming</td><td>1,128</td><td>0.2%</td><td></td><td>50</td><td>Vermont</td><td>881</td><td>0.2%</td></tr>
<tr><td></td><td></td><td></td><td></td><td></td><td></td><td>District of Columbia</td><td>2,541</td><td>0.5%</td></tr>
</table>

Source: CQ Press using data from American Hospital Association (Chicago, IL)
"Hospital Statistics" (2011 edition)

*Average total of inpatients receiving care in all nonfederal, short-term general, and other special hospitals whose facilities and services are available to the public. Excludes newborns.

Average Stay in Community Hospitals in 2009

National Average = 5.4 Days*

ALPHA ORDER

RANK	STATE	DAYS
28	Alabama	5.2
14	Alaska	5.9
46	Arizona	4.5
35	Arkansas	5.1
35	California	5.1
41	Colorado	5.0
17	Connecticut	5.8
14	Delaware	5.9
41	Florida	5.0
9	Georgia	6.3
6	Hawaii	6.9
44	Idaho	4.8
41	Illinois	5.0
28	Indiana	5.2
12	Iowa	6.2
8	Kansas	6.4
28	Kentucky	5.2
21	Louisiana	5.5
21	Maine	5.5
46	Maryland	4.5
35	Massachusetts	5.1
28	Michigan	5.2
13	Minnesota	6.0
9	Mississippi	6.3
28	Missouri	5.2
2	Montana	8.6
5	Nebraska	7.4
26	Nevada	5.3
26	New Hampshire	5.3
35	New Jersey	5.1
45	New Mexico	4.6
6	New York	6.9
18	North Carolina	5.6
3	North Dakota	8.1
35	Ohio	5.1
24	Oklahoma	5.4
49	Oregon	4.4
24	Pennsylvania	5.4
28	Rhode Island	5.2
18	South Carolina	5.6
1	South Dakota	9.8
18	Tennessee	5.6
28	Texas	5.2
49	Utah	4.4
9	Vermont	6.3
21	Virginia	5.5
46	Washington	4.5
14	West Virginia	5.9
35	Wisconsin	5.1
4	Wyoming	7.9

RANK ORDER

RANK	STATE	DAYS
1	South Dakota	9.8
2	Montana	8.6
3	North Dakota	8.1
4	Wyoming	7.9
5	Nebraska	7.4
6	Hawaii	6.9
6	New York	6.9
8	Kansas	6.4
9	Georgia	6.3
9	Mississippi	6.3
9	Vermont	6.3
12	Iowa	6.2
13	Minnesota	6.0
14	Alaska	5.9
14	Delaware	5.9
14	West Virginia	5.9
17	Connecticut	5.8
18	North Carolina	5.6
18	South Carolina	5.6
18	Tennessee	5.6
21	Louisiana	5.5
21	Maine	5.5
21	Virginia	5.5
24	Oklahoma	5.4
24	Pennsylvania	5.4
26	Nevada	5.3
26	New Hampshire	5.3
28	Alabama	5.2
28	Indiana	5.2
28	Kentucky	5.2
28	Michigan	5.2
28	Missouri	5.2
28	Rhode Island	5.2
28	Texas	5.2
35	Arkansas	5.1
35	California	5.1
35	Massachusetts	5.1
35	New Jersey	5.1
35	Ohio	5.1
35	Wisconsin	5.1
41	Colorado	5.0
41	Florida	5.0
41	Illinois	5.0
44	Idaho	4.8
45	New Mexico	4.6
46	Arizona	4.5
46	Maryland	4.5
46	Washington	4.5
49	Oregon	4.4
49	Utah	4.4

	District of Columbia	6.7

Source: American Hospital Association (Chicago, IL)
   "Hospital Statistics" (2011 edition)
*All nonfederal, short-term general, and other special hospitals whose facilities and services are available to the public.

Occupancy Rate in Community Hospitals in 2009

National Rate = 65.5% of Community Hospital Beds Occupied*

ALPHA ORDER

RANK	STATE	RATE
30	Alabama	62.0
36	Alaska	60.6
19	Arizona	65.2
46	Arkansas	56.1
10	California	70.1
39	Colorado	59.2
1	Connecticut	81.0
3	Delaware	77.1
22	Florida	63.0
18	Georgia	65.3
8	Hawaii	71.3
50	Idaho	50.8
23	Illinois	62.9
41	Indiana	58.4
42	Iowa	58.3
49	Kansas	54.5
37	Kentucky	60.4
34	Louisiana	60.8
23	Maine	62.9
4	Maryland	75.0
5	Massachusetts	74.1
15	Michigan	67.1
17	Minnesota	65.5
47	Mississippi	55.3
32	Missouri	61.1
28	Montana	62.4
44	Nebraska	57.1
9	Nevada	70.2
26	New Hampshire	62.7
6	New Jersey	72.4
40	New Mexico	59.1
2	New York	79.3
11	North Carolina	69.5
31	North Dakota	61.2
28	Ohio	62.4
43	Oklahoma	58.1
34	Oregon	60.8
12	Pennsylvania	68.9
7	Rhode Island	71.4
20	South Carolina	65.0
16	South Dakota	66.5
26	Tennessee	62.7
38	Texas	60.0
47	Utah	55.3
14	Vermont	68.0
13	Virginia	68.4
21	Washington	64.4
33	West Virginia	61.0
25	Wisconsin	62.8
45	Wyoming	56.3

RANK ORDER

RANK	STATE	RATE
1	Connecticut	81.0
2	New York	79.3
3	Delaware	77.1
4	Maryland	75.0
5	Massachusetts	74.1
6	New Jersey	72.4
7	Rhode Island	71.4
8	Hawaii	71.3
9	Nevada	70.2
10	California	70.1
11	North Carolina	69.5
12	Pennsylvania	68.9
13	Virginia	68.4
14	Vermont	68.0
15	Michigan	67.1
16	South Dakota	66.5
17	Minnesota	65.5
18	Georgia	65.3
19	Arizona	65.2
20	South Carolina	65.0
21	Washington	64.4
22	Florida	63.0
23	Illinois	62.9
23	Maine	62.9
25	Wisconsin	62.8
26	New Hampshire	62.7
26	Tennessee	62.7
28	Montana	62.4
28	Ohio	62.4
30	Alabama	62.0
31	North Dakota	61.2
32	Missouri	61.1
33	West Virginia	61.0
34	Louisiana	60.8
34	Oregon	60.8
36	Alaska	60.6
37	Kentucky	60.4
38	Texas	60.0
39	Colorado	59.2
40	New Mexico	59.1
41	Indiana	58.4
42	Iowa	58.3
43	Oklahoma	58.1
44	Nebraska	57.1
45	Wyoming	56.3
46	Arkansas	56.1
47	Mississippi	55.3
47	Utah	55.3
49	Kansas	54.5
50	Idaho	50.8

District of Columbia	73.6

Source: CQ Press using data from American Hospital Association (Chicago, IL)
"Hospital Statistics" (2011 edition)

*Average daily census compared to number of community hospital beds. Community hospitals are all nonfederal, short-term general, and other special hospitals whose facilities and services are available to the public.

Outpatient Visits to Community Hospitals in 2009

National Total = 624,098,296 Visits*

ALPHA ORDER

RANK	STATE	VISITS	% of USA
23	Alabama	9,191,353	1.4%
48	Alaska	1,767,418	0.3%
28	Arizona	7,102,044	1.1%
35	Arkansas	5,047,981	0.8%
2	California	48,254,933	7.5%
25	Colorado	8,860,081	1.4%
27	Connccticut	8,175,518	1.3%
49	Delaware	1,744,484	0.3%
8	Florida	24,873,618	3.9%
15	Georgia	14,390,335	2.2%
46	Hawaii	2,157,328	0.3%
42	Idaho	3,072,952	0.5%
6	Illinois	32,093,015	5.0%
13	Indiana	17,450,998	2.7%
20	Iowa	10,955,005	1.7%
29	Kansas	6,729,715	1.0%
22	Kentucky	10,119,606	1.6%
17	Louisiana	12,373,138	1.9%
32	Maine	5,760,429	0.9%
26	Maryland	8,293,899	1.3%
9	Massachusetts	21,354,335	3.3%
7	Michigan	29,297,777	4.6%
21	Minnesota	10,780,054	1.7%
37	Mississippi	4,684,822	0.7%
10	Missouri	19,213,984	3.0%
41	Montana	3,330,284	0.5%
38	Nebraska	4,658,108	0.7%
43	Nevada	2,809,649	0.4%
36	New Hampshire	4,724,846	0.7%
11	New Jersey	18,432,502	2.9%
39	New Mexico	4,643,668	0.7%
1	New York	54,244,821	8.4%
12	North Carolina	18,320,548	2.9%
45	North Dakota	2,362,500	0.4%
5	Ohio	34,240,945	5.3%
33	Oklahoma	5,570,902	0.9%
24	Oregon	8,899,999	1.4%
3	Pennsylvania	37,891,794	5.9%
44	Rhode Island	2,633,514	0.4%
31	South Carolina	6,319,670	1.0%
47	South Dakota	1,939,448	0.3%
18	Tennessee	11,583,346	1.8%
4	Texas	36,023,058	5.6%
34	Utah	5,474,372	0.9%
40	Vermont	3,355,609	0.5%
16	Virginia	14,158,853	2.2%
19	Washington	11,505,910	1.8%
30	West Virginia	6,684,643	1.0%
14	Wisconsin	14,927,668	2.3%
50	Wyoming	1,060,157	0.2%

RANK ORDER

RANK	STATE	VISITS	% of USA
1	New York	54,244,821	8.4%
2	California	48,254,933	7.5%
3	Pennsylvania	37,891,794	5.9%
4	Texas	36,023,058	5.6%
5	Ohio	34,240,945	5.3%
6	Illinois	32,093,015	5.0%
7	Michigan	29,297,777	4.6%
8	Florida	24,873,618	3.9%
9	Massachusetts	21,354,335	3.3%
10	Missouri	19,213,984	3.0%
11	New Jersey	18,432,502	2.9%
12	North Carolina	18,320,548	2.9%
13	Indiana	17,450,998	2.7%
14	Wisconsin	14,927,668	2.3%
15	Georgia	14,390,335	2.2%
16	Virginia	14,158,853	2.2%
17	Louisiana	12,373,138	1.9%
18	Tennessee	11,583,346	1.8%
19	Washington	11,505,910	1.8%
20	Iowa	10,955,005	1.7%
21	Minnesota	10,780,054	1.7%
22	Kentucky	10,119,606	1.6%
23	Alabama	9,191,353	1.4%
24	Oregon	8,899,999	1.4%
25	Colorado	8,860,081	1.4%
26	Maryland	8,293,899	1.3%
27	Connecticut	8,175,518	1.3%
28	Arizona	7,102,044	1.1%
29	Kansas	6,729,715	1.0%
30	West Virginia	6,684,643	1.0%
31	South Carolina	6,319,670	1.0%
32	Maine	5,760,429	0.9%
33	Oklahoma	5,570,902	0.9%
34	Utah	5,474,372	0.9%
35	Arkansas	5,047,981	0.8%
36	New Hampshire	4,724,846	0.7%
37	Mississippi	4,684,822	0.7%
38	Nebraska	4,658,108	0.7%
39	New Mexico	4,643,668	0.7%
40	Vermont	3,355,609	0.5%
41	Montana	3,330,284	0.5%
42	Idaho	3,072,952	0.5%
43	Nevada	2,809,649	0.4%
44	Rhode Island	2,633,514	0.4%
45	North Dakota	2,362,500	0.4%
46	Hawaii	2,157,328	0.3%
47	South Dakota	1,939,448	0.3%
48	Alaska	1,767,418	0.3%
49	Delaware	1,744,484	0.3%
50	Wyoming	1,060,157	0.2%
	District of Columbia	2,411,806	0.4%

Source: American Hospital Association (Chicago, IL)
  "Hospital Statistics" (2011 edition)
*All nonfederal, short-term general, and other special hospitals whose facilities and services are available to the public. Includes emergency and other visits.

Emergency Outpatient Visits to Community Hospitals in 2009

National Total = 127,298,193 Visits*

ALPHA ORDER

RANK	STATE	VISITS	% of USA
21	Alabama	2,286,343	1.8%
48	Alaska	296,524	0.2%
23	Arizona	2,137,007	1.7%
30	Arkansas	1,355,032	1.1%
1	California	10,554,310	8.3%
27	Colorado	1,725,417	1.4%
29	Connecticut	1,607,670	1.3%
43	Delaware	392,660	0.3%
4	Florida	7,477,209	5.9%
10	Georgia	4,081,812	3.2%
44	Hawaii	383,778	0.3%
41	Idaho	514,299	0.4%
7	Illinois	5,312,763	4.2%
15	Indiana	3,004,721	2.4%
32	Iowa	1,230,737	1.0%
34	Kansas	1,042,407	0.8%
20	Kentucky	2,321,519	1.8%
18	Louisiana	2,450,514	1.9%
38	Maine	792,592	0.6%
19	Maryland	2,429,724	1.9%
14	Massachusetts	3,116,535	2.4%
8	Michigan	4,538,588	3.6%
25	Minnesota	1,873,419	1.5%
28	Mississippi	1,720,780	1.4%
16	Missouri	2,894,040	2.3%
46	Montana	357,066	0.3%
39	Nebraska	688,519	0.5%
37	Nevada	820,980	0.6%
40	New Hampshire	627,769	0.5%
11	New Jersey	3,484,463	2.7%
36	New Mexico	829,138	0.7%
3	New York	8,542,392	6.7%
9	North Carolina	4,249,375	3.3%
47	North Dakota	303,190	0.2%
5	Ohio	6,207,290	4.9%
26	Oklahoma	1,743,802	1.4%
31	Oregon	1,312,068	1.0%
6	Pennsylvania	6,009,572	4.7%
42	Rhode Island	502,224	0.4%
22	South Carolina	2,171,925	1.7%
49	South Dakota	240,618	0.2%
12	Tennessee	3,301,872	2.6%
2	Texas	9,438,151	7.4%
35	Utah	865,286	0.7%
45	Vermont	357,793	0.3%
13	Virginia	3,199,466	2.5%
17	Washington	2,509,243	2.0%
33	West Virginia	1,221,485	1.0%
24	Wisconsin	2,080,601	1.6%
50	Wyoming	236,213	0.2%

RANK ORDER

RANK	STATE	VISITS	% of USA
1	California	10,554,310	8.3%
2	Texas	9,438,151	7.4%
3	New York	8,542,392	6.7%
4	Florida	7,477,209	5.9%
5	Ohio	6,207,290	4.9%
6	Pennsylvania	6,009,572	4.7%
7	Illinois	5,312,763	4.2%
8	Michigan	4,538,588	3.6%
9	North Carolina	4,249,375	3.3%
10	Georgia	4,081,812	3.2%
11	New Jersey	3,484,463	2.7%
12	Tennessee	3,301,872	2.6%
13	Virginia	3,199,466	2.5%
14	Massachusetts	3,116,535	2.4%
15	Indiana	3,004,721	2.4%
16	Missouri	2,894,040	2.3%
17	Washington	2,509,243	2.0%
18	Louisiana	2,450,514	1.9%
19	Maryland	2,429,724	1.9%
20	Kentucky	2,321,519	1.8%
21	Alabama	2,286,343	1.8%
22	South Carolina	2,171,925	1.7%
23	Arizona	2,137,007	1.7%
24	Wisconsin	2,080,601	1.6%
25	Minnesota	1,873,419	1.5%
26	Oklahoma	1,743,802	1.4%
27	Colorado	1,725,417	1.4%
28	Mississippi	1,720,780	1.4%
29	Connecticut	1,607,670	1.3%
30	Arkansas	1,355,032	1.1%
31	Oregon	1,312,068	1.0%
32	Iowa	1,230,737	1.0%
33	West Virginia	1,221,485	1.0%
34	Kansas	1,042,407	0.8%
35	Utah	865,286	0.7%
36	New Mexico	829,138	0.7%
37	Nevada	820,980	0.6%
38	Maine	792,592	0.6%
39	Nebraska	688,519	0.5%
40	New Hampshire	627,769	0.5%
41	Idaho	514,299	0.4%
42	Rhode Island	502,224	0.4%
43	Delaware	392,660	0.3%
44	Hawaii	383,778	0.3%
45	Vermont	357,793	0.3%
46	Montana	357,066	0.3%
47	North Dakota	303,190	0.2%
48	Alaska	296,524	0.2%
49	South Dakota	240,618	0.2%
50	Wyoming	236,213	0.2%
	District of Columbia	457,292	0.4%

Source: American Hospital Association (Chicago, IL)
"Hospital Statistics" (2011 edition)
*All nonfederal, short-term general, and other special hospitals whose facilities and services are available to the public.

Medicare and Medicaid Certified Facilities in 2011

National Total = 288,846 Facilities*

ALPHA ORDER

RANK	STATE	FACILITIES	% of USA
19	Alabama	4,853	1.7%
48	Alaska	680	0.2%
17	Arizona	5,378	1.9%
33	Arkansas	3,050	1.1%
2	California	26,325	9.1%
28	Colorado	3,857	1.3%
31	Connecticut	3,405	1.2%
46	Delaware	959	0.3%
3	Florida	21,685	7.5%
9	Georgia	9,070	3.1%
44	Hawaii	981	0.3%
39	Idaho	1,457	0.5%
6	Illinois	12,449	4.3%
11	Indiana	7,245	2.5%
27	Iowa	4,216	1.5%
29	Kansas	3,580	1.2%
20	Kentucky	4,704	1.6%
16	Louisiana	5,961	2.1%
40	Maine	1,422	0.5%
22	Maryland	4,643	1.6%
18	Massachusetts	4,924	1.7%
8	Michigan	9,506	3.3%
21	Minnesota	4,690	1.6%
30	Mississippi	3,447	1.2%
12	Missouri	6,908	2.4%
43	Montana	1,049	0.4%
34	Nebraska	2,568	0.9%
37	Nevada	1,875	0.6%
42	New Hampshire	1,214	0.4%
13	New Jersey	6,882	2.4%
38	New Mexico	1,834	0.6%
5	New York	13,141	4.5%
10	North Carolina	8,738	3.0%
47	North Dakota	924	0.3%
4	Ohio	13,147	4.6%
26	Oklahoma	4,528	1.6%
32	Oregon	3,072	1.1%
7	Pennsylvania	10,784	3.7%
45	Rhode Island	977	0.3%
24	South Carolina	4,591	1.6%
41	South Dakota	1,217	0.4%
14	Tennessee	6,702	2.3%
1	Texas	28,431	9.8%
36	Utah	1,949	0.7%
49	Vermont	643	0.2%
15	Virginia	6,329	2.2%
23	Washington	4,594	1.6%
35	West Virginia	2,424	0.8%
25	Wisconsin	4,578	1.6%
50	Wyoming	583	0.2%

RANK ORDER

RANK	STATE	FACILITIES	% of USA
1	Texas	28,431	9.8%
2	California	26,325	9.1%
3	Florida	21,685	7.5%
4	Ohio	13,147	4.6%
5	New York	13,141	4.5%
6	Illinois	12,449	4.3%
7	Pennsylvania	10,784	3.7%
8	Michigan	9,506	3.3%
9	Georgia	9,070	3.1%
10	North Carolina	8,738	3.0%
11	Indiana	7,245	2.5%
12	Missouri	6,908	2.4%
13	New Jersey	6,882	2.4%
14	Tennessee	6,702	2.3%
15	Virginia	6,329	2.2%
16	Louisiana	5,961	2.1%
17	Arizona	5,378	1.9%
18	Massachusetts	4,924	1.7%
19	Alabama	4,853	1.7%
20	Kentucky	4,704	1.6%
21	Minnesota	4,690	1.6%
22	Maryland	4,643	1.6%
23	Washington	4,594	1.6%
24	South Carolina	4,591	1.6%
25	Wisconsin	4,578	1.6%
26	Oklahoma	4,528	1.6%
27	Iowa	4,216	1.5%
28	Colorado	3,857	1.3%
29	Kansas	3,580	1.2%
30	Mississippi	3,447	1.2%
31	Connecticut	3,405	1.2%
32	Oregon	3,072	1.1%
33	Arkansas	3,050	1.1%
34	Nebraska	2,568	0.9%
35	West Virginia	2,424	0.8%
36	Utah	1,949	0.7%
37	Nevada	1,875	0.6%
38	New Mexico	1,834	0.6%
39	Idaho	1,457	0.5%
40	Maine	1,422	0.5%
41	South Dakota	1,217	0.4%
42	New Hampshire	1,214	0.4%
43	Montana	1,049	0.4%
44	Hawaii	981	0.3%
45	Rhode Island	977	0.3%
46	Delaware	959	0.3%
47	North Dakota	924	0.3%
48	Alaska	680	0.2%
49	Vermont	643	0.2%
50	Wyoming	583	0.2%
	District of Columbia	677	0.2%

Source: U.S. Department of Health and Human Services, Centers for Medicare and Medicaid Services
OSCAR Report 10 (January 24, 2011)

*Certified by CMS to participate in the Medicare/Medicaid programs. All provider groups including hospitals, home health agencies, rural health centers, community mental health centers, nursing facilities, outpatient physical therapy facilities, hospices, and laboratories. National total does not include 1,580 certified facilities in U.S. territories.

Medicare and Medicaid Certified Hospitals in 2011

National Total = 6,116 Hospitals*

ALPHA ORDER				RANK ORDER			
RANK	STATE	HOSPITALS	% of USA	RANK	STATE	HOSPITALS	% of USA
19	Alabama	127	2.1%	1	Texas	588	9.6%
47	Alaska	25	0.4%	2	California	418	6.8%
25	Arizona	103	1.7%	3	Florida	244	4.0%
26	Arkansas	101	1.7%	4	Pennsylvania	237	3.9%
2	California	418	6.8%	5	Louisiana	226	3.7%
28	Colorado	98	1.6%	5	Ohio	226	3.7%
42	Connecticut	44	0.7%	7	New York	223	3.6%
50	Delaware	12	0.2%	8	Illinois	207	3.4%
3	Florida	244	4.0%	9	Georgia	177	2.9%
9	Georgia	177	2.9%	10	Michigan	172	2.8%
46	Hawaii	27	0.4%	11	Indiana	168	2.7%
39	Idaho	51	0.8%	12	Oklahoma	154	2.5%
8	Illinois	207	3.4%	13	Kansas	153	2.5%
11	Indiana	168	2.7%	14	Missouri	150	2.5%
20	Iowa	122	2.0%	15	Tennessee	149	2.4%
13	Kansas	153	2.5%	16	Wisconsin	146	2.4%
21	Kentucky	117	1.9%	17	Minnesota	145	2.4%
5	Louisiana	226	3.7%	18	North Carolina	133	2.2%
43	Maine	41	0.7%	19	Alabama	127	2.1%
33	Maryland	63	1.0%	20	Iowa	122	2.0%
24	Massachusetts	108	1.8%	21	Kentucky	117	1.9%
10	Michigan	172	2.8%	22	Virginia	116	1.9%
17	Minnesota	145	2.4%	23	Mississippi	111	1.8%
23	Mississippi	111	1.8%	24	Massachusetts	108	1.8%
14	Missouri	150	2.5%	25	Arizona	103	1.7%
32	Montana	64	1.0%	26	Arkansas	101	1.7%
30	Nebraska	96	1.6%	27	New Jersey	100	1.6%
38	Nevada	52	0.9%	28	Colorado	98	1.6%
44	New Hampshire	30	0.5%	28	Washington	98	1.6%
27	New Jersey	100	1.6%	30	Nebraska	96	1.6%
37	New Mexico	53	0.9%	31	South Carolina	80	1.3%
7	New York	223	3.6%	32	Montana	64	1.0%
18	North Carolina	133	2.2%	33	Maryland	63	1.0%
41	North Dakota	49	0.8%	33	South Dakota	63	1.0%
5	Ohio	226	3.7%	35	Oregon	62	1.0%
12	Oklahoma	154	2.5%	35	West Virginia	62	1.0%
35	Oregon	62	1.0%	37	New Mexico	53	0.9%
4	Pennsylvania	237	3.9%	38	Nevada	52	0.9%
48	Rhode Island	15	0.2%	39	Idaho	51	0.8%
31	South Carolina	80	1.3%	39	Utah	51	0.8%
33	South Dakota	63	1.0%	41	North Dakota	49	0.8%
15	Tennessee	149	2.4%	42	Connecticut	44	0.7%
1	Texas	588	9.6%	43	Maine	41	0.7%
39	Utah	51	0.8%	44	New Hampshire	30	0.5%
48	Vermont	15	0.2%	44	Wyoming	30	0.5%
22	Virginia	116	1.9%	46	Hawaii	27	0.4%
28	Washington	98	1.6%	47	Alaska	25	0.4%
35	West Virginia	62	1.0%	48	Rhode Island	15	0.2%
16	Wisconsin	146	2.4%	48	Vermont	15	0.2%
44	Wyoming	30	0.5%	50	Delaware	12	0.2%
					District of Columbia	14	0.2%

Source: U.S. Department of Health and Human Services, Centers for Medicare and Medicaid Services
   OSCAR Report 10 (January 24, 2011)

*Certified by CMS to participate in the Medicare/Medicaid programs. Excludes licensed facilities that do not accept federal funding and facilities managed by the Department of Veterans Affairs. National total does not include 62 certified hospitals in U.S. territories.

Beds in Medicare and Medicaid Certified Hospitals in 2011

National Total = 918,145 Beds*

ALPHA ORDER				RANK ORDER			
RANK	STATE	BEDS	% of USA	RANK	STATE	BEDS	% of USA
18	Alabama	19,324	2.1%	1	California	79,238	8.6%
49	Alaska	1,556	0.2%	2	Texas	69,251	7.5%
21	Arizona	15,968	1.7%	3	New York	63,783	6.9%
29	Arkansas	11,614	1.3%	4	Florida	60,715	6.6%
1	California	79,238	8.6%	5	Ohio	44,461	4.8%
28	Colorado	12,581	1.4%	6	Illinois	40,294	4.4%
32	Connecticut	10,445	1.1%	7	Pennsylvania	35,588	3.9%
47	Delaware	2,693	0.3%	8	Michigan	28,131	3.1%
4	Florida	60,715	6.6%	9	New Jersey	26,649	2.9%
11	Georgia	24,672	2.7%	10	North Carolina	26,566	2.9%
46	Hawaii	2,763	0.3%	11	Georgia	24,672	2.7%
42	Idaho	3,497	0.4%	12	Tennessee	24,433	2.7%
6	Illinois	40,294	4.4%	13	Missouri	23,878	2.6%
17	Indiana	19,347	2.1%	14	Louisiana	20,634	2.2%
31	Iowa	10,450	1.1%	15	Massachusetts	19,783	2.2%
30	Kansas	11,207	1.2%	16	Virginia	19,592	2.1%
20	Kentucky	17,463	1.9%	17	Indiana	19,347	2.1%
14	Louisiana	20,634	2.2%	18	Alabama	19,324	2.1%
39	Maine	3,979	0.4%	19	Wisconsin	17,623	1.9%
23	Maryland	14,884	1.6%	20	Kentucky	17,463	1.9%
15	Massachusetts	19,783	2.2%	21	Arizona	15,968	1.7%
8	Michigan	28,131	3.1%	22	Minnesota	15,520	1.7%
22	Minnesota	15,520	1.7%	23	Maryland	14,884	1.6%
27	Mississippi	13,039	1.4%	24	Oklahoma	14,650	1.6%
13	Missouri	23,878	2.6%	25	South Carolina	13,709	1.5%
44	Montana	3,131	0.3%	26	Washington	13,461	1.5%
35	Nebraska	6,662	0.7%	27	Mississippi	13,039	1.4%
36	Nevada	6,535	0.7%	28	Colorado	12,581	1.4%
41	New Hampshire	3,529	0.4%	29	Arkansas	11,614	1.3%
9	New Jersey	26,649	2.9%	30	Kansas	11,207	1.2%
38	New Mexico	4,801	0.5%	31	Iowa	10,450	1.1%
3	New York	63,783	6.9%	32	Connecticut	10,445	1.1%
10	North Carolina	26,566	2.9%	33	West Virginia	8,899	1.0%
45	North Dakota	3,107	0.3%	34	Oregon	8,075	0.9%
5	Ohio	44,461	4.8%	35	Nebraska	6,662	0.7%
24	Oklahoma	14,650	1.6%	36	Nevada	6,535	0.7%
34	Oregon	8,075	0.9%	37	Utah	5,458	0.6%
7	Pennsylvania	35,588	3.9%	38	New Mexico	4,801	0.5%
40	Rhode Island	3,657	0.4%	39	Maine	3,979	0.4%
25	South Carolina	13,709	1.5%	40	Rhode Island	3,657	0.4%
43	South Dakota	3,360	0.4%	41	New Hampshire	3,529	0.4%
12	Tennessee	24,433	2.7%	42	Idaho	3,497	0.4%
2	Texas	69,251	7.5%	43	South Dakota	3,360	0.4%
37	Utah	5,458	0.6%	44	Montana	3,131	0.3%
48	Vermont	1,788	0.2%	45	North Dakota	3,107	0.3%
16	Virginia	19,592	2.1%	46	Hawaii	2,763	0.3%
26	Washington	13,461	1.5%	47	Delaware	2,693	0.3%
33	West Virginia	8,899	1.0%	48	Vermont	1,788	0.2%
19	Wisconsin	17,623	1.9%	49	Alaska	1,556	0.2%
50	Wyoming	1,549	0.2%	50	Wyoming	1,549	0.2%
					District of Columbia	4,153	0.5%

Source: U.S. Department of Health and Human Services, Centers for Medicare and Medicaid Services
   CASPER Report 10B (January 06, 2010)
*Beds in hospitals certified by CMS to participate in the Medicare/Medicaid programs. Excludes licensed facilities that do not
accept federal funding and facilities managed by the Department of Veterans Affairs. National total does not include 11,336
beds in U.S. territories.

Medicare and Medicaid Certified Children's Hospitals in 2011

National Total = 76 Hospitals*

ALPHA ORDER

RANK ORDER

RANK	STATE	HOSPITALS	% of USA		RANK	STATE	HOSPITALS	% of USA
8	Alabama	2	2.6%		1	California	10	13.2%
32	Alaska	0	0.0%		2	Texas	8	10.5%
8	Arizona	2	2.6%		3	Ohio	6	7.9%
21	Arkansas	1	1.3%		4	Pennsylvania	5	6.6%
1	California	10	13.2%		5	Minnesota	3	3.9%
21	Colorado	1	1.3%		5	Missouri	3	3.9%
21	Connecticut	1	1.3%		5	Virginia	3	3.9%
21	Delaware	1	1.3%		8	Alabama	2	2.6%
8	Florida	2	2.6%		8	Arizona	2	2.6%
8	Georgia	2	2.6%		8	Florida	2	2.6%
21	Hawaii	1	1.3%		8	Georgia	2	2.6%
32	Idaho	0	0.0%		8	Illinois	2	2.6%
8	Illinois	2	2.6%		8	Maryland	2	2.6%
32	Indiana	0	0.0%		8	Massachusetts	2	2.6%
32	Iowa	0	0.0%		8	Nebraska	2	2.6%
21	Kansas	1	1.3%		8	New Jersey	2	2.6%
32	Kentucky	0	0.0%		8	Oklahoma	2	2.6%
21	Louisiana	1	1.3%		8	Tennessee	2	2.6%
32	Maine	0	0.0%		8	Washington	2	2.6%
8	Maryland	2	2.6%		8	Wisconsin	2	2.6%
8	Massachusetts	2	2.6%		21	Arkansas	1	1.3%
21	Michigan	1	1.3%		21	Colorado	1	1.3%
5	Minnesota	3	3.9%		21	Connecticut	1	1.3%
32	Mississippi	0	0.0%		21	Delaware	1	1.3%
5	Missouri	3	3.9%		21	Hawaii	1	1.3%
32	Montana	0	0.0%		21	Kansas	1	1.3%
8	Nebraska	2	2.6%		21	Louisiana	1	1.3%
32	Nevada	0	0.0%		21	Michigan	1	1.3%
32	New Hampshire	0	0.0%		21	New York	1	1.3%
8	New Jersey	2	2.6%		21	South Dakota	1	1.3%
32	New Mexico	0	0.0%		21	Utah	1	1.3%
21	New York	1	1.3%		32	Alaska	0	0.0%
32	North Carolina	0	0.0%		32	Idaho	0	0.0%
32	North Dakota	0	0.0%		32	Indiana	0	0.0%
3	Ohio	6	7.9%		32	Iowa	0	0.0%
8	Oklahoma	2	2.6%		32	Kentucky	0	0.0%
32	Oregon	0	0.0%		32	Maine	0	0.0%
4	Pennsylvania	5	6.6%		32	Mississippi	0	0.0%
32	Rhode Island	0	0.0%		32	Montana	0	0.0%
32	South Carolina	0	0.0%		32	Nevada	0	0.0%
21	South Dakota	1	1.3%		32	New Hampshire	0	0.0%
8	Tennessee	2	2.6%		32	New Mexico	0	0.0%
2	Texas	8	10.5%		32	North Carolina	0	0.0%
21	Utah	1	1.3%		32	North Dakota	0	0.0%
32	Vermont	0	0.0%		32	Oregon	0	0.0%
5	Virginia	3	3.9%		32	Rhode Island	0	0.0%
8	Washington	2	2.6%		32	South Carolina	0	0.0%
32	West Virginia	0	0.0%		32	Vermont	0	0.0%
8	Wisconsin	2	2.6%		32	West Virginia	0	0.0%
32	Wyoming	0	0.0%		32	Wyoming	0	0.0%
						District of Columbia	1	1.3%

Source: U.S. Department of Health and Human Services, Centers for Medicare and Medicaid Services
CASPER Report 10B (January 06, 2010)

*Certified by CMS to participate in the Medicare/Medicaid programs. National total does not include one facility in U.S. territories.
Excludes licensed facilities that do not accept federal funding and facilities managed by the Department of Veterans Affairs.

Beds in Medicare and Medicaid Certified Children's Hospitals in 2011

National Total = 12,608 Beds*

RANK	STATE	BEDS	% of USA		RANK	STATE	BEDS	% of USA
7	Alabama	434	3.4%		1	California	1,905	15.1%
32	Alaska	0	0.0%		2	Texas	1,385	11.0%
17	Arizona	250	2.0%		3	Ohio	1,356	10.8%
15	Arkansas	280	2.2%		4	Pennsylvania	845	6.7%
1	California	1,905	15.1%		5	Georgia	483	3.8%
16	Colorado	253	2.0%		6	Florida	467	3.7%
27	Connecticut	129	1.0%		7	Alabama	434	3.4%
24	Delaware	180	1.4%		8	Missouri	432	3.4%
6	Florida	467	3.7%		9	Massachusetts	421	3.3%
5	Georgia	483	3.8%		10	Illinois	339	2.7%
20	Hawaii	207	1.6%		10	Minnesota	339	2.7%
32	Idaho	0	0.0%		12	Wisconsin	338	2.7%
10	Illinois	339	2.7%		13	Washington	318	2.5%
32	Indiana	0	0.0%		14	Virginia	296	2.3%
32	Iowa	0	0.0%		15	Arkansas	280	2.2%
31	Kansas	34	0.3%		16	Colorado	253	2.0%
32	Kentucky	0	0.0%		17	Arizona	250	2.0%
21	Louisiana	201	1.6%		18	Utah	232	1.8%
32	Maine	0	0.0%		19	Michigan	228	1.8%
26	Maryland	150	1.2%		20	Hawaii	207	1.6%
9	Massachusetts	421	3.3%		21	Louisiana	201	1.6%
19	Michigan	228	1.8%		22	Nebraska	200	1.6%
10	Minnesota	339	2.7%		23	Tennessee	197	1.6%
32	Mississippi	0	0.0%		24	Delaware	180	1.4%
8	Missouri	432	3.4%		25	Oklahoma	160	1.3%
32	Montana	0	0.0%		26	Maryland	150	1.2%
22	Nebraska	200	1.6%		27	Connecticut	129	1.0%
32	Nevada	0	0.0%		28	South Dakota	114	0.9%
32	New Hampshire	0	0.0%		29	New Jersey	100	0.8%
29	New Jersey	100	0.8%		30	New York	92	0.7%
32	New Mexico	0	0.0%		31	Kansas	34	0.3%
30	New York	92	0.7%		32	Alaska	0	0.0%
32	North Carolina	0	0.0%		32	Idaho	0	0.0%
32	North Dakota	0	0.0%		32	Indiana	0	0.0%
3	Ohio	1,356	10.8%		32	Iowa	0	0.0%
25	Oklahoma	160	1.3%		32	Kentucky	0	0.0%
32	Oregon	0	0.0%		32	Maine	0	0.0%
4	Pennsylvania	845	6.7%		32	Mississippi	0	0.0%
32	Rhode Island	0	0.0%		32	Montana	0	0.0%
32	South Carolina	0	0.0%		32	Nevada	0	0.0%
28	South Dakota	114	0.9%		32	New Hampshire	0	0.0%
23	Tennessee	197	1.6%		32	New Mexico	0	0.0%
2	Texas	1,385	11.0%		32	North Carolina	0	0.0%
18	Utah	232	1.8%		32	North Dakota	0	0.0%
32	Vermont	0	0.0%		32	Oregon	0	0.0%
14	Virginia	296	2.3%		32	Rhode Island	0	0.0%
13	Washington	318	2.5%		32	South Carolina	0	0.0%
32	West Virginia	0	0.0%		32	Vermont	0	0.0%
12	Wisconsin	338	2.7%		32	West Virginia	0	0.0%
32	Wyoming	0	0.0%		32	Wyoming	0	0.0%
						District of Columbia	243	1.9%

ALPHA ORDER

RANK ORDER

Source: U.S. Department of Health and Human Services, Centers for Medicare and Medicaid Services
    CASPER Report 10B (January 06, 2010)
*Certified by CMS to participate in the Medicare/Medicaid programs. National total does not include 215 beds in one facility in
U.S. territories. Excludes licensed facilities that do not accept federal funding and facilities managed by the Department of
Veterans Affairs.

Medicare and Medicaid Certified Rehabilitation Hospitals in 2011

National Total = 233 Hospitals*

ALPHA ORDER

RANK	STATE	HOSPITALS	% of USA
9	Alabama	7	3.0%
40	Alaska	0	0.0%
9	Arizona	7	3.0%
6	Arkansas	8	3.4%
14	California	5	2.1%
22	Colorado	3	1.3%
31	Connecticut	1	0.4%
40	Delaware	0	0.0%
4	Florida	13	5.6%
22	Georgia	3	1.3%
31	Hawaii	1	0.4%
31	Idaho	1	0.4%
19	Illinois	4	1.7%
11	Indiana	6	2.6%
40	Iowa	0	0.0%
19	Kansas	4	1.7%
14	Kentucky	5	2.1%
2	Louisiana	21	9.0%
31	Maine	1	0.4%
26	Maryland	2	0.9%
6	Massachusetts	8	3.4%
19	Michigan	4	1.7%
40	Minnesota	0	0.0%
40	Mississippi	0	0.0%
14	Missouri	5	2.1%
40	Montana	0	0.0%
31	Nebraska	1	0.4%
22	Nevada	3	1.3%
26	New Hampshire	2	0.9%
6	New Jersey	8	3.4%
14	New Mexico	5	2.1%
40	New York	0	0.0%
26	North Carolina	2	0.9%
40	North Dakota	0	0.0%
22	Ohio	3	1.3%
26	Oklahoma	2	0.9%
40	Oregon	0	0.0%
3	Pennsylvania	16	6.9%
31	Rhode Island	1	0.4%
11	South Carolina	6	2.6%
40	South Dakota	0	0.0%
11	Tennessee	6	2.6%
1	Texas	49	21.0%
31	Utah	1	0.4%
40	Vermont	0	0.0%
5	Virginia	9	3.9%
31	Washington	1	0.4%
14	West Virginia	5	2.1%
26	Wisconsin	2	0.9%
31	Wyoming	1	0.4%

RANK ORDER

RANK	STATE	HOSPITALS	% of USA
1	Texas	49	21.0%
2	Louisiana	21	9.0%
3	Pennsylvania	16	6.9%
4	Florida	13	5.6%
5	Virginia	9	3.9%
6	Arkansas	8	3.4%
6	Massachusetts	8	3.4%
6	New Jersey	8	3.4%
9	Alabama	7	3.0%
9	Arizona	7	3.0%
11	Indiana	6	2.6%
11	South Carolina	6	2.6%
11	Tennessee	6	2.6%
14	California	5	2.1%
14	Kentucky	5	2.1%
14	Missouri	5	2.1%
14	New Mexico	5	2.1%
14	West Virginia	5	2.1%
19	Illinois	4	1.7%
19	Kansas	4	1.7%
19	Michigan	4	1.7%
22	Colorado	3	1.3%
22	Georgia	3	1.3%
22	Nevada	3	1.3%
22	Ohio	3	1.3%
26	Maryland	2	0.9%
26	New Hampshire	2	0.9%
26	North Carolina	2	0.9%
26	Oklahoma	2	0.9%
26	Wisconsin	2	0.9%
31	Connecticut	1	0.4%
31	Hawaii	1	0.4%
31	Idaho	1	0.4%
31	Maine	1	0.4%
31	Nebraska	1	0.4%
31	Rhode Island	1	0.4%
31	Utah	1	0.4%
31	Washington	1	0.4%
31	Wyoming	1	0.4%
40	Alaska	0	0.0%
40	Delaware	0	0.0%
40	Iowa	0	0.0%
40	Minnesota	0	0.0%
40	Mississippi	0	0.0%
40	Montana	0	0.0%
40	New York	0	0.0%
40	North Dakota	0	0.0%
40	Oregon	0	0.0%
40	South Dakota	0	0.0%
40	Vermont	0	0.0%
	District of Columbia	1	0.4%

Source: U.S. Department of Health and Human Services, Centers for Medicare and Medicaid Services
CASPER Report 10B (January 06, 2010)
*Certified by CMS to participate in the Medicare/Medicaid programs. Excludes licensed facilities that do not accept federal funding and facilities managed by the Department of Veterans Affairs. National total does not include two certified hospitals in U.S. territories.

Beds in Medicare and Medicaid Certified Rehabilitation Hospitals in 2011

National Total = 14,852 Beds*

ALPHA ORDER				RANK ORDER			
RANK	STATE	BEDS	% of USA	RANK	STATE	BEDS	% of USA
10	Alabama	392	2.6%	1	Texas	2,701	18.2%
40	Alaska	0	0.0%	2	Pennsylvania	1,395	9.4%
9	Arizona	396	2.7%	3	Florida	1,042	7.0%
7	Arkansas	463	3.1%	4	Massachusetts	1,040	7.0%
12	California	367	2.5%	5	New Jersey	783	5.3%
21	Colorado	226	1.5%	6	Louisiana	538	3.6%
37	Connecticut	60	0.4%	7	Arkansas	463	3.1%
40	Delaware	0	0.0%	8	Illinois	448	3.0%
3	Florida	1,042	7.0%	9	Arizona	396	2.7%
26	Georgia	168	1.1%	10	Alabama	392	2.6%
32	Hawaii	100	0.7%	11	Tennessee	370	2.5%
38	Idaho	46	0.3%	12	California	367	2.5%
8	Illinois	448	3.0%	13	South Carolina	355	2.4%
16	Indiana	290	2.0%	14	Virginia	353	2.4%
40	Iowa	0	0.0%	15	Missouri	297	2.0%
19	Kansas	257	1.7%	16	Indiana	290	2.0%
17	Kentucky	288	1.9%	17	Kentucky	288	1.9%
6	Louisiana	538	3.6%	18	West Virginia	280	1.9%
32	Maine	100	0.7%	19	Kansas	257	1.7%
28	Maryland	131	0.9%	20	Michigan	240	1.6%
4	Massachusetts	1,040	7.0%	21	Colorado	226	1.5%
20	Michigan	240	1.6%	22	North Carolina	213	1.4%
40	Minnesota	0	0.0%	23	New Mexico	212	1.4%
40	Mississippi	0	0.0%	24	Ohio	199	1.3%
15	Missouri	297	2.0%	25	Nevada	181	1.2%
40	Montana	0	0.0%	26	Georgia	168	1.1%
36	Nebraska	72	0.5%	27	New Hampshire	152	1.0%
25	Nevada	181	1.2%	28	Maryland	131	0.9%
27	New Hampshire	152	1.0%	29	Wisconsin	121	0.8%
5	New Jersey	783	5.3%	30	Oklahoma	107	0.7%
23	New Mexico	212	1.4%	31	Washington	102	0.7%
40	New York	0	0.0%	32	Hawaii	100	0.7%
22	North Carolina	213	1.4%	32	Maine	100	0.7%
40	North Dakota	0	0.0%	34	Utah	84	0.6%
24	Ohio	199	1.3%	35	Rhode Island	82	0.6%
30	Oklahoma	107	0.7%	36	Nebraska	72	0.5%
40	Oregon	0	0.0%	37	Connecticut	60	0.4%
2	Pennsylvania	1,395	9.4%	38	Idaho	46	0.3%
35	Rhode Island	82	0.6%	39	Wyoming	41	0.3%
13	South Carolina	355	2.4%	40	Alaska	0	0.0%
40	South Dakota	0	0.0%	40	Delaware	0	0.0%
11	Tennessee	370	2.5%	40	Iowa	0	0.0%
1	Texas	2,701	18.2%	40	Minnesota	0	0.0%
34	Utah	84	0.6%	40	Mississippi	0	0.0%
40	Vermont	0	0.0%	40	Montana	0	0.0%
14	Virginia	353	2.4%	40	New York	0	0.0%
31	Washington	102	0.7%	40	North Dakota	0	0.0%
18	West Virginia	280	1.9%	40	Oregon	0	0.0%
29	Wisconsin	121	0.8%	40	South Dakota	0	0.0%
39	Wyoming	41	0.3%	40	Vermont	0	0.0%
					District of Columbia	160	1.1%

Source: U.S. Department of Health and Human Services, Centers for Medicare and Medicaid Services
 CASPER Report 10B (January 06, 2010)
*Beds in hospitals certified by CMS to participate in the Medicare/Medicaid programs. Excludes licensed facilities that do not accept federal funding and facilities managed by the Department of Veterans Affairs. National total does not include 72 beds in U.S. territories.

Medicare and Medicaid Certified Psychiatric Hospitals in 2011

National Total = 510 Psychiatric Hospitals*

ALPHA ORDER

RANK	STATE	HOSPITALS	% of USA
16	Alabama	11	2.2%
42	Alaska	2	0.4%
25	Arizona	8	1.6%
21	Arkansas	9	1.8%
3	California	32	6.3%
21	Colorado	9	1.8%
29	Connecticut	6	1.2%
33	Delaware	4	0.8%
5	Florida	25	4.9%
9	Georgia	15	2.9%
48	Hawaii	1	0.2%
30	Idaho	5	1.0%
10	Illinois	14	2.7%
7	Indiana	23	4.5%
33	Iowa	4	0.8%
33	Kansas	4	0.8%
16	Kentucky	11	2.2%
1	Louisiana	38	7.5%
33	Maine	4	0.8%
21	Maryland	9	1.8%
10	Massachusetts	14	2.7%
14	Michigan	12	2.4%
25	Minnesota	8	1.6%
30	Mississippi	5	1.0%
13	Missouri	13	2.5%
42	Montana	2	0.4%
38	Nebraska	3	0.6%
25	Nevada	8	1.6%
42	New Hampshire	2	0.4%
8	New Jersey	17	3.3%
42	New Mexico	2	0.4%
4	New York	28	5.5%
19	North Carolina	10	2.0%
38	North Dakota	3	0.6%
10	Ohio	14	2.7%
19	Oklahoma	10	2.0%
38	Oregon	3	0.6%
6	Pennsylvania	24	4.7%
42	Rhode Island	2	0.4%
25	South Carolina	8	1.6%
48	South Dakota	1	0.2%
14	Tennessee	12	2.4%
2	Texas	37	7.3%
38	Utah	3	0.6%
48	Vermont	1	0.2%
21	Virginia	9	1.8%
30	Washington	5	1.0%
33	West Virginia	4	0.8%
16	Wisconsin	11	2.2%
42	Wyoming	2	0.4%

RANK ORDER

RANK	STATE	HOSPITALS	% of USA
1	Louisiana	38	7.5%
2	Texas	37	7.3%
3	California	32	6.3%
4	New York	28	5.5%
5	Florida	25	4.9%
6	Pennsylvania	24	4.7%
7	Indiana	23	4.5%
8	New Jersey	17	3.3%
9	Georgia	15	2.9%
10	Illinois	14	2.7%
10	Massachusetts	14	2.7%
10	Ohio	14	2.7%
13	Missouri	13	2.5%
14	Michigan	12	2.4%
14	Tennessee	12	2.4%
16	Alabama	11	2.2%
16	Kentucky	11	2.2%
16	Wisconsin	11	2.2%
19	North Carolina	10	2.0%
19	Oklahoma	10	2.0%
21	Arkansas	9	1.8%
21	Colorado	9	1.8%
21	Maryland	9	1.8%
21	Virginia	9	1.8%
25	Arizona	8	1.6%
25	Minnesota	8	1.6%
25	Nevada	8	1.6%
25	South Carolina	8	1.6%
29	Connecticut	6	1.2%
30	Idaho	5	1.0%
30	Mississippi	5	1.0%
30	Washington	5	1.0%
33	Delaware	4	0.8%
33	Iowa	4	0.8%
33	Kansas	4	0.8%
33	Maine	4	0.8%
33	West Virginia	4	0.8%
38	Nebraska	3	0.6%
38	North Dakota	3	0.6%
38	Oregon	3	0.6%
38	Utah	3	0.6%
42	Alaska	2	0.4%
42	Montana	2	0.4%
42	New Hampshire	2	0.4%
42	New Mexico	2	0.4%
42	Rhode Island	2	0.4%
42	Wyoming	2	0.4%
48	Hawaii	1	0.2%
48	South Dakota	1	0.2%
48	Vermont	1	0.2%
	District of Columbia	3	0.6%

Source: U.S. Department of Health and Human Services, Centers for Medicare and Medicaid Services
CASPER Report 10B (January 06, 2010)

*Certified by CMS to participate in the Medicare/Medicaid programs. Excludes licensed facilities that do not accept federal funding and facilities managed by the Department of Veterans Affairs. National total does not include three certified psychiatric hospitals in U.S. territories.

Beds in Medicare and Medicaid Certified Psychiatric Hospitals in 2011

National Total = 57,133 Beds*

ALPHA ORDER

RANK	STATE	BEDS	% of USA
26	Alabama	756	1.3%
42	Alaska	205	0.4%
25	Arizona	874	1.5%
22	Arkansas	919	1.6%
7	California	2,428	4.2%
23	Colorado	889	1.6%
21	Connecticut	1,022	1.8%
38	Delaware	312	0.5%
2	Florida	3,801	6.7%
10	Georgia	1,576	2.8%
50	Hawaii	88	0.2%
41	Idaho	263	0.5%
11	Illinois	1,573	2.8%
19	Indiana	1,091	1.9%
40	Iowa	287	0.5%
30	Kansas	561	1.0%
14	Kentucky	1,402	2.5%
8	Louisiana	2,074	3.6%
35	Maine	386	0.7%
9	Maryland	1,731	3.0%
13	Massachusetts	1,420	2.5%
12	Michigan	1,486	2.6%
33	Minnesota	458	0.8%
29	Mississippi	617	1.1%
23	Missouri	889	1.6%
45	Montana	153	0.3%
36	Nebraska	369	0.6%
28	Nevada	656	1.1%
37	New Hampshire	341	0.6%
6	New Jersey	2,877	5.0%
48	New Mexico	124	0.2%
1	New York	6,322	11.1%
4	North Carolina	3,310	5.8%
39	North Dakota	303	0.5%
15	Ohio	1,384	2.4%
31	Oklahoma	536	0.9%
44	Oregon	168	0.3%
3	Pennsylvania	3,472	6.1%
43	Rhode Island	177	0.3%
18	South Carolina	1,093	1.9%
47	South Dakota	133	0.2%
20	Tennessee	1,046	1.8%
5	Texas	3,017	5.3%
34	Utah	391	0.7%
46	Vermont	149	0.3%
27	Virginia	755	1.3%
16	Washington	1,241	2.2%
32	West Virginia	485	0.8%
17	Wisconsin	1,133	2.0%
49	Wyoming	98	0.2%

RANK ORDER

RANK	STATE	BEDS	% of USA
1	New York	6,322	11.1%
2	Florida	3,801	6.7%
3	Pennsylvania	3,472	6.1%
4	North Carolina	3,310	5.8%
5	Texas	3,017	5.3%
6	New Jersey	2,877	5.0%
7	California	2,428	4.2%
8	Louisiana	2,074	3.6%
9	Maryland	1,731	3.0%
10	Georgia	1,576	2.8%
11	Illinois	1,573	2.8%
12	Michigan	1,486	2.6%
13	Massachusetts	1,420	2.5%
14	Kentucky	1,402	2.5%
15	Ohio	1,384	2.4%
16	Washington	1,241	2.2%
17	Wisconsin	1,133	2.0%
18	South Carolina	1,093	1.9%
19	Indiana	1,091	1.9%
20	Tennessee	1,046	1.8%
21	Connecticut	1,022	1.8%
22	Arkansas	919	1.6%
23	Colorado	889	1.6%
23	Missouri	889	1.6%
25	Arizona	874	1.5%
26	Alabama	756	1.3%
27	Virginia	755	1.3%
28	Nevada	656	1.1%
29	Mississippi	617	1.1%
30	Kansas	561	1.0%
31	Oklahoma	536	0.9%
32	West Virginia	485	0.8%
33	Minnesota	458	0.8%
34	Utah	391	0.7%
35	Maine	386	0.7%
36	Nebraska	369	0.6%
37	New Hampshire	341	0.6%
38	Delaware	312	0.5%
39	North Dakota	303	0.5%
40	Iowa	287	0.5%
41	Idaho	263	0.5%
42	Alaska	205	0.4%
43	Rhode Island	177	0.3%
44	Oregon	168	0.3%
45	Montana	153	0.3%
46	Vermont	149	0.3%
47	South Dakota	133	0.2%
48	New Mexico	124	0.2%
49	Wyoming	98	0.2%
50	Hawaii	88	0.2%
	District of Columbia	292	0.5%

Source: U.S. Department of Health and Human Services, Centers for Medicare and Medicaid Services
   CASPER Report 10B (January 06, 2010)
*Beds in hospitals certified by CMS to participate in the Medicare/Medicaid programs. Excludes licensed facilities that do not accept federal funding and facilities managed by the Department of Veterans Affairs. National total does not include 292 beds in U.S. territories.

Medicare and Medicaid Certified Outpatient Surgery Centers in 2011

National Total = 5,300 Centers*

ALPHA ORDER

RANK	STATE	CENTERS	% of USA
35	Alabama	40	0.8%
49	Alaska	10	0.2%
10	Arizona	152	2.9%
26	Arkansas	60	1.1%
1	California	749	14.1%
15	Colorado	104	2.0%
33	Connecticut	45	0.8%
38	Delaware	25	0.5%
2	Florida	402	7.6%
5	Georgia	283	5.3%
45	Hawaii	13	0.2%
30	Idaho	51	1.0%
13	Illinois	118	2.2%
12	Indiana	119	2.2%
37	Iowa	26	0.5%
25	Kansas	62	1.2%
36	Kentucky	32	0.6%
19	Louisiana	80	1.5%
42	Maine	17	0.3%
3	Maryland	361	6.8%
24	Massachusetts	64	1.2%
17	Michigan	89	1.7%
27	Minnesota	55	1.0%
22	Mississippi	66	1.2%
14	Missouri	105	2.0%
42	Montana	17	0.3%
32	Nebraska	47	0.9%
28	Nevada	52	1.0%
39	New Hampshire	23	0.4%
7	New Jersey	228	4.3%
40	New Mexico	19	0.4%
16	New York	100	1.9%
18	North Carolina	84	1.6%
45	North Dakota	13	0.2%
9	Ohio	200	3.8%
31	Oklahoma	50	0.9%
19	Oregon	80	1.5%
6	Pennsylvania	235	4.4%
45	Rhode Island	13	0.2%
21	South Carolina	70	1.3%
44	South Dakota	16	0.3%
11	Tennessee	147	2.8%
4	Texas	359	6.8%
34	Utah	44	0.8%
50	Vermont	1	0.0%
28	Virginia	52	1.0%
8	Washington	223	4.2%
48	West Virginia	11	0.2%
23	Wisconsin	65	1.2%
40	Wyoming	19	0.4%

RANK ORDER

RANK	STATE	CENTERS	% of USA
1	California	749	14.1%
2	Florida	402	7.6%
3	Maryland	361	6.8%
4	Texas	359	6.8%
5	Georgia	283	5.3%
6	Pennsylvania	235	4.4%
7	New Jersey	228	4.3%
8	Washington	223	4.2%
9	Ohio	200	3.8%
10	Arizona	152	2.9%
11	Tennessee	147	2.8%
12	Indiana	119	2.2%
13	Illinois	118	2.2%
14	Missouri	105	2.0%
15	Colorado	104	2.0%
16	New York	100	1.9%
17	Michigan	89	1.7%
18	North Carolina	84	1.6%
19	Louisiana	80	1.5%
19	Oregon	80	1.5%
21	South Carolina	70	1.3%
22	Mississippi	66	1.2%
23	Wisconsin	65	1.2%
24	Massachusetts	64	1.2%
25	Kansas	62	1.2%
26	Arkansas	60	1.1%
27	Minnesota	55	1.0%
28	Nevada	52	1.0%
28	Virginia	52	1.0%
30	Idaho	51	1.0%
31	Oklahoma	50	0.9%
32	Nebraska	47	0.9%
33	Connecticut	45	0.8%
34	Utah	44	0.8%
35	Alabama	40	0.8%
36	Kentucky	32	0.6%
37	Iowa	26	0.5%
38	Delaware	25	0.5%
39	New Hampshire	23	0.4%
40	New Mexico	19	0.4%
40	Wyoming	19	0.4%
42	Maine	17	0.3%
42	Montana	17	0.3%
44	South Dakota	16	0.3%
45	Hawaii	13	0.2%
45	North Dakota	13	0.2%
45	Rhode Island	13	0.2%
48	West Virginia	11	0.2%
49	Alaska	10	0.2%
50	Vermont	1	0.0%
	District of Columbia	4	0.1%

Source: U.S. Department of Health and Human Services, Centers for Medicare and Medicaid Services
OSCAR Report 10 (January 24, 2011)

*Certified by CMS to participate in the Medicare/Medicaid programs. Excludes licensed facilities that do not accept federal funding and facilities managed by the Department of Veterans Affairs. National total does not include 21 certified outpatient surgery centers in U.S. territories. Also known as Ambulatory Surgical Centers.

Medicare and Medicaid Certified Community Mental Health Centers in 2011

National Total = 629 Centers*

ALPHA ORDER				RANK ORDER			
RANK	STATE	CENTERS	% of USA	RANK	STATE	CENTERS	% of USA
2	Alabama	61	9.7%	1	Florida	139	22.1%
40	Alaska	0	0.0%	2	Alabama	61	9.7%
30	Arizona	3	0.5%	3	Louisiana	54	8.6%
14	Arkansas	13	2.1%	4	Texas	43	6.8%
7	California	20	3.2%	5	New Jersey	25	4.0%
11	Colorado	14	2.2%	5	Washington	25	4.0%
27	Connecticut	5	0.8%	7	California	20	3.2%
40	Delaware	0	0.0%	7	North Carolina	20	3.2%
1	Florida	139	22.1%	9	Tennessee	19	3.0%
20	Georgia	10	1.6%	10	Pennsylvania	16	2.5%
40	Hawaii	0	0.0%	11	Colorado	14	2.2%
40	Idaho	0	0.0%	11	Minnesota	14	2.2%
18	Illinois	11	1.7%	11	New Mexico	14	2.2%
25	Indiana	7	1.1%	14	Arkansas	13	2.1%
27	Iowa	5	0.8%	14	Ohio	13	2.1%
23	Kansas	8	1.3%	16	Massachusetts	12	1.9%
21	Kentucky	9	1.4%	16	Oregon	12	1.9%
3	Louisiana	54	8.6%	18	Illinois	11	1.7%
40	Maine	0	0.0%	18	Missouri	11	1.7%
33	Maryland	2	0.3%	20	Georgia	10	1.6%
16	Massachusetts	12	1.9%	21	Kentucky	9	1.4%
25	Michigan	7	1.1%	21	Mississippi	9	1.4%
11	Minnesota	14	2.2%	23	Kansas	8	1.3%
21	Mississippi	9	1.4%	23	Oklahoma	8	1.3%
18	Missouri	11	1.7%	25	Indiana	7	1.1%
40	Montana	0	0.0%	25	Michigan	7	1.1%
38	Nebraska	1	0.2%	27	Connecticut	5	0.8%
33	Nevada	2	0.3%	27	Iowa	5	0.8%
40	New Hampshire	0	0.0%	29	New York	4	0.6%
5	New Jersey	25	4.0%	30	Arizona	3	0.5%
11	New Mexico	14	2.2%	30	South Carolina	3	0.5%
29	New York	4	0.6%	30	Wyoming	3	0.5%
7	North Carolina	20	3.2%	33	Maryland	2	0.3%
40	North Dakota	0	0.0%	33	Nevada	2	0.3%
14	Ohio	13	2.1%	33	Utah	2	0.3%
23	Oklahoma	8	1.3%	33	Virginia	2	0.3%
16	Oregon	12	1.9%	33	West Virginia	2	0.3%
10	Pennsylvania	16	2.5%	38	Nebraska	1	0.2%
40	Rhode Island	0	0.0%	38	South Dakota	1	0.2%
30	South Carolina	3	0.5%	40	Alaska	0	0.0%
38	South Dakota	1	0.2%	40	Delaware	0	0.0%
9	Tennessee	19	3.0%	40	Hawaii	0	0.0%
4	Texas	43	6.8%	40	Idaho	0	0.0%
33	Utah	2	0.3%	40	Maine	0	0.0%
40	Vermont	0	0.0%	40	Montana	0	0.0%
33	Virginia	2	0.3%	40	New Hampshire	0	0.0%
5	Washington	25	4.0%	40	North Dakota	0	0.0%
33	West Virginia	2	0.3%	40	Rhode Island	0	0.0%
40	Wisconsin	0	0.0%	40	Vermont	0	0.0%
30	Wyoming	3	0.5%	40	Wisconsin	0	0.0%
					District of Columbia	0	0.0%

Source: U.S. Department of Health and Human Services, Centers for Medicare and Medicaid Services
OSCAR Report 10 (January 24, 2011)
*Certified by CMS to participate in the Medicare/Medicaid programs. Excludes licensed facilities that do not accept federal funding and facilities managed by the Department of Veterans Affairs. National total does not include 13 certified mental health centers in U.S. territories.

Medicare and Medicaid Certified Outpatient Physical Therapy Facilities in 2011

National Total = 2,528 Facilities*

ALPHA ORDER					RANK ORDER			
RANK	STATE		FACILITIES	% of USA	RANK	STATE	FACILITIES	% of USA
26	Alabama		28	1.1%	1	Florida	319	12.6%
36	Alaska		11	0.4%	2	Texas	226	8.9%
29	Arizona		23	0.9%	3	Michigan	206	8.1%
28	Arkansas		24	0.9%	4	California	152	6.0%
4	California		152	6.0%	5	Ohio	119	4.7%
14	Colorado		54	2.1%	6	Virginia	116	4.6%
23	Connecticut		36	1.4%	7	Pennsylvania	100	4.0%
38	Delaware		9	0.4%	8	Kentucky	95	3.8%
1	Florida		319	12.6%	9	Maryland	84	3.3%
12	Georgia		73	2.9%	10	Illinois	79	3.1%
44	Hawaii		5	0.2%	11	Tennessee	74	2.9%
38	Idaho		9	0.4%	12	Georgia	73	2.9%
10	Illinois		79	3.1%	13	New Jersey	56	2.2%
14	Indiana		54	2.1%	14	Colorado	54	2.1%
24	Iowa		35	1.4%	14	Indiana	54	2.1%
29	Kansas		23	0.9%	14	Missouri	54	2.1%
8	Kentucky		95	3.8%	14	North Carolina	54	2.1%
18	Louisiana		49	1.9%	18	Louisiana	49	1.9%
34	Maine		16	0.6%	19	Oklahoma	48	1.9%
9	Maryland		84	3.3%	20	South Carolina	43	1.7%
33	Massachusetts		17	0.7%	21	Minnesota	39	1.5%
3	Michigan		206	8.1%	22	Wisconsin	37	1.5%
21	Minnesota		39	1.5%	23	Connecticut	36	1.4%
25	Mississippi		32	1.3%	24	Iowa	35	1.4%
14	Missouri		54	2.1%	25	Mississippi	32	1.3%
46	Montana		1	0.0%	26	Alabama	28	1.1%
42	Nebraska		7	0.3%	27	New Mexico	25	1.0%
31	Nevada		19	0.8%	28	Arkansas	24	0.9%
38	New Hampshire		9	0.4%	29	Arizona	23	0.9%
13	New Jersey		56	2.2%	29	Kansas	23	0.9%
27	New Mexico		25	1.0%	31	Nevada	19	0.8%
35	New York		15	0.6%	31	Washington	19	0.8%
14	North Carolina		54	2.1%	33	Massachusetts	17	0.7%
46	North Dakota		1	0.0%	34	Maine	16	0.6%
5	Ohio		119	4.7%	35	New York	15	0.6%
19	Oklahoma		48	1.9%	36	Alaska	11	0.4%
37	Oregon		10	0.4%	37	Oregon	10	0.4%
7	Pennsylvania		100	4.0%	38	Delaware	9	0.4%
45	Rhode Island		2	0.1%	38	Idaho	9	0.4%
20	South Carolina		43	1.7%	38	New Hampshire	9	0.4%
46	South Dakota		1	0.0%	38	West Virginia	9	0.4%
11	Tennessee		74	2.9%	42	Nebraska	7	0.3%
2	Texas		226	8.9%	43	Utah	6	0.2%
43	Utah		6	0.2%	44	Hawaii	5	0.2%
46	Vermont		1	0.0%	45	Rhode Island	2	0.1%
6	Virginia		116	4.6%	46	Montana	1	0.0%
31	Washington		19	0.8%	46	North Dakota	1	0.0%
38	West Virginia		9	0.4%	46	South Dakota	1	0.0%
22	Wisconsin		37	1.5%	46	Vermont	1	0.0%
46	Wyoming		1	0.0%	46	Wyoming	1	0.0%
						District of Columbia	3	0.1%

Source: U.S. Department of Health and Human Services, Centers for Medicare and Medicaid Services
OSCAR Report 10 (January 24, 2011)

*Certified by CMS to participate in the Medicare/Medicaid programs. Excludes licensed facilities that do not accept federal funding and facilities managed by the Department of Veterans Affairs. National total does not include four certified outpatient physical therapy facilities in U.S. territories.

Medicare and Medicaid Certified Rural Health Clinics in 2011

National Total = 3,849 Rural Health Clinics*

ALPHA ORDER					RANK ORDER			
RANK	STATE	CLINICS	% of USA		RANK	STATE	CLINICS	% of USA
18	Alabama	73	1.9%		1	Missouri	348	9.0%
43	Alaska	2	0.1%		2	Texas	317	8.2%
36	Arizona	17	0.4%		3	California	277	7.2%
19	Arkansas	72	1.9%		4	Illinois	221	5.7%
3	California	277	7.2%		5	Kansas	178	4.6%
26	Colorado	54	1.4%		6	Mississippi	167	4.3%
46	Connecticut	0	0.0%		7	Michigan	160	4.2%
46	Delaware	0	0.0%		8	Kentucky	149	3.9%
9	Florida	143	3.7%		9	Florida	143	3.7%
15	Georgia	89	2.3%		10	Iowa	141	3.7%
43	Hawaii	2	0.1%		11	Nebraska	135	3.5%
31	Idaho	44	1.1%		12	Washington	129	3.4%
4	Illinois	221	5.7%		13	South Carolina	111	2.9%
20	Indiana	63	1.6%		14	Louisiana	108	2.8%
10	Iowa	141	3.7%		15	Georgia	89	2.3%
5	Kansas	178	4.6%		16	North Carolina	82	2.1%
8	Kentucky	149	3.9%		17	Minnesota	81	2.1%
14	Louisiana	108	2.8%		18	Alabama	73	1.9%
33	Maine	40	1.0%		19	Arkansas	72	1.9%
46	Maryland	0	0.0%		20	Indiana	63	1.6%
45	Massachusetts	1	0.0%		21	Pennsylvania	62	1.6%
7	Michigan	160	4.2%		22	Oregon	61	1.6%
17	Minnesota	81	2.1%		23	North Dakota	58	1.5%
6	Mississippi	167	4.3%		24	South Dakota	57	1.5%
1	Missouri	348	9.0%		24	Tennessee	57	1.5%
28	Montana	52	1.4%		26	Colorado	54	1.4%
11	Nebraska	135	3.5%		26	West Virginia	54	1.4%
42	Nevada	7	0.2%		28	Montana	52	1.4%
40	New Hampshire	11	0.3%		29	Wisconsin	50	1.3%
46	New Jersey	0	0.0%		30	Virginia	49	1.3%
39	New Mexico	12	0.3%		31	Idaho	44	1.1%
41	New York	8	0.2%		32	Oklahoma	41	1.1%
16	North Carolina	82	2.1%		33	Maine	40	1.0%
23	North Dakota	58	1.5%		34	Utah	18	0.5%
37	Ohio	15	0.4%		34	Wyoming	18	0.5%
32	Oklahoma	41	1.1%		36	Arizona	17	0.4%
22	Oregon	61	1.6%		37	Ohio	15	0.4%
21	Pennsylvania	62	1.6%		37	Vermont	15	0.4%
46	Rhode Island	0	0.0%		39	New Mexico	12	0.3%
13	South Carolina	111	2.9%		40	New Hampshire	11	0.3%
24	South Dakota	57	1.5%		41	New York	8	0.2%
24	Tennessee	57	1.5%		42	Nevada	7	0.2%
2	Texas	317	8.2%		43	Alaska	2	0.1%
34	Utah	18	0.5%		43	Hawaii	2	0.1%
37	Vermont	15	0.4%		45	Massachusetts	1	0.0%
30	Virginia	49	1.3%		46	Connecticut	0	0.0%
12	Washington	129	3.4%		46	Delaware	0	0.0%
26	West Virginia	54	1.4%		46	Maryland	0	0.0%
29	Wisconsin	50	1.3%		46	New Jersey	0	0.0%
34	Wyoming	18	0.5%		46	Rhode Island	0	0.0%
						District of Columbia	0	0.0%

Source: U.S. Department of Health and Human Services, Centers for Medicare and Medicaid Services
   OSCAR Report 10 (January 24, 2011)

*Certified by CMS to participate in the Medicare/Medicaid programs. Excludes licensed facilities that do not accept federal funding and facilities managed by the Department of Veterans Affairs. There are no certified rural health centers in U.S. territories.

Medicare and Medicaid Certified Home Health Agencies in 2011

National Total = 11,443 Home Health Agencies*

ALPHA ORDER

RANK	STATE	AGENCIES	% of USA
19	Alabama	149	1.3%
48	Alaska	14	0.1%
24	Arizona	121	1.1%
16	Arkansas	171	1.5%
3	California	991	8.7%
18	Colorado	150	1.3%
29	Connecticut	84	0.7%
47	Delaware	20	0.2%
2	Florida	1,446	12.6%
25	Georgia	104	0.9%
48	Hawaii	14	0.1%
39	Idaho	46	0.4%
4	Illinois	685	6.0%
9	Indiana	237	2.1%
14	Iowa	177	1.5%
22	Kansas	131	1.1%
27	Kentucky	102	0.9%
10	Louisiana	220	1.9%
43	Maine	30	0.3%
37	Maryland	54	0.5%
20	Massachusetts	143	1.2%
5	Michigan	595	5.2%
11	Minnesota	205	1.8%
36	Mississippi	55	0.5%
15	Missouri	176	1.5%
42	Montana	33	0.3%
31	Nebraska	73	0.6%
25	Nevada	104	0.9%
41	New Hampshire	34	0.3%
38	New Jersey	51	0.4%
30	New Mexico	74	0.6%
13	New York	194	1.7%
16	North Carolina	171	1.5%
46	North Dakota	21	0.2%
6	Ohio	585	5.1%
8	Oklahoma	242	2.1%
34	Oregon	57	0.5%
7	Pennsylvania	382	3.3%
45	Rhode Island	23	0.2%
32	South Carolina	70	0.6%
40	South Dakota	39	0.3%
20	Tennessee	143	1.2%
1	Texas	2,428	21.2%
28	Utah	88	0.8%
50	Vermont	12	0.1%
12	Virginia	202	1.8%
33	Washington	59	0.5%
35	West Virginia	56	0.5%
23	Wisconsin	127	1.1%
44	Wyoming	28	0.2%

RANK ORDER

RANK	STATE	AGENCIES	% of USA
1	Texas	2,428	21.2%
2	Florida	1,446	12.6%
3	California	991	8.7%
4	Illinois	685	6.0%
5	Michigan	595	5.2%
6	Ohio	585	5.1%
7	Pennsylvania	382	3.3%
8	Oklahoma	242	2.1%
9	Indiana	237	2.1%
10	Louisiana	220	1.9%
11	Minnesota	205	1.8%
12	Virginia	202	1.8%
13	New York	194	1.7%
14	Iowa	177	1.5%
15	Missouri	176	1.5%
16	Arkansas	171	1.5%
16	North Carolina	171	1.5%
18	Colorado	150	1.3%
19	Alabama	149	1.3%
20	Massachusetts	143	1.2%
20	Tennessee	143	1.2%
22	Kansas	131	1.1%
23	Wisconsin	127	1.1%
24	Arizona	121	1.1%
25	Georgia	104	0.9%
25	Nevada	104	0.9%
27	Kentucky	102	0.9%
28	Utah	88	0.8%
29	Connecticut	84	0.7%
30	New Mexico	74	0.6%
31	Nebraska	73	0.6%
32	South Carolina	70	0.6%
33	Washington	59	0.5%
34	Oregon	57	0.5%
35	West Virginia	56	0.5%
36	Mississippi	55	0.5%
37	Maryland	54	0.5%
38	New Jersey	51	0.4%
39	Idaho	46	0.4%
40	South Dakota	39	0.3%
41	New Hampshire	34	0.3%
42	Montana	33	0.3%
43	Maine	30	0.3%
44	Wyoming	28	0.2%
45	Rhode Island	23	0.2%
46	North Dakota	21	0.2%
47	Delaware	20	0.2%
48	Alaska	14	0.1%
48	Hawaii	14	0.1%
50	Vermont	12	0.1%
	District of Columbia	27	0.2%

Source: U.S. Department of Health and Human Services, Centers for Medicare and Medicaid Services
    OSCAR Report 10 (January 24, 2011)

*Certified by CMS to participate in the Medicare/Medicaid programs. Excludes agencies that do not accept federal funding. National total does not include 52 certified home health agencies in U.S. territories. A home health agency provides health services to individuals in their homes for the purpose of promoting, maintaining, or restoring health or maximizing the level of independence, while minimizing the effects of disability and illness.

Medicare and Medicaid Certified Hospices in 2011

National Total = 3,481 Hospices*

ALPHA ORDER

RANK	STATE	HOSPICES	% of USA
8	Alabama	120	3.4%
50	Alaska	3	0.1%
21	Arizona	66	1.9%
26	Arkansas	52	1.5%
2	California	275	7.9%
26	Colorado	52	1.5%
34	Connecticut	32	0.9%
47	Delaware	9	0.3%
31	Florida	41	1.2%
4	Georgia	151	4.3%
47	Hawaii	9	0.3%
30	Idaho	42	1.2%
12	Illinois	101	2.9%
16	Indiana	82	2.4%
13	Iowa	83	2.4%
23	Kansas	59	1.7%
38	Kentucky	24	0.7%
6	Louisiana	133	3.8%
40	Maine	20	0.6%
37	Maryland	27	0.8%
19	Massachusetts	71	2.0%
10	Michigan	103	3.0%
21	Minnesota	66	1.9%
7	Mississippi	121	3.5%
11	Missouri	102	2.9%
36	Montana	29	0.8%
33	Nebraska	35	1.0%
40	Nevada	20	0.6%
39	New Hampshire	22	0.6%
24	New Jersey	58	1.7%
32	New Mexico	39	1.1%
28	New York	49	1.4%
13	North Carolina	83	2.4%
45	North Dakota	14	0.4%
9	Ohio	116	3.3%
5	Oklahoma	144	4.1%
29	Oregon	47	1.4%
3	Pennsylvania	177	5.1%
49	Rhode Island	8	0.2%
13	South Carolina	83	2.4%
44	South Dakota	15	0.4%
25	Tennessee	56	1.6%
1	Texas	342	9.8%
18	Utah	72	2.1%
46	Vermont	10	0.3%
17	Virginia	76	2.2%
34	Washington	32	0.9%
40	West Virginia	20	0.6%
20	Wisconsin	67	1.9%
43	Wyoming	19	0.5%

RANK ORDER

RANK	STATE	HOSPICES	% of USA
1	Texas	342	9.8%
2	California	275	7.9%
3	Pennsylvania	177	5.1%
4	Georgia	151	4.3%
5	Oklahoma	144	4.1%
6	Louisiana	133	3.8%
7	Mississippi	121	3.5%
8	Alabama	120	3.4%
9	Ohio	116	3.3%
10	Michigan	103	3.0%
11	Missouri	102	2.9%
12	Illinois	101	2.9%
13	Iowa	83	2.4%
13	North Carolina	83	2.4%
13	South Carolina	83	2.4%
16	Indiana	82	2.4%
17	Virginia	76	2.2%
18	Utah	72	2.1%
19	Massachusetts	71	2.0%
20	Wisconsin	67	1.9%
21	Arizona	66	1.9%
21	Minnesota	66	1.9%
23	Kansas	59	1.7%
24	New Jersey	58	1.7%
25	Tennessee	56	1.6%
26	Arkansas	52	1.5%
26	Colorado	52	1.5%
28	New York	49	1.4%
29	Oregon	47	1.4%
30	Idaho	42	1.2%
31	Florida	41	1.2%
32	New Mexico	39	1.1%
33	Nebraska	35	1.0%
34	Connecticut	32	0.9%
34	Washington	32	0.9%
36	Montana	29	0.8%
37	Maryland	27	0.8%
38	Kentucky	24	0.7%
39	New Hampshire	22	0.6%
40	Maine	20	0.6%
40	Nevada	20	0.6%
40	West Virginia	20	0.6%
43	Wyoming	19	0.5%
44	South Dakota	15	0.4%
45	North Dakota	14	0.4%
46	Vermont	10	0.3%
47	Delaware	9	0.3%
47	Hawaii	9	0.3%
49	Rhode Island	8	0.2%
50	Alaska	3	0.1%
	District of Columbia	4	0.1%

Source: U.S. Department of Health and Human Services, Centers for Medicare and Medicaid Services
  OSCAR Report 10 (January 24, 2011)
*Certified by CMS to participate in the Medicare/Medicaid programs. Excludes licensed facilities that do not accept federal funding and facilities managed by the Department of Veterans Affairs. National total does not include 41 certified hospices in U.S. territories. A hospice provides specialized services for terminally ill people and their families.

Hospice Patients in Residential Facilities in 2011

National Total = 91,126 Patients*

ALPHA ORDER

RANK	STATE	PATIENTS	% of USA
19	Alabama	1,524	1.7%
50	Alaska	4	0.0%
10	Arizona	2,902	3.2%
35	Arkansas	588	0.6%
6	California	4,059	4.5%
28	Colorado	1,075	1.2%
26	Connecticut	1,149	1.3%
41	Delaware	428	0.5%
1	Florida	8,815	9.7%
7	Georgia	3,446	3.8%
47	Hawaii	58	0.1%
46	Idaho	189	0.2%
5	Illinois	4,341	4.8%
14	Indiana	2,146	2.4%
24	Iowa	1,263	1.4%
29	Kansas	869	1.0%
33	Kentucky	619	0.7%
30	Louisiana	844	0.9%
18	Maine	1,622	1.8%
34	Maryland	603	0.7%
12	Massachusetts	2,542	2.8%
8	Michigan	3,289	3.6%
16	Minnesota	1,904	2.1%
36	Mississippi	532	0.6%
11	Missouri	2,620	2.9%
31	Montana	833	0.9%
37	Nebraska	530	0.6%
45	Nevada	193	0.2%
39	New Hampshire	446	0.5%
23	New Jersey	1,333	1.5%
42	New Mexico	414	0.5%
20	New York	1,505	1.7%
9	North Carolina	2,931	3.2%
43	North Dakota	237	0.3%
4	Ohio	6,228	6.8%
15	Oklahoma	1,965	2.2%
17	Oregon	1,844	2.0%
2	Pennsylvania	7,800	8.6%
27	Rhode Island	1,143	1.3%
32	South Carolina	783	0.9%
38	South Dakota	456	0.5%
22	Tennessee	1,340	1.5%
3	Texas	7,730	8.5%
40	Utah	435	0.5%
48	Vermont	55	0.1%
25	Virginia	1,217	1.3%
21	Washington	1,467	1.6%
44	West Virginia	210	0.2%
13	Wisconsin	2,450	2.7%
49	Wyoming	44	0.0%

RANK ORDER

RANK	STATE	PATIENTS	% of USA
1	Florida	8,815	9.7%
2	Pennsylvania	7,800	8.6%
3	Texas	7,730	8.5%
4	Ohio	6,228	6.8%
5	Illinois	4,341	4.8%
6	California	4,059	4.5%
7	Georgia	3,446	3.8%
8	Michigan	3,289	3.6%
9	North Carolina	2,931	3.2%
10	Arizona	2,902	3.2%
11	Missouri	2,620	2.9%
12	Massachusetts	2,542	2.8%
13	Wisconsin	2,450	2.7%
14	Indiana	2,146	2.4%
15	Oklahoma	1,965	2.2%
16	Minnesota	1,904	2.1%
17	Oregon	1,844	2.0%
18	Maine	1,622	1.8%
19	Alabama	1,524	1.7%
20	New York	1,505	1.7%
21	Washington	1,467	1.6%
22	Tennessee	1,340	1.5%
23	New Jersey	1,333	1.5%
24	Iowa	1,263	1.4%
25	Virginia	1,217	1.3%
26	Connecticut	1,149	1.3%
27	Rhode Island	1,143	1.3%
28	Colorado	1,075	1.2%
29	Kansas	869	1.0%
30	Louisiana	844	0.9%
31	Montana	833	0.9%
32	South Carolina	783	0.9%
33	Kentucky	619	0.7%
34	Maryland	603	0.7%
35	Arkansas	588	0.6%
36	Mississippi	532	0.6%
37	Nebraska	530	0.6%
38	South Dakota	456	0.5%
39	New Hampshire	446	0.5%
40	Utah	435	0.5%
41	Delaware	428	0.5%
42	New Mexico	414	0.5%
43	North Dakota	237	0.3%
44	West Virginia	210	0.2%
45	Nevada	193	0.2%
46	Idaho	189	0.2%
47	Hawaii	58	0.1%
48	Vermont	55	0.1%
49	Wyoming	44	0.0%
50	Alaska	4	0.0%
	District of Columbia	106	0.1%

Source: U.S. Department of Health and Human Services, Centers for Medicare and Medicaid Services
CASPER Report 10B (January 06, 2010)

*Patients in facilities certified by CMS to participate in the Medicare/Medicaid programs. Excludes licensed facilities that do not accept federal funding and facilities managed by the Department of Veterans Affairs. National total does not include 50 patients in U.S. territories. A hospice provides specialized services for terminally ill people and their families.

Medicare and Medicaid Certified Nursing Care Facilities in 2011

National Total = 15,700 Nursing Care Facilities*

ALPHA ORDER					RANK ORDER			
RANK	STATE	FACILITIES	% of USA		RANK	STATE	FACILITIES	% of USA
28	Alabama	227	1.4%		1	California	1,239	7.9%
50	Alaska	15	0.1%		2	Texas	1,173	7.5%
33	Arizona	139	0.9%		3	Ohio	962	6.1%
25	Arkansas	233	1.5%		4	Illinois	785	5.0%
1	California	1,239	7.9%		5	Pennsylvania	710	4.5%
30	Colorado	213	1.4%		6	Florida	679	4.3%
24	Connecticut	239	1.5%		7	New York	635	4.0%
47	Delaware	47	0.3%		8	Missouri	514	3.3%
6	Florida	679	4.3%		9	Indiana	506	3.2%
16	Georgia	361	2.3%		10	Iowa	443	2.8%
46	Hawaii	48	0.3%		11	Michigan	428	2.7%
42	Idaho	79	0.5%		12	Massachusetts	427	2.7%
4	Illinois	785	5.0%		13	North Carolina	424	2.7%
9	Indiana	506	3.2%		14	Wisconsin	392	2.5%
10	Iowa	443	2.8%		15	Minnesota	385	2.5%
18	Kansas	343	2.2%		16	Georgia	361	2.3%
22	Kentucky	285	1.8%		16	New Jersey	361	2.3%
23	Louisiana	281	1.8%		18	Kansas	343	2.2%
37	Maine	109	0.7%		19	Tennessee	320	2.0%
26	Maryland	231	1.5%		20	Oklahoma	315	2.0%
12	Massachusetts	427	2.7%		21	Virginia	286	1.8%
11	Michigan	428	2.7%		22	Kentucky	285	1.8%
15	Minnesota	385	2.5%		23	Louisiana	281	1.8%
31	Mississippi	203	1.3%		24	Connecticut	239	1.5%
8	Missouri	514	3.3%		25	Arkansas	233	1.5%
39	Montana	87	0.6%		26	Maryland	231	1.5%
29	Nebraska	222	1.4%		27	Washington	229	1.5%
45	Nevada	50	0.3%		28	Alabama	227	1.4%
43	New Hampshire	78	0.5%		29	Nebraska	222	1.4%
16	New Jersey	361	2.3%		30	Colorado	213	1.4%
44	New Mexico	70	0.4%		31	Mississippi	203	1.3%
7	New York	635	4.0%		32	South Carolina	185	1.2%
13	North Carolina	424	2.7%		33	Arizona	139	0.9%
41	North Dakota	85	0.5%		34	Oregon	137	0.9%
3	Ohio	962	6.1%		35	West Virginia	127	0.8%
20	Oklahoma	315	2.0%		36	South Dakota	110	0.7%
34	Oregon	137	0.9%		37	Maine	109	0.7%
5	Pennsylvania	710	4.5%		38	Utah	100	0.6%
40	Rhode Island	86	0.5%		39	Montana	87	0.6%
32	South Carolina	185	1.2%		40	Rhode Island	86	0.5%
36	South Dakota	110	0.7%		41	North Dakota	85	0.5%
19	Tennessee	320	2.0%		42	Idaho	79	0.5%
2	Texas	1,173	7.5%		43	New Hampshire	78	0.5%
38	Utah	100	0.6%		44	New Mexico	70	0.4%
48	Vermont	40	0.3%		45	Nevada	50	0.3%
21	Virginia	286	1.8%		46	Hawaii	48	0.3%
27	Washington	229	1.5%		47	Delaware	47	0.3%
35	West Virginia	127	0.8%		48	Vermont	40	0.3%
14	Wisconsin	392	2.5%		49	Wyoming	38	0.2%
49	Wyoming	38	0.2%		50	Alaska	15	0.1%
						District of Columbia	19	0.1%

Source: U.S. Department of Health and Human Services, Centers for Medicare and Medicaid Services
CASPER Report 10B (January 06, 2010)
*Certified by CMS to participate in the Medicare/Medicaid programs. Excludes licensed facilities that do not accept federal funding and facilities managed by the Department of Veterans Affairs. National total does not include nine certified nursing facilities in U.S. territories.

Beds in Medicare and Medicaid Certified Nursing Care Facilities in 2011

National Total = 1,672,440 Beds*

ALPHA ORDER					RANK ORDER			
RANK	STATE	BEDS	% of USA		RANK	STATE	BEDS	% of USA
24	Alabama	26,604	1.6%		1	Texas	127,277	7.6%
50	Alaska	682	0.0%		2	California	120,728	7.2%
32	Arizona	16,096	1.0%		3	New York	117,994	7.1%
26	Arkansas	24,439	1.5%		4	Illinois	96,178	5.8%
2	California	120,728	7.2%		5	Ohio	92,860	5.6%
29	Colorado	20,290	1.2%		6	Pennsylvania	88,801	5.3%
21	Connecticut	28,831	1.7%		7	Florida	82,056	4.9%
46	Delaware	4,911	0.3%		8	Missouri	52,196	3.1%
7	Florida	82,056	4.9%		9	New Jersey	51,118	3.1%
14	Georgia	39,989	2.4%		10	Indiana	49,077	2.9%
47	Hawaii	4,175	0.2%		11	Massachusetts	48,438	2.9%
44	Idaho	6,153	0.4%		12	Michigan	46,897	2.8%
4	Illinois	96,178	5.8%		13	North Carolina	43,688	2.6%
10	Indiana	49,077	2.9%		14	Georgia	39,989	2.4%
20	Iowa	31,714	1.9%		15	Tennessee	37,150	2.2%
27	Kansas	23,078	1.4%		16	Wisconsin	35,952	2.1%
25	Kentucky	25,945	1.6%		17	Louisiana	34,965	2.1%
17	Louisiana	34,965	2.1%		18	Minnesota	32,178	1.9%
40	Maine	7,109	0.4%		19	Virginia	31,875	1.9%
23	Maryland	28,687	1.7%		20	Iowa	31,714	1.9%
11	Massachusetts	48,438	2.9%		21	Connecticut	28,831	1.7%
12	Michigan	46,897	2.8%		22	Oklahoma	28,739	1.7%
18	Minnesota	32,178	1.9%		23	Maryland	28,687	1.7%
31	Mississippi	18,583	1.1%		24	Alabama	26,604	1.6%
8	Missouri	52,196	3.1%		25	Kentucky	25,945	1.6%
41	Montana	6,976	0.4%		26	Arkansas	24,439	1.5%
33	Nebraska	15,731	0.9%		27	Kansas	23,078	1.4%
45	Nevada	5,862	0.4%		28	Washington	21,785	1.3%
39	New Hampshire	7,673	0.5%		29	Colorado	20,290	1.2%
9	New Jersey	51,118	3.1%		30	South Carolina	18,864	1.1%
42	New Mexico	6,767	0.4%		31	Mississippi	18,583	1.1%
3	New York	117,994	7.1%		32	Arizona	16,096	1.0%
13	North Carolina	43,688	2.6%		33	Nebraska	15,731	0.9%
43	North Dakota	6,438	0.4%		34	Oregon	12,208	0.7%
5	Ohio	92,860	5.6%		35	West Virginia	10,768	0.6%
22	Oklahoma	28,739	1.7%		36	Rhode Island	8,784	0.5%
34	Oregon	12,208	0.7%		37	Utah	8,258	0.5%
6	Pennsylvania	88,801	5.3%		38	South Dakota	7,927	0.5%
36	Rhode Island	8,784	0.5%		39	New Hampshire	7,673	0.5%
30	South Carolina	18,864	1.1%		40	Maine	7,109	0.4%
38	South Dakota	7,927	0.5%		41	Montana	6,976	0.4%
15	Tennessee	37,150	2.2%		42	New Mexico	6,767	0.4%
1	Texas	127,277	7.6%		43	North Dakota	6,438	0.4%
37	Utah	8,258	0.5%		44	Idaho	6,153	0.4%
48	Vermont	3,266	0.2%		45	Nevada	5,862	0.4%
19	Virginia	31,875	1.9%		46	Delaware	4,911	0.3%
28	Washington	21,785	1.3%		47	Hawaii	4,175	0.2%
35	West Virginia	10,768	0.6%		48	Vermont	3,266	0.2%
16	Wisconsin	35,952	2.1%		49	Wyoming	2,965	0.2%
49	Wyoming	2,965	0.2%		50	Alaska	682	0.0%
						District of Columbia	2,715	0.2%

Source: U.S. Department of Health and Human Services, Centers for Medicare and Medicaid Services
CASPER Report 10B (January 06, 2010)

*Beds in nursing care facilities certified by CMS to participate in the Medicare/Medicaid programs. National total does not include 351 beds in U.S. territories.

Rate of Beds in Medicare and Medicaid Certified Nursing Care Facilities in 2011

National Rate = 297 Beds per 1,000 Population 85 Years and Older*

ALPHA ORDER

RANK	STATE	RATE
23	Alabama	324
48	Alaska	144
49	Arizona	134
3	Arkansas	428
42	California	200
30	Colorado	301
13	Connecticut	374
28	Delaware	303
47	Florida	159
22	Georgia	334
50	Hawaii	131
41	Idaho	244
7	Illinois	412
5	Indiana	417
6	Iowa	416
12	Kansas	381
16	Kentucky	355
1	Louisiana	497
39	Maine	250
24	Maryland	321
20	Massachusetts	342
38	Michigan	256
28	Minnesota	303
14	Mississippi	372
2	Missouri	437
18	Montana	346
9	Nebraska	398
45	Nevada	181
26	New Hampshire	310
31	New Jersey	297
43	New Mexico	194
27	New York	305
32	North Carolina	293
15	North Dakota	371
8	Ohio	408
4	Oklahoma	419
46	Oregon	164
33	Pennsylvania	287
19	Rhode Island	345
40	South Carolina	246
10	South Dakota	392
17	Tennessee	354
11	Texas	385
37	Utah	257
36	Vermont	262
35	Virginia	267
44	Washington	193
34	West Virginia	282
25	Wisconsin	313
21	Wyoming	337

RANK ORDER

RANK	STATE	RATE
1	Louisiana	497
2	Missouri	437
3	Arkansas	428
4	Oklahoma	419
5	Indiana	417
6	Iowa	416
7	Illinois	412
8	Ohio	408
9	Nebraska	398
10	South Dakota	392
11	Texas	385
12	Kansas	381
13	Connecticut	374
14	Mississippi	372
15	North Dakota	371
16	Kentucky	355
17	Tennessee	354
18	Montana	346
19	Rhode Island	345
20	Massachusetts	342
21	Wyoming	337
22	Georgia	334
23	Alabama	324
24	Maryland	321
25	Wisconsin	313
26	New Hampshire	310
27	New York	305
28	Delaware	303
28	Minnesota	303
30	Colorado	301
31	New Jersey	297
32	North Carolina	293
33	Pennsylvania	287
34	West Virginia	282
35	Virginia	267
36	Vermont	262
37	Utah	257
38	Michigan	256
39	Maine	250
40	South Carolina	246
41	Idaho	244
42	California	200
43	New Mexico	194
44	Washington	193
45	Nevada	181
46	Oregon	164
47	Florida	159
48	Alaska	144
49	Arizona	134
50	Hawaii	131

District of Columbia	280

Source: CQ Press using data from U.S. Department of Health and Human Services, Centers for Medicare and Medicaid Services
CASPER Report 10B (January 06, 2010)

*Beds in nursing care facilities certified by CMS to participate in the Medicare/Medicaid programs. National rate does not include beds or population in U.S. territories. Calculated using 2009 Census population estimates.

Nursing Home Occupancy Rate in 2009

National Rate = 82.2% of Beds in Nursing Homes Occupied

ALPHA ORDER

RANK	STATE	RATE
23	Alabama	86.3
17	Alaska	88.4
38	Arizona	74.1
41	Arkansas	72.9
30	California	84.4
34	Colorado	82.0
13	Connecticut	89.6
25	Delaware	85.9
20	Florida	87.5
21	Georgia	87.3
7	Hawaii	90.6
43	Idaho	71.6
38	Illinois	74.1
46	Indiana	68.2
37	Iowa	77.5
40	Kansas	74.0
11	Kentucky	89.7
44	Louisiana	70.4
3	Maine	91.2
24	Maryland	86.0
19	Massachusetts	88.0
28	Michigan	85.3
2	Minnesota	91.3
18	Mississippi	88.3
47	Missouri	67.9
42	Montana	72.0
36	Nebraska	77.9
33	Nevada	82.2
11	New Hampshire	89.7
14	New Jersey	89.5
32	New Mexico	82.4
9	New York	90.2
29	North Carolina	85.2
5	North Dakota	91.1
25	Ohio	85.9
49	Oklahoma	65.6
50	Oregon	62.6
6	Pennsylvania	90.7
3	Rhode Island	91.2
10	South Carolina	89.9
1	South Dakota	93.9
27	Tennessee	85.7
45	Texas	70.2
48	Utah	66.8
8	Vermont	90.5
15	Virginia	88.8
31	Washington	82.5
16	West Virginia	88.7
22	Wisconsin	86.7
35	Wyoming	80.0

RANK ORDER

RANK	STATE	RATE
1	South Dakota	93.9
2	Minnesota	91.3
3	Maine	91.2
3	Rhode Island	91.2
5	North Dakota	91.1
6	Pennsylvania	90.7
7	Hawaii	90.6
8	Vermont	90.5
9	New York	90.2
10	South Carolina	89.9
11	Kentucky	89.7
11	New Hampshire	89.7
13	Connecticut	89.6
14	New Jersey	89.5
15	Virginia	88.8
16	West Virginia	88.7
17	Alaska	88.4
18	Mississippi	88.3
19	Massachusetts	88.0
20	Florida	87.5
21	Georgia	87.3
22	Wisconsin	86.7
23	Alabama	86.3
24	Maryland	86.0
25	Delaware	85.9
25	Ohio	85.9
27	Tennessee	85.7
28	Michigan	85.3
29	North Carolina	85.2
30	California	84.4
31	Washington	82.5
32	New Mexico	82.4
33	Nevada	82.2
34	Colorado	82.0
35	Wyoming	80.0
36	Nebraska	77.9
37	Iowa	77.5
38	Arizona	74.1
38	Illinois	74.1
40	Kansas	74.0
41	Arkansas	72.9
42	Montana	72.0
43	Idaho	71.6
44	Louisiana	70.4
45	Texas	70.2
46	Indiana	68.2
47	Missouri	67.9
48	Utah	66.8
49	Oklahoma	65.6
50	Oregon	62.6
	District of Columbia	91.5

Source: U.S. Department of Health and Human Services, Centers for Medicare and Medicaid Services
"Health, United States, 2009" web update (www.cdc.gov/nchs/data/hus/hus09.pdf)

Nursing Home Resident Rate in 2009

National Rate = 249 Residents per 1,000 Population Age 85 and Older*

ALPHA ORDER

RANK	STATE	RATE
20	Alabama	283
47	Alaska	133
50	Arizona	99
15	Arkansas	312
41	California	171
34	Colorado	242
3	Connecticut	341
29	Delaware	263
46	Florida	139
18	Georgia	292
48	Hawaii	121
40	Idaho	175
8	Illinois	324
5	Indiana	333
4	Iowa	339
12	Kansas	315
10	Kentucky	319
1	Louisiana	357
37	Maine	228
23	Maryland	280
16	Massachusetts	305
39	Michigan	220
20	Minnesota	283
7	Mississippi	326
12	Missouri	315
31	Montana	252
10	Nebraska	319
45	Nevada	145
22	New Hampshire	281
28	New Jersey	266
44	New Mexico	160
19	New York	284
31	North Carolina	252
5	North Dakota	333
2	Ohio	353
23	Oklahoma	280
49	Oregon	104
30	Pennsylvania	261
12	Rhode Island	315
38	South Carolina	224
9	South Dakota	321
17	Tennessee	304
26	Texas	274
42	Utah	167
35	Vermont	239
36	Virginia	238
43	Washington	161
31	West Virginia	252
25	Wisconsin	275
27	Wyoming	270

RANK ORDER

RANK	STATE	RATE
1	Louisiana	357
2	Ohio	353
3	Connecticut	341
4	Iowa	339
5	Indiana	333
5	North Dakota	333
7	Mississippi	326
8	Illinois	324
9	South Dakota	321
10	Kentucky	319
10	Nebraska	319
12	Kansas	315
12	Missouri	315
12	Rhode Island	315
15	Arkansas	312
16	Massachusetts	305
17	Tennessee	304
18	Georgia	292
19	New York	284
20	Alabama	283
20	Minnesota	283
22	New Hampshire	281
23	Maryland	280
23	Oklahoma	280
25	Wisconsin	275
26	Texas	274
27	Wyoming	270
28	New Jersey	266
29	Delaware	263
30	Pennsylvania	261
31	Montana	252
31	North Carolina	252
31	West Virginia	252
34	Colorado	242
35	Vermont	239
36	Virginia	238
37	Maine	228
38	South Carolina	224
39	Michigan	220
40	Idaho	175
41	California	171
42	Utah	167
43	Washington	161
44	New Mexico	160
45	Nevada	145
46	Florida	139
47	Alaska	133
48	Hawaii	121
49	Oregon	104
50	Arizona	99

	District of Columbia	261

Source: CQ Press using data from U.S. Department of Health and Human Services, Centers for Medicare and Medicaid Services
"Health, United States, 2009" web update (www.cdc.gov/nchs/data/hus/hus09.pdf)
*Number of nursing home residents (all ages) per 1,000 resident population 85 years of age and over.

Nursing Home Population in 2009

National Total = 1,401,718

ALPHA ORDER

RANK	STATE	POPULATION	% of USA
24	Alabama	23,186	1.7%
50	Alaska	633	0.0%
33	Arizona	11,908	0.8%
28	Arkansas	17,801	1.3%
2	California	102,747	7.3%
31	Colorado	16,288	1.2%
19	Connecticut	26,253	1.9%
46	Delaware	4,256	0.3%
7	Florida	71,657	5.1%
14	Georgia	34,899	2.5%
47	Hawaii	3,841	0.3%
45	Idaho	4,419	0.3%
6	Illinois	75,673	5.4%
11	Indiana	39,190	2.8%
20	Iowa	25,814	1.8%
26	Kansas	19,029	1.4%
23	Kentucky	23,318	1.7%
21	Louisiana	25,077	1.8%
38	Maine	6,485	0.5%
22	Maryland	25,025	1.8%
9	Massachusetts	43,227	3.1%
10	Michigan	40,306	2.9%
17	Minnesota	30,073	2.1%
30	Mississippi	16,294	1.2%
12	Missouri	37,588	2.7%
43	Montana	5,077	0.4%
32	Nebraska	12,627	0.9%
44	Nevada	4,699	0.3%
37	New Hampshire	6,941	0.5%
8	New Jersey	45,788	3.3%
41	New Mexico	5,569	0.4%
1	New York	109,867	7.8%
13	North Carolina	37,587	2.7%
40	North Dakota	5,777	0.4%
5	Ohio	80,185	5.7%
25	Oklahoma	19,209	1.4%
36	Oregon	7,708	0.5%
4	Pennsylvania	80,562	5.7%
35	Rhode Island	8,040	0.6%
29	South Carolina	17,148	1.2%
39	South Dakota	6,476	0.5%
15	Tennessee	31,876	2.3%
3	Texas	90,534	6.5%
42	Utah	5,358	0.4%
48	Vermont	2,980	0.2%
18	Virginia	28,392	2.0%
27	Washington	18,188	1.3%
34	West Virginia	9,613	0.7%
16	Wisconsin	31,619	2.3%
49	Wyoming	2,380	0.2%

RANK ORDER

RANK	STATE	POPULATION	% of USA
1	New York	109,867	7.8%
2	California	102,747	7.3%
3	Texas	90,534	6.5%
4	Pennsylvania	80,562	5.7%
5	Ohio	80,185	5.7%
6	Illinois	75,673	5.4%
7	Florida	71,657	5.1%
8	New Jersey	45,788	3.3%
9	Massachusetts	43,227	3.1%
10	Michigan	40,306	2.9%
11	Indiana	39,190	2.8%
12	Missouri	37,588	2.7%
13	North Carolina	37,587	2.7%
14	Georgia	34,899	2.5%
15	Tennessee	31,876	2.3%
16	Wisconsin	31,619	2.3%
17	Minnesota	30,073	2.1%
18	Virginia	28,392	2.0%
19	Connecticut	26,253	1.9%
20	Iowa	25,814	1.8%
21	Louisiana	25,077	1.8%
22	Maryland	25,025	1.8%
23	Kentucky	23,318	1.7%
24	Alabama	23,186	1.7%
25	Oklahoma	19,209	1.4%
26	Kansas	19,029	1.4%
27	Washington	18,188	1.3%
28	Arkansas	17,801	1.3%
29	South Carolina	17,148	1.2%
30	Mississippi	16,294	1.2%
31	Colorado	16,288	1.2%
32	Nebraska	12,627	0.9%
33	Arizona	11,908	0.8%
34	West Virginia	9,613	0.7%
35	Rhode Island	8,040	0.6%
36	Oregon	7,708	0.5%
37	New Hampshire	6,941	0.5%
38	Maine	6,485	0.5%
39	South Dakota	6,476	0.5%
40	North Dakota	5,777	0.4%
41	New Mexico	5,569	0.4%
42	Utah	5,358	0.4%
43	Montana	5,077	0.4%
44	Nevada	4,699	0.3%
45	Idaho	4,419	0.3%
46	Delaware	4,256	0.3%
47	Hawaii	3,841	0.3%
48	Vermont	2,980	0.2%
49	Wyoming	2,380	0.2%
50	Alaska	633	0.0%
	District of Columbia	2,531	0.2%

Source: U.S. Department of Health and Human Services, Centers for Medicare and Medicaid Services
"Health, United States, 2009" web update (www.cdc.gov/nchs/data/hus/hus09.pdf)

Health Care Establishments in 2008

National Total = 635,808 Establishments*

ALPHA ORDER					RANK ORDER			
RANK	STATE	ESTABLISH'S	% of USA		RANK	STATE	ESTABLISH'S	% of USA
27	Alabama	8,207	1.3%		1	California	81,493	12.8%
46	Alaska	1,657	0.3%		2	Texas	46,307	7.3%
15	Arizona	13,620	2.1%		3	Florida	44,723	7.0%
33	Arkansas	5,573	0.9%		4	New York	43,914	6.9%
1	California	81,493	12.8%		5	Pennsylvania	27,704	4.4%
20	Colorado	11,221	1.8%		6	Illinois	25,595	4.0%
28	Connecticut	8,003	1.3%		7	Ohio	22,497	3.5%
45	Delaware	1,835	0.3%		8	Michigan	21,457	3.4%
3	Florida	44,723	7.0%		9	New Jersey	21,447	3.4%
11	Georgia	16,945	2.7%		10	North Carolina	16,951	2.7%
41	Hawaii	2,862	0.5%		11	Georgia	16,945	2.7%
38	Idaho	3,575	0.6%		12	Washington	14,124	2.2%
6	Illinois	25,595	4.0%		13	Virginia	13,932	2.2%
18	Indiana	11,798	1.9%		14	Massachusetts	13,660	2.1%
30	Iowa	5,982	0.9%		15	Arizona	13,620	2.1%
31	Kansas	5,886	0.9%		16	Maryland	12,547	2.0%
25	Kentucky	8,426	1.3%		17	Missouri	12,159	1.9%
24	Louisiana	9,078	1.4%		18	Indiana	11,798	1.9%
40	Maine	3,494	0.5%		19	Tennessee	11,645	1.8%
16	Maryland	12,547	2.0%		20	Colorado	11,221	1.8%
14	Massachusetts	13,660	2.1%		21	Minnesota	10,701	1.7%
8	Michigan	21,457	3.4%		22	Wisconsin	10,651	1.7%
21	Minnesota	10,701	1.7%		23	Oregon	9,284	1.5%
35	Mississippi	4,536	0.7%		24	Louisiana	9,078	1.4%
17	Missouri	12,159	1.9%		25	Kentucky	8,426	1.3%
44	Montana	2,366	0.4%		26	Oklahoma	8,259	1.3%
37	Nebraska	3,726	0.6%		27	Alabama	8,207	1.3%
34	Nevada	5,272	0.8%		28	Connecticut	8,003	1.3%
43	New Hampshire	2,574	0.4%		29	South Carolina	7,451	1.2%
9	New Jersey	21,447	3.4%		30	Iowa	5,982	0.9%
39	New Mexico	3,556	0.6%		31	Kansas	5,886	0.9%
4	New York	43,914	6.9%		32	Utah	5,586	0.9%
10	North Carolina	16,951	2.7%		33	Arkansas	5,573	0.9%
49	North Dakota	1,291	0.2%		34	Nevada	5,272	0.8%
7	Ohio	22,497	3.5%		35	Mississippi	4,536	0.7%
26	Oklahoma	8,259	1.3%		36	West Virginia	3,785	0.6%
23	Oregon	9,284	1.5%		37	Nebraska	3,726	0.6%
5	Pennsylvania	27,704	4.4%		38	Idaho	3,575	0.6%
42	Rhode Island	2,683	0.4%		39	New Mexico	3,556	0.6%
29	South Carolina	7,451	1.2%		40	Maine	3,494	0.5%
47	South Dakota	1,633	0.3%		41	Hawaii	2,862	0.5%
19	Tennessee	11,645	1.8%		42	Rhode Island	2,683	0.4%
2	Texas	46,307	7.3%		43	New Hampshire	2,574	0.4%
32	Utah	5,586	0.9%		44	Montana	2,366	0.4%
48	Vermont	1,510	0.2%		45	Delaware	1,835	0.3%
13	Virginia	13,932	2.2%		46	Alaska	1,657	0.3%
12	Washington	14,124	2.2%		47	South Dakota	1,633	0.3%
36	West Virginia	3,785	0.6%		48	Vermont	1,510	0.2%
22	Wisconsin	10,651	1.7%		49	North Dakota	1,291	0.2%
50	Wyoming	1,283	0.2%		50	Wyoming	1,283	0.2%
						District of Columbia	1,344	0.2%

Source: U.S. Bureau of the Census
  "County Business Patterns 2008 (NAICS)" (http://censtats.census.gov/cbpnaic/cbpnaic.shtml)
*Includes establishments exempt from as well as subject to the federal income tax. Includes those establishments within the
North American Industry Classification System (NAICS) classifications 621 (ambulatory health care services), 622 (hospitals),
and 623 (nursing and residential care facilities). Does not include classification 624 (social assistance facilities).

IV. Finance

Average Medical Malpractice Payment in 2006......... 234
Percent of Private-Sector Establishments That Offer
    Health Insurance: 2009 235
Percent of Private-Sector Establishments with Fewer
    Than 50 Employees That Offer Health Insurance:
    2009 236
Percent of Private-Sector Establishments with More
    Than 50 Employees That Offer Health Insurance:
    2009 237
Average Annual Single Coverage Health Insurance
    Premium per Enrolled Employee in 2009 238
Average Annual Employee Contribution for Single
    Coverage Health Insurance in 2009 239
Percent of Total Premiums for Single Coverage Health
    Insurance Paid by Employees in 2009 240
Average Annual Family Coverage Health Insurance
    Premium per Enrolled Employee in 2009 241
Average Annual Employee Contribution for Family
    Coverage Health Insurance in 2009 242
Percent of Total Premiums for Family Coverage Health
    Insurance Paid by Employees in 2009 243
Persons Not Covered by Health Insurance in 2009 244
Percent of Population Not Covered by Health Insurance
    in 2009 245
Numerical Change in Persons Uninsured: 2005 to 2009 .. 246
Percent Change in Persons Uninsured: 2005 to 2009..... 247
Change in Percent of Population Uninsured: 2005 to
    2009 248
Percent of Children Not Covered by Health Insurance
    in 2009 249
Persons Covered by Health Insurance in 2009.......... 250
Percent of Population Covered by Health Insurance
    in 2009 251
Percent of Population Covered by Private Health
    Insurance in 2009............................. 252
Percent of Population Covered by Employment-Based
    Health Insurance in 2009 253
Percent of Population Covered by Direct-Purchase
    Health Insurance in 2009 254

Percent of Population Covered by Government Health
    Insurance in 2009............................. 255
Percent of Population Covered by Military Health Care
    in 2009 256
Percent of Children Covered by Health Insurance
    in 2009 257
Percent of Children Covered by Private Health
    Insurance in 2009............................. 258
Percent of Children Covered by Employment-Based
    Health Insurance in 2009 259
Percent of Children Covered by Direct-Purchase Health
    Insurance in 2009............................. 260
Percent of Children Covered by Government Health
    Insurance in 2009............................. 261
Percent of Children Covered by Military Health Care
    in 2009 262
Percent of Children Covered by Medicaid in 2009 263
The Children's Health Insurance Program (CHIP)
    Enrollment in 2009............................ 264
Percent Change in the Children's Health Insurance
    Program (CHIP) Enrollment: 2008 to 2009......... 265
Percent of Children Enrolled in the Children's Health
    Insurance Program (CHIP) in 2009 266
Expenditures for the Children's Health Insurance
    Program (CHIP) in 2009 267
Per Capita Expenditures for the Children's Health
    Insurance Program (CHIP) in 2009 268
Expenditures per Participant in the Children's Health
    Insurance Program (CHIP) in 2009 269
Health Maintenance Organizations (HMOs) in 2009..... 270
Enrollees in Health Maintenance Organizations (HMOs)
    in 2009 271
Percent Change in Enrollees in Health Maintenance
    Organizations (HMOs): 2008 to 2009 272
Percent of Population Enrolled in Health Maintenance
    Organizations (HMOs) in 2009 273
Percent of Insured Population Enrolled in Health
    Maintenance Organizations (HMOs) in 2009 274
Medicare Enrollees in 2009 275

Percent Change in Medicare Enrollees: 2008 to 2009 276
Percent of Population Enrolled in Medicare in 2009 277
Percent of Medicare Enrollees in Managed Care
    Programs in 2009 278
Percent of Physicians Participating in Medicare in 2010 .. 279
Enrollees in Medicare Prescription Drug Program
    in 2010 280
Percent of Medicare Enrollees Participating in the
    Medicare Prescription Drug Program in 2010 281
Medicare Program Payments in 2009 282
Per Capita Medicare Program Payments in 2009 283
Medicare Program Payments per Enrollee in 2009 284
Medicaid Enrollment in 2009 285
Percent of Population Enrolled in Medicaid in 2009 286
Medicaid Managed Care Enrollment in 2009 287
Percent of Medicaid Enrollees in Managed Care in 2009 .. 288
Estimated Medicaid Expenditures in 2010 289
Estimated Per Capita Medicaid Expenditures in 2010 290
Estimated Medicaid Expenditures as a Percent of Total
    Expenditures in 2010 291
Percent Change in Medicaid Expenditures: 2009 to
    2010 292
Medicaid Expenditures in 2009 293
Per Capita Medicaid Expenditures in 2009 294
Medicaid Expenditures per Beneficiary in 2009 295
Federal Medicaid Matching Fund Rate for 2011 296
State and Local Government Expenditures for Hospitals
    in 2008 297
Per Capita State and Local Government Expenditures for
    Hospitals in 2008 298
Percent of State and Local Government Expenditures
    Used for Hospitals in 2008 299
State and Local Government Expenditures for Health
    Programs in 2008 300
Per Capita State and Local Government Expenditures for
    Health Programs in 2008 301
Percent of State and Local Government Expenditures
    Used for Health Programs in 2008 302
Estimated Tobacco Settlement Revenues in Fiscal
    Year 2011 303
Annual Smoking-Related Health Costs in 2010 304
Personal Health Care Expenditures in 2004 305
Health Care Expenditures as a Percent of Gross State
    Product in 2004 306
Per Capita Personal Health Care Expenditures in 2004 ... 307

Average Annual Growth in Personal Health Care
    Expenditures: 1991 to 2004 308
Expenditures for Hospital Care in 2004 309
Percent of Total Personal Health Care Expenditures
    Spent on Hospital Care in 2004 310
Per Capita Expenditures for Hospital Care in 2004 311
Expenditures for Physician and Clinical Services
    in 2004 312
Percent of Total Personal Health Care Expenditures
    Spent on Physician and Clinical Services in 2004 313
Per Capita Expenditures for Physician and Clinical
    Services in 2004 314
Expenditures for Dental Services in 2004 315
Percent of Total Personal Health Care Expenditures
    Spent on Dental Services in 2004 316
Per Capita Expenditures for Dental Care in 2004 317
Expenditures for Other Professional Health Care
    Services in 2004 318
Percent of Total Personal Health Care Expenditures
    Spent on Other Professional Health Care Services
    in 2004 319
Per Capita Expenditures for Other Professional Health
    Care Services in 2004 320
Expenditures for Nursing Home Care in 2004 321
Percent of Total Personal Health Care Expenditures
    Spent on Nursing Home Care in 2004 322
Per Capita Expenditures for Nursing Home Care in 2004 .. 323
Expenditures for Home Health Care in 2004 324
Percent of Total Personal Health Care Expenditures
    Spent on Home Health Care in 2004 325
Per Capita Expenditures for Home Health Care
    in 2004 326
Expenditures for Drugs and Other Medical Nondurables
    in 2004 327
Percent of Total Personal Health Care Expenditures
    Spent on Drugs and Other Medical Nondurables
    in 2004 328
Per Capita Expenditures for Drugs and Other Medical
    Nondurables in 2004 329
Expenditures for Durable Medical Products in 2004 330
Percent of Total Personal Health Care Expenditures
    Spent on Durable Medical Products in 2004 331
Per Capita Expenditures for Durable Medical Products
    in 2004 332
Projected National Health Care Expenditures in 2011 333

Average Medical Malpractice Payment in 2006

National Average = $311,965*

ALPHA ORDER

RANK	STATE	AVERAGE PAYMENT
7	Alabama	$453,665
39	Alaska	240,511
30	Arizona	286,898
37	Arkansas	246,959
41	California	223,039
24	Colorado	312,138
4	Connecticut	500,289
3	Delaware	521,177
40	Florida**	240,363
29	Georgia	292,902
14	Hawaii	342,316
31	Idaho	281,751
1	Illinois	619,205
20	Indiana**	322,822
34	Iowa	274,281
48	Kansas**	155,285
32	Kentucky	280,599
43	Louisiana**	207,878
21	Maine	322,325
13	Maryland	347,477
6	Massachusetts	465,236
49	Michigan	138,433
5	Minnesota	480,822
35	Mississippi	258,806
18	Missouri	330,115
22	Montana	320,849
42	Nebraska**	213,081
15	Nevada	340,211
16	New Hampshire	336,032
11	New Jersey	401,144
45	New Mexico**	199,917
10	New York	405,558
12	North Carolina	366,966
27	North Dakota	301,422
25	Ohio	310,573
38	Oklahoma	245,127
26	Oregon	305,725
17	Pennsylvania**	332,376
19	Rhode Island	326,542
47	South Carolina**	174,454
8	South Dakota	422,033
23	Tennessee	317,305
46	Texas	175,644
36	Utah	247,349
50	Vermont	125,795
28	Virginia	295,840
33	Washington	277,493
44	West Virginia	204,794
2	Wisconsin**	524,041
9	Wyoming	413,553

RANK ORDER

RANK	STATE	AVERAGE PAYMENT
1	Illinois	$619,205
2	Wisconsin**	524,041
3	Delaware	521,177
4	Connecticut	500,289
5	Minnesota	480,822
6	Massachusetts	465,236
7	Alabama	453,665
8	South Dakota	422,033
9	Wyoming	413,553
10	New York	405,558
11	New Jersey	401,144
12	North Carolina	366,966
13	Maryland	347,477
14	Hawaii	342,316
15	Nevada	340,211
16	New Hampshire	336,032
17	Pennsylvania**	332,376
18	Missouri	330,115
19	Rhode Island	326,542
20	Indiana**	322,822
21	Maine	322,325
22	Montana	320,849
23	Tennessee	317,305
24	Colorado	312,138
25	Ohio	310,573
26	Oregon	305,725
27	North Dakota	301,422
28	Virginia	295,840
29	Georgia	292,902
30	Arizona	286,898
31	Idaho	281,751
32	Kentucky	280,599
33	Washington	277,493
34	Iowa	274,281
35	Mississippi	258,806
36	Utah	247,349
37	Arkansas	246,959
38	Oklahoma	245,127
39	Alaska	240,511
40	Florida**	240,363
41	California	223,039
42	Nebraska**	213,081
43	Louisiana**	207,878
44	West Virginia	204,794
45	New Mexico**	199,917
46	Texas	175,644
47	South Carolina**	174,454
48	Kansas**	155,285
49	Michigan	138,433
50	Vermont	125,795
	District of Columbia	331,628

Source: U.S. Department of Health and Human Services, Bureau of Health Professions
  "National Practitioner Data Bank, 2006 Annual Report" (http://www.npdb-hipdb.com/annualrpt.html)
*National figure includes U.S. territories and U.S. Armed Forces locations overseas.
**The figures for these states have not been adjusted for payments by state compensation funds and other similar funds.
Average payments for these states understate the actual average amounts received by claimants.

Percent of Private-Sector Establishments That Offer Health Insurance: 2009

National Percent = 55.0%

ALPHA ORDER				RANK ORDER		
RANK	STATE	PERCENT		RANK	STATE	PERCENT
12	Alabama	58.9		1	Hawaii	85.4
48	Alaska	40.5		2	New Jersey	65.2
30	Arizona	52.1		3	Connecticut	63.9
44	Arkansas	47.1		3	Ohio	63.9
16	California	56.0		5	Pennsylvania	63.0
20	Colorado	55.2		6	Massachusetts	61.6
3	Connecticut	63.9		7	Maryland	61.0
9	Delaware	60.0		8	Rhode Island	60.2
37	Florida	49.5		9	Delaware	60.0
27	Georgia	52.8		10	New Hampshire	59.7
1	Hawaii	85.4		11	New York	59.1
47	Idaho	45.0		12	Alabama	58.9
27	Illinois	52.8		13	Missouri	57.1
39	Indiana	49.1		14	Kentucky	56.6
35	Iowa	50.7		15	Vermont	56.4
17	Kansas	55.9		16	California	56.0
14	Kentucky	56.6		17	Kansas	55.9
42	Louisiana	48.1		18	Tennessee	55.5
24	Maine	53.8		19	Minnesota	55.4
7	Maryland	61.0		20	Colorado	55.2
6	Massachusetts	61.6		21	Nevada	55.0
23	Michigan	54.0		22	Virginia	54.1
19	Minnesota	55.4		23	Michigan	54.0
41	Mississippi	48.7		24	Maine	53.8
13	Missouri	57.1		25	Washington	53.6
50	Montana	39.5		26	South Carolina	53.3
46	Nebraska	45.4		27	Georgia	52.8
21	Nevada	55.0		27	Illinois	52.8
10	New Hampshire	59.7		27	Oregon	52.8
2	New Jersey	65.2		30	Arizona	52.1
33	New Mexico	51.0		31	North Carolina	51.6
11	New York	59.1		32	Wisconsin	51.4
31	North Carolina	51.6		33	New Mexico	51.0
38	North Dakota	49.2		34	Texas	50.9
3	Ohio	63.9		35	Iowa	50.7
43	Oklahoma	47.4		36	West Virginia	50.3
27	Oregon	52.8		37	Florida	49.5
5	Pennsylvania	63.0		38	North Dakota	49.2
8	Rhode Island	60.2		39	Indiana	49.1
26	South Carolina	53.3		40	South Dakota	48.8
40	South Dakota	48.8		41	Mississippi	48.7
18	Tennessee	55.5		42	Louisiana	48.1
34	Texas	50.9		43	Oklahoma	47.4
45	Utah	46.4		44	Arkansas	47.1
15	Vermont	56.4		45	Utah	46.4
22	Virginia	54.1		46	Nebraska	45.4
25	Washington	53.6		47	Idaho	45.0
36	West Virginia	50.3		48	Alaska	40.5
32	Wisconsin	51.4		48	Wyoming	40.5
48	Wyoming	40.5		50	Montana	39.5
					District of Columbia	74.1

Source: U.S. Department of Health and Human Services, Agency for Healthcare Research and Quality
"Private-Sector Data by Firm Size and State" (Table II Series, Medical Expenditures Panel Survey)
(http://www.meps.ahrq.gov/mepsweb/survey_comp/Insurance.jsp)

Percent of Private-Sector Establishments with Fewer Than 50 Employees That Offer Health Insurance: 2009
National Percent = 41.0%

ALPHA ORDER

RANK	STATE	PERCENT
16	Alabama	42.5
50	Alaska	25.8
36	Arizona	34.2
46	Arkansas	29.5
13	California	43.9
14	Colorado	43.0
3	Connecticut	51.6
12	Delaware	45.9
35	Florida	34.5
31	Georgia	36.3
1	Hawaii	81.1
41	Idaho	31.8
24	Illinois	38.5
46	Indiana	29.5
31	Iowa	36.3
21	Kansas	40.6
23	Kentucky	38.6
44	Louisiana	30.7
17	Maine	41.8
8	Maryland	49.0
9	Massachusetts	48.9
22	Michigan	40.4
15	Minnesota	42.6
43	Mississippi	31.2
20	Missouri	41.0
49	Montana	28.0
45	Nebraska	30.0
25	Nevada	38.1
10	New Hampshire	48.4
2	New Jersey	56.1
34	New Mexico	34.7
4	New York	50.1
38	North Carolina	33.8
25	North Dakota	38.1
6	Ohio	49.5
40	Oklahoma	32.0
19	Oregon	41.2
7	Pennsylvania	49.4
5	Rhode Island	49.6
33	South Carolina	35.5
27	South Dakota	37.5
29	Tennessee	36.9
36	Texas	34.2
42	Utah	31.4
11	Vermont	46.8
28	Virginia	37.1
18	Washington	41.7
39	West Virginia	32.1
30	Wisconsin	36.8
48	Wyoming	28.5

RANK ORDER

RANK	STATE	PERCENT
1	Hawaii	81.1
2	New Jersey	56.1
3	Connecticut	51.6
4	New York	50.1
5	Rhode Island	49.6
6	Ohio	49.5
7	Pennsylvania	49.4
8	Maryland	49.0
9	Massachusetts	48.9
10	New Hampshire	48.4
11	Vermont	46.8
12	Delaware	45.9
13	California	43.9
14	Colorado	43.0
15	Minnesota	42.6
16	Alabama	42.5
17	Maine	41.8
18	Washington	41.7
19	Oregon	41.2
20	Missouri	41.0
21	Kansas	40.6
22	Michigan	40.4
23	Kentucky	38.6
24	Illinois	38.5
25	Nevada	38.1
25	North Dakota	38.1
27	South Dakota	37.5
28	Virginia	37.1
29	Tennessee	36.9
30	Wisconsin	36.8
31	Georgia	36.3
31	Iowa	36.3
33	South Carolina	35.5
34	New Mexico	34.7
35	Florida	34.5
36	Arizona	34.2
36	Texas	34.2
38	North Carolina	33.8
39	West Virginia	32.1
40	Oklahoma	32.0
41	Idaho	31.8
42	Utah	31.4
43	Mississippi	31.2
44	Louisiana	30.7
45	Nebraska	30.0
46	Arkansas	29.5
46	Indiana	29.5
48	Wyoming	28.5
49	Montana	28.0
50	Alaska	25.8

District of Columbia	61.2

Source: U.S. Department of Health and Human Services, Agency for Healthcare Research and Quality
"Private-Sector Data by Firm Size and State" (Table II Series, Medical Expenditures Panel Survey)
(http://www.meps.ahrq.gov/mepsweb/survey_comp/Insurance.jsp)

Percent of Private-Sector Establishments with More Than 50 Employees That Offer Health Insurance: 2009
National Percent = 96.2%

ALPHA ORDER

RANK	STATE	PERCENT
37	Alabama	95.0
45	Alaska	93.8
12	Arizona	97.7
46	Arkansas	93.6
38	California	94.8
16	Colorado	97.1
3	Connecticut	98.6
50	Delaware	91.4
18	Florida	97.0
18	Georgia	97.0
14	Hawaii	97.5
35	Idaho	95.3
26	Illinois	96.1
24	Indiana	96.4
13	Iowa	97.6
29	Kansas	95.9
21	Kentucky	96.9
29	Louisiana	95.9
6	Maine	98.4
26	Maryland	96.1
1	Massachusetts	98.8
38	Michigan	94.8
40	Minnesota	94.7
36	Mississippi	95.2
26	Missouri	96.1
5	Montana	98.5
31	Nebraska	95.7
48	Nevada	92.7
8	New Hampshire	98.2
1	New Jersey	98.8
42	New Mexico	94.5
11	New York	98.0
16	North Carolina	97.1
25	North Dakota	96.2
18	Ohio	97.0
47	Oklahoma	93.1
40	Oregon	94.7
9	Pennsylvania	98.1
6	Rhode Island	98.4
32	South Carolina	95.5
23	South Dakota	96.6
22	Tennessee	96.8
44	Texas	94.0
43	Utah	94.3
3	Vermont	98.6
9	Virginia	98.1
15	Washington	97.4
32	West Virginia	95.5
32	Wisconsin	95.5
49	Wyoming	91.7

RANK ORDER

RANK	STATE	PERCENT
1	Massachusetts	98.8
1	New Jersey	98.8
3	Connecticut	98.6
3	Vermont	98.6
5	Montana	98.5
6	Maine	98.4
6	Rhode Island	98.4
8	New Hampshire	98.2
9	Pennsylvania	98.1
9	Virginia	98.1
11	New York	98.0
12	Arizona	97.7
13	Iowa	97.6
14	Hawaii	97.5
15	Washington	97.4
16	Colorado	97.1
16	North Carolina	97.1
18	Florida	97.0
18	Georgia	97.0
18	Ohio	97.0
21	Kentucky	96.9
22	Tennessee	96.8
23	South Dakota	96.6
24	Indiana	96.4
25	North Dakota	96.2
26	Illinois	96.1
26	Maryland	96.1
26	Missouri	96.1
29	Kansas	95.9
29	Louisiana	95.9
31	Nebraska	95.7
32	South Carolina	95.5
32	West Virginia	95.5
32	Wisconsin	95.5
35	Idaho	95.3
36	Mississippi	95.2
37	Alabama	95.0
38	California	94.8
38	Michigan	94.8
40	Minnesota	94.7
40	Oregon	94.7
42	New Mexico	94.5
43	Utah	94.3
44	Texas	94.0
45	Alaska	93.8
46	Arkansas	93.6
47	Oklahoma	93.1
48	Nevada	92.7
49	Wyoming	91.7
50	Delaware	91.4

	District of Columbia	97.5

Source: U.S. Department of Health and Human Services, Agency for Healthcare Research and Quality
  "Private-Sector Data by Firm Size and State" (Table II Series, Medical Expenditures Panel Survey)
  (http://www.meps.ahrq.gov/mepsweb/survey_comp/Insurance.jsp)

Average Annual Single Coverage Health Insurance Premium per Enrolled Employee in 2009
National Average = $4,669*

ALPHA ORDER

RANK	STATE	PREMIUM
24	Alabama	$4,647
1	Alaska	6,047
39	Arizona	4,358
50	Arkansas	3,717
25	California	4,631
29	Colorado	4,570
12	Connecticut	4,909
9	Delaware	4,955
35	Florida	4,488
21	Georgia	4,692
49	Hawaii	4,116
45	Idaho	4,248
18	Illinois	4,725
16	Indiana	4,849
37	Iowa	4,453
47	Kansas	4,236
40	Kentucky	4,336
15	Louisiana	4,861
6	Maine	5,119
14	Maryland	4,870
2	Massachusetts	5,268
11	Michigan	4,916
27	Minnesota	4,600
36	Mississippi	4,469
38	Missouri	4,393
31	Montana	4,546
41	Nebraska	4,315
26	Nevada	4,627
3	New Hampshire	5,227
13	New Jersey	4,901
32	New Mexico	4,535
5	New York	5,121
23	North Carolina	4,676
48	North Dakota	4,127
43	Ohio	4,261
46	Oklahoma	4,243
22	Oregon	4,680
17	Pennsylvania	4,749
7	Rhode Island	5,059
33	South Carolina	4,503
42	South Dakota	4,262
30	Tennessee	4,549
34	Texas	4,499
44	Utah	4,257
8	Vermont	5,001
28	Virginia	4,590
10	Washington	4,923
20	West Virginia	4,700
4	Wisconsin	5,132
19	Wyoming	4,703

RANK ORDER

RANK	STATE	PREMIUM
1	Alaska	$6,047
2	Massachusetts	5,268
3	New Hampshire	5,227
4	Wisconsin	5,132
5	New York	5,121
6	Maine	5,119
7	Rhode Island	5,059
8	Vermont	5,001
9	Delaware	4,955
10	Washington	4,923
11	Michigan	4,916
12	Connecticut	4,909
13	New Jersey	4,901
14	Maryland	4,870
15	Louisiana	4,861
16	Indiana	4,849
17	Pennsylvania	4,749
18	Illinois	4,725
19	Wyoming	4,703
20	West Virginia	4,700
21	Georgia	4,692
22	Oregon	4,680
23	North Carolina	4,676
24	Alabama	4,647
25	California	4,631
26	Nevada	4,627
27	Minnesota	4,600
28	Virginia	4,590
29	Colorado	4,570
30	Tennessee	4,549
31	Montana	4,546
32	New Mexico	4,535
33	South Carolina	4,503
34	Texas	4,499
35	Florida	4,488
36	Mississippi	4,469
37	Iowa	4,453
38	Missouri	4,393
39	Arizona	4,358
40	Kentucky	4,336
41	Nebraska	4,315
42	South Dakota	4,262
43	Ohio	4,261
44	Utah	4,257
45	Idaho	4,248
46	Oklahoma	4,243
47	Kansas	4,236
48	North Dakota	4,127
49	Hawaii	4,116
50	Arkansas	3,717

District of Columbia	5,082

Source: U.S. Department of Health and Human Services, Agency for Healthcare Research and Quality
   "Private-Sector Data by Firm Size and State" (Table II Series, Medical Expenditures Panel Survey)
   (http://www.meps.ahrq.gov/mepsweb/survey_comp/Insurance.jsp)
*Enrolled employees at private-sector establishments that offer health insurance coverage.

Average Annual Employee Contribution for Single Coverage Health Insurance in 2009
National Average = $957*

ALPHA ORDER

RANK	STATE	CONTRIBUTION
13	Alabama	$1,025
39	Alaska	842
38	Arizona	851
46	Arkansas	750
42	California	795
26	Colorado	971
7	Connecticut	1,082
4	Delaware	1,101
27	Florida	969
28	Georgia	963
50	Hawaii	461
45	Idaho	762
16	Illinois	1,008
9	Indiana	1,070
37	Iowa	855
25	Kansas	976
18	Kentucky	1,000
29	Louisiana	956
24	Maine	981
3	Maryland	1,105
1	Massachusetts	1,321
30	Michigan	946
21	Minnesota	994
21	Mississippi	994
19	Missouri	999
44	Montana	768
35	Nebraska	873
39	Nevada	842
5	New Hampshire	1,087
12	New Jersey	1,045
31	New Mexico	934
8	New York	1,075
20	North Carolina	998
36	North Dakota	860
10	Ohio	1,065
41	Oklahoma	815
49	Oregon	627
32	Pennsylvania	917
2	Rhode Island	1,207
33	South Carolina	898
34	South Dakota	890
15	Tennessee	1,010
23	Texas	991
43	Utah	772
16	Vermont	1,008
11	Virginia	1,060
48	Washington	640
6	West Virginia	1,085
14	Wisconsin	1,011
47	Wyoming	729

RANK ORDER

RANK	STATE	CONTRIBUTION
1	Massachusetts	$1,321
2	Rhode Island	1,207
3	Maryland	1,105
4	Delaware	1,101
5	New Hampshire	1,087
6	West Virginia	1,085
7	Connecticut	1,082
8	New York	1,075
9	Indiana	1,070
10	Ohio	1,065
11	Virginia	1,060
12	New Jersey	1,045
13	Alabama	1,025
14	Wisconsin	1,011
15	Tennessee	1,010
16	Illinois	1,008
16	Vermont	1,008
18	Kentucky	1,000
19	Missouri	999
20	North Carolina	998
21	Minnesota	994
21	Mississippi	994
23	Texas	991
24	Maine	981
25	Kansas	976
26	Colorado	971
27	Florida	969
28	Georgia	963
29	Louisiana	956
30	Michigan	946
31	New Mexico	934
32	Pennsylvania	917
33	South Carolina	898
34	South Dakota	890
35	Nebraska	873
36	North Dakota	860
37	Iowa	855
38	Arizona	851
39	Alaska	842
39	Nevada	842
41	Oklahoma	815
42	California	795
43	Utah	772
44	Montana	768
45	Idaho	762
46	Arkansas	750
47	Wyoming	729
48	Washington	640
49	Oregon	627
50	Hawaii	461
	District of Columbia	906

Source: U.S. Department of Health and Human Services, Agency for Healthcare Research and Quality
"Private-Sector Data by Firm Size and State" (Table II Series, Medical Expenditures Panel Survey)
(http://www.meps.ahrq.gov/mepsweb/survey_comp/Insurance.jsp)
*Enrolled employees at private-sector establishments that offer health insurance coverage.

Percent of Total Premiums for Single Coverage
Health Insurance Paid by Employees in 2009
National Average = 20.5%*

ALPHA ORDER

RANK	STATE	PERCENT
13	Alabama	22.1
47	Alaska	13.9
35	Arizona	19.5
29	Arkansas	20.2
44	California	17.2
22	Colorado	21.2
15	Connecticut	22.0
10	Delaware	22.2
17	Florida	21.6
28	Georgia	20.5
50	Hawaii	11.2
43	Idaho	17.9
20	Illinois	21.3
13	Indiana	22.1
37	Iowa	19.2
7	Kansas	23.0
4	Kentucky	23.1
33	Louisiana	19.7
37	Maine	19.2
8	Maryland	22.7
1	Massachusetts	25.1
37	Michigan	19.2
17	Minnesota	21.6
10	Mississippi	22.2
8	Missouri	22.7
45	Montana	16.9
29	Nebraska	20.2
41	Nevada	18.2
26	New Hampshire	20.8
20	New Jersey	21.3
27	New Mexico	20.6
23	New York	21.0
19	North Carolina	21.4
24	North Dakota	20.9
2	Ohio	25.0
37	Oklahoma	19.2
48	Oregon	13.4
36	Pennsylvania	19.3
3	Rhode Island	23.9
32	South Carolina	19.9
24	South Dakota	20.9
10	Tennessee	22.2
15	Texas	22.0
42	Utah	18.1
29	Vermont	20.2
4	Virginia	23.1
49	Washington	13.0
4	West Virginia	23.1
33	Wisconsin	19.7
46	Wyoming	15.5

RANK ORDER

RANK	STATE	PERCENT
1	Massachusetts	25.1
2	Ohio	25.0
3	Rhode Island	23.9
4	Kentucky	23.1
4	Virginia	23.1
4	West Virginia	23.1
7	Kansas	23.0
8	Maryland	22.7
8	Missouri	22.7
10	Delaware	22.2
10	Mississippi	22.2
10	Tennessee	22.2
13	Alabama	22.1
13	Indiana	22.1
15	Connecticut	22.0
15	Texas	22.0
17	Florida	21.6
17	Minnesota	21.6
19	North Carolina	21.4
20	Illinois	21.3
20	New Jersey	21.3
22	Colorado	21.2
23	New York	21.0
24	North Dakota	20.9
24	South Dakota	20.9
26	New Hampshire	20.8
27	New Mexico	20.6
28	Georgia	20.5
29	Arkansas	20.2
29	Nebraska	20.2
29	Vermont	20.2
32	South Carolina	19.9
33	Louisiana	19.7
33	Wisconsin	19.7
35	Arizona	19.5
36	Pennsylvania	19.3
37	Iowa	19.2
37	Maine	19.2
37	Michigan	19.2
37	Oklahoma	19.2
41	Nevada	18.2
42	Utah	18.1
43	Idaho	17.9
44	California	17.2
45	Montana	16.9
46	Wyoming	15.5
47	Alaska	13.9
48	Oregon	13.4
49	Washington	13.0
50	Hawaii	11.2

	District of Columbia	17.8

Source: U.S. Department of Health and Human Services, Agency for Healthcare Research and Quality
   "Private-Sector Data by Firm Size and State" (Table II Series, Medical Expenditures Panel Survey)
      (http://www.meps.ahrq.gov/mepsweb/survey_comp/Insurance.jsp)
*Enrolled employees at private-sector establishments that offer health insurance coverage.

Average Annual Family Coverage Health Insurance Premium per Enrolled Employee in 2009
National Average = $13,027*

ALPHA ORDER

RANK	STATE	PREMIUM
40	Alabama	$11,978
5	Alaska	14,182
24	Arizona	12,813
50	Arkansas	10,969
30	California	12,631
15	Colorado	13,360
6	Connecticut	14,064
29	Delaware	12,682
21	Florida	12,912
25	Georgia	12,792
45	Hawaii	11,826
41	Idaho	11,887
12	Illinois	13,708
22	Indiana	12,872
39	Iowa	12,036
44	Kansas	11,829
34	Kentucky	12,407
7	Louisiana	13,846
14	Maine	13,522
8	Maryland	13,833
1	Massachusetts	14,723
19	Michigan	13,160
18	Minnesota	13,202
32	Mississippi	12,590
35	Missouri	12,353
49	Montana	11,365
37	Nebraska	12,227
28	Nevada	12,700
9	New Hampshire	13,822
11	New Jersey	13,750
23	New Mexico	12,848
10	New York	13,757
20	North Carolina	13,087
47	North Dakota	11,590
42	Ohio	11,870
48	Oklahoma	11,417
26	Oregon	12,783
16	Pennsylvania	13,229
13	Rhode Island	13,608
36	South Carolina	12,343
46	South Dakota	11,596
38	Tennessee	12,134
17	Texas	13,221
43	Utah	11,869
3	Vermont	14,558
31	Virginia	12,622
27	Washington	12,758
33	West Virginia	12,554
2	Wisconsin	14,656
4	Wyoming	14,319

RANK ORDER

RANK	STATE	PREMIUM
1	Massachusetts	$14,723
2	Wisconsin	14,656
3	Vermont	14,558
4	Wyoming	14,319
5	Alaska	14,182
6	Connecticut	14,064
7	Louisiana	13,846
8	Maryland	13,833
9	New Hampshire	13,822
10	New York	13,757
11	New Jersey	13,750
12	Illinois	13,708
13	Rhode Island	13,608
14	Maine	13,522
15	Colorado	13,360
16	Pennsylvania	13,229
17	Texas	13,221
18	Minnesota	13,202
19	Michigan	13,160
20	North Carolina	13,087
21	Florida	12,912
22	Indiana	12,872
23	New Mexico	12,848
24	Arizona	12,813
25	Georgia	12,792
26	Oregon	12,783
27	Washington	12,758
28	Nevada	12,700
29	Delaware	12,682
30	California	12,631
31	Virginia	12,622
32	Mississippi	12,590
33	West Virginia	12,554
34	Kentucky	12,407
35	Missouri	12,353
36	South Carolina	12,343
37	Nebraska	12,227
38	Tennessee	12,134
39	Iowa	12,036
40	Alabama	11,978
41	Idaho	11,887
42	Ohio	11,870
43	Utah	11,869
44	Kansas	11,829
45	Hawaii	11,826
46	South Dakota	11,596
47	North Dakota	11,590
48	Oklahoma	11,417
49	Montana	11,365
50	Arkansas	10,969

	District of Columbia	14,222

Source: U.S. Department of Health and Human Services, Agency for Healthcare Research and Quality
   "Private-Sector Data by Firm Size and State" (Table II Series, Medical Expenditures Panel Survey)
      (http://www.meps.ahrq.gov/mepsweb/survey_comp/Insurance.jsp)
*Enrolled employees at private-sector establishments that offer health insurance coverage.

Average Annual Employee Contribution for Family Coverage Health Insurance in 2009
National Average = $3,474*

ALPHA ORDER				RANK ORDER		
RANK	STATE	CONTRIBUTION		RANK	STATE	CONTRIBUTION
33	Alabama	$3,320		1	Florida	$4,275
2	Alaska	4,151		2	Alaska	4,151
18	Arizona	3,617		3	Louisiana	4,108
43	Arkansas	2,923		4	Massachusetts	4,088
24	California	3,483		5	Texas	4,024
31	Colorado	3,370		6	North Carolina	3,936
23	Connecticut	3,511		7	Mississippi	3,907
27	Delaware	3,423		8	Montana	3,898
1	Florida	4,275		9	Maine	3,857
19	Georgia	3,597		10	Vermont	3,793
46	Hawaii	2,868		11	Virginia	3,792
35	Idaho	3,233		12	Tennessee	3,790
29	Illinois	3,396		13	Minnesota	3,712
34	Indiana	3,257		14	Rhode Island	3,689
37	Iowa	3,184		15	Maryland	3,671
39	Kansas	3,132		16	Ohio	3,667
28	Kentucky	3,408		17	Missouri	3,644
3	Louisiana	4,108		18	Arizona	3,617
9	Maine	3,857		19	Georgia	3,597
15	Maryland	3,671		20	New Mexico	3,578
4	Massachusetts	4,088		21	Nebraska	3,532
47	Michigan	2,819		22	New Hampshire	3,527
13	Minnesota	3,712		23	Connecticut	3,511
7	Mississippi	3,907		24	California	3,483
17	Missouri	3,644		25	Washington	3,476
8	Montana	3,898		26	South Carolina	3,433
21	Nebraska	3,532		27	Delaware	3,423
45	Nevada	2,881		28	Kentucky	3,408
22	New Hampshire	3,527		29	Illinois	3,396
38	New Jersey	3,135		30	South Dakota	3,377
20	New Mexico	3,578		31	Colorado	3,370
41	New York	3,034		32	Wyoming	3,326
6	North Carolina	3,936		33	Alabama	3,320
36	North Dakota	3,210		34	Indiana	3,257
16	Ohio	3,667		35	Idaho	3,233
40	Oklahoma	3,086		36	North Dakota	3,210
48	Oregon	2,792		37	Iowa	3,184
50	Pennsylvania	2,774		38	New Jersey	3,135
14	Rhode Island	3,689		39	Kansas	3,132
26	South Carolina	3,433		40	Oklahoma	3,086
30	South Dakota	3,377		41	New York	3,034
12	Tennessee	3,790		42	Utah	3,006
5	Texas	4,024		43	Arkansas	2,923
42	Utah	3,006		44	Wisconsin	2,899
10	Vermont	3,793		45	Nevada	2,881
11	Virginia	3,792		46	Hawaii	2,868
25	Washington	3,476		47	Michigan	2,819
49	West Virginia	2,783		48	Oregon	2,792
44	Wisconsin	2,899		49	West Virginia	2,783
32	Wyoming	3,326		50	Pennsylvania	2,774
					District of Columbia	3,623

Source: U.S. Department of Health and Human Services, Agency for Healthcare Research and Quality
"Private-Sector Data by Firm Size and State" (Table II Series, Medical Expenditures Panel Survey)
(http://www.meps.ahrq.gov/mepsweb/survey_comp/Insurance.jsp)
*Enrolled employees at private-sector establishments that offer health insurance coverage.

Percent of Total Premiums for Family Coverage
Health Insurance Paid by Employees in 2009
National Average = 26.7%*

ALPHA ORDER

RANK	STATE	PERCENT
21	Alabama	27.7
11	Alaska	29.3
15	Arizona	28.2
30	Arkansas	26.6
23	California	27.6
38	Colorado	25.2
39	Connecticut	25.0
28	Delaware	27.0
2	Florida	33.1
16	Georgia	28.1
41	Hawaii	24.2
25	Idaho	27.2
40	Illinois	24.8
36	Indiana	25.3
31	Iowa	26.5
31	Kansas	26.5
24	Kentucky	27.5
9	Louisiana	29.7
14	Maine	28.5
31	Maryland	26.5
19	Massachusetts	27.8
48	Michigan	21.4
16	Minnesota	28.1
4	Mississippi	31.0
10	Missouri	29.5
1	Montana	34.3
13	Nebraska	28.9
44	Nevada	22.7
35	New Hampshire	25.5
43	New Jersey	22.8
18	New Mexico	27.9
46	New York	22.1
7	North Carolina	30.1
21	North Dakota	27.7
5	Ohio	30.9
28	Oklahoma	27.0
47	Oregon	21.8
49	Pennsylvania	21.0
27	Rhode Island	27.1
19	South Carolina	27.8
12	South Dakota	29.1
3	Tennessee	31.2
6	Texas	30.4
36	Utah	25.3
34	Vermont	26.1
8	Virginia	30.0
25	Washington	27.2
45	West Virginia	22.2
50	Wisconsin	19.8
42	Wyoming	23.2

RANK ORDER

RANK	STATE	PERCENT
1	Montana	34.3
2	Florida	33.1
3	Tennessee	31.2
4	Mississippi	31.0
5	Ohio	30.9
6	Texas	30.4
7	North Carolina	30.1
8	Virginia	30.0
9	Louisiana	29.7
10	Missouri	29.5
11	Alaska	29.3
12	South Dakota	29.1
13	Nebraska	28.9
14	Maine	28.5
15	Arizona	28.2
16	Georgia	28.1
16	Minnesota	28.1
18	New Mexico	27.9
19	Massachusetts	27.8
19	South Carolina	27.8
21	Alabama	27.7
21	North Dakota	27.7
23	California	27.6
24	Kentucky	27.5
25	Idaho	27.2
25	Washington	27.2
27	Rhode Island	27.1
28	Delaware	27.0
28	Oklahoma	27.0
30	Arkansas	26.6
31	Iowa	26.5
31	Kansas	26.5
31	Maryland	26.5
34	Vermont	26.1
35	New Hampshire	25.5
36	Indiana	25.3
36	Utah	25.3
38	Colorado	25.2
39	Connecticut	25.0
40	Illinois	24.8
41	Hawaii	24.2
42	Wyoming	23.2
43	New Jersey	22.8
44	Nevada	22.7
45	West Virginia	22.2
46	New York	22.1
47	Oregon	21.8
48	Michigan	21.4
49	Pennsylvania	21.0
50	Wisconsin	19.8

| | District of Columbia | 25.5 |

Source: U.S. Department of Health and Human Services, Agency for Healthcare Research and Quality
   "Private-Sector Data by Firm Size and State" (Table II Series, Medical Expenditures Panel Survey)
   (http://www.meps.ahrq.gov/mepsweb/survey_comp/Insurance.jsp)
*Enrolled employees at private-sector establishments that offer health insurance coverage.

Persons Not Covered by Health Insurance in 2009

National Total = 50,674,000 Uninsured

ALPHA ORDER

RANK	STATE	UNINSURED	% of USA
19	Alabama	789,000	1.6%
44	Alaska	122,000	0.2%
12	Arizona	1,273,000	2.5%
26	Arkansas	548,000	1.1%
1	California	7,345,000	14.5%
21	Colorado	762,000	1.5%
32	Connecticut	418,000	0.8%
45	Delaware	118,000	0.2%
3	Florida	4,118,000	8.1%
5	Georgia	1,985,000	3.9%
47	Hawaii	102,000	0.2%
38	Idaho	232,000	0.5%
6	Illinois	1,891,000	3.7%
16	Indiana	902,000	1.8%
35	Iowa	342,000	0.7%
34	Kansas	365,000	0.7%
23	Kentucky	694,000	1.4%
22	Louisiana	711,000	1.4%
42	Maine	133,000	0.3%
18	Maryland	793,000	1.6%
36	Massachusetts	295,000	0.6%
11	Michigan	1,350,000	2.7%
30	Minnesota	456,000	0.9%
29	Mississippi	502,000	1.0%
15	Missouri	914,000	1.8%
40	Montana	149,000	0.3%
39	Nebraska	205,000	0.4%
27	Nevada	546,000	1.1%
41	New Hampshire	138,000	0.3%
10	New Jersey	1,371,000	2.7%
31	New Mexico	430,000	0.8%
4	New York	2,837,000	5.6%
7	North Carolina	1,685,000	3.3%
49	North Dakota	67,000	0.1%
8	Ohio	1,643,000	3.2%
25	Oklahoma	659,000	1.3%
24	Oregon	678,000	1.3%
9	Pennsylvania	1,409,000	2.8%
43	Rhode Island	127,000	0.3%
20	South Carolina	766,000	1.5%
46	South Dakota	108,000	0.2%
14	Tennessee	963,000	1.9%
2	Texas	6,433,000	12.7%
33	Utah	415,000	0.8%
50	Vermont	61,000	0.1%
13	Virginia	1,014,000	2.0%
17	Washington	869,000	1.7%
37	West Virginia	253,000	0.5%
28	Wisconsin	527,000	1.0%
48	Wyoming	86,000	0.2%

RANK ORDER

RANK	STATE	UNINSURED	% of USA
1	California	7,345,000	14.5%
2	Texas	6,433,000	12.7%
3	Florida	4,118,000	8.1%
4	New York	2,837,000	5.6%
5	Georgia	1,985,000	3.9%
6	Illinois	1,891,000	3.7%
7	North Carolina	1,685,000	3.3%
8	Ohio	1,643,000	3.2%
9	Pennsylvania	1,409,000	2.8%
10	New Jersey	1,371,000	2.7%
11	Michigan	1,350,000	2.7%
12	Arizona	1,273,000	2.5%
13	Virginia	1,014,000	2.0%
14	Tennessee	963,000	1.9%
15	Missouri	914,000	1.8%
16	Indiana	902,000	1.8%
17	Washington	869,000	1.7%
18	Maryland	793,000	1.6%
19	Alabama	789,000	1.6%
20	South Carolina	766,000	1.5%
21	Colorado	762,000	1.5%
22	Louisiana	711,000	1.4%
23	Kentucky	694,000	1.4%
24	Oregon	678,000	1.3%
25	Oklahoma	659,000	1.3%
26	Arkansas	548,000	1.1%
27	Nevada	546,000	1.1%
28	Wisconsin	527,000	1.0%
29	Mississippi	502,000	1.0%
30	Minnesota	456,000	0.9%
31	New Mexico	430,000	0.8%
32	Connecticut	418,000	0.8%
33	Utah	415,000	0.8%
34	Kansas	365,000	0.7%
35	Iowa	342,000	0.7%
36	Massachusetts	295,000	0.6%
37	West Virginia	253,000	0.5%
38	Idaho	232,000	0.5%
39	Nebraska	205,000	0.4%
40	Montana	149,000	0.3%
41	New Hampshire	138,000	0.3%
42	Maine	133,000	0.3%
43	Rhode Island	127,000	0.3%
44	Alaska	122,000	0.2%
45	Delaware	118,000	0.2%
46	South Dakota	108,000	0.2%
47	Hawaii	102,000	0.2%
48	Wyoming	86,000	0.2%
49	North Dakota	67,000	0.1%
50	Vermont	61,000	0.1%
	District of Columbia	74,000	0.1%

Source: U.S. Bureau of the Census
"Income, Poverty, and Health Insurance Coverage: 2009"
(http://www.census.gov/hhes/www/hlthins/data/incpovhlth/index.html)

Percent of Population Not Covered by Health Insurance in 2009

National Percent = 15.8% of Population*

ALPHA ORDER

RANK	STATE	PERCENT
26	Alabama	13.6
7	Alaska	18.6
4	Arizona	19.1
11	Arkansas	17.7
5	California	18.9
16	Colorado	15.9
41	Connecticut	10.5
38	Delaware	11.8
3	Florida	20.9
7	Georgia	18.6
49	Hawaii	7.8
20	Idaho	14.9
25	Illinois	13.7
32	Indiana	12.6
45	Iowa	10.0
31	Kansas	12.7
18	Kentucky	15.3
9	Louisiana	18.2
46	Maine	9.8
30	Maryland	13.2
50	Massachusetts	5.1
34	Michigan	12.4
48	Minnesota	8.6
10	Mississippi	18.1
28	Missouri	13.5
17	Montana	15.7
35	Nebraska	12.2
5	Nevada	18.9
42	New Hampshire	10.4
19	New Jersey	15.2
2	New Mexico	22.6
24	New York	14.0
13	North Carolina	16.6
40	North Dakota	10.8
33	Ohio	12.5
13	Oklahoma	16.6
12	Oregon	16.9
43	Pennsylvania	10.3
39	Rhode Island	11.6
15	South Carolina	16.4
37	South Dakota	12.0
20	Tennessee	14.9
1	Texas	25.5
26	Utah	13.6
44	Vermont	10.1
29	Virginia	13.4
35	Washington	12.2
22	West Virginia	14.4
47	Wisconsin	9.1
23	Wyoming	14.3

RANK ORDER

RANK	STATE	PERCENT
1	Texas	25.5
2	New Mexico	22.6
3	Florida	20.9
4	Arizona	19.1
5	California	18.9
5	Nevada	18.9
7	Alaska	18.6
7	Georgia	18.6
9	Louisiana	18.2
10	Mississippi	18.1
11	Arkansas	17.7
12	Oregon	16.9
13	North Carolina	16.6
13	Oklahoma	16.6
15	South Carolina	16.4
16	Colorado	15.9
17	Montana	15.7
18	Kentucky	15.3
19	New Jersey	15.2
20	Idaho	14.9
20	Tennessee	14.9
22	West Virginia	14.4
23	Wyoming	14.3
24	New York	14.0
25	Illinois	13.7
26	Alabama	13.6
26	Utah	13.6
28	Missouri	13.5
29	Virginia	13.4
30	Maryland	13.2
31	Kansas	12.7
32	Indiana	12.6
33	Ohio	12.5
34	Michigan	12.4
35	Nebraska	12.2
35	Washington	12.2
37	South Dakota	12.0
38	Delaware	11.8
39	Rhode Island	11.6
40	North Dakota	10.8
41	Connecticut	10.5
42	New Hampshire	10.4
43	Pennsylvania	10.3
44	Vermont	10.1
45	Iowa	10.0
46	Maine	9.8
47	Wisconsin	9.1
48	Minnesota	8.6
49	Hawaii	7.8
50	Massachusetts	5.1

District of Columbia	10.6

Source: U.S. Bureau of the Census
   "Income, Poverty, and Health Insurance Coverage: 2009"
   (http://www.census.gov/hhes/www/hlthins/data/incpovhlth/index.html)
*Three-year average for 2007 through 2009.

Numerical Change in Persons Uninsured: 2005 to 2009

National Change = 5,859,000 Increase

ALPHA ORDER

RANK	STATE	GAIN/LOSS
14	Alabama	132,000
39	Alaska	9,000
19	Arizona	90,000
22	Arkansas	66,000
2	California	588,000
46	Colorado	(10,000)
28	Connecticut	37,000
36	Delaware	15,000
3	Florida	502,000
7	Georgia	331,000
45	Hawaii	(8,000)
32	Idaho	19,000
13	Illinois	161,000
21	Indiana	70,000
18	Iowa	101,000
20	Kansas	87,000
11	Kentucky	196,000
48	Louisiana	(14,000)
44	Maine	(3,000)
25	Maryland	47,000
50	Massachusetts	(288,000)
8	Michigan	317,000
24	Minnesota	48,000
32	Mississippi	19,000
9	Missouri	246,000
41	Montana	4,000
31	Nebraska	20,000
15	Nevada	128,000
37	New Hampshire	12,000
17	New Jersey	106,000
28	New Mexico	37,000
5	New York	363,000
4	North Carolina	373,000
43	North Dakota	(2,000)
6	Ohio	355,000
30	Oklahoma	32,000
16	Oregon	112,000
10	Pennsylvania	213,000
40	Rhode Island	5,000
26	South Carolina	45,000
34	South Dakota	18,000
12	Tennessee	165,000
1	Texas	1,039,000
42	Utah	1,000
47	Vermont	(11,000)
23	Virginia	63,000
27	Washington	41,000
49	West Virginia	(51,000)
34	Wisconsin	18,000
38	Wyoming	11,000

RANK ORDER

RANK	STATE	GAIN/LOSS
1	Texas	1,039,000
2	California	588,000
3	Florida	502,000
4	North Carolina	373,000
5	New York	363,000
6	Ohio	355,000
7	Georgia	331,000
8	Michigan	317,000
9	Missouri	246,000
10	Pennsylvania	213,000
11	Kentucky	196,000
12	Tennessee	165,000
13	Illinois	161,000
14	Alabama	132,000
15	Nevada	128,000
16	Oregon	112,000
17	New Jersey	106,000
18	Iowa	101,000
19	Arizona	90,000
20	Kansas	87,000
21	Indiana	70,000
22	Arkansas	66,000
23	Virginia	63,000
24	Minnesota	48,000
25	Maryland	47,000
26	South Carolina	45,000
27	Washington	41,000
28	Connecticut	37,000
28	New Mexico	37,000
30	Oklahoma	32,000
31	Nebraska	20,000
32	Idaho	19,000
32	Mississippi	19,000
34	South Dakota	18,000
34	Wisconsin	18,000
36	Delaware	15,000
37	New Hampshire	12,000
38	Wyoming	11,000
39	Alaska	9,000
40	Rhode Island	5,000
41	Montana	4,000
42	Utah	1,000
43	North Dakota	(2,000)
44	Maine	(3,000)
45	Hawaii	(8,000)
46	Colorado	(10,000)
47	Vermont	(11,000)
48	Louisiana	(14,000)
49	West Virginia	(51,000)
50	Massachusetts	(288,000)

District of Columbia — 3,000

Source: CQ Press using data from U.S. Bureau of the Census
"Income, Poverty, and Health Insurance Coverage: 2009 and 2005"
(http://www.census.gov/hhes/www/hlthins/data/incpovhlth/index.html)

Percent Change in Persons Uninsured: 2005 to 2009

National Percent Change = 13.1% Increase

ALPHA ORDER				RANK ORDER		
RANK	STATE	PERCENT CHANGE		RANK	STATE	PERCENT CHANGE
10	Alabama	20.1		1	Iowa	41.9
31	Alaska	8.0		2	Kentucky	39.4
32	Arizona	7.6		3	Missouri	36.8
20	Arkansas	13.7		4	Kansas	31.3
28	California	8.7		5	Michigan	30.7
43	Colorado	(1.3)		6	Nevada	30.6
23	Connecticut	9.7		7	North Carolina	28.4
18	Delaware	14.6		8	Ohio	27.6
19	Florida	13.9		9	Tennessee	20.7
11	Georgia	20.0		10	Alabama	20.1
47	Hawaii	(7.3)		11	Georgia	20.0
27	Idaho	8.9		11	South Dakota	20.0
26	Illinois	9.3		13	Oregon	19.8
29	Indiana	8.4		14	Texas	19.3
1	Iowa	41.9		15	Pennsylvania	17.8
4	Kansas	31.3		16	New York	14.7
2	Kentucky	39.4		16	Wyoming	14.7
44	Louisiana	(1.9)		18	Delaware	14.6
45	Maine	(2.2)		19	Florida	13.9
34	Maryland	6.3		20	Arkansas	13.7
50	Massachusetts	(49.4)		21	Minnesota	11.8
5	Michigan	30.7		22	Nebraska	10.8
21	Minnesota	11.8		23	Connecticut	9.7
39	Mississippi	3.9		24	New Hampshire	9.5
3	Missouri	36.8		25	New Mexico	9.4
41	Montana	2.8		26	Illinois	9.3
22	Nebraska	10.8		27	Idaho	8.9
6	Nevada	30.6		28	California	8.7
24	New Hampshire	9.5		29	Indiana	8.4
29	New Jersey	8.4		29	New Jersey	8.4
25	New Mexico	9.4		31	Alaska	8.0
16	New York	14.7		32	Arizona	7.6
7	North Carolina	28.4		33	Virginia	6.6
46	North Dakota	(2.9)		34	Maryland	6.3
8	Ohio	27.6		35	South Carolina	6.2
36	Oklahoma	5.1		36	Oklahoma	5.1
13	Oregon	19.8		37	Washington	5.0
15	Pennsylvania	17.8		38	Rhode Island	4.1
38	Rhode Island	4.1		39	Mississippi	3.9
35	South Carolina	6.2		40	Wisconsin	3.5
11	South Dakota	20.0		41	Montana	2.8
9	Tennessee	20.7		42	Utah	0.2
14	Texas	19.3		43	Colorado	(1.3)
42	Utah	0.2		44	Louisiana	(1.9)
48	Vermont	(15.3)		45	Maine	(2.2)
33	Virginia	6.6		46	North Dakota	(2.9)
37	Washington	5.0		47	Hawaii	(7.3)
49	West Virginia	(16.8)		48	Vermont	(15.3)
40	Wisconsin	3.5		49	West Virginia	(16.8)
16	Wyoming	14.7		50	Massachusetts	(49.4)

District of Columbia   4.2

Source: CQ Press using data from U.S. Bureau of the Census
"Income, Poverty, and Health Insurance Coverage: 2009 and 2005"
(http://www.census.gov/hhes/www/hlthins/data/incpovhlth/index.html)

Change in Percent of Population Uninsured: 2005 to 2009

National Percent Change = 0.6% Increase*

ALPHA ORDER

RANK	STATE	PERCENT CHANGE
33	Alabama	(4.9)
15	Alaska	4.5
10	Arizona	5.5
18	Arkansas	2.9
24	California	0.5
36	Colorado	(5.9)
32	Connecticut	(4.5)
40	Delaware	(7.1)
8	Florida	6.6
9	Georgia	6.3
49	Hawaii	(17.9)
42	Idaho	(9.7)
30	Illinois	(3.5)
43	Indiana	(11.3)
21	Iowa	2.0
1	Kansas	16.5
3	Kentucky	12.5
29	Louisiana	(2.7)
35	Maine	(5.8)
39	Maryland	(6.4)
50	Massachusetts	(52.3)
4	Michigan	9.7
27	Minnesota	(1.1)
14	Mississippi	4.6
2	Missouri	13.4
48	Montana	(16.0)
7	Nebraska	7.0
19	Nevada	2.7
25	New Hampshire	0.0
13	New Jersey	4.8
6	New Mexico	7.1
23	New York	0.7
20	North Carolina	2.5
31	North Dakota	(3.6)
16	Ohio	4.2
47	Oklahoma	(14.9)
22	Oregon	1.2
41	Pennsylvania	(8.0)
10	Rhode Island	5.5
12	South Carolina	5.1
26	South Dakota	(0.8)
5	Tennessee	8.8
17	Texas	3.7
38	Utah	(6.2)
34	Vermont	(5.6)
28	Virginia	(1.5)
45	Washington	(13.5)
46	West Virginia	(14.8)
44	Wisconsin	(11.7)
36	Wyoming	(5.9)

RANK ORDER

RANK	STATE	PERCENT CHANGE
1	Kansas	16.5
2	Missouri	13.4
3	Kentucky	12.5
4	Michigan	9.7
5	Tennessee	8.8
6	New Mexico	7.1
7	Nebraska	7.0
8	Florida	6.6
9	Georgia	6.3
10	Arizona	5.5
10	Rhode Island	5.5
12	South Carolina	5.1
13	New Jersey	4.8
14	Mississippi	4.6
15	Alaska	4.5
16	Ohio	4.2
17	Texas	3.7
18	Arkansas	2.9
19	Nevada	2.7
20	North Carolina	2.5
21	Iowa	2.0
22	Oregon	1.2
23	New York	0.7
24	California	0.5
25	New Hampshire	0.0
26	South Dakota	(0.8)
27	Minnesota	(1.1)
28	Virginia	(1.5)
29	Louisiana	(2.7)
30	Illinois	(3.5)
31	North Dakota	(3.6)
32	Connecticut	(4.5)
33	Alabama	(4.9)
34	Vermont	(5.6)
35	Maine	(5.8)
36	Colorado	(5.9)
36	Wyoming	(5.9)
38	Utah	(6.2)
39	Maryland	(6.4)
40	Delaware	(7.1)
41	Pennsylvania	(8.0)
42	Idaho	(9.7)
43	Indiana	(11.3)
44	Wisconsin	(11.7)
45	Washington	(13.5)
46	West Virginia	(14.8)
47	Oklahoma	(14.9)
48	Montana	(16.0)
49	Hawaii	(17.9)
50	Massachusetts	(52.3)

District of Columbia   (21.5)

Source: CQ Press using data from U.S. Bureau of the Census
"Income, Poverty, and Health Insurance Coverage: 2009"
(http://www.census.gov/hhes/www/hlthins/data/incpovhlth/index.html)
*Based on three-year averages for 2007 through 2009 and 2003 through 2005.

Percent of Children Not Covered by Health Insurance in 2009

National Percent = 16.7% of Children*

<table>
<tr><td colspan="3">ALPHA ORDER</td><td colspan="3">RANK ORDER</td></tr>
<tr><td>RANK</td><td>STATE</td><td>PERCENT</td><td>RANK</td><td>STATE</td><td>PERCENT</td></tr>
<tr><td>15</td><td>Alabama</td><td>16.9</td><td>1</td><td>Texas</td><td>26.1</td></tr>
<tr><td>11</td><td>Alaska</td><td>17.7</td><td>2</td><td>Florida</td><td>22.4</td></tr>
<tr><td>7</td><td>Arizona</td><td>19.6</td><td>3</td><td>New Mexico</td><td>21.7</td></tr>
<tr><td>8</td><td>Arkansas</td><td>19.2</td><td>4</td><td>Nevada</td><td>20.8</td></tr>
<tr><td>6</td><td>California</td><td>20.0</td><td>5</td><td>Georgia</td><td>20.5</td></tr>
<tr><td>22</td><td>Colorado</td><td>15.3</td><td>6</td><td>California</td><td>20.0</td></tr>
<tr><td>39</td><td>Connecticut</td><td>12.0</td><td>7</td><td>Arizona</td><td>19.6</td></tr>
<tr><td>34</td><td>Delaware</td><td>13.4</td><td>8</td><td>Arkansas</td><td>19.2</td></tr>
<tr><td>2</td><td>Florida</td><td>22.4</td><td>9</td><td>Oklahoma</td><td>18.1</td></tr>
<tr><td>5</td><td>Georgia</td><td>20.5</td><td>10</td><td>North Carolina</td><td>18.0</td></tr>
<tr><td>49</td><td>Hawaii</td><td>8.2</td><td>11</td><td>Alaska</td><td>17.7</td></tr>
<tr><td>24</td><td>Idaho</td><td>15.2</td><td>11</td><td>Oregon</td><td>17.7</td></tr>
<tr><td>25</td><td>Illinois</td><td>14.8</td><td>13</td><td>Mississippi</td><td>17.6</td></tr>
<tr><td>29</td><td>Indiana</td><td>14.2</td><td>14</td><td>South Carolina</td><td>17.0</td></tr>
<tr><td>41</td><td>Iowa</td><td>11.4</td><td>15</td><td>Alabama</td><td>16.9</td></tr>
<tr><td>35</td><td>Kansas</td><td>13.3</td><td>16</td><td>Kentucky</td><td>16.2</td></tr>
<tr><td>16</td><td>Kentucky</td><td>16.2</td><td>17</td><td>Louisiana</td><td>16.0</td></tr>
<tr><td>17</td><td>Louisiana</td><td>16.0</td><td>18</td><td>New Jersey</td><td>15.8</td></tr>
<tr><td>45</td><td>Maine</td><td>10.2</td><td>18</td><td>Wyoming</td><td>15.8</td></tr>
<tr><td>30</td><td>Maryland</td><td>14.0</td><td>20</td><td>Montana</td><td>15.4</td></tr>
<tr><td>50</td><td>Massachusetts</td><td>4.4</td><td>20</td><td>Tennessee</td><td>15.4</td></tr>
<tr><td>32</td><td>Michigan</td><td>13.8</td><td>22</td><td>Colorado</td><td>15.3</td></tr>
<tr><td>48</td><td>Minnesota</td><td>8.8</td><td>22</td><td>Missouri</td><td>15.3</td></tr>
<tr><td>13</td><td>Mississippi</td><td>17.6</td><td>24</td><td>Idaho</td><td>15.2</td></tr>
<tr><td>22</td><td>Missouri</td><td>15.3</td><td>25</td><td>Illinois</td><td>14.8</td></tr>
<tr><td>20</td><td>Montana</td><td>15.4</td><td>25</td><td>New York</td><td>14.8</td></tr>
<tr><td>40</td><td>Nebraska</td><td>11.5</td><td>25</td><td>Utah</td><td>14.8</td></tr>
<tr><td>4</td><td>Nevada</td><td>20.8</td><td>28</td><td>Ohio</td><td>14.3</td></tr>
<tr><td>44</td><td>New Hampshire</td><td>10.5</td><td>29</td><td>Indiana</td><td>14.2</td></tr>
<tr><td>18</td><td>New Jersey</td><td>15.8</td><td>30</td><td>Maryland</td><td>14.0</td></tr>
<tr><td>3</td><td>New Mexico</td><td>21.7</td><td>30</td><td>West Virginia</td><td>14.0</td></tr>
<tr><td>25</td><td>New York</td><td>14.8</td><td>32</td><td>Michigan</td><td>13.8</td></tr>
<tr><td>10</td><td>North Carolina</td><td>18.0</td><td>33</td><td>South Dakota</td><td>13.5</td></tr>
<tr><td>43</td><td>North Dakota</td><td>10.7</td><td>34</td><td>Delaware</td><td>13.4</td></tr>
<tr><td>28</td><td>Ohio</td><td>14.3</td><td>35</td><td>Kansas</td><td>13.3</td></tr>
<tr><td>9</td><td>Oklahoma</td><td>18.1</td><td>36</td><td>Virginia</td><td>13.0</td></tr>
<tr><td>11</td><td>Oregon</td><td>17.7</td><td>37</td><td>Washington</td><td>12.9</td></tr>
<tr><td>41</td><td>Pennsylvania</td><td>11.4</td><td>38</td><td>Rhode Island</td><td>12.3</td></tr>
<tr><td>38</td><td>Rhode Island</td><td>12.3</td><td>39</td><td>Connecticut</td><td>12.0</td></tr>
<tr><td>14</td><td>South Carolina</td><td>17.0</td><td>40</td><td>Nebraska</td><td>11.5</td></tr>
<tr><td>33</td><td>South Dakota</td><td>13.5</td><td>41</td><td>Iowa</td><td>11.4</td></tr>
<tr><td>20</td><td>Tennessee</td><td>15.4</td><td>41</td><td>Pennsylvania</td><td>11.4</td></tr>
<tr><td>1</td><td>Texas</td><td>26.1</td><td>43</td><td>North Dakota</td><td>10.7</td></tr>
<tr><td>25</td><td>Utah</td><td>14.8</td><td>44</td><td>New Hampshire</td><td>10.5</td></tr>
<tr><td>46</td><td>Vermont</td><td>9.9</td><td>45</td><td>Maine</td><td>10.2</td></tr>
<tr><td>36</td><td>Virginia</td><td>13.0</td><td>46</td><td>Vermont</td><td>9.9</td></tr>
<tr><td>37</td><td>Washington</td><td>12.9</td><td>47</td><td>Wisconsin</td><td>9.5</td></tr>
<tr><td>30</td><td>West Virginia</td><td>14.0</td><td>48</td><td>Minnesota</td><td>8.8</td></tr>
<tr><td>47</td><td>Wisconsin</td><td>9.5</td><td>49</td><td>Hawaii</td><td>8.2</td></tr>
<tr><td>18</td><td>Wyoming</td><td>15.8</td><td>50</td><td>Massachusetts</td><td>4.4</td></tr>
<tr><td></td><td></td><td></td><td></td><td>District of Columbia</td><td>12.4</td></tr>
</table>

Source: U.S. Bureau of the Census
"Health Insurance Coverage Status by State for All People: 2009" (http://www.census.gov/hhes/www/hlthins/index.html)
*Children under 18 years old.

Persons Covered by Health Insurance in 2009

National Total = 253,606,000 Insured

RANK	STATE	INSURED	% of USA
ALPHA ORDER			
23	Alabama	3,880,000	1.5%
47	Alaska	568,000	0.2%
17	Arizona	5,239,000	2.1%
34	Arkansas	2,304,000	0.9%
1	California	29,449,000	11.6%
22	Colorado	4,209,000	1.7%
28	Connecticut	3,062,000	1.2%
45	Delaware	766,000	0.3%
4	Florida	14,287,000	5.6%
9	Georgia	7,687,000	3.0%
42	Hawaii	1,149,000	0.5%
39	Idaho	1,294,000	0.5%
6	Illinois	10,875,000	4.3%
15	Indiana	5,462,000	2.2%
30	Iowa	2,654,000	1.0%
32	Kansas	2,380,000	0.9%
26	Kentucky	3,588,000	1.4%
24	Louisiana	3,741,000	1.5%
41	Maine	1,167,000	0.5%
20	Maryland	4,874,000	1.9%
13	Massachusetts	6,337,000	2.5%
8	Michigan	8,465,000	3.3%
21	Minnesota	4,747,000	1.9%
33	Mississippi	2,349,000	0.9%
18	Missouri	5,055,000	2.0%
44	Montana	823,000	0.3%
36	Nebraska	1,574,000	0.6%
35	Nevada	2,086,000	0.8%
40	New Hampshire	1,176,000	0.5%
11	New Jersey	7,309,000	2.9%
38	New Mexico	1,548,000	0.6%
3	New York	16,347,000	6.4%
10	North Carolina	7,663,000	3.0%
48	North Dakota	565,000	0.2%
7	Ohio	9,819,000	3.9%
29	Oklahoma	2,977,000	1.2%
27	Oregon	3,156,000	1.2%
5	Pennsylvania	11,004,000	4.3%
43	Rhode Island	906,000	0.4%
25	South Carolina	3,740,000	1.5%
46	South Dakota	693,000	0.3%
16	Tennessee	5,290,000	2.1%
2	Texas	18,224,000	7.2%
31	Utah	2,385,000	0.9%
49	Vermont	557,000	0.2%
12	Virginia	6,764,000	2.7%
14	Washington	5,845,000	2.3%
37	West Virginia	1,552,000	0.6%
19	Wisconsin	5,037,000	2.0%
50	Wyoming	455,000	0.2%

RANK	STATE	INSURED	% of USA
RANK ORDER			
1	California	29,449,000	11.6%
2	Texas	18,224,000	7.2%
3	New York	16,347,000	6.4%
4	Florida	14,287,000	5.6%
5	Pennsylvania	11,004,000	4.3%
6	Illinois	10,875,000	4.3%
7	Ohio	9,819,000	3.9%
8	Michigan	8,465,000	3.3%
9	Georgia	7,687,000	3.0%
10	North Carolina	7,663,000	3.0%
11	New Jersey	7,309,000	2.9%
12	Virginia	6,764,000	2.7%
13	Massachusetts	6,337,000	2.5%
14	Washington	5,845,000	2.3%
15	Indiana	5,462,000	2.2%
16	Tennessee	5,290,000	2.1%
17	Arizona	5,239,000	2.1%
18	Missouri	5,055,000	2.0%
19	Wisconsin	5,037,000	2.0%
20	Maryland	4,874,000	1.9%
21	Minnesota	4,747,000	1.9%
22	Colorado	4,209,000	1.7%
23	Alabama	3,880,000	1.5%
24	Louisiana	3,741,000	1.5%
25	South Carolina	3,740,000	1.5%
26	Kentucky	3,588,000	1.4%
27	Oregon	3,156,000	1.2%
28	Connecticut	3,062,000	1.2%
29	Oklahoma	2,977,000	1.2%
30	Iowa	2,654,000	1.0%
31	Utah	2,385,000	0.9%
32	Kansas	2,380,000	0.9%
33	Mississippi	2,349,000	0.9%
34	Arkansas	2,304,000	0.9%
35	Nevada	2,086,000	0.8%
36	Nebraska	1,574,000	0.6%
37	West Virginia	1,552,000	0.6%
38	New Mexico	1,548,000	0.6%
39	Idaho	1,294,000	0.5%
40	New Hampshire	1,176,000	0.5%
41	Maine	1,167,000	0.5%
42	Hawaii	1,149,000	0.5%
43	Rhode Island	906,000	0.4%
44	Montana	823,000	0.3%
45	Delaware	766,000	0.3%
46	South Dakota	693,000	0.3%
47	Alaska	568,000	0.2%
48	North Dakota	565,000	0.2%
49	Vermont	557,000	0.2%
50	Wyoming	455,000	0.2%
	District of Columbia	522,000	0.2%

Source: U.S. Bureau of the Census
"Health Insurance Coverage Status by State for All People: 2009" (http://www.census.gov/hhes/www/hlthins/index.html)

Percent of Population Covered by Health Insurance in 2009

National Percent = 83.3% of Population

ALPHA ORDER				RANK ORDER		
RANK	STATE	PERCENT		RANK	STATE	PERCENT
36	Alabama	83.1		1	Massachusetts	95.6
39	Alaska	82.3		2	Hawaii	91.8
44	Arizona	80.4		3	Minnesota	91.2
43	Arkansas	80.8		4	Wisconsin	90.5
45	California	80.0		5	Vermont	90.1
28	Colorado	84.7		6	Maine	89.8
12	Connecticut	88.0		7	New Hampshire	89.5
17	Delaware	86.6		8	North Dakota	89.3
49	Florida	77.6		9	Iowa	88.6
46	Georgia	79.5		9	Pennsylvania	88.6
2	Hawaii	91.8		11	Nebraska	88.5
27	Idaho	84.8		12	Connecticut	88.0
24	Illinois	85.2		13	Rhode Island	87.7
22	Indiana	85.8		14	Washington	87.1
9	Iowa	88.6		15	Virginia	87.0
16	Kansas	86.7		16	Kansas	86.7
35	Kentucky	83.8		17	Delaware	86.6
34	Louisiana	84.0		18	South Dakota	86.5
6	Maine	89.8		19	Michigan	86.2
20	Maryland	86.0		20	Maryland	86.0
1	Massachusetts	95.6		20	West Virginia	86.0
19	Michigan	86.2		22	Indiana	85.8
3	Minnesota	91.2		23	Ohio	85.7
38	Mississippi	82.4		24	Illinois	85.2
28	Missouri	84.7		24	New York	85.2
30	Montana	84.6		24	Utah	85.2
11	Nebraska	88.5		27	Idaho	84.8
47	Nevada	79.2		28	Colorado	84.7
7	New Hampshire	89.5		28	Missouri	84.7
32	New Jersey	84.2		30	Montana	84.6
48	New Mexico	78.3		30	Tennessee	84.6
24	New York	85.2		32	New Jersey	84.2
41	North Carolina	82.0		32	Wyoming	84.2
8	North Dakota	89.3		34	Louisiana	84.0
23	Ohio	85.7		35	Kentucky	83.8
42	Oklahoma	81.9		36	Alabama	83.1
39	Oregon	82.3		37	South Carolina	83.0
9	Pennsylvania	88.6		38	Mississippi	82.4
13	Rhode Island	87.7		39	Alaska	82.3
37	South Carolina	83.0		39	Oregon	82.3
18	South Dakota	86.5		41	North Carolina	82.0
30	Tennessee	84.6		42	Oklahoma	81.9
50	Texas	73.9		43	Arkansas	80.8
24	Utah	85.2		44	Arizona	80.4
5	Vermont	90.1		45	California	80.0
15	Virginia	87.0		46	Georgia	79.5
14	Washington	87.1		47	Nevada	79.2
20	West Virginia	86.0		48	New Mexico	78.3
4	Wisconsin	90.5		49	Florida	77.6
32	Wyoming	84.2		50	Texas	73.9
					District of Columbia	87.6

Source: U.S. Bureau of the Census
"Health Insurance Coverage Status by State for All People: 2009" (http://www.census.gov/hhes/www/hlthins/index.html)

Percent of Population Covered by Private Health Insurance in 2009

National Percent = 63.9% of Population*

ALPHA ORDER

RANK	STATE	PERCENT
34	Alabama	62.6
39	Alaska	60.9
46	Arizona	56.7
47	Arkansas	55.3
44	California	58.1
18	Colorado	69.5
3	Connecticut	75.3
23	Delaware	67.9
45	Florida	57.4
42	Georgia	60.8
13	Hawaii	71.0
21	Idaho	68.5
28	Illinois	66.5
31	Indiana	65.8
4	Iowa	75.2
14	Kansas	70.8
34	Kentucky	62.6
33	Louisiana	62.7
30	Maine	65.9
10	Maryland	73.0
5	Massachusetts	74.8
17	Michigan	69.9
5	Minnesota	74.8
49	Mississippi	53.1
25	Missouri	67.3
28	Montana	66.5
8	Nebraska	74.1
32	Nevada	64.0
2	New Hampshire	76.5
11	New Jersey	71.3
50	New Mexico	51.2
39	New York	60.9
38	North Carolina	61.7
1	North Dakota	78.0
21	Ohio	68.5
39	Oklahoma	60.9
27	Oregon	67.1
12	Pennsylvania	71.2
25	Rhode Island	67.3
37	South Carolina	62.2
14	South Dakota	70.8
43	Tennessee	59.9
48	Texas	53.8
9	Utah	73.4
23	Vermont	67.9
16	Virginia	70.0
19	Washington	69.1
36	West Virginia	62.3
7	Wisconsin	74.4
20	Wyoming	68.7

RANK ORDER

RANK	STATE	PERCENT
1	North Dakota	78.0
2	New Hampshire	76.5
3	Connecticut	75.3
4	Iowa	75.2
5	Massachusetts	74.8
5	Minnesota	74.8
7	Wisconsin	74.4
8	Nebraska	74.1
9	Utah	73.4
10	Maryland	73.0
11	New Jersey	71.3
12	Pennsylvania	71.2
13	Hawaii	71.0
14	Kansas	70.8
14	South Dakota	70.8
16	Virginia	70.0
17	Michigan	69.9
18	Colorado	69.5
19	Washington	69.1
20	Wyoming	68.7
21	Idaho	68.5
21	Ohio	68.5
23	Delaware	67.9
23	Vermont	67.9
25	Missouri	67.3
25	Rhode Island	67.3
27	Oregon	67.1
28	Illinois	66.5
28	Montana	66.5
30	Maine	65.9
31	Indiana	65.8
32	Nevada	64.0
33	Louisiana	62.7
34	Alabama	62.6
34	Kentucky	62.6
36	West Virginia	62.3
37	South Carolina	62.2
38	North Carolina	61.7
39	Alaska	60.9
39	New York	60.9
39	Oklahoma	60.9
42	Georgia	60.8
43	Tennessee	59.9
44	California	58.1
45	Florida	57.4
46	Arizona	56.7
47	Arkansas	55.3
48	Texas	53.8
49	Mississippi	53.1
50	New Mexico	51.2
	District of Columbia	63.7

Source: U.S. Bureau of the Census
"Health Insurance Coverage Status by State for All People: 2009" (http://www.census.gov/hhes/www/hlthins/index.html)
*Private health insurance is coverage by a health plan provided through an employer or union or purchased by an individual from a private health insurance company.

Percent of Population Covered by Employment-Based Health Insurance in 2009
National Percent = 55.8% of Population*

ALPHA ORDER

RANK	STATE	PERCENT
30	Alabama	56.4
27	Alaska	56.9
47	Arizona	47.8
48	Arkansas	47.2
44	California	49.8
19	Colorado	59.5
4	Connecticut	66.3
14	Delaware	61.6
45	Florida	48.2
37	Georgia	54.4
7	Hawaii	65.1
31	Idaho	55.9
23	Illinois	57.9
22	Indiana	58.1
11	Iowa	62.2
25	Kansas	57.6
31	Kentucky	55.9
34	Louisiana	55.4
34	Maine	55.4
2	Maryland	66.7
3	Massachusetts	66.5
9	Michigan	63.1
11	Minnesota	62.2
50	Mississippi	44.7
26	Missouri	57.1
43	Montana	50.0
15	Nebraska	61.3
24	Nevada	57.8
1	New Hampshire	68.3
5	New Jersey	65.3
49	New Mexico	45.0
40	New York	53.7
39	North Carolina	53.8
17	North Dakota	59.8
16	Ohio	60.7
41	Oklahoma	53.6
36	Oregon	54.9
13	Pennsylvania	61.8
20	Rhode Island	59.0
38	South Carolina	54.0
33	South Dakota	55.8
42	Tennessee	51.3
45	Texas	48.2
5	Utah	65.3
21	Vermont	58.9
10	Virginia	63.0
18	Washington	59.7
28	West Virginia	56.8
8	Wisconsin	63.8
29	Wyoming	56.5

RANK ORDER

RANK	STATE	PERCENT
1	New Hampshire	68.3
2	Maryland	66.7
3	Massachusetts	66.5
4	Connecticut	66.3
5	New Jersey	65.3
5	Utah	65.3
7	Hawaii	65.1
8	Wisconsin	63.8
9	Michigan	63.1
10	Virginia	63.0
11	Iowa	62.2
11	Minnesota	62.2
13	Pennsylvania	61.8
14	Delaware	61.6
15	Nebraska	61.3
16	Ohio	60.7
17	North Dakota	59.8
18	Washington	59.7
19	Colorado	59.5
20	Rhode Island	59.0
21	Vermont	58.9
22	Indiana	58.1
23	Illinois	57.9
24	Nevada	57.8
25	Kansas	57.6
26	Missouri	57.1
27	Alaska	56.9
28	West Virginia	56.8
29	Wyoming	56.5
30	Alabama	56.4
31	Idaho	55.9
31	Kentucky	55.9
33	South Dakota	55.8
34	Louisiana	55.4
34	Maine	55.4
36	Oregon	54.9
37	Georgia	54.4
38	South Carolina	54.0
39	North Carolina	53.8
40	New York	53.7
41	Oklahoma	53.6
42	Tennessee	51.3
43	Montana	50.0
44	California	49.8
45	Florida	48.2
45	Texas	48.2
47	Arizona	47.8
48	Arkansas	47.2
49	New Mexico	45.0
50	Mississippi	44.7

District of Columbia — 56.7

Source: U.S. Bureau of the Census
"Health Insurance Coverage Status by State for All People: 2009" (http://www.census.gov/hhes/www/hlthins/index.html)
*Employment-based health insurance is private insurance coverage offered through one's own employment or a relative's. It may be offered by an employer or by a union.

Percent of Population Covered by Direct-Purchase Health Insurance in 2009

National Percent = 8.9% of Population*

<table>
<thead>
<tr><th colspan="3">ALPHA ORDER</th><th colspan="3">RANK ORDER</th></tr>
<tr><th>RANK</th><th>STATE</th><th>PERCENT</th><th>RANK</th><th>STATE</th><th>PERCENT</th></tr>
</thead>
<tbody>
<tr><td>35</td><td>Alabama</td><td>8.0</td><td>1</td><td>North Dakota</td><td>20.3</td></tr>
<tr><td>50</td><td>Alaska</td><td>5.3</td><td>2</td><td>South Dakota</td><td>16.2</td></tr>
<tr><td>13</td><td>Arizona</td><td>10.6</td><td>3</td><td>Nebraska</td><td>15.6</td></tr>
<tr><td>28</td><td>Arkansas</td><td>8.8</td><td>4</td><td>Idaho</td><td>15.4</td></tr>
<tr><td>33</td><td>California</td><td>8.4</td><td>4</td><td>Montana</td><td>15.4</td></tr>
<tr><td>13</td><td>Colorado</td><td>10.6</td><td>6</td><td>Iowa</td><td>14.1</td></tr>
<tr><td>21</td><td>Connecticut</td><td>9.6</td><td>6</td><td>Oregon</td><td>14.1</td></tr>
<tr><td>37</td><td>Delaware</td><td>7.7</td><td>8</td><td>Minnesota</td><td>13.9</td></tr>
<tr><td>16</td><td>Florida</td><td>10.5</td><td>9</td><td>Kansas</td><td>13.0</td></tr>
<tr><td>38</td><td>Georgia</td><td>7.5</td><td>10</td><td>Wyoming</td><td>12.3</td></tr>
<tr><td>45</td><td>Hawaii</td><td>6.8</td><td>11</td><td>Missouri</td><td>11.6</td></tr>
<tr><td>4</td><td>Idaho</td><td>15.4</td><td>12</td><td>Wisconsin</td><td>11.0</td></tr>
<tr><td>20</td><td>Illinois</td><td>10.0</td><td>13</td><td>Arizona</td><td>10.6</td></tr>
<tr><td>18</td><td>Indiana</td><td>10.3</td><td>13</td><td>Colorado</td><td>10.6</td></tr>
<tr><td>6</td><td>Iowa</td><td>14.1</td><td>13</td><td>Maine</td><td>10.6</td></tr>
<tr><td>9</td><td>Kansas</td><td>13.0</td><td>16</td><td>Florida</td><td>10.5</td></tr>
<tr><td>40</td><td>Kentucky</td><td>7.3</td><td>17</td><td>Pennsylvania</td><td>10.4</td></tr>
<tr><td>34</td><td>Louisiana</td><td>8.3</td><td>18</td><td>Indiana</td><td>10.3</td></tr>
<tr><td>13</td><td>Maine</td><td>10.6</td><td>19</td><td>Washington</td><td>10.2</td></tr>
<tr><td>43</td><td>Maryland</td><td>6.9</td><td>20</td><td>Illinois</td><td>10.0</td></tr>
<tr><td>31</td><td>Massachusetts</td><td>8.6</td><td>21</td><td>Connecticut</td><td>9.6</td></tr>
<tr><td>41</td><td>Michigan</td><td>7.1</td><td>21</td><td>Vermont</td><td>9.6</td></tr>
<tr><td>8</td><td>Minnesota</td><td>13.9</td><td>23</td><td>South Carolina</td><td>9.3</td></tr>
<tr><td>26</td><td>Mississippi</td><td>8.9</td><td>24</td><td>Ohio</td><td>9.2</td></tr>
<tr><td>11</td><td>Missouri</td><td>11.6</td><td>25</td><td>New Hampshire</td><td>9.0</td></tr>
<tr><td>4</td><td>Montana</td><td>15.4</td><td>26</td><td>Mississippi</td><td>8.9</td></tr>
<tr><td>3</td><td>Nebraska</td><td>15.6</td><td>26</td><td>Tennessee</td><td>8.9</td></tr>
<tr><td>47</td><td>Nevada</td><td>6.5</td><td>28</td><td>Arkansas</td><td>8.8</td></tr>
<tr><td>25</td><td>New Hampshire</td><td>9.0</td><td>28</td><td>North Carolina</td><td>8.8</td></tr>
<tr><td>41</td><td>New Jersey</td><td>7.1</td><td>28</td><td>Utah</td><td>8.8</td></tr>
<tr><td>43</td><td>New Mexico</td><td>6.9</td><td>31</td><td>Massachusetts</td><td>8.6</td></tr>
<tr><td>45</td><td>New York</td><td>6.8</td><td>32</td><td>Rhode Island</td><td>8.5</td></tr>
<tr><td>28</td><td>North Carolina</td><td>8.8</td><td>33</td><td>California</td><td>8.4</td></tr>
<tr><td>1</td><td>North Dakota</td><td>20.3</td><td>34</td><td>Louisiana</td><td>8.3</td></tr>
<tr><td>24</td><td>Ohio</td><td>9.2</td><td>35</td><td>Alabama</td><td>8.0</td></tr>
<tr><td>36</td><td>Oklahoma</td><td>7.9</td><td>36</td><td>Oklahoma</td><td>7.9</td></tr>
<tr><td>6</td><td>Oregon</td><td>14.1</td><td>37</td><td>Delaware</td><td>7.7</td></tr>
<tr><td>17</td><td>Pennsylvania</td><td>10.4</td><td>38</td><td>Georgia</td><td>7.5</td></tr>
<tr><td>32</td><td>Rhode Island</td><td>8.5</td><td>39</td><td>Virginia</td><td>7.4</td></tr>
<tr><td>23</td><td>South Carolina</td><td>9.3</td><td>40</td><td>Kentucky</td><td>7.3</td></tr>
<tr><td>2</td><td>South Dakota</td><td>16.2</td><td>41</td><td>Michigan</td><td>7.1</td></tr>
<tr><td>26</td><td>Tennessee</td><td>8.9</td><td>41</td><td>New Jersey</td><td>7.1</td></tr>
<tr><td>48</td><td>Texas</td><td>6.2</td><td>43</td><td>Maryland</td><td>6.9</td></tr>
<tr><td>28</td><td>Utah</td><td>8.8</td><td>43</td><td>New Mexico</td><td>6.9</td></tr>
<tr><td>21</td><td>Vermont</td><td>9.6</td><td>45</td><td>Hawaii</td><td>6.8</td></tr>
<tr><td>39</td><td>Virginia</td><td>7.4</td><td>45</td><td>New York</td><td>6.8</td></tr>
<tr><td>19</td><td>Washington</td><td>10.2</td><td>47</td><td>Nevada</td><td>6.5</td></tr>
<tr><td>49</td><td>West Virginia</td><td>6.0</td><td>48</td><td>Texas</td><td>6.2</td></tr>
<tr><td>12</td><td>Wisconsin</td><td>11.0</td><td>49</td><td>West Virginia</td><td>6.0</td></tr>
<tr><td>10</td><td>Wyoming</td><td>12.3</td><td>50</td><td>Alaska</td><td>5.3</td></tr>
<tr><td></td><td></td><td></td><td></td><td>District of Columbia</td><td>8.1</td></tr>
</tbody>
</table>

Source: U.S. Bureau of the Census
   "Health Insurance Coverage Status by State for All People: 2009" (http://www.census.gov/hhes/www/hlthins/index.html)
*Direct-purchase health insurance is private insurance coverage through a plan purchased by an individual from a private company.

Percent of Population Covered by Government Health Insurance in 2009

National Percent = 30.6% of Population*

ALPHA ORDER

RANK	STATE	PERCENT
11	Alabama	34.3
15	Alaska	32.9
13	Arizona	34.0
8	Arkansas	35.6
28	California	30.3
44	Colorado	26.0
45	Connecticut	24.7
23	Delaware	31.9
17	Florida	32.6
42	Georgia	26.8
5	Hawaii	37.1
41	Idaho	27.0
36	Illinois	29.1
24	Indiana	31.8
40	Iowa	27.7
30	Kansas	29.9
14	Kentucky	33.1
25	Louisiana	31.1
1	Maine	40.4
47	Maryland	24.2
9	Massachusetts	35.3
37	Michigan	28.9
34	Minnesota	29.2
2	Mississippi	40.2
30	Missouri	29.9
18	Montana	32.5
32	Nebraska	29.3
46	Nevada	24.6
48	New Hampshire	23.6
49	New Jersey	23.0
5	New Mexico	37.1
10	New York	35.1
19	North Carolina	32.2
43	North Dakota	26.3
34	Ohio	29.2
12	Oklahoma	34.2
32	Oregon	29.3
25	Pennsylvania	31.1
16	Rhode Island	32.7
19	South Carolina	32.2
19	South Dakota	32.2
7	Tennessee	35.8
38	Texas	28.1
50	Utah	20.3
4	Vermont	38.1
29	Virginia	30.1
22	Washington	32.1
3	West Virginia	40.1
27	Wisconsin	31.0
39	Wyoming	27.8

RANK ORDER

RANK	STATE	PERCENT
1	Maine	40.4
2	Mississippi	40.2
3	West Virginia	40.1
4	Vermont	38.1
5	Hawaii	37.1
5	New Mexico	37.1
7	Tennessee	35.8
8	Arkansas	35.6
9	Massachusetts	35.3
10	New York	35.1
11	Alabama	34.3
12	Oklahoma	34.2
13	Arizona	34.0
14	Kentucky	33.1
15	Alaska	32.9
16	Rhode Island	32.7
17	Florida	32.6
18	Montana	32.5
19	North Carolina	32.2
19	South Carolina	32.2
19	South Dakota	32.2
22	Washington	32.1
23	Delaware	31.9
24	Indiana	31.8
25	Louisiana	31.1
25	Pennsylvania	31.1
27	Wisconsin	31.0
28	California	30.3
29	Virginia	30.1
30	Kansas	29.9
30	Missouri	29.9
32	Nebraska	29.3
32	Oregon	29.3
34	Minnesota	29.2
34	Ohio	29.2
36	Illinois	29.1
37	Michigan	28.9
38	Texas	28.1
39	Wyoming	27.8
40	Iowa	27.7
41	Idaho	27.0
42	Georgia	26.8
43	North Dakota	26.3
44	Colorado	26.0
45	Connecticut	24.7
46	Nevada	24.6
47	Maryland	24.2
48	New Hampshire	23.6
49	New Jersey	23.0
50	Utah	20.3
	District of Columbia	33.3

Source: U.S. Bureau of the Census
   "Health Insurance Coverage Status by State for All People: 2009" (http://www.census.gov/hhes/www/hlthins/index.html)
*Includes Medicaid, Medicare, the Children's Health Insurance Program (CHIP), and military health care.

Percent of Population Covered by Military Health Care in 2009

National Percent = 4.1% of Population*

ALPHA ORDER

RANK	STATE	PERCENT
32	Alabama	3.7
1	Alaska	14.3
30	Arizona	4.0
18	Arkansas	5.8
39	California	2.8
20	Colorado	5.6
46	Connecticut	2.2
34	Delaware	3.2
14	Florida	6.3
21	Georgia	5.3
2	Hawaii	10.0
31	Idaho	3.9
44	Illinois	2.5
33	Indiana	3.3
37	Iowa	2.9
7	Kansas	7.5
24	Kentucky	4.8
37	Louisiana	2.9
13	Maine	6.5
27	Maryland	4.4
46	Massachusetts	2.2
48	Michigan	1.7
40	Minnesota	2.6
25	Mississippi	4.5
29	Missouri	4.1
18	Montana	5.8
9	Nebraska	7.2
12	Nevada	6.6
36	New Hampshire	3.0
50	New Jersey	0.8
11	New Mexico	6.7
49	New York	1.3
14	North Carolina	6.3
16	North Dakota	6.0
40	Ohio	2.6
4	Oklahoma	8.2
25	Oregon	4.5
40	Pennsylvania	2.6
44	Rhode Island	2.5
23	South Carolina	5.2
5	South Dakota	7.8
9	Tennessee	7.2
28	Texas	4.3
34	Utah	3.2
21	Vermont	5.3
3	Virginia	9.9
6	Washington	7.7
17	West Virginia	5.9
40	Wisconsin	2.6
8	Wyoming	7.3

RANK ORDER

RANK	STATE	PERCENT
1	Alaska	14.3
2	Hawaii	10.0
3	Virginia	9.9
4	Oklahoma	8.2
5	South Dakota	7.8
6	Washington	7.7
7	Kansas	7.5
8	Wyoming	7.3
9	Nebraska	7.2
9	Tennessee	7.2
11	New Mexico	6.7
12	Nevada	6.6
13	Maine	6.5
14	Florida	6.3
14	North Carolina	6.3
16	North Dakota	6.0
17	West Virginia	5.9
18	Arkansas	5.8
18	Montana	5.8
20	Colorado	5.6
21	Georgia	5.3
21	Vermont	5.3
23	South Carolina	5.2
24	Kentucky	4.8
25	Mississippi	4.5
25	Oregon	4.5
27	Maryland	4.4
28	Texas	4.3
29	Missouri	4.1
30	Arizona	4.0
31	Idaho	3.9
32	Alabama	3.7
33	Indiana	3.3
34	Delaware	3.2
34	Utah	3.2
36	New Hampshire	3.0
37	Iowa	2.9
37	Louisiana	2.9
39	California	2.8
40	Minnesota	2.6
40	Ohio	2.6
40	Pennsylvania	2.6
40	Wisconsin	2.6
44	Illinois	2.5
44	Rhode Island	2.5
46	Connecticut	2.2
46	Massachusetts	2.2
48	Michigan	1.7
49	New York	1.3
50	New Jersey	0.8

District of Columbia	1.7

Source: U.S. Bureau of the Census
   "Health Insurance Coverage Status by State for All People: 2009" (http://www.census.gov/hhes/www/hlthins/index.html)
*Includes CHAMPUS (Comprehensive Health and Medical Plan for Uniformed Services)/Tricare, Veterans, and military health care.

Percent of Children Covered by Health Insurance in 2009

National Percent = 90.0% of Children*

ALPHA ORDER

RANK	STATE	PERCENT
21	Alabama	92.1
34	Alaska	90.1
47	Arizona	86.6
41	Arkansas	88.5
37	California	89.3
31	Colorado	90.4
20	Connecticut	92.3
28	Delaware	91.2
50	Florida	82.1
39	Georgia	88.7
2	Hawaii	96.5
35	Idaho	89.8
29	Illinois	90.9
26	Indiana	91.4
10	Iowa	94.1
22	Kansas	91.9
23	Kentucky	91.8
24	Louisiana	91.6
4	Maine	96.0
17	Maryland	93.0
1	Massachusetts	97.1
8	Michigan	94.4
7	Minnesota	94.5
38	Mississippi	89.1
33	Missouri	90.3
36	Montana	89.6
15	Nebraska	93.3
46	Nevada	86.7
3	New Hampshire	96.2
30	New Jersey	90.8
48	New Mexico	86.0
18	New York	92.5
42	North Carolina	88.2
10	North Dakota	94.1
27	Ohio	91.3
45	Oklahoma	87.4
43	Oregon	88.1
16	Pennsylvania	93.2
12	Rhode Island	94.0
44	South Carolina	87.7
24	South Dakota	91.6
14	Tennessee	93.4
49	Texas	83.5
39	Utah	88.7
8	Vermont	94.4
18	Virginia	92.5
6	Washington	95.2
13	West Virginia	93.8
5	Wisconsin	95.3
31	Wyoming	90.4

RANK ORDER

RANK	STATE	PERCENT
1	Massachusetts	97.1
2	Hawaii	96.5
3	New Hampshire	96.2
4	Maine	96.0
5	Wisconsin	95.3
6	Washington	95.2
7	Minnesota	94.5
8	Michigan	94.4
8	Vermont	94.4
10	Iowa	94.1
10	North Dakota	94.1
12	Rhode Island	94.0
13	West Virginia	93.8
14	Tennessee	93.4
15	Nebraska	93.3
16	Pennsylvania	93.2
17	Maryland	93.0
18	New York	92.5
18	Virginia	92.5
20	Connecticut	92.3
21	Alabama	92.1
22	Kansas	91.9
23	Kentucky	91.8
24	Louisiana	91.6
24	South Dakota	91.6
26	Indiana	91.4
27	Ohio	91.3
28	Delaware	91.2
29	Illinois	90.9
30	New Jersey	90.8
31	Colorado	90.4
31	Wyoming	90.4
33	Missouri	90.3
34	Alaska	90.1
35	Idaho	89.8
36	Montana	89.6
37	California	89.3
38	Mississippi	89.1
39	Georgia	88.7
39	Utah	88.7
41	Arkansas	88.5
42	North Carolina	88.2
43	Oregon	88.1
44	South Carolina	87.7
45	Oklahoma	87.4
46	Nevada	86.7
47	Arizona	86.6
48	New Mexico	86.0
49	Texas	83.5
50	Florida	82.1

District of Columbia   92.0

Source: U.S. Bureau of the Census
   "Health Insurance Coverage Status by State for All People: 2009" (http://www.census.gov/hhes/www/hlthins/index.html)
*Children under 18 covered by either private or government health insurance.

Percent of Children Covered by Private Health Insurance in 2009

National Percent = 60.4% of Children*

ALPHA ORDER

RANK	STATE	PERCENT
43	Alabama	54.8
41	Alaska	55.9
46	Arizona	51.5
47	Arkansas	50.1
44	California	54.2
20	Colorado	66.0
2	Connecticut	76.4
21	Delaware	65.9
42	Florida	55.1
30	Georgia	59.9
18	Hawaii	66.3
17	Idaho	66.6
31	Illinois	59.4
33	Indiana	59.3
8	Iowa	72.0
23	Kansas	64.9
39	Kentucky	58.0
38	Louisiana	58.2
29	Maine	62.3
8	Maryland	72.0
6	Massachusetts	72.5
11	Michigan	70.3
10	Minnesota	71.6
49	Mississippi	45.4
24	Missouri	64.8
31	Montana	59.4
12	Nebraska	70.1
22	Nevada	65.2
1	New Hampshire	78.7
6	New Jersey	72.5
50	New Mexico	42.2
36	New York	58.5
40	North Carolina	57.2
3	North Dakota	74.8
18	Ohio	66.3
45	Oklahoma	52.2
25	Oregon	63.7
16	Pennsylvania	67.3
28	Rhode Island	62.4
26	South Carolina	63.0
15	South Dakota	67.8
36	Tennessee	58.5
48	Texas	48.5
4	Utah	73.8
35	Vermont	59.1
12	Virginia	70.1
27	Washington	62.9
33	West Virginia	59.3
5	Wisconsin	73.6
14	Wyoming	68.5

RANK ORDER

RANK	STATE	PERCENT
1	New Hampshire	78.7
2	Connecticut	76.4
3	North Dakota	74.8
4	Utah	73.8
5	Wisconsin	73.6
6	Massachusetts	72.5
6	New Jersey	72.5
8	Iowa	72.0
8	Maryland	72.0
10	Minnesota	71.6
11	Michigan	70.3
12	Nebraska	70.1
12	Virginia	70.1
14	Wyoming	68.5
15	South Dakota	67.8
16	Pennsylvania	67.3
17	Idaho	66.6
18	Hawaii	66.3
18	Ohio	66.3
20	Colorado	66.0
21	Delaware	65.9
22	Nevada	65.2
23	Kansas	64.9
24	Missouri	64.8
25	Oregon	63.7
26	South Carolina	63.0
27	Washington	62.9
28	Rhode Island	62.4
29	Maine	62.3
30	Georgia	59.9
31	Illinois	59.4
31	Montana	59.4
33	Indiana	59.3
33	West Virginia	59.3
35	Vermont	59.1
36	New York	58.5
36	Tennessee	58.5
38	Louisiana	58.2
39	Kentucky	58.0
40	North Carolina	57.2
41	Alaska	55.9
42	Florida	55.1
43	Alabama	54.8
44	California	54.2
45	Oklahoma	52.2
46	Arizona	51.5
47	Arkansas	50.1
48	Texas	48.5
49	Mississippi	45.4
50	New Mexico	42.2

	District of Columbia	45.1

Source: U.S. Bureau of the Census
"Health Insurance Coverage Status by State for All People: 2009" (http://www.census.gov/hhes/www/hlthins/index.html)
*Children under 18. Private health insurance is coverage by a health plan provided through an employer or union or purchased by an individual from a private health insurance company.

Percent of Children Covered by Employment-Based Health Insurance in 2009

National Percent = 55.8% of Children*

<table>
<tr><td colspan="3">ALPHA ORDER</td><td colspan="3">RANK ORDER</td></tr>
<tr><td>RANK</td><td>STATE</td><td>PERCENT</td><td>RANK</td><td>STATE</td><td>PERCENT</td></tr>
<tr><td>37</td><td>Alabama</td><td>53.7</td><td>1</td><td>New Hampshire</td><td>72.7</td></tr>
<tr><td>39</td><td>Alaska</td><td>52.9</td><td>2</td><td>Connecticut</td><td>70.7</td></tr>
<tr><td>46</td><td>Arizona</td><td>46.6</td><td>3</td><td>New Jersey</td><td>70.2</td></tr>
<tr><td>47</td><td>Arkansas</td><td>46.5</td><td>4</td><td>Wisconsin</td><td>69.6</td></tr>
<tr><td>44</td><td>California</td><td>49.0</td><td>5</td><td>Utah</td><td>68.5</td></tr>
<tr><td>20</td><td>Colorado</td><td>60.3</td><td>6</td><td>Massachusetts</td><td>68.3</td></tr>
<tr><td>2</td><td>Connecticut</td><td>70.7</td><td>7</td><td>Maryland</td><td>67.7</td></tr>
<tr><td>15</td><td>Delaware</td><td>62.1</td><td>8</td><td>North Dakota</td><td>67.4</td></tr>
<tr><td>43</td><td>Florida</td><td>49.4</td><td>9</td><td>Minnesota</td><td>67.3</td></tr>
<tr><td>30</td><td>Georgia</td><td>56.0</td><td>10</td><td>Michigan</td><td>66.2</td></tr>
<tr><td>17</td><td>Hawaii</td><td>61.5</td><td>11</td><td>Virginia</td><td>65.6</td></tr>
<tr><td>27</td><td>Idaho</td><td>57.1</td><td>12</td><td>Iowa</td><td>65.0</td></tr>
<tr><td>30</td><td>Illinois</td><td>56.0</td><td>13</td><td>Pennsylvania</td><td>63.7</td></tr>
<tr><td>34</td><td>Indiana</td><td>55.8</td><td>14</td><td>Nebraska</td><td>63.4</td></tr>
<tr><td>12</td><td>Iowa</td><td>65.0</td><td>15</td><td>Delaware</td><td>62.1</td></tr>
<tr><td>23</td><td>Kansas</td><td>59.4</td><td>16</td><td>South Dakota</td><td>61.9</td></tr>
<tr><td>35</td><td>Kentucky</td><td>54.3</td><td>17</td><td>Hawaii</td><td>61.5</td></tr>
<tr><td>41</td><td>Louisiana</td><td>51.5</td><td>18</td><td>Ohio</td><td>61.3</td></tr>
<tr><td>25</td><td>Maine</td><td>58.1</td><td>19</td><td>Nevada</td><td>61.1</td></tr>
<tr><td>7</td><td>Maryland</td><td>67.7</td><td>20</td><td>Colorado</td><td>60.3</td></tr>
<tr><td>6</td><td>Massachusetts</td><td>68.3</td><td>21</td><td>Missouri</td><td>60.0</td></tr>
<tr><td>10</td><td>Michigan</td><td>66.2</td><td>22</td><td>Wyoming</td><td>59.6</td></tr>
<tr><td>9</td><td>Minnesota</td><td>67.3</td><td>23</td><td>Kansas</td><td>59.4</td></tr>
<tr><td>49</td><td>Mississippi</td><td>41.6</td><td>24</td><td>Rhode Island</td><td>59.2</td></tr>
<tr><td>21</td><td>Missouri</td><td>60.0</td><td>25</td><td>Maine</td><td>58.1</td></tr>
<tr><td>42</td><td>Montana</td><td>51.1</td><td>26</td><td>South Carolina</td><td>57.2</td></tr>
<tr><td>14</td><td>Nebraska</td><td>63.4</td><td>27</td><td>Idaho</td><td>57.1</td></tr>
<tr><td>19</td><td>Nevada</td><td>61.1</td><td>28</td><td>West Virginia</td><td>56.9</td></tr>
<tr><td>1</td><td>New Hampshire</td><td>72.7</td><td>29</td><td>Vermont</td><td>56.7</td></tr>
<tr><td>3</td><td>New Jersey</td><td>70.2</td><td>30</td><td>Georgia</td><td>56.0</td></tr>
<tr><td>50</td><td>New Mexico</td><td>40.5</td><td>30</td><td>Illinois</td><td>56.0</td></tr>
<tr><td>37</td><td>New York</td><td>53.7</td><td>30</td><td>Oregon</td><td>56.0</td></tr>
<tr><td>40</td><td>North Carolina</td><td>52.8</td><td>30</td><td>Washington</td><td>56.0</td></tr>
<tr><td>8</td><td>North Dakota</td><td>67.4</td><td>34</td><td>Indiana</td><td>55.8</td></tr>
<tr><td>18</td><td>Ohio</td><td>61.3</td><td>35</td><td>Kentucky</td><td>54.3</td></tr>
<tr><td>44</td><td>Oklahoma</td><td>49.0</td><td>36</td><td>Tennessee</td><td>54.0</td></tr>
<tr><td>30</td><td>Oregon</td><td>56.0</td><td>37</td><td>Alabama</td><td>53.7</td></tr>
<tr><td>13</td><td>Pennsylvania</td><td>63.7</td><td>37</td><td>New York</td><td>53.7</td></tr>
<tr><td>24</td><td>Rhode Island</td><td>59.2</td><td>39</td><td>Alaska</td><td>52.9</td></tr>
<tr><td>26</td><td>South Carolina</td><td>57.2</td><td>40</td><td>North Carolina</td><td>52.8</td></tr>
<tr><td>16</td><td>South Dakota</td><td>61.9</td><td>41</td><td>Louisiana</td><td>51.5</td></tr>
<tr><td>36</td><td>Tennessee</td><td>54.0</td><td>42</td><td>Montana</td><td>51.1</td></tr>
<tr><td>48</td><td>Texas</td><td>45.1</td><td>43</td><td>Florida</td><td>49.4</td></tr>
<tr><td>5</td><td>Utah</td><td>68.5</td><td>44</td><td>California</td><td>49.0</td></tr>
<tr><td>29</td><td>Vermont</td><td>56.7</td><td>44</td><td>Oklahoma</td><td>49.0</td></tr>
<tr><td>11</td><td>Virginia</td><td>65.6</td><td>46</td><td>Arizona</td><td>46.6</td></tr>
<tr><td>30</td><td>Washington</td><td>56.0</td><td>47</td><td>Arkansas</td><td>46.5</td></tr>
<tr><td>28</td><td>West Virginia</td><td>56.9</td><td>48</td><td>Texas</td><td>45.1</td></tr>
<tr><td>4</td><td>Wisconsin</td><td>69.6</td><td>49</td><td>Mississippi</td><td>41.6</td></tr>
<tr><td>22</td><td>Wyoming</td><td>59.6</td><td>50</td><td>New Mexico</td><td>40.5</td></tr>
<tr><td></td><td></td><td></td><td></td><td>District of Columbia</td><td>43.4</td></tr>
</table>

Source: U.S. Bureau of the Census

"Health Insurance Coverage Status by State for All People: 2009" (http://www.census.gov/hhes/www/hlthins/index.html)
*Children under 18. Employment-based health insurance is private insurance coverage offered through one's own employment or a relative's. It may be offered by an employer or by a union.

Percent of Children Covered by Direct-Purchase Health Insurance in 2009

National Percent = 5.1% of Children*

ALPHA ORDER			RANK ORDER		
RANK	STATE	PERCENT	RANK	STATE	PERCENT
49	Alabama	2.4	1	Idaho	12.3
30	Alaska	4.6	2	North Dakota	10.7
14	Arizona	6.2	3	Montana	10.0
45	Arkansas	3.2	4	Oregon	9.9
17	California	5.6	5	Nebraska	8.4
16	Colorado	6.1	6	Iowa	7.6
23	Connecticut	5.2	6	Wyoming	7.6
44	Delaware	3.3	8	Washington	7.4
10	Florida	6.9	9	South Dakota	7.3
26	Georgia	5.0	10	Florida	6.9
28	Hawaii	4.8	11	Missouri	6.7
1	Idaho	12.3	12	Louisiana	6.6
32	Illinois	4.5	13	South Carolina	6.5
17	Indiana	5.6	14	Arizona	6.2
6	Iowa	7.6	14	Ohio	6.2
17	Kansas	5.6	16	Colorado	6.1
37	Kentucky	3.8	17	California	5.6
12	Louisiana	6.6	17	Indiana	5.6
42	Maine	3.4	17	Kansas	5.6
20	Maryland	5.5	20	Maryland	5.5
42	Massachusetts	3.4	20	Tennessee	5.5
34	Michigan	4.1	22	Minnesota	5.4
22	Minnesota	5.4	23	Connecticut	5.2
35	Mississippi	4.0	24	New Hampshire	5.1
11	Missouri	6.7	24	Virginia	5.1
3	Montana	10.0	26	Georgia	5.0
5	Nebraska	8.4	26	Utah	5.0
29	Nevada	4.7	28	Hawaii	4.8
24	New Hampshire	5.1	29	Nevada	4.7
41	New Jersey	3.5	30	Alaska	4.6
46	New Mexico	2.9	30	North Carolina	4.6
32	New York	4.5	32	Illinois	4.5
30	North Carolina	4.6	32	New York	4.5
2	North Dakota	10.7	34	Michigan	4.1
14	Ohio	6.2	35	Mississippi	4.0
35	Oklahoma	4.0	35	Oklahoma	4.0
4	Oregon	9.9	37	Kentucky	3.8
39	Pennsylvania	3.6	37	Wisconsin	3.8
47	Rhode Island	2.5	39	Pennsylvania	3.6
13	South Carolina	6.5	39	Texas	3.6
9	South Dakota	7.3	41	New Jersey	3.5
20	Tennessee	5.5	42	Maine	3.4
39	Texas	3.6	42	Massachusetts	3.4
26	Utah	5.0	44	Delaware	3.3
47	Vermont	2.5	45	Arkansas	3.2
24	Virginia	5.1	46	New Mexico	2.9
8	Washington	7.4	47	Rhode Island	2.5
50	West Virginia	0.7	47	Vermont	2.5
37	Wisconsin	3.8	49	Alabama	2.4
6	Wyoming	7.6	50	West Virginia	0.7
				District of Columbia	1.1

Source: U.S. Bureau of the Census
"Health Insurance Coverage Status by State for All People: 2009" (http://www.census.gov/hhes/www/hlthins/index.html)
*Children under 18. Direct-purchase health insurance is private insurance coverage through a plan purchased by an individual from a private company.

Percent of Children Covered by Government Health Insurance in 2009

National Percent = 36.8% of Children*

ALPHA ORDER				RANK ORDER		
RANK	STATE	PERCENT		RANK	STATE	PERCENT
4	Alabama	46.7		1	Mississippi	51.6
7	Alaska	46.1		2	New Mexico	50.0
13	Arizona	41.7		3	Vermont	47.4
6	Arkansas	46.4		4	Alabama	46.7
15	California	40.8		5	West Virginia	46.6
42	Colorado	30.4		6	Arkansas	46.4
49	Connecticut	21.3		7	Alaska	46.1
40	Delaware	31.1		7	Washington	46.1
28	Florida	34.2		9	Oklahoma	45.1
24	Georgia	36.0		10	Tennessee	44.9
11	Hawaii	44.3		11	Hawaii	44.3
40	Idaho	31.1		12	Maine	43.4
22	Illinois	37.0		13	Arizona	41.7
21	Indiana	38.3		14	New York	41.4
29	Iowa	33.5		15	California	40.8
26	Kansas	35.0		16	Kentucky	40.3
16	Kentucky	40.3		17	Texas	40.2
18	Louisiana	39.9		18	Louisiana	39.9
12	Maine	43.4		18	Rhode Island	39.9
44	Maryland	27.4		20	North Carolina	38.7
31	Massachusetts	33.1		21	Indiana	38.3
32	Michigan	32.5		22	Illinois	37.0
43	Minnesota	29.6		23	South Dakota	36.4
1	Mississippi	51.6		24	Georgia	36.0
26	Missouri	35.0		25	Montana	35.8
25	Montana	35.8		26	Kansas	35.0
30	Nebraska	33.2		26	Missouri	35.0
46	Nevada	26.9		28	Florida	34.2
48	New Hampshire	22.0		29	Iowa	33.5
47	New Jersey	23.7		30	Nebraska	33.2
2	New Mexico	50.0		31	Massachusetts	33.1
14	New York	41.4		32	Michigan	32.5
20	North Carolina	38.7		33	Oregon	32.4
45	North Dakota	27.3		33	Pennsylvania	32.4
38	Ohio	31.3		35	Wisconsin	32.1
9	Oklahoma	45.1		35	Wyoming	32.1
33	Oregon	32.4		37	South Carolina	31.4
33	Pennsylvania	32.4		38	Ohio	31.3
18	Rhode Island	39.9		39	Virginia	31.2
37	South Carolina	31.4		40	Delaware	31.1
23	South Dakota	36.4		40	Idaho	31.1
10	Tennessee	44.9		42	Colorado	30.4
17	Texas	40.2		43	Minnesota	29.6
50	Utah	20.2		44	Maryland	27.4
3	Vermont	47.4		45	North Dakota	27.3
39	Virginia	31.2		46	Nevada	26.9
7	Washington	46.1		47	New Jersey	23.7
5	West Virginia	46.6		48	New Hampshire	22.0
35	Wisconsin	32.1		49	Connecticut	21.3
35	Wyoming	32.1		50	Utah	20.2
					District of Columbia	54.6

Source: U.S. Bureau of the Census
"Health Insurance Coverage Status by State for All People: 2009" (http://www.census.gov/hhes/www/hlthins/index.html)
*Children under 18. Includes Medicaid, Medicare, the Children's Health Insurance Program (CHIP), and military health care.

Percent of Children Covered by Military Health Care in 2009

National Percent = 3.2% of Children*

ALPHA ORDER

RANK	STATE	PERCENT
33	Alabama	2.2
1	Alaska	18.0
31	Arizona	2.3
23	Arkansas	3.9
35	California	2.0
10	Colorado	5.5
39	Connecticut	1.5
38	Delaware	1.7
12	Florida	5.3
12	Georgia	5.3
2	Hawaii	11.5
28	Idaho	2.8
42	Illinois	1.4
43	Indiana	1.3
39	Iowa	1.5
5	Kansas	7.9
25	Kentucky	3.0
34	Louisiana	2.1
10	Maine	5.5
24	Maryland	3.8
46	Massachusetts	1.0
48	Michigan	0.6
36	Minnesota	1.9
27	Mississippi	2.9
25	Missouri	3.0
21	Montana	4.3
7	Nebraska	6.9
19	Nevada	4.5
39	New Hampshire	1.5
50	New Jersey	0.5
17	New Mexico	4.7
48	New York	0.6
8	North Carolina	6.6
14	North Dakota	5.2
43	Ohio	1.3
9	Oklahoma	6.3
30	Oregon	2.4
45	Pennsylvania	1.2
36	Rhode Island	1.9
17	South Carolina	4.7
21	South Dakota	4.3
4	Tennessee	8.8
28	Texas	2.8
31	Utah	2.3
16	Vermont	4.9
3	Virginia	9.0
6	Washington	7.6
20	West Virginia	4.4
47	Wisconsin	0.8
15	Wyoming	5.0

RANK ORDER

RANK	STATE	PERCENT
1	Alaska	18.0
2	Hawaii	11.5
3	Virginia	9.0
4	Tennessee	8.8
5	Kansas	7.9
6	Washington	7.6
7	Nebraska	6.9
8	North Carolina	6.6
9	Oklahoma	6.3
10	Colorado	5.5
10	Maine	5.5
12	Florida	5.3
12	Georgia	5.3
14	North Dakota	5.2
15	Wyoming	5.0
16	Vermont	4.9
17	New Mexico	4.7
17	South Carolina	4.7
19	Nevada	4.5
20	West Virginia	4.4
21	Montana	4.3
21	South Dakota	4.3
23	Arkansas	3.9
24	Maryland	3.8
25	Kentucky	3.0
25	Missouri	3.0
27	Mississippi	2.9
28	Idaho	2.8
28	Texas	2.8
30	Oregon	2.4
31	Arizona	2.3
31	Utah	2.3
33	Alabama	2.2
34	Louisiana	2.1
35	California	2.0
36	Minnesota	1.9
36	Rhode Island	1.9
38	Delaware	1.7
39	Connecticut	1.5
39	Iowa	1.5
39	New Hampshire	1.5
42	Illinois	1.4
43	Indiana	1.3
43	Ohio	1.3
45	Pennsylvania	1.2
46	Massachusetts	1.0
47	Wisconsin	0.8
48	Michigan	0.6
48	New York	0.6
50	New Jersey	0.5
	District of Columbia	1.4

Source: U.S. Bureau of the Census
"Health Insurance Coverage Status by State for All People: 2009" (http://www.census.gov/hhes/www/hlthins/index.html)
*Children under 18. Includes CHAMPUS (Comprehensive Health and Medical Plan for Uniformed Services)/Tricare, Veterans, and military health care.

Percent of Children Covered by Medicaid in 2009

National Percent = 33.8% of Children*

ALPHA ORDER				RANK ORDER		
RANK	STATE	PERCENT		RANK	STATE	PERCENT
3	Alabama	44.2		1	Mississippi	48.4
35	Alaska	28.5		2	New Mexico	45.9
10	Arizona	39.6		3	Alabama	44.2
5	Arkansas	42.7		4	Vermont	43.9
13	California	38.7		5	Arkansas	42.7
42	Colorado	24.9		6	West Virginia	41.4
49	Connecticut	19.3		7	Oklahoma	40.5
36	Delaware	28.0		8	New York	40.3
34	Florida	29.4		9	Maine	40.0
26	Georgia	31.4		10	Arizona	39.6
20	Hawaii	34.0		11	Washington	39.1
32	Idaho	30.0		12	Kentucky	38.9
19	Illinois	35.4		13	California	38.7
17	Indiana	37.1		14	Rhode Island	38.2
23	Iowa	32.1		15	Louisiana	38.1
38	Kansas	27.6		16	Texas	37.4
12	Kentucky	38.9		17	Indiana	37.1
15	Louisiana	38.1		18	Tennessee	36.9
9	Maine	40.0		19	Illinois	35.4
43	Maryland	23.5		20	Hawaii	34.0
22	Massachusetts	32.2		21	Missouri	32.5
24	Michigan	32.0		22	Massachusetts	32.2
37	Minnesota	27.7		23	Iowa	32.1
1	Mississippi	48.4		24	Michigan	32.0
21	Missouri	32.5		25	North Carolina	31.9
28	Montana	31.1		26	Georgia	31.4
40	Nebraska	26.9		26	Pennsylvania	31.4
45	Nevada	23.1		28	Montana	31.1
48	New Hampshire	20.3		28	South Dakota	31.1
44	New Jersey	23.2		30	Wisconsin	30.6
2	New Mexico	45.9		31	Oregon	30.2
8	New York	40.3		32	Idaho	30.0
25	North Carolina	31.9		33	Ohio	29.7
47	North Dakota	22.0		34	Florida	29.4
33	Ohio	29.7		35	Alaska	28.5
7	Oklahoma	40.5		36	Delaware	28.0
31	Oregon	30.2		37	Minnesota	27.7
26	Pennsylvania	31.4		38	Kansas	27.6
14	Rhode Island	38.2		38	Wyoming	27.6
41	South Carolina	26.6		40	Nebraska	26.9
28	South Dakota	31.1		41	South Carolina	26.6
18	Tennessee	36.9		42	Colorado	24.9
16	Texas	37.4		43	Maryland	23.5
50	Utah	17.9		44	New Jersey	23.2
4	Vermont	43.9		45	Nevada	23.1
46	Virginia	23.0		46	Virginia	23.0
11	Washington	39.1		47	North Dakota	22.0
6	West Virginia	41.4		48	New Hampshire	20.3
30	Wisconsin	30.6		49	Connecticut	19.3
38	Wyoming	27.6		50	Utah	17.9
					District of Columbia	53.0

Source: U.S. Bureau of the Census
   "Health Insurance Coverage Status by State for All People: 2009" (http://www.census.gov/hhes/www/hlthins/index.html)
*Children under 18. Medicaid is a form of government insurance.

The Children's Health Insurance Program (CHIP) Enrollment in 2009

National Total = 7,717,300 Children*

ALPHA ORDER

RANK	STATE	ENROLLMENT	% of USA
18	Alabama	110,200	1.4%
46	Alaska	11,700	0.2%
19	Arizona	105,100	1.4%
22	Arkansas	101,300	1.3%
1	California	1,748,100	22.7%
21	Colorado	102,400	1.3%
40	Connecticut	21,800	0.3%
45	Delaware	12,600	0.2%
4	Florida	417,400	5.4%
8	Georgia	254,400	3.3%
39	Hawaii	24,700	0.3%
33	Idaho	44,300	0.6%
5	Illinois	376,600	4.9%
14	Indiana	138,600	1.8%
30	Iowa	52,600	0.7%
31	Kansas	48,100	0.6%
26	Kentucky	73,100	0.9%
10	Louisiana	170,100	2.2%
36	Maine	31,300	0.4%
16	Maryland	124,600	1.6%
13	Massachusetts	143,000	1.9%
27	Michigan	72,000	0.9%
50	Minnesota	5,500	0.1%
23	Mississippi	86,800	1.1%
20	Missouri	103,700	1.3%
38	Montana	25,700	0.3%
31	Nebraska	48,100	0.6%
35	Nevada	34,000	0.4%
44	New Hampshire	13,200	0.2%
12	New Jersey	167,000	2.2%
42	New Mexico	16,100	0.2%
3	New York	532,600	6.9%
9	North Carolina	252,600	3.3%
49	North Dakota	7,000	0.1%
6	Ohio	265,700	3.4%
17	Oklahoma	123,700	1.6%
28	Oregon	62,100	0.8%
7	Pennsylvania	264,800	3.4%
41	Rhode Island	19,600	0.3%
24	South Carolina	85,000	1.1%
43	South Dakota	15,300	0.2%
25	Tennessee	83,300	1.1%
2	Texas	869,900	11.3%
29	Utah	59,800	0.8%
48	Vermont	7,100	0.1%
11	Virginia	167,600	2.2%
37	Washington	27,400	0.4%
34	West Virginia	38,200	0.5%
15	Wisconsin	132,900	1.7%
47	Wyoming	8,900	0.1%

RANK ORDER

RANK	STATE	ENROLLMENT	% of USA
1	California	1,748,100	22.7%
2	Texas	869,900	11.3%
3	New York	532,600	6.9%
4	Florida	417,400	5.4%
5	Illinois	376,600	4.9%
6	Ohio	265,700	3.4%
7	Pennsylvania	264,800	3.4%
8	Georgia	254,400	3.3%
9	North Carolina	252,600	3.3%
10	Louisiana	170,100	2.2%
11	Virginia	167,600	2.2%
12	New Jersey	167,000	2.2%
13	Massachusetts	143,000	1.9%
14	Indiana	138,600	1.8%
15	Wisconsin	132,900	1.7%
16	Maryland	124,600	1.6%
17	Oklahoma	123,700	1.6%
18	Alabama	110,200	1.4%
19	Arizona	105,100	1.4%
20	Missouri	103,700	1.3%
21	Colorado	102,400	1.3%
22	Arkansas	101,300	1.3%
23	Mississippi	86,800	1.1%
24	South Carolina	85,000	1.1%
25	Tennessee	83,300	1.1%
26	Kentucky	73,100	0.9%
27	Michigan	72,000	0.9%
28	Oregon	62,100	0.8%
29	Utah	59,800	0.8%
30	Iowa	52,600	0.7%
31	Kansas	48,100	0.6%
31	Nebraska	48,100	0.6%
33	Idaho	44,300	0.6%
34	West Virginia	38,200	0.5%
35	Nevada	34,000	0.4%
36	Maine	31,300	0.4%
37	Washington	27,400	0.4%
38	Montana	25,700	0.3%
39	Hawaii	24,700	0.3%
40	Connecticut	21,800	0.3%
41	Rhode Island	19,600	0.3%
42	New Mexico	16,100	0.2%
43	South Dakota	15,300	0.2%
44	New Hampshire	13,200	0.2%
45	Delaware	12,600	0.2%
46	Alaska	11,700	0.2%
47	Wyoming	8,900	0.1%
48	Vermont	7,100	0.1%
49	North Dakota	7,000	0.1%
50	Minnesota	5,500	0.1%
	District of Columbia	9,300	0.1%

Source: U.S. Department of Health and Human Services, Centers for Medicare and Medicaid Services
"The Children's Health Insurance Program Annual Enrollment Report" (http://www.cms.gov/NationalCHIPPolicy/)
*Figures for fiscal year 2009. The Children's Health Insurance Program (CHIP) was created in 1997 to help states expand health insurance to children whose families earn too much to qualify for Medicaid, yet not enough to afford private health insurance.

Percent Change in the Children's Health Insurance
Program (CHIP) Enrollment: 2008 to 2009
National Percent Change = 4.7% Increase*

ALPHA ORDER

RANK	STATE	PERCENT CHANGE
34	Alabama	(0.6)
50	Alaska	(37.5)
40	Arizona	(6.2)
14	Arkansas	8.4
24	California	3.3
27	Colorado	2.9
37	Connecticut	(2.1)
10	Delaware	12.6
5	Florida	17.8
46	Georgia	(18.3)
44	Hawaii	(14.2)
29	Idaho	1.8
20	Illinois	5.7
11	Indiana	10.9
23	Iowa	4.4
39	Kansas	(6.0)
15	Kentucky	7.9
8	Louisiana	15.0
31	Maine	1.1
40	Maryland	(6.2)
49	Massachusetts	(28.8)
19	Michigan	6.3
38	Minnesota	(2.2)
27	Mississippi	2.9
47	Missouri	(23.8)
9	Montana	13.3
36	Nebraska	(1.5)
43	Nevada	(11.9)
15	New Hampshire	7.9
12	New Jersey	10.0
18	New Mexico	7.7
26	New York	3.0
32	North Carolina	0.4
42	North Dakota	(8.1)
20	Ohio	5.7
22	Oklahoma	5.3
45	Oregon	(15.7)
25	Pennsylvania	3.2
48	Rhode Island	(24.7)
7	South Carolina	15.5
33	South Dakota	0.2
3	Tennessee	30.9
4	Texas	18.9
6	Utah	17.0
13	Vermont	9.3
15	Virginia	7.9
2	Washington	62.8
30	West Virginia	1.5
1	Wisconsin	151.0
35	Wyoming	(0.8)

RANK ORDER

RANK	STATE	PERCENT CHANGE
1	Wisconsin	151.0
2	Washington	62.8
3	Tennessee	30.9
4	Texas	18.9
5	Florida	17.8
6	Utah	17.0
7	South Carolina	15.5
8	Louisiana	15.0
9	Montana	13.3
10	Delaware	12.6
11	Indiana	10.9
12	New Jersey	10.0
13	Vermont	9.3
14	Arkansas	8.4
15	Kentucky	7.9
15	New Hampshire	7.9
15	Virginia	7.9
18	New Mexico	7.7
19	Michigan	6.3
20	Illinois	5.7
20	Ohio	5.7
22	Oklahoma	5.3
23	Iowa	4.4
24	California	3.3
25	Pennsylvania	3.2
26	New York	3.0
27	Colorado	2.9
27	Mississippi	2.9
29	Idaho	1.8
30	West Virginia	1.5
31	Maine	1.1
32	North Carolina	0.4
33	South Dakota	0.2
34	Alabama	(0.6)
35	Wyoming	(0.8)
36	Nebraska	(1.5)
37	Connecticut	(2.1)
38	Minnesota	(2.2)
39	Kansas	(6.0)
40	Arizona	(6.2)
40	Maryland	(6.2)
42	North Dakota	(8.1)
43	Nevada	(11.9)
44	Hawaii	(14.2)
45	Oregon	(15.7)
46	Georgia	(18.3)
47	Missouri	(23.8)
48	Rhode Island	(24.7)
49	Massachusetts	(28.8)
50	Alaska	(37.5)

	District of Columbia	6.3

Source: CQ Press using data from U.S. Department of Health and Human Services, Centers for Medicare and Medicaid Services
"The Children's Health Insurance Program Annual Enrollment Report" (http://www.cms.gov/NationalCHIPPolicy/)
*Figures for fiscal years. The Children's Health Insurance Program (CHIP) was created in 1997 to help states expand health
insurance to children whose families earn too much to qualify for Medicaid, yet not enough to afford private health insurance.

Percent of Children Enrolled in the Children's Health Insurance Program (CHIP) in 2009
National Percent = 10.4% of Children 17 Years and Younger*

ALPHA ORDER

RANK	STATE	PERCENT
18	Alabama	9.8
38	Alaska	6.4
39	Arizona	6.1
3	Arkansas	14.3
1	California	18.5
27	Colorado	8.3
48	Connecticut	2.7
39	Delaware	6.1
14	Florida	10.3
18	Georgia	9.8
26	Hawaii	8.5
13	Idaho	10.6
7	Illinois	11.9
24	Indiana	8.7
31	Iowa	7.4
36	Kansas	6.8
32	Kentucky	7.2
2	Louisiana	15.1
9	Maine	11.5
22	Maryland	9.2
16	Massachusetts	10.0
47	Michigan	3.1
50	Minnesota	0.4
10	Mississippi	11.3
32	Missouri	7.2
8	Montana	11.7
12	Nebraska	10.7
43	Nevada	5.0
45	New Hampshire	4.6
28	New Jersey	8.2
46	New Mexico	3.2
6	New York	12.0
11	North Carolina	11.1
44	North Dakota	4.9
18	Ohio	9.8
4	Oklahoma	13.5
34	Oregon	7.1
21	Pennsylvania	9.5
25	Rhode Island	8.6
29	South Carolina	7.9
30	South Dakota	7.7
41	Tennessee	5.6
5	Texas	12.6
35	Utah	6.9
41	Vermont	5.6
23	Virginia	9.1
49	Washington	1.7
17	West Virginia	9.9
15	Wisconsin	10.1
37	Wyoming	6.7

RANK ORDER

RANK	STATE	PERCENT
1	California	18.5
2	Louisiana	15.1
3	Arkansas	14.3
4	Oklahoma	13.5
5	Texas	12.6
6	New York	12.0
7	Illinois	11.9
8	Montana	11.7
9	Maine	11.5
10	Mississippi	11.3
11	North Carolina	11.1
12	Nebraska	10.7
13	Idaho	10.6
14	Florida	10.3
15	Wisconsin	10.1
16	Massachusetts	10.0
17	West Virginia	9.9
18	Alabama	9.8
18	Georgia	9.8
18	Ohio	9.8
21	Pennsylvania	9.5
22	Maryland	9.2
23	Virginia	9.1
24	Indiana	8.7
25	Rhode Island	8.6
26	Hawaii	8.5
27	Colorado	8.3
28	New Jersey	8.2
29	South Carolina	7.9
30	South Dakota	7.7
31	Iowa	7.4
32	Kentucky	7.2
32	Missouri	7.2
34	Oregon	7.1
35	Utah	6.9
36	Kansas	6.8
37	Wyoming	6.7
38	Alaska	6.4
39	Arizona	6.1
39	Delaware	6.1
41	Tennessee	5.6
41	Vermont	5.6
43	Nevada	5.0
44	North Dakota	4.9
45	New Hampshire	4.6
46	New Mexico	3.2
47	Michigan	3.1
48	Connecticut	2.7
49	Washington	1.7
50	Minnesota	0.4

District of Columbia 8.2

Source: CQ Press using data from U.S. Department of Health and Human Services, Centers for Medicare and Medicaid Services "The Children's Health Insurance Program Annual Enrollment Report" (http://www.cms.gov/NationalCHIPPolicy/)
*Figures for fiscal year 2009. The Children's Health Insurance Program (CHIP) was created in 1997 to help states expand health insurance to children whose families earn too much to qualify for Medicaid, yet not enough to afford private health insurance. Calculated using 2009 Census estimates for 17 and younger.

Expenditures for the Children's Health Insurance Program (CHIP) in 2009

National Total = $7,319,000,000*

ALPHA ORDER

RANK	STATE	EXPENDITURES	% of USA
19	Alabama	$116,400,000	1.6%
45	Alaska	16,200,000	0.2%
13	Arizona	194,300,000	2.7%
28	Arkansas	79,500,000	1.1%
1	California	1,139,200,000	15.6%
23	Colorado	102,300,000	1.4%
38	Connecticut	34,500,000	0.5%
48	Delaware	11,400,000	0.2%
5	Florida	286,400,000	3.9%
11	Georgia	225,600,000	3.1%
42	Hawaii	20,100,000	0.3%
33	Idaho	39,600,000	0.5%
8	Illinois	247,600,000	3.4%
27	Indiana	81,000,000	1.1%
30	Iowa	59,200,000	0.8%
32	Kansas	50,900,000	0.7%
22	Kentucky	110,400,000	1.5%
14	Louisiana	189,700,000	2.6%
36	Maine	34,800,000	0.5%
16	Maryland	154,900,000	2.1%
10	Massachusetts	227,400,000	3.1%
15	Michigan	186,900,000	2.6%
37	Minnesota	34,600,000	0.5%
17	Mississippi	148,600,000	2.0%
24	Missouri	100,900,000	1.4%
40	Montana	31,400,000	0.4%
35	Nebraska	36,700,000	0.5%
41	Nevada	22,700,000	0.3%
46	New Hampshire	13,300,000	0.2%
3	New Jersey	442,500,000	6.0%
6	New Mexico	283,000,000	3.9%
4	New York	345,300,000	4.7%
12	North Carolina	220,000,000	3.0%
47	North Dakota	13,100,000	0.2%
7	Ohio	252,000,000	3.4%
20	Oklahoma	116,000,000	1.6%
29	Oregon	74,400,000	1.0%
9	Pennsylvania	246,300,000	3.4%
43	Rhode Island	19,500,000	0.3%
26	South Carolina	84,200,000	1.2%
44	South Dakota	16,700,000	0.2%
21	Tennessee	113,700,000	1.6%
2	Texas	702,200,000	9.6%
31	Utah	55,600,000	0.8%
50	Vermont	6,000,000	0.1%
18	Virginia	148,400,000	2.0%
39	Washington	33,500,000	0.5%
34	West Virginia	38,200,000	0.5%
25	Wisconsin	91,000,000	1.2%
49	Wyoming	9,100,000	0.1%

RANK ORDER

RANK	STATE	EXPENDITURES	% of USA
1	California	$1,139,200,000	15.6%
2	Texas	702,200,000	9.6%
3	New Jersey	442,500,000	6.0%
4	New York	345,300,000	4.7%
5	Florida	286,400,000	3.9%
6	New Mexico	283,000,000	3.9%
7	Ohio	252,000,000	3.4%
8	Illinois	247,600,000	3.4%
9	Pennsylvania	246,300,000	3.4%
10	Massachusetts	227,400,000	3.1%
11	Georgia	225,600,000	3.1%
12	North Carolina	220,000,000	3.0%
13	Arizona	194,300,000	2.7%
14	Louisiana	189,700,000	2.6%
15	Michigan	186,900,000	2.6%
16	Maryland	154,900,000	2.1%
17	Mississippi	148,600,000	2.0%
18	Virginia	148,400,000	2.0%
19	Alabama	116,400,000	1.6%
20	Oklahoma	116,000,000	1.6%
21	Tennessee	113,700,000	1.6%
22	Kentucky	110,400,000	1.5%
23	Colorado	102,300,000	1.4%
24	Missouri	100,900,000	1.4%
25	Wisconsin	91,000,000	1.2%
26	South Carolina	84,200,000	1.2%
27	Indiana	81,000,000	1.1%
28	Arkansas	79,500,000	1.1%
29	Oregon	74,400,000	1.0%
30	Iowa	59,200,000	0.8%
31	Utah	55,600,000	0.8%
32	Kansas	50,900,000	0.7%
33	Idaho	39,600,000	0.5%
34	West Virginia	38,200,000	0.5%
35	Nebraska	36,700,000	0.5%
36	Maine	34,800,000	0.5%
37	Minnesota	34,600,000	0.5%
38	Connecticut	34,500,000	0.5%
39	Washington	33,500,000	0.5%
40	Montana	31,400,000	0.4%
41	Nevada	22,700,000	0.3%
42	Hawaii	20,100,000	0.3%
43	Rhode Island	19,500,000	0.3%
44	South Dakota	16,700,000	0.2%
45	Alaska	16,200,000	0.2%
46	New Hampshire	13,300,000	0.2%
47	North Dakota	13,100,000	0.2%
48	Delaware	11,400,000	0.2%
49	Wyoming	9,100,000	0.1%
50	Vermont	6,000,000	0.1%
	District of Columbia	11,200,000	0.2%

Source: U.S. Department of Health and Human Services, Centers for Medicare and Medicaid Services
"The Children's Health Insurance Program Annual Enrollment Report" (http://www.cms.gov/NationalCHIPPolicy/)
*Federal and state expenditures for fiscal year 2009. National total does not include funds spent in U.S. territories. The Children's Health Insurance Program (CHIP) was created in 1997 to help states expand health insurance to children whose families earn too much to qualify for Medicaid, yet not enough to afford private health insurance.

Per Capita Expenditures for the Children's Health Insurance Program (CHIP) in 2009
National Per Capita = $23.84*

ALPHA ORDER

RANK	STATE	PER CAPITA
16	Alabama	$24.72
18	Alaska	23.19
9	Arizona	29.46
11	Arkansas	27.51
8	California	30.82
24	Colorado	20.36
46	Connecticut	9.81
43	Delaware	12.88
42	Florida	15.45
19	Georgia	22.95
41	Hawaii	15.52
14	Idaho	25.62
30	Illinois	19.18
44	Indiana	12.61
27	Iowa	19.68
35	Kansas	18.06
15	Kentucky	25.59
4	Louisiana	42.23
13	Maine	26.40
12	Maryland	27.18
5	Massachusetts	34.49
32	Michigan	18.75
49	Minnesota	6.57
3	Mississippi	50.34
38	Missouri	16.85
6	Montana	32.21
23	Nebraska	20.43
48	Nevada	8.59
45	New Hampshire	10.04
2	New Jersey	50.82
1	New Mexico	140.82
37	New York	17.67
17	North Carolina	23.45
25	North Dakota	20.25
20	Ohio	21.83
7	Oklahoma	31.46
29	Oregon	19.45
28	Pennsylvania	19.54
33	Rhode Island	18.51
34	South Carolina	18.46
22	South Dakota	20.56
35	Tennessee	18.06
10	Texas	28.33
26	Utah	19.97
47	Vermont	9.65
31	Virginia	18.83
50	Washington	5.03
21	West Virginia	20.99
40	Wisconsin	16.09
39	Wyoming	16.72

RANK ORDER

RANK	STATE	PER CAPITA
1	New Mexico	$140.82
2	New Jersey	50.82
3	Mississippi	50.34
4	Louisiana	42.23
5	Massachusetts	34.49
6	Montana	32.21
7	Oklahoma	31.46
8	California	30.82
9	Arizona	29.46
10	Texas	28.33
11	Arkansas	27.51
12	Maryland	27.18
13	Maine	26.40
14	Idaho	25.62
15	Kentucky	25.59
16	Alabama	24.72
17	North Carolina	23.45
18	Alaska	23.19
19	Georgia	22.95
20	Ohio	21.83
21	West Virginia	20.99
22	South Dakota	20.56
23	Nebraska	20.43
24	Colorado	20.36
25	North Dakota	20.25
26	Utah	19.97
27	Iowa	19.68
28	Pennsylvania	19.54
29	Oregon	19.45
30	Illinois	19.18
31	Virginia	18.83
32	Michigan	18.75
33	Rhode Island	18.51
34	South Carolina	18.46
35	Kansas	18.06
35	Tennessee	18.06
37	New York	17.67
38	Missouri	16.85
39	Wyoming	16.72
40	Wisconsin	16.09
41	Hawaii	15.52
42	Florida	15.45
43	Delaware	12.88
44	Indiana	12.61
45	New Hampshire	10.04
46	Connecticut	9.81
47	Vermont	9.65
48	Nevada	8.59
49	Minnesota	6.57
50	Washington	5.03

District of Columbia 18.68

Source: CQ Press using data from U.S. Department of Health and Human Services, Centers for Medicare and Medicaid Services "The Children's Health Insurance Program Annual Enrollment Report" (http://www.cms.gov/NationalCHIPPolicy/)

*Federal expenditures for fiscal year 2009. National figure does not include funds spent in U.S. territories. The Children's Health Insurance Program (CHIP) was created in 1997 to help states expand health insurance to children whose families earn too much to qualify for Medicaid, yet not enough to afford private health insurance.

Expenditures per Participant in the Children's Health Insurance Program (CHIP) in 2009
National Per Participant = $948*

ALPHA ORDER

RANK	STATE	PER PARTICIPANT
22	Alabama	$1,056
11	Alaska	1,385
6	Arizona	1,849
42	Arkansas	785
48	California	652
26	Colorado	999
9	Connecticut	1,583
34	Delaware	905
44	Florida	686
36	Georgia	887
40	Hawaii	814
35	Idaho	894
47	Illinois	657
50	Indiana	584
17	Iowa	1,125
21	Kansas	1,058
10	Kentucky	1,510
18	Louisiana	1,115
19	Maine	1,112
13	Maryland	1,243
8	Massachusetts	1,590
4	Michigan	2,596
2	Minnesota	6,291
7	Mississippi	1,712
29	Missouri	973
15	Montana	1,222
43	Nebraska	763
46	Nevada	668
24	New Hampshire	1,008
3	New Jersey	2,650
1	New Mexico	17,578
49	New York	648
38	North Carolina	871
5	North Dakota	1,871
30	Ohio	948
31	Oklahoma	938
16	Oregon	1,198
32	Pennsylvania	930
27	Rhode Island	995
28	South Carolina	991
20	South Dakota	1,092
12	Tennessee	1,365
41	Texas	807
32	Utah	930
39	Vermont	845
37	Virginia	885
14	Washington	1,223
25	West Virginia	1,000
45	Wisconsin	685
23	Wyoming	1,022

RANK ORDER

RANK	STATE	PER PARTICIPANT
1	New Mexico	$17,578
2	Minnesota	6,291
3	New Jersey	2,650
4	Michigan	2,596
5	North Dakota	1,871
6	Arizona	1,849
7	Mississippi	1,712
8	Massachusetts	1,590
9	Connecticut	1,583
10	Kentucky	1,510
11	Alaska	1,385
12	Tennessee	1,365
13	Maryland	1,243
14	Washington	1,223
15	Montana	1,222
16	Oregon	1,198
17	Iowa	1,125
18	Louisiana	1,115
19	Maine	1,112
20	South Dakota	1,092
21	Kansas	1,058
22	Alabama	1,056
23	Wyoming	1,022
24	New Hampshire	1,008
25	West Virginia	1,000
26	Colorado	999
27	Rhode Island	995
28	South Carolina	991
29	Missouri	973
30	Ohio	948
31	Oklahoma	938
32	Pennsylvania	930
32	Utah	930
34	Delaware	905
35	Idaho	894
36	Georgia	887
37	Virginia	885
38	North Carolina	871
39	Vermont	845
40	Hawaii	814
41	Texas	807
42	Arkansas	785
43	Nebraska	763
44	Florida	686
45	Wisconsin	685
46	Nevada	668
47	Illinois	657
48	California	652
49	New York	648
50	Indiana	584

District of Columbia	1,204

Source: CQ Press using data from U.S. Department of Health and Human Services, Centers for Medicare and Medicaid Services "The Children's Health Insurance Program Annual Enrollment Report" (http://www.cms.gov/NationalCHIPPolicy/)

*Federal expenditures for fiscal year 2009. National figure does not include funds spent in U.S. territories. The Children's Health Insurance Program (CHIP) was created in 1997 to help states expand health insurance to children whose families earn too much to qualify for Medicaid, yet not enough to afford private health insurance.

Health Maintenance Organizations (HMOs) in 2009

National Total = 462 HMOs*

ALPHA ORDER

RANK	STATE	HMOs	% of USA
31	Alabama	43	9.3%
50	Alaska	20	4.3%
6	Arizona	72	15.6%
25	Arkansas	51	11.0%
1	California	102	22.1%
20	Colorado	55	11.9%
28	Connecticut	46	10.0%
35	Delaware	41	8.9%
2	Florida	98	21.2%
9	Georgia	62	13.4%
40	Hawaii	35	7.6%
40	Idaho	35	7.6%
7	Illinois	65	14.1%
17	Indiana	57	12.3%
37	Iowa	38	8.2%
31	Kansas	43	9.3%
27	Kentucky	47	10.2%
28	Louisiana	46	10.0%
40	Maine	35	7.6%
24	Maryland	52	11.3%
16	Massachusetts	58	12.6%
14	Michigan	60	13.0%
30	Minnesota	45	9.7%
38	Mississippi	37	8.0%
15	Missouri	59	12.8%
47	Montana	26	5.6%
44	Nebraska	30	6.5%
20	Nevada	55	11.9%
43	New Hampshire	33	7.1%
19	New Jersey	56	12.1%
35	New Mexico	41	8.9%
3	New York	88	19.0%
20	North Carolina	55	11.9%
45	North Dakota	27	5.8%
8	Ohio	64	13.9%
31	Oklahoma	43	9.3%
23	Oregon	53	11.5%
5	Pennsylvania	73	15.8%
47	Rhode Island	26	5.6%
10	South Carolina	61	13.2%
38	South Dakota	37	8.0%
10	Tennessee	61	13.2%
4	Texas	83	18.0%
26	Utah	48	10.4%
49	Vermont	25	5.4%
10	Virginia	61	13.2%
17	Washington	57	12.3%
34	West Virginia	42	9.1%
10	Wisconsin	61	13.2%
45	Wyoming	27	5.8%

RANK ORDER

RANK	STATE	HMOs	% of USA
1	California	102	22.1%
2	Florida	98	21.2%
3	New York	88	19.0%
4	Texas	83	18.0%
5	Pennsylvania	73	15.8%
6	Arizona	72	15.6%
7	Illinois	65	14.1%
8	Ohio	64	13.9%
9	Georgia	62	13.4%
10	South Carolina	61	13.2%
10	Tennessee	61	13.2%
10	Virginia	61	13.2%
10	Wisconsin	61	13.2%
14	Michigan	60	13.0%
15	Missouri	59	12.8%
16	Massachusetts	58	12.6%
17	Indiana	57	12.3%
17	Washington	57	12.3%
19	New Jersey	56	12.1%
20	Colorado	55	11.9%
20	Nevada	55	11.9%
20	North Carolina	55	11.9%
23	Oregon	53	11.5%
24	Maryland	52	11.3%
25	Arkansas	51	11.0%
26	Utah	48	10.4%
27	Kentucky	47	10.2%
28	Connecticut	46	10.0%
28	Louisiana	46	10.0%
30	Minnesota	45	9.7%
31	Alabama	43	9.3%
31	Kansas	43	9.3%
31	Oklahoma	43	9.3%
34	West Virginia	42	9.1%
35	Delaware	41	8.9%
35	New Mexico	41	8.9%
37	Iowa	38	8.2%
38	Mississippi	37	8.0%
38	South Dakota	37	8.0%
40	Hawaii	35	7.6%
40	Idaho	35	7.6%
40	Maine	35	7.6%
43	New Hampshire	33	7.1%
44	Nebraska	30	6.5%
45	North Dakota	27	5.8%
45	Wyoming	27	5.8%
47	Montana	26	5.6%
47	Rhode Island	26	5.6%
49	Vermont	25	5.4%
50	Alaska	20	4.3%
	District of Columbia	38	8.2%

Source: Lance Wolkenbrod, Data Analyst

HealthLeaders - InterStudy (Nashville, TN, http://home.healthleaders-interstudy.com)

*As of January 2009. National total reflects the total HMOs nationwide and does not count HMOs in more than one state as multiple HMOs. The total for all HMO programs by state is 2,573.

Enrollees in Health Maintenance Organizations (HMOs) in 2009

National Total = 74,494,844 Enrollees*

ALPHA ORDER

RANK	STATE	ENROLLEES	% of USA
37	Alabama	257,584	0.3%
50	Alaska	8,825	0.0%
11	Arizona	1,836,849	2.5%
44	Arkansas	104,516	0.1%
1	California	16,489,216	22.1%
22	Colorado	916,295	1.2%
23	Connecticut	915,376	1.2%
36	Delaware	262,859	0.4%
3	Florida	4,123,318	5.5%
9	Georgia	2,346,939	3.2%
25	Hawaii	665,435	0.9%
43	Idaho	112,507	0.2%
16	Illinois	1,604,723	2.2%
18	Indiana	1,109,757	1.5%
33	Iowa	330,092	0.4%
32	Kansas	369,312	0.5%
30	Kentucky	443,904	0.6%
31	Louisiana	382,110	0.5%
41	Maine	143,367	0.2%
12	Maryland	1,781,237	2.4%
6	Massachusetts	2,991,311	4.0%
7	Michigan	2,848,966	3.8%
20	Minnesota	993,494	1.3%
45	Mississippi	60,868	0.1%
21	Missouri	928,378	1.2%
46	Montana	56,322	0.1%
40	Nebraska	150,259	0.2%
28	Nevada	510,864	0.7%
35	New Hampshire	271,608	0.4%
10	New Jersey	2,001,474	2.7%
26	New Mexico	611,926	0.8%
2	New York	6,195,912	8.3%
27	North Carolina	545,636	0.7%
48	North Dakota	21,556	0.0%
8	Ohio	2,477,375	3.3%
38	Oklahoma	256,128	0.3%
19	Oregon	1,099,721	1.5%
4	Pennsylvania	3,780,412	5.1%
39	Rhode Island	198,618	0.3%
29	South Carolina	503,594	0.7%
42	South Dakota	140,247	0.2%
15	Tennessee	1,607,946	2.2%
5	Texas	3,732,750	5.0%
24	Utah	836,248	1.1%
47	Vermont	48,531	0.1%
13	Virginia	1,694,815	2.3%
17	Washington	1,302,266	1.7%
34	West Virginia	285,232	0.4%
14	Wisconsin	1,672,688	2.2%
49	Wyoming	11,348	0.0%

RANK ORDER

RANK	STATE	ENROLLEES	% of USA
1	California	16,489,216	22.1%
2	New York	6,195,912	8.3%
3	Florida	4,123,318	5.5%
4	Pennsylvania	3,780,412	5.1%
5	Texas	3,732,750	5.0%
6	Massachusetts	2,991,311	4.0%
7	Michigan	2,848,966	3.8%
8	Ohio	2,477,375	3.3%
9	Georgia	2,346,939	3.2%
10	New Jersey	2,001,474	2.7%
11	Arizona	1,836,849	2.5%
12	Maryland	1,781,237	2.4%
13	Virginia	1,694,815	2.3%
14	Wisconsin	1,672,688	2.2%
15	Tennessee	1,607,946	2.2%
16	Illinois	1,604,723	2.2%
17	Washington	1,302,266	1.7%
18	Indiana	1,109,757	1.5%
19	Oregon	1,099,721	1.5%
20	Minnesota	993,494	1.3%
21	Missouri	928,378	1.2%
22	Colorado	916,295	1.2%
23	Connecticut	915,376	1.2%
24	Utah	836,248	1.1%
25	Hawaii	665,435	0.9%
26	New Mexico	611,926	0.8%
27	North Carolina	545,636	0.7%
28	Nevada	510,864	0.7%
29	South Carolina	503,594	0.7%
30	Kentucky	443,904	0.6%
31	Louisiana	382,110	0.5%
32	Kansas	369,312	0.5%
33	Iowa	330,092	0.4%
34	West Virginia	285,232	0.4%
35	New Hampshire	271,608	0.4%
36	Delaware	262,859	0.4%
37	Alabama	257,584	0.3%
38	Oklahoma	256,128	0.3%
39	Rhode Island	198,618	0.3%
40	Nebraska	150,259	0.2%
41	Maine	143,367	0.2%
42	South Dakota	140,247	0.2%
43	Idaho	112,507	0.2%
44	Arkansas	104,516	0.1%
45	Mississippi	60,868	0.1%
46	Montana	56,322	0.1%
47	Vermont	48,531	0.1%
48	North Dakota	21,556	0.0%
49	Wyoming	11,348	0.0%
50	Alaska	8,825	0.0%
	District of Columbia	274,160	0.4%

Source: Lance Wolkenbrod, Data Analyst
    HealthLeaders - InterStudy (Nashville, TN, http://home.healthleaders-interstudy.com)
*As of January 2009.

Percent Change in Enrollees in Health Maintenance Organizations (HMOs): 2008 to 2009
National Percent Change = 1.2% Decrease*

ALPHA ORDER

RANK	STATE	PERCENT CHANGE
7	Alabama	9.5
16	Alaska	2.2
33	Arizona	(6.6)
10	Arkansas	5.6
20	California	0.2
43	Colorado	(13.5)
27	Connecticut	(2.0)
2	Delaware	35.1
37	Florida	(9.6)
11	Georgia	5.3
8	Hawaii	8.5
5	Idaho	11.0
41	Illinois	(12.9)
30	Indiana	(4.7)
3	Iowa	24.8
46	Kansas	(19.7)
14	Kentucky	3.5
25	Louisiana	(1.6)
45	Maine	(18.0)
15	Maryland	2.6
13	Massachusetts	4.7
22	Michigan	(0.2)
39	Minnesota	(11.4)
35	Mississippi	(7.6)
38	Missouri	(9.7)
24	Montana	(1.3)
1	Nebraska	64.4
34	Nevada	(7.0)
42	New Hampshire	(13.2)
36	New Jersey	(9.3)
18	New Mexico	0.5
9	New York	6.6
48	North Carolina	(35.8)
4	North Dakota	16.4
12	Ohio	4.8
28	Oklahoma	(2.5)
17	Oregon	1.8
32	Pennsylvania	(5.9)
47	Rhode Island	(22.1)
26	South Carolina	(1.7)
31	South Dakota	(5.2)
44	Tennessee	(15.0)
29	Texas	(3.1)
40	Utah	(11.8)
49	Vermont	(43.5)
20	Virginia	0.2
19	Washington	0.3
23	West Virginia	(1.1)
6	Wisconsin	9.8
50	Wyoming	(53.6)

RANK ORDER

RANK	STATE	PERCENT CHANGE
1	Nebraska	64.4
2	Delaware	35.1
3	Iowa	24.8
4	North Dakota	16.4
5	Idaho	11.0
6	Wisconsin	9.8
7	Alabama	9.5
8	Hawaii	8.5
9	New York	6.6
10	Arkansas	5.6
11	Georgia	5.3
12	Ohio	4.8
13	Massachusetts	4.7
14	Kentucky	3.5
15	Maryland	2.6
16	Alaska	2.2
17	Oregon	1.8
18	New Mexico	0.5
19	Washington	0.3
20	California	0.2
20	Virginia	0.2
22	Michigan	(0.2)
23	West Virginia	(1.1)
24	Montana	(1.3)
25	Louisiana	(1.6)
26	South Carolina	(1.7)
27	Connecticut	(2.0)
28	Oklahoma	(2.5)
29	Texas	(3.1)
30	Indiana	(4.7)
31	South Dakota	(5.2)
32	Pennsylvania	(5.9)
33	Arizona	(6.6)
34	Nevada	(7.0)
35	Mississippi	(7.6)
36	New Jersey	(9.3)
37	Florida	(9.6)
38	Missouri	(9.7)
39	Minnesota	(11.4)
40	Utah	(11.8)
41	Illinois	(12.9)
42	New Hampshire	(13.2)
43	Colorado	(13.5)
44	Tennessee	(15.0)
45	Maine	(18.0)
46	Kansas	(19.7)
47	Rhode Island	(22.1)
48	North Carolina	(35.8)
49	Vermont	(43.5)
50	Wyoming	(53.6)

District of Columbia (12.5)

Source: CQ Press using data from Lance Wolkenbrod, Data Analyst
HealthLeaders - InterStudy (Nashville, TN, http://home.healthleaders-interstudy.com)
*As of January 2009. National figure does not include enrollees in U.S. territories.

Percent of Population Enrolled in Health Maintenance Organizations (HMOs) in 2009
National Percent = 24.2% Enrolled in HMOs*

ALPHA ORDER

RANK	STATE	PERCENT
45	Alabama	5.5
50	Alaska	1.3
13	Arizona	28.3
46	Arkansas	3.7
3	California	44.9
26	Colorado	18.6
14	Connecticut	26.1
9	Delaware	30.1
18	Florida	22.5
16	Georgia	24.2
1	Hawaii	51.7
41	Idaho	7.4
33	Illinois	12.4
27	Indiana	17.4
35	Iowa	11.0
32	Kansas	13.2
37	Kentucky	10.4
38	Louisiana	8.7
36	Maine	10.9
5	Maryland	31.6
2	Massachusetts	46.0
12	Michigan	28.5
24	Minnesota	19.0
48	Mississippi	2.1
29	Missouri	15.7
44	Montana	5.8
39	Nebraska	8.4
23	Nevada	19.6
21	New Hampshire	20.6
17	New Jersey	23.1
6	New Mexico	30.8
4	New York	31.8
43	North Carolina	5.9
47	North Dakota	3.4
20	Ohio	21.6
42	Oklahoma	7.0
11	Oregon	29.0
8	Pennsylvania	30.4
25	Rhode Island	18.9
34	South Carolina	11.2
27	South Dakota	17.4
15	Tennessee	25.9
31	Texas	15.3
7	Utah	30.6
40	Vermont	7.8
19	Virginia	21.8
22	Washington	19.9
29	West Virginia	15.7
10	Wisconsin	29.7
48	Wyoming	2.1

RANK ORDER

RANK	STATE	PERCENT
1	Hawaii	51.7
2	Massachusetts	46.0
3	California	44.9
4	New York	31.8
5	Maryland	31.6
6	New Mexico	30.8
7	Utah	30.6
8	Pennsylvania	30.4
9	Delaware	30.1
10	Wisconsin	29.7
11	Oregon	29.0
12	Michigan	28.5
13	Arizona	28.3
14	Connecticut	26.1
15	Tennessee	25.9
16	Georgia	24.2
17	New Jersey	23.1
18	Florida	22.5
19	Virginia	21.8
20	Ohio	21.6
21	New Hampshire	20.6
22	Washington	19.9
23	Nevada	19.6
24	Minnesota	19.0
25	Rhode Island	18.9
26	Colorado	18.6
27	Indiana	17.4
27	South Dakota	17.4
29	Missouri	15.7
29	West Virginia	15.7
31	Texas	15.3
32	Kansas	13.2
33	Illinois	12.4
34	South Carolina	11.2
35	Iowa	11.0
36	Maine	10.9
37	Kentucky	10.4
38	Louisiana	8.7
39	Nebraska	8.4
40	Vermont	7.8
41	Idaho	7.4
42	Oklahoma	7.0
43	North Carolina	5.9
44	Montana	5.8
45	Alabama	5.5
46	Arkansas	3.7
47	North Dakota	3.4
48	Mississippi	2.1
48	Wyoming	2.1
50	Alaska	1.3
	District of Columbia	46.3

Source: Lance Wolkenbrod, Data Analyst
        HealthLeaders - InterStudy (Nashville, TN, http://home.healthleaders-interstudy.com)
*As of January 2009.

Percent of Insured Population Enrolled in
Health Maintenance Organizations (HMOs) in 2009
National Percent = 29.2% of Insured Are Enrolled in HMOs*

ALPHA ORDER

RANK	STATE	PERCENT
45	Alabama	6.2
50	Alaska	1.6
7	Arizona	34.9
46	Arkansas	4.5
2	California	55.2
24	Colorado	22.2
16	Connecticut	29.6
11	Delaware	34.2
17	Florida	28.6
15	Georgia	29.9
1	Hawaii	57.4
40	Idaho	8.8
33	Illinois	14.5
28	Indiana	20.1
36	Iowa	12.2
32	Kansas	15.4
35	Kentucky	12.4
38	Louisiana	11.0
37	Maine	12.1
6	Maryland	36.6
3	Massachusetts	49.3
13	Michigan	32.9
26	Minnesota	21.2
48	Mississippi	2.5
31	Missouri	18.1
44	Montana	6.9
39	Nebraska	9.6
21	Nevada	24.4
22	New Hampshire	23.3
18	New Jersey	27.3
4	New Mexico	40.5
5	New York	37.3
43	North Carolina	7.0
47	North Dakota	3.9
20	Ohio	24.6
42	Oklahoma	8.4
9	Oregon	34.4
9	Pennsylvania	34.4
25	Rhode Island	21.6
34	South Carolina	13.4
28	South Dakota	20.1
14	Tennessee	30.6
27	Texas	20.6
7	Utah	34.9
41	Vermont	8.7
19	Virginia	25.0
23	Washington	22.7
30	West Virginia	18.7
12	Wisconsin	33.3
48	Wyoming	2.5

RANK ORDER

RANK	STATE	PERCENT
1	Hawaii	57.4
2	California	55.2
3	Massachusetts	49.3
4	New Mexico	40.5
5	New York	37.3
6	Maryland	36.6
7	Arizona	34.9
7	Utah	34.9
9	Oregon	34.4
9	Pennsylvania	34.4
11	Delaware	34.2
12	Wisconsin	33.3
13	Michigan	32.9
14	Tennessee	30.6
15	Georgia	29.9
16	Connecticut	29.6
17	Florida	28.6
18	New Jersey	27.3
19	Virginia	25.0
20	Ohio	24.6
21	Nevada	24.4
22	New Hampshire	23.3
23	Washington	22.7
24	Colorado	22.2
25	Rhode Island	21.6
26	Minnesota	21.2
27	Texas	20.6
28	Indiana	20.1
28	South Dakota	20.1
30	West Virginia	18.7
31	Missouri	18.1
32	Kansas	15.4
33	Illinois	14.5
34	South Carolina	13.4
35	Kentucky	12.4
36	Iowa	12.2
37	Maine	12.1
38	Louisiana	11.0
39	Nebraska	9.6
40	Idaho	8.8
41	Vermont	8.7
42	Oklahoma	8.4
43	North Carolina	7.0
44	Montana	6.9
45	Alabama	6.2
46	Arkansas	4.5
47	North Dakota	3.9
48	Mississippi	2.5
48	Wyoming	2.5
50	Alaska	1.6

District of Columbia   51.4

Source: CQ Press using data from Lance Wolkenbrod, Data Analyst
   HealthLeaders - InterStudy (Nashville, TN, http://home.healthleaders-interstudy.com)
*As of January 2009. Calculated using estimated number of insured as of 2008 from the U.S. Census Bureau.

Medicare Enrollees in 2009

National Total = 46,520,716 Enrollees*

ALPHA ORDER

RANK	STATE	ENROLLEES	% of USA
20	Alabama	827,594	1.8%
50	Alaska	62,707	0.1%
18	Arizona	899,487	1.9%
30	Arkansas	520,377	1.1%
1	California	4,619,642	9.9%
27	Colorado	601,992	1.3%
29	Connecticut	558,107	1.2%
45	Delaware	145,065	0.3%
2	Florida	3,289,117	7.1%
11	Georgia	1,193,887	2.6%
42	Hawaii	200,305	0.4%
40	Idaho	221,962	0.5%
7	Illinois	1,806,475	3.9%
16	Indiana	985,107	2.1%
31	Iowa	511,615	1.1%
33	Kansas	425,444	0.9%
24	Kentucky	743,418	1.6%
25	Louisiana	671,294	1.4%
39	Maine	259,090	0.6%
22	Maryland	764,123	1.6%
13	Massachusetts	1,039,299	2.2%
8	Michigan	1,614,512	3.5%
21	Minnesota	766,806	1.6%
32	Mississippi	487,978	1.0%
15	Missouri	985,325	2.1%
44	Montana	164,635	0.4%
37	Nebraska	275,617	0.6%
35	Nevada	343,026	0.7%
41	New Hampshire	217,378	0.5%
10	New Jersey	1,304,311	2.8%
36	New Mexico	303,827	0.7%
3	New York	2,937,045	6.3%
9	North Carolina	1,447,965	3.1%
47	North Dakota	107,998	0.2%
6	Ohio	1,870,284	4.0%
28	Oklahoma	591,793	1.3%
26	Oregon	602,246	1.3%
5	Pennsylvania	2,252,011	4.8%
43	Rhode Island	180,233	0.4%
23	South Carolina	748,651	1.6%
46	South Dakota	134,470	0.3%
14	Tennessee	1,031,204	2.2%
4	Texas	2,899,787	6.2%
38	Utah	273,860	0.6%
48	Vermont	107,950	0.2%
12	Virginia	1,109,909	2.4%
17	Washington	938,166	2.0%
34	West Virginia	377,244	0.8%
19	Wisconsin	891,742	1.9%
49	Wyoming	78,223	0.2%

RANK ORDER

RANK	STATE	ENROLLEES	% of USA
1	California	4,619,642	9.9%
2	Florida	3,289,117	7.1%
3	New York	2,937,045	6.3%
4	Texas	2,899,787	6.2%
5	Pennsylvania	2,252,011	4.8%
6	Ohio	1,870,284	4.0%
7	Illinois	1,806,475	3.9%
8	Michigan	1,614,512	3.5%
9	North Carolina	1,447,965	3.1%
10	New Jersey	1,304,311	2.8%
11	Georgia	1,193,887	2.6%
12	Virginia	1,109,909	2.4%
13	Massachusetts	1,039,299	2.2%
14	Tennessee	1,031,204	2.2%
15	Missouri	985,325	2.1%
16	Indiana	985,107	2.1%
17	Washington	938,166	2.0%
18	Arizona	899,487	1.9%
19	Wisconsin	891,742	1.9%
20	Alabama	827,594	1.8%
21	Minnesota	766,806	1.6%
22	Maryland	764,123	1.6%
23	South Carolina	748,651	1.6%
24	Kentucky	743,418	1.6%
25	Louisiana	671,294	1.4%
26	Oregon	602,246	1.3%
27	Colorado	601,992	1.3%
28	Oklahoma	591,793	1.3%
29	Connecticut	558,107	1.2%
30	Arkansas	520,377	1.1%
31	Iowa	511,615	1.1%
32	Mississippi	487,978	1.0%
33	Kansas	425,444	0.9%
34	West Virginia	377,244	0.8%
35	Nevada	343,026	0.7%
36	New Mexico	303,827	0.7%
37	Nebraska	275,617	0.6%
38	Utah	273,860	0.6%
39	Maine	259,090	0.6%
40	Idaho	221,962	0.5%
41	New Hampshire	217,378	0.5%
42	Hawaii	200,305	0.4%
43	Rhode Island	180,233	0.4%
44	Montana	164,635	0.4%
45	Delaware	145,065	0.3%
46	South Dakota	134,470	0.3%
47	North Dakota	107,998	0.2%
48	Vermont	107,950	0.2%
49	Wyoming	78,223	0.2%
50	Alaska	62,707	0.1%
	District of Columbia	76,694	0.2%

Source: U.S. Department of Health and Human Services, Centers for Medicare and Medicaid Services
    "2010 Data Compendium" (http://www.cms.hhs.gov/DataCompendium/)
*Includes aged and disabled enrollees. Total includes 653,166 enrollees in Puerto Rico and other outlying areas, foreign countries, or whose address is unknown.

Percent Change in Medicare Enrollees: 2008 to 2009

National Percent Change = 2.4% Increase*

ALPHA ORDER

RANK	STATE	PERCENT CHANGE
26	Alabama	2.3
1	Alaska	4.9
9	Arizona	3.4
26	Arkansas	2.3
15	California	2.9
2	Colorado	3.9
41	Connecticut	1.7
18	Delaware	2.8
24	Florida	2.4
6	Georgia	3.6
11	Hawaii	3.2
6	Idaho	3.6
37	Illinois	1.8
31	Indiana	2.2
49	Iowa	1.1
37	Kansas	1.8
33	Kentucky	2.1
26	Louisiana	2.3
26	Maine	2.3
22	Maryland	2.6
35	Massachusetts	2.0
31	Michigan	2.2
24	Minnesota	2.4
37	Mississippi	1.8
35	Missouri	2.0
22	Montana	2.6
43	Nebraska	1.6
2	Nevada	3.9
20	New Hampshire	2.7
41	New Jersey	1.7
11	New Mexico	3.2
43	New York	1.6
13	North Carolina	3.1
48	North Dakota	1.2
43	Ohio	1.6
26	Oklahoma	2.3
13	Oregon	3.1
46	Pennsylvania	1.4
47	Rhode Island	1.3
9	South Carolina	3.4
37	South Dakota	1.8
20	Tennessee	2.7
8	Texas	3.5
5	Utah	3.7
15	Vermont	2.9
15	Virginia	2.9
2	Washington	3.9
49	West Virginia	1.1
33	Wisconsin	2.1
18	Wyoming	2.8

RANK ORDER

RANK	STATE	PERCENT CHANGE
1	Alaska	4.9
2	Colorado	3.9
2	Nevada	3.9
2	Washington	3.9
5	Utah	3.7
6	Georgia	3.6
6	Idaho	3.6
8	Texas	3.5
9	Arizona	3.4
9	South Carolina	3.4
11	Hawaii	3.2
11	New Mexico	3.2
13	North Carolina	3.1
13	Oregon	3.1
15	California	2.9
15	Vermont	2.9
15	Virginia	2.9
18	Delaware	2.8
18	Wyoming	2.8
20	New Hampshire	2.7
20	Tennessee	2.7
22	Maryland	2.6
22	Montana	2.6
24	Florida	2.4
24	Minnesota	2.4
26	Alabama	2.3
26	Arkansas	2.3
26	Louisiana	2.3
26	Maine	2.3
26	Oklahoma	2.3
31	Indiana	2.2
31	Michigan	2.2
33	Kentucky	2.1
33	Wisconsin	2.1
35	Massachusetts	2.0
35	Missouri	2.0
37	Illinois	1.8
37	Kansas	1.8
37	Mississippi	1.8
37	South Dakota	1.8
41	Connecticut	1.7
41	New Jersey	1.7
43	Nebraska	1.6
43	New York	1.6
43	Ohio	1.6
46	Pennsylvania	1.4
47	Rhode Island	1.3
48	North Dakota	1.2
49	Iowa	1.1
49	West Virginia	1.1

	District of Columbia	2.1

Source: CQ Press using data from U.S. Department of Health and Human Services, Centers for Medicare and Medicaid Services "2010 Data Compendium" (http://www.cms.hhs.gov/DataCompendium/)

*Includes aged and disabled enrollees. National rate includes enrollees in Puerto Rico and other outlying areas, foreign countries, or whose address is unknown.

Percent of Population Enrolled in Medicare in 2009

National Percent = 14.8% of Population*

ALPHA ORDER			RANK ORDER		
RANK	STATE	PERCENT	RANK	STATE	PERCENT
6	Alabama	17.6	1	West Virginia	20.7
50	Alaska	9.0	2	Maine	19.7
42	Arizona	13.6	3	Arkansas	18.0
3	Arkansas	18.0	4	Pennsylvania	17.9
45	California	12.5	5	Florida	17.7
47	Colorado	12.0	6	Alabama	17.6
23	Connecticut	15.9	7	Vermont	17.4
18	Delaware	16.4	8	Kentucky	17.2
5	Florida	17.7	9	Rhode Island	17.1
46	Georgia	12.1	10	Iowa	17.0
27	Hawaii	15.5	11	Montana	16.9
38	Idaho	14.4	12	North Dakota	16.7
41	Illinois	14.0	13	South Dakota	16.6
30	Indiana	15.3	14	Mississippi	16.5
10	Iowa	17.0	15	Missouri	16.5
32	Kansas	15.1	16	South Carolina	16.4
8	Kentucky	17.2	17	New Hampshire	16.4
35	Louisiana	14.9	18	Delaware	16.4
2	Maine	19.7	19	Tennessee	16.4
43	Maryland	13.4	20	Ohio	16.2
25	Massachusetts	15.8	21	Michigan	16.2
21	Michigan	16.2	22	Oklahoma	16.1
36	Minnesota	14.6	23	Connecticut	15.9
14	Mississippi	16.5	24	Wisconsin	15.8
15	Missouri	16.5	25	Massachusetts	15.8
11	Montana	16.9	26	Oregon	15.7
29	Nebraska	15.3	27	Hawaii	15.5
44	Nevada	13.0	28	North Carolina	15.4
17	New Hampshire	16.4	29	Nebraska	15.3
34	New Jersey	15.0	30	Indiana	15.3
31	New Mexico	15.1	31	New Mexico	15.1
33	New York	15.0	32	Kansas	15.1
28	North Carolina	15.4	33	New York	15.0
12	North Dakota	16.7	34	New Jersey	15.0
20	Ohio	16.2	35	Louisiana	14.9
22	Oklahoma	16.1	36	Minnesota	14.6
26	Oregon	15.7	37	Wyoming	14.4
4	Pennsylvania	17.9	38	Idaho	14.4
9	Rhode Island	17.1	39	Virginia	14.1
16	South Carolina	16.4	40	Washington	14.1
13	South Dakota	16.6	41	Illinois	14.0
19	Tennessee	16.4	42	Arizona	13.6
48	Texas	11.7	43	Maryland	13.4
49	Utah	9.8	44	Nevada	13.0
7	Vermont	17.4	45	California	12.5
39	Virginia	14.1	46	Georgia	12.1
40	Washington	14.1	47	Colorado	12.0
1	West Virginia	20.7	48	Texas	11.7
24	Wisconsin	15.8	49	Utah	9.8
37	Wyoming	14.4	50	Alaska	9.0
				District of Columbia	12.8

Source: U.S. Department of Health and Human Services, Centers for Medicare and Medicaid Services
    "2010 Data Compendium" (http://www.cms.hhs.gov/DataCompendium/)
*Includes aged and disabled enrollees. National rate includes only residents of the 50 states and the District of Columbia.

Percent of Medicare Enrollees in Managed Care Programs in 2009

National Percent = 21.3% of Medicare Enrollees*

ALPHA ORDER				RANK ORDER		
RANK	STATE	PERCENT		RANK	STATE	PERCENT
22	Alabama	22.7		1	Oregon	42.0
50	Alaska	1.2		2	Hawaii	40.6
5	Arizona	37.0		3	Pennsylvania	38.9
35	Arkansas	13.9		4	Minnesota	38.0
7	California	35.1		5	Arizona	37.0
8	Colorado	33.5		6	Rhode Island	36.2
28	Connecticut	17.4		7	California	35.1
48	Delaware	4.9		8	Colorado	33.5
12	Florida	29.3		9	Utah	32.2
29	Georgia	15.4		10	Nevada	30.7
2	Hawaii	40.6		11	New York	29.5
13	Idaho	28.5		12	Florida	29.3
41	Illinois	9.9		13	Idaho	28.5
29	Indiana	15.4		14	Wisconsin	27.9
36	Iowa	13.0		15	Ohio	26.9
40	Kansas	10.9		16	Michigan	25.7
29	Kentucky	15.4		17	New Mexico	25.0
21	Louisiana	23.1		18	Washington	24.7
39	Maine	11.0		19	West Virginia	23.7
43	Maryland	8.0		20	Tennessee	23.6
24	Massachusetts	19.5		21	Louisiana	23.1
16	Michigan	25.7		22	Alabama	22.7
4	Minnesota	38.0		23	Missouri	20.2
42	Mississippi	9.6		24	Massachusetts	19.5
23	Missouri	20.2		25	Texas	18.8
27	Montana	17.6		26	North Carolina	17.8
38	Nebraska	11.8		27	Montana	17.6
10	Nevada	30.7		28	Connecticut	17.4
46	New Hampshire	6.6		29	Georgia	15.4
37	New Jersey	12.3		29	Indiana	15.4
17	New Mexico	25.0		29	Kentucky	15.4
11	New York	29.5		32	South Carolina	15.3
26	North Carolina	17.8		33	Oklahoma	14.7
44	North Dakota	7.9		34	Virginia	14.1
15	Ohio	26.9		35	Arkansas	13.9
33	Oklahoma	14.7		36	Iowa	13.0
1	Oregon	42.0		37	New Jersey	12.3
3	Pennsylvania	38.9		38	Nebraska	11.8
6	Rhode Island	36.2		39	Maine	11.0
32	South Carolina	15.3		40	Kansas	10.9
45	South Dakota	7.5		41	Illinois	9.9
20	Tennessee	23.6		42	Mississippi	9.6
25	Texas	18.8		43	Maryland	8.0
9	Utah	32.2		44	North Dakota	7.9
49	Vermont	4.2		45	South Dakota	7.5
34	Virginia	14.1		46	New Hampshire	6.6
18	Washington	24.7		47	Wyoming	5.9
19	West Virginia	23.7		48	Delaware	4.9
14	Wisconsin	27.9		49	Vermont	4.2
47	Wyoming	5.9		50	Alaska	1.2

District of Columbia   10.5

Source: U.S. Department of Health and Human Services, Centers for Medicare and Medicaid Services
"Health Care Financing Review, 2010 Statistical Supplement" (http://cms.hhs.gov/MedicareMedicaidStatSupp)
*As of December 2009. National rate is a weighted average calculated by the editors. Includes Medicare Advantage and Employer Direct Plans. Regional Preferred Provider Organizations, Special Needs Plans, and employer only plans are also included.

Percent of Physicians Participating in Medicare in 2010

National Percent = 95.8% of Physicians Participate in Medicare*

ALPHA ORDER

RANK	STATE	PERCENT
11	Alabama	97.7
49	Alaska	91.2
44	Arizona	93.8
7	Arkansas	98.0
47	California	92.7
42	Colorado	94.2
30	Connecticut	96.6
3	Delaware	98.5
34	Florida	96.4
40	Georgia	95.3
32	Hawaii	96.5
48	Idaho	92.4
30	Illinois	96.6
20	Indiana	97.1
28	Iowa	96.7
9	Kansas	97.9
20	Kentucky	97.1
28	Louisiana	96.7
4	Maine	98.3
11	Maryland	97.7
2	Massachusetts	98.6
4	Michigan	98.3
50	Minnesota	81.6
35	Mississippi	96.1
36	Missouri	95.9
39	Montana	95.4
15	Nebraska	97.3
15	Nevada	97.3
26	New Hampshire	97.0
44	New Jersey	93.8
32	New Mexico	96.5
38	New York	95.5
20	North Carolina	97.1
13	North Dakota	97.5
14	Ohio	97.4
26	Oklahoma	97.0
37	Oregon	95.7
6	Pennsylvania	98.2
1	Rhode Island	98.7
20	South Carolina	97.1
42	South Dakota	94.2
17	Tennessee	97.2
40	Texas	95.3
7	Utah	98.0
20	Vermont	97.1
17	Virginia	97.2
17	Washington	97.2
10	West Virginia	97.8
20	Wisconsin	97.1
46	Wyoming	93.5

RANK ORDER

RANK	STATE	PERCENT
1	Rhode Island	98.7
2	Massachusetts	98.6
3	Delaware	98.5
4	Maine	98.3
4	Michigan	98.3
6	Pennsylvania	98.2
7	Arkansas	98.0
7	Utah	98.0
9	Kansas	97.9
10	West Virginia	97.8
11	Alabama	97.7
11	Maryland	97.7
13	North Dakota	97.5
14	Ohio	97.4
15	Nebraska	97.3
15	Nevada	97.3
17	Tennessee	97.2
17	Virginia	97.2
17	Washington	97.2
20	Indiana	97.1
20	Kentucky	97.1
20	North Carolina	97.1
20	South Carolina	97.1
20	Vermont	97.1
20	Wisconsin	97.1
26	New Hampshire	97.0
26	Oklahoma	97.0
28	Iowa	96.7
28	Louisiana	96.7
30	Connecticut	96.6
30	Illinois	96.6
32	Hawaii	96.5
32	New Mexico	96.5
34	Florida	96.4
35	Mississippi	96.1
36	Missouri	95.9
37	Oregon	95.7
38	New York	95.5
39	Montana	95.4
40	Georgia	95.3
40	Texas	95.3
42	Colorado	94.2
42	South Dakota	94.2
44	Arizona	93.8
44	New Jersey	93.8
46	Wyoming	93.5
47	California	92.7
48	Idaho	92.4
49	Alaska	91.2
50	Minnesota	81.6

District of Columbia	95.7

Source: U.S. Department of Health and Human Services, Centers for Medicare and Medicaid Services
  "2010 Data Compendium" (http://www.cms.hhs.gov/DataCompendium/)
*As of January 2010. Refers to Medicare Part B. Physicians include MDs, DOs, limited license practitioners, and non-physician practitioners.

Enrollees in Medicare Prescription Drug Program in 2010

National Total = 27,972,325 Enrollees*

ALPHA ORDER

RANK	STATE	ENROLLEES	% of USA
22	Alabama	475,770	1.7%
50	Alaska	24,751	0.1%
19	Arizona	525,439	1.9%
30	Arkansas	319,594	1.1%
1	California	3,255,498	11.6%
26	Colorado	358,393	1.3%
32	Connecticut	311,030	1.1%
46	Delaware	74,434	0.3%
2	Florida	1,999,398	7.1%
10	Georgia	741,648	2.7%
40	Hawaii	135,610	0.5%
41	Idaho	132,411	0.5%
7	Illinois	1,013,467	3.6%
16	Indiana	571,370	2.0%
29	Iowa	343,638	1.2%
33	Kansas	267,890	1.0%
21	Kentucky	477,746	1.7%
23	Louisiana	418,676	1.5%
38	Maine	164,779	0.6%
27	Maryland	354,822	1.3%
14	Massachusetts	606,749	2.2%
9	Michigan	780,985	2.8%
17	Minnesota	533,397	1.9%
31	Mississippi	318,802	1.1%
13	Missouri	620,024	2.2%
44	Montana	95,887	0.3%
37	Nebraska	178,990	0.6%
35	Nevada	193,503	0.7%
43	New Hampshire	102,866	0.4%
11	New Jersey	691,611	2.5%
36	New Mexico	190,905	0.7%
3	New York	1,769,195	6.3%
8	North Carolina	870,180	3.1%
47	North Dakota	74,389	0.3%
6	Ohio	1,036,335	3.7%
28	Oklahoma	354,527	1.3%
25	Oregon	395,623	1.4%
5	Pennsylvania	1,426,852	5.1%
42	Rhode Island	122,492	0.4%
24	South Carolina	413,396	1.5%
45	South Dakota	87,815	0.3%
12	Tennessee	672,260	2.4%
4	Texas	1,678,418	6.0%
39	Utah	157,046	0.6%
48	Vermont	61,683	0.2%
15	Virginia	592,018	2.1%
18	Washington	526,954	1.9%
34	West Virginia	231,194	0.8%
20	Wisconsin	487,879	1.7%
49	Wyoming	42,739	0.2%

RANK ORDER

RANK	STATE	ENROLLEES	% of USA
1	California	3,255,498	11.6%
2	Florida	1,999,398	7.1%
3	New York	1,769,195	6.3%
4	Texas	1,678,418	6.0%
5	Pennsylvania	1,426,852	5.1%
6	Ohio	1,036,335	3.7%
7	Illinois	1,013,467	3.6%
8	North Carolina	870,180	3.1%
9	Michigan	780,985	2.8%
10	Georgia	741,648	2.7%
11	New Jersey	691,611	2.5%
12	Tennessee	672,260	2.4%
13	Missouri	620,024	2.2%
14	Massachusetts	606,749	2.2%
15	Virginia	592,018	2.1%
16	Indiana	571,370	2.0%
17	Minnesota	533,397	1.9%
18	Washington	526,954	1.9%
19	Arizona	525,439	1.9%
20	Wisconsin	487,879	1.7%
21	Kentucky	477,746	1.7%
22	Alabama	475,770	1.7%
23	Louisiana	418,676	1.5%
24	South Carolina	413,396	1.5%
25	Oregon	395,623	1.4%
26	Colorado	358,393	1.3%
27	Maryland	354,822	1.3%
28	Oklahoma	354,527	1.3%
29	Iowa	343,638	1.2%
30	Arkansas	319,594	1.1%
31	Mississippi	318,802	1.1%
32	Connecticut	311,030	1.1%
33	Kansas	267,890	1.0%
34	West Virginia	231,194	0.8%
35	Nevada	193,503	0.7%
36	New Mexico	190,905	0.7%
37	Nebraska	178,990	0.6%
38	Maine	164,779	0.6%
39	Utah	157,046	0.6%
40	Hawaii	135,610	0.5%
41	Idaho	132,411	0.5%
42	Rhode Island	122,492	0.4%
43	New Hampshire	102,866	0.4%
44	Montana	95,887	0.3%
45	South Dakota	87,815	0.3%
46	Delaware	74,434	0.3%
47	North Dakota	74,389	0.3%
48	Vermont	61,683	0.2%
49	Wyoming	42,739	0.2%
50	Alaska	24,751	0.1%
	District of Columbia	37,153	0.1%

Source: U.S. Department of Health and Human Services, Centers for Medicare and Medicaid Services
"2010 Data Compendium" (http://www.cms.hhs.gov/DataCompendium/)
*Total includes 654,094 enrollees in U.S. territories.

Percent of Medicare Enrollees Participating in the Medicare Prescription Drug Program in 2010
National Percent = 58.7%*

ALPHA ORDER

RANK	STATE	PERCENT
32	Alabama	56.5
50	Alaska	37.6
20	Arizona	60.4
21	Arkansas	60.2
1	California	68.7
27	Colorado	57.9
38	Connecticut	54.8
46	Delaware	50.0
23	Florida	60.0
22	Georgia	60.1
6	Hawaii	65.7
27	Idaho	57.9
36	Illinois	55.1
30	Indiana	56.8
5	Iowa	66.5
15	Kansas	61.9
12	Kentucky	62.9
17	Louisiana	61.2
14	Maine	62.2
49	Maryland	45.2
29	Massachusetts	57.3
47	Michigan	47.2
3	Minnesota	68.0
7	Mississippi	64.3
15	Missouri	61.9
31	Montana	56.6
10	Nebraska	64.1
37	Nevada	54.9
47	New Hampshire	47.2
44	New Jersey	52.1
18	New Mexico	61.1
24	New York	59.2
26	North Carolina	58.6
2	North Dakota	68.5
39	Ohio	54.6
25	Oklahoma	58.9
7	Oregon	64.3
13	Pennsylvania	62.7
4	Rhode Island	67.1
41	South Carolina	53.7
7	South Dakota	64.3
11	Tennessee	63.8
33	Texas	56.1
34	Utah	55.7
35	Vermont	55.3
45	Virginia	51.9
40	Washington	54.5
19	West Virginia	60.6
41	Wisconsin	53.7
43	Wyoming	53.3

RANK ORDER

RANK	STATE	PERCENT
1	California	68.7
2	North Dakota	68.5
3	Minnesota	68.0
4	Rhode Island	67.1
5	Iowa	66.5
6	Hawaii	65.7
7	Mississippi	64.3
7	Oregon	64.3
7	South Dakota	64.3
10	Nebraska	64.1
11	Tennessee	63.8
12	Kentucky	62.9
13	Pennsylvania	62.7
14	Maine	62.2
15	Kansas	61.9
15	Missouri	61.9
17	Louisiana	61.2
18	New Mexico	61.1
19	West Virginia	60.6
20	Arizona	60.4
21	Arkansas	60.2
22	Georgia	60.1
23	Florida	60.0
24	New York	59.2
25	Oklahoma	58.9
26	North Carolina	58.6
27	Colorado	57.9
27	Idaho	57.9
29	Massachusetts	57.3
30	Indiana	56.8
31	Montana	56.6
32	Alabama	56.5
33	Texas	56.1
34	Utah	55.7
35	Vermont	55.3
36	Illinois	55.1
37	Nevada	54.9
38	Connecticut	54.8
39	Ohio	54.6
40	Washington	54.5
41	South Carolina	53.7
41	Wisconsin	53.7
43	Wyoming	53.3
44	New Jersey	52.1
45	Virginia	51.9
46	Delaware	50.0
47	Michigan	47.2
47	New Hampshire	47.2
49	Maryland	45.2
50	Alaska	37.6

District of Columbia	47.5

Source: U.S. Department of Health and Human Services, Centers for Medicare and Medicaid Services
   "2010 Data Compendium" (http://www.cms.hhs.gov/DataCompendium/)
*National figure includes enrollees in U.S. territories.

Medicare Program Payments in 2009

National Total = $316,915,000,000*

ALPHA ORDER

RANK	STATE	PAYMENTS	% of USA
18	Alabama	$5,471,000,000	1.7%
50	Alaska	477,000,000	0.2%
24	Arizona	4,751,000,000	1.5%
29	Arkansas	3,435,000,000	1.1%
1	California	28,389,000,000	9.0%
31	Colorado	3,214,000,000	1.0%
25	Connecticut	4,635,000,000	1.5%
41	Delaware	1,272,000,000	0.4%
2	Florida	25,292,000,000	8.0%
11	Georgia	8,484,000,000	2.7%
47	Hawaii	702,000,000	0.2%
42	Idaho	1,104,000,000	0.3%
5	Illinois	15,334,000,000	4.8%
15	Indiana	7,183,000,000	2.3%
30	Iowa	3,224,000,000	1.0%
32	Kansas	3,038,000,000	1.0%
19	Kentucky	5,380,000,000	1.7%
20	Louisiana	5,342,000,000	1.7%
37	Maine	1,689,000,000	0.5%
14	Maryland	7,336,000,000	2.3%
12	Massachusetts	8,441,000,000	2.7%
8	Michigan	12,180,000,000	3.8%
27	Minnesota	4,153,000,000	1.3%
28	Mississippi	4,150,000,000	1.3%
17	Missouri	6,743,000,000	2.1%
44	Montana	907,000,000	0.3%
36	Nebraska	1,954,000,000	0.6%
35	Nevada	2,083,000,000	0.7%
38	New Hampshire	1,586,000,000	0.5%
9	New Jersey	11,895,000,000	3.8%
39	New Mexico	1,543,000,000	0.5%
4	New York	20,896,000,000	6.6%
10	North Carolina	10,006,000,000	3.2%
48	North Dakota	652,000,000	0.2%
6	Ohio	12,651,000,000	4.0%
26	Oklahoma	4,446,000,000	1.4%
34	Oregon	2,315,000,000	0.7%
7	Pennsylvania	12,567,000,000	4.0%
43	Rhode Island	988,000,000	0.3%
21	South Carolina	5,330,000,000	1.7%
45	South Dakota	859,000,000	0.3%
16	Tennessee	6,892,000,000	2.2%
3	Texas	24,514,000,000	7.7%
40	Utah	1,370,000,000	0.4%
46	Vermont	772,000,000	0.2%
13	Virginia	7,414,000,000	2.3%
22	Washington	5,217,000,000	1.6%
33	West Virginia	2,382,000,000	0.8%
23	Wisconsin	5,002,000,000	1.6%
49	Wyoming	507,000,000	0.2%

RANK ORDER

RANK	STATE	PAYMENTS	% of USA
1	California	$28,389,000,000	9.0%
2	Florida	25,292,000,000	8.0%
3	Texas	24,514,000,000	7.7%
4	New York	20,896,000,000	6.6%
5	Illinois	15,334,000,000	4.8%
6	Ohio	12,651,000,000	4.0%
7	Pennsylvania	12,567,000,000	4.0%
8	Michigan	12,180,000,000	3.8%
9	New Jersey	11,895,000,000	3.8%
10	North Carolina	10,006,000,000	3.2%
11	Georgia	8,484,000,000	2.7%
12	Massachusetts	8,441,000,000	2.7%
13	Virginia	7,414,000,000	2.3%
14	Maryland	7,336,000,000	2.3%
15	Indiana	7,183,000,000	2.3%
16	Tennessee	6,892,000,000	2.2%
17	Missouri	6,743,000,000	2.1%
18	Alabama	5,471,000,000	1.7%
19	Kentucky	5,380,000,000	1.7%
20	Louisiana	5,342,000,000	1.7%
21	South Carolina	5,330,000,000	1.7%
22	Washington	5,217,000,000	1.6%
23	Wisconsin	5,002,000,000	1.6%
24	Arizona	4,751,000,000	1.5%
25	Connecticut	4,635,000,000	1.5%
26	Oklahoma	4,446,000,000	1.4%
27	Minnesota	4,153,000,000	1.3%
28	Mississippi	4,150,000,000	1.3%
29	Arkansas	3,435,000,000	1.1%
30	Iowa	3,224,000,000	1.0%
31	Colorado	3,214,000,000	1.0%
32	Kansas	3,038,000,000	1.0%
33	West Virginia	2,382,000,000	0.8%
34	Oregon	2,315,000,000	0.7%
35	Nevada	2,083,000,000	0.7%
36	Nebraska	1,954,000,000	0.6%
37	Maine	1,689,000,000	0.5%
38	New Hampshire	1,586,000,000	0.5%
39	New Mexico	1,543,000,000	0.5%
40	Utah	1,370,000,000	0.4%
41	Delaware	1,272,000,000	0.4%
42	Idaho	1,104,000,000	0.3%
43	Rhode Island	988,000,000	0.3%
44	Montana	907,000,000	0.3%
45	South Dakota	859,000,000	0.3%
46	Vermont	772,000,000	0.2%
47	Hawaii	702,000,000	0.2%
48	North Dakota	652,000,000	0.2%
49	Wyoming	507,000,000	0.2%
50	Alaska	477,000,000	0.2%
	District of Columbia	747,000,000	0.2%

Source: U.S. Department of Health and Human Services, Centers for Medicare and Medicaid Services
   "Health Care Financing Review, 2010 Statistical Supplement" (http://cms.hhs.gov/MedicareMedicaidStatSupp)
*Figures for calendar year 2009. Includes payments to aged and disabled enrollees. Total does not include payments to beneficiaries in Puerto Rico and other outlying areas.

Per Capita Medicare Program Payments in 2009

National Per Capita = $1,032*

ALPHA ORDER				RANK ORDER		
RANK	STATE	PER CAPITA		RANK	STATE	PER CAPITA
19	Alabama	$1,162		1	Delaware	$1,437
46	Alaska	683		2	Mississippi	1,406
44	Arizona	720		3	New Jersey	1,366
15	Arkansas	1,189		4	Florida	1,364
42	California	768		5	Connecticut	1,317
47	Colorado	640		6	West Virginia	1,309
5	Connecticut	1,317		7	Maryland	1,287
1	Delaware	1,437		8	Maine	1,281
4	Florida	1,364		9	Massachusetts	1,280
38	Georgia	863		10	Kentucky	1,247
49	Hawaii	542		11	Vermont	1,242
45	Idaho	714		12	Michigan	1,222
17	Illinois	1,188		13	Oklahoma	1,206
21	Indiana	1,118		14	New Hampshire	1,197
26	Iowa	1,072		15	Arkansas	1,189
25	Kansas	1,078		15	Louisiana	1,189
10	Kentucky	1,247		17	Illinois	1,188
15	Louisiana	1,189		18	South Carolina	1,169
8	Maine	1,281		19	Alabama	1,162
7	Maryland	1,287		20	Missouri	1,126
9	Massachusetts	1,280		21	Indiana	1,118
12	Michigan	1,222		22	Ohio	1,096
39	Minnesota	789		23	Tennessee	1,095
2	Mississippi	1,406		24	Nebraska	1,088
20	Missouri	1,126		25	Kansas	1,078
36	Montana	930		26	Iowa	1,072
24	Nebraska	1,088		27	New York	1,069
40	Nevada	788		28	North Carolina	1,067
14	New Hampshire	1,197		29	South Dakota	1,057
3	New Jersey	1,366		30	North Dakota	1,008
42	New Mexico	768		31	Pennsylvania	997
27	New York	1,069		32	Texas	989
28	North Carolina	1,067		33	Virginia	941
30	North Dakota	1,008		34	Rhode Island	938
22	Ohio	1,096		35	Wyoming	932
13	Oklahoma	1,206		36	Montana	930
48	Oregon	605		37	Wisconsin	885
31	Pennsylvania	997		38	Georgia	863
34	Rhode Island	938		39	Minnesota	789
18	South Carolina	1,169		40	Nevada	788
29	South Dakota	1,057		41	Washington	783
23	Tennessee	1,095		42	California	768
32	Texas	989		42	New Mexico	768
50	Utah	492		44	Arizona	720
11	Vermont	1,242		45	Idaho	714
33	Virginia	941		46	Alaska	683
41	Washington	783		47	Colorado	640
6	West Virginia	1,309		48	Oregon	605
37	Wisconsin	885		49	Hawaii	542
35	Wyoming	932		50	Utah	492
					District of Columbia	1,246

Source: CQ Press using data from U.S. Department of Health and Human Services, Centers for Medicare and Medicaid Services
"Health Care Financing Review, 2010 Statistical Supplement" (http://cms.hhs.gov/MedicareMedicaidStatSupp)
*Figures for calendar year 2009. Includes payments to aged and disabled enrollees. National rate does not include payments or enrollees in Puerto Rico and other outlying areas.

Medicare Program Payments per Enrollee in 2009

National Rate = $9,121*

ALPHA ORDER				RANK ORDER		
RANK	STATE	PER ENROLLEE		RANK	STATE	PER ENROLLEE
24	Alabama	$8,496		1	Florida	$10,894
36	Alaska	7,744		2	Texas	10,413
27	Arizona	8,405		3	Louisiana	10,338
34	Arkansas	7,847		4	New Jersey	10,327
11	California	9,411		5	Maryland	10,322
31	Colorado	7,998		6	Michigan	10,085
9	Connecticut	9,968		7	New York	10,014
14	Delaware	9,139		8	Massachusetts	9,988
1	Florida	10,894		9	Connecticut	9,968
28	Georgia	8,320		10	Mississippi	9,479
50	Hawaii	5,802		11	California	9,411
43	Idaho	6,929		12	Illinois	9,367
12	Illinois	9,367		13	Ohio	9,202
17	Indiana	8,650		14	Delaware	9,139
42	Iowa	7,257		15	Pennsylvania	9,036
30	Kansas	8,071		16	Oklahoma	8,826
23	Kentucky	8,517		17	Indiana	8,650
3	Louisiana	10,338		17	Rhode Island	8,650
41	Maine	7,264		19	Minnesota	8,647
5	Maryland	10,322		20	Tennessee	8,642
8	Massachusetts	9,988		21	Nevada	8,619
6	Michigan	10,085		22	Missouri	8,528
19	Minnesota	8,647		23	Kentucky	8,517
10	Mississippi	9,479		24	Alabama	8,496
22	Missouri	8,528		25	South Carolina	8,453
47	Montana	6,576		26	North Carolina	8,433
33	Nebraska	7,906		27	Arizona	8,405
21	Nevada	8,619		28	Georgia	8,320
32	New Hampshire	7,951		29	West Virginia	8,200
4	New Jersey	10,327		30	Kansas	8,071
45	New Mexico	6,782		31	Colorado	7,998
7	New York	10,014		32	New Hampshire	7,951
26	North Carolina	8,433		33	Nebraska	7,906
49	North Dakota	6,453		34	Arkansas	7,847
13	Ohio	9,202		35	Wisconsin	7,815
16	Oklahoma	8,826		36	Alaska	7,744
48	Oregon	6,561		36	Virginia	7,744
15	Pennsylvania	9,036		38	Washington	7,376
17	Rhode Island	8,650		39	Utah	7,352
25	South Carolina	8,453		40	Vermont	7,338
44	South Dakota	6,927		41	Maine	7,264
20	Tennessee	8,642		42	Iowa	7,257
2	Texas	10,413		43	Idaho	6,929
39	Utah	7,352		44	South Dakota	6,927
40	Vermont	7,338		45	New Mexico	6,782
36	Virginia	7,744		46	Wyoming	6,774
38	Washington	7,376		47	Montana	6,576
29	West Virginia	8,200		48	Oregon	6,561
35	Wisconsin	7,815		49	North Dakota	6,453
46	Wyoming	6,774		50	Hawaii	5,802
					District of Columbia	10,910

Source: U.S. Department of Health and Human Services, Centers for Medicare and Medicaid Services
   "Health Care Financing Review, 2010 Statistical Supplement" (http://cms.hhs.gov/MedicareMedicaidStatSupp)
*Figures for calendar year 2009. Includes payments to aged and disabled enrollees. National figure does not include enrollees in managed care plans in the denominator used to calculate average payments. National rate also does not include payments or enrollees in Puerto Rico and other outlying areas.

Medicaid Enrollment in 2009

National Total = 52,355,471 Enrollees*

ALPHA ORDER

RANK	STATE	ENROLLEES	% of USA
22	Alabama	825,655	1.6%
47	Alaska	107,440	0.2%
11	Arizona	1,312,189	2.5%
28	Arkansas	655,766	1.3%
1	California	7,131,538	13.6%
31	Colorado	494,699	0.9%
32	Connecticut	474,288	0.9%
43	Delaware	173,846	0.3%
4	Florida	2,589,982	4.9%
10	Georgia	1,443,271	2.8%
37	Hawaii	248,984	0.5%
41	Idaho	206,846	0.4%
5	Illinois	2,344,100	4.5%
17	Indiana	1,041,295	2.0%
33	Iowa	414,201	0.8%
35	Kansas	291,720	0.6%
23	Kentucky	789,371	1.5%
14	Louisiana	1,147,955	2.2%
36	Maine	279,439	0.5%
21	Maryland	830,172	1.6%
12	Massachusetts	1,227,224	2.3%
8	Michigan	1,732,487	3.3%
26	Minnesota	682,193	1.3%
25	Mississippi	692,296	1.3%
19	Missouri	900,302	1.7%
48	Montana	90,392	0.2%
40	Nebraska	225,523	0.4%
39	Nevada	230,067	0.4%
45	New Hampshire	128,858	0.2%
18	New Jersey	1,006,067	1.9%
30	New Mexico	497,782	1.0%
2	New York	4,557,053	8.7%
9	North Carolina	1,537,651	2.9%
50	North Dakota	63,752	0.1%
6	Ohio	2,028,863	3.9%
27	Oklahoma	656,221	1.3%
29	Oregon	513,079	1.0%
7	Pennsylvania	1,976,439	3.8%
42	Rhode Island	181,572	0.3%
24	South Carolina	776,610	1.5%
46	South Dakota	115,597	0.2%
13	Tennessee	1,184,092	2.3%
3	Texas	3,513,243	6.7%
38	Utah	247,040	0.5%
44	Vermont	155,283	0.3%
20	Virginia	854,858	1.6%
16	Washington	1,074,361	2.1%
34	West Virginia	330,565	0.6%
15	Wisconsin	1,102,516	2.1%
49	Wyoming	67,366	0.1%

RANK ORDER

RANK	STATE	ENROLLEES	% of USA
1	California	7,131,538	13.6%
2	New York	4,557,053	8.7%
3	Texas	3,513,243	6.7%
4	Florida	2,589,982	4.9%
5	Illinois	2,344,100	4.5%
6	Ohio	2,028,863	3.9%
7	Pennsylvania	1,976,439	3.8%
8	Michigan	1,732,487	3.3%
9	North Carolina	1,537,651	2.9%
10	Georgia	1,443,271	2.8%
11	Arizona	1,312,189	2.5%
12	Massachusetts	1,227,224	2.3%
13	Tennessee	1,184,092	2.3%
14	Louisiana	1,147,955	2.2%
15	Wisconsin	1,102,516	2.1%
16	Washington	1,074,361	2.1%
17	Indiana	1,041,295	2.0%
18	New Jersey	1,006,067	1.9%
19	Missouri	900,302	1.7%
20	Virginia	854,858	1.6%
21	Maryland	830,172	1.6%
22	Alabama	825,655	1.6%
23	Kentucky	789,371	1.5%
24	South Carolina	776,610	1.5%
25	Mississippi	692,296	1.3%
26	Minnesota	682,193	1.3%
27	Oklahoma	656,221	1.3%
28	Arkansas	655,766	1.3%
29	Oregon	513,079	1.0%
30	New Mexico	497,782	1.0%
31	Colorado	494,699	0.9%
32	Connecticut	474,288	0.9%
33	Iowa	414,201	0.8%
34	West Virginia	330,565	0.6%
35	Kansas	291,720	0.6%
36	Maine	279,439	0.5%
37	Hawaii	248,984	0.5%
38	Utah	247,040	0.5%
39	Nevada	230,067	0.4%
40	Nebraska	225,523	0.4%
41	Idaho	206,846	0.4%
42	Rhode Island	181,572	0.3%
43	Delaware	173,846	0.3%
44	Vermont	155,283	0.3%
45	New Hampshire	128,858	0.2%
46	South Dakota	115,597	0.2%
47	Alaska	107,440	0.2%
48	Montana	90,392	0.2%
49	Wyoming	67,366	0.1%
50	North Dakota	63,752	0.1%
	District of Columbia	161,041	0.3%

Source: U.S. Department of Health and Human Services, Centers for Medicare and Medicaid Services
    "2009 Medicaid Managed Care Enrollment Report" (http://www.cms.hhs.gov/MedicaidDataSourcesGenInfo/)
*Unduplicated enrollment as of December 31, 2009. National total includes 1,042,150 Medicaid enrollees in Puerto Rico and the Virgin Islands.

Percent of Population Enrolled in Medicaid in 2009

National Percent = 16.7% of Population*

ALPHA ORDER

RANK	STATE	PERCENT
20	Alabama	17.5
28	Alaska	15.4
8	Arizona	19.9
6	Arkansas	22.7
11	California	19.3
46	Colorado	9.8
36	Connecticut	13.5
9	Delaware	19.6
34	Florida	14.0
30	Georgia	14.7
12	Hawaii	19.2
37	Idaho	13.4
16	Illinois	18.2
25	Indiana	16.2
35	Iowa	13.8
44	Kansas	10.3
15	Kentucky	18.3
1	Louisiana	25.6
7	Maine	21.2
31	Maryland	14.6
14	Massachusetts	18.6
21	Michigan	17.4
39	Minnesota	13.0
4	Mississippi	23.5
29	Missouri	15.0
48	Montana	9.3
40	Nebraska	12.6
50	Nevada	8.7
47	New Hampshire	9.7
42	New Jersey	11.6
3	New Mexico	24.8
5	New York	23.3
24	North Carolina	16.4
45	North Dakota	9.9
19	Ohio	17.6
18	Oklahoma	17.8
37	Oregon	13.4
27	Pennsylvania	15.7
22	Rhode Island	17.2
23	South Carolina	17.0
32	South Dakota	14.2
13	Tennessee	18.8
32	Texas	14.2
49	Utah	8.9
2	Vermont	25.0
43	Virginia	10.8
26	Washington	16.1
16	West Virginia	18.2
10	Wisconsin	19.5
41	Wyoming	12.4

RANK ORDER

RANK	STATE	PERCENT
1	Louisiana	25.6
2	Vermont	25.0
3	New Mexico	24.8
4	Mississippi	23.5
5	New York	23.3
6	Arkansas	22.7
7	Maine	21.2
8	Arizona	19.9
9	Delaware	19.6
10	Wisconsin	19.5
11	California	19.3
12	Hawaii	19.2
13	Tennessee	18.8
14	Massachusetts	18.6
15	Kentucky	18.3
16	Illinois	18.2
16	West Virginia	18.2
18	Oklahoma	17.8
19	Ohio	17.6
20	Alabama	17.5
21	Michigan	17.4
22	Rhode Island	17.2
23	South Carolina	17.0
24	North Carolina	16.4
25	Indiana	16.2
26	Washington	16.1
27	Pennsylvania	15.7
28	Alaska	15.4
29	Missouri	15.0
30	Georgia	14.7
31	Maryland	14.6
32	South Dakota	14.2
32	Texas	14.2
34	Florida	14.0
35	Iowa	13.8
36	Connecticut	13.5
37	Idaho	13.4
37	Oregon	13.4
39	Minnesota	13.0
40	Nebraska	12.6
41	Wyoming	12.4
42	New Jersey	11.6
43	Virginia	10.8
44	Kansas	10.3
45	North Dakota	9.9
46	Colorado	9.8
47	New Hampshire	9.7
48	Montana	9.3
49	Utah	8.9
50	Nevada	8.7

District of Columbia 26.9

Source: CQ Press using data from U.S. Department of Health and Human Services, Centers for Medicare and Medicaid Services "2009 Medicaid Managed Care Enrollment Report" (http://www.cms.hhs.gov/MedicaidDataSourcesGenInfo/)
*Unduplicated enrollment as of December 31, 2009. National percent does not include recipients or population in U.S. territories.

Medicaid Managed Care Enrollment in 2009

National Total = 38,170,114 Enrollees*

ALPHA ORDER					RANK ORDER			
RANK	STATE	ENROLLEES	% of USA		RANK	STATE	ENROLLEES	% of USA
24	Alabama	577,070	1.5%		1	California	3,846,902	10.1%
48	Alaska	0	0.0%		2	New York	3,101,548	8.1%
10	Arizona	1,185,016	3.1%		3	Texas	2,305,082	6.0%
27	Arkansas	521,717	1.4%		4	Florida	1,773,637	4.6%
1	California	3,846,902	10.1%		5	Pennsylvania	1,633,390	4.3%
28	Colorado	471,648	1.2%		6	Michigan	1,527,952	4.0%
32	Connecticut	357,264	0.9%		7	Ohio	1,484,354	3.9%
43	Delaware	132,642	0.3%		8	Illinois	1,319,700	3.5%
4	Florida	1,773,637	4.6%		9	Georgia	1,286,812	3.4%
9	Georgia	1,286,812	3.4%		10	Arizona	1,185,016	3.1%
35	Hawaii	245,863	0.6%		11	Tennessee	1,184,092	3.1%
39	Idaho	178,267	0.5%		12	North Carolina	1,161,772	3.0%
8	Illinois	1,319,700	3.5%		13	Washington	997,980	2.6%
17	Indiana	772,781	2.0%		14	Missouri	896,189	2.3%
33	Iowa	345,141	0.9%		15	Massachusetts	790,625	2.1%
34	Kansas	265,463	0.7%		16	South Carolina	776,610	2.0%
20	Kentucky	694,251	1.8%		17	Indiana	772,781	2.0%
19	Louisiana	744,142	1.9%		18	New Jersey	766,674	2.0%
40	Maine	177,654	0.5%		19	Louisiana	744,142	1.9%
21	Maryland	670,812	1.8%		20	Kentucky	694,251	1.8%
15	Massachusetts	790,625	2.1%		21	Maryland	670,812	1.8%
6	Michigan	1,527,952	4.0%		22	Wisconsin	666,208	1.7%
30	Minnesota	443,301	1.2%		23	Oklahoma	587,530	1.5%
26	Mississippi	532,941	1.4%		24	Alabama	577,070	1.5%
14	Missouri	896,189	2.3%		25	Virginia	559,398	1.5%
46	Montana	56,239	0.1%		26	Mississippi	532,941	1.4%
38	Nebraska	194,135	0.5%		27	Arkansas	521,717	1.4%
37	Nevada	200,481	0.5%		28	Colorado	471,648	1.2%
48	New Hampshire	0	0.0%		29	Oregon	448,580	1.2%
18	New Jersey	766,674	2.0%		30	Minnesota	443,301	1.2%
31	New Mexico	358,773	0.9%		31	New Mexico	358,773	0.9%
2	New York	3,101,548	8.1%		32	Connecticut	357,264	0.9%
12	North Carolina	1,161,772	3.0%		33	Iowa	345,141	0.9%
47	North Dakota	40,961	0.1%		34	Kansas	265,463	0.7%
7	Ohio	1,484,354	3.9%		35	Hawaii	245,863	0.6%
23	Oklahoma	587,530	1.5%		36	Utah	213,195	0.6%
29	Oregon	448,580	1.2%		37	Nevada	200,481	0.5%
5	Pennsylvania	1,633,390	4.3%		38	Nebraska	194,135	0.5%
44	Rhode Island	115,326	0.3%		39	Idaho	178,267	0.5%
16	South Carolina	776,610	2.0%		40	Maine	177,654	0.5%
45	South Dakota	87,267	0.2%		41	West Virginia	161,690	0.4%
11	Tennessee	1,184,092	3.1%		42	Vermont	151,334	0.4%
3	Texas	2,305,082	6.0%		43	Delaware	132,642	0.3%
36	Utah	213,195	0.6%		44	Rhode Island	115,326	0.3%
42	Vermont	151,334	0.4%		45	South Dakota	87,267	0.2%
25	Virginia	559,398	1.5%		46	Montana	56,239	0.1%
13	Washington	997,980	2.6%		47	North Dakota	40,961	0.1%
41	West Virginia	161,690	0.4%		48	Alaska	0	0.0%
22	Wisconsin	666,208	1.7%		48	New Hampshire	0	0.0%
48	Wyoming	0	0.0%		48	Wyoming	0	0.0%
						District of Columbia	157,011	0.4%

Source: U.S. Department of Health and Human Services, Centers for Medicare and Medicaid Services
 "2009 Medicaid Managed Care Enrollment Report" (http://www.cms.hhs.gov/MedicaidDataSourcesGenInfo/)
*Unduplicated enrollment as of December 31, 2009. Enrollment in state health care reform programs that expand eligibility beyond
traditional Medicaid standards. National total includes 1,002,694 Medicaid managed care enrollees in Puerto Rico.

Percent of Medicaid Enrollees in Managed Care in 2009

National Percent = 72.9% of Medicaid Enrollees*

ALPHA ORDER

RANK	STATE	PERCENT
32	Alabama	69.9
48	Alaska	0.0
9	Arizona	90.3
22	Arkansas	79.6
46	California	53.9
6	Colorado	95.3
28	Connecticut	75.3
24	Delaware	76.3
33	Florida	68.5
11	Georgia	89.2
4	Hawaii	98.8
17	Idaho	86.2
45	Illinois	56.3
29	Indiana	74.2
19	Iowa	83.3
8	Kansas	91.0
13	Kentucky	88.0
38	Louisiana	64.8
41	Maine	63.6
21	Maryland	80.8
39	Massachusetts	64.4
12	Michigan	88.2
37	Minnesota	65.0
23	Mississippi	77.0
3	Missouri	99.5
43	Montana	62.2
18	Nebraska	86.1
15	Nevada	87.1
48	New Hampshire	0.0
25	New Jersey	76.2
31	New Mexico	72.1
34	New York	68.1
26	North Carolina	75.6
40	North Dakota	64.3
30	Ohio	73.2
10	Oklahoma	89.5
14	Oregon	87.4
20	Pennsylvania	82.6
42	Rhode Island	63.5
1	South Carolina	100.0
27	South Dakota	75.5
1	Tennessee	100.0
35	Texas	65.6
16	Utah	86.3
5	Vermont	97.5
36	Virginia	65.4
7	Washington	92.9
47	West Virginia	48.9
44	Wisconsin	60.4
48	Wyoming	0.0

RANK ORDER

RANK	STATE	PERCENT
1	South Carolina	100.0
1	Tennessee	100.0
3	Missouri	99.5
4	Hawaii	98.8
5	Vermont	97.5
6	Colorado	95.3
7	Washington	92.9
8	Kansas	91.0
9	Arizona	90.3
10	Oklahoma	89.5
11	Georgia	89.2
12	Michigan	88.2
13	Kentucky	88.0
14	Oregon	87.4
15	Nevada	87.1
16	Utah	86.3
17	Idaho	86.2
18	Nebraska	86.1
19	Iowa	83.3
20	Pennsylvania	82.6
21	Maryland	80.8
22	Arkansas	79.6
23	Mississippi	77.0
24	Delaware	76.3
25	New Jersey	76.2
26	North Carolina	75.6
27	South Dakota	75.5
28	Connecticut	75.3
29	Indiana	74.2
30	Ohio	73.2
31	New Mexico	72.1
32	Alabama	69.9
33	Florida	68.5
34	New York	68.1
35	Texas	65.6
36	Virginia	65.4
37	Minnesota	65.0
38	Louisiana	64.8
39	Massachusetts	64.4
40	North Dakota	64.3
41	Maine	63.6
42	Rhode Island	63.5
43	Montana	62.2
44	Wisconsin	60.4
45	Illinois	56.3
46	California	53.9
47	West Virginia	48.9
48	Alaska	0.0
48	New Hampshire	0.0
48	Wyoming	0.0
	District of Columbia	97.5

Source: U.S. Department of Health and Human Services, Centers for Medicare and Medicaid Services
    "2009 Medicaid Managed Care Enrollment Report" (http://www.cms.hhs.gov/MedicaidDataSourcesGenInfo/)
*Unduplicated enrollment as of December 31, 2009. Enrollment in state health care reform programs that expand eligibility beyond traditional Medicaid standards. National percent includes Medicaid enrollees in Puerto Rico and the Virgin Islands.

Estimated Medicaid Expenditures in 2010

National Total = $353,837,000,000*

ALPHA ORDER				RANK ORDER			
RANK	STATE	EXPENDITURES	% of USA	RANK	STATE	EXPENDITURES	% of USA
26	Alabama	$4,857,000,000	1.4%	1	California	$48,326,000,000	13.7%
46	Alaska	1,120,000,000	0.3%	2	New York	37,025,000,000	10.5%
14	Arizona	7,663,000,000	2.2%	3	Pennsylvania	19,427,000,000	5.5%
30	Arkansas	4,161,000,000	1.2%	4	Florida	18,810,000,000	5.3%
1	California	48,326,000,000	13.7%	5	Illinois	15,551,000,000	4.4%
27	Colorado	4,770,000,000	1.3%	6	Ohio	12,654,000,000	3.6%
25	Connecticut	4,980,000,000	1.4%	7	North Carolina	11,796,000,000	3.3%
44	Delaware	1,258,000,000	0.4%	8	Michigan	11,529,000,000	3.3%
4	Florida	18,810,000,000	5.3%	9	New Jersey	10,254,000,000	2.9%
13	Georgia	7,674,000,000	2.2%	10	Massachusetts	9,465,000,000	2.7%
41	Hawaii	1,456,000,000	0.4%	11	Missouri	8,071,000,000	2.3%
40	Idaho	1,506,000,000	0.4%	12	Tennessee	7,684,000,000	2.2%
5	Illinois	15,551,000,000	4.4%	13	Georgia	7,674,000,000	2.2%
22	Indiana	6,172,000,000	1.7%	14	Arizona	7,663,000,000	2.2%
32	Iowa	3,370,000,000	1.0%	15	Washington	7,440,000,000	2.1%
35	Kansas	2,509,000,000	0.7%	16	Texas	7,322,000,000	2.1%
23	Kentucky	5,693,000,000	1.6%	17	Minnesota	6,774,000,000	1.9%
19	Louisiana	6,626,000,000	1.9%	18	Maryland	6,661,000,000	1.9%
36	Maine	2,395,000,000	0.7%	19	Louisiana	6,626,000,000	1.9%
18	Maryland	6,661,000,000	1.9%	20	Wisconsin	6,586,000,000	1.9%
10	Massachusetts	9,465,000,000	2.7%	21	Virginia	6,554,000,000	1.9%
8	Michigan	11,529,000,000	3.3%	22	Indiana	6,172,000,000	1.7%
17	Minnesota	6,774,000,000	1.9%	23	Kentucky	5,693,000,000	1.6%
28	Mississippi	4,255,000,000	1.2%	24	South Carolina	5,005,000,000	1.4%
11	Missouri	8,071,000,000	2.3%	25	Connecticut	4,980,000,000	1.4%
47	Montana	930,000,000	0.3%	26	Alabama	4,857,000,000	1.4%
39	Nebraska	1,649,000,000	0.5%	27	Colorado	4,770,000,000	1.3%
43	Nevada	1,364,000,000	0.4%	28	Mississippi	4,255,000,000	1.2%
42	New Hampshire	1,374,000,000	0.4%	29	Oklahoma	4,203,000,000	1.2%
9	New Jersey	10,254,000,000	2.9%	30	Arkansas	4,161,000,000	1.2%
33	New Mexico	3,363,000,000	1.0%	31	Oregon	3,948,000,000	1.1%
2	New York	37,025,000,000	10.5%	32	Iowa	3,370,000,000	1.0%
7	North Carolina	11,796,000,000	3.3%	33	New Mexico	3,363,000,000	1.0%
49	North Dakota	665,000,000	0.2%	34	West Virginia	2,551,000,000	0.7%
6	Ohio	12,654,000,000	3.6%	35	Kansas	2,509,000,000	0.7%
29	Oklahoma	4,203,000,000	1.2%	36	Maine	2,395,000,000	0.7%
31	Oregon	3,948,000,000	1.1%	37	Rhode Island	1,958,000,000	0.6%
3	Pennsylvania	19,427,000,000	5.5%	38	Utah	1,811,000,000	0.5%
37	Rhode Island	1,958,000,000	0.6%	39	Nebraska	1,649,000,000	0.5%
24	South Carolina	5,005,000,000	1.4%	40	Idaho	1,506,000,000	0.4%
48	South Dakota	850,000,000	0.2%	41	Hawaii	1,456,000,000	0.4%
12	Tennessee	7,684,000,000	2.2%	42	New Hampshire	1,374,000,000	0.4%
16	Texas	7,322,000,000	2.1%	43	Nevada	1,364,000,000	0.4%
38	Utah	1,811,000,000	0.5%	44	Delaware	1,258,000,000	0.4%
45	Vermont	1,213,000,000	0.3%	45	Vermont	1,213,000,000	0.3%
21	Virginia	6,554,000,000	1.9%	46	Alaska	1,120,000,000	0.3%
15	Washington	7,440,000,000	2.1%	47	Montana	930,000,000	0.3%
34	West Virginia	2,551,000,000	0.7%	48	South Dakota	850,000,000	0.2%
20	Wisconsin	6,586,000,000	1.9%	49	North Dakota	665,000,000	0.2%
50	Wyoming	559,000,000	0.2%	50	Wyoming	559,000,000	0.2%
					District of Columbia**	NA	NA

Source: National Association of State Budget Officers
   "2009 State Expenditure Report" (http://www.nasbo.org)
*Estimates for fiscal year 2010.
**Not available.

Estimated Per Capita Medicaid Expenditures in 2010

National Per Capita = $1,153*

ALPHA ORDER				RANK ORDER		
RANK	STATE	PER CAPITA		RANK	STATE	PER CAPITA
36	Alabama	$1,031		1	Vermont	$1,951
6	Alaska	1,603		2	New York	1,895
25	Arizona	1,162		3	Rhode Island	1,859
10	Arkansas	1,440		4	Maine	1,817
17	California	1,307		5	New Mexico	1,673
43	Colorado	949		6	Alaska	1,603
13	Connecticut	1,415		7	Pennsylvania	1,541
12	Delaware	1,421		8	Louisiana	1,475
39	Florida	1,015		9	Mississippi	1,441
47	Georgia	781		10	Arkansas	1,440
28	Hawaii	1,124		11	Massachusetts	1,435
40	Idaho	974		12	Delaware	1,421
21	Illinois	1,205		13	Connecticut	1,415
41	Indiana	961		14	West Virginia	1,402
29	Iowa	1,120		15	Missouri	1,348
45	Kansas	890		16	Kentucky	1,320
16	Kentucky	1,320		17	California	1,307
8	Louisiana	1,475		18	Minnesota	1,286
4	Maine	1,817		19	North Carolina	1,257
23	Maryland	1,169		20	Tennessee	1,220
11	Massachusetts	1,435		21	Illinois	1,205
26	Michigan	1,156		22	New Jersey	1,178
18	Minnesota	1,286		23	Maryland	1,169
9	Mississippi	1,441		24	Wisconsin	1,165
15	Missouri	1,348		25	Arizona	1,162
42	Montana	954		26	Michigan	1,156
44	Nebraska	918		27	Oklahoma	1,140
49	Nevada	516		28	Hawaii	1,124
34	New Hampshire	1,037		29	Iowa	1,120
22	New Jersey	1,178		30	Washington	1,116
5	New Mexico	1,673		31	South Carolina	1,097
2	New York	1,895		32	Ohio	1,096
19	North Carolina	1,257		33	South Dakota	1,046
37	North Dakota	1,028		34	New Hampshire	1,037
32	Ohio	1,096		35	Oregon	1,032
27	Oklahoma	1,140		36	Alabama	1,031
35	Oregon	1,032		37	North Dakota	1,028
7	Pennsylvania	1,541		38	Wyoming	1,027
3	Rhode Island	1,859		39	Florida	1,015
31	South Carolina	1,097		40	Idaho	974
33	South Dakota	1,046		41	Indiana	961
20	Tennessee	1,220		42	Montana	954
50	Texas	295		43	Colorado	949
48	Utah	650		44	Nebraska	918
1	Vermont	1,951		45	Kansas	890
46	Virginia	831		46	Virginia	831
30	Washington	1,116		47	Georgia	781
14	West Virginia	1,402		48	Utah	650
24	Wisconsin	1,165		49	Nevada	516
38	Wyoming	1,027		50	Texas	295
					District of Columbia**	NA

Source: CQ Press using data from National Association of State Budget Officers
   "2009 State Expenditure Report" (http://www.nasbo.org)
*Estimates for fiscal year 2010. Calculated using 2009 Census population estimates.
**Not available.

Estimated Medicaid Expenditures as a Percent of Total Expenditures in 2010

National Percent = 21.8%*

<table>
<tr><td colspan="3">ALPHA ORDER</td><td colspan="3">RANK ORDER</td></tr>
<tr><th>RANK</th><th>STATE</th><th>PERCENT</th><th>RANK</th><th>STATE</th><th>PERCENT</th></tr>
<tr><td>28</td><td>Alabama</td><td>19.9</td><td>1</td><td>North Carolina</td><td>37.1</td></tr>
<tr><td>48</td><td>Alaska</td><td>11.5</td><td>2</td><td>Illinois</td><td>32.8</td></tr>
<tr><td>7</td><td>Arizona</td><td>27.9</td><td>3</td><td>Missouri</td><td>32.5</td></tr>
<tr><td>27</td><td>Arkansas</td><td>20.5</td><td>4</td><td>Maine</td><td>29.0</td></tr>
<tr><td>18</td><td>California</td><td>22.2</td><td>5</td><td>Florida</td><td>28.3</td></tr>
<tr><td>38</td><td>Colorado</td><td>16.4</td><td>5</td><td>New York</td><td>28.3</td></tr>
<tr><td>32</td><td>Connecticut</td><td>19.1</td><td>7</td><td>Arizona</td><td>27.9</td></tr>
<tr><td>42</td><td>Delaware</td><td>14.4</td><td>8</td><td>Pennsylvania</td><td>27.6</td></tr>
<tr><td>5</td><td>Florida</td><td>28.3</td><td>9</td><td>Tennessee</td><td>26.4</td></tr>
<tr><td>28</td><td>Georgia</td><td>19.9</td><td>10</td><td>Michigan</td><td>25.2</td></tr>
<tr><td>46</td><td>Hawaii</td><td>13.3</td><td>11</td><td>New Hampshire</td><td>25.1</td></tr>
<tr><td>24</td><td>Idaho</td><td>21.1</td><td>12</td><td>Rhode Island</td><td>24.0</td></tr>
<tr><td>2</td><td>Illinois</td><td>32.8</td><td>13</td><td>New Mexico</td><td>23.4</td></tr>
<tr><td>14</td><td>Indiana</td><td>23.1</td><td>14</td><td>Indiana</td><td>23.1</td></tr>
<tr><td>33</td><td>Iowa</td><td>18.2</td><td>15</td><td>Washington</td><td>22.9</td></tr>
<tr><td>35</td><td>Kansas</td><td>17.3</td><td>16</td><td>South Dakota</td><td>22.6</td></tr>
<tr><td>20</td><td>Kentucky</td><td>22.0</td><td>17</td><td>Louisiana</td><td>22.4</td></tr>
<tr><td>17</td><td>Louisiana</td><td>22.4</td><td>18</td><td>California</td><td>22.2</td></tr>
<tr><td>4</td><td>Maine</td><td>29.0</td><td>18</td><td>South Carolina</td><td>22.2</td></tr>
<tr><td>28</td><td>Maryland</td><td>19.9</td><td>20</td><td>Kentucky</td><td>22.0</td></tr>
<tr><td>34</td><td>Massachusetts</td><td>17.7</td><td>20</td><td>Mississippi</td><td>22.0</td></tr>
<tr><td>10</td><td>Michigan</td><td>25.2</td><td>20</td><td>Ohio</td><td>22.0</td></tr>
<tr><td>23</td><td>Minnesota</td><td>21.5</td><td>23</td><td>Minnesota</td><td>21.5</td></tr>
<tr><td>20</td><td>Mississippi</td><td>22.0</td><td>24</td><td>Idaho</td><td>21.1</td></tr>
<tr><td>3</td><td>Missouri</td><td>32.5</td><td>25</td><td>New Jersey</td><td>20.9</td></tr>
<tr><td>41</td><td>Montana</td><td>15.4</td><td>26</td><td>Vermont</td><td>20.8</td></tr>
<tr><td>37</td><td>Nebraska</td><td>17.2</td><td>27</td><td>Arkansas</td><td>20.5</td></tr>
<tr><td>35</td><td>Nevada</td><td>17.3</td><td>28</td><td>Alabama</td><td>19.9</td></tr>
<tr><td>11</td><td>New Hampshire</td><td>25.1</td><td>28</td><td>Georgia</td><td>19.9</td></tr>
<tr><td>25</td><td>New Jersey</td><td>20.9</td><td>28</td><td>Maryland</td><td>19.9</td></tr>
<tr><td>13</td><td>New Mexico</td><td>23.4</td><td>31</td><td>Oklahoma</td><td>19.5</td></tr>
<tr><td>5</td><td>New York</td><td>28.3</td><td>32</td><td>Connecticut</td><td>19.1</td></tr>
<tr><td>1</td><td>North Carolina</td><td>37.1</td><td>33</td><td>Iowa</td><td>18.2</td></tr>
<tr><td>43</td><td>North Dakota</td><td>14.1</td><td>34</td><td>Massachusetts</td><td>17.7</td></tr>
<tr><td>20</td><td>Ohio</td><td>22.0</td><td>35</td><td>Kansas</td><td>17.3</td></tr>
<tr><td>31</td><td>Oklahoma</td><td>19.5</td><td>35</td><td>Nevada</td><td>17.3</td></tr>
<tr><td>43</td><td>Oregon</td><td>14.1</td><td>37</td><td>Nebraska</td><td>17.2</td></tr>
<tr><td>8</td><td>Pennsylvania</td><td>27.6</td><td>38</td><td>Colorado</td><td>16.4</td></tr>
<tr><td>12</td><td>Rhode Island</td><td>24.0</td><td>38</td><td>Wisconsin</td><td>16.4</td></tr>
<tr><td>18</td><td>South Carolina</td><td>22.2</td><td>40</td><td>Virginia</td><td>16.1</td></tr>
<tr><td>16</td><td>South Dakota</td><td>22.6</td><td>41</td><td>Montana</td><td>15.4</td></tr>
<tr><td>9</td><td>Tennessee</td><td>26.4</td><td>42</td><td>Delaware</td><td>14.4</td></tr>
<tr><td>49</td><td>Texas</td><td>7.5</td><td>43</td><td>North Dakota</td><td>14.1</td></tr>
<tr><td>45</td><td>Utah</td><td>14.0</td><td>43</td><td>Oregon</td><td>14.1</td></tr>
<tr><td>26</td><td>Vermont</td><td>20.8</td><td>45</td><td>Utah</td><td>14.0</td></tr>
<tr><td>40</td><td>Virginia</td><td>16.1</td><td>46</td><td>Hawaii</td><td>13.3</td></tr>
<tr><td>15</td><td>Washington</td><td>22.9</td><td>47</td><td>West Virginia</td><td>12.6</td></tr>
<tr><td>47</td><td>West Virginia</td><td>12.6</td><td>48</td><td>Alaska</td><td>11.5</td></tr>
<tr><td>38</td><td>Wisconsin</td><td>16.4</td><td>49</td><td>Texas</td><td>7.5</td></tr>
<tr><td>50</td><td>Wyoming</td><td>7.3</td><td>50</td><td>Wyoming</td><td>7.3</td></tr>
<tr><td></td><td></td><td></td><td colspan="2">District of Columbia**</td><td>NA</td></tr>
</table>

Source: National Association of State Budget Officers
"2009 State Expenditure Report" (http://www.nasbo.org)
*Estimates for fiscal year 2010.
**Not available.

Percent Change in Medicaid Expenditures: 2009 to 2010

National Percent Change = 8.2% Increase*

RANK	STATE	PERCENT CHANGE
47	Alabama	(3.8)
14	Alaska	10.0
48	Arizona	(3.9)
6	Arkansas	16.3
1	California	20.1
4	Colorado	17.7
49	Connecticut	(7.5)
5	Delaware	16.8
3	Florida	18.4
43	Georgia	1.1
16	Hawaii	9.4
32	Idaho	4.5
20	Illinois	8.4
12	Indiana	10.3
23	Iowa	7.6
36	Kansas	3.5
37	Kentucky	3.3
24	Louisiana	7.4
45	Maine	(0.9)
25	Maryland	7.2
18	Massachusetts	9.1
16	Michigan	9.4
42	Minnesota	2.2
46	Mississippi	(1.2)
21	Missouri	7.9
11	Montana	10.6
40	Nebraska	2.5
41	Nevada	2.3
33	New Hampshire	4.2
27	New Jersey	5.9
29	New Mexico	5.6
7	New York	14.2
14	North Carolina	10.0
2	North Dakota	20.0
50	Ohio	(9.9)
27	Oklahoma	5.9
8	Oregon	12.6
44	Pennsylvania	0.8
26	Rhode Island	6.9
38	South Carolina	3.2
10	South Dakota	10.7
35	Tennessee	4.0
18	Texas	9.1
30	Utah	5.1
13	Vermont	10.2
22	Virginia	7.8
39	Washington	3.0
31	West Virginia	4.8
9	Wisconsin	11.1
34	Wyoming	4.1

RANK	STATE	PERCENT CHANGE
1	California	20.1
2	North Dakota	20.0
3	Florida	18.4
4	Colorado	17.7
5	Delaware	16.8
6	Arkansas	16.3
7	New York	14.2
8	Oregon	12.6
9	Wisconsin	11.1
10	South Dakota	10.7
11	Montana	10.6
12	Indiana	10.3
13	Vermont	10.2
14	Alaska	10.0
14	North Carolina	10.0
16	Hawaii	9.4
16	Michigan	9.4
18	Massachusetts	9.1
18	Texas	9.1
20	Illinois	8.4
21	Missouri	7.9
22	Virginia	7.8
23	Iowa	7.6
24	Louisiana	7.4
25	Maryland	7.2
26	Rhode Island	6.9
27	New Jersey	5.9
27	Oklahoma	5.9
29	New Mexico	5.6
30	Utah	5.1
31	West Virginia	4.8
32	Idaho	4.5
33	New Hampshire	4.2
34	Wyoming	4.1
35	Tennessee	4.0
36	Kansas	3.5
37	Kentucky	3.3
38	South Carolina	3.2
39	Washington	3.0
40	Nebraska	2.5
41	Nevada	2.3
42	Minnesota	2.2
43	Georgia	1.1
44	Pennsylvania	0.8
45	Maine	(0.9)
46	Mississippi	(1.2)
47	Alabama	(3.8)
48	Arizona	(3.9)
49	Connecticut	(7.5)
50	Ohio	(9.9)
	District of Columbia**	NA

Source: National Association of State Budget Officers
   "2009 State Expenditure Report" (http://www.nasbo.org)
*Estimates for fiscal year 2010.
**Not available.

Medicaid Expenditures in 2009

National Total = $360,316,236,711*

ALPHA ORDER

RANK	STATE	EXPENDITURES	% of USA
26	Alabama	$4,388,967,084	1.2%
46	Alaska	1,065,133,940	0.3%
12	Arizona	8,664,547,751	2.4%
31	Arkansas	3,387,530,449	0.9%
2	California	40,847,829,842	11.3%
30	Colorado	3,533,332,167	1.0%
23	Connecticut	5,667,612,721	1.6%
44	Delaware	1,211,409,046	0.3%
5	Florida	14,990,559,595	4.2%
14	Georgia	7,499,071,546	2.1%
42	Hawaii	1,275,749,588	0.4%
43	Idaho	1,251,982,777	0.3%
7	Illinois	13,011,894,799	3.6%
21	Indiana	5,864,429,697	1.6%
33	Iowa	2,895,657,819	0.8%
35	Kansas	2,422,912,043	0.7%
24	Kentucky	5,362,501,971	1.5%
20	Louisiana	6,271,680,348	1.7%
34	Maine	2,491,609,104	0.7%
19	Maryland	6,340,703,178	1.8%
8	Massachusetts	12,324,081,045	3.4%
10	Michigan	10,527,467,060	2.9%
15	Minnesota	7,300,893,418	2.0%
27	Mississippi	3,926,907,637	1.1%
13	Missouri	7,648,493,348	2.1%
47	Montana	867,917,221	0.2%
39	Nebraska	1,575,671,426	0.4%
40	Nevada	1,376,535,435	0.4%
41	New Hampshire	1,307,557,646	0.4%
11	New Jersey	9,481,301,639	2.6%
32	New Mexico	3,244,639,530	0.9%
1	New York	47,678,723,205	13.2%
9	North Carolina	10,888,466,523	3.0%
49	North Dakota	567,171,228	0.2%
6	Ohio	14,003,331,113	3.9%
28	Oklahoma	3,766,999,610	1.0%
29	Oregon	3,630,207,539	1.0%
4	Pennsylvania	17,113,120,743	4.7%
37	Rhode Island	1,874,745,061	0.5%
25	South Carolina	4,546,369,802	1.3%
48	South Dakota	708,098,958	0.2%
16	Tennessee	7,246,891,973	2.0%
3	Texas	23,000,014,985	6.4%
38	Utah	1,596,851,204	0.4%
45	Vermont	1,189,152,604	0.3%
22	Virginia	5,692,752,496	1.6%
17	Washington	6,554,567,723	1.8%
36	West Virginia	2,420,608,803	0.7%
18	Wisconsin	6,537,704,026	1.8%
50	Wyoming	518,684,497	0.1%

RANK ORDER

RANK	STATE	EXPENDITURES	% of USA
1	New York	$47,678,723,205	13.2%
2	California	40,847,829,842	11.3%
3	Texas	23,000,014,985	6.4%
4	Pennsylvania	17,113,120,743	4.7%
5	Florida	14,990,559,595	4.2%
6	Ohio	14,003,331,113	3.9%
7	Illinois	13,011,894,799	3.6%
8	Massachusetts	12,324,081,045	3.4%
9	North Carolina	10,888,466,523	3.0%
10	Michigan	10,527,467,060	2.9%
11	New Jersey	9,481,301,639	2.6%
12	Arizona	8,664,547,751	2.4%
13	Missouri	7,648,493,348	2.1%
14	Georgia	7,499,071,546	2.1%
15	Minnesota	7,300,893,418	2.0%
16	Tennessee	7,246,891,973	2.0%
17	Washington	6,554,567,723	1.8%
18	Wisconsin	6,537,704,026	1.8%
19	Maryland	6,340,703,178	1.8%
20	Louisiana	6,271,680,348	1.7%
21	Indiana	5,864,429,697	1.6%
22	Virginia	5,692,752,496	1.6%
23	Connecticut	5,667,612,721	1.6%
24	Kentucky	5,362,501,971	1.5%
25	South Carolina	4,546,369,802	1.3%
26	Alabama	4,388,967,084	1.2%
27	Mississippi	3,926,907,637	1.1%
28	Oklahoma	3,766,999,610	1.0%
29	Oregon	3,630,207,539	1.0%
30	Colorado	3,533,332,167	1.0%
31	Arkansas	3,387,530,449	0.9%
32	New Mexico	3,244,639,530	0.9%
33	Iowa	2,895,657,819	0.8%
34	Maine	2,491,609,104	0.7%
35	Kansas	2,422,912,043	0.7%
36	West Virginia	2,420,608,803	0.7%
37	Rhode Island	1,874,745,061	0.5%
38	Utah	1,596,851,204	0.4%
39	Nebraska	1,575,671,426	0.4%
40	Nevada	1,376,535,435	0.4%
41	New Hampshire	1,307,557,646	0.4%
42	Hawaii	1,275,749,588	0.4%
43	Idaho	1,251,982,777	0.3%
44	Delaware	1,211,409,046	0.3%
45	Vermont	1,189,152,604	0.3%
46	Alaska	1,065,133,940	0.3%
47	Montana	867,917,221	0.2%
48	South Dakota	708,098,958	0.2%
49	North Dakota	567,171,228	0.2%
50	Wyoming	518,684,497	0.1%
	District of Columbia	1,611,030,471	0.4%

Source: U.S. Department of Health and Human Services, Centers for Medicare and Medicaid Services
   "2009 Data Compendium" (http://www.cms.hhs.gov/DataCompendium/)
*For fiscal year 2009. National total includes $1,144,143,321 in expenditures in U.S. territories. Net expenditures reported from
Form CMS-64. Excludes ADM, Medicaid CHIP expansions, and CMS adjustments.

Per Capita Medicaid Expenditures in 2009

National Per Capita = $1,170*

ALPHA ORDER				RANK ORDER		
RANK	STATE	PER CAPITA		RANK	STATE	PER CAPITA
36	Alabama	$932		1	New York	$2,440
8	Alaska	1,525		2	Vermont	1,913
15	Arizona	1,314		3	Maine	1,890
19	Arkansas	1,172		4	Massachusetts	1,869
24	California	1,105		5	Rhode Island	1,780
48	Colorado	703		6	New Mexico	1,615
7	Connecticut	1,611		7	Connecticut	1,611
11	Delaware	1,369		8	Alaska	1,525
45	Florida	809		9	Louisiana	1,396
46	Georgia	763		10	Minnesota	1,386
31	Hawaii	985		11	Delaware	1,369
44	Idaho	810		12	Pennsylvania	1,358
28	Illinois	1,008		13	Mississippi	1,330
38	Indiana	913		13	West Virginia	1,330
33	Iowa	963		15	Arizona	1,314
43	Kansas	860		16	Missouri	1,277
17	Kentucky	1,243		17	Kentucky	1,243
9	Louisiana	1,396		18	Ohio	1,213
3	Maine	1,890		19	Arkansas	1,172
23	Maryland	1,113		20	North Carolina	1,161
4	Massachusetts	1,869		21	Wisconsin	1,156
26	Michigan	1,056		22	Tennessee	1,151
10	Minnesota	1,386		23	Maryland	1,113
13	Mississippi	1,330		24	California	1,105
16	Missouri	1,277		25	New Jersey	1,089
39	Montana	890		26	Michigan	1,056
40	Nebraska	877		27	Oklahoma	1,022
50	Nevada	521		28	Illinois	1,008
30	New Hampshire	987		29	South Carolina	997
25	New Jersey	1,089		30	New Hampshire	987
6	New Mexico	1,615		31	Hawaii	985
1	New York	2,440		32	Washington	984
20	North Carolina	1,161		33	Iowa	963
40	North Dakota	877		34	Wyoming	953
18	Ohio	1,213		35	Oregon	949
27	Oklahoma	1,022		36	Alabama	932
35	Oregon	949		37	Texas	928
12	Pennsylvania	1,358		38	Indiana	913
5	Rhode Island	1,780		39	Montana	890
29	South Carolina	997		40	Nebraska	877
42	South Dakota	872		40	North Dakota	877
22	Tennessee	1,151		42	South Dakota	872
37	Texas	928		43	Kansas	860
49	Utah	573		44	Idaho	810
2	Vermont	1,913		45	Florida	809
47	Virginia	722		46	Georgia	763
32	Washington	984		47	Virginia	722
13	West Virginia	1,330		48	Colorado	703
21	Wisconsin	1,156		49	Utah	573
34	Wyoming	953		50	Nevada	521

District of Columbia	2,687

Source: CQ Press using data from U.S. Department of Health and Human Services, Centers for Medicare and Medicaid Services
  "2009 Data Compendium" (http://www.cms.hhs.gov/DataCompendium/)
*Figures for fiscal year 2009. National figure does not include expenditures or population in U.S. territories. Net expenditures
reported from Form CMS-64. Excludes ADM, Medicaid CHIP expansions, and CMS adjustments.

Medicaid Expenditures per Beneficiary in 2009

National Rate = $7,000 per Beneficiary*

ALPHA ORDER			RANK ORDER		
RANK	STATE	PER BENEFICIARY	RANK	STATE	PER BENEFICIARY
47	Alabama	$5,316	1	Connecticut	$11,950
7	Alaska	9,914	2	Minnesota	10,702
28	Arizona	6,603	3	New York	10,463
49	Arkansas	5,166	4	Rhode Island	10,325
42	California	5,728	5	New Hampshire	10,147
19	Colorado	7,142	6	Massachusetts	10,042
1	Connecticut	11,060	7	Alaska	9,914
24	Delaware	6,968	8	Montana	9,602
40	Florida	5,788	9	New Jersey	9,424
48	Georgia	5,196	10	Maine	8,916
50	Hawaii	5,124	11	North Dakota	8,897
36	Idaho	6,053	12	Pennsylvania	8,659
45	Illinois	5,551	13	Missouri	8,495
44	Indiana	5,632	14	Kansas	8,306
22	Iowa	6,991	15	Wyoming	7,699
14	Kansas	8,306	16	Vermont	7,658
26	Kentucky	6,793	17	Maryland	7,638
46	Louisiana	5,463	18	West Virginia	7,323
10	Maine	8,916	19	Colorado	7,142
17	Maryland	7,638	20	North Carolina	7,081
6	Massachusetts	10,042	21	Oregon	7,075
35	Michigan	6,077	22	Iowa	6,991
2	Minnesota	10,702	23	Nebraska	6,987
43	Mississippi	5,672	24	Delaware	6,968
13	Missouri	8,495	25	Ohio	6,902
8	Montana	9,602	26	Kentucky	6,793
23	Nebraska	6,987	27	Virginia	6,659
37	Nevada	5,983	28	Arizona	6,603
5	New Hampshire	10,147	29	Texas	6,547
9	New Jersey	9,424	30	New Mexico	6,518
30	New Mexico	6,518	31	Utah	6,464
3	New York	10,463	32	South Dakota	6,126
20	North Carolina	7,081	33	Tennessee	6,120
11	North Dakota	8,897	34	Washington	6,101
25	Ohio	6,902	35	Michigan	6,077
41	Oklahoma	5,740	36	Idaho	6,053
21	Oregon	7,075	37	Nevada	5,983
12	Pennsylvania	8,659	38	Wisconsin	5,930
4	Rhode Island	10,325	39	South Carolina	5,854
39	South Carolina	5,854	40	Florida	5,788
32	South Dakota	6,126	41	Oklahoma	5,740
33	Tennessee	6,120	42	California	5,728
29	Texas	6,547	43	Mississippi	5,672
31	Utah	6,464	44	Indiana	5,632
16	Vermont	7,658	45	Illinois	5,551
27	Virginia	6,659	46	Louisiana	5,463
34	Washington	6,101	47	Alabama	5,316
18	West Virginia	7,323	48	Georgia	5,196
38	Wisconsin	5,930	49	Arkansas	5,166
15	Wyoming	7,699	50	Hawaii	5,124
				District of Columbia	10,004

Source: CQ Press using data from U.S. Department of Health and Human Services, Centers for Medicare and Medicaid Services
"2009 Data Compendium" (http://www.cms.hhs.gov/DataCompendium/)
*Figures for fiscal year 2009. National figure does not include expenditures or enrollees in U.S. territories. Net expenditures
reported from Form CMS-64. Excludes ADM, Medicaid CHIP expansions, and CMS adjustments.

Federal Medicaid Matching Fund Rate for 2011

National Average = 71.73% of States' Funds Matched by Federal Government*

ALPHA ORDER

RANK	STATE	RATE
9	Alabama	78.03
37	Alaska	65.00
10	Arizona	77.11
5	Arkansas	79.50
37	California	65.00
37	Colorado	65.00
37	Connecticut	65.00
34	Delaware	67.92
31	Florida	69.23
13	Georgia	76.31
36	Hawaii	65.34
7	Idaho	79.16
37	Illinois	65.00
11	Indiana	76.87
23	Iowa	72.50
28	Kansas	69.84
3	Kentucky	79.83
22	Louisiana	72.76
20	Maine	74.29
37	Maryland	65.00
37	Massachusetts	65.00
14	Michigan	76.30
37	Minnesota	65.00
1	Mississippi	81.93
19	Missouri	74.42
15	Montana	76.28
29	Nebraska	69.65
30	Nevada	69.34
37	New Hampshire	65.00
37	New Jersey	65.00
8	New Mexico	78.55
37	New York	65.00
16	North Carolina	75.70
32	North Dakota	68.78
17	Ohio	74.91
18	Oklahoma	74.72
21	Oregon	74.04
33	Pennsylvania	68.55
35	Rhode Island	66.48
6	South Carolina	79.17
25	South Dakota	71.39
12	Tennessee	76.45
26	Texas	70.75
4	Utah	79.69
27	Vermont	70.31
37	Virginia	65.00
37	Washington	65.00
2	West Virginia	80.83
24	Wisconsin	72.37
37	Wyoming	65.00

RANK ORDER

RANK	STATE	RATE
1	Mississippi	81.93
2	West Virginia	80.83
3	Kentucky	79.83
4	Utah	79.69
5	Arkansas	79.50
6	South Carolina	79.17
7	Idaho	79.16
8	New Mexico	78.55
9	Alabama	78.03
10	Arizona	77.11
11	Indiana	76.87
12	Tennessee	76.45
13	Georgia	76.31
14	Michigan	76.30
15	Montana	76.28
16	North Carolina	75.70
17	Ohio	74.91
18	Oklahoma	74.72
19	Missouri	74.42
20	Maine	74.29
21	Oregon	74.04
22	Louisiana	72.76
23	Iowa	72.50
24	Wisconsin	72.37
25	South Dakota	71.39
26	Texas	70.75
27	Vermont	70.31
28	Kansas	69.84
29	Nebraska	69.65
30	Nevada	69.34
31	Florida	69.23
32	North Dakota	68.78
33	Pennsylvania	68.55
34	Delaware	67.92
35	Rhode Island	66.48
36	Hawaii	65.34
37	Alaska	65.00
37	California	65.00
37	Colorado	65.00
37	Connecticut	65.00
37	Illinois	65.00
37	Maryland	65.00
37	Massachusetts	65.00
37	Minnesota	65.00
37	New Hampshire	65.00
37	New Jersey	65.00
37	New York	65.00
37	Virginia	65.00
37	Washington	65.00
37	Wyoming	65.00
	District of Columbia	79.00

Source: U.S. Department of Health and Human Services, Centers for Medicare and Medicaid Services
   "Enhanced Federal Medical Assistance Percentages" (Federal Register, Vol. 75, No. 217, Nov. 10, 2010, page 69083)
      (http://www.gpoaccess.gov/fr/index.html)
*For fiscal year 2012. These are "enhanced" matching rates established by the Children's Health Insurance Program, signed into law in August 1997. Sixty-five percent is the minimum. National average is a simple average of the 51 individual rates and is not weighted for population or funds.

State and Local Government Expenditures for Hospitals in 2008

National Total = $128,853,219,000*

ALPHA ORDER

RANK	STATE	EXPENDITURES	% of USA
8	Alabama	$3,859,596,000	3.0%
42	Alaska	257,290,000	0.2%
30	Arizona	1,216,225,000	0.9%
32	Arkansas	993,226,000	0.8%
1	California	17,959,444,000	13.9%
22	Colorado	1,921,834,000	1.5%
28	Connecticut	1,384,731,000	1.1%
47	Delaware	63,435,000	0.0%
4	Florida	7,732,181,000	6.0%
6	Georgia	5,115,679,000	4.0%
39	Hawaii	531,055,000	0.4%
37	Idaho	803,102,000	0.6%
20	Illinois	2,431,785,000	1.9%
14	Indiana	3,065,087,000	2.4%
21	Iowa	2,386,881,000	1.9%
25	Kansas	1,744,165,000	1.4%
26	Kentucky	1,628,928,000	1.3%
12	Louisiana	3,150,335,000	2.4%
43	Maine	130,920,000	0.1%
40	Maryland	495,169,000	0.4%
24	Massachusetts	1,769,174,000	1.4%
11	Michigan	3,264,001,000	2.5%
23	Minnesota	1,836,771,000	1.4%
16	Mississippi	2,866,961,000	2.2%
17	Missouri	2,676,462,000	2.1%
44	Montana	108,842,000	0.1%
36	Nebraska	875,576,000	0.7%
33	Nevada	955,148,000	0.7%
48	New Hampshire	60,361,000	0.0%
19	New Jersey	2,433,954,000	1.9%
34	New Mexico	881,308,000	0.7%
2	New York	12,264,482,000	9.5%
5	North Carolina	5,599,431,000	4.3%
50	North Dakota	18,459,000	0.0%
10	Ohio	3,436,343,000	2.7%
31	Oklahoma	1,073,846,000	0.8%
27	Oregon	1,422,258,000	1.1%
18	Pennsylvania	2,443,729,000	1.9%
46	Rhode Island	87,528,000	0.1%
7	South Carolina	4,502,158,000	3.5%
45	South Dakota	102,115,000	0.1%
15	Tennessee	2,891,705,000	2.2%
3	Texas	9,981,702,000	7.7%
35	Utah	877,647,000	0.7%
49	Vermont	20,092,000	0.0%
13	Virginia	3,080,774,000	2.4%
9	Washington	3,816,740,000	3.0%
41	West Virginia	355,043,000	0.3%
29	Wisconsin	1,273,838,000	1.0%
38	Wyoming	773,874,000	0.6%

RANK ORDER

RANK	STATE	EXPENDITURES	% of USA
1	California	$17,959,444,000	13.9%
2	New York	12,264,482,000	9.5%
3	Texas	9,981,702,000	7.7%
4	Florida	7,732,181,000	6.0%
5	North Carolina	5,599,431,000	4.3%
6	Georgia	5,115,679,000	4.0%
7	South Carolina	4,502,158,000	3.5%
8	Alabama	3,859,596,000	3.0%
9	Washington	3,816,740,000	3.0%
10	Ohio	3,436,343,000	2.7%
11	Michigan	3,264,001,000	2.5%
12	Louisiana	3,150,335,000	2.4%
13	Virginia	3,080,774,000	2.4%
14	Indiana	3,065,087,000	2.4%
15	Tennessee	2,891,705,000	2.2%
16	Mississippi	2,866,961,000	2.2%
17	Missouri	2,676,462,000	2.1%
18	Pennsylvania	2,443,729,000	1.9%
19	New Jersey	2,433,954,000	1.9%
20	Illinois	2,431,785,000	1.9%
21	Iowa	2,386,881,000	1.9%
22	Colorado	1,921,834,000	1.5%
23	Minnesota	1,836,771,000	1.4%
24	Massachusetts	1,769,174,000	1.4%
25	Kansas	1,744,165,000	1.4%
26	Kentucky	1,628,928,000	1.3%
27	Oregon	1,422,258,000	1.1%
28	Connecticut	1,384,731,000	1.1%
29	Wisconsin	1,273,838,000	1.0%
30	Arizona	1,216,225,000	0.9%
31	Oklahoma	1,073,846,000	0.8%
32	Arkansas	993,226,000	0.8%
33	Nevada	955,148,000	0.7%
34	New Mexico	881,308,000	0.7%
35	Utah	877,647,000	0.7%
36	Nebraska	875,576,000	0.7%
37	Idaho	803,102,000	0.6%
38	Wyoming	773,874,000	0.6%
39	Hawaii	531,055,000	0.4%
40	Maryland	495,169,000	0.4%
41	West Virginia	355,043,000	0.3%
42	Alaska	257,290,000	0.2%
43	Maine	130,920,000	0.1%
44	Montana	108,842,000	0.1%
45	South Dakota	102,115,000	0.1%
46	Rhode Island	87,528,000	0.1%
47	Delaware	63,435,000	0.0%
48	New Hampshire	60,361,000	0.0%
49	Vermont	20,092,000	0.0%
50	North Dakota	18,459,000	0.0%
	District of Columbia	231,829,000	0.2%

Source: U.S. Bureau of the Census, Governments Division
"2008 State and Local Government Finances" (http://www.census.gov/govs/estimate/index.html)
*Financing, construction, acquisition, maintenance or operation of hospital facilities, provision of hospital care, and support of public or private hospitals.

Per Capita State and Local Government Expenditures for Hospitals in 2008

National Per Capita = $423*

ALPHA ORDER

RANK	STATE	PER CAPITA
4	Alabama	$825
27	Alaska	374
41	Arizona	187
30	Arkansas	346
13	California	491
24	Colorado	389
22	Connecticut	395
47	Delaware	72
19	Florida	420
11	Georgia	528
20	Hawaii	412
12	Idaho	526
40	Illinois	189
15	Indiana	480
5	Iowa	797
8	Kansas	624
25	Kentucky	380
6	Louisiana	708
44	Maine	99
45	Maryland	88
36	Massachusetts	270
31	Michigan	326
29	Minnesota	351
3	Mississippi	975
17	Missouri	449
43	Montana	112
13	Nebraska	491
28	Nevada	365
48	New Hampshire	46
35	New Jersey	281
18	New Mexico	444
7	New York	630
9	North Carolina	606
50	North Dakota	29
33	Ohio	298
34	Oklahoma	295
26	Oregon	376
39	Pennsylvania	194
46	Rhode Island	83
2	South Carolina	1,000
42	South Dakota	127
16	Tennessee	463
21	Texas	411
32	Utah	322
49	Vermont	32
22	Virginia	395
10	Washington	581
38	West Virginia	196
37	Wisconsin	226
1	Wyoming	1,452

RANK ORDER

RANK	STATE	PER CAPITA
1	Wyoming	$1,452
2	South Carolina	1,000
3	Mississippi	975
4	Alabama	825
5	Iowa	797
6	Louisiana	708
7	New York	630
8	Kansas	624
9	North Carolina	606
10	Washington	581
11	Georgia	528
12	Idaho	526
13	California	491
13	Nebraska	491
15	Indiana	480
16	Tennessee	463
17	Missouri	449
18	New Mexico	444
19	Florida	420
20	Hawaii	412
21	Texas	411
22	Connecticut	395
22	Virginia	395
24	Colorado	389
25	Kentucky	380
26	Oregon	376
27	Alaska	374
28	Nevada	365
29	Minnesota	351
30	Arkansas	346
31	Michigan	326
32	Utah	322
33	Ohio	298
34	Oklahoma	295
35	New Jersey	281
36	Massachusetts	270
37	Wisconsin	226
38	West Virginia	196
39	Pennsylvania	194
40	Illinois	189
41	Arizona	187
42	South Dakota	127
43	Montana	112
44	Maine	99
45	Maryland	88
46	Rhode Island	83
47	Delaware	72
48	New Hampshire	46
49	Vermont	32
50	North Dakota	29
	District of Columbia	393

Source: CQ Press using data from U.S. Bureau of the Census, Governments Division
  "2008 State and Local Government Finances" (http://www.census.gov/govs/estimate/index.html)
*Financing, construction, acquisition, maintenance or operation of hospital facilities, provision of hospital care, and support of public or private hospitals.

Percent of State and Local Government Expenditures
Used for Hospitals in 2008
National Percent = 5.4%*

ALPHA ORDER

RANK	STATE	PERCENT
3	Alabama	11.8
41	Alaska	2.2
38	Arizona	2.8
18	Arkansas	5.6
21	California	5.4
21	Colorado	5.4
28	Connecticut	4.6
47	Delaware	0.8
18	Florida	5.6
9	Georgia	7.8
29	Hawaii	4.5
7	Idaho	8.3
40	Illinois	2.5
13	Indiana	6.9
5	Iowa	10.4
7	Kansas	8.3
20	Kentucky	5.5
10	Louisiana	7.6
44	Maine	1.3
45	Maryland	1.1
34	Massachusetts	3.1
29	Michigan	4.5
32	Minnesota	4.2
2	Mississippi	12.8
14	Missouri	6.8
43	Montana	1.5
15	Nebraska	6.4
24	Nevada	5.2
48	New Hampshire	0.7
34	New Jersey	3.1
25	New Mexico	5.1
17	New York	5.8
6	North Carolina	8.8
49	North Dakota	0.4
33	Ohio	4.0
29	Oklahoma	4.5
25	Oregon	5.1
39	Pennsylvania	2.6
46	Rhode Island	1.0
1	South Carolina	13.4
42	South Dakota	2.0
10	Tennessee	7.6
16	Texas	6.1
27	Utah	4.7
49	Vermont	0.4
21	Virginia	5.4
12	Washington	7.1
37	West Virginia	2.9
36	Wisconsin	3.0
4	Wyoming	11.4

RANK ORDER

RANK	STATE	PERCENT
1	South Carolina	13.4
2	Mississippi	12.8
3	Alabama	11.8
4	Wyoming	11.4
5	Iowa	10.4
6	North Carolina	8.8
7	Idaho	8.3
7	Kansas	8.3
9	Georgia	7.8
10	Louisiana	7.6
10	Tennessee	7.6
12	Washington	7.1
13	Indiana	6.9
14	Missouri	6.8
15	Nebraska	6.4
16	Texas	6.1
17	New York	5.8
18	Arkansas	5.6
18	Florida	5.6
20	Kentucky	5.5
21	California	5.4
21	Colorado	5.4
21	Virginia	5.4
24	Nevada	5.2
25	New Mexico	5.1
25	Oregon	5.1
27	Utah	4.7
28	Connecticut	4.6
29	Hawaii	4.5
29	Michigan	4.5
29	Oklahoma	4.5
32	Minnesota	4.2
33	Ohio	4.0
34	Massachusetts	3.1
34	New Jersey	3.1
36	Wisconsin	3.0
37	West Virginia	2.9
38	Arizona	2.8
39	Pennsylvania	2.6
40	Illinois	2.5
41	Alaska	2.2
42	South Dakota	2.0
43	Montana	1.5
44	Maine	1.3
45	Maryland	1.1
46	Rhode Island	1.0
47	Delaware	0.8
48	New Hampshire	0.7
49	North Dakota	0.4
49	Vermont	0.4

| | District of Columbia | 2.2 |

Source: CQ Press using data from U.S. Bureau of the Census, Governments Division
   "2008 State and Local Government Finances" (http://www.census.gov/govs/estimate/index.html)
*As a percent of direct general expenditures. Financing, construction, acquisition, maintenance or operation of hospital facilities, provision of hospital care, and support of public or private hospitals.

State and Local Government Expenditures for Health Programs in 2008

National Total = $79,704,063,000*

ALPHA ORDER					RANK ORDER			
RANK	STATE	EXPENDITURES	% of USA		RANK	STATE	EXPENDITURES	% of USA
22	Alabama	$1,042,598,000	1.3%		1	California	$13,940,626,000	17.5%
45	Alaska	200,183,000	0.3%		2	New York	5,799,382,000	7.3%
13	Arizona	1,792,075,000	2.2%		3	Florida	4,533,314,000	5.7%
43	Arkansas	281,486,000	0.4%		4	Ohio	4,183,392,000	5.2%
1	California	13,940,626,000	17.5%		5	Pennsylvania	4,047,874,000	5.1%
23	Colorado	959,756,000	1.2%		6	Michigan	3,640,833,000	4.6%
28	Connecticut	764,807,000	1.0%		7	Texas	3,481,006,000	4.4%
38	Delaware	417,650,000	0.5%		8	Illinois	2,897,613,000	3.6%
3	Florida	4,533,314,000	5.7%		9	North Carolina	2,880,289,000	3.6%
10	Georgia	2,298,100,000	2.9%		10	Georgia	2,298,100,000	2.9%
29	Hawaii	715,767,000	0.9%		11	Washington	2,238,653,000	2.8%
44	Idaho	205,416,000	0.3%		12	Wisconsin	1,837,620,000	2.3%
8	Illinois	2,897,613,000	3.6%		13	Arizona	1,792,075,000	2.2%
26	Indiana	808,918,000	1.0%		14	Maryland	1,725,140,000	2.2%
33	Iowa	507,921,000	0.6%		15	New Jersey	1,675,679,000	2.1%
35	Kansas	466,997,000	0.6%		16	Tennessee	1,590,361,000	2.0%
27	Kentucky	805,263,000	1.0%		17	Missouri	1,503,610,000	1.9%
25	Louisiana	815,890,000	1.0%		18	Virginia	1,343,634,000	1.7%
34	Maine	504,569,000	0.6%		19	South Carolina	1,187,273,000	1.5%
14	Maryland	1,725,140,000	2.2%		20	Massachusetts	1,167,756,000	1.5%
20	Massachusetts	1,167,756,000	1.5%		21	Minnesota	1,108,592,000	1.4%
6	Michigan	3,640,833,000	4.6%		22	Alabama	1,042,598,000	1.3%
21	Minnesota	1,108,592,000	1.4%		23	Colorado	959,756,000	1.2%
36	Mississippi	420,476,000	0.5%		24	Oregon	862,321,000	1.1%
17	Missouri	1,503,610,000	1.9%		25	Louisiana	815,890,000	1.0%
39	Montana	405,983,000	0.5%		26	Indiana	808,918,000	1.0%
37	Nebraska	418,479,000	0.5%		27	Kentucky	805,263,000	1.0%
40	Nevada	390,871,000	0.5%		28	Connecticut	764,807,000	1.0%
49	New Hampshire	152,090,000	0.2%		29	Hawaii	715,767,000	0.9%
15	New Jersey	1,675,679,000	2.1%		30	Oklahoma	689,642,000	0.9%
32	New Mexico	540,902,000	0.7%		31	Utah	566,334,000	0.7%
2	New York	5,799,382,000	7.3%		32	New Mexico	540,902,000	0.7%
9	North Carolina	2,880,289,000	3.6%		33	Iowa	507,921,000	0.6%
50	North Dakota	90,847,000	0.1%		34	Maine	504,569,000	0.6%
4	Ohio	4,183,392,000	5.2%		35	Kansas	466,997,000	0.6%
30	Oklahoma	689,642,000	0.9%		36	Mississippi	420,476,000	0.5%
24	Oregon	862,321,000	1.1%		37	Nebraska	418,479,000	0.5%
5	Pennsylvania	4,047,874,000	5.1%		38	Delaware	417,650,000	0.5%
46	Rhode Island	187,269,000	0.2%		39	Montana	405,983,000	0.5%
19	South Carolina	1,187,273,000	1.5%		40	Nevada	390,871,000	0.5%
48	South Dakota	155,562,000	0.2%		41	Wyoming	362,472,000	0.5%
16	Tennessee	1,590,361,000	2.0%		42	West Virginia	355,586,000	0.4%
7	Texas	3,481,006,000	4.4%		43	Arkansas	281,486,000	0.4%
31	Utah	566,334,000	0.7%		44	Idaho	205,416,000	0.3%
47	Vermont	171,578,000	0.2%		45	Alaska	200,183,000	0.3%
18	Virginia	1,343,634,000	1.7%		46	Rhode Island	187,269,000	0.2%
11	Washington	2,238,653,000	2.8%		47	Vermont	171,578,000	0.2%
42	West Virginia	355,586,000	0.4%		48	South Dakota	155,562,000	0.2%
12	Wisconsin	1,837,620,000	2.3%		49	New Hampshire	152,090,000	0.2%
41	Wyoming	362,472,000	0.5%		50	North Dakota	90,847,000	0.1%
						District of Columbia	563,608,000	0.7%

Source: U.S. Bureau of the Census, Governments Division
"2008 State and Local Government Finances" (http://www.census.gov/govs/estimate/index.html)
*Includes outpatient health services other than hospital care, research and education, categorical health programs, treatment and immunization clinics, nursing, and environmental health activities. Includes capital expenditures.

Per Capita State and Local Government Expenditures for
Health Programs in 2008
National Per Capita = $262*

ALPHA ORDER				RANK ORDER		
RANK	STATE	PER CAPITA		RANK	STATE	PER CAPITA
27	Alabama	$223		1	Wyoming	$680
15	Alaska	291		2	Hawaii	556
16	Arizona	276		3	Delaware	477
50	Arkansas	98		4	Montana	419
6	California	381		5	Maine	382
32	Colorado	194		6	California	381
28	Connecticut	218		7	Michigan	364
3	Delaware	477		8	Ohio	363
22	Florida	246		9	Washington	341
23	Georgia	237		10	Wisconsin	327
2	Hawaii	556		11	Pennsylvania	322
47	Idaho	134		12	North Carolina	311
26	Illinois	226		13	Maryland	305
48	Indiana	127		14	New York	298
41	Iowa	170		15	Alaska	291
42	Kansas	167		16	Arizona	276
36	Kentucky	188		16	Vermont	276
37	Louisiana	183		18	New Mexico	272
5	Maine	382		19	South Carolina	264
13	Maryland	305		20	Tennessee	255
38	Massachusetts	178		21	Missouri	252
7	Michigan	364		22	Florida	246
29	Minnesota	212		23	Georgia	237
44	Mississippi	143		24	Nebraska	235
21	Missouri	252		25	Oregon	228
4	Montana	419		26	Illinois	226
24	Nebraska	235		27	Alabama	223
43	Nevada	149		28	Connecticut	218
49	New Hampshire	115		29	Minnesota	212
33	New Jersey	193		30	Utah	208
18	New Mexico	272		31	West Virginia	196
14	New York	298		32	Colorado	194
12	North Carolina	311		33	New Jersey	193
46	North Dakota	142		33	South Dakota	193
8	Ohio	363		35	Oklahoma	189
35	Oklahoma	189		36	Kentucky	188
25	Oregon	228		37	Louisiana	183
11	Pennsylvania	322		38	Massachusetts	178
38	Rhode Island	178		38	Rhode Island	178
19	South Carolina	264		40	Virginia	172
33	South Dakota	193		41	Iowa	170
20	Tennessee	255		42	Kansas	167
44	Texas	143		43	Nevada	149
30	Utah	208		44	Mississippi	143
16	Vermont	276		44	Texas	143
40	Virginia	172		46	North Dakota	142
9	Washington	341		47	Idaho	134
31	West Virginia	196		48	Indiana	127
10	Wisconsin	327		49	New Hampshire	115
1	Wyoming	680		50	Arkansas	98
					District of Columbia	955

Source: CQ Press using data from U.S. Bureau of the Census, Governments Division
"2008 State and Local Government Finances" (http://www.census.gov/govs/estimate/index.html)
*Includes outpatient health services other than hospital care, research and education, categorical health programs, treatment and immunization clinics, nursing, and environmental health activities. Includes capital expenditures.

Percent of State and Local Government Expenditures
Used for Health Programs in 2008
National Percent = 3.3%*

ALPHA ORDER

RANK	STATE	PERCENT
20	Alabama	3.2
48	Alaska	1.7
14	Arizona	4.1
50	Arkansas	1.6
11	California	4.2
30	Colorado	2.7
33	Connecticut	2.5
4	Delaware	5.2
19	Florida	3.3
17	Georgia	3.5
1	Hawaii	6.1
38	Idaho	2.1
25	Illinois	3.0
46	Indiana	1.8
36	Iowa	2.2
36	Kansas	2.2
30	Kentucky	2.7
44	Louisiana	2.0
6	Maine	4.9
15	Maryland	3.8
38	Massachusetts	2.1
5	Michigan	5.0
33	Minnesota	2.5
45	Mississippi	1.9
15	Missouri	3.8
2	Montana	5.6
22	Nebraska	3.1
38	Nevada	2.1
48	New Hampshire	1.7
38	New Jersey	2.1
22	New Mexico	3.1
30	New York	2.7
8	North Carolina	4.5
46	North Dakota	1.8
7	Ohio	4.8
28	Oklahoma	2.9
22	Oregon	3.1
9	Pennsylvania	4.3
38	Rhode Island	2.1
17	South Carolina	3.5
25	South Dakota	3.0
11	Tennessee	4.2
38	Texas	2.1
25	Utah	3.0
20	Vermont	3.2
35	Virginia	2.4
11	Washington	4.2
28	West Virginia	2.9
9	Wisconsin	4.3
3	Wyoming	5.3

RANK ORDER

RANK	STATE	PERCENT
1	Hawaii	6.1
2	Montana	5.6
3	Wyoming	5.3
4	Delaware	5.2
5	Michigan	5.0
6	Maine	4.9
7	Ohio	4.8
8	North Carolina	4.5
9	Pennsylvania	4.3
9	Wisconsin	4.3
11	California	4.2
11	Tennessee	4.2
11	Washington	4.2
14	Arizona	4.1
15	Maryland	3.8
15	Missouri	3.8
17	Georgia	3.5
17	South Carolina	3.5
19	Florida	3.3
20	Alabama	3.2
20	Vermont	3.2
22	Nebraska	3.1
22	New Mexico	3.1
22	Oregon	3.1
25	Illinois	3.0
25	South Dakota	3.0
25	Utah	3.0
28	Oklahoma	2.9
28	West Virginia	2.9
30	Colorado	2.7
30	Kentucky	2.7
30	New York	2.7
33	Connecticut	2.5
33	Minnesota	2.5
35	Virginia	2.4
36	Iowa	2.2
36	Kansas	2.2
38	Idaho	2.1
38	Massachusetts	2.1
38	Nevada	2.1
38	New Jersey	2.1
38	Rhode Island	2.1
38	Texas	2.1
44	Louisiana	2.0
45	Mississippi	1.9
46	Indiana	1.8
46	North Dakota	1.8
48	Alaska	1.7
48	New Hampshire	1.7
50	Arkansas	1.6

	District of Columbia	5.3

Source: CQ Press using data from U.S. Bureau of the Census, Governments Division
     "2008 State and Local Government Finances" (http://www.census.gov/govs/estimate/index.html)
*As a percent of direct general expenditures. Includes outpatient health services other than hospital care, research and education, categorical health programs, treatment and immunization clinics, nursing, and environmental health activities. Includes capital expenditures.

Estimated Tobacco Settlement Revenues in Fiscal Year 2011

National Total = $7,400,000,000*

ALPHA ORDER					RANK ORDER			
RANK	STATE	REVENUES	% of USA		RANK	STATE	REVENUES	% of USA
26	Alabama	$97,000,000	1.3%		1	New York	$762,300,000	10.3%
45	Alaska	32,200,000	0.4%		2	California	760,100,000	10.3%
24	Arizona	106,300,000	1.4%		3	Texas	466,200,000	6.3%
35	Arkansas	52,500,000	0.7%		4	Florida	364,300,000	4.9%
2	California	760,100,000	10.3%		5	Pennsylvania	349,200,000	4.7%
27	Colorado	95,200,000	1.3%		6	Ohio	305,500,000	4.1%
21	Connecticut	129,800,000	1.8%		7	Illinois	283,400,000	3.8%
47	Delaware	28,000,000	0.4%		8	Michigan	265,300,000	3.6%
4	Florida	364,300,000	4.9%		9	Massachusetts	264,400,000	3.6%
16	Georgia	145,700,000	2.0%		10	New Jersey	239,900,000	3.2%
36	Hawaii	51,800,000	0.7%		11	Minnesota	166,500,000	2.3%
48	Idaho	26,200,000	0.4%		12	Washington	159,400,000	2.2%
7	Illinois	283,400,000	3.8%		13	Maryland	152,500,000	2.1%
20	Indiana	135,200,000	1.8%		14	Louisiana	147,200,000	2.0%
31	Iowa	69,600,000	0.9%		15	North Carolina	146,400,000	2.0%
33	Kansas	61,000,000	0.8%		16	Georgia	145,700,000	2.0%
25	Kentucky	105,200,000	1.4%		17	Tennessee	143,600,000	1.9%
14	Louisiana	147,200,000	2.0%		18	Missouri	140,200,000	1.9%
34	Maine	53,500,000	0.7%		19	Wisconsin	136,800,000	1.8%
13	Maryland	152,500,000	2.1%		20	Indiana	135,200,000	1.8%
9	Massachusetts	264,400,000	3.6%		21	Connecticut	129,800,000	1.8%
8	Michigan	265,300,000	3.6%		22	Virginia	121,200,000	1.6%
11	Minnesota	166,500,000	2.3%		23	Mississippi	112,600,000	1.5%
23	Mississippi	112,600,000	1.5%		24	Arizona	106,300,000	1.4%
18	Missouri	140,200,000	1.9%		25	Kentucky	105,200,000	1.4%
46	Montana	31,900,000	0.4%		26	Alabama	97,000,000	1.3%
41	Nebraska	39,300,000	0.5%		27	Colorado	95,200,000	1.3%
39	Nevada	42,200,000	0.6%		28	Oregon	83,000,000	1.1%
38	New Hampshire	44,400,000	0.6%		29	Oklahoma	82,000,000	1.1%
10	New Jersey	239,900,000	3.2%		30	South Carolina	76,500,000	1.0%
40	New Mexico	41,200,000	0.6%		31	Iowa	69,600,000	0.9%
1	New York	762,300,000	10.3%		32	West Virginia	67,200,000	0.9%
15	North Carolina	146,400,000	2.0%		33	Kansas	61,000,000	0.8%
44	North Dakota	33,800,000	0.5%		34	Maine	53,500,000	0.7%
6	Ohio	305,500,000	4.1%		35	Arkansas	52,500,000	0.7%
29	Oklahoma	82,000,000	1.1%		36	Hawaii	51,800,000	0.7%
28	Oregon	83,000,000	1.1%		37	Rhode Island	48,900,000	0.7%
5	Pennsylvania	349,200,000	4.7%		38	New Hampshire	44,400,000	0.6%
37	Rhode Island	48,900,000	0.7%		39	Nevada	42,200,000	0.6%
30	South Carolina	76,500,000	1.0%		40	New Mexico	41,200,000	0.6%
49	South Dakota	25,400,000	0.3%		41	Nebraska	39,300,000	0.5%
17	Tennessee	143,600,000	1.9%		42	Utah	38,900,000	0.5%
3	Texas	466,200,000	6.3%		43	Vermont	36,900,000	0.5%
42	Utah	38,900,000	0.5%		44	North Dakota	33,800,000	0.5%
43	Vermont	36,900,000	0.5%		45	Alaska	32,200,000	0.4%
22	Virginia	121,200,000	1.6%		46	Montana	31,900,000	0.4%
12	Washington	159,400,000	2.2%		47	Delaware	28,000,000	0.4%
32	West Virginia	67,200,000	0.9%		48	Idaho	26,200,000	0.4%
19	Wisconsin	136,800,000	1.8%		49	South Dakota	25,400,000	0.3%
50	Wyoming	19,700,000	0.3%		50	Wyoming	19,700,000	0.3%
						District of Columbia	40,000,000	0.5%

Source: Campaign for Tobacco-Free Kids
   "A Broken Promise to Our Children" (http://tobaccofreekids.org/reports/settlements/)
*For fiscal year 2011. Settlement originally reached in November 1998 and called for an estimated 25 years of payments.

Annual Smoking-Related Health Costs in 2010

National Estimate = $96,700,000,000*

ALPHA ORDER					RANK ORDER			
RANK	STATE	COSTS	% of USA		RANK	STATE	COSTS	% of USA
23	Alabama	$1,490,000,000	1.5%		1	California	$9,140,000,000	9.5%
49	Alaska	169,000,000	0.2%		2	New York	8,170,000,000	8.4%
26	Arizona	1,300,000,000	1.3%		3	Florida	6,320,000,000	6.5%
32	Arkansas	812,000,000	0.8%		4	Texas	5,830,000,000	6.0%
1	California	9,140,000,000	9.5%		5	Pennsylvania	5,190,000,000	5.4%
25	Colorado	1,310,000,000	1.4%		6	Ohio	4,370,000,000	4.5%
21	Connecticut	1,630,000,000	1.7%		7	Illinois	4,100,000,000	4.2%
44	Delaware	284,000,000	0.3%		8	Massachusetts	3,540,000,000	3.7%
3	Florida	6,320,000,000	6.5%		9	Michigan	3,400,000,000	3.5%
12	Georgia	2,250,000,000	2.3%		10	New Jersey	3,170,000,000	3.3%
42	Hawaii	336,000,000	0.3%		11	North Carolina	2,460,000,000	2.5%
43	Idaho	319,000,000	0.3%		12	Georgia	2,250,000,000	2.3%
7	Illinois	4,100,000,000	4.2%		13	Tennessee	2,160,000,000	2.2%
15	Indiana	2,080,000,000	2.2%		14	Missouri	2,130,000,000	2.2%
30	Iowa	1,010,000,000	1.0%		15	Indiana	2,080,000,000	2.2%
31	Kansas	927,000,000	1.0%		15	Virginia	2,080,000,000	2.2%
22	Kentucky	1,500,000,000	1.6%		17	Minnesota	2,060,000,000	2.1%
24	Louisiana	1,470,000,000	1.5%		18	Wisconsin	2,020,000,000	2.1%
35	Maine	602,000,000	0.6%		19	Maryland	1,960,000,000	2.0%
19	Maryland	1,960,000,000	2.0%		20	Washington	1,950,000,000	2.0%
8	Massachusetts	3,540,000,000	3.7%		21	Connecticut	1,630,000,000	1.7%
9	Michigan	3,400,000,000	3.5%		22	Kentucky	1,500,000,000	1.6%
17	Minnesota	2,060,000,000	2.1%		23	Alabama	1,490,000,000	1.5%
33	Mississippi	719,000,000	0.7%		24	Louisiana	1,470,000,000	1.5%
14	Missouri	2,130,000,000	2.2%		25	Colorado	1,310,000,000	1.4%
45	Montana	277,000,000	0.3%		26	Arizona	1,300,000,000	1.3%
38	Nebraska	537,000,000	0.6%		27	Oklahoma	1,160,000,000	1.2%
36	Nevada	565,000,000	0.6%		28	Oregon	1,110,000,000	1.1%
37	New Hampshire	564,000,000	0.6%		29	South Carolina	1,090,000,000	1.1%
10	New Jersey	3,170,000,000	3.3%		30	Iowa	1,010,000,000	1.0%
40	New Mexico	461,000,000	0.5%		31	Kansas	927,000,000	1.0%
2	New York	8,170,000,000	8.4%		32	Arkansas	812,000,000	0.8%
11	North Carolina	2,460,000,000	2.5%		33	Mississippi	719,000,000	0.7%
47	North Dakota	247,000,000	0.3%		34	West Virginia	690,000,000	0.7%
6	Ohio	4,370,000,000	4.5%		35	Maine	602,000,000	0.6%
27	Oklahoma	1,160,000,000	1.2%		36	Nevada	565,000,000	0.6%
28	Oregon	1,110,000,000	1.1%		37	New Hampshire	564,000,000	0.6%
5	Pennsylvania	5,190,000,000	5.4%		38	Nebraska	537,000,000	0.6%
39	Rhode Island	506,000,000	0.5%		39	Rhode Island	506,000,000	0.5%
29	South Carolina	1,090,000,000	1.1%		40	New Mexico	461,000,000	0.5%
46	South Dakota	274,000,000	0.3%		41	Utah	345,000,000	0.4%
13	Tennessee	2,160,000,000	2.2%		42	Hawaii	336,000,000	0.3%
4	Texas	5,830,000,000	6.0%		43	Idaho	319,000,000	0.3%
41	Utah	345,000,000	0.4%		44	Delaware	284,000,000	0.3%
48	Vermont	233,000,000	0.2%		45	Montana	277,000,000	0.3%
15	Virginia	2,080,000,000	2.2%		46	South Dakota	274,000,000	0.3%
20	Washington	1,950,000,000	2.0%		47	North Dakota	247,000,000	0.3%
34	West Virginia	690,000,000	0.7%		48	Vermont	233,000,000	0.2%
18	Wisconsin	2,020,000,000	2.1%		49	Alaska	169,000,000	0.2%
50	Wyoming	136,000,000	0.1%		50	Wyoming	136,000,000	0.1%
						District of Columbia	243,000,000	0.3%

Source: Campaign for Tobacco-Free Kids
"A Decade of Broken Promises" (http://tobaccofreekids.org/reports/settlements/)
*Estimate based on figures from Centers for Disease Control and Prevention.

Personal Health Care Expenditures in 2004

National Total = $1,551,255,000,000*

ALPHA ORDER

RANK	STATE	EXPENDITURES	% of USA
22	Alabama	$23,199,000,000	1.5%
46	Alaska	4,237,000,000	0.3%
21	Arizona	23,576,000,000	1.5%
33	Arkansas	13,357,000,000	0.9%
1	California	166,236,000,000	10.7%
26	Colorado	21,691,000,000	1.4%
25	Connecticut	22,167,000,000	1.4%
44	Delaware	5,226,000,000	0.3%
4	Florida	95,223,000,000	6.1%
12	Georgia	41,097,000,000	2.6%
42	Hawaii	6,222,000,000	0.4%
43	Idaho	6,197,000,000	0.4%
6	Illinois	67,292,000,000	4.3%
14	Indiana	32,951,000,000	2.1%
30	Iowa	15,892,000,000	1.0%
31	Kansas	14,736,000,000	0.9%
23	Kentucky	22,662,000,000	1.5%
24	Louisiana	22,658,000,000	1.5%
38	Maine	8,593,000,000	0.6%
19	Maryland	31,044,000,000	2.0%
11	Massachusetts	43,009,000,000	2.8%
8	Michigan	51,048,000,000	3.3%
20	Minnesota	29,524,000,000	1.9%
32	Mississippi	14,634,000,000	0.9%
17	Missouri	31,317,000,000	2.0%
45	Montana	4,706,000,000	0.3%
36	Nebraska	9,782,000,000	0.6%
35	Nevada	10,656,000,000	0.7%
40	New Hampshire	7,050,000,000	0.5%
9	New Jersey	50,384,000,000	3.2%
39	New Mexico	8,498,000,000	0.5%
2	New York	126,076,000,000	8.1%
10	North Carolina	44,281,000,000	2.9%
49	North Dakota	3,693,000,000	0.2%
7	Ohio	65,622,000,000	4.2%
29	Oklahoma	17,323,000,000	1.1%
28	Oregon	17,516,000,000	1.1%
5	Pennsylvania	73,441,000,000	4.7%
41	Rhode Island	6,682,000,000	0.4%
27	South Carolina	21,450,000,000	1.4%
47	South Dakota	4,103,000,000	0.3%
15	Tennessee	32,161,000,000	2.1%
3	Texas	103,600,000,000	6.7%
37	Utah	9,618,000,000	0.6%
48	Vermont	3,768,000,000	0.2%
13	Virginia	36,032,000,000	2.3%
16	Washington	31,600,000,000	2.0%
34	West Virginia	10,783,000,000	0.7%
18	Wisconsin	31,177,000,000	2.0%
50	Wyoming	2,662,000,000	0.2%

RANK ORDER

RANK	STATE	EXPENDITURES	% of USA
1	California	$166,236,000,000	10.7%
2	New York	126,076,000,000	8.1%
3	Texas	103,600,000,000	6.7%
4	Florida	95,223,000,000	6.1%
5	Pennsylvania	73,441,000,000	4.7%
6	Illinois	67,292,000,000	4.3%
7	Ohio	65,622,000,000	4.2%
8	Michigan	51,048,000,000	3.3%
9	New Jersey	50,384,000,000	3.2%
10	North Carolina	44,281,000,000	2.9%
11	Massachusetts	43,009,000,000	2.8%
12	Georgia	41,097,000,000	2.6%
13	Virginia	36,032,000,000	2.3%
14	Indiana	32,951,000,000	2.1%
15	Tennessee	32,161,000,000	2.1%
16	Washington	31,600,000,000	2.0%
17	Missouri	31,317,000,000	2.0%
18	Wisconsin	31,177,000,000	2.0%
19	Maryland	31,044,000,000	2.0%
20	Minnesota	29,524,000,000	1.9%
21	Arizona	23,576,000,000	1.5%
22	Alabama	23,199,000,000	1.5%
23	Kentucky	22,662,000,000	1.5%
24	Louisiana	22,658,000,000	1.5%
25	Connecticut	22,167,000,000	1.4%
26	Colorado	21,691,000,000	1.4%
27	South Carolina	21,450,000,000	1.4%
28	Oregon	17,516,000,000	1.1%
29	Oklahoma	17,323,000,000	1.1%
30	Iowa	15,892,000,000	1.0%
31	Kansas	14,736,000,000	0.9%
32	Mississippi	14,634,000,000	0.9%
33	Arkansas	13,357,000,000	0.9%
34	West Virginia	10,783,000,000	0.7%
35	Nevada	10,656,000,000	0.7%
36	Nebraska	9,782,000,000	0.6%
37	Utah	9,618,000,000	0.6%
38	Maine	8,593,000,000	0.6%
39	New Mexico	8,498,000,000	0.5%
40	New Hampshire	7,050,000,000	0.5%
41	Rhode Island	6,682,000,000	0.4%
42	Hawaii	6,222,000,000	0.4%
43	Idaho	6,197,000,000	0.4%
44	Delaware	5,226,000,000	0.3%
45	Montana	4,706,000,000	0.3%
46	Alaska	4,237,000,000	0.3%
47	South Dakota	4,103,000,000	0.3%
48	Vermont	3,768,000,000	0.2%
49	North Dakota	3,693,000,000	0.2%
50	Wyoming	2,662,000,000	0.2%
	District of Columbia	4,809,000,000	0.3%

Source: U.S. Department of Health and Human Services, Centers for Medicare and Medicaid Services
   "State Health Care Expenditures" (http://www.cms.hhs.gov/NationalHealthExpendData/)
*By state of residence. Includes hospital care, physician services, dental services, home health care, drugs, vision products, nursing home care, and other personal health care services and products.

Health Care Expenditures as a Percent of Gross State Product in 2004

National Percent = 13.3% of Total Gross State Product*

ALPHA ORDER				RANK ORDER		
RANK	STATE	PERCENT		RANK	STATE	PERCENT
7	Alabama	16.2		1	West Virginia	20.3
44	Alaska	11.6		2	Maine	19.4
36	Arizona	12.5		3	Mississippi	18.1
16	Arkansas	15.4		4	North Dakota	17.6
46	California	11.0		5	Kentucky	16.9
45	Colorado	11.1		6	Montana	16.7
40	Connecticut	12.1		7	Alabama	16.2
49	Delaware	9.7		7	Rhode Island	16.2
13	Florida	15.6		7	Vermont	16.2
38	Georgia	12.2		10	Pennsylvania	16.1
36	Hawaii	12.5		11	Missouri	15.7
32	Idaho	13.0		11	South Carolina	15.7
38	Illinois	12.2		13	Florida	15.6
20	Indiana	14.4		13	Tennessee	15.6
27	Iowa	13.7		15	Ohio	15.5
20	Kansas	14.4		16	Arkansas	15.4
5	Kentucky	16.9		17	Oklahoma	14.8
23	Louisiana	14.2		17	Wisconsin	14.8
2	Maine	19.4		19	Nebraska	14.5
31	Maryland	13.3		20	Indiana	14.4
24	Massachusetts	14.1		20	Kansas	14.4
29	Michigan	13.5		20	South Dakota	14.4
27	Minnesota	13.7		23	Louisiana	14.2
3	Mississippi	18.1		24	Massachusetts	14.1
11	Missouri	15.7		25	New York	13.9
6	Montana	16.7		26	North Carolina	13.8
19	Nebraska	14.5		27	Iowa	13.7
46	Nevada	11.0		27	Minnesota	13.7
29	New Hampshire	13.5		29	Michigan	13.5
42	New Jersey	11.8		29	New Hampshire	13.5
34	New Mexico	12.6		31	Maryland	13.3
25	New York	13.9		32	Idaho	13.0
26	North Carolina	13.8		32	Oregon	13.0
4	North Dakota	17.6		34	New Mexico	12.6
15	Ohio	15.5		34	Washington	12.6
17	Oklahoma	14.8		36	Arizona	12.5
32	Oregon	13.0		36	Hawaii	12.5
10	Pennsylvania	16.1		38	Georgia	12.2
7	Rhode Island	16.2		38	Illinois	12.2
11	South Carolina	15.7		40	Connecticut	12.1
20	South Dakota	14.4		40	Utah	12.1
13	Tennessee	15.6		42	New Jersey	11.8
43	Texas	11.7		43	Texas	11.7
40	Utah	12.1		44	Alaska	11.6
7	Vermont	16.2		45	Colorado	11.1
48	Virginia	10.9		46	California	11.0
34	Washington	12.6		46	Nevada	11.0
1	West Virginia	20.3		48	Virginia	10.9
17	Wisconsin	14.8		49	Delaware	9.7
50	Wyoming	9.4		50	Wyoming	9.4
					District of Columbia	8.1

Source: U.S. Department of Health and Human Services, Centers for Medicare and Medicaid Services
"State Health Care Expenditures" (http://www.cms.hhs.gov/NationalHealthExpendData/)
*By state of provider. Includes hospital care, physician services, dental services, home health care, drugs, vision products, nursing home care, and other personal health care services and products.

Per Capita Personal Health Care Expenditures in 2004

National Per Capita = $5,283*

ALPHA ORDER			RANK ORDER		
RANK	STATE	PER CAPITA	RANK	STATE	PER CAPITA
30	Alabama	$5,135	1	Massachusetts	$6,683
4	Alaska	6,450	2	Maine	6,540
49	Arizona	4,103	3	New York	6,535
40	Arkansas	4,863	4	Alaska	6,450
43	California	4,638	5	Connecticut	6,344
42	Colorado	4,717	6	Delaware	6,306
5	Connecticut	6,344	7	Rhode Island	6,193
6	Delaware	6,306	8	Vermont	6,069
18	Florida	5,483	9	West Virginia	5,954
45	Georgia	4,600	10	Pennsylvania	5,933
37	Hawaii	4,941	11	North Dakota	5,808
48	Idaho	4,444	12	New Jersey	5,807
27	Illinois	5,293	13	Minnesota	5,795
26	Indiana	5,295	14	Ohio	5,725
24	Iowa	5,380	15	Wisconsin	5,670
23	Kansas	5,382	16	Nebraska	5,599
19	Kentucky	5,473	17	Maryland	5,590
36	Louisiana	5,040	18	Florida	5,483
2	Maine	6,540	19	Kentucky	5,473
17	Maryland	5,590	20	Tennessee	5,464
1	Massachusetts	6,683	21	Missouri	5,444
35	Michigan	5,058	22	New Hampshire	5,432
13	Minnesota	5,795	23	Kansas	5,382
34	Mississippi	5,059	24	Iowa	5,380
21	Missouri	5,444	25	South Dakota	5,327
33	Montana	5,080	26	Indiana	5,295
16	Nebraska	5,599	27	Illinois	5,293
46	Nevada	4,569	28	Wyoming	5,265
22	New Hampshire	5,432	29	North Carolina	5,191
12	New Jersey	5,807	30	Alabama	5,135
47	New Mexico	4,471	31	South Carolina	5,114
3	New York	6,535	32	Washington	5,092
29	North Carolina	5,191	33	Montana	5,080
11	North Dakota	5,808	34	Mississippi	5,059
14	Ohio	5,725	35	Michigan	5,058
38	Oklahoma	4,917	36	Louisiana	5,040
39	Oregon	4,880	37	Hawaii	4,941
10	Pennsylvania	5,933	38	Oklahoma	4,917
7	Rhode Island	6,193	39	Oregon	4,880
31	South Carolina	5,114	40	Arkansas	4,863
25	South Dakota	5,327	41	Virginia	4,822
20	Tennessee	5,464	42	Colorado	4,717
44	Texas	4,601	43	California	4,638
50	Utah	3,972	44	Texas	4,601
8	Vermont	6,069	45	Georgia	4,600
41	Virginia	4,822	46	Nevada	4,569
32	Washington	5,092	47	New Mexico	4,471
9	West Virginia	5,954	48	Idaho	4,444
15	Wisconsin	5,670	49	Arizona	4,103
28	Wyoming	5,265	50	Utah	3,972
				District of Columbia	8,295

Source: U.S. Department of Health and Human Services, Centers for Medicare and Medicaid Services
     "State Health Care Expenditures" (http://www.cms.hhs.gov/NationalHealthExpendData/)
*By state of provider. Includes hospital care, physician services, dental services, home health care, drugs, vision products,
nursing home care, and other personal health care services and products.

Average Annual Growth in Personal Health Care Expenditures: 1991 to 2004

National Average = 6.7% Annual Growth*

ALPHA ORDER				RANK ORDER		
RANK	STATE	ANNUAL GROWTH		RANK	STATE	ANNUAL GROWTH
37	Alabama	6.4		1	Nevada	10.0
3	Alaska	8.4		2	North Carolina	8.6
10	Arizona	7.7		3	Alaska	8.4
30	Arkansas	6.9		3	Idaho	8.4
48	California	5.7		3	Vermont	8.4
10	Colorado	7.7		6	Maine	8.3
48	Connecticut	5.7		6	Utah	8.3
8	Delaware	8.0		8	Delaware	8.0
26	Florida	7.1		9	South Carolina	7.8
23	Georgia	7.2		10	Arizona	7.7
45	Hawaii	5.9		10	Colorado	7.7
3	Idaho	8.4		10	Oregon	7.7
44	Illinois	6.1		10	Wyoming	7.7
31	Indiana	6.8		14	Minnesota	7.6
37	Iowa	6.4		14	Mississippi	7.6
34	Kansas	6.6		14	Nebraska	7.6
18	Kentucky	7.5		14	New Hampshire	7.6
48	Louisiana	5.7		18	Kentucky	7.5
6	Maine	8.3		19	Tennessee	7.4
34	Maryland	6.6		19	Texas	7.4
40	Massachusetts	6.3		21	Montana	7.3
46	Michigan	5.8		21	Washington	7.3
14	Minnesota	7.6		23	Georgia	7.2
14	Mississippi	7.6		23	New Mexico	7.2
27	Missouri	7.0		23	Wisconsin	7.2
21	Montana	7.3		26	Florida	7.1
14	Nebraska	7.6		27	Missouri	7.0
1	Nevada	10.0		27	South Dakota	7.0
14	New Hampshire	7.6		27	Virginia	7.0
40	New Jersey	6.3		30	Arkansas	6.9
23	New Mexico	7.2		31	Indiana	6.8
40	New York	6.3		31	West Virginia	6.8
2	North Carolina	8.6		33	Oklahoma	6.7
40	North Dakota	6.3		34	Kansas	6.6
37	Ohio	6.4		34	Maryland	6.6
33	Oklahoma	6.7		34	Rhode Island	6.6
10	Oregon	7.7		37	Alabama	6.4
46	Pennsylvania	5.8		37	Iowa	6.4
34	Rhode Island	6.6		37	Ohio	6.4
9	South Carolina	7.8		40	Massachusetts	6.3
27	South Dakota	7.0		40	New Jersey	6.3
19	Tennessee	7.4		40	New York	6.3
19	Texas	7.4		40	North Dakota	6.3
6	Utah	8.3		44	Illinois	6.1
3	Vermont	8.4		45	Hawaii	5.9
27	Virginia	7.0		46	Michigan	5.8
21	Washington	7.3		46	Pennsylvania	5.8
31	West Virginia	6.8		48	California	5.7
23	Wisconsin	7.2		48	Connecticut	5.7
10	Wyoming	7.7		48	Louisiana	5.7
					District of Columbia	4.1

Source: U.S. Department of Health and Human Services, Centers for Medicare and Medicaid Services
"State Health Care Expenditures" (http://www.cms.hhs.gov/NationalHealthExpendData/)
*By state of residence. Includes hospital care, physician services, dental services, home health care, drugs, vision products, nursing home care, and other personal health care services and products.

Expenditures for Hospital Care in 2004

National Total = $566,886,000,000*

ALPHA ORDER

RANK	STATE	EXPENDITURES	% of USA
25	Alabama	$7,938,000,000	1.4%
47	Alaska	1,704,000,000	0.3%
22	Arizona	8,499,000,000	1.5%
33	Arkansas	5,092,000,000	0.9%
1	California	57,805,000,000	10.2%
26	Colorado	7,624,000,000	1.3%
27	Conncoticut	7,029,000,000	1.2%
45	Delaware	1,917,000,000	0.3%
4	Florida	31,494,000,000	5.6%
12	Georgia	14,613,000,000	2.6%
42	Hawaii	2,310,000,000	0.4%
43	Idaho	2,298,000,000	0.4%
6	Illinois	25,801,000,000	4.6%
15	Indiana	12,761,000,000	2.3%
29	Iowa	6,179,000,000	1.1%
32	Kansas	5,157,000,000	0.9%
24	Kentucky	8,283,000,000	1.5%
21	Louisiana	9,145,000,000	1.6%
39	Maine	3,035,000,000	0.5%
17	Maryland	11,559,000,000	2.0%
10	Massachusetts	16,865,000,000	3.0%
8	Michigan	20,206,000,000	3.6%
20	Minnesota	10,009,000,000	1.8%
30	Mississippi	6,129,000,000	1.1%
14	Missouri	12,993,000,000	2.3%
44	Montana	1,944,000,000	0.3%
35	Nebraska	3,938,000,000	0.7%
37	Nevada	3,459,000,000	0.6%
40	New Hampshire	2,519,000,000	0.4%
9	New Jersey	17,024,000,000	3.0%
38	New Mexico	3,315,000,000	0.6%
2	New York	45,569,000,000	8.0%
11	North Carolina	16,294,000,000	2.9%
48	North Dakota	1,533,000,000	0.3%
7	Ohio	24,822,000,000	4.4%
28	Oklahoma	6,659,000,000	1.2%
31	Oregon	5,998,000,000	1.1%
5	Pennsylvania	26,715,000,000	4.7%
41	Rhode Island	2,437,000,000	0.4%
23	South Carolina	8,316,000,000	1.5%
46	South Dakota	1,753,000,000	0.3%
18	Tennessee	10,744,000,000	1.9%
3	Texas	38,910,000,000	6.9%
36	Utah	3,468,000,000	0.6%
49	Vermont	1,446,000,000	0.3%
13	Virginia	13,361,000,000	2.4%
19	Washington	10,702,000,000	1.9%
34	West Virginia	4,432,000,000	0.8%
16	Wisconsin	11,625,000,000	2.1%
50	Wyoming	1,095,000,000	0.2%

RANK ORDER

RANK	STATE	EXPENDITURES	% of USA
1	California	$57,805,000,000	10.2%
2	New York	45,569,000,000	8.0%
3	Texas	38,910,000,000	6.9%
4	Florida	31,494,000,000	5.6%
5	Pennsylvania	26,715,000,000	4.7%
6	Illinois	25,801,000,000	4.6%
7	Ohio	24,822,000,000	4.4%
8	Michigan	20,206,000,000	3.6%
9	New Jersey	17,024,000,000	3.0%
10	Massachusetts	16,865,000,000	3.0%
11	North Carolina	16,294,000,000	2.9%
12	Georgia	14,613,000,000	2.6%
13	Virginia	13,361,000,000	2.4%
14	Missouri	12,993,000,000	2.3%
15	Indiana	12,761,000,000	2.3%
16	Wisconsin	11,625,000,000	2.1%
17	Maryland	11,559,000,000	2.0%
18	Tennessee	10,744,000,000	1.9%
19	Washington	10,702,000,000	1.9%
20	Minnesota	10,009,000,000	1.8%
21	Louisiana	9,145,000,000	1.6%
22	Arizona	8,499,000,000	1.5%
23	South Carolina	8,316,000,000	1.5%
24	Kentucky	8,283,000,000	1.5%
25	Alabama	7,938,000,000	1.4%
26	Colorado	7,624,000,000	1.3%
27	Connecticut	7,029,000,000	1.2%
28	Oklahoma	6,659,000,000	1.2%
29	Iowa	6,179,000,000	1.1%
30	Mississippi	6,129,000,000	1.1%
31	Oregon	5,998,000,000	1.1%
32	Kansas	5,157,000,000	0.9%
33	Arkansas	5,092,000,000	0.9%
34	West Virginia	4,432,000,000	0.8%
35	Nebraska	3,938,000,000	0.7%
36	Utah	3,468,000,000	0.6%
37	Nevada	3,459,000,000	0.6%
38	New Mexico	3,315,000,000	0.6%
39	Maine	3,035,000,000	0.5%
40	New Hampshire	2,519,000,000	0.4%
41	Rhode Island	2,437,000,000	0.4%
42	Hawaii	2,310,000,000	0.4%
43	Idaho	2,298,000,000	0.4%
44	Montana	1,944,000,000	0.3%
45	Delaware	1,917,000,000	0.3%
46	South Dakota	1,753,000,000	0.3%
47	Alaska	1,704,000,000	0.3%
48	North Dakota	1,533,000,000	0.3%
49	Vermont	1,446,000,000	0.3%
50	Wyoming	1,095,000,000	0.2%
	District of Columbia	2,366,000,000	0.4%

Source: U.S. Department of Health and Human Services, Centers for Medicare and Medicaid Services
"State Health Care Expenditures" (http://www.cms.hhs.gov/NationalHealthExpendData/)
*By state of residence.

Percent of Total Personal Health Care Expenditures
Spent on Hospital Care in 2004
National Percent = 36.5%*

ALPHA ORDER

RANK	STATE	PERCENT
42	Alabama	34.2
10	Alaska	40.2
35	Arizona	36.0
20	Arkansas	38.1
41	California	34.8
39	Colorado	35.1
50	Connecticut	31.7
29	Delaware	36.7
48	Florida	33.1
37	Georgia	35.6
25	Hawaii	37.1
25	Idaho	37.1
19	Illinois	38.3
16	Indiana	38.7
14	Iowa	38.9
40	Kansas	35.0
30	Kentucky	36.6
8	Louisiana	40.4
38	Maine	35.3
24	Maryland	37.2
12	Massachusetts	39.2
11	Michigan	39.6
44	Minnesota	33.9
2	Mississippi	41.9
3	Missouri	41.5
5	Montana	41.3
9	Nebraska	40.3
49	Nevada	32.5
36	New Hampshire	35.7
46	New Jersey	33.8
13	New Mexico	39.0
33	New York	36.1
28	North Carolina	36.8
3	North Dakota	41.5
21	Ohio	37.8
17	Oklahoma	38.4
42	Oregon	34.2
32	Pennsylvania	36.4
31	Rhode Island	36.5
15	South Carolina	38.8
1	South Dakota	42.7
47	Tennessee	33.4
22	Texas	37.6
33	Utah	36.1
17	Vermont	38.4
25	Virginia	37.1
44	Washington	33.9
6	West Virginia	41.1
23	Wisconsin	37.3
6	Wyoming	41.1

RANK ORDER

RANK	STATE	PERCENT
1	South Dakota	42.7
2	Mississippi	41.9
3	Missouri	41.5
3	North Dakota	41.5
5	Montana	41.3
6	West Virginia	41.1
6	Wyoming	41.1
8	Louisiana	40.4
9	Nebraska	40.3
10	Alaska	40.2
11	Michigan	39.6
12	Massachusetts	39.2
13	New Mexico	39.0
14	Iowa	38.9
15	South Carolina	38.8
16	Indiana	38.7
17	Oklahoma	38.4
17	Vermont	38.4
19	Illinois	38.3
20	Arkansas	38.1
21	Ohio	37.8
22	Texas	37.6
23	Wisconsin	37.3
24	Maryland	37.2
25	Hawaii	37.1
25	Idaho	37.1
25	Virginia	37.1
28	North Carolina	36.8
29	Delaware	36.7
30	Kentucky	36.6
31	Rhode Island	36.5
32	Pennsylvania	36.4
33	New York	36.1
33	Utah	36.1
35	Arizona	36.0
36	New Hampshire	35.7
37	Georgia	35.6
38	Maine	35.3
39	Colorado	35.1
40	Kansas	35.0
41	California	34.8
42	Alabama	34.2
42	Oregon	34.2
44	Minnesota	33.9
44	Washington	33.9
46	New Jersey	33.8
47	Tennessee	33.4
48	Florida	33.1
49	Nevada	32.5
50	Connecticut	31.7
	District of Columbia	49.2

Source: CQ Press using data from U.S. Department of Health and Human Services, Centers for Medicare and Medicaid Services
"State Health Care Expenditures" (http://www.cms.hhs.gov/NationalHealthExpendData/)
*By state of residence.

Per Capita Expenditures for Hospital Care in 2004

National Per Capita = $1,931*

<table>
<tr><td colspan="3">ALPHA ORDER</td><td colspan="3">RANK ORDER</td></tr>
<tr><td>RANK</td><td>STATE</td><td>PER CAPITA</td><td>RANK</td><td>STATE</td><td>PER CAPITA</td></tr>
<tr><td>39</td><td>Alabama</td><td>$1,757</td><td>1</td><td>Massachusetts</td><td>$2,620</td></tr>
<tr><td>2</td><td>Alaska</td><td>2,594</td><td>2</td><td>Alaska</td><td>2,594</td></tr>
<tr><td>49</td><td>Arizona</td><td>1,479</td><td>3</td><td>West Virginia</td><td>2,447</td></tr>
<tr><td>34</td><td>Arkansas</td><td>1,854</td><td>4</td><td>North Dakota</td><td>2,411</td></tr>
<tr><td>47</td><td>California</td><td>1,613</td><td>5</td><td>New York</td><td>2,362</td></tr>
<tr><td>44</td><td>Colorado</td><td>1,658</td><td>6</td><td>Vermont</td><td>2,329</td></tr>
<tr><td>24</td><td>Connecticut</td><td>2,012</td><td>7</td><td>Delaware</td><td>2,313</td></tr>
<tr><td>7</td><td>Delaware</td><td>2,313</td><td>8</td><td>Maine</td><td>2,310</td></tr>
<tr><td>37</td><td>Florida</td><td>1,813</td><td>9</td><td>South Dakota</td><td>2,276</td></tr>
<tr><td>46</td><td>Georgia</td><td>1,635</td><td>10</td><td>Missouri</td><td>2,259</td></tr>
<tr><td>35</td><td>Hawaii</td><td>1,834</td><td>10</td><td>Rhode Island</td><td>2,259</td></tr>
<tr><td>45</td><td>Idaho</td><td>1,648</td><td>12</td><td>Nebraska</td><td>2,254</td></tr>
<tr><td>23</td><td>Illinois</td><td>2,029</td><td>13</td><td>Ohio</td><td>2,166</td></tr>
<tr><td>21</td><td>Indiana</td><td>2,051</td><td>14</td><td>Wyoming</td><td>2,165</td></tr>
<tr><td>19</td><td>Iowa</td><td>2,092</td><td>15</td><td>Pennsylvania</td><td>2,158</td></tr>
<tr><td>33</td><td>Kansas</td><td>1,883</td><td>16</td><td>Mississippi</td><td>2,119</td></tr>
<tr><td>26</td><td>Kentucky</td><td>2,001</td><td>17</td><td>Wisconsin</td><td>2,114</td></tr>
<tr><td>22</td><td>Louisiana</td><td>2,034</td><td>18</td><td>Montana</td><td>2,099</td></tr>
<tr><td>8</td><td>Maine</td><td>2,310</td><td>19</td><td>Iowa</td><td>2,092</td></tr>
<tr><td>20</td><td>Maryland</td><td>2,081</td><td>20</td><td>Maryland</td><td>2,081</td></tr>
<tr><td>1</td><td>Massachusetts</td><td>2,620</td><td>21</td><td>Indiana</td><td>2,051</td></tr>
<tr><td>25</td><td>Michigan</td><td>2,002</td><td>22</td><td>Louisiana</td><td>2,034</td></tr>
<tr><td>28</td><td>Minnesota</td><td>1,965</td><td>23</td><td>Illinois</td><td>2,029</td></tr>
<tr><td>16</td><td>Mississippi</td><td>2,119</td><td>24</td><td>Connecticut</td><td>2,012</td></tr>
<tr><td>10</td><td>Missouri</td><td>2,259</td><td>25</td><td>Michigan</td><td>2,002</td></tr>
<tr><td>18</td><td>Montana</td><td>2,099</td><td>26</td><td>Kentucky</td><td>2,001</td></tr>
<tr><td>12</td><td>Nebraska</td><td>2,254</td><td>27</td><td>South Carolina</td><td>1,982</td></tr>
<tr><td>48</td><td>Nevada</td><td>1,483</td><td>28</td><td>Minnesota</td><td>1,965</td></tr>
<tr><td>30</td><td>New Hampshire</td><td>1,941</td><td>29</td><td>New Jersey</td><td>1,962</td></tr>
<tr><td>29</td><td>New Jersey</td><td>1,962</td><td>30</td><td>New Hampshire</td><td>1,941</td></tr>
<tr><td>40</td><td>New Mexico</td><td>1,744</td><td>31</td><td>North Carolina</td><td>1,910</td></tr>
<tr><td>5</td><td>New York</td><td>2,362</td><td>32</td><td>Oklahoma</td><td>1,890</td></tr>
<tr><td>31</td><td>North Carolina</td><td>1,910</td><td>33</td><td>Kansas</td><td>1,883</td></tr>
<tr><td>4</td><td>North Dakota</td><td>2,411</td><td>34</td><td>Arkansas</td><td>1,854</td></tr>
<tr><td>13</td><td>Ohio</td><td>2,166</td><td>35</td><td>Hawaii</td><td>1,834</td></tr>
<tr><td>32</td><td>Oklahoma</td><td>1,890</td><td>36</td><td>Tennessee</td><td>1,826</td></tr>
<tr><td>43</td><td>Oregon</td><td>1,671</td><td>37</td><td>Florida</td><td>1,813</td></tr>
<tr><td>15</td><td>Pennsylvania</td><td>2,158</td><td>38</td><td>Virginia</td><td>1,788</td></tr>
<tr><td>10</td><td>Rhode Island</td><td>2,259</td><td>39</td><td>Alabama</td><td>1,757</td></tr>
<tr><td>27</td><td>South Carolina</td><td>1,982</td><td>40</td><td>New Mexico</td><td>1,744</td></tr>
<tr><td>9</td><td>South Dakota</td><td>2,276</td><td>41</td><td>Texas</td><td>1,728</td></tr>
<tr><td>36</td><td>Tennessee</td><td>1,826</td><td>42</td><td>Washington</td><td>1,725</td></tr>
<tr><td>41</td><td>Texas</td><td>1,728</td><td>43</td><td>Oregon</td><td>1,671</td></tr>
<tr><td>50</td><td>Utah</td><td>1,432</td><td>44</td><td>Colorado</td><td>1,658</td></tr>
<tr><td>6</td><td>Vermont</td><td>2,329</td><td>45</td><td>Idaho</td><td>1,648</td></tr>
<tr><td>38</td><td>Virginia</td><td>1,788</td><td>46</td><td>Georgia</td><td>1,635</td></tr>
<tr><td>42</td><td>Washington</td><td>1,725</td><td>47</td><td>California</td><td>1,613</td></tr>
<tr><td>3</td><td>West Virginia</td><td>2,447</td><td>48</td><td>Nevada</td><td>1,483</td></tr>
<tr><td>17</td><td>Wisconsin</td><td>2,114</td><td>49</td><td>Arizona</td><td>1,479</td></tr>
<tr><td>14</td><td>Wyoming</td><td>2,165</td><td>50</td><td>Utah</td><td>1,432</td></tr>
<tr><td></td><td></td><td></td><td></td><td>District of Columbia</td><td>4,081</td></tr>
</table>

Source: U.S. Department of Health and Human Services, Centers for Medicare and Medicaid Services
   "State Health Care Expenditures" (http://www.cms.hhs.gov/NationalHealthExpendData/)
*By state of residence.

Expenditures for Physician and Clinical Services in 2004

National Total = $393,713,000,000*

ALPHA ORDER

RANK	STATE	EXPENDITURES	% of USA
23	Alabama	$6,200,000,000	1.6%
45	Alaska	1,220,000,000	0.3%
21	Arizona	6,855,000,000	1.7%
33	Arkansas	3,316,000,000	0.8%
1	California	49,417,000,000	12.6%
22	Colorado	6,375,000,000	1.6%
27	Connecticut	5,155,000,000	1.3%
44	Delaware	1,228,000,000	0.3%
3	Florida	26,439,000,000	6.7%
10	Georgia	11,227,000,000	2.9%
41	Hawaii	1,587,000,000	0.4%
42	Idaho	1,466,000,000	0.4%
5	Illinois	16,984,000,000	4.3%
18	Indiana	7,869,000,000	2.0%
31	Iowa	3,719,000,000	0.9%
30	Kansas	4,144,000,000	1.1%
24	Kentucky	5,748,000,000	1.5%
26	Louisiana	5,271,000,000	1.3%
38	Maine	2,075,000,000	0.5%
17	Maryland	7,891,000,000	2.0%
13	Massachusetts	9,116,000,000	2.3%
9	Michigan	11,757,000,000	3.0%
19	Minnesota	7,757,000,000	2.0%
34	Mississippi	3,219,000,000	0.8%
20	Missouri	6,891,000,000	1.8%
46	Montana	1,157,000,000	0.3%
37	Nebraska	2,287,000,000	0.6%
32	Nevada	3,386,000,000	0.9%
40	New Hampshire	1,757,000,000	0.4%
8	New Jersey	12,265,000,000	3.1%
39	New Mexico	1,925,000,000	0.5%
4	New York	25,643,000,000	6.5%
11	North Carolina	10,248,000,000	2.6%
49	North Dakota	763,000,000	0.2%
7	Ohio	15,322,000,000	3.9%
29	Oklahoma	4,305,000,000	1.1%
28	Oregon	5,142,000,000	1.3%
6	Pennsylvania	16,942,000,000	4.3%
43	Rhode Island	1,325,000,000	0.3%
25	South Carolina	5,491,000,000	1.4%
47	South Dakota	920,000,000	0.2%
14	Tennessee	9,069,000,000	2.3%
2	Texas	28,769,000,000	7.3%
36	Utah	2,393,000,000	0.6%
48	Vermont	874,000,000	0.2%
12	Virginia	9,220,000,000	2.3%
15	Washington	9,004,000,000	2.3%
35	West Virginia	2,444,000,000	0.6%
16	Wisconsin	8,441,000,000	2.1%
50	Wyoming	670,000,000	0.2%

RANK ORDER

RANK	STATE	EXPENDITURES	% of USA
1	California	$49,417,000,000	12.6%
2	Texas	28,769,000,000	7.3%
3	Florida	26,439,000,000	6.7%
4	New York	25,643,000,000	6.5%
5	Illinois	16,984,000,000	4.3%
6	Pennsylvania	16,942,000,000	4.3%
7	Ohio	15,322,000,000	3.9%
8	New Jersey	12,265,000,000	3.1%
9	Michigan	11,757,000,000	3.0%
10	Georgia	11,227,000,000	2.9%
11	North Carolina	10,248,000,000	2.6%
12	Virginia	9,220,000,000	2.3%
13	Massachusetts	9,116,000,000	2.3%
14	Tennessee	9,069,000,000	2.3%
15	Washington	9,004,000,000	2.3%
16	Wisconsin	8,441,000,000	2.1%
17	Maryland	7,891,000,000	2.0%
18	Indiana	7,869,000,000	2.0%
19	Minnesota	7,757,000,000	2.0%
20	Missouri	6,891,000,000	1.8%
21	Arizona	6,855,000,000	1.7%
22	Colorado	6,375,000,000	1.6%
23	Alabama	6,200,000,000	1.6%
24	Kentucky	5,748,000,000	1.5%
25	South Carolina	5,491,000,000	1.4%
26	Louisiana	5,271,000,000	1.3%
27	Connecticut	5,155,000,000	1.3%
28	Oregon	5,142,000,000	1.3%
29	Oklahoma	4,305,000,000	1.1%
30	Kansas	4,144,000,000	1.1%
31	Iowa	3,719,000,000	0.9%
32	Nevada	3,386,000,000	0.9%
33	Arkansas	3,316,000,000	0.8%
34	Mississippi	3,219,000,000	0.8%
35	West Virginia	2,444,000,000	0.6%
36	Utah	2,393,000,000	0.6%
37	Nebraska	2,287,000,000	0.6%
38	Maine	2,075,000,000	0.5%
39	New Mexico	1,925,000,000	0.5%
40	New Hampshire	1,757,000,000	0.4%
41	Hawaii	1,587,000,000	0.4%
42	Idaho	1,466,000,000	0.4%
43	Rhode Island	1,325,000,000	0.3%
44	Delaware	1,228,000,000	0.3%
45	Alaska	1,220,000,000	0.3%
46	Montana	1,157,000,000	0.3%
47	South Dakota	920,000,000	0.2%
48	Vermont	874,000,000	0.2%
49	North Dakota	763,000,000	0.2%
50	Wyoming	670,000,000	0.2%
	District of Columbia	1,024,000,000	0.3%

Source: U.S. Department of Health and Human Services, Centers for Medicare and Medicaid Services
"State Health Care Expenditures" (http://www.cms.hhs.gov/NationalHealthExpendData/)
*By state of residence. Includes private physician offices and clinics, independently billing laboratories, and clinics run by the U.S. Department of Veterans Affairs and the U.S. Indian Health Service.

Percent of Total Personal Health Care Expenditures
Spent on Physician and Clinical Services in 2004
National Percent = 25.4%*

ALPHA ORDER

RANK	STATE	PERCENT
14	Alabama	26.7
6	Alaska	28.8
5	Arizona	29.1
26	Arkansas	24.8
2	California	29.7
3	Colorado	29.4
35	Connecticut	23.3
32	Delaware	23.5
10	Florida	27.8
12	Georgia	27.3
18	Hawaii	25.5
31	Idaho	23.7
21	Illinois	25.2
30	Indiana	23.9
33	Iowa	23.4
9	Kansas	28.1
19	Kentucky	25.4
35	Louisiana	23.3
29	Maine	24.1
19	Maryland	25.4
47	Massachusetts	21.2
41	Michigan	23.0
15	Minnesota	26.3
45	Mississippi	22.0
45	Missouri	22.0
27	Montana	24.6
33	Nebraska	23.4
1	Nevada	31.8
23	New Hampshire	24.9
28	New Jersey	24.3
42	New Mexico	22.7
49	New York	20.3
39	North Carolina	23.1
48	North Dakota	20.7
35	Ohio	23.3
23	Oklahoma	24.9
3	Oregon	29.4
39	Pennsylvania	23.1
50	Rhode Island	19.8
16	South Carolina	25.6
44	South Dakota	22.4
8	Tennessee	28.2
10	Texas	27.8
23	Utah	24.9
38	Vermont	23.2
16	Virginia	25.6
7	Washington	28.5
42	West Virginia	22.7
13	Wisconsin	27.1
21	Wyoming	25.2

RANK ORDER

RANK	STATE	PERCENT
1	Nevada	31.8
2	California	29.7
3	Colorado	29.4
3	Oregon	29.4
5	Arizona	29.1
6	Alaska	28.8
7	Washington	28.5
8	Tennessee	28.2
9	Kansas	28.1
10	Florida	27.8
10	Texas	27.8
12	Georgia	27.3
13	Wisconsin	27.1
14	Alabama	26.7
15	Minnesota	26.3
16	South Carolina	25.6
16	Virginia	25.6
18	Hawaii	25.5
19	Kentucky	25.4
19	Maryland	25.4
21	Illinois	25.2
21	Wyoming	25.2
23	New Hampshire	24.9
23	Oklahoma	24.9
23	Utah	24.9
26	Arkansas	24.8
27	Montana	24.6
28	New Jersey	24.3
29	Maine	24.1
30	Indiana	23.9
31	Idaho	23.7
32	Delaware	23.5
33	Iowa	23.4
33	Nebraska	23.4
35	Connecticut	23.3
35	Louisiana	23.3
35	Ohio	23.3
38	Vermont	23.2
39	North Carolina	23.1
39	Pennsylvania	23.1
41	Michigan	23.0
42	New Mexico	22.7
42	West Virginia	22.7
44	South Dakota	22.4
45	Mississippi	22.0
45	Missouri	22.0
47	Massachusetts	21.2
48	North Dakota	20.7
49	New York	20.3
50	Rhode Island	19.8

District of Columbia 21.3

Source: CQ Press using data from U.S. Department of Health and Human Services, Centers for Medicare and Medicaid Services
"State Health Care Expenditures" (http://www.cms.hhs.gov/NationalHealthExpendData/)
*By state of residence. Includes private physician offices and clinics, independently billing laboratories, and clinics run by the
U.S. Department of Veterans Affairs and the U.S. Indian Health Service.

Per Capita Expenditures for Physician and Clinical Services in 2004

National Per Capita = $1,341*

ALPHA ORDER

RANK	STATE	PER CAPITA
20	Alabama	$1,372
1	Alaska	1,858
44	Arizona	1,193
39	Arkansas	1,207
19	California	1,379
18	Colorado	1,386
9	Connecticut	1,475
8	Delaware	1,482
6	Florida	1,522
34	Georgia	1,257
32	Hawaii	1,260
48	Idaho	1,051
25	Illinois	1,336
31	Indiana	1,264
33	Iowa	1,259
7	Kansas	1,513
17	Kentucky	1,388
45	Louisiana	1,173
2	Maine	1,579
13	Maryland	1,421
14	Massachusetts	1,416
46	Michigan	1,165
5	Minnesota	1,523
47	Mississippi	1,113
42	Missouri	1,198
35	Montana	1,249
28	Nebraska	1,309
10	Nevada	1,451
22	New Hampshire	1,354
15	New Jersey	1,414
49	New Mexico	1,013
26	New York	1,329
40	North Carolina	1,201
41	North Dakota	1,200
24	Ohio	1,337
38	Oklahoma	1,222
12	Oregon	1,433
21	Pennsylvania	1,369
37	Rhode Island	1,228
28	South Carolina	1,309
43	South Dakota	1,195
3	Tennessee	1,541
30	Texas	1,278
50	Utah	988
16	Vermont	1,408
36	Virginia	1,234
10	Washington	1,451
23	West Virginia	1,350
4	Wisconsin	1,535
27	Wyoming	1,326

RANK ORDER

RANK	STATE	PER CAPITA
1	Alaska	$1,858
2	Maine	1,579
3	Tennessee	1,541
4	Wisconsin	1,535
5	Minnesota	1,523
6	Florida	1,522
7	Kansas	1,513
8	Delaware	1,482
9	Connecticut	1,475
10	Nevada	1,451
10	Washington	1,451
12	Oregon	1,433
13	Maryland	1,421
14	Massachusetts	1,416
15	New Jersey	1,414
16	Vermont	1,408
17	Kentucky	1,388
18	Colorado	1,386
19	California	1,379
20	Alabama	1,372
21	Pennsylvania	1,369
22	New Hampshire	1,354
23	West Virginia	1,350
24	Ohio	1,337
25	Illinois	1,336
26	New York	1,329
27	Wyoming	1,326
28	Nebraska	1,309
28	South Carolina	1,309
30	Texas	1,278
31	Indiana	1,264
32	Hawaii	1,260
33	Iowa	1,259
34	Georgia	1,257
35	Montana	1,249
36	Virginia	1,234
37	Rhode Island	1,228
38	Oklahoma	1,222
39	Arkansas	1,207
40	North Carolina	1,201
41	North Dakota	1,200
42	Missouri	1,198
43	South Dakota	1,195
44	Arizona	1,193
45	Louisiana	1,173
46	Michigan	1,165
47	Mississippi	1,113
48	Idaho	1,051
49	New Mexico	1,013
50	Utah	988
	District of Columbia	1,767

Source: U.S. Department of Health and Human Services, Centers for Medicare and Medicaid Services
"State Health Care Expenditures" (http://www.cms.hhs.gov/NationalHealthExpendData/)
*By state of residence. Includes private physician offices and clinics, independently billing laboratories, and clinics run by the U.S. Department of Veterans Affairs and the U.S. Indian Health Service.

Expenditures for Dental Services in 2004

National Total = $81,476,000,000*

ALPHA ORDER					RANK ORDER			

ALPHA ORDER

RANK	STATE	EXPENDITURES	% of USA
26	Alabama	$977,000,000	1.2%
46	Alaska	241,000,000	0.3%
20	Arizona	1,457,000,000	1.8%
34	Arkansas	601,000,000	0.7%
1	California	11,625,000,000	14.3%
19	Colorado	1,537,000,000	1.9%
22	Connecticut	1,336,000,000	1.6%
44	Delaware	279,000,000	0.3%
4	Florida	4,494,000,000	5.5%
12	Georgia	2,257,000,000	2.8%
41	Hawaii	382,000,000	0.5%
37	Idaho	468,000,000	0.6%
5	Illinois	3,488,000,000	4.3%
17	Indiana	1,606,000,000	2.0%
30	Iowa	735,000,000	0.9%
31	Kansas	723,000,000	0.9%
27	Kentucky	876,000,000	1.1%
29	Louisiana	781,000,000	1.0%
42	Maine	363,000,000	0.4%
18	Maryland	1,553,000,000	1.9%
11	Massachusetts	2,276,000,000	2.8%
7	Michigan	3,147,000,000	3.9%
16	Minnesota	1,678,000,000	2.1%
35	Mississippi	507,000,000	0.6%
22	Missouri	1,336,000,000	1.6%
45	Montana	249,000,000	0.3%
39	Nebraska	423,000,000	0.5%
33	Nevada	679,000,000	0.8%
36	New Hampshire	471,000,000	0.6%
8	New Jersey	2,903,000,000	3.6%
38	New Mexico	425,000,000	0.5%
2	New York	5,445,000,000	6.7%
13	North Carolina	2,253,000,000	2.8%
49	North Dakota	174,000,000	0.2%
9	Ohio	2,901,000,000	3.6%
28	Oklahoma	842,000,000	1.0%
24	Oregon	1,269,000,000	1.6%
6	Pennsylvania	3,189,000,000	3.9%
43	Rhode Island	294,000,000	0.4%
25	South Carolina	1,003,000,000	1.2%
48	South Dakota	195,000,000	0.2%
21	Tennessee	1,428,000,000	1.8%
3	Texas	4,749,000,000	5.8%
32	Utah	718,000,000	0.9%
47	Vermont	198,000,000	0.2%
14	Virginia	2,043,000,000	2.5%
10	Washington	2,505,000,000	3.1%
40	West Virginia	384,000,000	0.5%
15	Wisconsin	1,694,000,000	2.1%
50	Wyoming	134,000,000	0.2%

RANK ORDER

RANK	STATE	EXPENDITURES	% of USA
1	California	$11,625,000,000	14.3%
2	New York	5,445,000,000	6.7%
3	Texas	4,749,000,000	5.8%
4	Florida	4,494,000,000	5.5%
5	Illinois	3,488,000,000	4.3%
6	Pennsylvania	3,189,000,000	3.9%
7	Michigan	3,147,000,000	3.9%
8	New Jersey	2,903,000,000	3.6%
9	Ohio	2,901,000,000	3.6%
10	Washington	2,505,000,000	3.1%
11	Massachusetts	2,276,000,000	2.8%
12	Georgia	2,257,000,000	2.8%
13	North Carolina	2,253,000,000	2.8%
14	Virginia	2,043,000,000	2.5%
15	Wisconsin	1,694,000,000	2.1%
16	Minnesota	1,678,000,000	2.1%
17	Indiana	1,606,000,000	2.0%
18	Maryland	1,553,000,000	1.9%
19	Colorado	1,537,000,000	1.9%
20	Arizona	1,457,000,000	1.8%
21	Tennessee	1,428,000,000	1.8%
22	Connecticut	1,336,000,000	1.6%
22	Missouri	1,336,000,000	1.6%
24	Oregon	1,269,000,000	1.6%
25	South Carolina	1,003,000,000	1.2%
26	Alabama	977,000,000	1.2%
27	Kentucky	876,000,000	1.1%
28	Oklahoma	842,000,000	1.0%
29	Louisiana	781,000,000	1.0%
30	Iowa	735,000,000	0.9%
31	Kansas	723,000,000	0.9%
32	Utah	718,000,000	0.9%
33	Nevada	679,000,000	0.8%
34	Arkansas	601,000,000	0.7%
35	Mississippi	507,000,000	0.6%
36	New Hampshire	471,000,000	0.6%
37	Idaho	468,000,000	0.6%
38	New Mexico	425,000,000	0.5%
39	Nebraska	423,000,000	0.5%
40	West Virginia	384,000,000	0.5%
41	Hawaii	382,000,000	0.5%
42	Maine	363,000,000	0.4%
43	Rhode Island	294,000,000	0.4%
44	Delaware	279,000,000	0.3%
45	Montana	249,000,000	0.3%
46	Alaska	241,000,000	0.3%
47	Vermont	198,000,000	0.2%
48	South Dakota	195,000,000	0.2%
49	North Dakota	174,000,000	0.2%
50	Wyoming	134,000,000	0.2%
	District of Columbia	183,000,000	0.2%

Source: U.S. Department of Health and Human Services, Centers for Medicare and Medicaid Services
    "State Health Care Expenditures" (http://www.cms.hhs.gov/NationalHealthExpendData/)
*By state of residence.

Percent of Total Personal Health Care Expenditures
Spent on Dental Services in 2004
National Percent = 5.3%*

<table>
<tr><td colspan="3">ALPHA ORDER</td><td colspan="3">RANK ORDER</td></tr>
<tr><td>RANK</td><td>STATE</td><td>PERCENT</td><td>RANK</td><td>STATE</td><td>PERCENT</td></tr>
<tr><td>45</td><td>Alabama</td><td>4.2</td><td>1</td><td>Washington</td><td>7.9</td></tr>
<tr><td>14</td><td>Alaska</td><td>5.7</td><td>2</td><td>Idaho</td><td>7.6</td></tr>
<tr><td>9</td><td>Arizona</td><td>6.2</td><td>3</td><td>Utah</td><td>7.5</td></tr>
<tr><td>37</td><td>Arkansas</td><td>4.5</td><td>4</td><td>Oregon</td><td>7.2</td></tr>
<tr><td>6</td><td>California</td><td>7.0</td><td>5</td><td>Colorado</td><td>7.1</td></tr>
<tr><td>5</td><td>Colorado</td><td>7.1</td><td>6</td><td>California</td><td>7.0</td></tr>
<tr><td>12</td><td>Connecticut</td><td>6.0</td><td>7</td><td>New Hampshire</td><td>6.7</td></tr>
<tr><td>19</td><td>Delaware</td><td>5.3</td><td>8</td><td>Nevada</td><td>6.4</td></tr>
<tr><td>32</td><td>Florida</td><td>4.7</td><td>9</td><td>Arizona</td><td>6.2</td></tr>
<tr><td>17</td><td>Georgia</td><td>5.5</td><td>9</td><td>Michigan</td><td>6.2</td></tr>
<tr><td>11</td><td>Hawaii</td><td>6.1</td><td>11</td><td>Hawaii</td><td>6.1</td></tr>
<tr><td>2</td><td>Idaho</td><td>7.6</td><td>12</td><td>Connecticut</td><td>6.0</td></tr>
<tr><td>23</td><td>Illinois</td><td>5.2</td><td>13</td><td>New Jersey</td><td>5.8</td></tr>
<tr><td>28</td><td>Indiana</td><td>4.9</td><td>14</td><td>Alaska</td><td>5.7</td></tr>
<tr><td>35</td><td>Iowa</td><td>4.6</td><td>14</td><td>Minnesota</td><td>5.7</td></tr>
<tr><td>28</td><td>Kansas</td><td>4.9</td><td>14</td><td>Virginia</td><td>5.7</td></tr>
<tr><td>47</td><td>Kentucky</td><td>3.9</td><td>17</td><td>Georgia</td><td>5.5</td></tr>
<tr><td>50</td><td>Louisiana</td><td>3.4</td><td>18</td><td>Wisconsin</td><td>5.4</td></tr>
<tr><td>45</td><td>Maine</td><td>4.2</td><td>19</td><td>Delaware</td><td>5.3</td></tr>
<tr><td>25</td><td>Maryland</td><td>5.0</td><td>19</td><td>Massachusetts</td><td>5.3</td></tr>
<tr><td>19</td><td>Massachusetts</td><td>5.3</td><td>19</td><td>Montana</td><td>5.3</td></tr>
<tr><td>9</td><td>Michigan</td><td>6.2</td><td>19</td><td>Vermont</td><td>5.3</td></tr>
<tr><td>14</td><td>Minnesota</td><td>5.7</td><td>23</td><td>Illinois</td><td>5.2</td></tr>
<tr><td>49</td><td>Mississippi</td><td>3.5</td><td>24</td><td>North Carolina</td><td>5.1</td></tr>
<tr><td>41</td><td>Missouri</td><td>4.3</td><td>25</td><td>Maryland</td><td>5.0</td></tr>
<tr><td>19</td><td>Montana</td><td>5.3</td><td>25</td><td>New Mexico</td><td>5.0</td></tr>
<tr><td>41</td><td>Nebraska</td><td>4.3</td><td>25</td><td>Wyoming</td><td>5.0</td></tr>
<tr><td>8</td><td>Nevada</td><td>6.4</td><td>28</td><td>Indiana</td><td>4.9</td></tr>
<tr><td>7</td><td>New Hampshire</td><td>6.7</td><td>28</td><td>Kansas</td><td>4.9</td></tr>
<tr><td>13</td><td>New Jersey</td><td>5.8</td><td>28</td><td>Oklahoma</td><td>4.9</td></tr>
<tr><td>25</td><td>New Mexico</td><td>5.0</td><td>31</td><td>South Dakota</td><td>4.8</td></tr>
<tr><td>41</td><td>New York</td><td>4.3</td><td>32</td><td>Florida</td><td>4.7</td></tr>
<tr><td>24</td><td>North Carolina</td><td>5.1</td><td>32</td><td>North Dakota</td><td>4.7</td></tr>
<tr><td>32</td><td>North Dakota</td><td>4.7</td><td>32</td><td>South Carolina</td><td>4.7</td></tr>
<tr><td>38</td><td>Ohio</td><td>4.4</td><td>35</td><td>Iowa</td><td>4.6</td></tr>
<tr><td>28</td><td>Oklahoma</td><td>4.9</td><td>35</td><td>Texas</td><td>4.6</td></tr>
<tr><td>4</td><td>Oregon</td><td>7.2</td><td>37</td><td>Arkansas</td><td>4.5</td></tr>
<tr><td>41</td><td>Pennsylvania</td><td>4.3</td><td>38</td><td>Ohio</td><td>4.4</td></tr>
<tr><td>38</td><td>Rhode Island</td><td>4.4</td><td>38</td><td>Rhode Island</td><td>4.4</td></tr>
<tr><td>32</td><td>South Carolina</td><td>4.7</td><td>38</td><td>Tennessee</td><td>4.4</td></tr>
<tr><td>31</td><td>South Dakota</td><td>4.8</td><td>41</td><td>Missouri</td><td>4.3</td></tr>
<tr><td>38</td><td>Tennessee</td><td>4.4</td><td>41</td><td>Nebraska</td><td>4.3</td></tr>
<tr><td>35</td><td>Texas</td><td>4.6</td><td>41</td><td>New York</td><td>4.3</td></tr>
<tr><td>3</td><td>Utah</td><td>7.5</td><td>41</td><td>Pennsylvania</td><td>4.3</td></tr>
<tr><td>19</td><td>Vermont</td><td>5.3</td><td>45</td><td>Alabama</td><td>4.2</td></tr>
<tr><td>14</td><td>Virginia</td><td>5.7</td><td>45</td><td>Maine</td><td>4.2</td></tr>
<tr><td>1</td><td>Washington</td><td>7.9</td><td>47</td><td>Kentucky</td><td>3.9</td></tr>
<tr><td>48</td><td>West Virginia</td><td>3.6</td><td>48</td><td>West Virginia</td><td>3.6</td></tr>
<tr><td>18</td><td>Wisconsin</td><td>5.4</td><td>49</td><td>Mississippi</td><td>3.5</td></tr>
<tr><td>25</td><td>Wyoming</td><td>5.0</td><td>50</td><td>Louisiana</td><td>3.4</td></tr>
<tr><td colspan="3"></td><td colspan="2">District of Columbia</td><td>3.8</td></tr>
</table>

Source: CQ Press using data from U.S. Department of Health and Human Services, Centers for Medicare and Medicaid Services
"State Health Care Expenditures" (http://www.cms.hhs.gov/NationalHealthExpendData/)
*By state of residence.

Per Capita Expenditures for Dental Care in 2004

National Per Capita = $277*

ALPHA ORDER			RANK ORDER		
RANK	STATE	PER CAPITA	RANK	STATE	PER CAPITA
45	Alabama	$216	1	Washington	$404
3	Alaska	366	2	Connecticut	382
33	Arizona	254	3	Alaska	366
44	Arkansas	219	4	New Hampshire	363
12	California	324	5	Massachusetts	354
10	Colorado	334	5	Oregon	354
2	Connecticut	382	7	Delaware	337
7	Delaware	337	8	Idaho	336
30	Florida	259	9	New Jersey	335
34	Georgia	253	10	Colorado	334
16	Hawaii	303	11	Minnesota	329
8	Idaho	336	12	California	324
22	Illinois	274	13	Vermont	319
31	Indiana	258	14	Michigan	312
37	Iowa	249	15	Wisconsin	308
28	Kansas	264	16	Hawaii	303
46	Kentucky	212	17	Utah	297
50	Louisiana	174	18	Nevada	291
21	Maine	276	19	New York	282
20	Maryland	280	20	Maryland	280
5	Massachusetts	354	21	Maine	276
14	Michigan	312	22	Illinois	274
11	Minnesota	329	22	North Dakota	274
49	Mississippi	175	24	Virginia	273
42	Missouri	232	25	Rhode Island	272
26	Montana	269	26	Montana	269
39	Nebraska	242	27	Wyoming	265
18	Nevada	291	28	Kansas	264
4	New Hampshire	363	28	North Carolina	264
9	New Jersey	335	30	Florida	259
43	New Mexico	224	31	Indiana	258
19	New York	282	31	Pennsylvania	258
28	North Carolina	264	33	Arizona	254
22	North Dakota	274	34	Georgia	253
34	Ohio	253	34	Ohio	253
40	Oklahoma	239	34	South Dakota	253
5	Oregon	354	37	Iowa	249
31	Pennsylvania	258	38	Tennessee	243
25	Rhode Island	272	39	Nebraska	242
40	South Carolina	239	40	Oklahoma	239
34	South Dakota	253	40	South Carolina	239
38	Tennessee	243	42	Missouri	232
48	Texas	211	43	New Mexico	224
17	Utah	297	44	Arkansas	219
13	Vermont	319	45	Alabama	216
24	Virginia	273	46	Kentucky	212
1	Washington	404	46	West Virginia	212
46	West Virginia	212	48	Texas	211
15	Wisconsin	308	49	Mississippi	175
27	Wyoming	265	50	Louisiana	174
				District of Columbia	315

Source: U.S. Department of Health and Human Services, Centers for Medicare and Medicaid Services
    "State Health Care Expenditures" (http://www.cms.hhs.gov/NationalHealthExpendData/)
*By state of residence.

Expenditures for Other Professional Health Care Services in 2004

National Total = $52,636,000,000*

ALPHA ORDER					RANK ORDER			
RANK	STATE	EXPENDITURES	% of USA		RANK	STATE	EXPENDITURES	% of USA
27	Alabama	$681,000,000	1.3%		1	California	$6,178,000,000	11.7%
46	Alaska	164,000,000	0.3%		2	New York	3,587,000,000	6.8%
22	Arizona	932,000,000	1.8%		3	Florida	3,529,000,000	6.7%
32	Arkansas	463,000,000	0.9%		4	Texas	3,177,000,000	6.0%
1	California	6,178,000,000	11.7%		5	Pennsylvania	2,613,000,000	5.0%
21	Colorado	939,000,000	1.8%		6	Illinois	2,365,000,000	4.5%
23	Connecticut	855,000,000	1.6%		7	Ohio	2,285,000,000	4.3%
43	Delaware	210,000,000	0.4%		8	New Jersey	1,919,000,000	3.6%
3	Florida	3,529,000,000	6.7%		9	Michigan	1,896,000,000	3.6%
13	Georgia	1,252,000,000	2.4%		10	Washington	1,363,000,000	2.6%
42	Hawaii	224,000,000	0.4%		11	North Carolina	1,336,000,000	2.5%
40	Idaho	303,000,000	0.6%		12	Massachusetts	1,289,000,000	2.4%
6	Illinois	2,365,000,000	4.5%		13	Georgia	1,252,000,000	2.4%
19	Indiana	1,002,000,000	1.9%		14	Virginia	1,123,000,000	2.1%
29	Iowa	557,000,000	1.1%		15	Tennessee	1,035,000,000	2.0%
31	Kansas	499,000,000	0.9%		16	Maryland	1,034,000,000	2.0%
24	Kentucky	796,000,000	1.5%		17	Wisconsin	1,031,000,000	2.0%
26	Louisiana	705,000,000	1.3%		18	Minnesota	1,005,000,000	1.9%
38	Maine	305,000,000	0.6%		19	Indiana	1,002,000,000	1.9%
16	Maryland	1,034,000,000	2.0%		20	Missouri	958,000,000	1.8%
12	Massachusetts	1,289,000,000	2.4%		21	Colorado	939,000,000	1.8%
9	Michigan	1,896,000,000	3.6%		22	Arizona	932,000,000	1.8%
18	Minnesota	1,005,000,000	1.9%		23	Connecticut	855,000,000	1.6%
35	Mississippi	351,000,000	0.7%		24	Kentucky	796,000,000	1.5%
20	Missouri	958,000,000	1.8%		25	Oregon	715,000,000	1.4%
45	Montana	172,000,000	0.3%		26	Louisiana	705,000,000	1.3%
39	Nebraska	304,000,000	0.6%		27	Alabama	681,000,000	1.3%
33	Nevada	370,000,000	0.7%		28	Oklahoma	561,000,000	1.1%
41	New Hampshire	229,000,000	0.4%		29	Iowa	557,000,000	1.1%
8	New Jersey	1,919,000,000	3.6%		30	South Carolina	534,000,000	1.0%
37	New Mexico	321,000,000	0.6%		31	Kansas	499,000,000	0.9%
2	New York	3,587,000,000	6.8%		32	Arkansas	463,000,000	0.9%
11	North Carolina	1,336,000,000	2.5%		33	Nevada	370,000,000	0.7%
50	North Dakota	103,000,000	0.2%		34	West Virginia	361,000,000	0.7%
7	Ohio	2,285,000,000	4.3%		35	Mississippi	351,000,000	0.7%
28	Oklahoma	561,000,000	1.1%		36	Utah	332,000,000	0.6%
25	Oregon	715,000,000	1.4%		37	New Mexico	321,000,000	0.6%
5	Pennsylvania	2,613,000,000	5.0%		38	Maine	305,000,000	0.6%
44	Rhode Island	193,000,000	0.4%		39	Nebraska	304,000,000	0.6%
30	South Carolina	534,000,000	1.0%		40	Idaho	303,000,000	0.6%
47	South Dakota	135,000,000	0.3%		41	New Hampshire	229,000,000	0.4%
15	Tennessee	1,035,000,000	2.0%		42	Hawaii	224,000,000	0.4%
4	Texas	3,177,000,000	6.0%		43	Delaware	210,000,000	0.4%
36	Utah	332,000,000	0.6%		44	Rhode Island	193,000,000	0.4%
48	Vermont	132,000,000	0.3%		45	Montana	172,000,000	0.3%
14	Virginia	1,123,000,000	2.1%		46	Alaska	164,000,000	0.3%
10	Washington	1,363,000,000	2.6%		47	South Dakota	135,000,000	0.3%
34	West Virginia	361,000,000	0.7%		48	Vermont	132,000,000	0.3%
17	Wisconsin	1,031,000,000	2.0%		49	Wyoming	117,000,000	0.2%
49	Wyoming	117,000,000	0.2%		50	North Dakota	103,000,000	0.2%
						District of Columbia	98,000,000	0.2%

Source: U.S. Department of Health and Human Services, Centers for Medicare and Medicaid Services
"State Health Care Expenditures" (http://www.cms.hhs.gov/NationalHealthExpendData/)
*By state of residence. Includes services of licensed professionals such as chiropractors, optometrists, podiatrists, and independently practicing nurses. Also includes Medicare ambulance services.

Percent of Total Personal Health Care Expenditures
Spent on Other Professional Health Care Services in 2004
National Percent = 3.4%*

ALPHA ORDER

RANK	STATE	PERCENT
45	Alabama	2.9
8	Alaska	3.9
6	Arizona	4.0
18	Arkansas	3.5
12	California	3.7
3	Colorado	4.3
8	Connecticut	3.9
6	Delaware	4.0
12	Florida	3.7
41	Georgia	3.0
16	Hawaii	3.6
1	Idaho	4.9
18	Illinois	3.5
41	Indiana	3.0
18	Iowa	3.5
27	Kansas	3.4
18	Kentucky	3.5
36	Louisiana	3.1
18	Maine	3.5
29	Maryland	3.3
41	Massachusetts	3.0
12	Michigan	3.7
27	Minnesota	3.4
50	Mississippi	2.4
36	Missouri	3.1
12	Montana	3.7
36	Nebraska	3.1
18	Nevada	3.5
33	New Hampshire	3.2
10	New Jersey	3.8
10	New Mexico	3.8
47	New York	2.8
41	North Carolina	3.0
47	North Dakota	2.8
18	Ohio	3.5
33	Oklahoma	3.2
5	Oregon	4.1
16	Pennsylvania	3.6
45	Rhode Island	2.9
49	South Carolina	2.5
29	South Dakota	3.3
33	Tennessee	3.2
36	Texas	3.1
18	Utah	3.5
18	Vermont	3.5
36	Virginia	3.1
3	Washington	4.3
29	West Virginia	3.3
29	Wisconsin	3.3
2	Wyoming	4.4

RANK ORDER

RANK	STATE	PERCENT
1	Idaho	4.9
2	Wyoming	4.4
3	Colorado	4.3
3	Washington	4.3
5	Oregon	4.1
6	Arizona	4.0
6	Delaware	4.0
8	Alaska	3.9
8	Connecticut	3.9
10	New Jersey	3.8
10	New Mexico	3.8
12	California	3.7
12	Florida	3.7
12	Michigan	3.7
12	Montana	3.7
16	Hawaii	3.6
16	Pennsylvania	3.6
18	Arkansas	3.5
18	Illinois	3.5
18	Iowa	3.5
18	Kentucky	3.5
18	Maine	3.5
18	Nevada	3.5
18	Ohio	3.5
18	Utah	3.5
18	Vermont	3.5
27	Kansas	3.4
27	Minnesota	3.4
29	Maryland	3.3
29	South Dakota	3.3
29	West Virginia	3.3
29	Wisconsin	3.3
33	New Hampshire	3.2
33	Oklahoma	3.2
33	Tennessee	3.2
36	Louisiana	3.1
36	Missouri	3.1
36	Nebraska	3.1
36	Texas	3.1
36	Virginia	3.1
41	Georgia	3.0
41	Indiana	3.0
41	Massachusetts	3.0
41	North Carolina	3.0
45	Alabama	2.9
45	Rhode Island	2.9
47	New York	2.8
47	North Dakota	2.8
49	South Carolina	2.5
50	Mississippi	2.4

District of Columbia   2.0

Source: CQ Press using data from U.S. Department of Health and Human Services, Centers for Medicare and Medicaid Services
"State Health Care Expenditures" (http://www.cms.hhs.gov/NationalHealthExpendData/)
*By state of residence. Includes services of licensed professionals such as chiropractors, optometrists, podiatrists, and
independently practicing nurses. Also includes Medicare ambulance services.

Per Capita Expenditures for Other Professional Health Care Services in 2004

National Per Capita = $179*

ALPHA ORDER

RANK	STATE	PER CAPITA
44	Alabama	$151
2	Alaska	249
37	Arizona	162
35	Arkansas	168
33	California	172
11	Colorado	204
3	Connecticut	245
1	Delaware	253
12	Florida	203
47	Georgia	140
27	Hawaii	178
8	Idaho	217
22	Illinois	186
39	Indiana	161
19	Iowa	188
26	Kansas	182
18	Kentucky	192
42	Louisiana	157
4	Maine	232
22	Maryland	186
13	Massachusetts	200
19	Michigan	188
17	Minnesota	197
50	Mississippi	121
36	Missouri	167
22	Montana	186
32	Nebraska	174
40	Nevada	159
29	New Hampshire	176
6	New Jersey	221
34	New Mexico	169
22	New York	186
42	North Carolina	157
37	North Dakota	162
14	Ohio	199
40	Oklahoma	159
14	Oregon	199
10	Pennsylvania	211
27	Rhode Island	178
49	South Carolina	127
29	South Dakota	176
29	Tennessee	176
46	Texas	141
48	Utah	137
9	Vermont	212
45	Virginia	150
7	Washington	220
14	West Virginia	199
21	Wisconsin	187
5	Wyoming	231

RANK ORDER

RANK	STATE	PER CAPITA
1	Delaware	$253
2	Alaska	249
3	Connecticut	245
4	Maine	232
5	Wyoming	231
6	New Jersey	221
7	Washington	220
8	Idaho	217
9	Vermont	212
10	Pennsylvania	211
11	Colorado	204
12	Florida	203
13	Massachusetts	200
14	Ohio	199
14	Oregon	199
14	West Virginia	199
17	Minnesota	197
18	Kentucky	192
19	Iowa	188
19	Michigan	188
21	Wisconsin	187
22	Illinois	186
22	Maryland	186
22	Montana	186
22	New York	186
26	Kansas	182
27	Hawaii	178
27	Rhode Island	178
29	New Hampshire	176
29	South Dakota	176
29	Tennessee	176
32	Nebraska	174
33	California	172
34	New Mexico	169
35	Arkansas	168
36	Missouri	167
37	Arizona	162
37	North Dakota	162
39	Indiana	161
40	Nevada	159
40	Oklahoma	159
42	Louisiana	157
42	North Carolina	157
44	Alabama	151
45	Virginia	150
46	Texas	141
47	Georgia	140
48	Utah	137
49	South Carolina	127
50	Mississippi	121

District of Columbia	170

Source: U.S. Department of Health and Human Services, Centers for Medicare and Medicaid Services
"State Health Care Expenditures" (http://www.cms.hhs.gov/NationalHealthExpendData/)
*By state of residence. Includes services of licensed professionals such as chiropractors, optometrists, podiatrists, and independently practicing nurses. Also includes Medicare ambulance services.

Expenditures for Nursing Home Care in 2004

National Total = $115,015,000,000*

ALPHA ORDER

RANK	STATE	EXPENDITURES	% of USA
25	Alabama	$1,475,000,000	1.3%
50	Alaska	80,000,000	0.1%
32	Arizona	1,023,000,000	0.9%
31	Arkansas	1,040,000,000	0.9%
2	California	8,424,000,000	7.3%
27	Colorado	1,178,000,000	1.0%
13	Connecticut	2,711,000,000	2.4%
40	Delaware	409,000,000	0.4%
5	Florida	6,503,000,000	5.7%
19	Georgia	2,272,000,000	2.0%
47	Hawaii	293,000,000	0.3%
44	Idaho	361,000,000	0.3%
7	Illinois	5,173,000,000	4.5%
12	Indiana	2,871,000,000	2.5%
22	Iowa	1,623,000,000	1.4%
29	Kansas	1,110,000,000	1.0%
24	Kentucky	1,526,000,000	1.3%
23	Louisiana	1,617,000,000	1.4%
36	Maine	630,000,000	0.5%
16	Maryland	2,419,000,000	2.1%
9	Massachusetts	4,124,000,000	3.6%
11	Michigan	3,193,000,000	2.8%
18	Minnesota	2,367,000,000	2.1%
30	Mississippi	1,094,000,000	1.0%
14	Missouri	2,479,000,000	2.2%
46	Montana	322,000,000	0.3%
34	Nebraska	860,000,000	0.7%
45	Nevada	341,000,000	0.3%
38	New Hampshire	548,000,000	0.5%
8	New Jersey	4,261,000,000	3.7%
43	New Mexico	372,000,000	0.3%
1	New York	13,364,000,000	11.6%
10	North Carolina	3,354,000,000	2.9%
42	North Dakota	387,000,000	0.3%
4	Ohio	6,834,000,000	5.9%
28	Oklahoma	1,157,000,000	1.0%
33	Oregon	897,000,000	0.8%
3	Pennsylvania	7,562,000,000	6.6%
37	Rhode Island	616,000,000	0.5%
26	South Carolina	1,236,000,000	1.1%
41	South Dakota	406,000,000	0.4%
20	Tennessee	2,211,000,000	1.9%
6	Texas	5,600,000,000	4.9%
39	Utah	428,000,000	0.4%
48	Vermont	235,000,000	0.2%
15	Virginia	2,448,000,000	2.1%
21	Washington	1,860,000,000	1.6%
35	West Virginia	716,000,000	0.6%
17	Wisconsin	2,405,000,000	2.1%
49	Wyoming	150,000,000	0.1%

RANK ORDER

RANK	STATE	EXPENDITURES	% of USA
1	New York	$13,364,000,000	11.6%
2	California	8,424,000,000	7.3%
3	Pennsylvania	7,562,000,000	6.6%
4	Ohio	6,834,000,000	5.9%
5	Florida	6,503,000,000	5.7%
6	Texas	5,600,000,000	4.9%
7	Illinois	5,173,000,000	4.5%
8	New Jersey	4,261,000,000	3.7%
9	Massachusetts	4,124,000,000	3.6%
10	North Carolina	3,354,000,000	2.9%
11	Michigan	3,193,000,000	2.8%
12	Indiana	2,871,000,000	2.5%
13	Connecticut	2,711,000,000	2.4%
14	Missouri	2,479,000,000	2.2%
15	Virginia	2,448,000,000	2.1%
16	Maryland	2,419,000,000	2.1%
17	Wisconsin	2,405,000,000	2.1%
18	Minnesota	2,367,000,000	2.1%
19	Georgia	2,272,000,000	2.0%
20	Tennessee	2,211,000,000	1.9%
21	Washington	1,860,000,000	1.6%
22	Iowa	1,623,000,000	1.4%
23	Louisiana	1,617,000,000	1.4%
24	Kentucky	1,526,000,000	1.3%
25	Alabama	1,475,000,000	1.3%
26	South Carolina	1,236,000,000	1.1%
27	Colorado	1,178,000,000	1.0%
28	Oklahoma	1,157,000,000	1.0%
29	Kansas	1,110,000,000	1.0%
30	Mississippi	1,094,000,000	1.0%
31	Arkansas	1,040,000,000	0.9%
32	Arizona	1,023,000,000	0.9%
33	Oregon	897,000,000	0.8%
34	Nebraska	860,000,000	0.7%
35	West Virginia	716,000,000	0.6%
36	Maine	630,000,000	0.5%
37	Rhode Island	616,000,000	0.5%
38	New Hampshire	548,000,000	0.5%
39	Utah	428,000,000	0.4%
40	Delaware	409,000,000	0.4%
41	South Dakota	406,000,000	0.4%
42	North Dakota	387,000,000	0.3%
43	New Mexico	372,000,000	0.3%
44	Idaho	361,000,000	0.3%
45	Nevada	341,000,000	0.3%
46	Montana	322,000,000	0.3%
47	Hawaii	293,000,000	0.3%
48	Vermont	235,000,000	0.2%
49	Wyoming	150,000,000	0.1%
50	Alaska	80,000,000	0.1%
	District of Columbia	452,000,000	0.4%

Source: U.S. Department of Health and Human Services, Centers for Medicare and Medicaid Services
"State Health Care Expenditures" (http://www.cms.hhs.gov/NationalHealthExpendData/)
*By state of residence. Includes all freestanding nursing homes. Does not include nursing home services provided in long-term care units of hospitals.

Percent of Total Personal Health Care Expenditures
Spent on Nursing Home Care in 2004
National Percent = 7.4%*

ALPHA ORDER

RANK	STATE	PERCENT
33	Alabama	6.4
50	Alaska	1.9
48	Arizona	4.3
15	Arkansas	7.8
43	California	5.1
41	Colorado	5.4
1	Connecticut	12.2
15	Delaware	7.8
27	Florida	6.8
40	Georgia	5.5
45	Hawaii	4.7
37	Idaho	5.8
19	Illinois	7.7
11	Indiana	8.7
6	Iowa	10.2
22	Kansas	7.5
30	Kentucky	6.7
25	Louisiana	7.1
24	Maine	7.3
15	Maryland	7.8
8	Massachusetts	9.6
34	Michigan	6.3
13	Minnesota	8.0
22	Mississippi	7.5
14	Missouri	7.9
27	Montana	6.8
10	Nebraska	8.8
49	Nevada	3.2
15	New Hampshire	7.8
12	New Jersey	8.5
46	New Mexico	4.4
2	New York	10.6
21	North Carolina	7.6
3	North Dakota	10.5
4	Ohio	10.4
30	Oklahoma	6.7
43	Oregon	5.1
5	Pennsylvania	10.3
9	Rhode Island	9.2
37	South Carolina	5.8
7	South Dakota	9.9
26	Tennessee	6.9
41	Texas	5.4
46	Utah	4.4
35	Vermont	6.2
27	Virginia	6.8
36	Washington	5.9
32	West Virginia	6.6
19	Wisconsin	7.7
39	Wyoming	5.6

RANK ORDER

RANK	STATE	PERCENT
1	Connecticut	12.2
2	New York	10.6
3	North Dakota	10.5
4	Ohio	10.4
5	Pennsylvania	10.3
6	Iowa	10.2
7	South Dakota	9.9
8	Massachusetts	9.6
9	Rhode Island	9.2
10	Nebraska	8.8
11	Indiana	8.7
12	New Jersey	8.5
13	Minnesota	8.0
14	Missouri	7.9
15	Arkansas	7.8
15	Delaware	7.8
15	Maryland	7.8
15	New Hampshire	7.8
19	Illinois	7.7
19	Wisconsin	7.7
21	North Carolina	7.6
22	Kansas	7.5
22	Mississippi	7.5
24	Maine	7.3
25	Louisiana	7.1
26	Tennessee	6.9
27	Florida	6.8
27	Montana	6.8
27	Virginia	6.8
30	Kentucky	6.7
30	Oklahoma	6.7
32	West Virginia	6.6
33	Alabama	6.4
34	Michigan	6.3
35	Vermont	6.2
36	Washington	5.9
37	Idaho	5.8
37	South Carolina	5.8
39	Wyoming	5.6
40	Georgia	5.5
41	Colorado	5.4
41	Texas	5.4
43	California	5.1
43	Oregon	5.1
45	Hawaii	4.7
46	New Mexico	4.4
46	Utah	4.4
48	Arizona	4.3
49	Nevada	3.2
50	Alaska	1.9

District of Columbia 9.4

Source: CQ Press using data from U.S. Department of Health and Human Services, Centers for Medicare and Medicaid Services "State Health Care Expenditures" (http://www.cms.hhs.gov/NationalHealthExpendData/)

*By state of residence. Includes all freestanding nursing homes. Does not include nursing home services provided in long-term care units of hospitals.

Per Capita Expenditures for Nursing Home Care in 2004

National Per Capita = $392*

<table>
<tr><td colspan="3">ALPHA ORDER</td><td colspan="3">RANK ORDER</td></tr>
<tr><td>RANK</td><td>STATE</td><td>PER CAPITA</td><td>RANK</td><td>STATE</td><td>PER CAPITA</td></tr>
<tr><td>34</td><td>Alabama</td><td>$326</td><td>1</td><td>Connecticut</td><td>$776</td></tr>
<tr><td>50</td><td>Alaska</td><td>122</td><td>2</td><td>New York</td><td>693</td></tr>
<tr><td>47</td><td>Arizona</td><td>178</td><td>3</td><td>Massachusetts</td><td>641</td></tr>
<tr><td>24</td><td>Arkansas</td><td>378</td><td>4</td><td>Pennsylvania</td><td>611</td></tr>
<tr><td>44</td><td>California</td><td>235</td><td>5</td><td>North Dakota</td><td>608</td></tr>
<tr><td>40</td><td>Colorado</td><td>256</td><td>6</td><td>Ohio</td><td>596</td></tr>
<tr><td>1</td><td>Connecticut</td><td>776</td><td>7</td><td>Rhode Island</td><td>570</td></tr>
<tr><td>10</td><td>Delaware</td><td>493</td><td>8</td><td>Iowa</td><td>549</td></tr>
<tr><td>28</td><td>Florida</td><td>374</td><td>9</td><td>South Dakota</td><td>527</td></tr>
<tr><td>41</td><td>Georgia</td><td>254</td><td>10</td><td>Delaware</td><td>493</td></tr>
<tr><td>45</td><td>Hawaii</td><td>233</td><td>11</td><td>Nebraska</td><td>492</td></tr>
<tr><td>39</td><td>Idaho</td><td>259</td><td>12</td><td>New Jersey</td><td>491</td></tr>
<tr><td>20</td><td>Illinois</td><td>407</td><td>13</td><td>Maine</td><td>480</td></tr>
<tr><td>15</td><td>Indiana</td><td>461</td><td>14</td><td>Minnesota</td><td>465</td></tr>
<tr><td>8</td><td>Iowa</td><td>549</td><td>15</td><td>Indiana</td><td>461</td></tr>
<tr><td>21</td><td>Kansas</td><td>406</td><td>16</td><td>Wisconsin</td><td>437</td></tr>
<tr><td>29</td><td>Kentucky</td><td>369</td><td>17</td><td>Maryland</td><td>436</td></tr>
<tr><td>30</td><td>Louisiana</td><td>360</td><td>18</td><td>Missouri</td><td>431</td></tr>
<tr><td>13</td><td>Maine</td><td>480</td><td>19</td><td>New Hampshire</td><td>422</td></tr>
<tr><td>17</td><td>Maryland</td><td>436</td><td>20</td><td>Illinois</td><td>407</td></tr>
<tr><td>3</td><td>Massachusetts</td><td>641</td><td>21</td><td>Kansas</td><td>406</td></tr>
<tr><td>35</td><td>Michigan</td><td>316</td><td>22</td><td>West Virginia</td><td>395</td></tr>
<tr><td>14</td><td>Minnesota</td><td>465</td><td>23</td><td>North Carolina</td><td>393</td></tr>
<tr><td>24</td><td>Mississippi</td><td>378</td><td>24</td><td>Arkansas</td><td>378</td></tr>
<tr><td>18</td><td>Missouri</td><td>431</td><td>24</td><td>Mississippi</td><td>378</td></tr>
<tr><td>31</td><td>Montana</td><td>348</td><td>24</td><td>Vermont</td><td>378</td></tr>
<tr><td>11</td><td>Nebraska</td><td>492</td><td>27</td><td>Tennessee</td><td>376</td></tr>
<tr><td>49</td><td>Nevada</td><td>146</td><td>28</td><td>Florida</td><td>374</td></tr>
<tr><td>19</td><td>New Hampshire</td><td>422</td><td>29</td><td>Kentucky</td><td>369</td></tr>
<tr><td>12</td><td>New Jersey</td><td>491</td><td>30</td><td>Louisiana</td><td>360</td></tr>
<tr><td>46</td><td>New Mexico</td><td>196</td><td>31</td><td>Montana</td><td>348</td></tr>
<tr><td>2</td><td>New York</td><td>693</td><td>32</td><td>Oklahoma</td><td>329</td></tr>
<tr><td>23</td><td>North Carolina</td><td>393</td><td>33</td><td>Virginia</td><td>328</td></tr>
<tr><td>5</td><td>North Dakota</td><td>608</td><td>34</td><td>Alabama</td><td>326</td></tr>
<tr><td>6</td><td>Ohio</td><td>596</td><td>35</td><td>Michigan</td><td>316</td></tr>
<tr><td>32</td><td>Oklahoma</td><td>329</td><td>36</td><td>Washington</td><td>300</td></tr>
<tr><td>42</td><td>Oregon</td><td>250</td><td>37</td><td>Wyoming</td><td>297</td></tr>
<tr><td>4</td><td>Pennsylvania</td><td>611</td><td>38</td><td>South Carolina</td><td>295</td></tr>
<tr><td>7</td><td>Rhode Island</td><td>570</td><td>39</td><td>Idaho</td><td>259</td></tr>
<tr><td>38</td><td>South Carolina</td><td>295</td><td>40</td><td>Colorado</td><td>256</td></tr>
<tr><td>9</td><td>South Dakota</td><td>527</td><td>41</td><td>Georgia</td><td>254</td></tr>
<tr><td>27</td><td>Tennessee</td><td>376</td><td>42</td><td>Oregon</td><td>250</td></tr>
<tr><td>43</td><td>Texas</td><td>249</td><td>43</td><td>Texas</td><td>249</td></tr>
<tr><td>48</td><td>Utah</td><td>177</td><td>44</td><td>California</td><td>235</td></tr>
<tr><td>24</td><td>Vermont</td><td>378</td><td>45</td><td>Hawaii</td><td>233</td></tr>
<tr><td>33</td><td>Virginia</td><td>328</td><td>46</td><td>New Mexico</td><td>196</td></tr>
<tr><td>36</td><td>Washington</td><td>300</td><td>47</td><td>Arizona</td><td>178</td></tr>
<tr><td>22</td><td>West Virginia</td><td>395</td><td>48</td><td>Utah</td><td>177</td></tr>
<tr><td>16</td><td>Wisconsin</td><td>437</td><td>49</td><td>Nevada</td><td>146</td></tr>
<tr><td>37</td><td>Wyoming</td><td>297</td><td>50</td><td>Alaska</td><td>122</td></tr>
<tr><td></td><td></td><td></td><td></td><td>District of Columbia</td><td>780</td></tr>
</table>

Source: U.S. Department of Health and Human Services, Centers for Medicare and Medicaid Services
"State Health Care Expenditures" (http://www.cms.hhs.gov/NationalHealthExpendData/)
*By state of residence. Includes all freestanding nursing homes. Does not include nursing home services provided in long-term care units of hospitals.

Expenditures for Home Health Care in 2004

National Total = $42,710,000,000*

RANK	STATE	EXPENDITURES	% of USA
18	Alabama	$661,000,000	1.5%
47	Alaska	64,000,000	0.1%
19	Arizona	656,000,000	1.5%
31	Arkansas	325,000,000	0.8%
2	California	5,537,000,000	13.0%
30	Colorado	367,000,000	0.9%
15	Connecticut	708,000,000	1.7%
43	Delaware	94,000,000	0.2%
4	Florida	2,876,000,000	6.7%
12	Georgia	876,000,000	2.1%
42	Hawaii	105,000,000	0.2%
41	Idaho	115,000,000	0.3%
11	Illinois	1,269,000,000	3.0%
25	Indiana	509,000,000	1.2%
32	Iowa	310,000,000	0.7%
34	Kansas	241,000,000	0.6%
23	Kentucky	531,000,000	1.2%
21	Louisiana	624,000,000	1.5%
38	Maine	173,000,000	0.4%
24	Maryland	511,000,000	1.2%
5	Massachusetts	1,743,000,000	4.1%
10	Michigan	1,326,000,000	3.1%
17	Minnesota	679,000,000	1.6%
26	Mississippi	484,000,000	1.1%
15	Missouri	708,000,000	1.7%
45	Montana	89,000,000	0.2%
46	Nebraska	79,000,000	0.2%
35	Nevada	231,000,000	0.5%
39	New Hampshire	168,000,000	0.4%
8	New Jersey	1,427,000,000	3.3%
28	New Mexico	451,000,000	1.1%
1	New York	6,021,000,000	14.1%
9	North Carolina	1,413,000,000	3.3%
50	North Dakota	18,000,000	0.0%
7	Ohio	1,519,000,000	3.6%
27	Oklahoma	464,000,000	1.1%
36	Oregon	201,000,000	0.5%
6	Pennsylvania	1,527,000,000	3.6%
40	Rhode Island	116,000,000	0.3%
29	South Carolina	422,000,000	1.0%
49	South Dakota	20,000,000	0.0%
14	Tennessee	738,000,000	1.7%
3	Texas	3,604,000,000	8.4%
33	Utah	245,000,000	0.6%
43	Vermont	94,000,000	0.2%
22	Virginia	605,000,000	1.4%
13	Washington	823,000,000	1.9%
37	West Virginia	197,000,000	0.5%
20	Wisconsin	642,000,000	1.5%
48	Wyoming	28,000,000	0.1%

RANK	STATE	EXPENDITURES	% of USA
1	New York	$6,021,000,000	14.1%
2	California	5,537,000,000	13.0%
3	Texas	3,604,000,000	8.4%
4	Florida	2,876,000,000	6.7%
5	Massachusetts	1,743,000,000	4.1%
6	Pennsylvania	1,527,000,000	3.6%
7	Ohio	1,519,000,000	3.6%
8	New Jersey	1,427,000,000	3.3%
9	North Carolina	1,413,000,000	3.3%
10	Michigan	1,326,000,000	3.1%
11	Illinois	1,269,000,000	3.0%
12	Georgia	876,000,000	2.1%
13	Washington	823,000,000	1.9%
14	Tennessee	738,000,000	1.7%
15	Connecticut	708,000,000	1.7%
15	Missouri	708,000,000	1.7%
17	Minnesota	679,000,000	1.6%
18	Alabama	661,000,000	1.5%
19	Arizona	656,000,000	1.5%
20	Wisconsin	642,000,000	1.5%
21	Louisiana	624,000,000	1.5%
22	Virginia	605,000,000	1.4%
23	Kentucky	531,000,000	1.2%
24	Maryland	511,000,000	1.2%
25	Indiana	509,000,000	1.2%
26	Mississippi	484,000,000	1.1%
27	Oklahoma	464,000,000	1.1%
28	New Mexico	451,000,000	1.1%
29	South Carolina	422,000,000	1.0%
30	Colorado	367,000,000	0.9%
31	Arkansas	325,000,000	0.8%
32	Iowa	310,000,000	0.7%
33	Utah	245,000,000	0.6%
34	Kansas	241,000,000	0.6%
35	Nevada	231,000,000	0.5%
36	Oregon	201,000,000	0.5%
37	West Virginia	197,000,000	0.5%
38	Maine	173,000,000	0.4%
39	New Hampshire	168,000,000	0.4%
40	Rhode Island	116,000,000	0.3%
41	Idaho	115,000,000	0.3%
42	Hawaii	105,000,000	0.2%
43	Delaware	94,000,000	0.2%
43	Vermont	94,000,000	0.2%
45	Montana	89,000,000	0.2%
46	Nebraska	79,000,000	0.2%
47	Alaska	64,000,000	0.1%
48	Wyoming	28,000,000	0.1%
49	South Dakota	20,000,000	0.0%
50	North Dakota	18,000,000	0.0%
	District of Columbia	78,000,000	0.2%

Source: U.S. Department of Health and Human Services, Centers for Medicare and Medicaid Services
"State Health Care Expenditures" (http://www.cms.hhs.gov/NationalHealthExpendData/)
*By state of residence. Includes spending for services and products by public and private freestanding home health agencies.
Excludes home health care services provided by hospital-based agencies which are included in hospital expenditures.

Percent of Total Personal Health Care Expenditures
Spent on Home Health Care in 2004
National Percent = 2.8%*

ALPHA ORDER

RANK	STATE	PERCENT
10	Alabama	2.8
44	Alaska	1.5
10	Arizona	2.8
19	Arkansas	2.4
5	California	3.3
38	Colorado	1.7
7	Conncoticut	3.2
36	Delaware	1.8
9	Florida	3.0
27	Georgia	2.1
38	Hawaii	1.7
33	Idaho	1.9
33	Illinois	1.9
44	Indiana	1.5
30	Iowa	2.0
42	Kansas	1.6
21	Kentucky	2.3
10	Louisiana	2.8
30	Maine	2.0
42	Maryland	1.6
3	Massachusetts	4.1
15	Michigan	2.6
21	Minnesota	2.3
5	Mississippi	3.3
21	Missouri	2.3
33	Montana	1.9
48	Nebraska	0.8
26	Nevada	2.2
19	New Hampshire	2.4
10	New Jersey	2.8
1	New Mexico	5.3
2	New York	4.8
7	North Carolina	3.2
49	North Dakota	0.5
21	Ohio	2.3
14	Oklahoma	2.7
46	Oregon	1.1
27	Pennsylvania	2.1
38	Rhode Island	1.7
30	South Carolina	2.0
49	South Dakota	0.5
21	Tennessee	2.3
4	Texas	3.5
17	Utah	2.5
17	Vermont	2.5
38	Virginia	1.7
15	Washington	2.6
36	West Virginia	1.8
27	Wisconsin	2.1
46	Wyoming	1.1

RANK ORDER

RANK	STATE	PERCENT
1	New Mexico	5.3
2	New York	4.8
3	Massachusetts	4.1
4	Texas	3.5
5	California	3.3
5	Mississippi	3.3
7	Conncoticut	3.2
7	North Carolina	3.2
9	Florida	3.0
10	Alabama	2.8
10	Arizona	2.8
10	Louisiana	2.8
10	New Jersey	2.8
14	Oklahoma	2.7
15	Michigan	2.6
15	Washington	2.6
17	Utah	2.5
17	Vermont	2.5
19	Arkansas	2.4
19	New Hampshire	2.4
21	Kentucky	2.3
21	Minnesota	2.3
21	Missouri	2.3
21	Ohio	2.3
21	Tennessee	2.3
26	Nevada	2.2
27	Georgia	2.1
27	Pennsylvania	2.1
27	Wisconsin	2.1
30	Iowa	2.0
30	Maine	2.0
30	South Carolina	2.0
33	Idaho	1.9
33	Illinois	1.9
33	Montana	1.9
36	Delaware	1.8
36	West Virginia	1.8
38	Colorado	1.7
38	Hawaii	1.7
38	Rhode Island	1.7
38	Virginia	1.7
42	Kansas	1.6
42	Maryland	1.6
44	Alaska	1.5
44	Indiana	1.5
46	Oregon	1.1
46	Wyoming	1.1
48	Nebraska	0.8
49	North Dakota	0.5
49	South Dakota	0.5

	District of Columbia	1.6

Source: CQ Press using data from U.S. Department of Health and Human Services, Centers for Medicare and Medicaid Services
"State Health Care Expenditures" (http://www.cms.hhs.gov/NationalHealthExpendData/)
*By state of residence. Includes spending for services and products by public and private freestanding home health agencies.
Excludes home health care services provided by hospital-based agencies which are included in hospital expenditures.

Per Capita Expenditures for Home Health Care in 2004

National Per Capita = $145*

ALPHA ORDER				RANK ORDER		
RANK	STATE	PER CAPITA		RANK	STATE	PER CAPITA
12	Alabama	$146		1	New York	$312
36	Alaska	98		2	Massachusetts	271
27	Arizona	114		3	New Mexico	237
25	Arkansas	118		4	Connecticut	203
10	California	154		5	Mississippi	167
45	Colorado	80		6	Florida	166
4	Connecticut	203		6	North Carolina	166
28	Delaware	113		8	New Jersey	164
6	Florida	166		9	Texas	160
36	Georgia	98		10	California	154
41	Hawaii	84		11	Vermont	152
42	Idaho	82		12	Alabama	146
34	Illinois	100		13	Louisiana	139
42	Indiana	82		14	Minnesota	133
31	Iowa	105		14	Ohio	133
40	Kansas	88		14	Washington	133
21	Kentucky	128		17	Maine	132
13	Louisiana	139		17	Oklahoma	132
17	Maine	132		19	Michigan	131
39	Maryland	92		20	New Hampshire	130
2	Massachusetts	271		21	Kentucky	128
19	Michigan	131		22	Tennessee	125
14	Minnesota	133		23	Missouri	123
5	Mississippi	167		23	Pennsylvania	123
23	Missouri	123		25	Arkansas	118
38	Montana	96		26	Wisconsin	117
48	Nebraska	45		27	Arizona	114
35	Nevada	99		28	Delaware	113
20	New Hampshire	130		29	West Virginia	109
8	New Jersey	164		30	Rhode Island	107
3	New Mexico	237		31	Iowa	105
1	New York	312		32	South Carolina	101
6	North Carolina	166		32	Utah	101
49	North Dakota	28		34	Illinois	100
14	Ohio	133		35	Nevada	99
17	Oklahoma	132		36	Alaska	98
46	Oregon	56		36	Georgia	98
23	Pennsylvania	123		38	Montana	96
30	Rhode Island	107		39	Maryland	92
32	South Carolina	101		40	Kansas	88
50	South Dakota	26		41	Hawaii	84
22	Tennessee	125		42	Idaho	82
9	Texas	160		42	Indiana	82
32	Utah	101		44	Virginia	81
11	Vermont	152		45	Colorado	80
44	Virginia	81		46	Oregon	56
14	Washington	133		47	Wyoming	55
29	West Virginia	109		48	Nebraska	45
26	Wisconsin	117		49	North Dakota	28
47	Wyoming	55		50	South Dakota	26

	District of Columbia	134

Source: U.S. Department of Health and Human Services, Centers for Medicare and Medicaid Services
   "State Health Care Expenditures" (http://www.cms.hhs.gov/NationalHealthExpendData/)
*By state of residence. Includes spending for services and products by public and private freestanding home health agencies.
Excludes home health care services provided by hospital-based agencies which are included in hospital expenditures.

Expenditures for Drugs and Other Medical Nondurables in 2004

National Total = $222,412,000,000*

<table>
<tr><td colspan="4">ALPHA ORDER</td><td colspan="4">RANK ORDER</td></tr>
<tr><th>RANK</th><th>STATE</th><th>EXPENDITURES</th><th>% of USA</th><th>RANK</th><th>STATE</th><th>EXPENDITURES</th><th>% of USA</th></tr>
<tr><td>18</td><td>Alabama</td><td>$4,241,000,000</td><td>1.9%</td><td>1</td><td>California</td><td>$20,799,000,000</td><td>9.4%</td></tr>
<tr><td>49</td><td>Alaska</td><td>418,000,000</td><td>0.2%</td><td>2</td><td>New York</td><td>17,722,000,000</td><td>8.0%</td></tr>
<tr><td>24</td><td>Arizona</td><td>3,378,000,000</td><td>1.5%</td><td>3</td><td>Florida</td><td>15,545,000,000</td><td>7.0%</td></tr>
<tr><td>32</td><td>Arkansas</td><td>1,938,000,000</td><td>0.9%</td><td>4</td><td>Texas</td><td>13,870,000,000</td><td>6.2%</td></tr>
<tr><td>1</td><td>California</td><td>20,799,000,000</td><td>9.4%</td><td>5</td><td>Pennsylvania</td><td>11,086,000,000</td><td>5.0%</td></tr>
<tr><td>28</td><td>Colorado</td><td>2,346,000,000</td><td>1.1%</td><td>6</td><td>Ohio</td><td>9,205,000,000</td><td>4.1%</td></tr>
<tr><td>26</td><td>Connecticut</td><td>3,246,000,000</td><td>1.5%</td><td>7</td><td>Illinois</td><td>9,098,000,000</td><td>4.1%</td></tr>
<tr><td>44</td><td>Delaware</td><td>769,000,000</td><td>0.3%</td><td>8</td><td>New Jersey</td><td>8,317,000,000</td><td>3.7%</td></tr>
<tr><td>3</td><td>Florida</td><td>15,545,000,000</td><td>7.0%</td><td>9</td><td>Michigan</td><td>7,790,000,000</td><td>3.5%</td></tr>
<tr><td>11</td><td>Georgia</td><td>6,493,000,000</td><td>2.9%</td><td>10</td><td>North Carolina</td><td>7,445,000,000</td><td>3.3%</td></tr>
<tr><td>42</td><td>Hawaii</td><td>925,000,000</td><td>0.4%</td><td>11</td><td>Georgia</td><td>6,493,000,000</td><td>2.9%</td></tr>
<tr><td>43</td><td>Idaho</td><td>834,000,000</td><td>0.4%</td><td>12</td><td>Tennessee</td><td>5,785,000,000</td><td>2.6%</td></tr>
<tr><td>7</td><td>Illinois</td><td>9,098,000,000</td><td>4.1%</td><td>13</td><td>Virginia</td><td>5,651,000,000</td><td>2.5%</td></tr>
<tr><td>15</td><td>Indiana</td><td>4,951,000,000</td><td>2.2%</td><td>14</td><td>Massachusetts</td><td>5,462,000,000</td><td>2.5%</td></tr>
<tr><td>31</td><td>Iowa</td><td>2,021,000,000</td><td>0.9%</td><td>15</td><td>Indiana</td><td>4,951,000,000</td><td>2.2%</td></tr>
<tr><td>33</td><td>Kansas</td><td>1,897,000,000</td><td>0.9%</td><td>16</td><td>Missouri</td><td>4,664,000,000</td><td>2.1%</td></tr>
<tr><td>19</td><td>Kentucky</td><td>3,917,000,000</td><td>1.8%</td><td>17</td><td>Maryland</td><td>4,595,000,000</td><td>2.1%</td></tr>
<tr><td>23</td><td>Louisiana</td><td>3,586,000,000</td><td>1.6%</td><td>18</td><td>Alabama</td><td>4,241,000,000</td><td>1.9%</td></tr>
<tr><td>40</td><td>Maine</td><td>1,052,000,000</td><td>0.5%</td><td>19</td><td>Kentucky</td><td>3,917,000,000</td><td>1.8%</td></tr>
<tr><td>17</td><td>Maryland</td><td>4,595,000,000</td><td>2.1%</td><td>20</td><td>Wisconsin</td><td>3,831,000,000</td><td>1.7%</td></tr>
<tr><td>14</td><td>Massachusetts</td><td>5,462,000,000</td><td>2.5%</td><td>21</td><td>Washington</td><td>3,792,000,000</td><td>1.7%</td></tr>
<tr><td>9</td><td>Michigan</td><td>7,790,000,000</td><td>3.5%</td><td>22</td><td>Minnesota</td><td>3,639,000,000</td><td>1.6%</td></tr>
<tr><td>22</td><td>Minnesota</td><td>3,639,000,000</td><td>1.6%</td><td>23</td><td>Louisiana</td><td>3,586,000,000</td><td>1.6%</td></tr>
<tr><td>29</td><td>Mississippi</td><td>2,208,000,000</td><td>1.0%</td><td>24</td><td>Arizona</td><td>3,378,000,000</td><td>1.5%</td></tr>
<tr><td>16</td><td>Missouri</td><td>4,664,000,000</td><td>2.1%</td><td>25</td><td>South Carolina</td><td>3,369,000,000</td><td>1.5%</td></tr>
<tr><td>46</td><td>Montana</td><td>499,000,000</td><td>0.2%</td><td>26</td><td>Connecticut</td><td>3,246,000,000</td><td>1.5%</td></tr>
<tr><td>37</td><td>Nebraska</td><td>1,288,000,000</td><td>0.6%</td><td>27</td><td>Oklahoma</td><td>2,472,000,000</td><td>1.1%</td></tr>
<tr><td>34</td><td>Nevada</td><td>1,786,000,000</td><td>0.8%</td><td>28</td><td>Colorado</td><td>2,346,000,000</td><td>1.1%</td></tr>
<tr><td>41</td><td>New Hampshire</td><td>962,000,000</td><td>0.4%</td><td>29</td><td>Mississippi</td><td>2,208,000,000</td><td>1.0%</td></tr>
<tr><td>8</td><td>New Jersey</td><td>8,317,000,000</td><td>3.7%</td><td>30</td><td>Oregon</td><td>2,042,000,000</td><td>0.9%</td></tr>
<tr><td>38</td><td>New Mexico</td><td>1,127,000,000</td><td>0.5%</td><td>31</td><td>Iowa</td><td>2,021,000,000</td><td>0.9%</td></tr>
<tr><td>2</td><td>New York</td><td>17,722,000,000</td><td>8.0%</td><td>32</td><td>Arkansas</td><td>1,938,000,000</td><td>0.9%</td></tr>
<tr><td>10</td><td>North Carolina</td><td>7,445,000,000</td><td>3.3%</td><td>33</td><td>Kansas</td><td>1,897,000,000</td><td>0.9%</td></tr>
<tr><td>45</td><td>North Dakota</td><td>537,000,000</td><td>0.2%</td><td>34</td><td>Nevada</td><td>1,786,000,000</td><td>0.8%</td></tr>
<tr><td>6</td><td>Ohio</td><td>9,205,000,000</td><td>4.1%</td><td>35</td><td>West Virginia</td><td>1,627,000,000</td><td>0.7%</td></tr>
<tr><td>27</td><td>Oklahoma</td><td>2,472,000,000</td><td>1.1%</td><td>36</td><td>Utah</td><td>1,592,000,000</td><td>0.7%</td></tr>
<tr><td>30</td><td>Oregon</td><td>2,042,000,000</td><td>0.9%</td><td>37</td><td>Nebraska</td><td>1,288,000,000</td><td>0.6%</td></tr>
<tr><td>5</td><td>Pennsylvania</td><td>11,086,000,000</td><td>5.0%</td><td>38</td><td>New Mexico</td><td>1,127,000,000</td><td>0.5%</td></tr>
<tr><td>39</td><td>Rhode Island</td><td>1,066,000,000</td><td>0.5%</td><td>39</td><td>Rhode Island</td><td>1,066,000,000</td><td>0.5%</td></tr>
<tr><td>25</td><td>South Carolina</td><td>3,369,000,000</td><td>1.5%</td><td>40</td><td>Maine</td><td>1,052,000,000</td><td>0.5%</td></tr>
<tr><td>48</td><td>South Dakota</td><td>440,000,000</td><td>0.2%</td><td>41</td><td>New Hampshire</td><td>962,000,000</td><td>0.4%</td></tr>
<tr><td>12</td><td>Tennessee</td><td>5,785,000,000</td><td>2.6%</td><td>42</td><td>Hawaii</td><td>925,000,000</td><td>0.4%</td></tr>
<tr><td>4</td><td>Texas</td><td>13,870,000,000</td><td>6.2%</td><td>43</td><td>Idaho</td><td>834,000,000</td><td>0.4%</td></tr>
<tr><td>36</td><td>Utah</td><td>1,592,000,000</td><td>0.7%</td><td>44</td><td>Delaware</td><td>769,000,000</td><td>0.3%</td></tr>
<tr><td>47</td><td>Vermont</td><td>444,000,000</td><td>0.2%</td><td>45</td><td>North Dakota</td><td>537,000,000</td><td>0.2%</td></tr>
<tr><td>13</td><td>Virginia</td><td>5,651,000,000</td><td>2.5%</td><td>46</td><td>Montana</td><td>499,000,000</td><td>0.2%</td></tr>
<tr><td>21</td><td>Washington</td><td>3,792,000,000</td><td>1.7%</td><td>47</td><td>Vermont</td><td>444,000,000</td><td>0.2%</td></tr>
<tr><td>35</td><td>West Virginia</td><td>1,627,000,000</td><td>0.7%</td><td>48</td><td>South Dakota</td><td>440,000,000</td><td>0.2%</td></tr>
<tr><td>20</td><td>Wisconsin</td><td>3,831,000,000</td><td>1.7%</td><td>49</td><td>Alaska</td><td>418,000,000</td><td>0.2%</td></tr>
<tr><td>50</td><td>Wyoming</td><td>302,000,000</td><td>0.1%</td><td>50</td><td>Wyoming</td><td>302,000,000</td><td>0.1%</td></tr>
<tr><td></td><td></td><td></td><td></td><td></td><td>District of Columbia</td><td>345,000,000</td><td>0.2%</td></tr>
</table>

Source: U.S. Department of Health and Human Services, Centers for Medicare and Medicaid Services
   "State Health Care Expenditures" (http://www.cms.hhs.gov/NationalHealthExpendData/)
*Purchases in retail outlets. By state of residence. Includes prescription drugs, over-the-counter drugs, and sundries.

Percent of Total Personal Health Care Expenditures
Spent on Drugs and Other Medical Nondurables in 2004
National Percent = 14.3%*

ALPHA ORDER

RANK	STATE	PERCENT
1	Alabama	18.3
50	Alaska	9.9
26	Arizona	14.3
24	Arkansas	14.5
39	California	12.5
47	Colorado	10.8
23	Connecticut	14.6
22	Delaware	14.7
8	Florida	16.3
10	Georgia	15.8
19	Hawaii	14.9
31	Idaho	13.5
31	Illinois	13.5
18	Indiana	15.0
37	Iowa	12.7
36	Kansas	12.9
3	Kentucky	17.3
10	Louisiana	15.8
42	Maine	12.2
21	Maryland	14.8
37	Massachusetts	12.7
14	Michigan	15.3
40	Minnesota	12.3
15	Mississippi	15.1
19	Missouri	14.9
49	Montana	10.6
35	Nebraska	13.2
4	Nevada	16.8
30	New Hampshire	13.6
7	New Jersey	16.5
34	New Mexico	13.3
28	New York	14.1
4	North Carolina	16.8
24	North Dakota	14.5
29	Ohio	14.0
26	Oklahoma	14.3
45	Oregon	11.7
15	Pennsylvania	15.1
9	Rhode Island	16.0
12	South Carolina	15.7
48	South Dakota	10.7
2	Tennessee	18.0
33	Texas	13.4
6	Utah	16.6
44	Vermont	11.8
12	Virginia	15.7
43	Washington	12.0
15	West Virginia	15.1
40	Wisconsin	12.3
46	Wyoming	11.3

RANK ORDER

RANK	STATE	PERCENT
1	Alabama	18.3
2	Tennessee	18.0
3	Kentucky	17.3
4	Nevada	16.8
4	North Carolina	16.8
6	Utah	16.6
7	New Jersey	16.5
8	Florida	16.3
9	Rhode Island	16.0
10	Georgia	15.8
10	Louisiana	15.8
12	South Carolina	15.7
12	Virginia	15.7
14	Michigan	15.3
15	Mississippi	15.1
15	Pennsylvania	15.1
15	West Virginia	15.1
18	Indiana	15.0
19	Hawaii	14.9
19	Missouri	14.9
21	Maryland	14.8
22	Delaware	14.7
23	Connecticut	14.6
24	Arkansas	14.5
24	North Dakota	14.5
26	Arizona	14.3
26	Oklahoma	14.3
28	New York	14.1
29	Ohio	14.0
30	New Hampshire	13.6
31	Idaho	13.5
31	Illinois	13.5
33	Texas	13.4
34	New Mexico	13.3
35	Nebraska	13.2
36	Kansas	12.9
37	Iowa	12.7
37	Massachusetts	12.7
39	California	12.5
40	Minnesota	12.3
40	Wisconsin	12.3
42	Maine	12.2
43	Washington	12.0
44	Vermont	11.8
45	Oregon	11.7
46	Wyoming	11.3
47	Colorado	10.8
48	South Dakota	10.7
49	Montana	10.6
50	Alaska	9.9

District of Columbia	7.2

Source: CQ Press using data from U.S. Department of Health and Human Services, Centers for Medicare and Medicaid Services
"State Health Care Expenditures" (http://www.cms.hhs.gov/NationalHealthExpendData/)
*Purchases in retail outlets. By state of residence. Includes prescription drugs, over-the-counter drugs, and sundries.

Per Capita Expenditures for Drugs and Other Medical Nondurables in 2004

National Per Capita = $757*

ALPHA ORDER			RANK ORDER		
RANK	STATE	PER CAPITA	RANK	STATE	PER CAPITA
5	Alabama	$939	1	Rhode Island	$988
39	Alaska	636	2	Tennessee	983
45	Arizona	588	3	New Jersey	959
33	Arkansas	705	4	Kentucky	946
46	California	580	5	Alabama	939
50	Colorado	510	6	Connecticut	929
6	Connecticut	929	7	Delaware	928
7	Delaware	928	8	New York	919
11	Florida	895	9	West Virginia	898
29	Georgia	727	10	Pennsylvania	896
28	Hawaii	734	11	Florida	895
42	Idaho	598	12	North Carolina	873
30	Illinois	716	13	Massachusetts	849
21	Indiana	796	14	North Dakota	845
37	Iowa	684	15	Maryland	827
36	Kansas	693	16	Missouri	811
4	Kentucky	946	17	Ohio	803
20	Louisiana	798	17	South Carolina	803
19	Maine	800	19	Maine	800
15	Maryland	827	20	Louisiana	798
13	Massachusetts	849	21	Indiana	796
22	Michigan	772	22	Michigan	772
32	Minnesota	714	23	Nevada	766
24	Mississippi	763	24	Mississippi	763
16	Missouri	811	25	Virginia	756
49	Montana	539	26	New Hampshire	741
27	Nebraska	737	27	Nebraska	737
23	Nevada	766	28	Hawaii	734
26	New Hampshire	741	29	Georgia	727
3	New Jersey	959	30	Illinois	716
44	New Mexico	593	31	Vermont	715
8	New York	919	32	Minnesota	714
12	North Carolina	873	33	Arkansas	705
14	North Dakota	845	34	Oklahoma	702
17	Ohio	803	35	Wisconsin	697
34	Oklahoma	702	36	Kansas	693
48	Oregon	569	37	Iowa	684
10	Pennsylvania	896	38	Utah	658
1	Rhode Island	988	39	Alaska	636
17	South Carolina	803	40	Texas	616
47	South Dakota	572	41	Washington	611
2	Tennessee	983	42	Idaho	598
40	Texas	616	43	Wyoming	597
38	Utah	658	44	New Mexico	593
31	Vermont	715	45	Arizona	588
25	Virginia	756	46	California	580
41	Washington	611	47	South Dakota	572
9	West Virginia	898	48	Oregon	569
35	Wisconsin	697	49	Montana	539
43	Wyoming	597	50	Colorado	510
				District of Columbia	594

Source: U.S. Department of Health and Human Services, Centers for Medicare and Medicaid Services
"State Health Care Expenditures" (http://www.cms.hhs.gov/NationalHealthExpendData/)
*Purchases in retail outlets. By state of residence. Includes prescription drugs, over-the-counter drugs, and sundries.

Expenditures for Durable Medical Products in 2004

National Total = $23,128,000,000*

ALPHA ORDER

RANK	STATE	EXPENDITURES	% of USA
24	Alabama	$316,000,000	1.4%
46	Alaska	61,000,000	0.3%
21	Arizona	422,000,000	1.8%
36	Arkansas	164,000,000	0.7%
1	California	2,552,000,000	11.0%
18	Colorado	440,000,000	1.9%
23	Connecticut	317,000,000	1.4%
44	Delaware	78,000,000	0.3%
4	Florida	1,574,000,000	6.8%
11	Georgia	619,000,000	2.7%
39	Hawaii	118,000,000	0.5%
41	Idaho	101,000,000	0.4%
6	Illinois	987,000,000	4.3%
16	Indiana	470,000,000	2.0%
29	Iowa	261,000,000	1.1%
32	Kansas	215,000,000	0.9%
25	Kentucky	281,000,000	1.2%
28	Louisiana	272,000,000	1.2%
42	Maine	92,000,000	0.4%
13	Maryland	503,000,000	2.2%
14	Massachusetts	501,000,000	2.2%
9	Michigan	779,000,000	3.4%
17	Minnesota	456,000,000	2.0%
34	Mississippi	172,000,000	0.7%
20	Missouri	424,000,000	1.8%
43	Montana	85,000,000	0.4%
29	Nebraska	261,000,000	1.1%
33	Nevada	211,000,000	0.9%
40	New Hampshire	116,000,000	0.5%
7	New Jersey	964,000,000	4.2%
37	New Mexico	141,000,000	0.6%
2	New York	1,685,000,000	7.3%
12	North Carolina	524,000,000	2.3%
48	North Dakota	55,000,000	0.2%
8	Ohio	880,000,000	3.8%
31	Oklahoma	239,000,000	1.0%
26	Oregon	279,000,000	1.2%
5	Pennsylvania	1,026,000,000	4.4%
45	Rhode Island	62,000,000	0.3%
27	South Carolina	275,000,000	1.2%
47	South Dakota	60,000,000	0.3%
19	Tennessee	431,000,000	1.9%
3	Texas	1,678,000,000	7.3%
35	Utah	171,000,000	0.7%
50	Vermont	44,000,000	0.2%
10	Virginia	630,000,000	2.7%
15	Washington	485,000,000	2.1%
38	West Virginia	129,000,000	0.6%
22	Wisconsin	419,000,000	1.8%
49	Wyoming	47,000,000	0.2%

RANK ORDER

RANK	STATE	EXPENDITURES	% of USA
1	California	$2,552,000,000	11.0%
2	New York	1,685,000,000	7.3%
3	Texas	1,678,000,000	7.3%
4	Florida	1,574,000,000	6.8%
5	Pennsylvania	1,026,000,000	4.4%
6	Illinois	987,000,000	4.3%
7	New Jersey	964,000,000	4.2%
8	Ohio	880,000,000	3.8%
9	Michigan	779,000,000	3.4%
10	Virginia	630,000,000	2.7%
11	Georgia	619,000,000	2.7%
12	North Carolina	524,000,000	2.3%
13	Maryland	503,000,000	2.2%
14	Massachusetts	501,000,000	2.2%
15	Washington	485,000,000	2.1%
16	Indiana	470,000,000	2.0%
17	Minnesota	456,000,000	2.0%
18	Colorado	440,000,000	1.9%
19	Tennessee	431,000,000	1.9%
20	Missouri	424,000,000	1.8%
21	Arizona	422,000,000	1.8%
22	Wisconsin	419,000,000	1.8%
23	Connecticut	317,000,000	1.4%
24	Alabama	316,000,000	1.4%
25	Kentucky	281,000,000	1.2%
26	Oregon	279,000,000	1.2%
27	South Carolina	275,000,000	1.2%
28	Louisiana	272,000,000	1.2%
29	Iowa	261,000,000	1.1%
29	Nebraska	261,000,000	1.1%
31	Oklahoma	239,000,000	1.0%
32	Kansas	215,000,000	0.9%
33	Nevada	211,000,000	0.9%
34	Mississippi	172,000,000	0.7%
35	Utah	171,000,000	0.7%
36	Arkansas	164,000,000	0.7%
37	New Mexico	141,000,000	0.6%
38	West Virginia	129,000,000	0.6%
39	Hawaii	118,000,000	0.5%
40	New Hampshire	116,000,000	0.5%
41	Idaho	101,000,000	0.4%
42	Maine	92,000,000	0.4%
43	Montana	85,000,000	0.4%
44	Delaware	78,000,000	0.3%
45	Rhode Island	62,000,000	0.3%
46	Alaska	61,000,000	0.3%
47	South Dakota	60,000,000	0.3%
48	North Dakota	55,000,000	0.2%
49	Wyoming	47,000,000	0.2%
50	Vermont	44,000,000	0.2%
	District of Columbia	59,000,000	0.3%

Source: U.S. Department of Health and Human Services, Centers for Medicare and Medicaid Services
"State Health Care Expenditures" (http://www.cms.hhs.gov/NationalHealthExpendData/)
*By state of residence. Includes eyeglasses, hearing aids, surgical appliances and supplies, bulk and cylinder oxygen, and medical equipment rentals.

Percent of Total Personal Health Care Expenditures
Spent on Durable Medical Products in 2004
National Percent = 1.5%*

ALPHA ORDER

RANK	STATE	PERCENT
29	Alabama	1.4
29	Alaska	1.4
6	Arizona	1.8
41	Arkansas	1.2
19	California	1.5
2	Colorado	2.0
29	Connecticut	1.4
19	Delaware	1.5
10	Florida	1.7
19	Georgia	1.5
4	Hawaii	1.9
13	Idaho	1.6
19	Illinois	1.5
29	Indiana	1.4
13	Iowa	1.6
19	Kansas	1.5
41	Kentucky	1.2
41	Louisiana	1.2
49	Maine	1.1
13	Maryland	1.6
41	Massachusetts	1.2
19	Michigan	1.5
19	Minnesota	1.5
41	Mississippi	1.2
29	Missouri	1.4
6	Montana	1.8
1	Nebraska	2.7
2	Nevada	2.0
13	New Hampshire	1.6
4	New Jersey	1.9
10	New Mexico	1.7
36	New York	1.3
41	North Carolina	1.2
19	North Dakota	1.5
36	Ohio	1.3
29	Oklahoma	1.4
13	Oregon	1.6
29	Pennsylvania	1.4
50	Rhode Island	0.9
36	South Carolina	1.3
19	South Dakota	1.5
36	Tennessee	1.3
13	Texas	1.6
6	Utah	1.8
41	Vermont	1.2
10	Virginia	1.7
19	Washington	1.5
41	West Virginia	1.2
36	Wisconsin	1.3
6	Wyoming	1.8

RANK ORDER

RANK	STATE	PERCENT
1	Nebraska	2.7
2	Colorado	2.0
2	Nevada	2.0
4	Hawaii	1.9
4	New Jersey	1.9
6	Arizona	1.8
6	Montana	1.8
6	Utah	1.8
6	Wyoming	1.8
10	Florida	1.7
10	New Mexico	1.7
10	Virginia	1.7
13	Idaho	1.6
13	Iowa	1.6
13	Maryland	1.6
13	New Hampshire	1.6
13	Oregon	1.6
13	Texas	1.6
19	California	1.5
19	Delaware	1.5
19	Georgia	1.5
19	Illinois	1.5
19	Kansas	1.5
19	Michigan	1.5
19	Minnesota	1.5
19	North Dakota	1.5
19	South Dakota	1.5
19	Washington	1.5
29	Alabama	1.4
29	Alaska	1.4
29	Connecticut	1.4
29	Indiana	1.4
29	Missouri	1.4
29	Oklahoma	1.4
29	Pennsylvania	1.4
36	New York	1.3
36	Ohio	1.3
36	South Carolina	1.3
36	Tennessee	1.3
36	Wisconsin	1.3
41	Arkansas	1.2
41	Kentucky	1.2
41	Louisiana	1.2
41	Massachusetts	1.2
41	Mississippi	1.2
41	North Carolina	1.2
41	Vermont	1.2
41	West Virginia	1.2
49	Maine	1.1
50	Rhode Island	0.9

District of Columbia — 1.2

Source: CQ Press using data from U.S. Department of Health and Human Services, Centers for Medicare and Medicaid Services
   "State Health Care Expenditures" (http://www.cms.hhs.gov/NationalHealthExpendData/)
*By state of residence. Includes eyeglasses, hearing aids, surgical appliances and supplies, bulk and cylinder oxygen, and medical equipment rentals.

Per Capita Expenditures for Durable Medical Products in 2004

National Per Capita = $79*

ALPHA ORDER				RANK ORDER		
RANK	STATE	PER CAPITA		RANK	STATE	PER CAPITA
40	Alabama	$70		1	Nebraska	$149
6	Alaska	93		2	New Jersey	111
30	Arizona	74		3	Colorado	96
47	Arkansas	60		4	Delaware	95
37	California	71		5	Hawaii	94
3	Colorado	96		6	Alaska	93
9	Connecticut	91		7	Montana	92
4	Delaware	95		7	Wyoming	92
9	Florida	91		9	Connecticut	91
42	Georgia	69		9	Florida	91
5	Hawaii	94		9	Maryland	91
35	Idaho	72		12	Nevada	90
20	Illinois	78		12	New Hampshire	90
28	Indiana	76		14	Minnesota	89
15	Iowa	88		15	Iowa	88
20	Kansas	78		16	New York	87
43	Kentucky	68		17	North Dakota	86
47	Louisiana	60		18	Virginia	84
40	Maine	70		19	Pennsylvania	83
9	Maryland	91		20	Illinois	78
20	Massachusetts	78		20	Kansas	78
25	Michigan	77		20	Massachusetts	78
14	Minnesota	89		20	Oregon	78
47	Mississippi	60		20	Washington	78
30	Missouri	74		25	Michigan	77
7	Montana	92		25	Ohio	77
1	Nebraska	149		25	South Dakota	77
12	Nevada	90		28	Indiana	76
12	New Hampshire	90		28	Wisconsin	76
2	New Jersey	111		30	Arizona	74
30	New Mexico	74		30	Missouri	74
16	New York	87		30	New Mexico	74
46	North Carolina	61		30	Texas	74
17	North Dakota	86		34	Tennessee	73
25	Ohio	77		35	Idaho	72
43	Oklahoma	68		35	Vermont	72
20	Oregon	78		37	California	71
19	Pennsylvania	83		37	Utah	71
50	Rhode Island	57		37	West Virginia	71
45	South Carolina	66		40	Alabama	70
25	South Dakota	77		40	Maine	70
34	Tennessee	73		42	Georgia	69
30	Texas	74		43	Kentucky	68
37	Utah	71		43	Oklahoma	68
35	Vermont	72		45	South Carolina	66
18	Virginia	84		46	North Carolina	61
20	Washington	78		47	Arkansas	60
37	West Virginia	71		47	Louisiana	60
28	Wisconsin	76		47	Mississippi	60
7	Wyoming	92		50	Rhode Island	57
					District of Columbia	102

Source: U.S. Department of Health and Human Services, Centers for Medicare and Medicaid Services
"State Health Care Expenditures" (http://www.cms.hhs.gov/NationalHealthExpendData/)
*By state of residence. Includes eyeglasses, hearing aids, surgical appliances and supplies, bulk and cylinder oxygen, and medical equipment rentals.

Projected National Health Care Expenditures in 2011

Total Health Care Expenditures = $2,702,900,000,000*

The 2004 health care expenditures broken down to the state level and shown on pages 305 to 332 were released in February of 2007 and are the most recent state health expenditure data available from the Centers for Medicare and Medicaid Services (CMS).

Given the high level of interest in health care finance data, we have assembled a table showing the most recent national level health care expenditure projections.

	PROJECTED EXPENDITURES IN 2011	PROJECTED PERCENT CHANGE: 2010 TO 2011
Total Health Care Expenditures	$2,702,900,000,000	5.2
Per Capita Total Health Care Expenditures	$8,804	
Personal Health Care Expenditures	$2,244,600,000,000	4.8
Per Capita Personal Health Care Expenditures	$7,311	
Hospital Care Expenditures	$827,300,000,000	4.9
Per Capita Hospital Care Expenditures	$2,695	
Physician Services Expenditures	$556,100,000,000	3.8
Per Capita Physician Services Expenditures	$1,811	
Dental Services Expenditures	$111,800,000,000	3.6
Per Capita Dental Services Expenditures	$364	
Other Professional Services	$74,600,000,000	4.4
Per Capita Other Professional Services	$243	
Home Health Care Expenditures	$82,800,000,000	7.4
Per Capita Home Health Care Expenditures	$270	
Prescription Drugs	$274,500,000,000	5.6
Per Capita Prescription Drugs	$894	
Nursing Home Care	$156,200,000,000	4.6
Per Capita Nursing Home Care	$509	
Other Personal Care Expenditures	$90,300,000,000	9.9
Per Capita Other Personal Care Expenditures	$294	

Source: U.S. Department of Health and Human Services, Centers for Medicare and Medicaid Services
"National Health Care Expenditures Projections: 2009-2019"
(http://www.cms.gov/NationalHealthExpendData/downloads/proj2009.pdf)
*Per Capita figures calculated by CQ Press using 2009 Census population estimates. For definitions see the corresponding 2004 state tables in this chapter.

V. Incidence of Disease

Estimated New Cancer Cases in 2010 336
Estimated Rate of New Cancer Cases in 2010 337
Age-Adjusted Cancer Incidence Rates for Males in 2006 . . 338
Age-Adjusted Cancer Incidence Rates for Females
    in 2006 339
Estimated New Cases of Bladder Cancer in 2010 340
Estimated Rate of New Bladder Cancer Cases in 2010 . . . 341
Estimated New Female Breast Cancer Cases in 2010 342
Age-Adjusted Incidence Rate of Female Breast Cancer
    Cases in 2006 343
Percent of Women 40 and Older Who Have Had a
    Mammogram in the Past Two Years: 2008 344
Estimated New Colon and Rectum Cancer Cases
    in 2010 345
Estimated Rate of New Colon and Rectum Cancer
    Cases in 2010 346
Percent of Adults Who Have Ever Had a Sigmoidoscopy
    or Colonoscopy Exam: 2008 347
Estimated New Leukemia Cases in 2010 348
Estimated Rate of New Leukemia Cases in 2010 349
Estimated New Lung Cancer Cases in 2010 350
Estimated Rate of New Lung Cancer Cases in 2010 351
Estimated New Non-Hodgkin's Lymphoma Cases
    in 2010 352
Estimated Rate of New Non-Hodgkin's Lymphoma
    Cases in 2010 353
Estimated New Prostate Cancer Cases in 2010 354
Age-Adjusted Incidence Rate of Prostate Cancer
    Cases in 2006 355
Percent of Males Receiving PSA Test for Prostate
    Cancer: 2008 356
Estimated New Skin Melanoma Cases in 2010 357
Estimated Rate of New Skin Melanoma Cases in 2010 . . . 358
Estimated New Cervical Cancer Cases in 2010 359
Estimated Rate of New Cervical Cancer Cases in 2010 . . . 360
Percent of Women 18 Years Old and Older Who Have
    Had a Pap Smear in the Past Three Years: 2008 361
Estimated New Uterine Cancer Cases in 2010 362
Estimated Rate of New Uterine Cancer Cases in 2010 363

AIDS Cases Reported in 2008 364
AIDS Rate in 2008 365
AIDS Cases Reported through December 2008 366
AIDS Cases in Children 12 Years and Younger through
    December 2008 367
Chickenpox (Varicella) Cases Reported in 2010 368
Chickenpox (Varicella) Rate in 2010 369
E. Coli Cases Reported in 2010 370
E. Coli Rate in 2010 371
Hepatitis A and B Cases Reported in 2010 372
Hepatitis A and B Rate in 2010 373
Hepatitis C Cases Reported in 2010 374
Hepatitis C Rate in 2010 375
Legionellosis Cases Reported in 2010 376
Legionellosis Rate in 2010 377
Lyme Disease Cases Reported in 2010 378
Lyme Disease Rate in 2010 379
Malaria Cases Reported in 2010 380
Malaria Rate in 2010 381
Meningococcal Infections Reported in 2010 382
Meningococcal Infection Rate in 2010 383
Rabies (Animal) Cases Reported in 2010 384
Rabies (Animal) Rate in 2010 385
Spotted Fever Rickettsiosis Reported in 2010 386
Rocky Mountain Spotted Fever Rate in 2010 387
Salmonellosis Cases Reported in 2010 388
Salmonellosis Rate in 2010 389
Shigellosis Cases Reported in 2010 390
Shigellosis Rate in 2010 391
West Nile Virus Disease Cases Reported in 2010 392
West Nile Disease Rate in 2010 393
Whooping Cough (Pertussis) Cases Reported in 2010 394
Whooping Cough (Pertussis) Rate in 2010 395
Percent of Children Aged 19 to 35 Months Fully
    Immunized in 2009 396
Percent of Adults Aged 65 Years and Older Who
    Received Flu Shots in 2009 397
Percent of Adults Aged 65 Years and Older Who Have
    Had a Pneumonia Vaccine: 2009 398

Sexually Transmitted Diseases in 2009 399
Sexually Transmitted Disease Rate in 2009 400
Chlamydia Cases Reported in 2009 401
Chlamydia Rate in 2009 402
Gonorrhea Cases Reported in 2009 403
Gonorrhea Rate in 2009 404
Syphilis Cases Reported in 2009 405
Syphilis Rate in 2009 406

Percent of Adults Who Have Asthma: 2009 407
Percent of Adults Who Have Been Told They Have
    Arthritis: 2009 408
Percent of Adults Who Have Been Told They Have
    Diabetes: 2009 409
Percent of Adults Reporting Serious Psychological
    Distress: 2007 410

Estimated New Cancer Cases in 2010

National Estimated Total = 1,529,560 New Cases*

ALPHA ORDER

RANK	STATE	CASES	% of USA
23	Alabama	23,640	1.5%
49	Alaska	2,860	0.2%
18	Arizona	29,780	1.9%
31	Arkansas	15,320	1.0%
1	California	157,320	10.3%
25	Colorado	21,340	1.4%
27	Connecticut	20,750	1.4%
45	Delaware	4,890	0.3%
2	Florida	107,000	7.0%
11	Georgia	40,480	2.6%
42	Hawaii	6,670	0.4%
41	Idaho	7,220	0.5%
7	Illinois	63,890	4.2%
16	Indiana	33,020	2.2%
30	Iowa	17,260	1.1%
33	Kansas	13,550	0.9%
22	Kentucky	24,240	1.6%
26	Louisiana	20,950	1.4%
39	Maine	8,650	0.6%
20	Maryland	27,700	1.8%
13	Massachusetts	36,040	2.4%
8	Michigan	55,660	3.6%
21	Minnesota	25,080	1.6%
32	Mississippi	14,330	0.9%
17	Missouri	31,160	2.0%
44	Montana	5,570	0.4%
37	Nebraska	9,230	0.6%
34	Nevada	12,230	0.8%
40	New Hampshire	7,810	0.5%
9	New Jersey	48,100	3.1%
38	New Mexico	9,210	0.6%
3	New York	103,340	6.8%
10	North Carolina	45,120	2.9%
48	North Dakota	3,300	0.2%
6	Ohio	64,450	4.2%
29	Oklahoma	18,670	1.2%
27	Oregon	20,750	1.4%
5	Pennsylvania	75,260	4.9%
43	Rhode Island	5,970	0.4%
24	South Carolina	23,240	1.5%
46	South Dakota	4,220	0.3%
15	Tennessee	33,070	2.2%
4	Texas	101,120	6.6%
36	Utah	9,970	0.7%
47	Vermont	3,720	0.2%
12	Virginia	36,410	2.4%
14	Washington	34,500	2.3%
35	West Virginia	10,610	0.7%
19	Wisconsin	29,610	1.9%
50	Wyoming	2,540	0.2%

RANK ORDER

RANK	STATE	CASES	% of USA
1	California	157,320	10.3%
2	Florida	107,000	7.0%
3	New York	103,340	6.8%
4	Texas	101,120	6.6%
5	Pennsylvania	75,260	4.9%
6	Ohio	64,450	4.2%
7	Illinois	63,890	4.2%
8	Michigan	55,660	3.6%
9	New Jersey	48,100	3.1%
10	North Carolina	45,120	2.9%
11	Georgia	40,480	2.6%
12	Virginia	36,410	2.4%
13	Massachusetts	36,040	2.4%
14	Washington	34,500	2.3%
15	Tennessee	33,070	2.2%
16	Indiana	33,020	2.2%
17	Missouri	31,160	2.0%
18	Arizona	29,780	1.9%
19	Wisconsin	29,610	1.9%
20	Maryland	27,700	1.8%
21	Minnesota	25,080	1.6%
22	Kentucky	24,240	1.6%
23	Alabama	23,640	1.5%
24	South Carolina	23,240	1.5%
25	Colorado	21,340	1.4%
26	Louisiana	20,950	1.4%
27	Connecticut	20,750	1.4%
27	Oregon	20,750	1.4%
29	Oklahoma	18,670	1.2%
30	Iowa	17,260	1.1%
31	Arkansas	15,320	1.0%
32	Mississippi	14,330	0.9%
33	Kansas	13,550	0.9%
34	Nevada	12,230	0.8%
35	West Virginia	10,610	0.7%
36	Utah	9,970	0.7%
37	Nebraska	9,230	0.6%
38	New Mexico	9,210	0.6%
39	Maine	8,650	0.6%
40	New Hampshire	7,810	0.5%
41	Idaho	7,220	0.5%
42	Hawaii	6,670	0.4%
43	Rhode Island	5,970	0.4%
44	Montana	5,570	0.4%
45	Delaware	4,890	0.3%
46	South Dakota	4,220	0.3%
47	Vermont	3,720	0.2%
48	North Dakota	3,300	0.2%
49	Alaska	2,860	0.2%
50	Wyoming	2,540	0.2%
	District of Columbia	2,760	0.2%

Source: American Cancer Society

"Cancer Facts & Figures 2010" (Copyright 2010, American Cancer Society, http://www.cancer.org/docroot/stt/stt_0.asp)
*These estimates are offered as a rough guide and should not be regarded as definitive. They are calculated by the American Cancer Society using a model based on 1995-2006 incidence rates. Totals do not include basal and squamous cell skin cancers or in situ carcinomas except urinary bladder.

Estimated Rate of New Cancer Cases in 2010

National Estimated Rate = 498.2 New Cases per 100,000 Population*

ALPHA ORDER				RANK ORDER		
RANK	STATE	RATE		RANK	STATE	RATE
31	Alabama	502.0		1	Maine	656.1
48	Alaska	409.5		2	Vermont	598.3
44	Arizona	451.5		3	Pennsylvania	597.1
18	Arkansas	530.2		4	Connecticut	589.8
45	California	425.6		5	New Hampshire	589.6
46	Colorado	424.7		6	West Virginia	583.0
4	Connecticut	589.8		7	Florida	577.2
14	Delaware	552.5		8	Iowa	573.8
7	Florida	577.2		9	Montana	571.3
47	Georgia	411.8		10	Rhode Island	566.8
25	Hawaii	515.0		11	Kentucky	561.9
38	Idaho	467.1		12	Ohio	558.4
32	Illinois	494.9		13	Michigan	558.3
26	Indiana	514.1		14	Delaware	552.5
8	Iowa	573.8		15	New Jersey	552.4
36	Kansas	480.7		16	Massachusetts	546.6
11	Kentucky	561.9		17	Oregon	542.4
40	Louisiana	466.4		18	Arkansas	530.2
1	Maine	656.1		19	New York	528.8
33	Maryland	486.0		20	Tennessee	525.2
16	Massachusetts	546.6		21	Wisconsin	523.6
13	Michigan	558.3		22	Missouri	520.4
37	Minnesota	476.2		23	South Dakota	519.5
34	Mississippi	485.4		24	Washington	517.7
22	Missouri	520.4		25	Hawaii	515.0
9	Montana	571.3		26	Indiana	514.1
27	Nebraska	513.7		27	Nebraska	513.7
41	Nevada	462.7		28	North Dakota	510.2
5	New Hampshire	589.6		29	South Carolina	509.5
15	New Jersey	552.4		30	Oklahoma	506.4
43	New Mexico	458.3		31	Alabama	502.0
19	New York	528.8		32	Illinois	494.9
35	North Carolina	481.0		33	Maryland	486.0
28	North Dakota	510.2		34	Mississippi	485.4
12	Ohio	558.4		35	North Carolina	481.0
30	Oklahoma	506.4		36	Kansas	480.7
17	Oregon	542.4		37	Minnesota	476.2
3	Pennsylvania	597.1		38	Idaho	467.1
10	Rhode Island	566.8		39	Wyoming	466.7
29	South Carolina	509.5		40	Louisiana	466.4
23	South Dakota	519.5		41	Nevada	462.7
20	Tennessee	525.2		42	Virginia	461.9
49	Texas	408.0		43	New Mexico	458.3
50	Utah	358.0		44	Arizona	451.5
2	Vermont	598.3		45	California	425.6
42	Virginia	461.9		46	Colorado	424.7
24	Washington	517.7		47	Georgia	411.8
6	West Virginia	583.0		48	Alaska	409.5
21	Wisconsin	523.6		49	Texas	408.0
39	Wyoming	466.7		50	Utah	358.0
					District of Columbia	460.3

Source: CQ Press using data from American Cancer Society
  "Cancer Facts & Figures 2009" (Copyright 2009, American Cancer Society, http://www.cancer.org/docroot/stt/stt_0.asp)
*These estimates are offered as a rough guide and should not be regarded as definitive. They are calculated by the American Cancer Society using a model based on 1995-2006 incidence rates. Totals do not include basal and squamous cell skin cancers or in situ carcinomas except urinary bladder. Rates calculated using 2009 Census resident population estimates.

Age-Adjusted Cancer Incidence Rates for Males in 2006

National Rate = 556.5 New Cases per 100,000 Male Population*

ALPHA ORDER

RANK	STATE	RATE
23	Alabama	561.2
38	Alaska	529.4
46	Arizona	465.9
20	Arkansas	562.8
41	California	510.1
42	Colorado	501.5
10	Connecticut	591.0
5	Delaware	607.7
35	Florida	537.3
19	Georgia	566.4
44	Hawaii	486.7
34	Idaho	538.4
13	Illinois	579.8
27	Indiana	551.3
24	Iowa	558.9
25	Kansas	557.2
4	Kentucky	608.4
2	Louisiana	619.2
1	Maine	620.9
NA	Maryland**	NA
9	Massachusetts	591.8
7	Michigan	597.5
17	Minnesota	567.2
16	Mississippi	574.7
31	Missouri	544.3
32	Montana	541.9
21	Nebraska	561.8
36	Nevada	531.2
12	New Hampshire	584.3
6	New Jersey	603.9
45	New Mexico	480.5
15	New York	577.5
26	North Carolina	553.4
28	North Dakota	549.3
NA	Ohio**	NA
22	Oklahoma	561.4
39	Oregon	529.3
8	Pennsylvania	592.7
3	Rhode Island	608.9
11	South Carolina	587.4
30	South Dakota	547.8
29	Tennessee	548.3
33	Texas	539.6
43	Utah	486.8
NA	Vermont**	NA
37	Virginia	529.5
18	Washington	566.9
14	West Virginia	578.6
NA	Wisconsin**	NA
40	Wyoming	516.5

RANK ORDER

RANK	STATE	RATE
1	Maine	620.9
2	Louisiana	619.2
3	Rhode Island	608.9
4	Kentucky	608.4
5	Delaware	607.7
6	New Jersey	603.9
7	Michigan	597.5
8	Pennsylvania	592.7
9	Massachusetts	591.8
10	Connecticut	591.0
11	South Carolina	587.4
12	New Hampshire	584.3
13	Illinois	579.8
14	West Virginia	578.6
15	New York	577.5
16	Mississippi	574.7
17	Minnesota	567.2
18	Washington	566.9
19	Georgia	566.4
20	Arkansas	562.8
21	Nebraska	561.8
22	Oklahoma	561.4
23	Alabama	561.2
24	Iowa	558.9
25	Kansas	557.2
26	North Carolina	553.4
27	Indiana	551.3
28	North Dakota	549.3
29	Tennessee	548.3
30	South Dakota	547.8
31	Missouri	544.3
32	Montana	541.9
33	Texas	539.6
34	Idaho	538.4
35	Florida	537.3
36	Nevada	531.2
37	Virginia	529.5
38	Alaska	529.4
39	Oregon	529.3
40	Wyoming	516.5
41	California	510.1
42	Colorado	501.5
43	Utah	486.8
44	Hawaii	486.7
45	New Mexico	480.5
46	Arizona	465.9
NA	Maryland**	NA
NA	Ohio**	NA
NA	Vermont**	NA
NA	Wisconsin**	NA

	District of Columbia	556.0

Source: American Cancer Society
"Cancer Facts & Figures 2010" (Copyright 2010, American Cancer Society, http://www.cancer.org/docroot/stt/stt_0.asp)
*For 2002 to 2006. Age-adjusted to the 2000 U.S. standard population.
**Not available.

Age-Adjusted Cancer Incidence Rates for Females in 2006

National Rate = 414.8 New Cases per 100,000 Female Population*

ALPHA ORDER

RANK	STATE	RATE
43	Alabama	379.6
19	Alaska	417.7
45	Arizona	364.0
40	Arkansas	383.5
35	California	393.3
34	Colorado	394.1
2	Connecticut	455.5
10	Delaware	440.8
27	Florida	404.2
37	Georgia	392.4
41	Hawaii	383.0
29	Idaho	401.7
16	Illinois	429.1
23	Indiana	415.1
15	Iowa	429.2
20	Kansas	417.2
7	Kentucky	446.4
25	Louisiana	409.6
1	Maine	465.8
NA	Maryland**	NA
5	Massachusetts	452.9
11	Michigan	437.9
22	Minnesota	416.4
42	Mississippi	382.1
20	Missouri	417.2
26	Montana	406.3
18	Nebraska	418.2
24	Nevada	412.0
3	New Hampshire	455.3
6	New Jersey	449.5
44	New Mexico	366.1
13	New York	434.4
31	North Carolina	398.1
28	North Dakota	402.7
NA	Ohio**	NA
17	Oklahoma	422.2
14	Oregon	429.7
8	Pennsylvania	444.6
3	Rhode Island	455.3
32	South Carolina	397.5
33	South Dakota	395.3
30	Tennessee	400.6
38	Texas	389.9
46	Utah	346.6
NA	Vermont**	NA
39	Virginia	385.8
9	Washington	443.3
12	West Virginia	437.1
NA	Wisconsin**	NA
36	Wyoming	392.9

RANK ORDER

RANK	STATE	RATE
1	Maine	465.8
2	Connecticut	455.5
3	New Hampshire	455.3
3	Rhode Island	455.3
5	Massachusetts	452.9
6	New Jersey	449.5
7	Kentucky	446.4
8	Pennsylvania	444.6
9	Washington	443.3
10	Delaware	440.8
11	Michigan	437.9
12	West Virginia	437.1
13	New York	434.4
14	Oregon	429.7
15	Iowa	429.2
16	Illinois	429.1
17	Oklahoma	422.2
18	Nebraska	418.2
19	Alaska	417.7
20	Kansas	417.2
20	Missouri	417.2
22	Minnesota	416.4
23	Indiana	415.1
24	Nevada	412.0
25	Louisiana	409.6
26	Montana	406.3
27	Florida	404.2
28	North Dakota	402.7
29	Idaho	401.7
30	Tennessee	400.6
31	North Carolina	398.1
32	South Carolina	397.5
33	South Dakota	395.3
34	Colorado	394.1
35	California	393.3
36	Wyoming	392.9
37	Georgia	392.4
38	Texas	389.9
39	Virginia	385.8
40	Arkansas	383.5
41	Hawaii	383.0
42	Mississippi	382.1
43	Alabama	379.6
44	New Mexico	366.1
45	Arizona	364.0
46	Utah	346.6
NA	Maryland**	NA
NA	Ohio**	NA
NA	Vermont**	NA
NA	Wisconsin**	NA

District of Columbia   412.1

Source: American Cancer Society
"Cancer Facts & Figures 2010" (Copyright 2010, American Cancer Society, http://www.cancer.org/docroot/stt/stt_0.asp)
*For 2002 to 2006. Age-adjusted to the 2000 U.S. standard population.
**Not available.

Estimated New Cases of Bladder Cancer in 2010

National Estimated Total = 70,530 New Cases*

ALPHA ORDER

RANK ORDER

RANK	STATE	CASES	% of USA
27	Alabama	920	1.3%
49	Alaska	140	0.2%
13	Arizona	1,530	2.2%
32	Arkansas	610	0.9%
1	California	6,620	9.4%
25	Colorado	960	1.4%
22	Connecticut	1,110	1.6%
44	Delaware	250	0.4%
2	Florida	5,600	7.9%
17	Georgia	1,470	2.1%
47	Hawaii	200	0.3%
40	Idaho	380	0.5%
6	Illinois	3,050	4.3%
15	Indiana	1,510	2.1%
29	Iowa	840	1.2%
33	Kansas	550	0.8%
24	Kentucky	1,030	1.5%
28	Louisiana	850	1.2%
34	Maine	530	0.8%
20	Maryland	1,180	1.7%
10	Massachusetts	2,000	2.8%
8	Michigan	2,790	4.0%
21	Minnesota	1,160	1.6%
36	Mississippi	510	0.7%
18	Missouri	1,360	1.9%
43	Montana	280	0.4%
38	Nebraska	420	0.6%
31	Nevada	620	0.9%
37	New Hampshire	430	0.6%
9	New Jersey	2,510	3.6%
41	New Mexico	350	0.5%
3	New York	5,230	7.4%
11	North Carolina	1,890	2.7%
48	North Dakota	180	0.3%
7	Ohio	2,970	4.2%
30	Oklahoma	770	1.1%
23	Oregon	1,040	1.5%
4	Pennsylvania	4,050	5.7%
41	Rhode Island	350	0.5%
26	South Carolina	950	1.3%
45	South Dakota	230	0.3%
19	Tennessee	1,350	1.9%
5	Texas	3,650	5.2%
39	Utah	390	0.6%
46	Vermont	210	0.3%
14	Virginia	1,520	2.2%
12	Washington	1,720	2.4%
34	West Virginia	530	0.8%
15	Wisconsin	1,510	2.1%
50	Wyoming	130	0.2%

RANK	STATE	CASES	% of USA
1	California	6,620	9.4%
2	Florida	5,600	7.9%
3	New York	5,230	7.4%
4	Pennsylvania	4,050	5.7%
5	Texas	3,650	5.2%
6	Illinois	3,050	4.3%
7	Ohio	2,970	4.2%
8	Michigan	2,790	4.0%
9	New Jersey	2,510	3.6%
10	Massachusetts	2,000	2.8%
11	North Carolina	1,890	2.7%
12	Washington	1,720	2.4%
13	Arizona	1,530	2.2%
14	Virginia	1,520	2.2%
15	Indiana	1,510	2.1%
15	Wisconsin	1,510	2.1%
17	Georgia	1,470	2.1%
18	Missouri	1,360	1.9%
19	Tennessee	1,350	1.9%
20	Maryland	1,180	1.7%
21	Minnesota	1,160	1.6%
22	Connecticut	1,110	1.6%
23	Oregon	1,040	1.5%
24	Kentucky	1,030	1.5%
25	Colorado	960	1.4%
26	South Carolina	950	1.3%
27	Alabama	920	1.3%
28	Louisiana	850	1.2%
29	Iowa	840	1.2%
30	Oklahoma	770	1.1%
31	Nevada	620	0.9%
32	Arkansas	610	0.9%
33	Kansas	550	0.8%
34	Maine	530	0.8%
34	West Virginia	530	0.8%
36	Mississippi	510	0.7%
37	New Hampshire	430	0.6%
38	Nebraska	420	0.6%
39	Utah	390	0.6%
40	Idaho	380	0.5%
41	New Mexico	350	0.5%
41	Rhode Island	350	0.5%
43	Montana	280	0.4%
44	Delaware	250	0.4%
45	South Dakota	230	0.3%
46	Vermont	210	0.3%
47	Hawaii	200	0.3%
48	North Dakota	180	0.3%
49	Alaska	140	0.2%
50	Wyoming	130	0.2%
	District of Columbia	90	0.1%

Source: American Cancer Society
    "Cancer Facts & Figures 2010" (Copyright 2010, American Cancer Society, http://www.cancer.org/docroot/stt/stt_0.asp)
*These estimates are offered as a rough guide and should be interpreted with caution. They are calculated by the American Cancer Society using a model based on 1995-2006 incidence rates.

Estimated Rate of New Bladder Cancer Cases in 2010

National Estimated Rate = 23.0 New Cases per 100,000 Population*

ALPHA ORDER			RANK ORDER		
RANK	STATE	RATE	RANK	STATE	RATE
39	Alabama	19.5	1	Maine	40.2
38	Alaska	20.0	2	Vermont	33.8
29	Arizona	23.2	3	Rhode Island	33.2
33	Arkansas	21.1	4	New Hampshire	32.5
44	California	17.9	5	Pennsylvania	32.1
42	Colorado	19.1	6	Connecticut	31.5
6	Connecticut	31.5	7	Massachusetts	30.3
13	Delaware	28.2	8	Florida	30.2
8	Florida	30.2	9	West Virginia	29.1
48	Georgia	15.0	10	New Jersey	28.8
47	Hawaii	15.4	11	Montana	28.7
22	Idaho	24.6	12	South Dakota	28.3
25	Illinois	23.6	13	Delaware	28.2
26	Indiana	23.5	14	Michigan	28.0
15	Iowa	27.9	15	Iowa	27.9
39	Kansas	19.5	16	North Dakota	27.8
23	Kentucky	23.9	17	Oregon	27.2
43	Louisiana	18.9	18	New York	26.8
1	Maine	40.2	19	Wisconsin	26.7
36	Maryland	20.7	20	Washington	25.8
7	Massachusetts	30.3	21	Ohio	25.7
14	Michigan	28.0	22	Idaho	24.6
31	Minnesota	22.0	23	Kentucky	23.9
46	Mississippi	17.3	23	Wyoming	23.9
30	Missouri	22.7	25	Illinois	23.6
11	Montana	28.7	26	Indiana	23.5
28	Nebraska	23.4	26	Nevada	23.5
26	Nevada	23.5	28	Nebraska	23.4
4	New Hampshire	32.5	29	Arizona	23.2
10	New Jersey	28.8	30	Missouri	22.7
45	New Mexico	17.4	31	Minnesota	22.0
18	New York	26.8	32	Tennessee	21.4
37	North Carolina	20.1	33	Arkansas	21.1
16	North Dakota	27.8	34	Oklahoma	20.9
21	Ohio	25.7	35	South Carolina	20.8
34	Oklahoma	20.9	36	Maryland	20.7
17	Oregon	27.2	37	North Carolina	20.1
5	Pennsylvania	32.1	38	Alaska	20.0
3	Rhode Island	33.2	39	Alabama	19.5
35	South Carolina	20.8	39	Kansas	19.5
12	South Dakota	28.3	41	Virginia	19.3
32	Tennessee	21.4	42	Colorado	19.1
49	Texas	14.7	43	Louisiana	18.9
50	Utah	14.0	44	California	17.9
2	Vermont	33.8	45	New Mexico	17.4
41	Virginia	19.3	46	Mississippi	17.3
20	Washington	25.8	47	Hawaii	15.4
9	West Virginia	29.1	48	Georgia	15.0
19	Wisconsin	26.7	49	Texas	14.7
23	Wyoming	23.9	50	Utah	14.0
				District of Columbia	15.0

Source: CQ Press using data from American Cancer Society
"Cancer Facts & Figures 2010" (Copyright 2010, American Cancer Society, http://www.cancer.org/docroot/stt/stt_0.asp)
*These estimates are offered as a rough guide and should be interpreted with caution. They are calculated by the American Cancer Society using a model based on 1995-2006 incidence rates.   Rates calculated using 2009 Census resident population estimates.

Estimated New Female Breast Cancer Cases in 2010

National Estimated Total = 207,090 New Cases*

ALPHA ORDER

RANK	STATE	CASES	% of USA
21	Alabama	3,450	1.7%
48	Alaska	410	0.2%
19	Arizona	3,950	1.9%
33	Arkansas	1,770	0.9%
1	California	21,130	10.2%
25	Colorado	3,100	1.5%
26	Connecticut	2,960	1.4%
44	Delaware	690	0.3%
3	Florida	14,080	6.8%
11	Georgia	6,130	3.0%
41	Hawaii	910	0.4%
41	Idaho	910	0.4%
6	Illinois	8,770	4.2%
16	Indiana	4,350	2.1%
30	Iowa	2,020	1.0%
32	Kansas	1,780	0.9%
23	Kentucky	3,290	1.6%
28	Louisiana	2,530	1.2%
38	Maine	1,160	0.6%
17	Maryland	4,150	2.0%
13	Massachusetts	5,320	2.6%
8	Michigan	7,340	3.5%
22	Minnesota	3,330	1.6%
31	Mississippi	1,970	1.0%
20	Missouri	3,880	1.9%
45	Montana	680	0.3%
38	Nebraska	1,160	0.6%
34	Nevada	1,350	0.7%
40	New Hampshire	990	0.5%
9	New Jersey	6,820	3.3%
37	New Mexico	1,180	0.6%
2	New York	14,610	7.1%
10	North Carolina	6,500	3.1%
49	North Dakota	400	0.2%
7	Ohio	8,280	4.0%
29	Oklahoma	2,300	1.1%
27	Oregon	2,910	1.4%
5	Pennsylvania	10,000	4.8%
43	Rhode Island	790	0.4%
24	South Carolina	3,260	1.6%
46	South Dakota	530	0.3%
15	Tennessee	4,700	2.3%
4	Texas	12,920	6.2%
36	Utah	1,260	0.6%
47	Vermont	520	0.3%
12	Virginia	5,470	2.6%
14	Washington	4,900	2.4%
35	West Virginia	1,310	0.6%
18	Wisconsin	4,120	2.0%
50	Wyoming	330	0.2%

RANK ORDER

RANK	STATE	CASES	% of USA
1	California	21,130	10.2%
2	New York	14,610	7.1%
3	Florida	14,080	6.8%
4	Texas	12,920	6.2%
5	Pennsylvania	10,000	4.8%
6	Illinois	8,770	4.2%
7	Ohio	8,280	4.0%
8	Michigan	7,340	3.5%
9	New Jersey	6,820	3.3%
10	North Carolina	6,500	3.1%
11	Georgia	6,130	3.0%
12	Virginia	5,470	2.6%
13	Massachusetts	5,320	2.6%
14	Washington	4,900	2.4%
15	Tennessee	4,700	2.3%
16	Indiana	4,350	2.1%
17	Maryland	4,150	2.0%
18	Wisconsin	4,120	2.0%
19	Arizona	3,950	1.9%
20	Missouri	3,880	1.9%
21	Alabama	3,450	1.7%
22	Minnesota	3,330	1.6%
23	Kentucky	3,290	1.6%
24	South Carolina	3,260	1.6%
25	Colorado	3,100	1.5%
26	Connecticut	2,960	1.4%
27	Oregon	2,910	1.4%
28	Louisiana	2,530	1.2%
29	Oklahoma	2,300	1.1%
30	Iowa	2,020	1.0%
31	Mississippi	1,970	1.0%
32	Kansas	1,780	0.9%
33	Arkansas	1,770	0.9%
34	Nevada	1,350	0.7%
35	West Virginia	1,310	0.6%
36	Utah	1,260	0.6%
37	New Mexico	1,180	0.6%
38	Maine	1,160	0.6%
38	Nebraska	1,160	0.6%
40	New Hampshire	990	0.5%
41	Hawaii	910	0.4%
41	Idaho	910	0.4%
43	Rhode Island	790	0.4%
44	Delaware	690	0.3%
45	Montana	680	0.3%
46	South Dakota	530	0.3%
47	Vermont	520	0.3%
48	Alaska	410	0.2%
49	North Dakota	400	0.2%
50	Wyoming	330	0.2%
	District of Columbia	390	0.2%

Source: American Cancer Society
   "Cancer Facts & Figures 2010" (Copyright 2010, American Cancer Society, http://www.cancer.org/docroot/stt/stt_0.asp)
*These estimates are offered as a rough guide and should be interpreted with caution. They are calculated by the American Cancer Society using a model based on 1995-2006 incidence rates.

Age-Adjusted Incidence Rate of Female Breast Cancer Cases in 2006

National Rate = 121.8 New Cases per 100,000 Female Population*

ALPHA ORDER

RANK	STATE	RATE
39	Alabama	114.6
10	Alaska	126.4
45	Arizona	108.8
41	Arkansas	113.1
22	California	122.3
19	Colorado	123.1
1	Connocticut	135.0
18	Delaware	123.9
40	Florida	114.1
32	Georgia	118.5
24	Hawaii	121.4
34	Idaho	117.5
19	Illinois	123.1
36	Indiana	115.3
17	Iowa	124.0
13	Kansas	126.1
27	Kentucky	119.8
28	Louisiana	119.6
6	Maine	128.6
NA	Maryland**	NA
3	Massachusetts	132.2
16	Michigan	124.2
10	Minnesota	126.4
46	Mississippi	108.2
23	Missouri	121.9
28	Montana	119.6
10	Nebraska	126.4
42	Nevada	112.1
5	New Hampshire	131.2
8	New Jersey	128.0
44	New Mexico	109.6
14	New York	124.5
26	North Carolina	120.3
21	North Dakota	122.8
NA	Ohio**	NA
9	Oklahoma	127.2
4	Oregon	131.9
14	Pennsylvania	124.5
7	Rhode Island	128.3
31	South Carolina	119.2
28	South Dakota	119.6
35	Tennessee	116.4
37	Texas	114.9
43	Utah	110.0
NA	Vermont**	NA
25	Virginia	120.7
2	Washington	134.8
38	West Virginia	114.7
NA	Wisconsin**	NA
33	Wyoming	117.8

RANK ORDER

RANK	STATE	RATE
1	Connecticut	135.0
2	Washington	134.8
3	Massachusetts	132.2
4	Oregon	131.9
5	New Hampshire	131.2
6	Maine	128.6
7	Rhode Island	128.3
8	New Jersey	128.0
9	Oklahoma	127.2
10	Alaska	126.4
10	Minnesota	126.4
10	Nebraska	126.4
13	Kansas	126.1
14	New York	124.5
14	Pennsylvania	124.5
16	Michigan	124.2
17	Iowa	124.0
18	Delaware	123.9
19	Colorado	123.1
19	Illinois	123.1
21	North Dakota	122.8
22	California	122.3
23	Missouri	121.9
24	Hawaii	121.4
25	Virginia	120.7
26	North Carolina	120.3
27	Kentucky	119.8
28	Louisiana	119.6
28	Montana	119.6
28	South Dakota	119.6
31	South Carolina	119.2
32	Georgia	118.5
33	Wyoming	117.8
34	Idaho	117.5
35	Tennessee	116.4
36	Indiana	115.3
37	Texas	114.9
38	West Virginia	114.7
39	Alabama	114.6
40	Florida	114.1
41	Arkansas	113.1
42	Nevada	112.1
43	Utah	110.0
44	New Mexico	109.6
45	Arizona	108.8
46	Mississippi	108.2
NA	Maryland**	NA
NA	Ohio**	NA
NA	Vermont**	NA
NA	Wisconsin**	NA
	District of Columbia	132.7

Source: American Cancer Society
"Cancer Facts & Figures 2010" (Copyright 2010, American Cancer Society, http://www.cancer.org/docroot/stt/stt_0.asp)
*For 2002 to 2006. Age-adjusted to the 2000 U.S. standard population.
**Not available.

Percent of Women 40 and Older Who Have Had a Mammogram in the Past Two Years: 2008
National Median = 76.0% of Women*

ALPHA ORDER

RANK	STATE	PERCENT
34	Alabama	74.1
49	Alaska	67.6
17	Arizona	77.4
42	Arkansas	70.9
12	California	78.9
38	Colorado	72.7
2	Connecticut	84.1
5	Delaware	82.3
9	Florida	79.3
12	Georgia	78.9
14	Hawaii	78.7
46	Idaho	68.1
27	Illinois	75.8
35	Indiana	73.9
20	Iowa	76.5
31	Kansas	74.9
30	Kentucky	75.0
25	Louisiana	76.0
3	Maine	83.3
18	Maryland	77.0
1	Massachusetts	84.9
10	Michigan	79.2
11	Minnesota	79.1
44	Mississippi	69.0
37	Missouri	73.5
41	Montana	71.8
38	Nebraska	72.7
47	Nevada	68.0
4	New Hampshire	83.0
25	New Jersey	76.0
43	New Mexico	70.8
8	New York	79.9
15	North Carolina	78.5
19	North Dakota	76.9
27	Ohio	75.8
45	Oklahoma	68.9
24	Oregon	76.2
21	Pennsylvania	76.4
6	Rhode Island	81.8
31	South Carolina	74.9
29	South Dakota	75.4
33	Tennessee	74.3
40	Texas	72.6
48	Utah	67.8
7	Vermont	80.0
16	Virginia	78.2
22	Washington	76.3
36	West Virginia	73.7
22	Wisconsin	76.3
50	Wyoming	67.2

RANK ORDER

RANK	STATE	PERCENT
1	Massachusetts	84.9
2	Connecticut	84.1
3	Maine	83.3
4	New Hampshire	83.0
5	Delaware	82.3
6	Rhode Island	81.8
7	Vermont	80.0
8	New York	79.9
9	Florida	79.3
10	Michigan	79.2
11	Minnesota	79.1
12	California	78.9
12	Georgia	78.9
14	Hawaii	78.7
15	North Carolina	78.5
16	Virginia	78.2
17	Arizona	77.4
18	Maryland	77.0
19	North Dakota	76.9
20	Iowa	76.5
21	Pennsylvania	76.4
22	Washington	76.3
22	Wisconsin	76.3
24	Oregon	76.2
25	Louisiana	76.0
25	New Jersey	76.0
27	Illinois	75.8
27	Ohio	75.8
29	South Dakota	75.4
30	Kentucky	75.0
31	Kansas	74.9
31	South Carolina	74.9
33	Tennessee	74.3
34	Alabama	74.1
35	Indiana	73.9
36	West Virginia	73.7
37	Missouri	73.5
38	Colorado	72.7
38	Nebraska	72.7
40	Texas	72.6
41	Montana	71.8
42	Arkansas	70.9
43	New Mexico	70.8
44	Mississippi	69.0
45	Oklahoma	68.9
46	Idaho	68.1
47	Nevada	68.0
48	Utah	67.8
49	Alaska	67.6
50	Wyoming	67.2
	District of Columbia	80.8

Source: U.S. Department of Health and Human Services, Centers for Disease Control and Prevention
"2008 Behavioral Risk Factor Surveillance Summary Prevalence Data" (http://apps.nccd.cdc.gov/brfss/)
*Percent of women 40 years and older.

Estimated New Colon and Rectum Cancer Cases in 2010

National Estimated Total = 142,570 New Cases*

ALPHA ORDER

RANK	STATE	CASES	% of USA
23	Alabama	2,300	1.6%
49	Alaska	260	0.2%
20	Arizona	2,620	1.8%
31	Arkansas	1,500	1.1%
1	California	13,950	9.8%
26	Colorado	1,770	1.2%
26	Connecticut	1,770	1.2%
46	Delaware	440	0.3%
2	Florida	10,500	7.4%
11	Georgia	3,840	2.7%
41	Hawaii	680	0.5%
42	Idaho	600	0.4%
6	Illinois	6,340	4.4%
13	Indiana	3,330	2.3%
28	Iowa	1,760	1.2%
33	Kansas	1,270	0.9%
22	Kentucky	2,370	1.7%
25	Louisiana	2,060	1.4%
37	Maine	800	0.6%
19	Maryland	2,630	1.8%
15	Massachusetts	3,120	2.2%
8	Michigan	5,170	3.6%
21	Minnesota	2,410	1.7%
32	Mississippi	1,480	1.0%
16	Missouri	3,080	2.2%
44	Montana	490	0.3%
36	Nebraska	910	0.6%
34	Nevada	1,090	0.8%
40	New Hampshire	720	0.5%
9	New Jersey	4,430	3.1%
38	New Mexico	790	0.6%
3	New York	9,780	6.9%
10	North Carolina	4,220	3.0%
47	North Dakota	340	0.2%
7	Ohio	5,960	4.2%
29	Oklahoma	1,730	1.2%
30	Oregon	1,710	1.2%
5	Pennsylvania	7,440	5.2%
43	Rhode Island	540	0.4%
24	South Carolina	2,140	1.5%
45	South Dakota	450	0.3%
14	Tennessee	3,130	2.2%
4	Texas	9,190	6.4%
39	Utah	740	0.5%
48	Vermont	320	0.2%
12	Virginia	3,370	2.4%
18	Washington	2,740	1.9%
35	West Virginia	1,060	0.7%
17	Wisconsin	2,760	1.9%
50	Wyoming	220	0.2%

RANK ORDER

RANK	STATE	CASES	% of USA
1	California	13,950	9.8%
2	Florida	10,500	7.4%
3	New York	9,780	6.9%
4	Texas	9,190	6.4%
5	Pennsylvania	7,440	5.2%
6	Illinois	6,340	4.4%
7	Ohio	5,960	4.2%
8	Michigan	5,170	3.6%
9	New Jersey	4,430	3.1%
10	North Carolina	4,220	3.0%
11	Georgia	3,840	2.7%
12	Virginia	3,370	2.4%
13	Indiana	3,330	2.3%
14	Tennessee	3,130	2.2%
15	Massachusetts	3,120	2.2%
16	Missouri	3,080	2.2%
17	Wisconsin	2,760	1.9%
18	Washington	2,740	1.9%
19	Maryland	2,630	1.8%
20	Arizona	2,620	1.8%
21	Minnesota	2,410	1.7%
22	Kentucky	2,370	1.7%
23	Alabama	2,300	1.6%
24	South Carolina	2,140	1.5%
25	Louisiana	2,060	1.4%
26	Colorado	1,770	1.2%
26	Connecticut	1,770	1.2%
28	Iowa	1,760	1.2%
29	Oklahoma	1,730	1.2%
30	Oregon	1,710	1.2%
31	Arkansas	1,500	1.1%
32	Mississippi	1,480	1.0%
33	Kansas	1,270	0.9%
34	Nevada	1,090	0.8%
35	West Virginia	1,060	0.7%
36	Nebraska	910	0.6%
37	Maine	800	0.6%
38	New Mexico	790	0.6%
39	Utah	740	0.5%
40	New Hampshire	720	0.5%
41	Hawaii	680	0.5%
42	Idaho	600	0.4%
43	Rhode Island	540	0.4%
44	Montana	490	0.3%
45	South Dakota	450	0.3%
46	Delaware	440	0.3%
47	North Dakota	340	0.2%
48	Vermont	320	0.2%
49	Alaska	260	0.2%
50	Wyoming	220	0.2%
	District of Columbia	260	0.2%

Source: American Cancer Society
    "Cancer Facts & Figures 2010" (Copyright 2010, American Cancer Society, http://www.cancer.org/docroot/stt/stt_0.asp)
*These estimates are offered as a rough guide and should be interpreted with caution. They are calculated by the American
Cancer Society using a model based on 1995-2006 incidence rates.

Estimated Rate of New Colon and Rectum Cancer Cases in 2010

National Estimated Rate = 46.4 New Cases per 100,000 Population*

ALPHA ORDER

RANK	STATE	RATE
27	Alabama	48.8
47	Alaska	37.2
42	Arizona	39.7
11	Arkansas	51.9
46	California	37.7
49	Colorado	35.2
20	Connecticut	50.3
24	Delaware	49.7
5	Florida	56.6
44	Georgia	39.1
10	Hawaii	52.5
45	Idaho	38.8
26	Illinois	49.1
13	Indiana	51.8
3	Iowa	58.5
35	Kansas	45.1
7	Kentucky	54.9
33	Louisiana	45.9
1	Maine	60.7
32	Maryland	46.1
29	Massachusetts	47.3
11	Michigan	51.9
34	Minnesota	45.8
22	Mississippi	50.1
16	Missouri	51.4
20	Montana	50.3
19	Nebraska	50.7
39	Nevada	41.2
8	New Hampshire	54.4
18	New Jersey	50.9
43	New Mexico	39.3
23	New York	50.0
36	North Carolina	45.0
9	North Dakota	52.6
14	Ohio	51.6
30	Oklahoma	46.9
37	Oregon	44.7
2	Pennsylvania	59.0
17	Rhode Island	51.3
30	South Carolina	46.9
6	South Dakota	55.4
24	Tennessee	49.7
48	Texas	37.1
50	Utah	26.6
15	Vermont	51.5
38	Virginia	42.8
40	Washington	41.1
4	West Virginia	58.2
27	Wisconsin	48.8
41	Wyoming	40.4

RANK ORDER

RANK	STATE	RATE
1	Maine	60.7
2	Pennsylvania	59.0
3	Iowa	58.5
4	West Virginia	58.2
5	Florida	56.6
6	South Dakota	55.4
7	Kentucky	54.9
8	New Hampshire	54.4
9	North Dakota	52.6
10	Hawaii	52.5
11	Arkansas	51.9
11	Michigan	51.9
13	Indiana	51.8
14	Ohio	51.6
15	Vermont	51.5
16	Missouri	51.4
17	Rhode Island	51.3
18	New Jersey	50.9
19	Nebraska	50.7
20	Connecticut	50.3
20	Montana	50.3
22	Mississippi	50.1
23	New York	50.0
24	Delaware	49.7
24	Tennessee	49.7
26	Illinois	49.1
27	Alabama	48.8
27	Wisconsin	48.8
29	Massachusetts	47.3
30	Oklahoma	46.9
30	South Carolina	46.9
32	Maryland	46.1
33	Louisiana	45.9
34	Minnesota	45.8
35	Kansas	45.1
36	North Carolina	45.0
37	Oregon	44.7
38	Virginia	42.8
39	Nevada	41.2
40	Washington	41.1
41	Wyoming	40.4
42	Arizona	39.7
43	New Mexico	39.3
44	Georgia	39.1
45	Idaho	38.8
46	California	37.7
47	Alaska	37.2
48	Texas	37.1
49	Colorado	35.2
50	Utah	26.6
	District of Columbia	43.4

Source: CQ Press using data from American Cancer Society
    "Cancer Facts & Figures 2010" (Copyright 2010, American Cancer Society, http://www.cancer.org/docroot/stt/stt_0.asp)
*These estimates are offered as a rough guide and should be interpreted with caution. They are calculated by the American Cancer Society using a model based on 1995-2006 incidence rates. Rates calculated using 2009 Census resident population estimates.

Percent of Adults Who Have Ever Had a Sigmoidoscopy or Colonoscopy Exam: 2008
National Median = 62.2% of Adults*

ALPHA ORDER			RANK ORDER		
RANK	STATE	PERCENT	RANK	STATE	PERCENT
30	Alabama	60.7	1	Delaware	74.3
38	Alaska	58.0	2	Maine	72.6
20	Arizona	63.8	3	New Hampshire	71.7
47	Arkansas	55.3	4	Massachusetts	71.4
32	California	59.8	5	Maryland	71.3
26	Colorado	61.9	6	Minnesota	71.0
9	Connecticut	69.5	7	Virginia	69.9
1	Delaware	74.3	8	Vermont	69.6
19	Florida	64.2	9	Connecticut	69.5
25	Georgia	62.2	10	Rhode Island	69.4
31	Hawaii	60.1	11	Michigan	68.6
46	Idaho	55.6	12	Utah	67.2
35	Illinois	59.1	12	Wisconsin	67.2
34	Indiana	59.3	14	Oregon	66.8
20	Iowa	63.8	15	North Carolina	66.6
27	Kansas	61.7	16	Washington	66.2
22	Kentucky	63.7	17	New York	65.5
50	Louisiana	52.6	17	South Carolina	65.5
2	Maine	72.6	19	Florida	64.2
5	Maryland	71.3	20	Arizona	63.8
4	Massachusetts	71.4	20	Iowa	63.8
11	Michigan	68.6	22	Kentucky	63.7
6	Minnesota	71.0	23	Pennsylvania	62.5
41	Mississippi	56.4	24	South Dakota	62.4
28	Missouri	61.4	25	Georgia	62.2
40	Montana	56.5	26	Colorado	61.9
37	Nebraska	58.6	27	Kansas	61.7
45	Nevada	55.7	28	Missouri	61.4
3	New Hampshire	71.7	29	Ohio	60.8
36	New Jersey	58.7	30	Alabama	60.7
44	New Mexico	55.9	31	Hawaii	60.1
17	New York	65.5	32	California	59.8
15	North Carolina	66.6	33	Tennessee	59.5
39	North Dakota	57.9	34	Indiana	59.3
29	Ohio	60.8	35	Illinois	59.1
48	Oklahoma	55.2	36	New Jersey	58.7
14	Oregon	66.8	37	Nebraska	58.6
23	Pennsylvania	62.5	38	Alaska	58.0
10	Rhode Island	69.4	39	North Dakota	57.9
17	South Carolina	65.5	40	Montana	56.5
24	South Dakota	62.4	41	Mississippi	56.4
33	Tennessee	59.5	42	Texas	56.2
42	Texas	56.2	43	Wyoming	56.0
12	Utah	67.2	44	New Mexico	55.9
8	Vermont	69.6	45	Nevada	55.7
7	Virginia	69.9	46	Idaho	55.6
16	Washington	66.2	47	Arkansas	55.3
49	West Virginia	54.7	48	Oklahoma	55.2
12	Wisconsin	67.2	49	West Virginia	54.7
43	Wyoming	56.0	50	Louisiana	52.6
				District of Columbia	68.6

Source: U.S. Department of Health and Human Services, Centers for Disease Control and Prevention
"2008 Behavioral Risk Factor Surveillance Summary Prevalence Data" (http://apps.nccd.cdc.gov/brfss/)
*Persons 50 and older.

Estimated New Leukemia Cases in 2010

National Estimated Total = 43,050 New Cases*

ALPHA ORDER

RANK	STATE	CASES	% of USA
26	Alabama	560	1.3%
49	Alaska	70	0.2%
20	Arizona	760	1.8%
31	Arkansas	420	1.0%
1	California	4,460	10.4%
21	Colorado	650	1.5%
30	Connecticut	510	1.2%
46	Delaware	120	0.3%
2	Florida	3,330	7.7%
11	Georgia	1,040	2.4%
42	Hawaii	160	0.4%
40	Idaho	230	0.5%
6	Illinois	1,860	4.3%
15	Indiana	890	2.1%
26	Iowa	560	1.3%
32	Kansas	400	0.9%
22	Kentucky	630	1.5%
24	Louisiana	590	1.4%
39	Maine	260	0.6%
23	Maryland	620	1.4%
14	Massachusetts	910	2.1%
8	Michigan	1,600	3.7%
19	Minnesota	830	1.9%
33	Mississippi	340	0.8%
17	Missouri	870	2.0%
42	Montana	160	0.4%
36	Nebraska	290	0.7%
34	Nevada	320	0.7%
41	New Hampshire	200	0.5%
9	New Jersey	1,330	3.1%
37	New Mexico	280	0.7%
4	New York	2,980	6.9%
10	North Carolina	1,150	2.7%
47	North Dakota	100	0.2%
7	Ohio	1,810	4.2%
26	Oklahoma	560	1.3%
29	Oregon	530	1.2%
5	Pennsylvania	2,070	4.8%
42	Rhode Island	160	0.4%
24	South Carolina	590	1.4%
45	South Dakota	130	0.3%
18	Tennessee	850	2.0%
3	Texas	3,240	7.5%
35	Utah	310	0.7%
48	Vermont	90	0.2%
16	Virginia	880	2.0%
12	Washington	1,000	2.3%
37	West Virginia	280	0.7%
13	Wisconsin	940	2.2%
49	Wyoming	70	0.2%

RANK ORDER

RANK	STATE	CASES	% of USA
1	California	4,460	10.4%
2	Florida	3,330	7.7%
3	Texas	3,240	7.5%
4	New York	2,980	6.9%
5	Pennsylvania	2,070	4.8%
6	Illinois	1,860	4.3%
7	Ohio	1,810	4.2%
8	Michigan	1,600	3.7%
9	New Jersey	1,330	3.1%
10	North Carolina	1,150	2.7%
11	Georgia	1,040	2.4%
12	Washington	1,000	2.3%
13	Wisconsin	940	2.2%
14	Massachusetts	910	2.1%
15	Indiana	890	2.1%
16	Virginia	880	2.0%
17	Missouri	870	2.0%
18	Tennessee	850	2.0%
19	Minnesota	830	1.9%
20	Arizona	760	1.8%
21	Colorado	650	1.5%
22	Kentucky	630	1.5%
23	Maryland	620	1.4%
24	Louisiana	590	1.4%
24	South Carolina	590	1.4%
26	Alabama	560	1.3%
26	Iowa	560	1.3%
26	Oklahoma	560	1.3%
29	Oregon	530	1.2%
30	Connecticut	510	1.2%
31	Arkansas	420	1.0%
32	Kansas	400	0.9%
33	Mississippi	340	0.8%
34	Nevada	320	0.7%
35	Utah	310	0.7%
36	Nebraska	290	0.7%
37	New Mexico	280	0.7%
37	West Virginia	280	0.7%
39	Maine	260	0.6%
40	Idaho	230	0.5%
41	New Hampshire	200	0.5%
42	Hawaii	160	0.4%
42	Montana	160	0.4%
42	Rhode Island	160	0.4%
45	South Dakota	130	0.3%
46	Delaware	120	0.3%
47	North Dakota	100	0.2%
48	Vermont	90	0.2%
49	Alaska	70	0.2%
49	Wyoming	70	0.2%
	District of Columbia	60	0.1%

Source: American Cancer Society
   "Cancer Facts & Figures 2010" (Copyright 2010, American Cancer Society, http://www.cancer.org/docroot/stt/stt_0.asp)
*These estimates are offered as a rough guide and should be interpreted with caution. They are calculated by the American Cancer Society using a model based on 1995-2006 incidence rates.

Estimated Rate of New Leukemia Cases in 2010

National Estimated Rate = 14.0 New Cases per 100,000 Population*

ALPHA ORDER

RANK	STATE	RATE
43	Alabama	11.9
50	Alaska	10.0
44	Arizona	11.5
22	Arkansas	14.5
41	California	12.1
36	Colorado	12.9
22	Connecticut	14.5
32	Delaware	13.6
3	Florida	18.0
49	Georgia	10.6
39	Hawaii	12.4
20	Idaho	14.9
26	Illinois	14.4
28	Indiana	13.9
2	Iowa	18.6
27	Kansas	14.2
21	Kentucky	14.6
34	Louisiana	13.1
1	Maine	19.7
48	Maryland	10.9
31	Massachusetts	13.8
8	Michigan	16.0
10	Minnesota	15.8
44	Mississippi	11.5
22	Missouri	14.5
5	Montana	16.4
7	Nebraska	16.1
41	Nevada	12.1
18	New Hampshire	15.1
14	New Jersey	15.3
28	New Mexico	13.9
15	New York	15.2
40	North Carolina	12.3
12	North Dakota	15.5
11	Ohio	15.7
15	Oklahoma	15.2
28	Oregon	13.9
5	Pennsylvania	16.4
15	Rhode Island	15.2
36	South Carolina	12.9
8	South Dakota	16.0
33	Tennessee	13.5
34	Texas	13.1
47	Utah	11.1
22	Vermont	14.5
46	Virginia	11.2
19	Washington	15.0
13	West Virginia	15.4
4	Wisconsin	16.6
36	Wyoming	12.9

RANK ORDER

RANK	STATE	RATE
1	Maine	19.7
2	Iowa	18.6
3	Florida	18.0
4	Wisconsin	16.6
5	Montana	16.4
5	Pennsylvania	16.4
7	Nebraska	16.1
8	Michigan	16.0
8	South Dakota	16.0
10	Minnesota	15.8
11	Ohio	15.7
12	North Dakota	15.5
13	West Virginia	15.4
14	New Jersey	15.3
15	New York	15.2
15	Oklahoma	15.2
15	Rhode Island	15.2
18	New Hampshire	15.1
19	Washington	15.0
20	Idaho	14.9
21	Kentucky	14.6
22	Arkansas	14.5
22	Connecticut	14.5
22	Missouri	14.5
22	Vermont	14.5
26	Illinois	14.4
27	Kansas	14.2
28	Indiana	13.9
28	New Mexico	13.9
28	Oregon	13.9
31	Massachusetts	13.8
32	Delaware	13.6
33	Tennessee	13.5
34	Louisiana	13.1
34	Texas	13.1
36	Colorado	12.9
36	South Carolina	12.9
36	Wyoming	12.9
39	Hawaii	12.4
40	North Carolina	12.3
41	California	12.1
41	Nevada	12.1
43	Alabama	11.9
44	Arizona	11.5
44	Mississippi	11.5
46	Virginia	11.2
47	Utah	11.1
48	Maryland	10.9
49	Georgia	10.6
50	Alaska	10.0

District of Columbia   10.0

Source: CQ Press using data from American Cancer Society
"Cancer Facts & Figures 2010" (Copyright 2010, American Cancer Society, http://www.cancer.org/docroot/stt/stt_0.asp)
*These estimates are offered as a rough guide and should be interpreted with caution. They are calculated by the American Cancer Society using a model based on 1995-2006 incidence rates. Rates calculated using 2009 Census resident population estimates.

Estimated New Lung Cancer Cases in 2010

National Estimated Total = 222,520 New Cases*

ALPHA ORDER

RANK	STATE	CASES	% of USA
20	Alabama	4,160	1.9%
49	Alaska	360	0.2%
21	Arizona	4,030	1.8%
29	Arkansas	2,620	1.2%
1	California	18,490	8.3%
32	Colorado	2,270	1.0%
28	Connecticut	2,640	1.2%
42	Delaware	800	0.4%
2	Florida	18,390	8.3%
10	Georgia	6,280	2.8%
43	Hawaii	770	0.3%
40	Idaho	860	0.4%
7	Illinois	9,190	4.1%
14	Indiana	5,430	2.4%
30	Iowa	2,450	1.1%
34	Kansas	1,990	0.9%
17	Kentucky	4,780	2.1%
24	Louisiana	3,320	1.5%
36	Maine	1,370	0.6%
19	Maryland	4,170	1.9%
16	Massachusetts	5,020	2.3%
8	Michigan	8,150	3.7%
26	Minnesota	3,150	1.4%
31	Mississippi	2,360	1.1%
15	Missouri	5,360	2.4%
44	Montana	740	0.3%
37	Nebraska	1,200	0.5%
35	Nevada	1,920	0.9%
38	New Hampshire	1,070	0.5%
11	New Jersey	6,260	2.8%
39	New Mexico	920	0.4%
4	New York	13,720	6.2%
9	North Carolina	7,520	3.4%
48	North Dakota	410	0.2%
5	Ohio	10,710	4.8%
25	Oklahoma	3,250	1.5%
27	Oregon	2,810	1.3%
6	Pennsylvania	10,520	4.7%
41	Rhode Island	840	0.4%
23	South Carolina	3,970	1.8%
46	South Dakota	540	0.2%
12	Tennessee	5,980	2.7%
3	Texas	14,030	6.3%
45	Utah	620	0.3%
47	Vermont	490	0.2%
13	Virginia	5,510	2.5%
18	Washington	4,320	1.9%
33	West Virginia	2,070	0.9%
22	Wisconsin	3,990	1.8%
50	Wyoming	320	0.1%

RANK ORDER

RANK	STATE	CASES	% of USA
1	California	18,490	8.3%
2	Florida	18,390	8.3%
3	Texas	14,030	6.3%
4	New York	13,720	6.2%
5	Ohio	10,710	4.8%
6	Pennsylvania	10,520	4.7%
7	Illinois	9,190	4.1%
8	Michigan	8,150	3.7%
9	North Carolina	7,520	3.4%
10	Georgia	6,280	2.8%
11	New Jersey	6,260	2.8%
12	Tennessee	5,980	2.7%
13	Virginia	5,510	2.5%
14	Indiana	5,430	2.4%
15	Missouri	5,360	2.4%
16	Massachusetts	5,020	2.3%
17	Kentucky	4,780	2.1%
18	Washington	4,320	1.9%
19	Maryland	4,170	1.9%
20	Alabama	4,160	1.9%
21	Arizona	4,030	1.8%
22	Wisconsin	3,990	1.8%
23	South Carolina	3,970	1.8%
24	Louisiana	3,320	1.5%
25	Oklahoma	3,250	1.5%
26	Minnesota	3,150	1.4%
27	Oregon	2,810	1.3%
28	Connecticut	2,640	1.2%
29	Arkansas	2,620	1.2%
30	Iowa	2,450	1.1%
31	Mississippi	2,360	1.1%
32	Colorado	2,270	1.0%
33	West Virginia	2,070	0.9%
34	Kansas	1,990	0.9%
35	Nevada	1,920	0.9%
36	Maine	1,370	0.6%
37	Nebraska	1,200	0.5%
38	New Hampshire	1,070	0.5%
39	New Mexico	920	0.4%
40	Idaho	860	0.4%
41	Rhode Island	840	0.4%
42	Delaware	800	0.4%
43	Hawaii	770	0.3%
44	Montana	740	0.3%
45	Utah	620	0.3%
46	South Dakota	540	0.2%
47	Vermont	490	0.2%
48	North Dakota	410	0.2%
49	Alaska	360	0.2%
50	Wyoming	320	0.1%
	District of Columbia	360	0.2%

Source: American Cancer Society
"Cancer Facts & Figures 2010" (Copyright 2010, American Cancer Society, http://www.cancer.org/docroot/stt/stt_0.asp)
*These estimates are offered as a rough guide and should be interpreted with caution. They are calculated by the American Cancer Society using a model based on 1995-2006 incidence rates.

Estimated Rate of New Lung Cancer Cases in 2010

National Estimated Rate = 72.5 New Cases per 100,000 Population*

ALPHA ORDER

RANK	STATE	RATE
10	Alabama	88.3
46	Alaska	51.5
40	Arizona	61.1
7	Arkansas	90.7
47	California	50.0
49	Colorado	45.2
24	Connecticut	75.0
8	Delaware	90.4
4	Florida	99.2
38	Georgia	63.9
42	Hawaii	59.5
45	Idaho	55.6
30	Illinois	71.2
13	Indiana	84.5
16	Iowa	81.5
31	Kansas	70.6
2	Kentucky	110.8
25	Louisiana	73.9
3	Maine	103.9
27	Maryland	73.2
22	Massachusetts	76.1
15	Michigan	81.7
41	Minnesota	59.8
19	Mississippi	79.9
9	Missouri	89.5
23	Montana	75.9
35	Nebraska	66.8
28	Nevada	72.6
17	New Hampshire	80.8
29	New Jersey	71.9
48	New Mexico	45.8
33	New York	70.2
18	North Carolina	80.2
39	North Dakota	63.4
6	Ohio	92.8
11	Oklahoma	88.1
26	Oregon	73.5
14	Pennsylvania	83.5
20	Rhode Island	79.8
12	South Carolina	87.0
36	South Dakota	66.5
5	Tennessee	95.0
44	Texas	56.6
50	Utah	22.3
21	Vermont	78.8
34	Virginia	69.9
37	Washington	64.8
1	West Virginia	113.8
31	Wisconsin	70.6
43	Wyoming	58.8

RANK ORDER

RANK	STATE	RATE
1	West Virginia	113.8
2	Kentucky	110.8
3	Maine	103.9
4	Florida	99.2
5	Tennessee	95.0
6	Ohio	92.8
7	Arkansas	90.7
8	Delaware	90.4
9	Missouri	89.5
10	Alabama	88.3
11	Oklahoma	88.1
12	South Carolina	87.0
13	Indiana	84.5
14	Pennsylvania	83.5
15	Michigan	81.7
16	Iowa	81.5
17	New Hampshire	80.8
18	North Carolina	80.2
19	Mississippi	79.9
20	Rhode Island	79.8
21	Vermont	78.8
22	Massachusetts	76.1
23	Montana	75.9
24	Connecticut	75.0
25	Louisiana	73.9
26	Oregon	73.5
27	Maryland	73.2
28	Nevada	72.6
29	New Jersey	71.9
30	Illinois	71.2
31	Kansas	70.6
31	Wisconsin	70.6
33	New York	70.2
34	Virginia	69.9
35	Nebraska	66.8
36	South Dakota	66.5
37	Washington	64.8
38	Georgia	63.9
39	North Dakota	63.4
40	Arizona	61.1
41	Minnesota	59.8
42	Hawaii	59.5
43	Wyoming	58.8
44	Texas	56.6
45	Idaho	55.6
46	Alaska	51.5
47	California	50.0
48	New Mexico	45.8
49	Colorado	45.2
50	Utah	22.3

District of Columbia 60.0

Source: CQ Press using data from American Cancer Society
"Cancer Facts & Figures 2010" (Copyright 2010, American Cancer Society, http://www.cancer.org/docroot/stt/stt_0.asp)
*These estimates are offered as a rough guide and should be interpreted with caution. They are calculated by the American Cancer Society using a model based on 1995-2006 incidence rates. Rates calculated using 2009 Census resident population estimates.

Estimated New Non-Hodgkin's Lymphoma Cases in 2010

National Estimated Total = 65,540 New Cases*

ALPHA ORDER

RANK	STATE	CASES	% of USA
24	Alabama	940	1.4%
49	Alaska	130	0.2%
19	Arizona	1,210	1.8%
31	Arkansas	640	1.0%
1	California	7,010	10.7%
26	Colorado	920	1.4%
28	Connecticut	860	1.3%
45	Delaware	200	0.3%
3	Florida	4,660	7.1%
11	Georgia	1,600	2.4%
44	Hawaii	230	0.4%
40	Idaho	310	0.5%
7	Illinois	2,690	4.1%
15	Indiana	1,370	2.1%
30	Iowa	750	1.1%
32	Kansas	590	0.9%
22	Kentucky	1,030	1.6%
26	Louisiana	920	1.4%
39	Maine	360	0.5%
20	Maryland	1,110	1.7%
14	Massachusetts	1,460	2.2%
8	Michigan	2,400	3.7%
21	Minnesota	1,100	1.7%
33	Mississippi	540	0.8%
18	Missouri	1,260	1.9%
42	Montana	240	0.4%
37	Nebraska	410	0.6%
34	Nevada	480	0.7%
40	New Hampshire	310	0.5%
9	New Jersey	2,130	3.2%
38	New Mexico	370	0.6%
2	New York	4,680	7.1%
10	North Carolina	1,800	2.7%
47	North Dakota	150	0.2%
6	Ohio	2,720	4.2%
29	Oklahoma	810	1.2%
25	Oregon	930	1.4%
5	Pennsylvania	3,430	5.2%
42	Rhode Island	240	0.4%
23	South Carolina	950	1.4%
46	South Dakota	180	0.3%
16	Tennessee	1,360	2.1%
4	Texas	4,410	6.7%
36	Utah	430	0.7%
47	Vermont	150	0.2%
13	Virginia	1,470	2.2%
11	Washington	1,600	2.4%
35	West Virginia	450	0.7%
17	Wisconsin	1,340	2.0%
50	Wyoming	110	0.2%

RANK ORDER

RANK	STATE	CASES	% of USA
1	California	7,010	10.7%
2	New York	4,680	7.1%
3	Florida	4,660	7.1%
4	Texas	4,410	6.7%
5	Pennsylvania	3,430	5.2%
6	Ohio	2,720	4.2%
7	Illinois	2,690	4.1%
8	Michigan	2,400	3.7%
9	New Jersey	2,130	3.2%
10	North Carolina	1,800	2.7%
11	Georgia	1,600	2.4%
11	Washington	1,600	2.4%
13	Virginia	1,470	2.2%
14	Massachusetts	1,460	2.2%
15	Indiana	1,370	2.1%
16	Tennessee	1,360	2.1%
17	Wisconsin	1,340	2.0%
18	Missouri	1,260	1.9%
19	Arizona	1,210	1.8%
20	Maryland	1,110	1.7%
21	Minnesota	1,100	1.7%
22	Kentucky	1,030	1.6%
23	South Carolina	950	1.4%
24	Alabama	940	1.4%
25	Oregon	930	1.4%
26	Colorado	920	1.4%
26	Louisiana	920	1.4%
28	Connecticut	860	1.3%
29	Oklahoma	810	1.2%
30	Iowa	750	1.1%
31	Arkansas	640	1.0%
32	Kansas	590	0.9%
33	Mississippi	540	0.8%
34	Nevada	480	0.7%
35	West Virginia	450	0.7%
36	Utah	430	0.7%
37	Nebraska	410	0.6%
38	New Mexico	370	0.6%
39	Maine	360	0.5%
40	Idaho	310	0.5%
40	New Hampshire	310	0.5%
42	Montana	240	0.4%
42	Rhode Island	240	0.4%
44	Hawaii	230	0.4%
45	Delaware	200	0.3%
46	South Dakota	180	0.3%
47	North Dakota	150	0.2%
47	Vermont	150	0.2%
49	Alaska	130	0.2%
50	Wyoming	110	0.2%
	District of Columbia	100	0.2%

Source: American Cancer Society
"Cancer Facts & Figures 2010" (Copyright 2010, American Cancer Society, http://www.cancer.org/docroot/stt/stt_0.asp)
*These estimates are offered as a rough guide and should be interpreted with caution. They are calculated by the American Cancer Society using a model based on 1995-2006 incidence rates.

Estimated Rate of New Non-Hodgkin's Lymphoma Cases in 2010

National Estimated Rate = 21.3 New Cases per 100,000 Population*

ALPHA ORDER				RANK ORDER		
RANK	STATE	RATE		RANK	STATE	RATE
36	Alabama	20.0		1	Maine	27.3
40	Alaska	18.6		2	Pennsylvania	27.2
43	Arizona	18.3		3	Florida	25.1
23	Arkansas	22.1		4	Iowa	24.9
39	California	19.0		5	West Virginia	24.7
43	Colorado	18.3		6	Montana	24.6
8	Connecticut	24.4		7	New Jersey	24.5
21	Delaware	22.6		8	Connecticut	24.4
3	Florida	25.1		9	Oregon	24.3
49	Georgia	16.3		10	Michigan	24.1
47	Hawaii	17.8		10	Vermont	24.1
35	Idaho	20.1		12	Washington	24.0
31	Illinois	20.8		13	Kentucky	23.9
27	Indiana	21.3		13	New York	23.9
4	Iowa	24.9		15	Wisconsin	23.7
29	Kansas	20.9		16	Ohio	23.6
13	Kentucky	23.9		17	New Hampshire	23.4
33	Louisiana	20.5		18	North Dakota	23.2
1	Maine	27.3		19	Nebraska	22.8
37	Maryland	19.5		19	Rhode Island	22.8
23	Massachusetts	22.1		21	Delaware	22.6
10	Michigan	24.1		22	South Dakota	22.2
29	Minnesota	20.9		23	Arkansas	22.1
43	Mississippi	18.3		23	Massachusetts	22.1
28	Missouri	21.0		25	Oklahoma	22.0
6	Montana	24.6		26	Tennessee	21.6
19	Nebraska	22.8		27	Indiana	21.3
46	Nevada	18.2		28	Missouri	21.0
17	New Hampshire	23.4		29	Kansas	20.9
7	New Jersey	24.5		29	Minnesota	20.9
42	New Mexico	18.4		31	Illinois	20.8
13	New York	23.9		31	South Carolina	20.8
38	North Carolina	19.2		33	Louisiana	20.5
18	North Dakota	23.2		34	Wyoming	20.2
16	Ohio	23.6		35	Idaho	20.1
25	Oklahoma	22.0		36	Alabama	20.0
9	Oregon	24.3		37	Maryland	19.5
2	Pennsylvania	27.2		38	North Carolina	19.2
19	Rhode Island	22.8		39	California	19.0
31	South Carolina	20.8		40	Alaska	18.6
22	South Dakota	22.2		40	Virginia	18.6
26	Tennessee	21.6		42	New Mexico	18.4
47	Texas	17.8		43	Arizona	18.3
50	Utah	15.4		43	Colorado	18.3
10	Vermont	24.1		43	Mississippi	18.3
40	Virginia	18.6		46	Nevada	18.2
12	Washington	24.0		47	Hawaii	17.8
5	West Virginia	24.7		47	Texas	17.8
15	Wisconsin	23.7		49	Georgia	16.3
34	Wyoming	20.2		50	Utah	15.4
					District of Columbia	16.7

Source: CQ Press using data from American Cancer Society
"Cancer Facts & Figures 2010" (Copyright 2010, American Cancer Society, http://www.cancer.org/docroot/stt/stt_0.asp)
*These estimates are offered as a rough guide and should be interpreted with caution. They are calculated by the American Cancer Society using a model based on 1995-2006 incidence rates. Rates calculated using 2009 Census resident population estimates.

Estimated New Prostate Cancer Cases in 2010

National Estimated Total = 217,730 New Cases*

ALPHA ORDER

RANK	STATE	CASES	% of USA
25	Alabama	3,300	1.5%
49	Alaska	440	0.2%
20	Arizona	3,850	1.8%
31	Arkansas	2,330	1.1%
1	California	22,640	10.4%
23	Colorado	3,430	1.6%
28	Connecticut	2,940	1.4%
46	Delaware	710	0.3%
3	Florida	14,610	6.7%
11	Georgia	6,380	2.9%
42	Hawaii	1,060	0.5%
40	Idaho	1,300	0.6%
6	Illinois	8,730	4.0%
17	Indiana	4,160	1.9%
30	Iowa	2,420	1.1%
35	Kansas	1,630	0.7%
26	Kentucky	3,180	1.5%
24	Louisiana	3,410	1.6%
39	Maine	1,410	0.6%
18	Maryland	4,010	1.8%
14	Massachusetts	4,820	2.2%
7	Michigan	8,490	3.9%
19	Minnesota	3,870	1.8%
32	Mississippi	2,260	1.0%
21	Missouri	3,600	1.7%
43	Montana	960	0.4%
37	Nebraska	1,470	0.7%
33	Nevada	1,750	0.8%
41	New Hampshire	1,100	0.5%
10	New Jersey	6,790	3.1%
36	New Mexico	1,610	0.7%
2	New York	14,840	6.8%
9	North Carolina	6,910	3.2%
48	North Dakota	580	0.3%
8	Ohio	8,010	3.7%
29	Oklahoma	2,440	1.1%
27	Oregon	3,010	1.4%
5	Pennsylvania	9,800	4.5%
45	Rhode Island	740	0.3%
21	South Carolina	3,600	1.7%
44	South Dakota	760	0.3%
16	Tennessee	4,600	2.1%
4	Texas	13,740	6.3%
34	Utah	1,730	0.8%
47	Vermont	600	0.3%
12	Virginia	5,550	2.5%
13	Washington	5,220	2.4%
38	West Virginia	1,440	0.7%
15	Wisconsin	4,670	2.1%
50	Wyoming	420	0.2%

RANK ORDER

RANK	STATE	CASES	% of USA
1	California	22,640	10.4%
2	New York	14,840	6.8%
3	Florida	14,610	6.7%
4	Texas	13,740	6.3%
5	Pennsylvania	9,800	4.5%
6	Illinois	8,730	4.0%
7	Michigan	8,490	3.9%
8	Ohio	8,010	3.7%
9	North Carolina	6,910	3.2%
10	New Jersey	6,790	3.1%
11	Georgia	6,380	2.9%
12	Virginia	5,550	2.5%
13	Washington	5,220	2.4%
14	Massachusetts	4,820	2.2%
15	Wisconsin	4,670	2.1%
16	Tennessee	4,600	2.1%
17	Indiana	4,160	1.9%
18	Maryland	4,010	1.8%
19	Minnesota	3,870	1.8%
20	Arizona	3,850	1.8%
21	Missouri	3,600	1.7%
21	South Carolina	3,600	1.7%
23	Colorado	3,430	1.6%
24	Louisiana	3,410	1.6%
25	Alabama	3,300	1.5%
26	Kentucky	3,180	1.5%
27	Oregon	3,010	1.4%
28	Connecticut	2,940	1.4%
29	Oklahoma	2,440	1.1%
30	Iowa	2,420	1.1%
31	Arkansas	2,330	1.1%
32	Mississippi	2,260	1.0%
33	Nevada	1,750	0.8%
34	Utah	1,730	0.8%
35	Kansas	1,630	0.7%
36	New Mexico	1,610	0.7%
37	Nebraska	1,470	0.7%
38	West Virginia	1,440	0.7%
39	Maine	1,410	0.6%
40	Idaho	1,300	0.6%
41	New Hampshire	1,100	0.5%
42	Hawaii	1,060	0.5%
43	Montana	960	0.4%
44	South Dakota	760	0.3%
45	Rhode Island	740	0.3%
46	Delaware	710	0.3%
47	Vermont	600	0.3%
48	North Dakota	580	0.3%
49	Alaska	440	0.2%
50	Wyoming	420	0.2%
	District of Columbia	450	0.2%

Source: American Cancer Society

"Cancer Facts & Figures 2010" (Copyright 2010, American Cancer Society, http://www.cancer.org/docroot/stt/stt_0.asp)
*These estimates are offered as a rough guide and should be interpreted with caution. They are calculated by the American Cancer Society using a model based on 1995-2006 incidence rates.

Age-Adjusted Incidence Rate of Prostate Cancer Cases in 2006

National Rate = 155.5 New Cases per 100,000 Male Population*

ALPHA ORDER

RANK	STATE	RATE
28	Alabama	154.2
39	Alaska	141.4
46	Arizona	118.9
20	Arkansas	161.3
32	California	149.0
26	Colorado	156.4
17	Connecticut	164.6
3	Delaware	179.9
41	Florida	138.4
19	Georgia	162.4
45	Hawaii	128.6
14	Idaho	165.8
24	Illinois	157.9
42	Indiana	135.9
35	Iowa	144.9
22	Kansas	159.6
38	Kentucky	142.5
6	Louisiana	176.8
16	Maine	164.8
NA	Maryland**	NA
17	Massachusetts	164.6
4	Michigan	179.4
1	Minnesota	184.6
12	Mississippi	166.7
44	Missouri	129.3
7	Montana	174.5
25	Nebraska	157.6
36	Nevada	144.2
23	New Hampshire	159.5
5	New Jersey	177.9
34	New Mexico	146.1
13	New York	166.3
29	North Carolina	153.2
10	North Dakota	169.5
NA	Ohio**	NA
31	Oklahoma	150.0
33	Oregon	148.0
21	Pennsylvania	159.7
30	Rhode Island	152.2
8	South Carolina	171.5
9	South Dakota	171.0
43	Tennessee	132.7
37	Texas	144.0
2	Utah	182.2
NA	Vermont**	NA
27	Virginia	155.0
15	Washington	165.3
40	West Virginia	138.6
NA	Wisconsin**	NA
11	Wyoming	168.0

RANK ORDER

RANK	STATE	RATE
1	Minnesota	184.6
2	Utah	182.2
3	Delaware	179.9
4	Michigan	179.4
5	New Jersey	177.9
6	Louisiana	176.8
7	Montana	174.5
8	South Carolina	171.5
9	South Dakota	171.0
10	North Dakota	169.5
11	Wyoming	168.0
12	Mississippi	166.7
13	New York	166.3
14	Idaho	165.8
15	Washington	165.3
16	Maine	164.8
17	Connecticut	164.6
17	Massachusetts	164.6
19	Georgia	162.4
20	Arkansas	161.3
21	Pennsylvania	159.7
22	Kansas	159.6
23	New Hampshire	159.5
24	Illinois	157.9
25	Nebraska	157.6
26	Colorado	156.4
27	Virginia	155.0
28	Alabama	154.2
29	North Carolina	153.2
30	Rhode Island	152.2
31	Oklahoma	150.0
32	California	149.0
33	Oregon	148.0
34	New Mexico	146.1
35	Iowa	144.9
36	Nevada	144.2
37	Texas	144.0
38	Kentucky	142.5
39	Alaska	141.4
40	West Virginia	138.6
41	Florida	138.4
42	Indiana	135.9
43	Tennessee	132.7
44	Missouri	129.3
45	Hawaii	128.6
46	Arizona	118.9
NA	Maryland**	NA
NA	Ohio**	NA
NA	Vermont**	NA
NA	Wisconsin**	NA
	District of Columbia	175.2

Source: American Cancer Society

"Cancer Facts & Figures 2010" (Copyright 2010, American Cancer Society, http://www.cancer.org/docroot/stt/stt_0.asp)

*For 2002 to 2006. Age-adjusted to the 2000 U.S. standard population.

**Not available.

Percent of Males Receiving PSA Test for Prostate Cancer: 2008

National Median = 54.8% of Men*

ALPHA ORDER				RANK ORDER		
RANK	STATE	PERCENT		RANK	STATE	PERCENT
3	Alabama	61.5		1	Wyoming	64.6
47	Alaska	48.4		2	Florida	64.1
7	Arizona	59.3		3	Alabama	61.5
16	Arkansas	57.4		4	Georgia	61.0
46	California	48.8		5	Rhode Island	60.4
29	Colorado	54.5		6	North Carolina	60.2
15	Connecticut	57.8		7	Arizona	59.3
18	Delaware	57.1		8	Michigan	59.2
2	Florida	64.1		9	Virginia	58.9
4	Georgia	61.0		10	South Carolina	58.8
50	Hawaii	44.9		11	Maryland	58.6
35	Idaho	52.9		12	Massachusetts	58.5
38	Illinois	52.6		12	New York	58.5
22	Indiana	55.3		14	South Dakota	58.2
38	Iowa	52.6		15	Connecticut	57.8
19	Kansas	57.0		16	Arkansas	57.4
36	Kentucky	52.8		17	Maine	57.2
44	Louisiana	49.5		18	Delaware	57.1
17	Maine	57.2		19	Kansas	57.0
11	Maryland	58.6		20	West Virginia	56.7
12	Massachusetts	58.5		21	Montana	55.6
8	Michigan	59.2		22	Indiana	55.3
45	Minnesota	49.4		23	New Hampshire	55.2
29	Mississippi	54.5		24	Nevada	54.8
26	Missouri	54.6		24	Pennsylvania	54.8
21	Montana	55.6		26	Missouri	54.6
32	Nebraska	53.8		26	North Dakota	54.6
24	Nevada	54.8		26	Ohio	54.6
23	New Hampshire	55.2		29	Colorado	54.5
31	New Jersey	54.3		29	Mississippi	54.5
43	New Mexico	50.6		31	New Jersey	54.3
12	New York	58.5		32	Nebraska	53.8
6	North Carolina	60.2		33	Oregon	53.5
26	North Dakota	54.6		34	Oklahoma	53.3
26	Ohio	54.6		35	Idaho	52.9
34	Oklahoma	53.3		36	Kentucky	52.8
33	Oregon	53.5		36	Texas	52.8
24	Pennsylvania	54.8		38	Illinois	52.6
5	Rhode Island	60.4		38	Iowa	52.6
10	South Carolina	58.8		38	Washington	52.6
14	South Dakota	58.2		41	Wisconsin	51.7
48	Tennessee	48.1		42	Vermont	51.5
36	Texas	52.8		43	New Mexico	50.6
49	Utah	47.7		44	Louisiana	49.5
42	Vermont	51.5		45	Minnesota	49.4
9	Virginia	58.9		46	California	48.8
38	Washington	52.6		47	Alaska	48.4
20	West Virginia	56.7		48	Tennessee	48.1
41	Wisconsin	51.7		49	Utah	47.7
1	Wyoming	64.6		50	Hawaii	44.9
					District of Columbia	61.7

Source: U.S. Department of Health and Human Services, Centers for Disease Control and Prevention
   "2008 Behavioral Risk Factor Surveillance Summary Prevalence Data" (http://apps.nccd.cdc.gov/brfss/)
*Men 40 and older receiving prostate-specific antigen (PSA) test within the past two years.

Estimated New Skin Melanoma Cases in 2010

National Estimated Total = 68,130 New Cases*

RANK	STATE (ALPHA ORDER)	CASES	% of USA		RANK	STATE (RANK ORDER)	CASES	% of USA
20	Alabama	1,210	1.8%		1	California	8,030	11.8%
50	Alaska	80	0.1%		2	Florida	4,980	7.3%
17	Arizona	1,430	2.1%		3	New York	4,050	5.9%
34	Arkansas	460	0.7%		4	Texas	3,570	5.2%
1	California	8,030	11.8%		5	Pennsylvania	3,550	5.2%
23	Colorado	1,180	1.7%		6	New Jersey	2,650	3.9%
24	Connecticut	1,090	1.6%		7	Michigan	2,240	3.3%
44	Delaware	210	0.3%		8	Ohio	2,200	3.2%
2	Florida	4,980	7.3%		9	North Carolina	2,130	3.1%
11	Georgia	2,020	3.0%		10	Illinois	2,060	3.0%
42	Hawaii	310	0.5%		11	Georgia	2,020	3.0%
41	Idaho	360	0.5%		12	Washington	1,930	2.8%
10	Illinois	2,060	3.0%		13	Virginia	1,810	2.7%
21	Indiana	1,200	1.8%		14	Massachusetts	1,770	2.6%
28	Iowa	900	1.3%		15	Tennessee	1,720	2.5%
29	Kansas	650	1.0%		16	Kentucky	1,440	2.1%
16	Kentucky	1,440	2.1%		17	Arizona	1,430	2.1%
32	Louisiana	600	0.9%		18	Missouri	1,320	1.9%
38	Maine	410	0.6%		19	Maryland	1,290	1.9%
19	Maryland	1,290	1.9%		20	Alabama	1,210	1.8%
14	Massachusetts	1,770	2.6%		21	Indiana	1,200	1.8%
7	Michigan	2,240	3.3%		21	Oregon	1,200	1.8%
27	Minnesota	970	1.4%		23	Colorado	1,180	1.7%
33	Mississippi	470	0.7%		24	Connecticut	1,090	1.6%
18	Missouri	1,320	1.9%		25	South Carolina	1,060	1.6%
45	Montana	200	0.3%		26	Wisconsin	1,050	1.5%
35	Nebraska	450	0.7%		27	Minnesota	970	1.4%
38	Nevada	410	0.6%		28	Iowa	900	1.3%
40	New Hampshire	390	0.6%		29	Kansas	650	1.0%
6	New Jersey	2,650	3.9%		30	Oklahoma	640	0.9%
37	New Mexico	420	0.6%		31	Utah	610	0.9%
3	New York	4,050	5.9%		32	Louisiana	600	0.9%
9	North Carolina	2,130	3.1%		33	Mississippi	470	0.7%
48	North Dakota	120	0.2%		34	Arkansas	460	0.7%
8	Ohio	2,200	3.2%		35	Nebraska	450	0.7%
30	Oklahoma	640	0.9%		36	West Virginia	440	0.6%
21	Oregon	1,200	1.8%		37	New Mexico	420	0.6%
5	Pennsylvania	3,550	5.2%		38	Maine	410	0.6%
43	Rhode Island	290	0.4%		38	Nevada	410	0.6%
25	South Carolina	1,060	1.6%		40	New Hampshire	390	0.6%
47	South Dakota	170	0.2%		41	Idaho	360	0.5%
15	Tennessee	1,720	2.5%		42	Hawaii	310	0.5%
4	Texas	3,570	5.2%		43	Rhode Island	290	0.4%
31	Utah	610	0.9%		44	Delaware	210	0.3%
46	Vermont	190	0.3%		45	Montana	200	0.3%
13	Virginia	1,810	2.7%		46	Vermont	190	0.3%
12	Washington	1,930	2.8%		47	South Dakota	170	0.2%
36	West Virginia	440	0.6%		48	North Dakota	120	0.2%
26	Wisconsin	1,050	1.5%		49	Wyoming	110	0.2%
49	Wyoming	110	0.2%		50	Alaska	80	0.1%
						District of Columbia	70	0.1%

Source: American Cancer Society
 "Cancer Facts & Figures 2010" (Copyright 2010, American Cancer Society, http://www.cancer.org/docroot/stt/stt_0.asp)
*These estimates are offered as a rough guide and should be interpreted with caution. They are calculated by the American Cancer Society using a model based on 1995-2006 incidence rates.

Estimated Rate of New Skin Melanoma Cases in 2010

National Estimated Rate = 22.2 New Cases per 100,000 Population*

ALPHA ORDER			RANK ORDER		
RANK	STATE	RATE	RANK	STATE	RATE
15	Alabama	25.7	1	Kentucky	33.4
50	Alaska	11.5	2	Oregon	31.4
30	Arizona	21.7	3	Maine	31.1
45	Arkansas	15.9	4	Connecticut	31.0
30	California	21.7	5	Vermont	30.6
20	Colorado	23.5	6	New Jersey	30.4
4	Connecticut	31.0	7	Iowa	29.9
19	Delaware	23.7	8	New Hampshire	29.4
13	Florida	26.9	9	Washington	29.0
35	Georgia	20.6	10	Pennsylvania	28.2
18	Hawaii	23.9	11	Rhode Island	27.5
21	Idaho	23.3	12	Tennessee	27.3
44	Illinois	16.0	13	Florida	26.9
39	Indiana	18.7	14	Massachusetts	26.8
7	Iowa	29.9	15	Alabama	25.7
23	Kansas	23.1	16	Nebraska	25.0
1	Kentucky	33.4	17	West Virginia	24.2
49	Louisiana	13.4	18	Hawaii	23.9
3	Maine	31.1	19	Delaware	23.7
26	Maryland	22.6	20	Colorado	23.5
14	Massachusetts	26.8	21	Idaho	23.3
27	Michigan	22.5	22	South Carolina	23.2
42	Minnesota	18.4	23	Kansas	23.1
45	Mississippi	15.9	24	Virginia	23.0
28	Missouri	22.0	25	North Carolina	22.7
36	Montana	20.5	26	Maryland	22.6
16	Nebraska	25.0	27	Michigan	22.5
47	Nevada	15.5	28	Missouri	22.0
8	New Hampshire	29.4	29	Utah	21.9
6	New Jersey	30.4	30	Arizona	21.7
32	New Mexico	20.9	30	California	21.7
34	New York	20.7	32	New Mexico	20.9
25	North Carolina	22.7	32	South Dakota	20.9
40	North Dakota	18.6	34	New York	20.7
38	Ohio	19.1	35	Georgia	20.6
43	Oklahoma	17.4	36	Montana	20.5
2	Oregon	31.4	37	Wyoming	20.2
10	Pennsylvania	28.2	38	Ohio	19.1
11	Rhode Island	27.5	39	Indiana	18.7
22	South Carolina	23.2	40	North Dakota	18.6
32	South Dakota	20.9	40	Wisconsin	18.6
12	Tennessee	27.3	42	Minnesota	18.4
48	Texas	14.4	43	Oklahoma	17.4
29	Utah	21.9	44	Illinois	16.0
5	Vermont	30.6	45	Arkansas	15.9
24	Virginia	23.0	45	Mississippi	15.9
9	Washington	29.0	47	Nevada	15.5
17	West Virginia	24.2	48	Texas	14.4
40	Wisconsin	18.6	49	Louisiana	13.4
37	Wyoming	20.2	50	Alaska	11.5
				District of Columbia	11.7

Source: CQ Press using data from American Cancer Society

"Cancer Facts & Figures 2010" (Copyright 2010, American Cancer Society, http://www.cancer.org/docroot/stt/stt_0.asp)
*These estimates are offered as a rough guide and should be interpreted with caution. They are calculated by the American Cancer Society using a model based on 1995-2006 incidence rates. Rates calculated using 2009 Census resident population estimates.

Estimated New Cervical Cancer Cases in 2010

National Estimated Total = 12,200 New Cases*

ALPHA ORDER					RANK ORDER			
RANK	STATE		CASES	% of USA	RANK	STATE	CASES	% of USA
19	Alabama		200	1.6%	1	California	1,540	12.6%
NA	Alaska**		NA	NA	2	Texas	1,070	8.8%
16	Arizona		210	1.7%	3	Florida	940	7.7%
27	Arkansas		140	1.1%	4	New York	930	7.6%
1	California		1,540	12.6%	5	Pennsylvania	540	4.4%
25	Colorado		150	1.2%	6	Illinois	490	4.0%
32	Connecticut		120	1.0%	7	New Jersey	420	3.4%
NA	Delaware**		NA	NA	8	Ohio	410	3.4%
3	Florida		940	7.7%	9	Georgia	390	3.2%
9	Georgia		390	3.2%	10	North Carolina	360	3.0%
40	Hawaii		50	0.4%	11	Michigan	330	2.7%
38	Idaho		60	0.5%	12	Virginia	280	2.3%
6	Illinois		490	4.0%	13	Tennessee	270	2.2%
14	Indiana		230	1.9%	14	Indiana	230	1.9%
33	Iowa		100	0.8%	15	Washington	220	1.8%
34	Kansas		90	0.7%	16	Arizona	210	1.7%
16	Kentucky		210	1.7%	16	Kentucky	210	1.7%
23	Louisiana		180	1.5%	16	Missouri	210	1.7%
40	Maine		50	0.4%	19	Alabama	200	1.6%
19	Maryland		200	1.6%	19	Maryland	200	1.6%
19	Massachusetts		200	1.6%	19	Massachusetts	200	1.6%
11	Michigan		330	2.7%	19	Wisconsin	200	1.6%
27	Minnesota		140	1.1%	23	Louisiana	180	1.5%
29	Mississippi		130	1.1%	24	South Carolina	170	1.4%
16	Missouri		210	1.7%	25	Colorado	150	1.2%
NA	Montana**		NA	NA	25	Oklahoma	150	1.2%
38	Nebraska		60	0.5%	27	Arkansas	140	1.1%
29	Nevada		130	1.1%	27	Minnesota	140	1.1%
NA	New Hampshire**		NA	NA	29	Mississippi	130	1.1%
7	New Jersey		420	3.4%	29	Nevada	130	1.1%
34	New Mexico		90	0.7%	29	Oregon	130	1.1%
4	New York		930	7.6%	32	Connecticut	120	1.0%
10	North Carolina		360	3.0%	33	Iowa	100	0.8%
NA	North Dakota**		NA	NA	34	Kansas	90	0.7%
8	Ohio		410	3.4%	34	New Mexico	90	0.7%
25	Oklahoma		150	1.2%	36	Utah	80	0.7%
29	Oregon		130	1.1%	36	West Virginia	80	0.7%
5	Pennsylvania		540	4.4%	38	Idaho	60	0.5%
NA	Rhode Island**		NA	NA	38	Nebraska	60	0.5%
24	South Carolina		170	1.4%	40	Hawaii	50	0.4%
NA	South Dakota**		NA	NA	40	Maine	50	0.4%
13	Tennessee		270	2.2%	NA	Alaska**	NA	NA
2	Texas		1,070	8.8%	NA	Delaware**	NA	NA
36	Utah		80	0.7%	NA	Montana**	NA	NA
NA	Vermont**		NA	NA	NA	New Hampshire**	NA	NA
12	Virginia		280	2.3%	NA	North Dakota**	NA	NA
15	Washington		220	1.8%	NA	Rhode Island**	NA	NA
36	West Virginia		80	0.7%	NA	South Dakota**	NA	NA
19	Wisconsin		200	1.6%	NA	Vermont**	NA	NA
NA	Wyoming**		NA	NA	NA	Wyoming**	NA	NA
						District of Columbia**	NA	NA

Source: American Cancer Society

"Cancer Facts & Figures 2010" (Copyright 2010, American Cancer Society, http://www.cancer.org/docroot/stt/stt_0.asp)

*These estimates are offered as a rough guide and should be interpreted with caution. They are calculated by the American Cancer Society using a model based on 1995-2006 incidence rates.

**Not available.

Estimated Rate of New Cervical Cancer Cases in 2010

National Estimated Rate = 7.8 New Cases per 100,000 Female Population*

ALPHA ORDER

RANK	STATE	RATE
14	Alabama	8.2
NA	Alaska**	NA
36	Arizona	6.4
4	Arkansas	9.5
13	California	8.3
38	Colorado	6.0
30	Connecticut	6.7
NA	Delaware**	NA
1	Florida	10.0
16	Georgia	7.8
16	Hawaii	7.8
16	Idaho	7.8
20	Illinois	7.5
24	Indiana	7.1
32	Iowa	6.6
37	Kansas	6.3
3	Kentucky	9.6
16	Louisiana	7.8
22	Maine	7.4
29	Maryland	6.8
39	Massachusetts	5.9
35	Michigan	6.5
41	Minnesota	5.3
10	Mississippi	8.5
27	Missouri	6.9
NA	Montana**	NA
32	Nebraska	6.6
1	Nevada	10.0
NA	New Hampshire**	NA
4	New Jersey	9.5
7	New Mexico	8.9
6	New York	9.3
20	North Carolina	7.5
NA	North Dakota**	NA
27	Ohio	6.9
15	Oklahoma	8.0
30	Oregon	6.7
11	Pennsylvania	8.4
NA	Rhode Island**	NA
23	South Carolina	7.3
NA	South Dakota**	NA
11	Tennessee	8.4
8	Texas	8.6
40	Utah	5.8
NA	Vermont**	NA
25	Virginia	7.0
32	Washington	6.6
8	West Virginia	8.6
25	Wisconsin	7.0
NA	Wyoming**	NA

RANK ORDER

RANK	STATE	RATE
1	Florida	10.0
1	Nevada	10.0
3	Kentucky	9.6
4	Arkansas	9.5
4	New Jersey	9.5
6	New York	9.3
7	New Mexico	8.9
8	Texas	8.6
8	West Virginia	8.6
10	Mississippi	8.5
11	Pennsylvania	8.4
11	Tennessee	8.4
13	California	8.3
14	Alabama	8.2
15	Oklahoma	8.0
16	Georgia	7.8
16	Hawaii	7.8
16	Idaho	7.8
16	Louisiana	7.8
20	Illinois	7.5
20	North Carolina	7.5
22	Maine	7.4
23	South Carolina	7.3
24	Indiana	7.1
25	Virginia	7.0
25	Wisconsin	7.0
27	Missouri	6.9
27	Ohio	6.9
29	Maryland	6.8
30	Connecticut	6.7
30	Oregon	6.7
32	Iowa	6.6
32	Nebraska	6.6
32	Washington	6.6
35	Michigan	6.5
36	Arizona	6.4
37	Kansas	6.3
38	Colorado	6.0
39	Massachusetts	5.9
40	Utah	5.8
41	Minnesota	5.3
NA	Alaska**	NA
NA	Delaware**	NA
NA	Montana**	NA
NA	New Hampshire**	NA
NA	North Dakota**	NA
NA	Rhode Island**	NA
NA	South Dakota**	NA
NA	Vermont**	NA
NA	Wyoming**	NA
	District of Columbia**	NA

Source: CQ Press using data from American Cancer Society
"Cancer Facts & Figures 2010" (Copyright 2010, American Cancer Society, http://www.cancer.org/docroot/stt/stt_0.asp)
*These estimates are offered as a rough guide and should be interpreted with caution. They are calculated by the American Cancer Society using a model based on 1995-2006 incidence rates. Rates calculated using 2009 Census female population estimates.
**Not available.

Percent of Women 18 Years Old and Older
Who Have Had a Pap Smear within the Past Three Years: 2008
National Median = 82.9% of Women 18 Years and Older*

ALPHA ORDER

RANK	STATE	PERCENT
39	Alabama	81.3
20	Alaska	83.6
32	Arizona	82.3
40	Arkansas	80.8
12	California	84.1
13	Colorado	84.0
16	Connecticut	83.9
10	Delaware	84.5
21	Florida	83.3
1	Georgia	87.6
26	Hawaii	82.8
48	Idaho	76.8
18	Illinois	83.8
45	Indiana	78.7
13	Iowa	84.0
13	Kansas	84.0
34	Kentucky	81.7
49	Louisiana	76.7
4	Maine	86.3
11	Maryland	84.2
1	Massachusetts	87.6
43	Michigan	80.1
8	Minnesota	86.0
30	Mississippi	82.6
25	Missouri	82.9
36	Montana	81.5
18	Nebraska	83.8
47	Nevada	78.2
5	New Hampshire	86.1
44	New Jersey	79.9
42	New Mexico	80.7
21	New York	83.3
3	North Carolina	86.9
26	North Dakota	82.8
28	Ohio	82.7
38	Oklahoma	81.4
34	Oregon	81.7
33	Pennsylvania	82.0
5	Rhode Island	86.1
5	South Carolina	86.1
31	South Dakota	82.5
16	Tennessee	83.9
36	Texas	81.5
50	Utah	74.2
9	Vermont	85.9
23	Virginia	83.2
28	Washington	82.7
40	West Virginia	80.8
24	Wisconsin	83.1
46	Wyoming	78.4

RANK ORDER

RANK	STATE	PERCENT
1	Georgia	87.6
1	Massachusetts	87.6
3	North Carolina	86.9
4	Maine	86.3
5	New Hampshire	86.1
5	Rhode Island	86.1
5	South Carolina	86.1
8	Minnesota	86.0
9	Vermont	85.9
10	Delaware	84.5
11	Maryland	84.2
12	California	84.1
13	Colorado	84.0
13	Iowa	84.0
13	Kansas	84.0
16	Connecticut	83.9
16	Tennessee	83.9
18	Illinois	83.8
18	Nebraska	83.8
20	Alaska	83.6
21	Florida	83.3
21	New York	83.3
23	Virginia	83.2
24	Wisconsin	83.1
25	Missouri	82.9
26	Hawaii	82.8
26	North Dakota	82.8
28	Ohio	82.7
28	Washington	82.7
30	Mississippi	82.6
31	South Dakota	82.5
32	Arizona	82.3
33	Pennsylvania	82.0
34	Kentucky	81.7
34	Oregon	81.7
36	Montana	81.5
36	Texas	81.5
38	Oklahoma	81.4
39	Alabama	81.3
40	Arkansas	80.8
40	West Virginia	80.8
42	New Mexico	80.7
43	Michigan	80.1
44	New Jersey	79.9
45	Indiana	78.7
46	Wyoming	78.4
47	Nevada	78.2
48	Idaho	76.8
49	Louisiana	76.7
50	Utah	74.2

District of Columbia	88.9

Source: U.S. Department of Health and Human Services, Centers for Disease Control and Prevention
   "2008 Behavioral Risk Factor Surveillance Summary Prevalence Data" (http://apps.nccd.cdc.gov/brfss/)
*A Pap test is a test for cancer, especially of the female genital tract such as cancer of the cervix. Named after George Papanicolaou (1883-1962), American anatomist.

Estimated New Uterine Cancer Cases in 2010

National Estimated Total = 43,470 New Cases*

ALPHA ORDER

RANK	STATE	CASES	% of USA
28	Alabama	520	1.2%
49	Alaska	70	0.2%
21	Arizona	710	1.6%
32	Arkansas	330	0.8%
1	California	4,470	10.3%
25	Colorado	570	1.3%
22	Connecticut	650	1.5%
45	Delaware	140	0.3%
3	Florida	2,710	6.2%
16	Georgia	950	2.2%
41	Hawaii	220	0.5%
42	Idaho	200	0.5%
7	Illinois	1,960	4.5%
15	Indiana	960	2.2%
27	Iowa	550	1.3%
31	Kansas	410	0.9%
23	Kentucky	610	1.4%
30	Louisiana	440	1.0%
37	Maine	280	0.6%
19	Maryland	810	1.9%
11	Massachusetts	1,150	2.6%
8	Michigan	1,700	3.9%
18	Minnesota	850	2.0%
34	Mississippi	300	0.7%
17	Missouri	910	2.1%
44	Montana	150	0.3%
35	Nebraska	290	0.7%
35	Nevada	290	0.7%
39	New Hampshire	240	0.6%
9	New Jersey	1,580	3.6%
40	New Mexico	230	0.5%
2	New York	3,430	7.9%
10	North Carolina	1,190	2.7%
48	North Dakota	100	0.2%
6	Ohio	2,010	4.6%
29	Oklahoma	460	1.1%
24	Oregon	600	1.4%
4	Pennsylvania	2,450	5.6%
43	Rhode Island	190	0.4%
26	South Carolina	560	1.3%
46	South Dakota	130	0.3%
20	Tennessee	750	1.7%
5	Texas	2,420	5.6%
37	Utah	280	0.6%
47	Vermont	110	0.3%
12	Virginia	1,040	2.4%
14	Washington	1,010	2.3%
32	West Virginia	330	0.8%
12	Wisconsin	1,040	2.4%
49	Wyoming	70	0.2%

RANK ORDER

RANK	STATE	CASES	% of USA
1	California	4,470	10.3%
2	New York	3,430	7.9%
3	Florida	2,710	6.2%
4	Pennsylvania	2,450	5.6%
5	Texas	2,420	5.6%
6	Ohio	2,010	4.6%
7	Illinois	1,960	4.5%
8	Michigan	1,700	3.9%
9	New Jersey	1,580	3.6%
10	North Carolina	1,190	2.7%
11	Massachusetts	1,150	2.6%
12	Virginia	1,040	2.4%
12	Wisconsin	1,040	2.4%
14	Washington	1,010	2.3%
15	Indiana	960	2.2%
16	Georgia	950	2.2%
17	Missouri	910	2.1%
18	Minnesota	850	2.0%
19	Maryland	810	1.9%
20	Tennessee	750	1.7%
21	Arizona	710	1.6%
22	Connecticut	650	1.5%
23	Kentucky	610	1.4%
24	Oregon	600	1.4%
25	Colorado	570	1.3%
26	South Carolina	560	1.3%
27	Iowa	550	1.3%
28	Alabama	520	1.2%
29	Oklahoma	460	1.1%
30	Louisiana	440	1.0%
31	Kansas	410	0.9%
32	Arkansas	330	0.8%
32	West Virginia	330	0.8%
34	Mississippi	300	0.7%
35	Nebraska	290	0.7%
35	Nevada	290	0.7%
37	Maine	280	0.6%
37	Utah	280	0.6%
39	New Hampshire	240	0.6%
40	New Mexico	230	0.5%
41	Hawaii	220	0.5%
42	Idaho	200	0.5%
43	Rhode Island	190	0.4%
44	Montana	150	0.3%
45	Delaware	140	0.3%
46	South Dakota	130	0.3%
47	Vermont	110	0.3%
48	North Dakota	100	0.2%
49	Alaska	70	0.2%
49	Wyoming	70	0.2%
	District of Columbia	80	0.2%

Source: American Cancer Society

"Cancer Facts & Figures 2010" (Copyright 2010, American Cancer Society, http://www.cancer.org/docroot/stt/stt_0.asp)
*These estimates are offered as a rough guide and should be interpreted with caution. They are calculated by the American Cancer Society using a model based on 1995-2006 incidence rates.

Estimated Rate of New Uterine Cancer Cases in 2010

National Estimated Rate = 27.9 New Cases per 100,000 Female Population*

ALPHA ORDER				RANK ORDER		
RANK	STATE	RATE		RANK	STATE	RATE
44	Alabama	21.4		1	Maine	41.5
45	Alaska	20.8		2	Pennsylvania	37.9
43	Arizona	21.6		3	Wisconsin	36.5
41	Arkansas	22.4		4	Connecticut	36.1
36	California	24.2		4	Iowa	36.1
39	Colorado	22.9		6	New Hampshire	35.7
4	Connecticut	36.1		7	New Jersey	35.6
22	Delaware	30.7		7	West Virginia	35.6
28	Florida	28.8		9	Rhode Island	35.1
50	Georgia	19.0		10	Vermont	34.8
11	Hawaii	34.3		11	Hawaii	34.3
32	Idaho	26.0		12	New York	34.2
24	Illinois	29.9		13	Ohio	34.0
26	Indiana	29.5		14	Massachusetts	33.9
4	Iowa	36.1		15	Michigan	33.6
27	Kansas	28.9		16	Minnesota	32.1
29	Kentucky	27.8		17	Nebraska	32.0
49	Louisiana	19.1		17	South Dakota	32.0
1	Maine	41.5		19	North Dakota	31.1
30	Maryland	27.6		19	Oregon	31.1
14	Massachusetts	33.9		21	Montana	30.8
15	Michigan	33.6		22	Delaware	30.7
16	Minnesota	32.1		23	Washington	30.3
47	Mississippi	19.7		24	Illinois	29.9
25	Missouri	29.7		25	Missouri	29.7
21	Montana	30.8		26	Indiana	29.5
17	Nebraska	32.0		27	Kansas	28.9
41	Nevada	22.4		28	Florida	28.8
6	New Hampshire	35.7		29	Kentucky	27.8
7	New Jersey	35.6		30	Maryland	27.6
40	New Mexico	22.7		31	Wyoming	26.2
12	New York	34.2		32	Idaho	26.0
34	North Carolina	24.8		33	Virginia	25.9
19	North Dakota	31.1		34	North Carolina	24.8
13	Ohio	34.0		35	Oklahoma	24.7
35	Oklahoma	24.7		36	California	24.2
19	Oregon	31.1		37	South Carolina	23.9
2	Pennsylvania	37.9		38	Tennessee	23.2
9	Rhode Island	35.1		39	Colorado	22.9
37	South Carolina	23.9		40	New Mexico	22.7
17	South Dakota	32.0		41	Arkansas	22.4
38	Tennessee	23.2		41	Nevada	22.4
48	Texas	19.5		43	Arizona	21.6
46	Utah	20.2		44	Alabama	21.4
10	Vermont	34.8		45	Alaska	20.8
33	Virginia	25.9		46	Utah	20.2
23	Washington	30.3		47	Mississippi	19.7
7	West Virginia	35.6		48	Texas	19.5
3	Wisconsin	36.5		49	Louisiana	19.1
31	Wyoming	26.2		50	Georgia	19.0
					District of Columbia	25.3

Source: CQ Press using data from American Cancer Society
    "Cancer Facts & Figures 2010" (Copyright 2010, American Cancer Society, http://www.cancer.org/docroot/stt/stt_0.asp)
*These estimates are offered as a rough guide and should be interpreted with caution. They are calculated by the American Cancer Society using a model based on 1995-2006 incidence rates. Rates calculated using 2009 Census female population estimates.

AIDS Cases Reported in 2008

National Total = 37,151 New AIDS Cases*

RANK	STATE	CASES	% of USA
20	Alabama	406	1.1%
46	Alaska	22	0.1%
17	Arizona	589	1.6%
32	Arkansas	151	0.4%
1	California	4,835	13.0%
24	Colorado	369	1.0%
25	Connecticut	354	1.0%
33	Delaware	146	0.4%
2	Florida	4,766	12.8%
5	Georgia	1,908	5.1%
41	Hawaii	39	0.1%
43	Idaho	33	0.1%
9	Illinois	1,305	3.5%
19	Indiana	416	1.1%
39	Iowa	75	0.2%
34	Kansas	110	0.3%
27	Kentucky	294	0.8%
11	Louisiana	1,060	2.9%
42	Maine	36	0.1%
6	Maryland	1,557	4.2%
22	Massachusetts	380	1.0%
12	Michigan	699	1.9%
29	Minnesota	210	0.6%
23	Mississippi	370	1.0%
18	Missouri	500	1.3%
44	Montana	29	0.1%
38	Nebraska	76	0.2%
26	Nevada	321	0.9%
45	New Hampshire	27	0.1%
7	New Jersey	1,527	4.1%
35	New Mexico	100	0.3%
3	New York	4,571	12.3%
10	North Carolina	1,157	3.1%
47	North Dakota	16	0.0%
14	Ohio	667	1.8%
30	Oklahoma	172	0.5%
28	Oregon	211	0.6%
8	Pennsylvania	1,402	3.8%
37	Rhode Island	78	0.2%
13	South Carolina	696	1.9%
49	South Dakota	11	0.0%
16	Tennessee	597	1.6%
4	Texas	2,924	7.9%
39	Utah	75	0.2%
49	Vermont	11	0.0%
15	Virginia	634	1.7%
21	Washington	405	1.1%
36	West Virginia	81	0.2%
31	Wisconsin	167	0.4%
48	Wyoming	15	0.0%

RANK	STATE	CASES	% of USA
1	California	4,835	13.0%
2	Florida	4,766	12.8%
3	New York	4,571	12.3%
4	Texas	2,924	7.9%
5	Georgia	1,908	5.1%
6	Maryland	1,557	4.2%
7	New Jersey	1,527	4.1%
8	Pennsylvania	1,402	3.8%
9	Illinois	1,305	3.5%
10	North Carolina	1,157	3.1%
11	Louisiana	1,060	2.9%
12	Michigan	699	1.9%
13	South Carolina	696	1.9%
14	Ohio	667	1.8%
15	Virginia	634	1.7%
16	Tennessee	597	1.6%
17	Arizona	589	1.6%
18	Missouri	500	1.3%
19	Indiana	416	1.1%
20	Alabama	406	1.1%
21	Washington	405	1.1%
22	Massachusetts	380	1.0%
23	Mississippi	370	1.0%
24	Colorado	369	1.0%
25	Connecticut	354	1.0%
26	Nevada	321	0.9%
27	Kentucky	294	0.8%
28	Oregon	211	0.6%
29	Minnesota	210	0.6%
30	Oklahoma	172	0.5%
31	Wisconsin	167	0.4%
32	Arkansas	151	0.4%
33	Delaware	146	0.4%
34	Kansas	110	0.3%
35	New Mexico	100	0.3%
36	West Virginia	81	0.2%
37	Rhode Island	78	0.2%
38	Nebraska	76	0.2%
39	Iowa	75	0.2%
39	Utah	75	0.2%
41	Hawaii	39	0.1%
42	Maine	36	0.1%
43	Idaho	33	0.1%
44	Montana	29	0.1%
45	New Hampshire	27	0.1%
46	Alaska	22	0.1%
47	North Dakota	16	0.0%
48	Wyoming	15	0.0%
49	South Dakota	11	0.0%
49	Vermont	11	0.0%
	District of Columbia	552	1.5%

Source: U.S. Department of Health and Human Services, Centers for Disease Control and Prevention

"HIV/AIDS Surveillance Report, 2008" (Vol. 20, http://www.cdc.gov/hiv/topics/surveillance/resources/reports/index.htm)

*AIDS is Acquired Immunodeficiency Syndrome. It is a specific group of diseases or conditions which are indicative of severe immunosuppression related to infection with the Human Immunodeficiency Virus (HIV). National total does not include 819 new cases in Puerto Rico, 1 in the Northern Mariana Islands, and 14 in the Virgin Islands.

AIDS Rate in 2008

National Rate = 12.2 New AIDS Cases Reported per 100,000 Population*

ALPHA ORDER

RANK	STATE	RATE
19	Alabama	8.7
38	Alaska	3.2
18	Arizona	9.1
31	Arkansas	5.3
9	California	13.2
22	Colorado	7.5
15	Connecticut	10.1
7	Delaware	16.8
2	Florida	26.0
5	Georgia	19.7
39	Hawaii	3.0
47	Idaho	2.1
15	Illinois	10.1
26	Indiana	6.5
45	Iowa	2.5
37	Kansas	3.9
25	Kentucky	6.9
3	Louisiana	24.0
43	Maine	2.7
1	Maryland	27.6
28	Massachusetts	5.8
24	Michigan	7.0
36	Minnesota	4.0
10	Mississippi	12.6
20	Missouri	8.5
39	Montana	3.0
35	Nebraska	4.3
12	Nevada	12.4
47	New Hampshire	2.1
6	New Jersey	17.6
32	New Mexico	5.1
4	New York	23.5
11	North Carolina	12.5
46	North Dakota	2.4
28	Ohio	5.8
33	Oklahoma	4.7
30	Oregon	5.6
14	Pennsylvania	11.3
23	Rhode Island	7.4
8	South Carolina	15.5
50	South Dakota	1.4
17	Tennessee	9.6
13	Texas	12.0
43	Utah	2.7
49	Vermont	1.8
21	Virginia	8.2
27	Washington	6.2
34	West Virginia	4.5
39	Wisconsin	3.0
42	Wyoming	2.9

RANK ORDER

RANK	STATE	RATE
1	Maryland	27.6
2	Florida	26.0
3	Louisiana	24.0
4	New York	23.5
5	Georgia	19.7
6	New Jersey	17.6
7	Delaware	16.8
8	South Carolina	15.5
9	California	13.2
10	Mississippi	12.6
11	North Carolina	12.5
12	Nevada	12.4
13	Texas	12.0
14	Pennsylvania	11.3
15	Connecticut	10.1
15	Illinois	10.1
17	Tennessee	9.6
18	Arizona	9.1
19	Alabama	8.7
20	Missouri	8.5
21	Virginia	8.2
22	Colorado	7.5
23	Rhode Island	7.4
24	Michigan	7.0
25	Kentucky	6.9
26	Indiana	6.5
27	Washington	6.2
28	Massachusetts	5.8
28	Ohio	5.8
30	Oregon	5.6
31	Arkansas	5.3
32	New Mexico	5.1
33	Oklahoma	4.7
34	West Virginia	4.5
35	Nebraska	4.3
36	Minnesota	4.0
37	Kansas	3.9
38	Alaska	3.2
39	Hawaii	3.0
39	Montana	3.0
39	Wisconsin	3.0
42	Wyoming	2.9
43	Maine	2.7
43	Utah	2.7
45	Iowa	2.5
46	North Dakota	2.4
47	Idaho	2.1
47	New Hampshire	2.1
49	Vermont	1.8
50	South Dakota	1.4

District of Columbia   93.3

Source: U.S. Department of Health and Human Services, Centers for Disease Control and Prevention
"HIV/AIDS Surveillance Report, 2008" (Vol. 20, http://www.cdc.gov/hiv/topics/surveillance/resources/reports/index.htm)
*AIDS is Acquired Immunodeficiency Syndrome. It is a specific group of diseases or conditions which are indicative of severe immunosuppression related to infection with the Human Immunodeficiency Virus (HIV). National rate does not include cases or population in U.S. territories.

AIDS Cases Reported through December 2008

National Total = 1,073,128 Reported AIDS Cases*

ALPHA ORDER

RANK	STATE	CASES	% of USA
22	Alabama	9,738	0.9%
44	Alaska	730	0.1%
21	Arizona	11,747	1.1%
32	Arkansas	4,436	0.4%
2	California	160,293	14.9%
23	Colorado	9,639	0.9%
16	Connecticut	16,127	1.5%
33	Delaware	4,028	0.4%
3	Florida	117,612	11.0%
6	Georgia	38,300	3.6%
34	Hawaii	3,189	0.3%
45	Idaho	676	0.1%
8	Illinois	37,880	3.5%
24	Indiana	9,186	0.9%
39	Iowa	1,936	0.2%
35	Kansas	3,121	0.3%
30	Kentucky	5,344	0.5%
11	Louisiana	20,319	1.9%
42	Maine	1,228	0.1%
9	Maryland	35,725	3.3%
10	Massachusetts	21,314	2.0%
15	Michigan	16,866	1.6%
29	Minnesota	5,422	0.5%
25	Mississippi	7,557	0.7%
20	Missouri	12,447	1.2%
47	Montana	466	0.0%
41	Nebraska	1,679	0.2%
27	Nevada	6,547	0.6%
43	New Hampshire	1,199	0.1%
5	New Jersey	54,557	5.1%
36	New Mexico	2,903	0.3%
1	New York	192,753	18.0%
12	North Carolina	19,539	1.8%
50	North Dakota	173	0.0%
14	Ohio	17,129	1.6%
28	Oklahoma	5,437	0.5%
26	Oregon	6,554	0.6%
7	Pennsylvania	38,217	3.6%
37	Rhode Island	2,846	0.3%
17	South Carolina	15,176	1.4%
48	South Dakota	297	0.0%
18	Tennessee	14,021	1.3%
4	Texas	77,070	7.2%
38	Utah	2,494	0.2%
46	Vermont	505	0.0%
13	Virginia	19,029	1.8%
19	Washington	12,826	1.2%
40	West Virginia	1,718	0.2%
31	Wisconsin	4,999	0.5%
49	Wyoming	266	0.0%

RANK ORDER

RANK	STATE	CASES	% of USA
1	New York	192,753	18.0%
2	California	160,293	14.9%
3	Florida	117,612	11.0%
4	Texas	77,070	7.2%
5	New Jersey	54,557	5.1%
6	Georgia	38,300	3.6%
7	Pennsylvania	38,217	3.6%
8	Illinois	37,880	3.5%
9	Maryland	35,725	3.3%
10	Massachusetts	21,314	2.0%
11	Louisiana	20,319	1.9%
12	North Carolina	19,539	1.8%
13	Virginia	19,029	1.8%
14	Ohio	17,129	1.6%
15	Michigan	16,866	1.6%
16	Connecticut	16,127	1.5%
17	South Carolina	15,176	1.4%
18	Tennessee	14,021	1.3%
19	Washington	12,826	1.2%
20	Missouri	12,447	1.2%
21	Arizona	11,747	1.1%
22	Alabama	9,738	0.9%
23	Colorado	9,639	0.9%
24	Indiana	9,186	0.9%
25	Mississippi	7,557	0.7%
26	Oregon	6,554	0.6%
27	Nevada	6,547	0.6%
28	Oklahoma	5,437	0.5%
29	Minnesota	5,422	0.5%
30	Kentucky	5,344	0.5%
31	Wisconsin	4,999	0.5%
32	Arkansas	4,436	0.4%
33	Delaware	4,028	0.4%
34	Hawaii	3,189	0.3%
35	Kansas	3,121	0.3%
36	New Mexico	2,903	0.3%
37	Rhode Island	2,846	0.3%
38	Utah	2,494	0.2%
39	Iowa	1,936	0.2%
40	West Virginia	1,718	0.2%
41	Nebraska	1,679	0.2%
42	Maine	1,228	0.1%
43	New Hampshire	1,199	0.1%
44	Alaska	730	0.1%
45	Idaho	676	0.1%
46	Vermont	505	0.0%
47	Montana	466	0.0%
48	South Dakota	297	0.0%
49	Wyoming	266	0.0%
50	North Dakota	173	0.0%
	District of Columbia	19,864	1.9%

Source: U.S. Department of Health and Human Services, Centers for Disease Control and Prevention
"HIV/AIDS Surveillance Report, 2008" (Vol. 20, http://www.cdc.gov/hiv/topics/surveillance/resources/reports/index.htm)
*Cumulative through December 2008. AIDS is Acquired Immunodeficiency Syndrome. It is a specific group of diseases or conditions which are indicative of severe immunosuppression related to infection with the Human Immunodeficiency Virus (HIV). National total does not include 32,463 cases in Puerto Rico, 710 cases in the Virgin Islands, and 89 cases in other U.S. territories.

AIDS Cases in Children 12 Years and Younger through December 2008

National Total = 9,349 Juvenile AIDS Cases*

ALPHA ORDER

RANK	STATE	CASES	% of USA
18	Alabama	76	0.8%
44	Alaska	7	0.1%
23	Arizona	47	0.5%
24	Arkansas	37	0.4%
4	California	687	7.3%
28	Colorado	32	0.3%
12	Connecticut	184	2.0%
32	Delaware	27	0.3%
2	Florida	1,571	16.8%
9	Georgia	245	2.6%
36	Hawaii	17	0.2%
48	Idaho	2	0.0%
8	Illinois	288	3.1%
22	Indiana	57	0.6%
38	Iowa	13	0.1%
37	Kansas	15	0.2%
24	Kentucky	37	0.4%
14	Louisiana	135	1.4%
43	Maine	8	0.1%
7	Maryland	330	3.5%
10	Massachusetts	226	2.4%
16	Michigan	117	1.3%
30	Minnesota	28	0.3%
20	Mississippi	59	0.6%
19	Missouri	62	0.7%
47	Montana	3	0.0%
39	Nebraska	12	0.1%
29	Nevada	29	0.3%
41	New Hampshire	10	0.1%
3	New Jersey	801	8.6%
42	New Mexico	9	0.1%
1	New York	2,390	25.6%
15	North Carolina	126	1.3%
48	North Dakota	2	0.0%
13	Ohio	149	1.6%
32	Oklahoma	27	0.3%
35	Oregon	19	0.2%
6	Pennsylvania	375	4.0%
30	Rhode Island	28	0.3%
17	South Carolina	109	1.2%
45	South Dakota	6	0.1%
20	Tennessee	59	0.6%
5	Texas	396	4.2%
34	Utah	20	0.2%
45	Vermont	6	0.1%
11	Virginia	186	2.0%
26	Washington	35	0.4%
39	West Virginia	12	0.1%
27	Wisconsin	34	0.4%
48	Wyoming	2	0.0%

RANK ORDER

RANK	STATE	CASES	% of USA
1	New York	2,390	25.6%
2	Florida	1,571	16.8%
3	New Jersey	801	8.6%
4	California	687	7.3%
5	Texas	396	4.2%
6	Pennsylvania	375	4.0%
7	Maryland	330	3.5%
8	Illinois	288	3.1%
9	Georgia	245	2.6%
10	Massachusetts	226	2.4%
11	Virginia	186	2.0%
12	Connecticut	184	2.0%
13	Ohio	149	1.6%
14	Louisiana	135	1.4%
15	North Carolina	126	1.3%
16	Michigan	117	1.3%
17	South Carolina	109	1.2%
18	Alabama	76	0.8%
19	Missouri	62	0.7%
20	Mississippi	59	0.6%
20	Tennessee	59	0.6%
22	Indiana	57	0.6%
23	Arizona	47	0.5%
24	Arkansas	37	0.4%
24	Kentucky	37	0.4%
26	Washington	35	0.4%
27	Wisconsin	34	0.4%
28	Colorado	32	0.3%
29	Nevada	29	0.3%
30	Minnesota	28	0.3%
30	Rhode Island	28	0.3%
32	Delaware	27	0.3%
32	Oklahoma	27	0.3%
34	Utah	20	0.2%
35	Oregon	19	0.2%
36	Hawaii	17	0.2%
37	Kansas	15	0.2%
38	Iowa	13	0.1%
39	Nebraska	12	0.1%
39	West Virginia	12	0.1%
41	New Hampshire	10	0.1%
42	New Mexico	9	0.1%
43	Maine	8	0.1%
44	Alaska	7	0.1%
45	South Dakota	6	0.1%
45	Vermont	6	0.1%
47	Montana	3	0.0%
48	Idaho	2	0.0%
48	North Dakota	2	0.0%
48	Wyoming	2	0.0%
	District of Columbia	192	2.1%

Source: U.S. Department of Health and Human Services, Centers for Disease Control and Prevention
"HIV/AIDS Surveillance Report, 2008" (Vol. 20, http://www.cdc.gov/hiv/topics/surveillance/resources/reports/index.htm)
*Cumulative through December 2008. AIDS is Acquired Immunodeficiency Syndrome. It is a specific group of diseases or conditions which are indicative of severe immunosuppression related to infection with the Human Immunodeficiency Virus (HIV). National total does not include 406 cases in Puerto Rico, 19 cases in the Virgin Islands, and 1 case in Guam.

Chickenpox (Varicella) Cases Reported in 2010

National Total = 16,207 Cases*

ALPHA ORDER

RANK	STATE	CASES	% of USA
16	Alabama	291	1.8%
29	Alaska	45	0.3%
36	Arizona	0	0.0%
21	Arkansas	129	0.8%
36	California	0	0.0%
12	Colorado	407	2.5%
15	Connecticut	292	1.8%
32	Delaware	25	0.2%
7	Florida	994	6.1%
NA	Georgia**	NA	NA
31	Hawaii	32	0.2%
NA	Idaho**	NA	NA
5	Illinois	1,164	7.2%
13	Indiana	406	2.5%
NA	Iowa**	NA	NA
19	Kansas	228	1.4%
NA	Kentucky**	NA	NA
24	Louisiana	88	0.5%
18	Maine	241	1.5%
NA	Maryland**	NA	NA
35	Massachusetts	2	0.0%
3	Michigan	1,432	8.8%
36	Minnesota	0	0.0%
34	Mississippi	7	0.0%
10	Missouri	474	2.9%
20	Montana	185	1.1%
NA	Nebraska**	NA	NA
NA	Nevada**	NA	NA
22	New Hampshire	114	0.7%
9	New Jersey	508	3.1%
23	New Mexico	95	0.6%
2	New York	2,110	13.0%
NA	North Carolina**	NA	NA
28	North Dakota	47	0.3%
4	Ohio	1,350	8.3%
NA	Oklahoma**	NA	NA
NA	Oregon**	NA	NA
6	Pennsylvania	1,109	6.8%
30	Rhode Island	34	0.2%
25	South Carolina	77	0.5%
27	South Dakota	55	0.3%
NA	Tennessee**	NA	NA
1	Texas	2,545	15.7%
17	Utah	273	1.7%
26	Vermont	72	0.4%
8	Virginia	523	3.2%
NA	Washington**	NA	NA
11	West Virginia	434	2.7%
14	Wisconsin	379	2.3%
33	Wyoming	21	0.1%

RANK ORDER

RANK	STATE	CASES	% of USA
1	Texas	2,545	15.7%
2	New York	2,110	13.0%
3	Michigan	1,432	8.8%
4	Ohio	1,350	8.3%
5	Illinois	1,164	7.2%
6	Pennsylvania	1,109	6.8%
7	Florida	994	6.1%
8	Virginia	523	3.2%
9	New Jersey	508	3.1%
10	Missouri	474	2.9%
11	West Virginia	434	2.7%
12	Colorado	407	2.5%
13	Indiana	406	2.5%
14	Wisconsin	379	2.3%
15	Connecticut	292	1.8%
16	Alabama	291	1.8%
17	Utah	273	1.7%
18	Maine	241	1.5%
19	Kansas	228	1.4%
20	Montana	185	1.1%
21	Arkansas	129	0.8%
22	New Hampshire	114	0.7%
23	New Mexico	95	0.6%
24	Louisiana	88	0.5%
25	South Carolina	77	0.5%
26	Vermont	72	0.4%
27	South Dakota	55	0.3%
28	North Dakota	47	0.3%
29	Alaska	45	0.3%
30	Rhode Island	34	0.2%
31	Hawaii	32	0.2%
32	Delaware	25	0.2%
33	Wyoming	21	0.1%
34	Mississippi	7	0.0%
35	Massachusetts	2	0.0%
36	Arizona	0	0.0%
36	California	0	0.0%
36	Minnesota	0	0.0%
NA	Georgia**	NA	NA
NA	Idaho**	NA	NA
NA	Iowa**	NA	NA
NA	Kentucky**	NA	NA
NA	Maryland**	NA	NA
NA	Nebraska**	NA	NA
NA	Nevada**	NA	NA
NA	North Carolina**	NA	NA
NA	Oklahoma**	NA	NA
NA	Oregon**	NA	NA
NA	Tennessee**	NA	NA
NA	Washington**	NA	NA
	District of Columbia	19	0.1%

Source: U.S. Department of Health and Human Services, National Center for Health Statistics
"Morbidity and Mortality Weekly Report" (January 7, 2011, Vol. 59, Nos. 51 & 52, http://www.cdc.gov/mmwr/)
*Provisional data. An illness with acute onset of generalized maculo-papulovesicular rash without other apparent cause.
**Not notifiable.

Chickenpox (Varicella) Rate in 2010

National Rate = 5.3 Cases per 100,000 Population*

ALPHA ORDER				RANK ORDER		
RANK	STATE	RATE		RANK	STATE	RATE
23	Alabama	6.2		1	West Virginia	23.8
21	Alaska	6.4		2	Montana	19.0
35	Arizona	0.0		3	Maine	18.3
27	Arkansas	4.5		4	Michigan	14.4
35	California	0.0		5	Ohio	11.7
14	Colorado	8.1		6	Vermont	11.6
13	Connecticut	8.3		7	New York	10.8
30	Delaware	2.8		8	Texas	10.3
25	Florida	5.4		9	Utah	9.8
NA	Georgia**	NA		10	Illinois	9.0
31	Hawaii	2.5		11	Pennsylvania	8.8
NA	Idaho**	NA		12	New Hampshire	8.6
10	Illinois	9.0		13	Connecticut	8.3
22	Indiana	6.3		14	Colorado	8.1
NA	Iowa**	NA		14	Kansas	8.1
14	Kansas	8.1		16	Missouri	7.9
NA	Kentucky**	NA		17	North Dakota	7.3
32	Louisiana	2.0		18	South Dakota	6.8
3	Maine	18.3		19	Wisconsin	6.7
NA	Maryland**	NA		20	Virginia	6.6
35	Massachusetts	0.0		21	Alaska	6.4
4	Michigan	14.4		22	Indiana	6.3
35	Minnesota	0.0		23	Alabama	6.2
34	Mississippi	0.2		24	New Jersey	5.8
16	Missouri	7.9		25	Florida	5.4
2	Montana	19.0		26	New Mexico	4.7
NA	Nebraska**	NA		27	Arkansas	4.5
NA	Nevada**	NA		28	Wyoming	3.9
12	New Hampshire	8.6		29	Rhode Island	3.2
24	New Jersey	5.8		30	Delaware	2.8
26	New Mexico	4.7		31	Hawaii	2.5
7	New York	10.8		32	Louisiana	2.0
NA	North Carolina**	NA		33	South Carolina	1.7
17	North Dakota	7.3		34	Mississippi	0.2
5	Ohio	11.7		35	Arizona	0.0
NA	Oklahoma**	NA		35	California	0.0
NA	Oregon**	NA		35	Massachusetts	0.0
11	Pennsylvania	8.8		35	Minnesota	0.0
29	Rhode Island	3.2		NA	Georgia**	NA
33	South Carolina	1.7		NA	Idaho**	NA
18	South Dakota	6.8		NA	Iowa**	NA
NA	Tennessee**	NA		NA	Kentucky**	NA
8	Texas	10.3		NA	Maryland**	NA
9	Utah	9.8		NA	Nebraska**	NA
6	Vermont	11.6		NA	Nevada**	NA
20	Virginia	6.6		NA	North Carolina**	NA
NA	Washington**	NA		NA	Oklahoma**	NA
1	West Virginia	23.8		NA	Oregon**	NA
19	Wisconsin	6.7		NA	Tennessee**	NA
28	Wyoming	3.9		NA	Washington**	NA

District of Columbia 3.2

Source: CQ Press using data from U.S. Department of Health and Human Services, National Center for Health Statistics
    "Morbidity and Mortality Weekly Report" (January 7, 2011, Vol. 59, Nos. 51 & 52, http://www.cdc.gov/mmwr/)
*Provisional data. An illness with acute onset of generalized maculo-papulovesicular rash without other apparent cause. Rates
calculated using 2009 population estimates.
**Not notifiable.

E. Coli Cases Reported in 2010

National Total = 4,757 Cases*

RANK	STATE	CASES	% of USA		RANK	STATE	CASES	% of USA
30	Alabama	55	1.2%		1	California	322	6.8%
49	Alaska	2	0.0%		2	New York	282	5.9%
21	Arizona	98	2.1%		3	Florida	263	5.5%
32	Arkansas	47	1.0%		4	Missouri	246	5.2%
1	California	322	6.8%		5	Wisconsin	223	4.7%
7	Colorado	209	4.4%		6	Washington	220	4.6%
29	Connecticut	57	1.2%		7	Colorado	209	4.4%
48	Delaware	6	0.1%		8	Iowa	169	3.6%
3	Florida	263	5.5%		8	Texas	169	3.6%
19	Georgia	103	2.2%		10	Pennsylvania	164	3.4%
43	Hawaii	19	0.4%		11	Michigan	150	3.2%
17	Idaho	114	2.4%		12	Ohio	138	2.9%
14	Illinois	123	2.6%		13	Virginia	136	2.9%
23	Indiana	88	1.8%		14	Illinois	123	2.6%
8	Iowa	169	3.6%		15	Oregon	118	2.5%
27	Kansas	74	1.6%		16	Tennessee	117	2.5%
28	Kentucky	68	1.4%		17	Idaho	114	2.4%
43	Louisiana	19	0.4%		18	Maryland	107	2.2%
41	Maine	21	0.4%		19	Georgia	103	2.2%
18	Maryland	107	2.2%		20	New Jersey	102	2.1%
26	Massachusetts	79	1.7%		21	Arizona	98	2.1%
11	Michigan	150	3.2%		22	North Carolina	97	2.0%
37	Minnesota	31	0.7%		23	Indiana	88	1.8%
38	Mississippi	30	0.6%		24	Utah	82	1.7%
4	Missouri	246	5.2%		25	Nebraska	81	1.7%
34	Montana	42	0.9%		26	Massachusetts	79	1.7%
25	Nebraska	81	1.7%		27	Kansas	74	1.6%
36	Nevada	33	0.7%		28	Kentucky	68	1.4%
42	New Hampshire	20	0.4%		29	Connecticut	57	1.2%
20	New Jersey	102	2.1%		30	Alabama	55	1.2%
32	New Mexico	47	1.0%		31	Oklahoma	48	1.0%
2	New York	282	5.9%		32	Arkansas	47	1.0%
22	North Carolina	97	2.0%		32	New Mexico	47	1.0%
46	North Dakota	17	0.4%		34	Montana	42	0.9%
12	Ohio	138	2.9%		35	South Dakota	34	0.7%
31	Oklahoma	48	1.0%		36	Nevada	33	0.7%
15	Oregon	118	2.5%		37	Minnesota	31	0.7%
10	Pennsylvania	164	3.4%		38	Mississippi	30	0.6%
49	Rhode Island	2	0.0%		39	West Virginia	23	0.5%
40	South Carolina	22	0.5%		40	South Carolina	22	0.5%
35	South Dakota	34	0.7%		41	Maine	21	0.4%
16	Tennessee	117	2.5%		42	New Hampshire	20	0.4%
8	Texas	169	3.6%		43	Hawaii	19	0.4%
24	Utah	82	1.7%		43	Louisiana	19	0.4%
43	Vermont	19	0.4%		43	Vermont	19	0.4%
13	Virginia	136	2.9%		46	North Dakota	17	0.4%
6	Washington	220	4.6%		47	Wyoming	15	0.3%
39	West Virginia	23	0.5%		48	Delaware	6	0.1%
5	Wisconsin	223	4.7%		49	Alaska	2	0.0%
47	Wyoming	15	0.3%		49	Rhode Island	2	0.0%
						District of Columbia	6	0.1%

Source: U.S. Department of Health and Human Services, National Center for Health Statistics
"Morbidity and Mortality Weekly Report" (January 7, 2011, Vol. 59, Nos. 51 & 52, http://www.cdc.gov/mmwr/)
*Escherichia Coli is a common bacterium that normally inhabits the intestinal tracts of humans and animals but can cause infection in other parts of the body, especially the urinary tract. One strain, sometimes transmitted in hamburger meat, can cause serious infection resulting in sickness and death.

E. Coli Rate in 2010

National Rate = 1.5 Cases per 100,000 Population*

ALPHA ORDER

RANK	STATE	RATE
34	Alabama	1.2
49	Alaska	0.3
24	Arizona	1.5
20	Arkansas	1.6
43	California	0.9
5	Colorado	4.2
20	Connecticut	1.6
44	Delaware	0.7
28	Florida	1.4
39	Georgia	1.0
24	Hawaii	1.5
1	Idaho	7.4
39	Illinois	1.0
28	Indiana	1.4
2	Iowa	5.6
14	Kansas	2.6
20	Kentucky	1.6
48	Louisiana	0.4
20	Maine	1.6
17	Maryland	1.9
34	Massachusetts	1.2
24	Michigan	1.5
46	Minnesota	0.6
39	Mississippi	1.0
7	Missouri	4.1
4	Montana	4.3
3	Nebraska	4.5
34	Nevada	1.2
24	New Hampshire	1.5
34	New Jersey	1.2
16	New Mexico	2.3
28	New York	1.4
39	North Carolina	1.0
14	North Dakota	2.6
34	Ohio	1.2
31	Oklahoma	1.3
10	Oregon	3.1
31	Pennsylvania	1.3
50	Rhode Island	0.2
47	South Carolina	0.5
5	South Dakota	4.2
17	Tennessee	1.9
44	Texas	0.7
12	Utah	2.9
10	Vermont	3.1
19	Virginia	1.7
9	Washington	3.3
31	West Virginia	1.3
8	Wisconsin	3.9
13	Wyoming	2.8

RANK ORDER

RANK	STATE	RATE
1	Idaho	7.4
2	Iowa	5.6
3	Nebraska	4.5
4	Montana	4.3
5	Colorado	4.2
5	South Dakota	4.2
7	Missouri	4.1
8	Wisconsin	3.9
9	Washington	3.3
10	Oregon	3.1
10	Vermont	3.1
12	Utah	2.9
13	Wyoming	2.8
14	Kansas	2.6
14	North Dakota	2.6
16	New Mexico	2.3
17	Maryland	1.9
17	Tennessee	1.9
19	Virginia	1.7
20	Arkansas	1.6
20	Connecticut	1.6
20	Kentucky	1.6
20	Maine	1.6
24	Arizona	1.5
24	Hawaii	1.5
24	Michigan	1.5
24	New Hampshire	1.5
28	Florida	1.4
28	Indiana	1.4
28	New York	1.4
31	Oklahoma	1.3
31	Pennsylvania	1.3
31	West Virginia	1.3
34	Alabama	1.2
34	Massachusetts	1.2
34	Nevada	1.2
34	New Jersey	1.2
34	Ohio	1.2
39	Georgia	1.0
39	Illinois	1.0
39	Mississippi	1.0
39	North Carolina	1.0
43	California	0.9
44	Delaware	0.7
44	Texas	0.7
46	Minnesota	0.6
47	South Carolina	0.5
48	Louisiana	0.4
49	Alaska	0.3
50	Rhode Island	0.2
	District of Columbia	1.0

Source: CQ Press using data from U.S. Department of Health and Human Services, National Center for Health Statistics "Morbidity and Mortality Weekly Report" (January 7, 2011, Vol. 59, Nos. 51 & 52, http://www.cdc.gov/mmwr/)
*Escherichia Coli is a common bacterium that normally inhabits the intestinal tracts of humans and animals but can cause infection in other parts of the body, especially the urinary tract. One strain, sometimes transmitted in hamburger meat, can cause serious infection resulting in sickness and death. Rates calculated using 2009 population estimates.

Hepatitis A and B Cases Reported in 2010

National Total = 8,937 Cases*

ALPHA ORDER					RANK ORDER			
RANK	STATE		CASES	% of USA	RANK	STATE	CASES	% of USA
23	Alabama		74	0.8%	1	New York	4,628	51.8%
41	Alaska		10	0.1%	2	Florida	442	4.9%
15	Arizona		97	1.1%	3	California	431	4.8%
31	Arkansas		43	0.5%	4	Texas	426	4.8%
3	California		431	4.8%	5	Michigan	195	2.2%
22	Colorado		75	0.8%	6	Georgia	190	2.1%
30	Connecticut		49	0.5%	7	Kentucky	155	1.7%
33	Delaware		30	0.3%	8	North Carolina	150	1.7%
2	Florida		442	4.9%	9	Tennessee	148	1.7%
6	Georgia		190	2.1%	9	Virginia	148	1.7%
45	Hawaii		7	0.1%	11	Illinois	136	1.5%
40	Idaho		14	0.2%	12	Ohio	135	1.5%
11	Illinois		136	1.5%	13	Pennsylvania	126	1.4%
24	Indiana		72	0.8%	14	Wisconsin	121	1.4%
34	Iowa		25	0.3%	15	Arizona	97	1.1%
37	Kansas		21	0.2%	15	Maryland	97	1.1%
7	Kentucky		155	1.7%	17	Missouri	96	1.1%
26	Louisiana		60	0.7%	18	Oklahoma	95	1.1%
38	Maine		20	0.2%	19	New Jersey	81	0.9%
15	Maryland		97	1.1%	20	West Virginia	80	0.9%
28	Massachusetts		53	0.6%	21	South Carolina	79	0.9%
5	Michigan		195	2.2%	22	Colorado	75	0.8%
36	Minnesota		23	0.3%	23	Alabama	74	0.8%
32	Mississippi		37	0.4%	24	Indiana	72	0.8%
17	Missouri		96	1.1%	25	Washington	68	0.8%
47	Montana		5	0.1%	26	Louisiana	60	0.7%
34	Nebraska		25	0.3%	27	Oregon	57	0.6%
29	Nevada		52	0.6%	28	Massachusetts	53	0.6%
43	New Hampshire		9	0.1%	29	Nevada	52	0.6%
19	New Jersey		81	0.9%	30	Connecticut	49	0.5%
41	New Mexico		10	0.1%	31	Arkansas	43	0.5%
1	New York		4,628	51.8%	32	Mississippi	37	0.4%
8	North Carolina		150	1.7%	33	Delaware	30	0.3%
48	North Dakota		3	0.0%	34	Iowa	25	0.3%
12	Ohio		135	1.5%	34	Nebraska	25	0.3%
18	Oklahoma		95	1.1%	36	Minnesota	23	0.3%
27	Oregon		57	0.6%	37	Kansas	21	0.2%
13	Pennsylvania		126	1.4%	38	Maine	20	0.2%
44	Rhode Island		8	0.1%	39	Utah	17	0.2%
21	South Carolina		79	0.9%	40	Idaho	14	0.2%
49	South Dakota		2	0.0%	41	Alaska	10	0.1%
9	Tennessee		148	1.7%	41	New Mexico	10	0.1%
4	Texas		426	4.8%	43	New Hampshire	9	0.1%
39	Utah		17	0.2%	44	Rhode Island	8	0.1%
49	Vermont		2	0.0%	45	Hawaii	7	0.1%
9	Virginia		148	1.7%	46	Wyoming	6	0.1%
25	Washington		68	0.8%	47	Montana	5	0.1%
20	West Virginia		80	0.9%	48	North Dakota	3	0.0%
14	Wisconsin		121	1.4%	49	South Dakota	2	0.0%
46	Wyoming		6	0.1%	49	Vermont	2	0.0%
						District of Columbia	4	0.0%

Source: U.S. Department of Health and Human Services, National Center for Health Statistics
   "Morbidity and Mortality Weekly Report" (January 7, 2011, Vol. 59, Nos. 51 & 52, http://www.cdc.gov/mmwr/)
*Provisional data. An inflammation of the liver.

Hepatitis A and B Rate in 2010

National Rate = 2.9 Cases per 100,000 Population*

ALPHA ORDER				RANK ORDER		
RANK	STATE	RATE		RANK	STATE	RATE
16	Alabama	1.6		1	New York	23.7
24	Alaska	1.4		2	West Virginia	4.4
19	Arizona	1.5		3	Kentucky	3.6
19	Arkansas	1.5		4	Delaware	3.4
29	California	1.2		5	Oklahoma	2.6
19	Colorado	1.5		6	Florida	2.4
24	Conncotiout	1.4		6	Tennessee	2.4
4	Delaware	3.4		8	Wisconsin	2.1
6	Florida	2.4		9	Michigan	2.0
11	Georgia	1.9		9	Nevada	2.0
44	Hawaii	0.5		11	Georgia	1.9
36	Idaho	0.9		11	Virginia	1.9
31	Illinois	1.1		13	Maryland	1.7
31	Indiana	1.1		13	South Carolina	1.7
38	Iowa	0.8		13	Texas	1.7
41	Kansas	0.7		16	Alabama	1.6
3	Kentucky	3.6		16	Missouri	1.6
27	Louisiana	1.3		16	North Carolina	1.6
19	Maine	1.5		19	Arizona	1.5
13	Maryland	1.7		19	Arkansas	1.5
38	Massachusetts	0.8		19	Colorado	1.5
9	Michigan	2.0		19	Maine	1.5
48	Minnesota	0.4		19	Oregon	1.5
27	Mississippi	1.3		24	Alaska	1.4
16	Missouri	1.6		24	Connecticut	1.4
44	Montana	0.5		24	Nebraska	1.4
24	Nebraska	1.4		27	Louisiana	1.3
9	Nevada	2.0		27	Mississippi	1.3
41	New Hampshire	0.7		29	California	1.2
36	New Jersey	0.9		29	Ohio	1.2
44	New Mexico	0.5		31	Illinois	1.1
1	New York	23.7		31	Indiana	1.1
16	North Carolina	1.6		31	Wyoming	1.1
44	North Dakota	0.5		34	Pennsylvania	1.0
29	Ohio	1.2		34	Washington	1.0
5	Oklahoma	2.6		36	Idaho	0.9
19	Oregon	1.5		36	New Jersey	0.9
34	Pennsylvania	1.0		38	Iowa	0.8
38	Rhode Island	0.8		38	Massachusetts	0.8
13	South Carolina	1.7		38	Rhode Island	0.8
50	South Dakota	0.2		41	Kansas	0.7
6	Tennessee	2.4		41	New Hampshire	0.7
13	Texas	1.7		43	Utah	0.6
43	Utah	0.6		44	Hawaii	0.5
49	Vermont	0.3		44	Montana	0.5
11	Virginia	1.9		44	New Mexico	0.5
34	Washington	1.0		44	North Dakota	0.5
2	West Virginia	4.4		48	Minnesota	0.4
8	Wisconsin	2.1		49	Vermont	0.3
31	Wyoming	1.1		50	South Dakota	0.2
					District of Columbia	0.7

Source: CQ Press using data from U.S. Department of Health and Human Services, National Center for Health Statistics
  "Morbidity and Mortality Weekly Report" (January 7, 2011, Vol. 59, Nos. 51 & 52, http://www.cdc.gov/mmwr/)
*Provisional data. An inflammation of the liver. Rates calculated using 2009 population estimates.

Hepatitis C Cases Reported in 2010

National Total = 3,254 Cases*

ALPHA ORDER

RANK	STATE	CASES	% of USA
30	Alabama	7	0.2%
NA	Alaska**	NA	NA
NA	Arizona**	NA	NA
38	Arkansas	0	0.0%
13	California	22	0.7%
19	Colorado	12	0.4%
7	Connecticut	33	1.0%
NA	Delaware**	NA	NA
4	Florida	56	1.7%
16	Georgia	15	0.5%
NA	Hawaii**	NA	NA
23	Idaho	11	0.3%
33	Illinois	2	0.1%
12	Indiana	24	0.7%
38	Iowa	0	0.0%
33	Kansas	2	0.1%
2	Kentucky	108	3.3%
26	Louisiana	9	0.3%
38	Maine	0	0.0%
11	Maryland	28	0.9%
19	Massachusetts	12	0.4%
3	Michigan	76	2.3%
19	Minnesota	12	0.4%
NA	Mississippi**	NA	NA
28	Missouri	8	0.2%
32	Montana	3	0.1%
33	Nebraska	2	0.1%
30	Nevada	7	0.2%
NA	New Hampshire**	NA	NA
16	New Jersey	15	0.5%
23	New Mexico	11	0.3%
1	New York	2,502	76.9%
6	North Carolina	42	1.3%
38	North Dakota	0	0.0%
26	Ohio	9	0.3%
7	Oklahoma	33	1.0%
16	Oregon	15	0.5%
10	Pennsylvania	31	1.0%
NA	Rhode Island**	NA	NA
37	South Carolina	1	0.0%
38	South Dakota	0	0.0%
5	Tennessee	43	1.3%
9	Texas	32	1.0%
25	Utah	10	0.3%
33	Vermont	2	0.1%
19	Virginia	12	0.4%
14	Washington	20	0.6%
15	West Virginia	17	0.5%
28	Wisconsin	8	0.2%
38	Wyoming	0	0.0%

RANK ORDER

RANK	STATE	CASES	% of USA
1	New York	2,502	76.9%
2	Kentucky	108	3.3%
3	Michigan	76	2.3%
4	Florida	56	1.7%
5	Tennessee	43	1.3%
6	North Carolina	42	1.3%
7	Connecticut	33	1.0%
7	Oklahoma	33	1.0%
9	Texas	32	1.0%
10	Pennsylvania	31	1.0%
11	Maryland	28	0.9%
12	Indiana	24	0.7%
13	California	22	0.7%
14	Washington	20	0.6%
15	West Virginia	17	0.5%
16	Georgia	15	0.5%
16	New Jersey	15	0.5%
16	Oregon	15	0.5%
19	Colorado	12	0.4%
19	Massachusetts	12	0.4%
19	Minnesota	12	0.4%
19	Virginia	12	0.4%
23	Idaho	11	0.3%
23	New Mexico	11	0.3%
25	Utah	10	0.3%
26	Louisiana	9	0.3%
26	Ohio	9	0.3%
28	Missouri	8	0.2%
28	Wisconsin	8	0.2%
30	Alabama	7	0.2%
30	Nevada	7	0.2%
32	Montana	3	0.1%
33	Illinois	2	0.1%
33	Kansas	2	0.1%
33	Nebraska	2	0.1%
33	Vermont	2	0.1%
37	South Carolina	1	0.0%
38	Arkansas	0	0.0%
38	Iowa	0	0.0%
38	Maine	0	0.0%
38	North Dakota	0	0.0%
38	South Dakota	0	0.0%
38	Wyoming	0	0.0%
NA	Alaska**	NA	NA
NA	Arizona**	NA	NA
NA	Delaware**	NA	NA
NA	Hawaii**	NA	NA
NA	Mississippi**	NA	NA
NA	New Hampshire**	NA	NA
NA	Rhode Island**	NA	NA
	District of Columbia	2	0.1%

Source: U.S. Department of Health and Human Services, National Center for Health Statistics
    "Morbidity and Mortality Weekly Report" (January 7, 2011, Vol. 59, Nos. 51 & 52, http://www.cdc.gov/mmwr/)
*Provisional data. An inflammation of the liver.
**Not available.

Hepatitis C Rate in 2010

National Rate = 1.1 Cases per 100,000 Population*

ALPHA ORDER				RANK ORDER		
RANK	STATE	RATE		RANK	STATE	RATE
28	Alabama	0.1		1	New York	12.8
NA	Alaska**	NA		2	Kentucky	2.5
NA	Arizona**	NA		3	Connecticut	0.9
36	Arkansas	0.0		3	Oklahoma	0.9
28	California	0.1		3	West Virginia	0.9
20	Colorado	0.2		6	Michigan	0.8
3	Connecticut	0.9		7	Idaho	0.7
NA	Delaware**	NA		7	Tennessee	0.7
15	Florida	0.3		9	Maryland	0.5
20	Georgia	0.2		9	New Mexico	0.5
NA	Hawaii**	NA		11	Indiana	0.4
7	Idaho	0.7		11	North Carolina	0.4
36	Illinois	0.0		11	Oregon	0.4
11	Indiana	0.4		11	Utah	0.4
36	Iowa	0.0		15	Florida	0.3
28	Kansas	0.1		15	Montana	0.3
2	Kentucky	2.5		15	Nevada	0.3
20	Louisiana	0.2		15	Vermont	0.3
36	Maine	0.0		15	Washington	0.3
9	Maryland	0.5		20	Colorado	0.2
20	Massachusetts	0.2		20	Georgia	0.2
6	Michigan	0.8		20	Louisiana	0.2
20	Minnesota	0.2		20	Massachusetts	0.2
NA	Mississippi**	NA		20	Minnesota	0.2
28	Missouri	0.1		20	New Jersey	0.2
15	Montana	0.3		20	Pennsylvania	0.2
28	Nebraska	0.1		20	Virginia	0.2
15	Nevada	0.3		28	Alabama	0.1
NA	New Hampshire**	NA		28	California	0.1
20	New Jersey	0.2		28	Kansas	0.1
9	New Mexico	0.5		28	Missouri	0.1
1	New York	12.8		28	Nebraska	0.1
11	North Carolina	0.4		28	Ohio	0.1
36	North Dakota	0.0		28	Texas	0.1
28	Ohio	0.1		28	Wisconsin	0.1
3	Oklahoma	0.9		36	Arkansas	0.0
11	Oregon	0.4		36	Illinois	0.0
20	Pennsylvania	0.2		36	Iowa	0.0
NA	Rhode Island**	NA		36	Maine	0.0
36	South Carolina	0.0		36	North Dakota	0.0
36	South Dakota	0.0		36	South Carolina	0.0
7	Tennessee	0.7		36	South Dakota	0.0
28	Texas	0.1		36	Wyoming	0.0
11	Utah	0.4		NA	Alaska**	NA
15	Vermont	0.3		NA	Arizona**	NA
20	Virginia	0.2		NA	Delaware**	NA
15	Washington	0.3		NA	Hawaii**	NA
3	West Virginia	0.9		NA	Mississippi**	NA
28	Wisconsin	0.1		NA	New Hampshire**	NA
36	Wyoming	0.0		NA	Rhode Island**	NA

District of Columbia   0.3

Source: CQ Press using data from U.S. Department of Health and Human Services, National Center for Health Statistics
"Morbidity and Mortality Weekly Report" (January 7, 2011, Vol. 59, Nos. 51 & 52, http://www.cdc.gov/mmwr/)
*Provisional data. An inflammation of the liver. Rates calculated using 2009 population estimates.

Legionellosis Cases Reported in 2010

National Total = 3,161 Cases*

ALPHA ORDER

RANK	STATE	CASES	% of USA
26	Alabama	22	0.7%
49	Alaska	2	0.1%
16	Arizona	62	2.0%
34	Arkansas	14	0.4%
4	California	218	6.9%
22	Colorado	34	1.1%
19	Connecticut	53	1.7%
30	Delaware	17	0.5%
5	Florida	175	5.5%
18	Georgia	57	1.8%
50	Hawaii	1	0.0%
45	Idaho	8	0.3%
7	Illinois	121	3.8%
11	Indiana	103	3.3%
31	Iowa	15	0.5%
38	Kansas	12	0.4%
23	Kentucky	27	0.9%
39	Louisiana	10	0.3%
36	Maine	13	0.4%
9	Maryland	114	3.6%
8	Massachusetts	119	3.8%
6	Michigan	172	5.4%
20	Minnesota	39	1.2%
39	Mississippi	10	0.3%
20	Missouri	39	1.2%
47	Montana	5	0.2%
41	Nebraska	9	0.3%
28	Nevada	20	0.6%
27	New Hampshire	21	0.7%
12	New Jersey	93	2.9%
41	New Mexico	9	0.3%
1	New York	438	13.9%
17	North Carolina	59	1.9%
46	North Dakota	7	0.2%
3	Ohio	232	7.3%
36	Oklahoma	13	0.4%
31	Oregon	15	0.5%
2	Pennsylvania	321	10.2%
24	Rhode Island	23	0.7%
34	South Carolina	14	0.4%
41	South Dakota	9	0.3%
14	Tennessee	72	2.3%
10	Texas	109	3.4%
28	Utah	20	0.6%
41	Vermont	9	0.3%
13	Virginia	79	2.5%
24	Washington	23	0.7%
31	West Virginia	15	0.5%
15	Wisconsin	67	2.1%
47	Wyoming	5	0.2%

RANK ORDER

RANK	STATE	CASES	% of USA
1	New York	438	13.9%
2	Pennsylvania	321	10.2%
3	Ohio	232	7.3%
4	California	218	6.9%
5	Florida	175	5.5%
6	Michigan	172	5.4%
7	Illinois	121	3.8%
8	Massachusetts	119	3.8%
9	Maryland	114	3.6%
10	Texas	109	3.4%
11	Indiana	103	3.3%
12	New Jersey	93	2.9%
13	Virginia	79	2.5%
14	Tennessee	72	2.3%
15	Wisconsin	67	2.1%
16	Arizona	62	2.0%
17	North Carolina	59	1.9%
18	Georgia	57	1.8%
19	Connecticut	53	1.7%
20	Minnesota	39	1.2%
20	Missouri	39	1.2%
22	Colorado	34	1.1%
23	Kentucky	27	0.9%
24	Rhode Island	23	0.7%
24	Washington	23	0.7%
26	Alabama	22	0.7%
27	New Hampshire	21	0.7%
28	Nevada	20	0.6%
28	Utah	20	0.6%
30	Delaware	17	0.5%
31	Iowa	15	0.5%
31	Oregon	15	0.5%
31	West Virginia	15	0.5%
34	Arkansas	14	0.4%
34	South Carolina	14	0.4%
36	Maine	13	0.4%
36	Oklahoma	13	0.4%
38	Kansas	12	0.4%
39	Louisiana	10	0.3%
39	Mississippi	10	0.3%
41	Nebraska	9	0.3%
41	New Mexico	9	0.3%
41	South Dakota	9	0.3%
41	Vermont	9	0.3%
45	Idaho	8	0.3%
46	North Dakota	7	0.2%
47	Montana	5	0.2%
47	Wyoming	5	0.2%
49	Alaska	2	0.1%
50	Hawaii	1	0.0%
	District of Columbia	17	0.5%

Source: U.S. Department of Health and Human Services, National Center for Health Statistics
"Morbidity and Mortality Weekly Report" (January 7, 2011, Vol. 59, Nos. 51 & 52, http://www.cdc.gov/mmwr/)
*Provisional data. A pneumonia-like disease (Legionnaire's Disease).

Legionellosis Rate in 2010

National Rate = 1.0 Cases per 100,000 Population*

RANK	STATE	RATE
34	Alabama	0.5
45	Alaska	0.3
20	Arizona	0.9
34	Arkansas	0.5
30	California	0.6
26	Colorado	0.7
11	Connecticut	1.5
6	Delaware	1.9
20	Florida	0.9
30	Georgia	0.6
50	Hawaii	0.1
34	Idaho	0.5
20	Illinois	0.9
9	Indiana	1.6
34	Iowa	0.5
40	Kansas	0.4
30	Kentucky	0.6
49	Louisiana	0.2
18	Maine	1.0
4	Maryland	2.0
7	Massachusetts	1.8
8	Michigan	1.7
26	Minnesota	0.7
45	Mississippi	0.3
26	Missouri	0.7
34	Montana	0.5
34	Nebraska	0.5
24	Nevada	0.8
9	New Hampshire	1.6
14	New Jersey	1.1
40	New Mexico	0.4
2	New York	2.2
30	North Carolina	0.6
14	North Dakota	1.1
4	Ohio	2.0
40	Oklahoma	0.4
40	Oregon	0.4
1	Pennsylvania	2.5
2	Rhode Island	2.2
45	South Carolina	0.3
14	South Dakota	1.1
14	Tennessee	1.1
40	Texas	0.4
26	Utah	0.7
12	Vermont	1.4
18	Virginia	1.0
45	Washington	0.3
24	West Virginia	0.8
13	Wisconsin	1.2
20	Wyoming	0.9

RANK	STATE	RATE
1	Pennsylvania	2.5
2	New York	2.2
2	Rhode Island	2.2
4	Maryland	2.0
4	Ohio	2.0
6	Delaware	1.9
7	Massachusetts	1.8
8	Michigan	1.7
9	Indiana	1.6
9	New Hampshire	1.6
11	Connecticut	1.5
12	Vermont	1.4
13	Wisconsin	1.2
14	New Jersey	1.1
14	North Dakota	1.1
14	South Dakota	1.1
14	Tennessee	1.1
18	Maine	1.0
18	Virginia	1.0
20	Arizona	0.9
20	Florida	0.9
20	Illinois	0.9
20	Wyoming	0.9
24	Nevada	0.8
24	West Virginia	0.8
26	Colorado	0.7
26	Minnesota	0.7
26	Missouri	0.7
26	Utah	0.7
30	California	0.6
30	Georgia	0.6
30	Kentucky	0.6
30	North Carolina	0.6
34	Alabama	0.5
34	Arkansas	0.5
34	Idaho	0.5
34	Iowa	0.5
34	Montana	0.5
34	Nebraska	0.5
40	Kansas	0.4
40	New Mexico	0.4
40	Oklahoma	0.4
40	Oregon	0.4
40	Texas	0.4
45	Alaska	0.3
45	Mississippi	0.3
45	South Carolina	0.3
45	Washington	0.3
49	Louisiana	0.2
50	Hawaii	0.1

	District of Columbia	2.8

Source: CQ Press using data from U.S. Department of Health and Human Services, National Center for Health Statistics
"Morbidity and Mortality Weekly Report" (January 7, 2011, Vol. 59, Nos. 51 & 52, http://www.cdc.gov/mmwr/)
*Provisional data. A pneumonia-like disease (Legionnaire's Disease). Rates calculated using 2009 population estimates.

Lyme Disease Cases Reported in 2010

National Total = 27,895 Cases*

RANK	STATE	CASES	% of USA
38	Alabama	2	0.0%
32	Alaska	6	0.0%
38	Arizona	2	0.0%
45	Arkansas	0	0.0%
14	California	137	0.5%
37	Colorado	3	0.0%
6	Connecticut	2,659	9.5%
11	Delaware	620	2.2%
18	Florida	108	0.4%
29	Georgia	11	0.0%
NA	Hawaii**	NA	NA
31	Idaho	8	0.0%
16	Illinois	123	0.4%
22	Indiana	70	0.3%
21	Iowa	80	0.3%
32	Kansas	6	0.0%
34	Kentucky	5	0.0%
38	Louisiana	2	0.0%
10	Maine	726	2.6%
7	Maryland	1,594	5.7%
3	Massachusetts	2,988	10.7%
19	Michigan	95	0.3%
45	Minnesota	0	0.0%
45	Mississippi	0	0.0%
43	Missouri	1	0.0%
36	Montana	4	0.0%
30	Nebraska	9	0.0%
38	Nevada	2	0.0%
8	New Hampshire	1,240	4.4%
2	New Jersey	3,270	11.7%
34	New Mexico	5	0.0%
4	New York	2,950	10.6%
20	North Carolina	85	0.3%
27	North Dakota	23	0.1%
24	Ohio	43	0.2%
45	Oklahoma	0	0.0%
23	Oregon	50	0.2%
1	Pennsylvania	6,277	22.5%
13	Rhode Island	153	0.5%
26	South Carolina	28	0.1%
43	South Dakota	1	0.0%
25	Tennessee	37	0.1%
17	Texas	110	0.4%
38	Utah	2	0.0%
12	Vermont	339	1.2%
9	Virginia	1,136	4.1%
28	Washington	14	0.1%
15	West Virginia	135	0.5%
5	Wisconsin	2,704	9.7%
45	Wyoming	0	0.0%

RANK	STATE	CASES	% of USA
1	Pennsylvania	6,277	22.5%
2	New Jersey	3,270	11.7%
3	Massachusetts	2,988	10.7%
4	New York	2,950	10.6%
5	Wisconsin	2,704	9.7%
6	Connecticut	2,659	9.5%
7	Maryland	1,594	5.7%
8	New Hampshire	1,240	4.4%
9	Virginia	1,136	4.1%
10	Maine	726	2.6%
11	Delaware	620	2.2%
12	Vermont	339	1.2%
13	Rhode Island	153	0.5%
14	California	137	0.5%
15	West Virginia	135	0.5%
16	Illinois	123	0.4%
17	Texas	110	0.4%
18	Florida	108	0.4%
19	Michigan	95	0.3%
20	North Carolina	85	0.3%
21	Iowa	80	0.3%
22	Indiana	70	0.3%
23	Oregon	50	0.2%
24	Ohio	43	0.2%
25	Tennessee	37	0.1%
26	South Carolina	28	0.1%
27	North Dakota	23	0.1%
28	Washington	14	0.1%
29	Georgia	11	0.0%
30	Nebraska	9	0.0%
31	Idaho	8	0.0%
32	Alaska	6	0.0%
32	Kansas	6	0.0%
34	Kentucky	5	0.0%
34	New Mexico	5	0.0%
36	Montana	4	0.0%
37	Colorado	3	0.0%
38	Alabama	2	0.0%
38	Arizona	2	0.0%
38	Louisiana	2	0.0%
38	Nevada	2	0.0%
38	Utah	2	0.0%
43	Missouri	1	0.0%
43	South Dakota	1	0.0%
45	Arkansas	0	0.0%
45	Minnesota	0	0.0%
45	Mississippi	0	0.0%
45	Oklahoma	0	0.0%
45	Wyoming	0	0.0%
NA	Hawaii**	NA	NA
	District of Columbia	32	0.1%

Source: U.S. Department of Health and Human Services, National Center for Health Statistics
  "Morbidity and Mortality Weekly Report" (January 7, 2011, Vol. 59, Nos. 51 & 52, http://www.cdc.gov/mmwr/)
*Provisional data. Caused by ticks-lesions, followed by arthritis of large joints, myalgia, malaise, and neurologic and cardiac manifestations. Named after Old Lyme, CT, where the disease was first reported.
**Not notifiable.

Lyme Disease Rate in 2010

National Rate = 9.1 Cases per 100,000 Population*

ALPHA ORDER			RANK ORDER		
RANK	STATE	RATE	RANK	STATE	RATE
41	Alabama	0.0	1	New Hampshire	93.6
21	Alaska	0.9	2	Connecticut	75.6
41	Arizona	0.0	3	Delaware	70.0
41	Arkansas	0.0	4	Maine	55.1
28	California	0.4	5	Vermont	54.5
35	Colorado	0.1	6	Pennsylvania	49.8
2	Connecticut	75.6	7	Wisconsin	47.8
3	Delaware	70.0	8	Massachusetts	45.3
23	Florida	0.6	9	New Jersey	37.6
35	Georgia	0.1	10	Maryland	28.0
NA	Hawaii**	NA	11	New York	15.1
26	Idaho	0.5	12	Rhode Island	14.5
19	Illinois	1.0	13	Virginia	14.4
18	Indiana	1.1	14	West Virginia	7.4
16	Iowa	2.7	15	North Dakota	3.6
32	Kansas	0.2	16	Iowa	2.7
35	Kentucky	0.1	17	Oregon	1.3
41	Louisiana	0.0	18	Indiana	1.1
4	Maine	55.1	19	Illinois	1.0
10	Maryland	28.0	19	Michigan	1.0
8	Massachusetts	45.3	21	Alaska	0.9
19	Michigan	1.0	21	North Carolina	0.9
41	Minnesota	0.0	23	Florida	0.6
41	Mississippi	0.0	23	South Carolina	0.6
41	Missouri	0.0	23	Tennessee	0.6
28	Montana	0.4	26	Idaho	0.5
26	Nebraska	0.5	26	Nebraska	0.5
35	Nevada	0.1	28	California	0.4
1	New Hampshire	93.6	28	Montana	0.4
9	New Jersey	37.6	28	Ohio	0.4
32	New Mexico	0.2	28	Texas	0.4
11	New York	15.1	32	Kansas	0.2
21	North Carolina	0.9	32	New Mexico	0.2
15	North Dakota	3.6	32	Washington	0.2
28	Ohio	0.4	35	Colorado	0.1
41	Oklahoma	0.0	35	Georgia	0.1
17	Oregon	1.3	35	Kentucky	0.1
6	Pennsylvania	49.8	35	Nevada	0.1
12	Rhode Island	14.5	35	South Dakota	0.1
23	South Carolina	0.6	35	Utah	0.1
35	South Dakota	0.1	41	Alabama	0.0
23	Tennessee	0.6	41	Arizona	0.0
28	Texas	0.4	41	Arkansas	0.0
35	Utah	0.1	41	Louisiana	0.0
5	Vermont	54.5	41	Minnesota	0.0
13	Virginia	14.4	41	Mississippi	0.0
32	Washington	0.2	41	Missouri	0.0
14	West Virginia	7.4	41	Oklahoma	0.0
7	Wisconsin	47.8	41	Wyoming	0.0
41	Wyoming	0.0	NA	Hawaii**	NA
				District of Columbia	5.3

Source: CQ Press using data from U.S. Department of Health and Human Services, National Center for Health Statistics
    "Morbidity and Mortality Weekly Report" (January 7, 2011, Vol. 59, Nos. 51 & 52, http://www.cdc.gov/mmwr/)
*Provisional data. Caused by ticks-lesions, followed by arthritis of large joints, myalgia, malaise, and neurologic and cardiac
manifestations. Named after Old Lyme, CT, where the disease was first reported. Rates calculated using 2009 population estimates.
**Not notifiable.

Malaria Cases Reported in 2010

National Total = 1,458 Cases*

ALPHA ORDER

RANK	STATE	CASES	% of USA
25	Alabama	9	0.6%
30	Alaska	5	0.3%
15	Arizona	27	1.9%
42	Arkansas	2	0.1%
3	California	122	8.4%
17	Colorado	21	1.4%
45	Connecticut	1	0.1%
42	Delaware	2	0.1%
2	Florida	138	9.5%
10	Georgia	47	3.2%
45	Hawaii	1	0.1%
35	Idaho	4	0.3%
8	Illinois	52	3.6%
23	Indiana	10	0.7%
20	Iowa	13	0.9%
20	Kansas	13	0.9%
26	Kentucky	8	0.5%
30	Louisiana	5	0.3%
28	Maine	6	0.4%
4	Maryland	98	6.7%
10	Massachusetts	47	3.2%
14	Michigan	31	2.1%
36	Minnesota	3	0.2%
42	Mississippi	2	0.1%
16	Missouri	22	1.5%
36	Montana	3	0.2%
18	Nebraska	15	1.0%
28	Nevada	6	0.4%
30	New Hampshire	5	0.3%
45	New Jersey	1	0.1%
45	New Mexico	1	0.1%
1	New York	329	22.6%
9	North Carolina	49	3.4%
45	North Dakota	1	0.1%
12	Ohio	42	2.9%
30	Oklahoma	5	0.3%
19	Oregon	14	1.0%
7	Pennsylvania	60	4.1%
27	Rhode Island	7	0.5%
30	South Carolina	5	0.3%
36	South Dakota	3	0.2%
22	Tennessee	12	0.8%
5	Texas	78	5.3%
36	Utah	3	0.2%
36	Vermont	3	0.2%
6	Virginia	64	4.4%
13	Washington	39	2.7%
36	West Virginia	3	0.2%
23	Wisconsin	10	0.7%
50	Wyoming	0	0.0%

RANK ORDER

RANK	STATE	CASES	% of USA
1	New York	329	22.6%
2	Florida	138	9.5%
3	California	122	8.4%
4	Maryland	98	6.7%
5	Texas	78	5.3%
6	Virginia	64	4.4%
7	Pennsylvania	60	4.1%
8	Illinois	52	3.6%
9	North Carolina	49	3.4%
10	Georgia	47	3.2%
10	Massachusetts	47	3.2%
12	Ohio	42	2.9%
13	Washington	39	2.7%
14	Michigan	31	2.1%
15	Arizona	27	1.9%
16	Missouri	22	1.5%
17	Colorado	21	1.4%
18	Nebraska	15	1.0%
19	Oregon	14	1.0%
20	Iowa	13	0.9%
20	Kansas	13	0.9%
22	Tennessee	12	0.8%
23	Indiana	10	0.7%
23	Wisconsin	10	0.7%
25	Alabama	9	0.6%
26	Kentucky	8	0.5%
27	Rhode Island	7	0.5%
28	Maine	6	0.4%
28	Nevada	6	0.4%
30	Alaska	5	0.3%
30	Louisiana	5	0.3%
30	New Hampshire	5	0.3%
30	Oklahoma	5	0.3%
30	South Carolina	5	0.3%
35	Idaho	4	0.3%
36	Minnesota	3	0.2%
36	Montana	3	0.2%
36	South Dakota	3	0.2%
36	Utah	3	0.2%
36	Vermont	3	0.2%
36	West Virginia	3	0.2%
42	Arkansas	2	0.1%
42	Delaware	2	0.1%
42	Mississippi	2	0.1%
45	Connecticut	1	0.1%
45	Hawaii	1	0.1%
45	New Jersey	1	0.1%
45	New Mexico	1	0.1%
45	North Dakota	1	0.1%
50	Wyoming	0	0.0%
	District of Columbia	11	0.8%

Source: U.S. Department of Health and Human Services, National Center for Health Statistics
   "Morbidity and Mortality Weekly Report" (January 7, 2011, Vol. 59, Nos. 51 & 52, http://www.cdc.gov/mmwr/)
*Provisional data. Infectious disease usually transmitted by bites of infected mosquitoes. Symptoms include high fever, shaking, chills, sweating, and anemia.

Malaria Rate in 2010

National Rate = 0.5 Cases per 100,000 Population*

ALPHA ORDER

RANK	STATE	RATE
30	Alabama	0.2
5	Alaska	0.7
16	Arizona	0.4
39	Arkansas	0.1
25	California	0.3
16	Colorado	0.4
47	Connecticut	0.0
30	Delaware	0.2
5	Florida	0.7
10	Georgia	0.5
39	Hawaii	0.1
25	Idaho	0.3
16	Illinois	0.4
30	Indiana	0.2
16	Iowa	0.4
10	Kansas	0.5
30	Kentucky	0.2
39	Louisiana	0.1
10	Maine	0.5
1	Maryland	1.7
5	Massachusetts	0.7
25	Michigan	0.3
39	Minnesota	0.1
39	Mississippi	0.1
16	Missouri	0.4
25	Montana	0.3
3	Nebraska	0.8
30	Nevada	0.2
16	New Hampshire	0.4
47	New Jersey	0.0
47	New Mexico	0.0
1	New York	1.7
10	North Carolina	0.5
30	North Dakota	0.2
16	Ohio	0.4
39	Oklahoma	0.1
16	Oregon	0.4
10	Pennsylvania	0.5
5	Rhode Island	0.7
39	South Carolina	0.1
16	South Dakota	0.4
30	Tennessee	0.2
25	Texas	0.3
39	Utah	0.1
10	Vermont	0.5
3	Virginia	0.8
9	Washington	0.6
30	West Virginia	0.2
30	Wisconsin	0.2
47	Wyoming	0.0

RANK ORDER

RANK	STATE	RATE
1	Maryland	1.7
1	New York	1.7
3	Nebraska	0.8
3	Virginia	0.8
5	Alaska	0.7
5	Florida	0.7
5	Massachusetts	0.7
5	Rhode Island	0.7
9	Washington	0.6
10	Georgia	0.5
10	Kansas	0.5
10	Maine	0.5
10	North Carolina	0.5
10	Pennsylvania	0.5
10	Vermont	0.5
16	Arizona	0.4
16	Colorado	0.4
16	Illinois	0.4
16	Iowa	0.4
16	Missouri	0.4
16	New Hampshire	0.4
16	Ohio	0.4
16	Oregon	0.4
16	South Dakota	0.4
25	California	0.3
25	Idaho	0.3
25	Michigan	0.3
25	Montana	0.3
25	Texas	0.3
30	Alabama	0.2
30	Delaware	0.2
30	Indiana	0.2
30	Kentucky	0.2
30	Nevada	0.2
30	North Dakota	0.2
30	Tennessee	0.2
30	West Virginia	0.2
30	Wisconsin	0.2
39	Arkansas	0.1
39	Hawaii	0.1
39	Louisiana	0.1
39	Minnesota	0.1
39	Mississippi	0.1
39	Oklahoma	0.1
39	South Carolina	0.1
39	Utah	0.1
47	Connecticut	0.0
47	New Jersey	0.0
47	New Mexico	0.0
47	Wyoming	0.0

District of Columbia   1.8

Source: CQ Press using data from U.S. Department of Health and Human Services, National Center for Health Statistics
"Morbidity and Mortality Weekly Report" (January 7, 2011, Vol. 59, Nos. 51 & 52, http://www.cdc.gov/mmwr/)
*Provisional data. Infectious disease usually transmitted by bites of infected mosquitoes. Symptoms include high fever, shaking, chills, sweating, and anemia. Rates calculated using 2009 population estimates.

Meningococcal Infections Reported in 2010

National Total = 749 Cases*

RANK	STATE	CASES	% of USA
27	Alabama	8	1.1%
39	Alaska	2	0.3%
21	Arizona	14	1.9%
30	Arkansas	6	0.8%
1	California	109	14.6%
12	Colorado	22	2.9%
37	Connecticut	3	0.4%
39	Delaware	2	0.3%
2	Florida	60	8.0%
22	Georgia	13	1.7%
45	Hawaii	1	0.1%
33	Idaho	5	0.7%
13	Illinois	20	2.7%
6	Indiana	28	3.7%
25	Iowa	10	1.3%
27	Kansas	8	1.1%
16	Kentucky	17	2.3%
19	Louisiana	15	2.0%
36	Maine	4	0.5%
26	Maryland	9	1.2%
30	Massachusetts	6	0.8%
11	Michigan	23	3.1%
39	Minnesota	2	0.3%
33	Mississippi	5	0.7%
8	Missouri	26	3.5%
39	Montana	2	0.3%
30	Nebraska	6	0.8%
27	Nevada	8	1.1%
48	New Hampshire	0	0.0%
16	New Jersey	17	2.3%
37	New Mexico	3	0.4%
6	New York	28	3.7%
19	North Carolina	15	2.0%
39	North Dakota	2	0.3%
4	Ohio	34	4.5%
18	Oklahoma	16	2.1%
5	Oregon	32	4.3%
8	Pennsylvania	26	3.5%
48	Rhode Island	0	0.0%
23	South Carolina	12	1.6%
48	South Dakota	0	0.0%
23	Tennessee	12	1.6%
3	Texas	47	6.3%
45	Utah	1	0.1%
33	Vermont	5	0.7%
14	Virginia	19	2.5%
15	Washington	18	2.4%
39	West Virginia	2	0.3%
10	Wisconsin	25	3.3%
45	Wyoming	1	0.1%

RANK	STATE	CASES	% of USA
1	California	109	14.6%
2	Florida	60	8.0%
3	Texas	47	6.3%
4	Ohio	34	4.5%
5	Oregon	32	4.3%
6	Indiana	28	3.7%
6	New York	28	3.7%
8	Missouri	26	3.5%
8	Pennsylvania	26	3.5%
10	Wisconsin	25	3.3%
11	Michigan	23	3.1%
12	Colorado	22	2.9%
13	Illinois	20	2.7%
14	Virginia	19	2.5%
15	Washington	18	2.4%
16	Kentucky	17	2.3%
16	New Jersey	17	2.3%
18	Oklahoma	16	2.1%
19	Louisiana	15	2.0%
19	North Carolina	15	2.0%
21	Arizona	14	1.9%
22	Georgia	13	1.7%
23	South Carolina	12	1.6%
23	Tennessee	12	1.6%
25	Iowa	10	1.3%
26	Maryland	9	1.2%
27	Alabama	8	1.1%
27	Kansas	8	1.1%
27	Nevada	8	1.1%
30	Arkansas	6	0.8%
30	Massachusetts	6	0.8%
30	Nebraska	6	0.8%
33	Idaho	5	0.7%
33	Mississippi	5	0.7%
33	Vermont	5	0.7%
36	Maine	4	0.5%
37	Connecticut	3	0.4%
37	New Mexico	3	0.4%
39	Alaska	2	0.3%
39	Delaware	2	0.3%
39	Minnesota	2	0.3%
39	Montana	2	0.3%
39	North Dakota	2	0.3%
39	West Virginia	2	0.3%
45	Hawaii	1	0.1%
45	Utah	1	0.1%
45	Wyoming	1	0.1%
48	New Hampshire	0	0.0%
48	Rhode Island	0	0.0%
48	South Dakota	0	0.0%
	District of Columbia	0	0.0%

Source: U.S. Department of Health and Human Services, National Center for Health Statistics
"Morbidity and Mortality Weekly Report" (January 7, 2011, Vol. 59, Nos. 51 & 52, http://www.cdc.gov/mmwr/)
*Provisional data. A bacterium (Neisseria meningitidis) that causes cerebrospinal meningitis.

Meningococcal Infection Rate in 2010

National Rate = 0.2 Cases per 100,000 Population*

ALPHA ORDER

RANK	STATE	RATE
23	Alabama	0.2
9	Alaska	0.3
23	Arizona	0.2
23	Arkansas	0.2
9	California	0.3
3	Colorado	0.4
39	Connecticut	0.1
23	Delaware	0.2
9	Florida	0.3
39	Georgia	0.1
39	Hawaii	0.1
9	Idaho	0.3
23	Illinois	0.2
3	Indiana	0.4
9	Iowa	0.3
9	Kansas	0.3
3	Kentucky	0.4
9	Louisiana	0.3
9	Maine	0.3
23	Maryland	0.2
39	Massachusetts	0.1
23	Michigan	0.2
46	Minnesota	0.0
23	Mississippi	0.2
3	Missouri	0.4
23	Montana	0.2
9	Nebraska	0.3
9	Nevada	0.3
46	New Hampshire	0.0
23	New Jersey	0.2
39	New Mexico	0.1
39	New York	0.1
23	North Carolina	0.2
9	North Dakota	0.3
9	Ohio	0.3
3	Oklahoma	0.4
1	Oregon	0.8
23	Pennsylvania	0.2
46	Rhode Island	0.0
9	South Carolina	0.3
46	South Dakota	0.0
23	Tennessee	0.2
23	Texas	0.2
46	Utah	0.0
1	Vermont	0.8
23	Virginia	0.2
9	Washington	0.3
39	West Virginia	0.1
3	Wisconsin	0.4
23	Wyoming	0.2

RANK ORDER

RANK	STATE	RATE
1	Oregon	0.8
1	Vermont	0.8
3	Colorado	0.4
3	Indiana	0.4
3	Kentucky	0.4
3	Missouri	0.4
3	Oklahoma	0.4
3	Wisconsin	0.4
9	Alaska	0.3
9	California	0.3
9	Florida	0.3
9	Idaho	0.3
9	Iowa	0.3
9	Kansas	0.3
9	Louisiana	0.3
9	Maine	0.3
9	Nebraska	0.3
9	Nevada	0.3
9	North Dakota	0.3
9	Ohio	0.3
9	South Carolina	0.3
9	Washington	0.3
23	Alabama	0.2
23	Arizona	0.2
23	Arkansas	0.2
23	Delaware	0.2
23	Illinois	0.2
23	Maryland	0.2
23	Michigan	0.2
23	Mississippi	0.2
23	Montana	0.2
23	New Jersey	0.2
23	North Carolina	0.2
23	Pennsylvania	0.2
23	Tennessee	0.2
23	Texas	0.2
23	Virginia	0.2
23	Wyoming	0.2
39	Connecticut	0.1
39	Georgia	0.1
39	Hawaii	0.1
39	Massachusetts	0.1
39	New Mexico	0.1
39	New York	0.1
39	West Virginia	0.1
46	Minnesota	0.0
46	New Hampshire	0.0
46	Rhode Island	0.0
46	South Dakota	0.0
46	Utah	0.0

| | District of Columbia | 0.0 |

Source: CQ Press using data from U.S. Department of Health and Human Services, National Center for Health Statistics
   "Morbidity and Mortality Weekly Report" (January 7, 2011, Vol. 59, Nos. 51 & 52, http://www.cdc.gov/mmwr/)
*Provisional data. A bacterium (Neisseria meningitidis) that causes cerebrospinal meningitis. Rates calculated using 2009
population estimates.

Rabies (Animal) Cases Reported in 2010

National Total = 3,180 Cases*

RANK	STATE	CASES	% of USA
17	Alabama	49	1.5%
31	Alaska	12	0.4%
36	Arizona	0	0.0%
21	Arkansas	28	0.9%
6	California	104	3.3%
36	Colorado	0	0.0%
14	Connecticut	59	1.9%
36	Delaware	0	0.0%
8	Florida	71	2.2%
36	Georgia	0	0.0%
36	Hawaii	0	0.0%
32	Idaho	11	0.3%
5	Illinois	114	3.6%
36	Indiana	0	0.0%
22	Iowa	26	0.8%
13	Kansas	60	1.9%
24	Kentucky	21	0.7%
36	Louisiana	0	0.0%
12	Maine	62	1.9%
4	Maryland	351	11.0%
36	Massachusetts	0	0.0%
10	Michigan	68	2.1%
22	Minnesota	26	0.8%
35	Mississippi	1	0.0%
11	Missouri	66	2.1%
26	Montana	17	0.5%
16	Nebraska	52	1.6%
34	Nevada	8	0.3%
28	New Hampshire	14	0.4%
36	New Jersey	0	0.0%
30	New Mexico	13	0.4%
1	New York	618	19.4%
36	North Carolina	0	0.0%
27	North Dakota	15	0.5%
18	Ohio	46	1.4%
19	Oklahoma	41	1.3%
28	Oregon	14	0.4%
3	Pennsylvania	390	12.3%
20	Rhode Island	31	1.0%
36	South Carolina	0	0.0%
36	South Dakota	0	0.0%
9	Tennessee	70	2.2%
36	Texas	0	0.0%
33	Utah	10	0.3%
15	Vermont	53	1.7%
2	Virginia	561	17.6%
36	Washington	0	0.0%
7	West Virginia	77	2.4%
36	Wisconsin	0	0.0%
24	Wyoming	21	0.7%

RANK	STATE	CASES	% of USA
1	New York	618	19.4%
2	Virginia	561	17.6%
3	Pennsylvania	390	12.3%
4	Maryland	351	11.0%
5	Illinois	114	3.6%
6	California	104	3.3%
7	West Virginia	77	2.4%
8	Florida	71	2.2%
9	Tennessee	70	2.2%
10	Michigan	68	2.1%
11	Missouri	66	2.1%
12	Maine	62	1.9%
13	Kansas	60	1.9%
14	Connecticut	59	1.9%
15	Vermont	53	1.7%
16	Nebraska	52	1.6%
17	Alabama	49	1.5%
18	Ohio	46	1.4%
19	Oklahoma	41	1.3%
20	Rhode Island	31	1.0%
21	Arkansas	28	0.9%
22	Iowa	26	0.8%
22	Minnesota	26	0.8%
24	Kentucky	21	0.7%
24	Wyoming	21	0.7%
26	Montana	17	0.5%
27	North Dakota	15	0.5%
28	New Hampshire	14	0.4%
28	Oregon	14	0.4%
30	New Mexico	13	0.4%
31	Alaska	12	0.4%
32	Idaho	11	0.3%
33	Utah	10	0.3%
34	Nevada	8	0.3%
35	Mississippi	1	0.0%
36	Arizona	0	0.0%
36	Colorado	0	0.0%
36	Delaware	0	0.0%
36	Georgia	0	0.0%
36	Hawaii	0	0.0%
36	Indiana	0	0.0%
36	Louisiana	0	0.0%
36	Massachusetts	0	0.0%
36	New Jersey	0	0.0%
36	North Carolina	0	0.0%
36	South Carolina	0	0.0%
36	South Dakota	0	0.0%
36	Texas	0	0.0%
36	Washington	0	0.0%
36	Wisconsin	0	0.0%
	District of Columbia	0	0.0%

Source: U.S. Department of Health and Human Services, National Center for Health Statistics
"Morbidity and Mortality Weekly Report" (January 7, 2011, Vol. 59, Nos. 51 & 52, http://www.cdc.gov/mmwr/)
*Provisional data. An acute, infectious, often fatal viral disease of most warm-blooded animals, especially wolves, cats, and dogs, that attacks the central nervous system and is transmitted by the bite of infected animals.

Rabies (Animal) Rate in 2010

National Rate = 1.0 Cases per 100,000 Human Population*

ALPHA ORDER

RANK	STATE	RATE
20	Alabama	1.0
13	Alaska	1.7
35	Arizona	0.0
20	Arkansas	1.0
33	California	0.3
35	Colorado	0.0
13	Connecticut	1.7
35	Delaware	0.0
29	Florida	0.4
35	Georgia	0.0
35	Hawaii	0.0
24	Idaho	0.7
22	Illinois	0.9
35	Indiana	0.0
22	Iowa	0.9
12	Kansas	2.1
27	Kentucky	0.5
35	Louisiana	0.0
4	Maine	4.7
3	Maryland	6.2
35	Massachusetts	0.0
24	Michigan	0.7
27	Minnesota	0.5
35	Mississippi	0.0
16	Missouri	1.1
13	Montana	1.7
9	Nebraska	2.9
33	Nevada	0.3
16	New Hampshire	1.1
35	New Jersey	0.0
26	New Mexico	0.6
7	New York	3.2
35	North Carolina	0.0
11	North Dakota	2.3
29	Ohio	0.4
16	Oklahoma	1.1
29	Oregon	0.4
8	Pennsylvania	3.1
9	Rhode Island	2.9
35	South Carolina	0.0
35	South Dakota	0.0
16	Tennessee	1.1
35	Texas	0.0
29	Utah	0.4
1	Vermont	8.5
2	Virginia	7.1
35	Washington	0.0
5	West Virginia	4.2
35	Wisconsin	0.0
6	Wyoming	3.9

RANK ORDER

RANK	STATE	RATE
1	Vermont	8.5
2	Virginia	7.1
3	Maryland	6.2
4	Maine	4.7
5	West Virginia	4.2
6	Wyoming	3.9
7	New York	3.2
8	Pennsylvania	3.1
9	Nebraska	2.9
9	Rhode Island	2.9
11	North Dakota	2.3
12	Kansas	2.1
13	Alaska	1.7
13	Connecticut	1.7
13	Montana	1.7
16	Missouri	1.1
16	New Hampshire	1.1
16	Oklahoma	1.1
16	Tennessee	1.1
20	Alabama	1.0
20	Arkansas	1.0
22	Illinois	0.9
22	Iowa	0.9
24	Idaho	0.7
24	Michigan	0.7
26	New Mexico	0.6
27	Kentucky	0.5
27	Minnesota	0.5
29	Florida	0.4
29	Ohio	0.4
29	Oregon	0.4
29	Utah	0.4
33	California	0.3
33	Nevada	0.3
35	Arizona	0.0
35	Colorado	0.0
35	Delaware	0.0
35	Georgia	0.0
35	Hawaii	0.0
35	Indiana	0.0
35	Louisiana	0.0
35	Massachusetts	0.0
35	Mississippi	0.0
35	New Jersey	0.0
35	North Carolina	0.0
35	South Carolina	0.0
35	South Dakota	0.0
35	Texas	0.0
35	Washington	0.0
35	Wisconsin	0.0

District of Columbia   0.0

Source: CQ Press using data from U.S. Department of Health and Human Services, National Center for Health Statistics
    "Morbidity and Mortality Weekly Report" (January 7, 2011, Vol. 59, Nos. 51 & 52, http://www.cdc.gov/mmwr/)
*Provisional data. An acute, infectious, often fatal viral disease of most warm-blooded animals, especially wolves, cats, and
dogs, that attacks the central nervous system and is transmitted by the bite of infected animals. Rates calculated using 2009
population estimates.

Spotted Fever Rickettsiosis Reported in 2010

National Total = 1,682 Cases*

ALPHA ORDER

RANK	STATE	CASES	% of USA
5	Alabama	82	4.9%
NA	Alaska**	NA	NA
20	Arizona	13	0.8%
6	Arkansas	66	3.9%
21	California	7	0.4%
28	Colorado	2	0.1%
39	Connecticut	0	0.0%
14	Delaware	22	1.3%
16	Florida	18	1.1%
7	Georgia	59	3.5%
NA	Hawaii**	NA	NA
23	Idaho	5	0.3%
11	Illinois	35	2.1%
10	Indiana	45	2.7%
25	Iowa	4	0.2%
28	Kansas	2	0.1%
22	Kentucky	6	0.4%
28	Louisiana	2	0.1%
28	Maine	2	0.1%
8	Maryland	57	3.4%
39	Massachusetts	0	0.0%
32	Michigan	1	0.1%
39	Minnesota	0	0.0%
17	Mississippi	16	1.0%
1	Missouri	343	20.4%
27	Montana	3	0.2%
23	Nebraska	5	0.3%
39	Nevada	0	0.0%
32	New Hampshire	1	0.1%
39	New Jersey	0	0.0%
32	New Mexico	1	0.1%
9	New York	51	3.0%
3	North Carolina	285	16.9%
32	North Dakota	1	0.1%
19	Ohio	14	0.8%
12	Oklahoma	29	1.7%
32	Oregon	1	0.1%
18	Pennsylvania	15	0.9%
39	Rhode Island	0	0.0%
15	South Carolina	19	1.1%
39	South Dakota	0	0.0%
2	Tennessee	301	17.9%
13	Texas	25	1.5%
32	Utah	1	0.1%
39	Vermont	0	0.0%
4	Virginia	137	8.1%
39	Washington	0	0.0%
39	West Virginia	0	0.0%
25	Wisconsin	4	0.2%
32	Wyoming	1	0.1%

RANK ORDER

RANK	STATE	CASES	% of USA
1	Missouri	343	20.4%
2	Tennessee	301	17.9%
3	North Carolina	285	16.9%
4	Virginia	137	8.1%
5	Alabama	82	4.9%
6	Arkansas	66	3.9%
7	Georgia	59	3.5%
8	Maryland	57	3.4%
9	New York	51	3.0%
10	Indiana	45	2.7%
11	Illinois	35	2.1%
12	Oklahoma	29	1.7%
13	Texas	25	1.5%
14	Delaware	22	1.3%
15	South Carolina	19	1.1%
16	Florida	18	1.1%
17	Mississippi	16	1.0%
18	Pennsylvania	15	0.9%
19	Ohio	14	0.8%
20	Arizona	13	0.8%
21	California	7	0.4%
22	Kentucky	6	0.4%
23	Idaho	5	0.3%
23	Nebraska	5	0.3%
25	Iowa	4	0.2%
25	Wisconsin	4	0.2%
27	Montana	3	0.2%
28	Colorado	2	0.1%
28	Kansas	2	0.1%
28	Louisiana	2	0.1%
28	Maine	2	0.1%
32	Michigan	1	0.1%
32	New Hampshire	1	0.1%
32	New Mexico	1	0.1%
32	North Dakota	1	0.1%
32	Oregon	1	0.1%
32	Utah	1	0.1%
32	Wyoming	1	0.1%
39	Connecticut	0	0.0%
39	Massachusetts	0	0.0%
39	Minnesota	0	0.0%
39	Nevada	0	0.0%
39	New Jersey	0	0.0%
39	Rhode Island	0	0.0%
39	South Dakota	0	0.0%
39	Vermont	0	0.0%
39	Washington	0	0.0%
39	West Virginia	0	0.0%
NA	Alaska**	NA	NA
NA	Hawaii**	NA	NA
	District of Columbia	1	0.1%

Source: U.S. Department of Health and Human Services, National Center for Health Statistics
"Morbidity and Mortality Weekly Report" (January 7, 2011, Vol. 59, Nos. 51 & 52, http://www.cdc.gov/mmwr/)
*Provisional data of confirmed and probable cases. A group of tickborne infections including Rocky Mountain Spotted Fever, an illness caused by Rickettsia rickettsii. Characterized by acute onset of fever, and may be accompanied by headache, malaise, myalgia, nausea/vomiting, or neurologic signs. A rash is often present on the palms and soles.
**Not notifiable.

Rocky Mountain Spotted Fever Rate in 2010

National Rate = 0.5 Cases per 100,000 Population*

ALPHA ORDER			RANK ORDER		
RANK	STATE	RATE	RANK	STATE	RATE
6	Alabama	1.7	1	Missouri	5.7
NA	Alaska**	NA	2	Tennessee	4.8
19	Arizona	0.2	3	North Carolina	3.0
5	Arkansas	2.3	4	Delaware	2.5
32	California	0.0	5	Arkansas	2.3
32	Colorado	0.0	6	Alabama	1.7
32	Connecticut	0.0	6	Virginia	1.7
4	Delaware	2.5	8	Maryland	1.0
23	Florida	0.1	9	Oklahoma	0.8
11	Georgia	0.6	10	Indiana	0.7
NA	Hawaii**	NA	11	Georgia	0.6
14	Idaho	0.3	12	Mississippi	0.5
14	Illinois	0.3	13	South Carolina	0.4
10	Indiana	0.7	14	Idaho	0.3
23	Iowa	0.1	14	Illinois	0.3
23	Kansas	0.1	14	Montana	0.3
23	Kentucky	0.1	14	Nebraska	0.3
32	Louisiana	0.0	14	New York	0.3
19	Maine	0.2	19	Arizona	0.2
8	Maryland	1.0	19	Maine	0.2
32	Massachusetts	0.0	19	North Dakota	0.2
32	Michigan	0.0	19	Wyoming	0.2
32	Minnesota	0.0	23	Florida	0.1
12	Mississippi	0.5	23	Iowa	0.1
1	Missouri	5.7	23	Kansas	0.1
14	Montana	0.3	23	Kentucky	0.1
14	Nebraska	0.3	23	New Hampshire	0.1
32	Nevada	0.0	23	Ohio	0.1
23	New Hampshire	0.1	23	Pennsylvania	0.1
32	New Jersey	0.0	23	Texas	0.1
32	New Mexico	0.0	23	Wisconsin	0.1
14	New York	0.3	32	California	0.0
3	North Carolina	3.0	32	Colorado	0.0
19	North Dakota	0.2	32	Connecticut	0.0
23	Ohio	0.1	32	Louisiana	0.0
9	Oklahoma	0.8	32	Massachusetts	0.0
32	Oregon	0.0	32	Michigan	0.0
23	Pennsylvania	0.1	32	Minnesota	0.0
32	Rhode Island	0.0	32	Nevada	0.0
13	South Carolina	0.4	32	New Jersey	0.0
32	South Dakota	0.0	32	New Mexico	0.0
2	Tennessee	4.8	32	Oregon	0.0
23	Texas	0.1	32	Rhode Island	0.0
32	Utah	0.0	32	South Dakota	0.0
32	Vermont	0.0	32	Utah	0.0
6	Virginia	1.7	32	Vermont	0.0
32	Washington	0.0	32	Washington	0.0
32	West Virginia	0.0	32	West Virginia	0.0
23	Wisconsin	0.1	NA	Alaska**	NA
19	Wyoming	0.2	NA	Hawaii**	NA
				District of Columbia	0.2

Source: CQ Press using data from U.S. Department of Health and Human Services, National Center for Health Statistics
  "Morbidity and Mortality Weekly Report" (January 7, 2011, Vol. 59, Nos. 51 & 52, http://www.cdc.gov/mmwr/)
*Provisional data of confirmed and probable cases. A group of tickborne infections including Rocky Mountain Spotted Fever, an illness caused by Rickettsia rickettsii. Characterized by acute onset of fever, and may be accompanied by headache, malaise, myalgia, nausea/vomiting, or neurologic signs. A rash is often present on the palms and soles. Rates calculated using 2009 population estimates. **Not notifiable.

Salmonellosis Cases Reported in 2010

National Total = 50,674 Cases*

ALPHA ORDER

RANK	STATE	CASES	% of USA
17	Alabama	1,045	2.1%
47	Alaska	79	0.2%
19	Arizona	929	1.8%
22	Arkansas	779	1.5%
2	California	4,882	9.6%
27	Colorado	584	1.2%
31	Connecticut	480	0.9%
40	Delaware	176	0.3%
1	Florida	6,299	12.4%
4	Georgia	2,753	5.4%
37	Hawaii	216	0.4%
41	Idaho	169	0.3%
8	Illinois	1,825	3.6%
26	Indiana	630	1.2%
29	Iowa	518	1.0%
32	Kansas	434	0.9%
28	Kentucky	566	1.1%
11	Louisiana	1,250	2.5%
45	Maine	128	0.3%
16	Maryland	1,076	2.1%
12	Massachusetts	1,228	2.4%
20	Michigan	913	1.8%
39	Minnesota	178	0.4%
13	Mississippi	1,195	2.4%
21	Missouri	851	1.7%
46	Montana	87	0.2%
36	Nebraska	247	0.5%
35	Nevada	288	0.6%
43	New Hampshire	162	0.3%
18	New Jersey	1,012	2.0%
33	New Mexico	322	0.6%
5	New York	2,713	5.4%
6	North Carolina	2,475	4.9%
49	North Dakota	52	0.1%
10	Ohio	1,311	2.6%
24	Oklahoma	650	1.3%
30	Oregon	504	1.0%
7	Pennsylvania	1,866	3.7%
44	Rhode Island	144	0.3%
9	South Carolina	1,662	3.3%
41	South Dakota	169	0.3%
15	Tennessee	1,083	2.1%
3	Texas	3,556	7.0%
34	Utah	310	0.6%
47	Vermont	79	0.2%
14	Virginia	1,130	2.2%
23	Washington	733	1.4%
38	West Virginia	180	0.4%
25	Wisconsin	635	1.3%
50	Wyoming	44	0.1%

RANK ORDER

RANK	STATE	CASES	% of USA
1	Florida	6,299	12.4%
2	California	4,882	9.6%
3	Texas	3,556	7.0%
4	Georgia	2,753	5.4%
5	New York	2,713	5.4%
6	North Carolina	2,475	4.9%
7	Pennsylvania	1,866	3.7%
8	Illinois	1,825	3.6%
9	South Carolina	1,662	3.3%
10	Ohio	1,311	2.6%
11	Louisiana	1,250	2.5%
12	Massachusetts	1,228	2.4%
13	Mississippi	1,195	2.4%
14	Virginia	1,130	2.2%
15	Tennessee	1,083	2.1%
16	Maryland	1,076	2.1%
17	Alabama	1,045	2.1%
18	New Jersey	1,012	2.0%
19	Arizona	929	1.8%
20	Michigan	913	1.8%
21	Missouri	851	1.7%
22	Arkansas	779	1.5%
23	Washington	733	1.4%
24	Oklahoma	650	1.3%
25	Wisconsin	635	1.3%
26	Indiana	630	1.2%
27	Colorado	584	1.2%
28	Kentucky	566	1.1%
29	Iowa	518	1.0%
30	Oregon	504	1.0%
31	Connecticut	480	0.9%
32	Kansas	434	0.9%
33	New Mexico	322	0.6%
34	Utah	310	0.6%
35	Nevada	288	0.6%
36	Nebraska	247	0.5%
37	Hawaii	216	0.4%
38	West Virginia	180	0.4%
39	Minnesota	178	0.4%
40	Delaware	176	0.3%
41	Idaho	169	0.3%
41	South Dakota	169	0.3%
43	New Hampshire	162	0.3%
44	Rhode Island	144	0.3%
45	Maine	128	0.3%
46	Montana	87	0.2%
47	Alaska	79	0.2%
47	Vermont	79	0.2%
49	North Dakota	52	0.1%
50	Wyoming	44	0.1%
	District of Columbia	77	0.2%

Source: U.S. Department of Health and Human Services, National Center for Health Statistics
    "Morbidity and Mortality Weekly Report" (January 7, 2011, Vol. 59, Nos. 51 & 52, http://www.cdc.gov/mmwr/)
*Provisional data. Any disease caused by a salmonella infection, which may be manifested as food poisoning with acute gastroenteritis, vomiting, and diarrhea.

Salmonellosis Rate in 2010

National Rate = 16.5 Cases per 100,000 Population*

ALPHA ORDER				RANK ORDER		
RANK	STATE	RATE		RANK	STATE	RATE
8	Alabama	22.2		1	Mississippi	40.5
37	Alaska	11.3		2	South Carolina	36.4
23	Arizona	14.1		3	Florida	34.0
6	Arkansas	27.0		4	Georgia	28.0
29	California	13.2		5	Louisiana	27.8
34	Colorado	11.6		6	Arkansas	27.0
20	Connecticut	13.6		7	North Carolina	26.4
10	Delaware	19.9		8	Alabama	22.2
3	Florida	34.0		9	South Dakota	20.8
4	Georgia	28.0		10	Delaware	19.9
16	Hawaii	16.7		11	Maryland	18.9
41	Idaho	10.9		12	Massachusetts	18.6
23	Illinois	14.1		13	Oklahoma	17.6
44	Indiana	9.8		14	Iowa	17.2
14	Iowa	17.2		14	Tennessee	17.2
18	Kansas	15.4		16	Hawaii	16.7
31	Kentucky	13.1		17	New Mexico	16.0
5	Louisiana	27.8		18	Kansas	15.4
45	Maine	9.7		19	Pennsylvania	14.8
11	Maryland	18.9		20	Texas	14.3
12	Massachusetts	18.6		20	Virginia	14.3
46	Michigan	9.2		22	Missouri	14.2
50	Minnesota	3.4		23	Arizona	14.1
1	Mississippi	40.5		23	Illinois	14.1
22	Missouri	14.2		25	New York	13.9
47	Montana	8.9		26	Nebraska	13.7
26	Nebraska	13.7		26	Rhode Island	13.7
41	Nevada	10.9		28	Connecticut	13.6
33	New Hampshire	12.2		29	California	13.2
34	New Jersey	11.6		29	Oregon	13.2
17	New Mexico	16.0		31	Kentucky	13.1
25	New York	13.9		32	Vermont	12.7
7	North Carolina	26.4		33	New Hampshire	12.2
49	North Dakota	8.0		34	Colorado	11.6
36	Ohio	11.4		34	New Jersey	11.6
13	Oklahoma	17.6		36	Ohio	11.4
29	Oregon	13.2		37	Alaska	11.3
19	Pennsylvania	14.8		38	Wisconsin	11.2
26	Rhode Island	13.7		39	Utah	11.1
2	South Carolina	36.4		40	Washington	11.0
9	South Dakota	20.8		41	Idaho	10.9
14	Tennessee	17.2		41	Nevada	10.9
20	Texas	14.3		43	West Virginia	9.9
39	Utah	11.1		44	Indiana	9.8
32	Vermont	12.7		45	Maine	9.7
20	Virginia	14.3		46	Michigan	9.2
40	Washington	11.0		47	Montana	8.9
43	West Virginia	9.9		48	Wyoming	8.1
38	Wisconsin	11.2		49	North Dakota	8.0
48	Wyoming	8.1		50	Minnesota	3.4
					District of Columbia	12.8

Source: CQ Press using data from U.S. Department of Health and Human Services, National Center for Health Statistics
    "Morbidity and Mortality Weekly Report" (January 7, 2011, Vol. 59, Nos. 51 & 52, http://www.cdc.gov/mmwr/)
*Provisional data. Any disease caused by a salmonella infection, which may be manifested as food poisoning with acute
gastroenteritis, vomiting, and diarrhea. Rates calculated using 2009 population estimates.

Shigellosis Cases Reported in 2010

National Total = 13,882 Cases*

ALPHA ORDER

RANK	STATE	CASES	% of USA
19	Alabama	226	1.6%
47	Alaska	1	0.0%
9	Arizona	437	3.1%
28	Arkansas	79	0.6%
4	California	1,065	7.7%
27	Colorado	99	0.7%
30	Connecticut	63	0.5%
38	Delaware	40	0.3%
3	Florida	1,214	8.7%
6	Georgia	784	5.6%
40	Hawaii	22	0.2%
39	Idaho	23	0.2%
5	Illinois	791	5.7%
36	Indiana	47	0.3%
32	Iowa	56	0.4%
12	Kansas	272	2.0%
20	Kentucky	219	1.6%
13	Louisiana	268	1.9%
44	Maine	8	0.1%
24	Maryland	133	1.0%
21	Massachusetts	207	1.5%
18	Michigan	247	1.8%
41	Minnesota	14	0.1%
32	Mississippi	56	0.4%
2	Missouri	1,581	11.4%
44	Montana	8	0.1%
32	Nebraska	56	0.4%
35	Nevada	48	0.3%
42	New Hampshire	12	0.1%
10	New Jersey	334	2.4%
22	New Mexico	149	1.1%
8	New York	503	3.6%
14	North Carolina	261	1.9%
49	North Dakota	0	0.0%
11	Ohio	309	2.2%
16	Oklahoma	252	1.8%
31	Oregon	58	0.4%
7	Pennsylvania	772	5.6%
43	Rhode Island	11	0.1%
29	South Carolina	68	0.5%
46	South Dakota	7	0.1%
15	Tennessee	255	1.8%
1	Texas	2,148	15.5%
37	Utah	43	0.3%
47	Vermont	1	0.0%
23	Virginia	142	1.0%
25	Washington	109	0.8%
25	West Virginia	109	0.8%
17	Wisconsin	248	1.8%
49	Wyoming	0	0.0%

RANK ORDER

RANK	STATE	CASES	% of USA
1	Texas	2,148	15.5%
2	Missouri	1,581	11.4%
3	Florida	1,214	8.7%
4	California	1,065	7.7%
5	Illinois	791	5.7%
6	Georgia	784	5.6%
7	Pennsylvania	772	5.6%
8	New York	503	3.6%
9	Arizona	437	3.1%
10	New Jersey	334	2.4%
11	Ohio	309	2.2%
12	Kansas	272	2.0%
13	Louisiana	268	1.9%
14	North Carolina	261	1.9%
15	Tennessee	255	1.8%
16	Oklahoma	252	1.8%
17	Wisconsin	248	1.8%
18	Michigan	247	1.8%
19	Alabama	226	1.6%
20	Kentucky	219	1.6%
21	Massachusetts	207	1.5%
22	New Mexico	149	1.1%
23	Virginia	142	1.0%
24	Maryland	133	1.0%
25	Washington	109	0.8%
25	West Virginia	109	0.8%
27	Colorado	99	0.7%
28	Arkansas	79	0.6%
29	South Carolina	68	0.5%
30	Connecticut	63	0.5%
31	Oregon	58	0.4%
32	Iowa	56	0.4%
32	Mississippi	56	0.4%
32	Nebraska	56	0.4%
35	Nevada	48	0.3%
36	Indiana	47	0.3%
37	Utah	43	0.3%
38	Delaware	40	0.3%
39	Idaho	23	0.2%
40	Hawaii	22	0.2%
41	Minnesota	14	0.1%
42	New Hampshire	12	0.1%
43	Rhode Island	11	0.1%
44	Maine	8	0.1%
44	Montana	8	0.1%
46	South Dakota	7	0.1%
47	Alaska	1	0.0%
47	Vermont	1	0.0%
49	North Dakota	0	0.0%
49	Wyoming	0	0.0%
	District of Columbia	27	0.2%

Source: U.S. Department of Health and Human Services, National Center for Health Statistics
    "Morbidity and Mortality Weekly Report" (January 7, 2011, Vol. 59, Nos. 51 & 52, http://www.cdc.gov/mmwr/)
*Provisional data. Dysentery caused by any of various species of shigellae, occurring most frequently in areas where poor sanitation and malnutrition are prevalent, and commonly affecting children and infants.

Shigellosis Rate in 2010

National Rate = 4.5 Cases per 100,000 Population*

ALPHA ORDER

RANK ORDER

RANK	STATE	RATE	RANK	STATE	RATE
14	Alabama	4.8	1	Missouri	26.4
48	Alaska	0.1	2	Kansas	9.6
7	Arizona	6.6	3	Texas	8.7
23	Arkansas	2.7	4	Georgia	8.0
21	California	2.9	5	New Mexico	7.4
28	Colorado	2.0	6	Oklahoma	6.8
31	Connecticut	1.8	7	Arizona	6.6
15	Delaware	4.5	8	Florida	6.5
8	Florida	6.5	9	Illinois	6.1
4	Georgia	8.0	9	Pennsylvania	6.1
34	Hawaii	1.7	11	Louisiana	6.0
36	Idaho	1.5	11	West Virginia	6.0
9	Illinois	6.1	13	Kentucky	5.1
44	Indiana	0.7	14	Alabama	4.8
29	Iowa	1.9	15	Delaware	4.5
2	Kansas	9.6	16	Wisconsin	4.4
13	Kentucky	5.1	17	Tennessee	4.1
11	Louisiana	6.0	18	New Jersey	3.8
45	Maine	0.6	19	Massachusetts	3.1
27	Maryland	2.3	19	Nebraska	3.1
19	Massachusetts	3.1	21	California	2.9
26	Michigan	2.5	22	North Carolina	2.8
46	Minnesota	0.3	23	Arkansas	2.7
29	Mississippi	1.9	23	Ohio	2.7
1	Missouri	26.4	25	New York	2.6
43	Montana	0.8	26	Michigan	2.5
19	Nebraska	3.1	27	Maryland	2.3
31	Nevada	1.8	28	Colorado	2.0
41	New Hampshire	0.9	29	Iowa	1.9
18	New Jersey	3.8	29	Mississippi	1.9
5	New Mexico	7.4	31	Connecticut	1.8
25	New York	2.6	31	Nevada	1.8
22	North Carolina	2.8	31	Virginia	1.8
49	North Dakota	0.0	34	Hawaii	1.7
23	Ohio	2.7	35	Washington	1.6
6	Oklahoma	6.8	36	Idaho	1.5
36	Oregon	1.5	36	Oregon	1.5
9	Pennsylvania	6.1	36	South Carolina	1.5
40	Rhode Island	1.0	36	Utah	1.5
36	South Carolina	1.5	40	Rhode Island	1.0
41	South Dakota	0.9	41	New Hampshire	0.9
17	Tennessee	4.1	41	South Dakota	0.9
3	Texas	8.7	43	Montana	0.8
36	Utah	1.5	44	Indiana	0.7
47	Vermont	0.2	45	Maine	0.6
31	Virginia	1.8	46	Minnesota	0.3
35	Washington	1.6	47	Vermont	0.2
11	West Virginia	6.0	48	Alaska	0.1
16	Wisconsin	4.4	49	North Dakota	0.0
49	Wyoming	0.0	49	Wyoming	0.0
				District of Columbia	4.5

Source: CQ Press using data from U.S. Department of Health and Human Services, National Center for Health Statistics
   "Morbidity and Mortality Weekly Report" (January 7, 2011, Vol. 59, Nos. 51 & 52, http://www.cdc.gov/mmwr/)
*Provisional data. Dysentery caused by any of various species of shigellae, occurring most frequently in areas where poor
sanitation and malnutrition are prevalent, and commonly affecting children and infants. Rates calculated using 2009 population
estimates.

West Nile Virus Disease Cases Reported in 2010

National Total = 987 Cases*

ALPHA ORDER

RANK	STATE	CASES	% of USA
30	Alabama	3	0.3%
40	Alaska	0	0.0%
1	Arizona	163	16.5%
23	Arkansas	7	0.7%
3	California	104	10.5%
5	Colorado	81	8.2%
21	Connecticut	8	0.8%
40	Delaware	0	0.0%
17	Florida	12	1.2%
16	Georgia	13	1.3%
40	Hawaii	0	0.0%
37	Idaho	1	0.1%
6	Illinois	61	6.2%
17	Indiana	12	1.2%
25	Iowa	6	0.6%
15	Kansas	17	1.7%
30	Kentucky	3	0.3%
13	Louisiana	20	2.0%
40	Maine	0	0.0%
11	Maryland	23	2.3%
23	Massachusetts	7	0.7%
10	Michigan	29	2.9%
21	Minnesota	8	0.8%
19	Mississippi	9	0.9%
30	Missouri	3	0.3%
40	Montana	0	0.0%
7	Nebraska	37	3.7%
33	Nevada	2	0.2%
37	New Hampshire	1	0.1%
8	New Jersey	30	3.0%
11	New Mexico	23	2.3%
2	New York	127	12.9%
40	North Carolina	0	0.0%
19	North Dakota	9	0.9%
27	Ohio	5	0.5%
40	Oklahoma	0	0.0%
40	Oregon	0	0.0%
8	Pennsylvania	30	3.0%
40	Rhode Island	0	0.0%
37	South Carolina	1	0.1%
13	South Dakota	20	2.0%
29	Tennessee	4	0.4%
4	Texas	89	9.0%
33	Utah	2	0.2%
40	Vermont	0	0.0%
27	Virginia	5	0.5%
33	Washington	2	0.2%
40	West Virginia	0	0.0%
33	Wisconsin	2	0.2%
25	Wyoming	6	0.6%

RANK ORDER

RANK	STATE	CASES	% of USA
1	Arizona	163	16.5%
2	New York	127	12.9%
3	California	104	10.5%
4	Texas	89	9.0%
5	Colorado	81	8.2%
6	Illinois	61	6.2%
7	Nebraska	37	3.7%
8	New Jersey	30	3.0%
8	Pennsylvania	30	3.0%
10	Michigan	29	2.9%
11	Maryland	23	2.3%
11	New Mexico	23	2.3%
13	Louisiana	20	2.0%
13	South Dakota	20	2.0%
15	Kansas	17	1.7%
16	Georgia	13	1.3%
17	Florida	12	1.2%
17	Indiana	12	1.2%
19	Mississippi	9	0.9%
19	North Dakota	9	0.9%
21	Connecticut	8	0.8%
21	Minnesota	8	0.8%
23	Arkansas	7	0.7%
23	Massachusetts	7	0.7%
25	Iowa	6	0.6%
25	Wyoming	6	0.6%
27	Ohio	5	0.5%
27	Virginia	5	0.5%
29	Tennessee	4	0.4%
30	Alabama	3	0.3%
30	Kentucky	3	0.3%
30	Missouri	3	0.3%
33	Nevada	2	0.2%
33	Utah	2	0.2%
33	Washington	2	0.2%
33	Wisconsin	2	0.2%
37	Idaho	1	0.1%
37	New Hampshire	1	0.1%
37	South Carolina	1	0.1%
40	Alaska	0	0.0%
40	Delaware	0	0.0%
40	Hawaii	0	0.0%
40	Maine	0	0.0%
40	Montana	0	0.0%
40	North Carolina	0	0.0%
40	Oklahoma	0	0.0%
40	Oregon	0	0.0%
40	Rhode Island	0	0.0%
40	Vermont	0	0.0%
40	West Virginia	0	0.0%
	District of Columbia	2	0.2%

Source: U.S. Department of Health and Human Services, National Center for Health Statistics
"Morbidity and Mortality Weekly Report" (January 7, 2011, Vol. 59, Nos. 51 & 52, http://www.cdc.gov/mmwr/)
*Provisional data. A flavivirus typically carried by mosquitoes.

West Nile Disease Rate in 2010

National Rate = 0.3 Cases per 100,000 Population*

<table>
<tr><td colspan="3">ALPHA ORDER</td><td colspan="3">RANK ORDER</td></tr>
<tr><td>RANK</td><td>STATE</td><td>RATE</td><td>RANK</td><td>STATE</td><td>RATE</td></tr>
<tr><td>24</td><td>Alabama</td><td>0.1</td><td>1</td><td>Arizona</td><td>2.5</td></tr>
<tr><td>36</td><td>Alaska</td><td>0.0</td><td>1</td><td>South Dakota</td><td>2.5</td></tr>
<tr><td>1</td><td>Arizona</td><td>2.5</td><td>3</td><td>Nebraska</td><td>2.1</td></tr>
<tr><td>18</td><td>Arkansas</td><td>0.2</td><td>4</td><td>Colorado</td><td>1.6</td></tr>
<tr><td>14</td><td>California</td><td>0.3</td><td>5</td><td>North Dakota</td><td>1.4</td></tr>
<tr><td>4</td><td>Colorado</td><td>1.6</td><td>6</td><td>New Mexico</td><td>1.1</td></tr>
<tr><td>18</td><td>Connecticut</td><td>0.2</td><td>6</td><td>Wyoming</td><td>1 1</td></tr>
<tr><td>36</td><td>Delaware</td><td>0.0</td><td>8</td><td>Kansas</td><td>0.6</td></tr>
<tr><td>24</td><td>Florida</td><td>0.1</td><td>8</td><td>New York</td><td>0.6</td></tr>
<tr><td>24</td><td>Georgia</td><td>0.1</td><td>10</td><td>Illinois</td><td>0.5</td></tr>
<tr><td>36</td><td>Hawaii</td><td>0.0</td><td>11</td><td>Louisiana</td><td>0.4</td></tr>
<tr><td>24</td><td>Idaho</td><td>0.1</td><td>11</td><td>Maryland</td><td>0.4</td></tr>
<tr><td>10</td><td>Illinois</td><td>0.5</td><td>11</td><td>Texas</td><td>0.4</td></tr>
<tr><td>18</td><td>Indiana</td><td>0.2</td><td>14</td><td>California</td><td>0.3</td></tr>
<tr><td>18</td><td>Iowa</td><td>0.2</td><td>14</td><td>Michigan</td><td>0.3</td></tr>
<tr><td>8</td><td>Kansas</td><td>0.6</td><td>14</td><td>Mississippi</td><td>0.3</td></tr>
<tr><td>24</td><td>Kentucky</td><td>0.1</td><td>14</td><td>New Jersey</td><td>0.3</td></tr>
<tr><td>11</td><td>Louisiana</td><td>0.4</td><td>18</td><td>Arkansas</td><td>0.2</td></tr>
<tr><td>36</td><td>Maine</td><td>0.0</td><td>18</td><td>Connecticut</td><td>0.2</td></tr>
<tr><td>11</td><td>Maryland</td><td>0.4</td><td>18</td><td>Indiana</td><td>0.2</td></tr>
<tr><td>24</td><td>Massachusetts</td><td>0.1</td><td>18</td><td>Iowa</td><td>0.2</td></tr>
<tr><td>14</td><td>Michigan</td><td>0.3</td><td>18</td><td>Minnesota</td><td>0.2</td></tr>
<tr><td>18</td><td>Minnesota</td><td>0.2</td><td>18</td><td>Pennsylvania</td><td>0.2</td></tr>
<tr><td>14</td><td>Mississippi</td><td>0.3</td><td>24</td><td>Alabama</td><td>0.1</td></tr>
<tr><td>24</td><td>Missouri</td><td>0.1</td><td>24</td><td>Florida</td><td>0.1</td></tr>
<tr><td>36</td><td>Montana</td><td>0.0</td><td>24</td><td>Georgia</td><td>0.1</td></tr>
<tr><td>3</td><td>Nebraska</td><td>2.1</td><td>24</td><td>Idaho</td><td>0.1</td></tr>
<tr><td>24</td><td>Nevada</td><td>0.1</td><td>24</td><td>Kentucky</td><td>0.1</td></tr>
<tr><td>24</td><td>New Hampshire</td><td>0.1</td><td>24</td><td>Massachusetts</td><td>0.1</td></tr>
<tr><td>14</td><td>New Jersey</td><td>0.3</td><td>24</td><td>Missouri</td><td>0.1</td></tr>
<tr><td>6</td><td>New Mexico</td><td>1.1</td><td>24</td><td>Nevada</td><td>0.1</td></tr>
<tr><td>8</td><td>New York</td><td>0.6</td><td>24</td><td>New Hampshire</td><td>0.1</td></tr>
<tr><td>36</td><td>North Carolina</td><td>0.0</td><td>24</td><td>Tennessee</td><td>0.1</td></tr>
<tr><td>5</td><td>North Dakota</td><td>1.4</td><td>24</td><td>Utah</td><td>0.1</td></tr>
<tr><td>36</td><td>Ohio</td><td>0.0</td><td>24</td><td>Virginia</td><td>0.1</td></tr>
<tr><td>36</td><td>Oklahoma</td><td>0.0</td><td>36</td><td>Alaska</td><td>0.0</td></tr>
<tr><td>36</td><td>Oregon</td><td>0.0</td><td>36</td><td>Delaware</td><td>0.0</td></tr>
<tr><td>18</td><td>Pennsylvania</td><td>0.2</td><td>36</td><td>Hawaii</td><td>0.0</td></tr>
<tr><td>36</td><td>Rhode Island</td><td>0.0</td><td>36</td><td>Maine</td><td>0.0</td></tr>
<tr><td>36</td><td>South Carolina</td><td>0.0</td><td>36</td><td>Montana</td><td>0.0</td></tr>
<tr><td>1</td><td>South Dakota</td><td>2.5</td><td>36</td><td>North Carolina</td><td>0.0</td></tr>
<tr><td>24</td><td>Tennessee</td><td>0.1</td><td>36</td><td>Ohio</td><td>0.0</td></tr>
<tr><td>11</td><td>Texas</td><td>0.4</td><td>36</td><td>Oklahoma</td><td>0.0</td></tr>
<tr><td>24</td><td>Utah</td><td>0.1</td><td>36</td><td>Oregon</td><td>0.0</td></tr>
<tr><td>36</td><td>Vermont</td><td>0.0</td><td>36</td><td>Rhode Island</td><td>0.0</td></tr>
<tr><td>24</td><td>Virginia</td><td>0.1</td><td>36</td><td>South Carolina</td><td>0.0</td></tr>
<tr><td>36</td><td>Washington</td><td>0.0</td><td>36</td><td>Vermont</td><td>0.0</td></tr>
<tr><td>36</td><td>West Virginia</td><td>0.0</td><td>36</td><td>Washington</td><td>0.0</td></tr>
<tr><td>36</td><td>Wisconsin</td><td>0.0</td><td>36</td><td>West Virginia</td><td>0.0</td></tr>
<tr><td>6</td><td>Wyoming</td><td>1.1</td><td>36</td><td>Wisconsin</td><td>0.0</td></tr>
<tr><td></td><td></td><td></td><td></td><td>District of Columbia</td><td>0.3</td></tr>
</table>

Source: CQ Press using data from U.S. Department of Health and Human Services, National Center for Health Statistics "Morbidity and Mortality Weekly Report" (January 7, 2011, Vol. 59, Nos. 51 & 52, http://www.cdc.gov/mmwr/)

*Provisional data. A flavivirus typically carried by mosquitoes. Rates calculated using 2009 population estimates.

Whooping Cough (Pertussis) Cases Reported in 2010

National Total = 21,291 Cases*

ALPHA ORDER

RANK	STATE	CASES	% of USA
26	Alabama	197	0.9%
42	Alaska	43	0.2%
15	Arizona	419	2.0%
28	Arkansas	183	0.9%
1	California	3,080	14.5%
9	Colorado	663	3.1%
36	Connecticut	108	0.5%
49	Delaware	15	0.1%
18	Florida	330	1.5%
23	Georgia	235	1.1%
41	Hawaii	46	0.2%
27	Idaho	186	0.9%
6	Illinois	919	4.3%
11	Indiana	606	2.8%
10	Iowa	632	3.0%
29	Kansas	163	0.8%
20	Kentucky	273	1.3%
43	Louisiana	41	0.2%
39	Maine	52	0.2%
31	Maryland	136	0.6%
21	Massachusetts	252	1.2%
4	Michigan	1,500	7.0%
8	Minnesota	739	3.5%
38	Mississippi	77	0.4%
12	Missouri	573	2.7%
35	Montana	116	0.5%
25	Nebraska	221	1.0%
44	Nevada	33	0.2%
47	New Hampshire	20	0.1%
30	New Jersey	137	0.6%
32	New Mexico	132	0.6%
7	New York	859	4.0%
32	North Carolina	132	0.6%
40	North Dakota	51	0.2%
3	Ohio	1,806	8.5%
37	Oklahoma	91	0.4%
19	Oregon	326	1.5%
5	Pennsylvania	950	4.5%
46	Rhode Island	27	0.1%
16	South Carolina	348	1.6%
45	South Dakota	28	0.1%
24	Tennessee	227	1.1%
2	Texas	2,608	12.2%
22	Utah	237	1.1%
48	Vermont	17	0.1%
17	Virginia	337	1.6%
14	Washington	480	2.3%
34	West Virginia	125	0.6%
13	Wisconsin	493	2.3%
50	Wyoming	10	0.0%

RANK ORDER

RANK	STATE	CASES	% of USA
1	California	3,080	14.5%
2	Texas	2,608	12.2%
3	Ohio	1,806	8.5%
4	Michigan	1,500	7.0%
5	Pennsylvania	950	4.5%
6	Illinois	919	4.3%
7	New York	859	4.0%
8	Minnesota	739	3.5%
9	Colorado	663	3.1%
10	Iowa	632	3.0%
11	Indiana	606	2.8%
12	Missouri	573	2.7%
13	Wisconsin	493	2.3%
14	Washington	480	2.3%
15	Arizona	419	2.0%
16	South Carolina	348	1.6%
17	Virginia	337	1.6%
18	Florida	330	1.5%
19	Oregon	326	1.5%
20	Kentucky	273	1.3%
21	Massachusetts	252	1.2%
22	Utah	237	1.1%
23	Georgia	235	1.1%
24	Tennessee	227	1.1%
25	Nebraska	221	1.0%
26	Alabama	197	0.9%
27	Idaho	186	0.9%
28	Arkansas	183	0.9%
29	Kansas	163	0.8%
30	New Jersey	137	0.6%
31	Maryland	136	0.6%
32	New Mexico	132	0.6%
32	North Carolina	132	0.6%
34	West Virginia	125	0.6%
35	Montana	116	0.5%
36	Connecticut	108	0.5%
37	Oklahoma	91	0.4%
38	Mississippi	77	0.4%
39	Maine	52	0.2%
40	North Dakota	51	0.2%
41	Hawaii	46	0.2%
42	Alaska	43	0.2%
43	Louisiana	41	0.2%
44	Nevada	33	0.2%
45	South Dakota	28	0.1%
46	Rhode Island	27	0.1%
47	New Hampshire	20	0.1%
48	Vermont	17	0.1%
49	Delaware	15	0.1%
50	Wyoming	10	0.0%
	District of Columbia	12	0.1%

Source: U.S. Department of Health and Human Services, National Center for Health Statistics
"Morbidity and Mortality Weekly Report" (January 7, 2011, Vol. 59, Nos. 51 & 52, http://www.cdc.gov/mmwr/)
*Provisional data. Acute, highly contagious infection of respiratory tract.

Whooping Cough (Pertussis) Rate in 2010

National Rate = 6.9 Cases per 100,000 Population*

ALPHA ORDER			RANK ORDER		
RANK	STATE	RATE	RANK	STATE	RATE
30	Alabama	4.2	1	Iowa	21.0
26	Alaska	6.2	2	Ohio	15.6
23	Arizona	6.4	3	Michigan	15.0
24	Arkansas	6.3	4	Minnesota	14.0
15	California	8.3	5	Colorado	13.2
5	Colorado	13.2	6	Nebraska	12.3
36	Connecticut	3.1	7	Idaho	12.0
45	Delaware	1.7	8	Montana	11.9
43	Florida	1.8	9	Texas	10.5
41	Georgia	2.4	10	Missouri	9.6
33	Hawaii	3.6	11	Indiana	9.4
7	Idaho	12.0	12	Wisconsin	8.7
20	Illinois	7.1	13	Oregon	8.5
11	Indiana	9.4	13	Utah	8.5
1	Iowa	21.0	15	California	8.3
27	Kansas	5.8	16	North Dakota	7.9
24	Kentucky	6.3	17	South Carolina	7.6
50	Louisiana	0.9	18	Pennsylvania	7.5
31	Maine	3.9	19	Washington	7.2
41	Maryland	2.4	20	Illinois	7.1
32	Massachusetts	3.8	21	West Virginia	6.9
3	Michigan	15.0	22	New Mexico	6.6
4	Minnesota	14.0	23	Arizona	6.4
38	Mississippi	2.6	24	Arkansas	6.3
10	Missouri	9.6	24	Kentucky	6.3
8	Montana	11.9	26	Alaska	6.2
6	Nebraska	12.3	27	Kansas	5.8
49	Nevada	1.2	28	New York	4.4
47	New Hampshire	1.5	29	Virginia	4.3
46	New Jersey	1.6	30	Alabama	4.2
22	New Mexico	6.6	31	Maine	3.9
28	New York	4.4	32	Massachusetts	3.8
48	North Carolina	1.4	33	Hawaii	3.6
16	North Dakota	7.9	33	Tennessee	3.6
2	Ohio	15.6	35	South Dakota	3.4
40	Oklahoma	2.5	36	Connecticut	3.1
13	Oregon	8.5	37	Vermont	2.7
18	Pennsylvania	7.5	38	Mississippi	2.6
38	Rhode Island	2.6	38	Rhode Island	2.6
17	South Carolina	7.6	40	Oklahoma	2.5
35	South Dakota	3.4	41	Georgia	2.4
33	Tennessee	3.6	41	Maryland	2.4
9	Texas	10.5	43	Florida	1.8
13	Utah	8.5	43	Wyoming	1.8
37	Vermont	2.7	45	Delaware	1.7
29	Virginia	4.3	46	New Jersey	1.6
19	Washington	7.2	47	New Hampshire	1.5
21	West Virginia	6.9	48	North Carolina	1.4
12	Wisconsin	8.7	49	Nevada	1.2
43	Wyoming	1.8	50	Louisiana	0.9
				District of Columbia	2.0

Source: CQ Press using data from U.S. Department of Health and Human Services, National Center for Health Statistics
"Morbidity and Mortality Weekly Report" (January 7, 2011, Vol. 59, Nos. 51 & 52, http://www.cdc.gov/mmwr/)
*Provisional data. Acute, highly contagious infection of respiratory tract. Rates calculated using 2009 population estimates.

Percent of Children Aged 19 to 35 Months Fully Immunized in 2009

National Percent = 70.5%*

ALPHA ORDER			RANK ORDER		
RANK	STATE	PERCENT	RANK	STATE	PERCENT
43	Alabama	63.9	1	Iowa	78.1
49	Alaska	56.6	2	Maryland	77.9
38	Arizona	66.4	3	North Dakota	77.0
46	Arkansas	61.5	4	North Carolina	76.7
17	California	72.2	5	Michigan	76.5
40	Colorado	66.1	6	Connecticut	76.0
6	Connecticut	76.0	6	Massachusetts	76.0
31	Delaware	69.2	8	Wisconsin	75.9
32	Florida	68.7	9	Mississippi	75.2
12	Georgia	73.1	10	Louisiana	74.9
21	Hawaii	71.0	11	New Hampshire	73.3
23	Idaho	70.5	12	Georgia	73.1
13	Illinois	72.8	13	Illinois	72.8
35	Indiana	67.3	14	Tennessee	72.5
1	Iowa	78.1	15	Ohio	72.4
18	Kansas	71.7	16	Maine	72.3
34	Kentucky	67.5	17	California	72.2
10	Louisiana	74.9	18	Kansas	71.7
16	Maine	72.3	19	Minnesota	71.6
2	Maryland	77.9	20	Texas	71.3
6	Massachusetts	76.0	21	Hawaii	71.0
5	Michigan	76.5	22	South Carolina	70.9
19	Minnesota	71.6	23	Idaho	70.5
9	Mississippi	75.2	24	New Mexico	70.2
50	Missouri	56.2	25	Oregon	69.9
45	Montana	61.7	26	Rhode Island	69.7
41	Nebraska	65.4	27	South Dakota	69.6
44	Nevada	62.6	27	Wyoming	69.6
11	New Hampshire	73.3	29	Pennsylvania	69.4
36	New Jersey	67.2	30	Utah	69.3
24	New Mexico	70.2	31	Delaware	69.2
36	New York	67.2	32	Florida	68.7
4	North Carolina	76.7	33	Virginia	68.6
3	North Dakota	77.0	34	Kentucky	67.5
15	Ohio	72.4	35	Indiana	67.3
39	Oklahoma	66.3	36	New Jersey	67.2
25	Oregon	69.9	36	New York	67.2
29	Pennsylvania	69.4	38	Arizona	66.4
26	Rhode Island	69.7	39	Oklahoma	66.3
22	South Carolina	70.9	40	Colorado	66.1
27	South Dakota	69.6	41	Nebraska	65.4
14	Tennessee	72.5	42	Washington	64.9
20	Texas	71.3	43	Alabama	63.9
30	Utah	69.3	44	Nevada	62.6
48	Vermont	59.9	45	Montana	61.7
33	Virginia	68.6	46	Arkansas	61.5
42	Washington	64.9	47	West Virginia	60.9
47	West Virginia	60.9	48	Vermont	59.9
8	Wisconsin	75.9	49	Alaska	56.6
27	Wyoming	69.6	50	Missouri	56.2
				District of Columbia	63.8

Source: U.S. Department of Health and Human Services, Centers for Disease Control and Prevention
"State Vaccination Coverage Levels" (MMWR, Vol. 59, No. 36, September 17, 2010, http://www.cdc.gov/mmwr/)
*Fully immunized (4:3:1:3:3:1:4 series) children received four doses of DTP/DT/DTaP (Diphtheria, Tetanus, Pertussis [Whooping Cough], Acellular Pertussis), three doses of OPV (Oral Poliovirus Vaccine), one dose of MCV (Measles-Containing Vaccine), three doses of Hib (Haemophilus influenzae type b), three doses of Hepatitis B vaccine, one dose of Varicella (chickenpox) vaccine, and four doses of PCV (pneumococcal conjugate vaccine). This differs from previous "fully" immunized tables.

Percent of Adults Aged 65 Years and Older Who Received Flu Shots in 2009

National Median = 70.1%*

ALPHA ORDER				RANK ORDER		
RANK	STATE	PERCENT		RANK	STATE	PERCENT
36	Alabama	68.1		1	Minnesota	76.8
50	Alaska	62.1		2	Rhode Island	75.7
17	Arizona	71.6		3	Colorado	75.2
21	Arkansas	70.7		4	South Dakota	75.0
44	California	65.1		5	Iowa	74.0
3	Colorado	75.2		6	Nebraska	73.9
7	Connecticut	73.7		7	Connecticut	73.7
17	Delaware	71.6		8	Massachusetts	73.0
45	Florida	64.8		9	Maine	72.9
43	Georgia	66.6		10	Pennsylvania	72.8
11	Hawaii	72.7		11	Hawaii	72.7
48	Idaho	64.1		12	Missouri	72.5
46	Illinois	64.7		13	Oklahoma	72.3
38	Indiana	67.7		14	Vermont	72.0
5	Iowa	74.0		14	Wisconsin	72.0
30	Kansas	69.4		16	New Hampshire	71.9
23	Kentucky	70.5		17	Arizona	71.6
36	Louisiana	68.1		17	Delaware	71.6
9	Maine	72.9		17	North Carolina	71.6
20	Maryland	71.5		20	Maryland	71.5
8	Massachusetts	73.0		21	Arkansas	70.7
31	Michigan	68.9		21	Wyoming	70.7
1	Minnesota	76.8		23	Kentucky	70.5
40	Mississippi	67.4		24	West Virginia	70.4
12	Missouri	72.5		25	Tennessee	70.1
33	Montana	68.7		25	Washington	70.1
6	Nebraska	73.9		27	Virginia	69.9
49	Nevada	63.5		28	North Dakota	69.7
16	New Hampshire	71.9		28	South Carolina	69.7
42	New Jersey	67.2		30	Kansas	69.4
35	New Mexico	68.3		31	Michigan	68.9
34	New York	68.6		32	Utah	68.8
17	North Carolina	71.6		33	Montana	68.7
28	North Dakota	69.7		34	New York	68.6
39	Ohio	67.5		35	New Mexico	68.3
13	Oklahoma	72.3		36	Alabama	68.1
47	Oregon	64.6		36	Louisiana	68.1
10	Pennsylvania	72.8		38	Indiana	67.7
2	Rhode Island	75.7		39	Ohio	67.5
28	South Carolina	69.7		40	Mississippi	67.4
4	South Dakota	75.0		41	Texas	67.3
25	Tennessee	70.1		42	New Jersey	67.2
41	Texas	67.3		43	Georgia	66.6
32	Utah	68.8		44	California	65.1
14	Vermont	72.0		45	Florida	64.8
27	Virginia	69.9		46	Illinois	64.7
25	Washington	70.1		47	Oregon	64.6
24	West Virginia	70.4		48	Idaho	64.1
14	Wisconsin	72.0		49	Nevada	63.5
21	Wyoming	70.7		50	Alaska	62.1
					District of Columbia	67.1

Source: U.S. Department of Health and Human Services, Centers for Disease Control and Prevention
"2009 Behavioral Risk Factor Surveillance Summary Prevalence Data" (http://apps.nccd.cdc.gov/brfss/)
*Percent of adults 65 years old and older who reported receiving influenza vaccine during the preceding 12 months.

Percent of Adults Aged 65 Years and Older
Who Have Had a Pneumonia Vaccine: 2009
National Median = 68.5%*

ALPHA ORDER

RANK	STATE	PERCENT
37	Alabama	66.3
37	Alaska	66.3
14	Arizona	70.5
34	Arkansas	67.3
50	California	59.9
1	Colorado	73.9
26	Connecticut	68.5
36	Delaware	66.5
47	Florida	63.3
46	Georgia	63.4
43	Hawaii	64.4
44	Idaho	64.0
47	Illinois	63.3
37	Indiana	66.3
17	Iowa	69.9
29	Kansas	67.7
35	Kentucky	66.8
21	Louisiana	69.3
6	Maine	71.4
24	Maryland	68.9
9	Massachusetts	71.3
32	Michigan	67.5
2	Minnesota	72.6
28	Mississippi	67.8
27	Missouri	68.3
4	Montana	71.8
22	Nebraska	69.1
29	Nevada	67.7
6	New Hampshire	71.4
49	New Jersey	62.4
31	New Mexico	67.6
40	New York	66.2
17	North Carolina	69.9
12	North Dakota	70.8
33	Ohio	67.4
3	Oklahoma	72.1
20	Oregon	69.5
15	Pennsylvania	70.0
10	Rhode Island	71.0
19	South Carolina	69.7
40	South Dakota	66.2
45	Tennessee	63.9
42	Texas	66.0
23	Utah	69.0
4	Vermont	71.8
12	Virginia	70.8
10	Washington	71.0
25	West Virginia	68.8
15	Wisconsin	70.0
6	Wyoming	71.4

RANK ORDER

RANK	STATE	PERCENT
1	Colorado	73.9
2	Minnesota	72.6
3	Oklahoma	72.1
4	Montana	71.8
4	Vermont	71.8
6	Maine	71.4
6	New Hampshire	71.4
6	Wyoming	71.4
9	Massachusetts	71.3
10	Rhode Island	71.0
10	Washington	71.0
12	North Dakota	70.8
12	Virginia	70.8
14	Arizona	70.5
15	Pennsylvania	70.0
15	Wisconsin	70.0
17	Iowa	69.9
17	North Carolina	69.9
19	South Carolina	69.7
20	Oregon	69.5
21	Louisiana	69.3
22	Nebraska	69.1
23	Utah	69.0
24	Maryland	68.9
25	West Virginia	68.8
26	Connecticut	68.5
27	Missouri	68.3
28	Mississippi	67.8
29	Kansas	67.7
29	Nevada	67.7
31	New Mexico	67.6
32	Michigan	67.5
33	Ohio	67.4
34	Arkansas	67.3
35	Kentucky	66.8
36	Delaware	66.5
37	Alabama	66.3
37	Alaska	66.3
37	Indiana	66.3
40	New York	66.2
40	South Dakota	66.2
42	Texas	66.0
43	Hawaii	64.4
44	Idaho	64.0
45	Tennessee	63.9
46	Georgia	63.4
47	Florida	63.3
47	Illinois	63.3
49	New Jersey	62.4
50	California	59.9
	District of Columbia	62.1

Source: U.S. Department of Health and Human Services, Centers for Disease Control and Prevention
"2009 Behavioral Risk Factor Surveillance Summary Prevalence Data" (http://apps.nccd.cdc.gov/brfss/)
*Percent of adults 65 years old and older who reported ever receiving a pneumonia vaccine.

Sexually Transmitted Diseases in 2009

National Total = 1,559,379 Cases*

ALPHA ORDER

RANK	STATE	CASES	% of USA
15	Alabama	33,844	2.2%
39	Alaska	6,156	0.4%
19	Arizona	29,483	1.9%
27	Arkansas	19,089	1.2%
1	California	171,925	11.0%
24	Colorado	22,926	1.5%
30	Connecticut	14,750	0.9%
40	Delaware	5,716	0.4%
4	Florida	94,851	6.1%
9	Georgia	54,468	3.5%
37	Hawaii	6,690	0.4%
43	Idaho	3,955	0.3%
5	Illinois	81,254	5.2%
21	Indiana	28,726	1.8%
34	Iowa	11,087	0.7%
31	Kansas	13,047	0.8%
28	Kentucky	17,212	1.1%
13	Louisiana	37,365	2.4%
46	Maine	2,578	0.2%
18	Maryland	30,456	2.0%
25	Massachusetts	21,532	1.4%
7	Michigan	60,648	3.9%
29	Minnesota	16,571	1.1%
17	Mississippi	31,067	2.0%
16	Missouri	32,529	2.1%
45	Montana	3,072	0.2%
36	Nebraska	6,824	0.4%
33	Nevada	11,862	0.8%
47	New Hampshire	2,229	0.1%
20	New Jersey	28,948	1.9%
35	New Mexico	10,636	0.7%
3	New York	110,255	7.1%
8	North Carolina	55,500	3.6%
48	North Dakota	2,112	0.1%
6	Ohio	64,587	4.1%
26	Oklahoma	19,793	1.3%
32	Oregon	12,667	0.8%
10	Pennsylvania	53,547	3.4%
42	Rhode Island	3,957	0.3%
14	South Carolina	35,096	2.3%
44	South Dakota	3,359	0.2%
12	Tennessee	38,040	2.4%
2	Texas	136,857	8.8%
38	Utah	6,517	0.4%
50	Vermont	1,236	0.1%
11	Virginia	38,992	2.5%
23	Washington	23,811	1.5%
41	West Virginia	4,087	0.3%
22	Wisconsin	26,157	1.7%
49	Wyoming	2,040	0.1%

RANK ORDER

RANK	STATE	CASES	% of USA
1	California	171,925	11.0%
2	Texas	136,857	8.8%
3	New York	110,255	7.1%
4	Florida	94,851	6.1%
5	Illinois	81,254	5.2%
6	Ohio	64,587	4.1%
7	Michigan	60,648	3.9%
8	North Carolina	55,500	3.6%
9	Georgia	54,468	3.5%
10	Pennsylvania	53,547	3.4%
11	Virginia	38,992	2.5%
12	Tennessee	38,040	2.4%
13	Louisiana	37,365	2.4%
14	South Carolina	35,096	2.3%
15	Alabama	33,844	2.2%
16	Missouri	32,529	2.1%
17	Mississippi	31,067	2.0%
18	Maryland	30,456	2.0%
19	Arizona	29,483	1.9%
20	New Jersey	28,948	1.9%
21	Indiana	28,726	1.8%
22	Wisconsin	26,157	1.7%
23	Washington	23,811	1.5%
24	Colorado	22,926	1.5%
25	Massachusetts	21,532	1.4%
26	Oklahoma	19,793	1.3%
27	Arkansas	19,089	1.2%
28	Kentucky	17,212	1.1%
29	Minnesota	16,571	1.1%
30	Connecticut	14,750	0.9%
31	Kansas	13,047	0.8%
32	Oregon	12,667	0.8%
33	Nevada	11,862	0.8%
34	Iowa	11,087	0.7%
35	New Mexico	10,636	0.7%
36	Nebraska	6,824	0.4%
37	Hawaii	6,690	0.4%
38	Utah	6,517	0.4%
39	Alaska	6,156	0.4%
40	Delaware	5,716	0.4%
41	West Virginia	4,087	0.3%
42	Rhode Island	3,957	0.3%
43	Idaho	3,955	0.3%
44	South Dakota	3,359	0.2%
45	Montana	3,072	0.2%
46	Maine	2,578	0.2%
47	New Hampshire	2,229	0.1%
48	North Dakota	2,112	0.1%
49	Wyoming	2,040	0.1%
50	Vermont	1,236	0.1%

District of Columbia — 9,273 — 0.6%

Source: CQ Press using data from U.S. Dept. of Health and Human Services, National Center for Health Statistics
"Sexually Transmitted Disease Surveillance 2009" (http://www.cdc.gov/STD/stats09/toc.htm)
*Includes chancroid, chlamydia, gonorrhea, and primary and secondary syphilis.

Sexually Transmitted Disease Rate in 2009

National Rate = 512.9 Cases per 100,000 Population*

ALPHA ORDER

RANK	STATE	RATE
5	Alabama	725.9
2	Alaska	897.0
28	Arizona	453.6
6	Arkansas	668.5
23	California	467.8
26	Colorado	464.2
31	Connecticut	421.4
7	Delaware	654.7
21	Florida	517.5
14	Georgia	562.3
20	Hawaii	519.4
45	Idaho	259.5
8	Illinois	629.8
29	Indiana	450.5
37	Iowa	369.3
24	Kansas	465.6
33	Kentucky	403.2
3	Louisiana	847.2
49	Maine	195.9
18	Maryland	540.6
41	Massachusetts	331.3
10	Michigan	606.3
44	Minnesota	317.5
1	Mississippi	1,057.2
16	Missouri	550.3
43	Montana	317.6
35	Nebraska	382.7
27	Nevada	456.2
50	New Hampshire	169.4
40	New Jersey	333.3
19	New Mexico	536.0
12	New York	565.7
11	North Carolina	601.9
42	North Dakota	329.2
14	Ohio	562.3
17	Oklahoma	543.5
39	Oregon	334.2
30	Pennsylvania	430.1
36	Rhode Island	376.5
4	South Carolina	783.4
32	South Dakota	417.7
9	Tennessee	612.1
13	Texas	562.6
46	Utah	238.2
48	Vermont	198.9
22	Virginia	501.9
38	Washington	363.6
47	West Virginia	225.2
25	Wisconsin	464.8
34	Wyoming	383.0

RANK ORDER

RANK	STATE	RATE
1	Mississippi	1,057.2
2	Alaska	897.0
3	Louisiana	847.2
4	South Carolina	783.4
5	Alabama	725.9
6	Arkansas	668.5
7	Delaware	654.7
8	Illinois	629.8
9	Tennessee	612.1
10	Michigan	606.3
11	North Carolina	601.9
12	New York	565.7
13	Texas	562.6
14	Georgia	562.3
14	Ohio	562.3
16	Missouri	550.3
17	Oklahoma	543.5
18	Maryland	540.6
19	New Mexico	536.0
20	Hawaii	519.4
21	Florida	517.5
22	Virginia	501.9
23	California	467.8
24	Kansas	465.6
25	Wisconsin	464.8
26	Colorado	464.2
27	Nevada	456.2
28	Arizona	453.6
29	Indiana	450.5
30	Pennsylvania	430.1
31	Connecticut	421.4
32	South Dakota	417.7
33	Kentucky	403.2
34	Wyoming	383.0
35	Nebraska	382.7
36	Rhode Island	376.5
37	Iowa	369.3
38	Washington	363.6
39	Oregon	334.2
40	New Jersey	333.3
41	Massachusetts	331.3
42	North Dakota	329.2
43	Montana	317.6
44	Minnesota	317.5
45	Idaho	259.5
46	Utah	238.2
47	West Virginia	225.2
48	Vermont	198.9
49	Maine	195.9
50	New Hampshire	169.4

District of Columbia	1,566.8

Source: CQ Press using data from U.S. Dept. of Health and Human Services, National Center for Health Statistics "Sexually Transmitted Disease Surveillance 2009" (http://www.cdc.gov/STD/stats09/toc.htm)
*Includes chancroid, chlamydia, gonorrhea, and primary and secondary syphilis.

Chlamydia Cases Reported in 2009

National Total = 1,244,180 Cases*

ALPHA ORDER

RANK	STATE	CASES	% of USA
16	Alabama	25,929	2.1%
39	Alaska	5,166	0.4%
15	Arizona	26,002	2.1%
27	Arkansas	14,354	1.2%
1	California	146,796	11.8%
24	Colorado	19,998	1.6%
30	Connecticut	12,127	1.0%
40	Delaware	4,718	0.4%
4	Florida	72,931	5.9%
10	Georgia	39,828	3.2%
37	Hawaii	6,026	0.5%
41	Idaho	3,842	0.3%
5	Illinois	60,542	4.9%
21	Indiana	21,732	1.7%
35	Iowa	9,406	0.8%
32	Kansas	10,510	0.8%
29	Kentucky	13,293	1.1%
13	Louisiana	27,628	2.2%
46	Maine	2,431	0.2%
19	Maryland	23,747	1.9%
25	Massachusetts	19,315	1.6%
7	Michigan	45,714	3.7%
28	Minnesota	14,197	1.1%
20	Mississippi	23,589	1.9%
17	Missouri	25,868	2.1%
45	Montana	2,988	0.2%
38	Nebraska	5,443	0.4%
33	Nevada	10,045	0.8%
47	New Hampshire	2,102	0.2%
18	New Jersey	23,974	1.9%
34	New Mexico	9,493	0.8%
3	New York	92,069	7.4%
9	North Carolina	41,045	3.3%
49	North Dakota	1,957	0.2%
6	Ohio	48,239	3.9%
26	Oklahoma	15,023	1.2%
31	Oregon	11,497	0.9%
8	Pennsylvania	43,068	3.5%
42	Rhode Island	3,615	0.3%
14	South Carolina	26,654	2.1%
44	South Dakota	3,015	0.2%
12	Tennessee	29,711	2.4%
2	Texas	105,910	8.5%
36	Utah	6,145	0.5%
50	Vermont	1,186	0.1%
11	Virginia	30,903	2.5%
22	Washington	21,387	1.7%
43	West Virginia	3,604	0.3%
23	Wisconsin	20,906	1.7%
48	Wyoming	1,963	0.2%

RANK ORDER

RANK	STATE	CASES	% of USA
1	California	146,796	11.8%
2	Texas	105,910	8.5%
3	New York	92,069	7.4%
4	Florida	72,931	5.9%
5	Illinois	60,542	4.9%
6	Ohio	48,239	3.9%
7	Michigan	45,714	3.7%
8	Pennsylvania	43,068	3.5%
9	North Carolina	41,045	3.3%
10	Georgia	39,828	3.2%
11	Virginia	30,903	2.5%
12	Tennessee	29,711	2.4%
13	Louisiana	27,628	2.2%
14	South Carolina	26,654	2.1%
15	Arizona	26,002	2.1%
16	Alabama	25,929	2.1%
17	Missouri	25,868	2.1%
18	New Jersey	23,974	1.9%
19	Maryland	23,747	1.9%
20	Mississippi	23,589	1.9%
21	Indiana	21,732	1.7%
22	Washington	21,387	1.7%
23	Wisconsin	20,906	1.7%
24	Colorado	19,998	1.6%
25	Massachusetts	19,315	1.6%
26	Oklahoma	15,023	1.2%
27	Arkansas	14,354	1.2%
28	Minnesota	14,197	1.1%
29	Kentucky	13,293	1.1%
30	Connecticut	12,127	1.0%
31	Oregon	11,497	0.9%
32	Kansas	10,510	0.8%
33	Nevada	10,045	0.8%
34	New Mexico	9,493	0.8%
35	Iowa	9,406	0.8%
36	Utah	6,145	0.5%
37	Hawaii	6,026	0.5%
38	Nebraska	5,443	0.4%
39	Alaska	5,166	0.4%
40	Delaware	4,718	0.4%
41	Idaho	3,842	0.3%
42	Rhode Island	3,615	0.3%
43	West Virginia	3,604	0.3%
44	South Dakota	3,015	0.2%
45	Montana	2,988	0.2%
46	Maine	2,431	0.2%
47	New Hampshire	2,102	0.2%
48	Wyoming	1,963	0.2%
49	North Dakota	1,957	0.2%
50	Vermont	1,186	0.1%
	District of Columbia	6,549	0.5%

Source: U.S. Department of Health and Human Services, National Center for Health Statistics
   "Sexually Transmitted Disease Surveillance 2009" (http://www.cdc.gov/STD/stats09/toc.htm)
*Any of several common, often asymptomatic, sexually transmitted diseases caused by the microorganism Chlamydia trachomatis, including nonspecific urethritis in men.

Chlamydia Rate in 2009

National Rate = 409.2 Cases per 100,000 Population*

ALPHA ORDER				RANK ORDER		
RANK	STATE	RATE		RANK	STATE	RATE
5	Alabama	556.2		1	Mississippi	802.7
2	Alaska	752.7		2	Alaska	752.7
22	Arizona	400.0		3	Louisiana	626.4
7	Arkansas	502.7		4	South Carolina	595.0
23	California	399.4		5	Alabama	556.2
21	Colorado	404.9		6	Delaware	540.4
31	Connecticut	346.4		7	Arkansas	502.7
6	Delaware	540.4		8	New Mexico	478.4
24	Florida	397.9		9	Tennessee	478.1
20	Georgia	411.2		10	New York	472.4
12	Hawaii	467.8		11	Illinois	469.3
45	Idaho	252.1		12	Hawaii	467.8
11	Illinois	469.3		13	Michigan	457.0
34	Indiana	340.8		14	North Carolina	445.1
36	Iowa	313.3		15	Missouri	437.6
27	Kansas	375.1		16	Texas	435.4
37	Kentucky	311.4		17	Maryland	421.5
3	Louisiana	626.4		18	Ohio	420.0
49	Maine	184.7		19	Oklahoma	412.5
17	Maryland	421.5		20	Georgia	411.2
42	Massachusetts	297.2		21	Colorado	404.9
13	Michigan	457.0		22	Arizona	400.0
44	Minnesota	272.0		23	California	399.4
1	Mississippi	802.7		24	Florida	397.9
15	Missouri	437.6		25	Virginia	397.8
38	Montana	308.9		26	Nevada	386.3
39	Nebraska	305.2		27	Kansas	375.1
26	Nevada	386.3		28	South Dakota	374.9
50	New Hampshire	159.7		29	Wisconsin	371.5
43	New Jersey	276.1		30	Wyoming	368.5
8	New Mexico	478.4		31	Connecticut	346.4
10	New York	472.4		32	Pennsylvania	346.0
14	North Carolina	445.1		33	Rhode Island	344.0
40	North Dakota	305.1		34	Indiana	340.8
18	Ohio	420.0		35	Washington	326.6
19	Oklahoma	412.5		36	Iowa	313.3
41	Oregon	303.3		37	Kentucky	311.4
32	Pennsylvania	346.0		38	Montana	308.9
33	Rhode Island	344.0		39	Nebraska	305.2
4	South Carolina	595.0		40	North Dakota	305.1
28	South Dakota	374.9		41	Oregon	303.3
9	Tennessee	478.1		42	Massachusetts	297.2
16	Texas	435.4		43	New Jersey	276.1
46	Utah	224.6		44	Minnesota	272.0
48	Vermont	190.9		45	Idaho	252.1
25	Virginia	397.8		46	Utah	224.6
35	Washington	326.6		47	West Virginia	198.6
47	West Virginia	198.6		48	Vermont	190.9
29	Wisconsin	371.5		49	Maine	184.7
30	Wyoming	368.5		50	New Hampshire	159.7
					District of Columbia	1,106.6

Source: U.S. Department of Health and Human Services, National Center for Health Statistics
"Sexually Transmitted Disease Surveillance 2009" (http://www.cdc.gov/STD/stats09/toc.htm)
*Any of several common, often asymptomatic, sexually transmitted diseases caused by the microorganism Chlamydia trachomatis, including nonspecific urethritis in men.

Gonorrhea Cases Reported in 2009

National Total = 301,174 Cases*

ALPHA ORDER

RANK	STATE	CASES	% of USA
15	Alabama	7,498	2.5%
37	Alaska	990	0.3%
25	Arizona	3,250	1.1%
23	Arkansas	4,460	1.5%
2	California	23,228	7.7%
26	Colorado	2,823	0.9%
27	Connecticut	2,558	0.8%
38	Delaware	971	0.3%
3	Florida	20,878	6.9%
9	Georgia	13,687	4.5%
39	Hawaii	631	0.2%
47	Idaho	110	0.0%
4	Illinois	19,962	6.6%
17	Indiana	6,835	2.3%
33	Iowa	1,658	0.6%
28	Kansas	2,505	0.8%
24	Kentucky	3,827	1.3%
11	Louisiana	8,996	3.0%
45	Maine	143	0.0%
19	Maryland	6,395	2.1%
31	Massachusetts	1,976	0.7%
7	Michigan	14,704	4.9%
29	Minnesota	2,303	0.8%
16	Mississippi	7,241	2.4%
18	Missouri	6,488	2.2%
48	Montana	80	0.0%
34	Nebraska	1,376	0.5%
32	Nevada	1,726	0.6%
46	New Hampshire	113	0.0%
21	New Jersey	4,762	1.6%
36	New Mexico	1,082	0.4%
5	New York	17,004	5.6%
8	North Carolina	13,870	4.6%
44	North Dakota	151	0.1%
6	Ohio	15,988	5.3%
22	Oklahoma	4,673	1.6%
35	Oregon	1,113	0.4%
10	Pennsylvania	10,138	3.4%
43	Rhode Island	322	0.1%
12	South Carolina	8,318	2.8%
41	South Dakota	344	0.1%
13	Tennessee	7,926	2.6%
1	Texas	29,295	9.7%
42	Utah	341	0.1%
50	Vermont	50	0.0%
14	Virginia	7,789	2.6%
30	Washington	2,285	0.8%
40	West Virginia	475	0.2%
20	Wisconsin	5,201	1.7%
49	Wyoming	74	0.0%

RANK ORDER

RANK	STATE	CASES	% of USA
1	Texas	29,295	9.7%
2	California	23,228	7.7%
3	Florida	20,878	6.9%
4	Illinois	19,962	6.6%
5	New York	17,004	5.6%
6	Ohio	15,988	5.3%
7	Michigan	14,704	4.9%
8	North Carolina	13,870	4.6%
9	Georgia	13,687	4.5%
10	Pennsylvania	10,138	3.4%
11	Louisiana	8,996	3.0%
12	South Carolina	8,318	2.8%
13	Tennessee	7,926	2.6%
14	Virginia	7,789	2.6%
15	Alabama	7,498	2.5%
16	Mississippi	7,241	2.4%
17	Indiana	6,835	2.3%
18	Missouri	6,488	2.2%
19	Maryland	6,395	2.1%
20	Wisconsin	5,201	1.7%
21	New Jersey	4,762	1.6%
22	Oklahoma	4,673	1.6%
23	Arkansas	4,460	1.5%
24	Kentucky	3,827	1.3%
25	Arizona	3,250	1.1%
26	Colorado	2,823	0.9%
27	Connecticut	2,558	0.8%
28	Kansas	2,505	0.8%
29	Minnesota	2,303	0.8%
30	Washington	2,285	0.8%
31	Massachusetts	1,976	0.7%
32	Nevada	1,726	0.6%
33	Iowa	1,658	0.6%
34	Nebraska	1,376	0.5%
35	Oregon	1,113	0.4%
36	New Mexico	1,082	0.4%
37	Alaska	990	0.3%
38	Delaware	971	0.3%
39	Hawaii	631	0.2%
40	West Virginia	475	0.2%
41	South Dakota	344	0.1%
42	Utah	341	0.1%
43	Rhode Island	322	0.1%
44	North Dakota	151	0.1%
45	Maine	143	0.0%
46	New Hampshire	113	0.0%
47	Idaho	110	0.0%
48	Montana	80	0.0%
49	Wyoming	74	0.0%
50	Vermont	50	0.0%
	District of Columbia	2,561	0.9%

Source: U.S. Department of Health and Human Services, National Center for Health Statistics
"Sexually Transmitted Disease Surveillance 2009" (http://www.cdc.gov/STD/stats09/toc.htm)
*Gonorrhea is a sexually transmitted disease caused by gonococcal bacteria that affects the mucous membrane chiefly of the genital and urinary tracts and is characterized by an acute purulent discharge and painful or difficult urination, though women often have no symptoms.

Gonorrhea Rate in 2009

National Rate = 99.1 Cases per 100,000 Population*

RANK	STATE	RATE
4	Alabama	160.8
9	Alaska	144.3
34	Arizona	50.0
5	Arkansas	156.2
29	California	63.2
30	Colorado	57.2
27	Connecticut	73.1
17	Delaware	111.2
15	Florida	113.9
10	Georgia	141.3
35	Hawaii	49.0
50	Idaho	7.2
6	Illinois	154.7
19	Indiana	107.2
31	Iowa	55.2
23	Kansas	89.4
22	Kentucky	89.6
2	Louisiana	204.0
46	Maine	10.9
16	Maryland	113.5
40	Massachusetts	30.4
8	Michigan	147.0
36	Minnesota	44.1
1	Mississippi	246.4
18	Missouri	109.8
48	Montana	8.3
26	Nebraska	77.2
28	Nevada	66.4
47	New Hampshire	8.6
32	New Jersey	54.8
33	New Mexico	54.5
24	New York	87.2
7	North Carolina	150.4
43	North Dakota	23.5
11	Ohio	139.2
12	Oklahoma	128.3
41	Oregon	29.4
25	Pennsylvania	81.4
39	Rhode Island	30.6
3	South Carolina	185.7
37	South Dakota	42.8
13	Tennessee	127.5
14	Texas	120.4
45	Utah	12.5
49	Vermont	8.0
20	Virginia	100.3
38	Washington	34.9
42	West Virginia	26.2
21	Wisconsin	92.4
44	Wyoming	13.9

RANK	STATE	RATE
1	Mississippi	246.4
2	Louisiana	204.0
3	South Carolina	185.7
4	Alabama	160.8
5	Arkansas	156.2
6	Illinois	154.7
7	North Carolina	150.4
8	Michigan	147.0
9	Alaska	144.3
10	Georgia	141.3
11	Ohio	139.2
12	Oklahoma	128.3
13	Tennessee	127.5
14	Texas	120.4
15	Florida	113.9
16	Maryland	113.5
17	Delaware	111.2
18	Missouri	109.8
19	Indiana	107.2
20	Virginia	100.3
21	Wisconsin	92.4
22	Kentucky	89.6
23	Kansas	89.4
24	New York	87.2
25	Pennsylvania	81.4
26	Nebraska	77.2
27	Connecticut	73.1
28	Nevada	66.4
29	California	63.2
30	Colorado	57.2
31	Iowa	55.2
32	New Jersey	54.8
33	New Mexico	54.5
34	Arizona	50.0
35	Hawaii	49.0
36	Minnesota	44.1
37	South Dakota	42.8
38	Washington	34.9
39	Rhode Island	30.6
40	Massachusetts	30.4
41	Oregon	29.4
42	West Virginia	26.2
43	North Dakota	23.5
44	Wyoming	13.9
45	Utah	12.5
46	Maine	10.9
47	New Hampshire	8.6
48	Montana	8.3
49	Vermont	8.0
50	Idaho	7.2

District of Columbia   432.7

Source: U.S. Department of Health and Human Services, National Center for Health Statistics
   "Sexually Transmitted Disease Surveillance 2009" (http://www.cdc.gov/STD/stats09/toc.htm)
*Gonorrhea is a sexually transmitted disease caused by gonococcal bacteria that affects the mucous membrane chiefly of the genital and urinary tracts and is characterized by an acute purulent discharge and painful or difficult urination, though women often have no symptoms.

Syphilis Cases Reported in 2009

National Total = 13,997 Cases*

ALPHA ORDER					RANK ORDER			
RANK	STATE		CASES	% of USA	RANK	STATE	CASES	% of USA
9	Alabama		417	3.0%	1	California	1,900	13.6%
48	Alaska		0	0.0%	2	Texas	1,644	11.7%
18	Arizona		231	1.7%	3	New York	1,182	8.4%
15	Arkansas		275	2.0%	4	Florida	1,041	7.4%
1	California		1,900	13.6%	5	Georgia	953	6.8%
25	Colorado		105	0.8%	6	Illinois	750	5.4%
30	Connecticut		65	0.5%	7	Louisiana	741	5.3%
37	Delaware		27	0.2%	8	North Carolina	579	4.1%
4	Florida		1,041	7.4%	9	Alabama	417	3.0%
5	Georgia		953	6.8%	10	Tennessee	403	2.9%
34	Hawaii		33	0.2%	11	Ohio	360	2.6%
46	Idaho		3	0.0%	12	Pennsylvania	341	2.4%
6	Illinois		750	5.4%	13	Maryland	314	2.2%
22	Indiana		158	1.1%	14	Virginia	299	2.1%
38	Iowa		23	0.2%	15	Arkansas	275	2.0%
35	Kansas		32	0.2%	16	Massachusetts	238	1.7%
27	Kentucky		92	0.7%	17	Mississippi	237	1.7%
7	Louisiana		741	5.3%	18	Arizona	231	1.7%
43	Maine		4	0.0%	19	Michigan	230	1.6%
13	Maryland		314	2.2%	20	New Jersey	212	1.5%
16	Massachusetts		238	1.7%	21	Missouri	173	1.2%
19	Michigan		230	1.6%	22	Indiana	158	1.1%
29	Minnesota		71	0.5%	23	Washington	139	1.0%
17	Mississippi		237	1.7%	24	South Carolina	123	0.9%
21	Missouri		173	1.2%	25	Colorado	105	0.8%
43	Montana		4	0.0%	26	Oklahoma	97	0.7%
42	Nebraska		5	0.0%	27	Kentucky	92	0.7%
28	Nevada		91	0.7%	28	Nevada	91	0.7%
40	New Hampshire		14	0.1%	29	Minnesota	71	0.5%
20	New Jersey		212	1.5%	30	Connecticut	65	0.5%
31	New Mexico		61	0.4%	31	New Mexico	61	0.4%
3	New York		1,182	8.4%	32	Oregon	57	0.4%
8	North Carolina		579	4.1%	33	Wisconsin	44	0.3%
43	North Dakota		4	0.0%	34	Hawaii	33	0.2%
11	Ohio		360	2.6%	35	Kansas	32	0.2%
26	Oklahoma		97	0.7%	36	Utah	31	0.2%
32	Oregon		57	0.4%	37	Delaware	27	0.2%
12	Pennsylvania		341	2.4%	38	Iowa	23	0.2%
39	Rhode Island		20	0.1%	39	Rhode Island	20	0.1%
24	South Carolina		123	0.9%	40	New Hampshire	14	0.1%
48	South Dakota		0	0.0%	41	West Virginia	8	0.1%
10	Tennessee		403	2.9%	42	Nebraska	5	0.0%
2	Texas		1,644	11.7%	43	Maine	4	0.0%
36	Utah		31	0.2%	43	Montana	4	0.0%
48	Vermont		0	0.0%	43	North Dakota	4	0.0%
14	Virginia		299	2.1%	46	Idaho	3	0.0%
23	Washington		139	1.0%	46	Wyoming	3	0.0%
41	West Virginia		8	0.1%	48	Alaska	0	0.0%
33	Wisconsin		44	0.3%	48	South Dakota	0	0.0%
46	Wyoming		3	0.0%	48	Vermont	0	0.0%
						District of Columbia	163	1.2%

Source: U.S. Department of Health and Human Services, National Center for Health Statistics
    "Sexually Transmitted Disease Surveillance 2009" (http://www.cdc.gov/STD/stats09/toc.htm)
*Includes only primary and secondary cases. Does not include 30,831 cases in other stages. A chronic infectious disease
caused by a spirochete (Treponema pallidum), either transmitted by direct contact, usually in sexual intercourse, or passed from
mother to child in utero, and progressing through three stages characterized respectively by local formation of chancres, ulcerous
skin eruptions, and systemic infection leading to general paresis.

Syphilis Rate in 2009

National Rate = 4.6 Cases per 100,000 Population*

ALPHA ORDER

RANK	STATE	RATE
4	Alabama	8.9
48	Alaska	0.0
16	Arizona	3.6
3	Arkansas	9.6
13	California	5.2
30	Colorado	2.1
32	Connecticut	1.9
18	Delaware	3.1
11	Florida	5.7
2	Georgia	9.8
25	Hawaii	2.6
47	Idaho	0.2
10	Illinois	5.8
26	Indiana	2.5
39	Iowa	0.8
36	Kansas	1.1
29	Kentucky	2.2
1	Louisiana	16.8
45	Maine	0.3
12	Maryland	5.6
15	Massachusetts	3.7
28	Michigan	2.3
35	Minnesota	1.4
5	Mississippi	8.1
21	Missouri	2.9
43	Montana	0.4
45	Nebraska	0.3
17	Nevada	3.5
36	New Hampshire	1.1
27	New Jersey	2.4
18	New Mexico	3.1
9	New York	6.1
8	North Carolina	6.3
41	North Dakota	0.6
18	Ohio	3.1
22	Oklahoma	2.7
34	Oregon	1.5
22	Pennsylvania	2.7
32	Rhode Island	1.9
22	South Carolina	2.7
48	South Dakota	0.0
7	Tennessee	6.5
6	Texas	6.8
36	Utah	1.1
48	Vermont	0.0
14	Virginia	3.8
30	Washington	2.1
43	West Virginia	0.4
39	Wisconsin	0.8
41	Wyoming	0.6

RANK ORDER

RANK	STATE	RATE
1	Louisiana	16.8
2	Georgia	9.8
3	Arkansas	9.6
4	Alabama	8.9
5	Mississippi	8.1
6	Texas	6.8
7	Tennessee	6.5
8	North Carolina	6.3
9	New York	6.1
10	Illinois	5.8
11	Florida	5.7
12	Maryland	5.6
13	California	5.2
14	Virginia	3.8
15	Massachusetts	3.7
16	Arizona	3.6
17	Nevada	3.5
18	Delaware	3.1
18	New Mexico	3.1
18	Ohio	3.1
21	Missouri	2.9
22	Oklahoma	2.7
22	Pennsylvania	2.7
22	South Carolina	2.7
25	Hawaii	2.6
26	Indiana	2.5
27	New Jersey	2.4
28	Michigan	2.3
29	Kentucky	2.2
30	Colorado	2.1
30	Washington	2.1
32	Connecticut	1.9
32	Rhode Island	1.9
34	Oregon	1.5
35	Minnesota	1.4
36	Kansas	1.1
36	New Hampshire	1.1
36	Utah	1.1
39	Iowa	0.8
39	Wisconsin	0.8
41	North Dakota	0.6
41	Wyoming	0.6
43	Montana	0.4
43	West Virginia	0.4
45	Maine	0.3
45	Nebraska	0.3
47	Idaho	0.2
48	Alaska	0.0
48	South Dakota	0.0
48	Vermont	0.0
	District of Columbia	27.5

Source: U.S. Department of Health and Human Services, National Center for Health Statistics
"Sexually Transmitted Disease Surveillance 2009" (http://www.cdc.gov/STD/stats09/toc.htm)
*Includes only primary and secondary cases. Does not include 30,831 cases in other stages. A chronic infectious disease caused by a spirochete (Treponema pallidum), either transmitted by direct contact, usually in sexual intercourse, or passed from mother to child in utero, and progressing through three stages characterized respectively by local formation of chancres, ulcerous skin eruptions, and systemic infection leading to general paresis.

Percent of Adults Who Have Asthma: 2009

National Median = 8.8% of Adults*

ALPHA ORDER

RANK	STATE	PERCENT
41	Alabama	7.6
20	Alaska	9.0
2	Arizona	10.8
41	Arkansas	7.6
35	California	7.8
31	Colorado	8.2
15	Connecticut	9.4
24	Delaware	8.8
45	Florida	6.9
45	Georgia	6.9
15	Hawaii	9.4
30	Idaho	8.4
20	Illinois	9.0
17	Indiana	9.1
47	Iowa	6.8
29	Kansas	8.5
6	Kentucky	10.2
50	Louisiana	6.3
2	Maine	10.8
17	Maryland	9.1
2	Massachusetts	10.8
8	Michigan	10.0
48	Minnesota	6.6
41	Mississippi	7.6
14	Missouri	9.5
32	Montana	8.1
41	Nebraska	7.6
20	Nevada	9.0
5	New Hampshire	10.3
39	New Jersey	7.7
28	New Mexico	8.6
12	New York	9.8
35	North Carolina	7.8
24	North Dakota	8.8
10	Ohio	9.9
8	Oklahoma	10.0
1	Oregon	11.1
17	Pennsylvania	9.1
7	Rhode Island	10.1
35	South Carolina	7.8
39	South Dakota	7.7
32	Tennessee	8.1
49	Texas	6.5
34	Utah	8.0
10	Vermont	9.9
35	Virginia	7.8
24	Washington	8.8
24	West Virginia	8.8
12	Wisconsin	9.8
23	Wyoming	8.9

RANK ORDER

RANK	STATE	PERCENT
1	Oregon	11.1
2	Arizona	10.8
2	Maine	10.8
2	Massachusetts	10.8
5	New Hampshire	10.3
6	Kentucky	10.2
7	Rhode Island	10.1
8	Michigan	10.0
8	Oklahoma	10.0
10	Ohio	9.9
10	Vermont	9.9
12	New York	9.8
12	Wisconsin	9.8
14	Missouri	9.5
15	Connecticut	9.4
15	Hawaii	9.4
17	Indiana	9.1
17	Maryland	9.1
17	Pennsylvania	9.1
20	Alaska	9.0
20	Illinois	9.0
20	Nevada	9.0
23	Wyoming	8.9
24	Delaware	8.8
24	North Dakota	8.8
24	Washington	8.8
24	West Virginia	8.8
28	New Mexico	8.6
29	Kansas	8.5
30	Idaho	8.4
31	Colorado	8.2
32	Montana	8.1
32	Tennessee	8.1
34	Utah	8.0
35	California	7.8
35	North Carolina	7.8
35	South Carolina	7.8
35	Virginia	7.8
39	New Jersey	7.7
39	South Dakota	7.7
41	Alabama	7.6
41	Arkansas	7.6
41	Mississippi	7.6
41	Nebraska	7.6
45	Florida	6.9
45	Georgia	6.9
47	Iowa	6.8
48	Minnesota	6.6
49	Texas	6.5
50	Louisiana	6.3
	District of Columbia	9.9

Source: U.S. Department of Health and Human Services, Centers for Disease Control and Prevention
  "2009 Behavioral Risk Factor Surveillance Summary Prevalence Data" (http://apps.nccd.cdc.gov/brfss/)
*Percent of adults who answered yes to the questions "Have you ever been told by a doctor, nurse, or other health professional that you had asthma?" and "Do you still have asthma?"

Percent of Adults Who Have Been Told They Have Arthritis: 2009

National Median = 26.0%*

<table>
<tr><th colspan="3">ALPHA ORDER</th><th colspan="3">RANK ORDER</th></tr>
<tr><th>RANK</th><th>STATE</th><th>PERCENT</th><th>RANK</th><th>STATE</th><th>PERCENT</th></tr>
<tr><td>2</td><td>Alabama</td><td>33.9</td><td>1</td><td>Kentucky</td><td>35.6</td></tr>
<tr><td>44</td><td>Alaska</td><td>23.5</td><td>2</td><td>Alabama</td><td>33.9</td></tr>
<tr><td>38</td><td>Arizona</td><td>24.3</td><td>2</td><td>West Virginia</td><td>33.9</td></tr>
<tr><td>4</td><td>Arkansas</td><td>31.3</td><td>4</td><td>Arkansas</td><td>31.3</td></tr>
<tr><td>50</td><td>California</td><td>20.3</td><td>4</td><td>Pennsylvania</td><td>31.3</td></tr>
<tr><td>41</td><td>Colorado</td><td>23.8</td><td>6</td><td>Missouri</td><td>31.0</td></tr>
<tr><td>36</td><td>Connecticut</td><td>24.9</td><td>7</td><td>Maine</td><td>30.9</td></tr>
<tr><td>17</td><td>Delaware</td><td>27.5</td><td>8</td><td>Michigan</td><td>30.8</td></tr>
<tr><td>21</td><td>Florida</td><td>27.0</td><td>8</td><td>Mississippi</td><td>30.8</td></tr>
<tr><td>42</td><td>Georgia</td><td>23.7</td><td>8</td><td>Ohio</td><td>30.8</td></tr>
<tr><td>48</td><td>Hawaii</td><td>21.2</td><td>11</td><td>South Carolina</td><td>30.7</td></tr>
<tr><td>42</td><td>Idaho</td><td>23.7</td><td>12</td><td>Oklahoma</td><td>30.4</td></tr>
<tr><td>24</td><td>Illinois</td><td>26.5</td><td>13</td><td>Indiana</td><td>29.3</td></tr>
<tr><td>13</td><td>Indiana</td><td>29.3</td><td>13</td><td>Rhode Island</td><td>29.3</td></tr>
<tr><td>34</td><td>Iowa</td><td>25.3</td><td>15</td><td>Vermont</td><td>28.6</td></tr>
<tr><td>40</td><td>Kansas</td><td>24.1</td><td>16</td><td>North Carolina</td><td>27.6</td></tr>
<tr><td>1</td><td>Kentucky</td><td>35.6</td><td>17</td><td>Delaware</td><td>27.5</td></tr>
<tr><td>26</td><td>Louisiana</td><td>26.0</td><td>17</td><td>Montana</td><td>27.5</td></tr>
<tr><td>7</td><td>Maine</td><td>30.9</td><td>19</td><td>North Dakota</td><td>27.4</td></tr>
<tr><td>27</td><td>Maryland</td><td>25.9</td><td>20</td><td>Oregon</td><td>27.2</td></tr>
<tr><td>37</td><td>Massachusetts</td><td>24.8</td><td>21</td><td>Florida</td><td>27.0</td></tr>
<tr><td>8</td><td>Michigan</td><td>30.8</td><td>21</td><td>New Hampshire</td><td>27.0</td></tr>
<tr><td>49</td><td>Minnesota</td><td>20.9</td><td>23</td><td>Wyoming</td><td>26.9</td></tr>
<tr><td>8</td><td>Mississippi</td><td>30.8</td><td>24</td><td>Illinois</td><td>26.5</td></tr>
<tr><td>6</td><td>Missouri</td><td>31.0</td><td>24</td><td>Washington</td><td>26.5</td></tr>
<tr><td>17</td><td>Montana</td><td>27.5</td><td>26</td><td>Louisiana</td><td>26.0</td></tr>
<tr><td>27</td><td>Nebraska</td><td>25.9</td><td>27</td><td>Maryland</td><td>25.9</td></tr>
<tr><td>38</td><td>Nevada</td><td>24.3</td><td>27</td><td>Nebraska</td><td>25.9</td></tr>
<tr><td>21</td><td>New Hampshire</td><td>27.0</td><td>27</td><td>Tennessee</td><td>25.9</td></tr>
<tr><td>45</td><td>New Jersey</td><td>22.7</td><td>27</td><td>Virginia</td><td>25.9</td></tr>
<tr><td>31</td><td>New Mexico</td><td>25.7</td><td>31</td><td>New Mexico</td><td>25.7</td></tr>
<tr><td>32</td><td>New York</td><td>25.6</td><td>32</td><td>New York</td><td>25.6</td></tr>
<tr><td>16</td><td>North Carolina</td><td>27.6</td><td>32</td><td>South Dakota</td><td>25.6</td></tr>
<tr><td>19</td><td>North Dakota</td><td>27.4</td><td>34</td><td>Iowa</td><td>25.3</td></tr>
<tr><td>8</td><td>Ohio</td><td>30.8</td><td>35</td><td>Wisconsin</td><td>25.2</td></tr>
<tr><td>12</td><td>Oklahoma</td><td>30.4</td><td>36</td><td>Connecticut</td><td>24.9</td></tr>
<tr><td>20</td><td>Oregon</td><td>27.2</td><td>37</td><td>Massachusetts</td><td>24.8</td></tr>
<tr><td>4</td><td>Pennsylvania</td><td>31.3</td><td>38</td><td>Arizona</td><td>24.3</td></tr>
<tr><td>13</td><td>Rhode Island</td><td>29.3</td><td>38</td><td>Nevada</td><td>24.3</td></tr>
<tr><td>11</td><td>South Carolina</td><td>30.7</td><td>40</td><td>Kansas</td><td>24.1</td></tr>
<tr><td>32</td><td>South Dakota</td><td>25.6</td><td>41</td><td>Colorado</td><td>23.8</td></tr>
<tr><td>27</td><td>Tennessee</td><td>25.9</td><td>42</td><td>Georgia</td><td>23.7</td></tr>
<tr><td>46</td><td>Texas</td><td>22.5</td><td>42</td><td>Idaho</td><td>23.7</td></tr>
<tr><td>47</td><td>Utah</td><td>21.4</td><td>44</td><td>Alaska</td><td>23.5</td></tr>
<tr><td>15</td><td>Vermont</td><td>28.6</td><td>45</td><td>New Jersey</td><td>22.7</td></tr>
<tr><td>27</td><td>Virginia</td><td>25.9</td><td>46</td><td>Texas</td><td>22.5</td></tr>
<tr><td>24</td><td>Washington</td><td>26.5</td><td>47</td><td>Utah</td><td>21.4</td></tr>
<tr><td>2</td><td>West Virginia</td><td>33.9</td><td>48</td><td>Hawaii</td><td>21.2</td></tr>
<tr><td>35</td><td>Wisconsin</td><td>25.2</td><td>49</td><td>Minnesota</td><td>20.9</td></tr>
<tr><td>23</td><td>Wyoming</td><td>26.9</td><td>50</td><td>California</td><td>20.3</td></tr>
<tr><td></td><td></td><td></td><td></td><td>District of Columbia</td><td>20.8</td></tr>
</table>

Source: U.S. Department of Health and Human Services, Centers for Disease Control and Prevention
    "2009 Behavioral Risk Factor Surveillance Summary Prevalence Data" (http://apps.nccd.cdc.gov/brfss/)
*Of population 18 years old and older.

Percent of Adults Who Have Been Told They Have Diabetes: 2009

National Median = 8.3% of Adults*

ALPHA ORDER			RANK ORDER		
RANK	STATE	PERCENT	RANK	STATE	PERCENT
2	Alabama	12.3	1	West Virginia	12.4
49	Alaska	5.8	2	Alabama	12.3
25	Arizona	8.4	3	Mississippi	11.6
10	Arkansas	10.1	4	Kentucky	11.5
18	California	9.1	5	Louisiana	11.1
49	Colorado	5.8	6	Oklahoma	11.0
45	Connecticut	6.7	7	Florida	10.7
31	Delaware	8.1	8	South Carolina	10.4
7	Florida	10.7	9	Tennessee	10.3
13	Georgia	9.5	10	Arkansas	10.1
23	Hawaii	8.5	10	Ohio	10.1
32	Idaho	8.0	12	North Carolina	9.6
28	Illinois	8.2	13	Georgia	9.5
14	Indiana	9.3	14	Indiana	9.3
37	Iowa	7.6	14	Maryland	9.3
23	Kansas	8.5	14	Michigan	9.3
4	Kentucky	11.5	14	Texas	9.3
5	Louisiana	11.1	18	California	9.1
26	Maine	8.3	18	Pennsylvania	9.1
14	Maryland	9.3	20	New York	8.9
33	Massachusetts	7.9	21	New Jersey	8.7
14	Michigan	9.3	22	New Mexico	8.6
46	Minnesota	6.4	23	Hawaii	8.5
3	Mississippi	11.6	23	Kansas	8.5
33	Missouri	7.9	25	Arizona	8.4
44	Montana	6.8	26	Maine	8.3
38	Nebraska	7.5	26	Oregon	8.3
33	Nevada	7.9	28	Illinois	8.2
41	New Hampshire	7.1	28	Virginia	8.2
21	New Jersey	8.7	28	Wisconsin	8.2
22	New Mexico	8.6	31	Delaware	8.1
20	New York	8.9	32	Idaho	8.0
12	North Carolina	9.6	33	Massachusetts	7.9
38	North Dakota	7.5	33	Missouri	7.9
10	Ohio	10.1	33	Nevada	7.9
6	Oklahoma	11.0	36	Washington	7.7
26	Oregon	8.3	37	Iowa	7.6
18	Pennsylvania	9.1	38	Nebraska	7.5
42	Rhode Island	7.0	38	North Dakota	7.5
8	South Carolina	10.4	40	South Dakota	7.3
40	South Dakota	7.3	41	New Hampshire	7.1
9	Tennessee	10.3	42	Rhode Island	7.0
14	Texas	9.3	42	Wyoming	7.0
48	Utah	6.1	44	Montana	6.8
47	Vermont	6.2	45	Connecticut	6.7
28	Virginia	8.2	46	Minnesota	6.4
36	Washington	7.7	47	Vermont	6.2
1	West Virginia	12.4	48	Utah	6.1
28	Wisconsin	8.2	49	Alaska	5.8
42	Wyoming	7.0	49	Colorado	5.8
				District of Columbia	7.5

Source: U.S. Department of Health and Human Services, Centers for Disease Control and Prevention
    "2009 Behavioral Risk Factor Surveillance Summary Prevalence Data" (http://apps.nccd.cdc.gov/brfss/)
*Of population 18 years old and older. Does not include pregnancy-related diabetes.

Percent of Adults Reporting Serious Psychological Distress: 2007

National Percent = 11.1% of Population*

ALPHA ORDER				RANK ORDER		
RANK	STATE	PERCENT		RANK	STATE	PERCENT
24	Alabama	11.5		1	West Virginia	14.4
28	Alaska	11.3		2	Oklahoma	14.0
18	Arizona	12.0		3	Tennessee	13.7
5	Arkansas	13.0		4	Kentucky	13.6
47	California	9.8		5	Arkansas	13.0
30	Colorado	11.2		5	Missouri	13.0
45	Connecticut	10.1		7	Indiana	12.8
39	Delaware	10.5		7	Rhode Island	12.8
44	Florida	10.2		9	Louisiana	12.7
16	Georgia	12.1		9	New Mexico	12.7
50	Hawaii	8.2		11	Utah	12.6
24	Idaho	11.5		11	Wyoming	12.6
43	Illinois	10.3		13	Maine	12.5
7	Indiana	12.8		14	North Dakota	12.3
27	Iowa	11.4		15	South Carolina	12.2
22	Kansas	11.9		16	Georgia	12.1
4	Kentucky	13.6		16	Nebraska	12.1
9	Louisiana	12.7		18	Arizona	12.0
13	Maine	12.5		18	Michigan	12.0
48	Maryland	9.7		18	Mississippi	12.0
41	Massachusetts	10.4		18	Nevada	12.0
18	Michigan	12.0		22	Kansas	11.9
35	Minnesota	10.9		23	Vermont	11.8
18	Mississippi	12.0		24	Alabama	11.5
5	Missouri	13.0		24	Idaho	11.5
28	Montana	11.3		24	Ohio	11.5
16	Nebraska	12.1		27	Iowa	11.4
18	Nevada	12.0		28	Alaska	11.3
30	New Hampshire	11.2		28	Montana	11.3
48	New Jersey	9.7		30	Colorado	11.2
9	New Mexico	12.7		30	New Hampshire	11.2
33	New York	11.0		32	Wisconsin	11.1
35	North Carolina	10.9		33	New York	11.0
14	North Dakota	12.3		33	Oregon	11.0
24	Ohio	11.5		35	Minnesota	10.9
2	Oklahoma	14.0		35	North Carolina	10.9
33	Oregon	11.0		35	Virginia	10.9
39	Pennsylvania	10.5		38	Texas	10.7
7	Rhode Island	12.8		39	Delaware	10.5
15	South Carolina	12.2		39	Pennsylvania	10.5
45	South Dakota	10.1		41	Massachusetts	10.4
3	Tennessee	13.7		41	Washington	10.4
38	Texas	10.7		43	Illinois	10.3
11	Utah	12.6		44	Florida	10.2
23	Vermont	11.8		45	Connecticut	10.1
35	Virginia	10.9		45	South Dakota	10.1
41	Washington	10.4		47	California	9.8
1	West Virginia	14.4		48	Maryland	9.7
32	Wisconsin	11.1		48	New Jersey	9.7
11	Wyoming	12.6		50	Hawaii	8.2
					District of Columbia	11.5

Source: U.S. Department of Health and Human Services, Substance Abuse and Mental Health Services Administration
"2006-2007 National Surveys on Drug Use and Health" (June 2009, http://www.oas.samhsa.gov/2k7state/toc.cfm)
*Population 18 years and older. Serious psychological distress was previously referred to as serious mental illness. It is defined as having a diagnosable mental, behavioral, or emotional disorder that resulted in functional impairment that substantially interfered with or limited one or more major life activities.

VI. Providers

Health Care Practitioners and Technicians in 2009 413
Rate of Health Care Practitioners and Technicians
    in 2009 414
Average Annual Wages of Health Care Practitioners and
    Technicians in 2009 415
Physicians in 2009 416
Rate of Physicians in 2009 417
Percent of Physicians Who Are Female: 2009 418
Percent of Physicians under 35 Years Old in 2009 419
Percent of Physicians 65 Years Old and Older in 2009 . . . 420
Physicians in Patient Care in 2009 421
Rate of Physicians in Patient Care in 2009 422
Physicians in Primary Care in 2009 423
Rate of Physicians in Primary Care in 2009 424
Percent of Physicians in Primary Care in 2009 425
Percent of Population Lacking Access to Primary Care
    in 2011 426
Physicians in General/Family Practice in 2009 427
Rate of Physicians in General/Family Practice in 2009 . . . 428
Average Annual Wages of Family and General
    Practitioners in 2009 429
Percent of Physicians Who Are Specialists in 2009 430
Physicians in Medical Specialties in 2009 431
Rate of Nonfederal Physicians in Medical Specialties
    in 2009 432
Physicians in Internal Medicine in 2009 433
Rate of Physicians in Internal Medicine in 2009 434
Physicians in Pediatrics in 2009 435
Rate of Physicians in Pediatrics in 2009 436
Physicians in Surgical Specialties in 2009 437
Rate of Physicians in Surgical Specialties in 2009 438
Average Annual Wages of Surgeons in 2009 439
Physicians in General Surgery in 2009 440
Rate of Physicians in General Surgery in 2009 441
Physicians in Obstetrics and Gynecology in 2009 442
Rate of Physicians in Obstetrics and Gynecology
    in 2009 443
Physicians in Ophthalmology in 2009 444
Rate of Physicians in Ophthalmology in 2009 445
Physicians in Orthopedic Surgery in 2009 446

Rate of Physicians in Orthopedic Surgery in 2009 447
Physicians in Plastic Surgery in 2009 448
Rate of Physicians in Plastic Surgery in 2009 449
Physicians in Other Specialties in 2009 450
Rate of Physicians in Other Specialties in 2009 451
Physicians in Anesthesiology in 2009 452
Rate of Physicians in Anesthesiology in 2009 453
Physicians in Psychiatry in 2009 454
Rate of Physicians in Psychiatry in 2009 455
Percent of Population Lacking Access to Mental Health
    Care in 2011 456
International Medical School Graduates in 2009 457
International Medical School Graduates as a Percent of
    Physicians in 2009 458
Osteopathic Physicians in 2010 459
Rate of Osteopathic Physicians in 2010 460
Podiatrists in 2009 461
Rate of Podiatrists in 2009 462
Average Annual Wages of Podiatrists in 2009 463
Doctors of Chiropractic in 2009 464
Rate of Doctors of Chiropractic in 2009 465
Average Annual Wages of Chiropractors in 2009 466
Physician Assistants in Clinical Practice in 2008 467
Rate of Physician Assistants in Clinical Practice in 2008 . . 468
Average Annual Wages of Physician Assistants in 2009 . . 469
Registered Nurses in 2009 470
Rate of Registered Nurses in 2009 471
Average Annual Wages of Registered Nurses in 2009 472
Licensed Practical and Licensed Vocational Nurses
    in 2009 473
Rate of Licensed Practical and Licensed Vocational
    Nurses in 2009 474
Average Annual Wages of Licensed Practical and
    Licensed Vocational Nurses in 2009 475
Physical Therapists in 2009 476
Rate of Physical Therapists in 2009 477
Average Annual Wages of Physical Therapists in 2009 . . . 478
Dentists in 2008 479
Rate of Dentists in 2008 480
Average Annual Wages of Dentists in 2009 481

Percent of Population Lacking Access to Dental Care
in 2011 482
Pharmacists in 2009 483
Rate of Pharmacists in 2009 484
Average Annual Wages of Pharmacists in 2009 485
Optometrists in 2009 486
Rate of Optometrists in 2009 487
Average Annual Wages of Optometrists in 2009 488
Emergency Medical Technicians and Paramedics
in 2009 489

Rate of Emergency Medical Technicians and Paramedics
in 2009 490
Average Annual Wages of Emergency Medical
Technicians and Paramedics in 2009 491
Employment in Health Care Support Industries in 2009 . . 492
Rate of Employees in Health Care Support Industries
in 2009 493
Average Annual Wages of Employees in Health Care
Support Industries in 2009 494

Health Care Practitioners and Technicians in 2009

National Total = 7,067,620 Practitioners and Technicians*

ALPHA ORDER

RANK	STATE	EMPLOYEES	% of USA
22	Alabama	111,870	1.6%
49	Alaska	13,840	0.2%
21	Arizona	121,640	1.7%
33	Arkansas	68,780	1.0%
1	California	641,610	9.1%
25	Colorado	108,460	1.5%
27	Connecticut	91,990	1.3%
43	Delaware	25,260	0.4%
4	Florida	414,550	5.9%
12	Georgia	191,510	2.7%
44	Hawaii	24,650	0.3%
41	Idaho	29,480	0.4%
7	Illinois	312,800	4.4%
16	Indiana	164,980	2.3%
30	Iowa	75,400	1.1%
31	Kansas	71,470	1.0%
24	Kentucky	109,350	1.5%
23	Louisiana	110,570	1.6%
39	Maine	36,110	0.5%
19	Maryland	143,890	2.0%
10	Massachusetts	220,040	3.1%
8	Michigan	237,600	3.4%
17	Minnesota	151,890	2.1%
32	Mississippi	70,160	1.0%
15	Missouri	167,010	2.4%
46	Montana	23,740	0.3%
34	Nebraska	51,340	0.7%
37	Nevada	42,860	0.6%
40	New Hampshire	34,770	0.5%
11	New Jersey	193,150	2.7%
38	New Mexico	40,040	0.6%
3	New York	459,630	6.5%
9	North Carolina	221,190	3.1%
47	North Dakota	19,420	0.3%
6	Ohio	312,860	4.4%
28	Oklahoma	86,620	1.2%
29	Oregon	79,580	1.1%
5	Pennsylvania	346,200	4.9%
42	Rhode Island	29,030	0.4%
26	South Carolina	100,160	1.4%
45	South Dakota	24,540	0.3%
14	Tennessee	170,490	2.4%
2	Texas	503,280	7.1%
35	Utah	50,750	0.7%
48	Vermont	16,230	0.2%
13	Virginia	173,270	2.5%
20	Washington	139,150	2.0%
36	West Virginia	49,060	0.7%
18	Wisconsin	149,600	2.1%
50	Wyoming	12,420	0.2%

RANK ORDER

RANK	STATE	EMPLOYEES	% of USA
1	California	641,610	9.1%
2	Texas	503,280	7.1%
3	New York	459,630	6.5%
4	Florida	414,550	5.9%
5	Pennsylvania	346,200	4.9%
6	Ohio	312,860	4.4%
7	Illinois	312,800	4.4%
8	Michigan	237,600	3.4%
9	North Carolina	221,190	3.1%
10	Massachusetts	220,040	3.1%
11	New Jersey	193,150	2.7%
12	Georgia	191,510	2.7%
13	Virginia	173,270	2.5%
14	Tennessee	170,490	2.4%
15	Missouri	167,010	2.4%
16	Indiana	164,980	2.3%
17	Minnesota	151,890	2.1%
18	Wisconsin	149,600	2.1%
19	Maryland	143,890	2.0%
20	Washington	139,150	2.0%
21	Arizona	121,640	1.7%
22	Alabama	111,870	1.6%
23	Louisiana	110,570	1.6%
24	Kentucky	109,350	1.5%
25	Colorado	108,460	1.5%
26	South Carolina	100,160	1.4%
27	Connecticut	91,990	1.3%
28	Oklahoma	86,620	1.2%
29	Oregon	79,580	1.1%
30	Iowa	75,400	1.1%
31	Kansas	71,470	1.0%
32	Mississippi	70,160	1.0%
33	Arkansas	68,780	1.0%
34	Nebraska	51,340	0.7%
35	Utah	50,750	0.7%
36	West Virginia	49,060	0.7%
37	Nevada	42,860	0.6%
38	New Mexico	40,040	0.6%
39	Maine	36,110	0.5%
40	New Hampshire	34,770	0.5%
41	Idaho	29,480	0.4%
42	Rhode Island	29,030	0.4%
43	Delaware	25,260	0.4%
44	Hawaii	24,650	0.3%
45	South Dakota	24,540	0.3%
46	Montana	23,740	0.3%
47	North Dakota	19,420	0.3%
48	Vermont	16,230	0.2%
49	Alaska	13,840	0.2%
50	Wyoming	12,420	0.2%
	District of Columbia	25,230	0.4%

Source: U.S. Department of Labor, Bureau of Labor Statistics
"Occupational Employment and Wages, 2009" (http://www.bls.gov/oes/)
*Does not include self-employed. Includes various doctors, dentists, nurses, therapists, optometrists, paramedics, and technicians. Does not include assistants and aides listed under health care support occupations. Veterinarians and veterinarian technicians have been subtracted from the totals.

Rate of Health Care Practitioners and Technicians in 2009

National Rate = 2,302 Practitioners and Technicians per 100,000 Population*

ALPHA ORDER

RANK	STATE	RATE
29	Alabama	2,376
43	Alaska	1,981
47	Arizona	1,844
27	Arkansas	2,380
49	California	1,736
38	Colorado	2,159
16	Connecticut	2,615
6	Delaware	2,854
34	Florida	2,236
44	Georgia	1,948
46	Hawaii	1,903
45	Idaho	1,907
25	Illinois	2,423
18	Indiana	2,569
22	Iowa	2,507
19	Kansas	2,536
20	Kentucky	2,535
23	Louisiana	2,461
10	Maine	2,739
21	Maryland	2,525
1	Massachusetts	3,337
26	Michigan	2,383
4	Minnesota	2,884
28	Mississippi	2,377
7	Missouri	2,789
24	Montana	2,435
5	Nebraska	2,858
50	Nevada	1,622
15	New Hampshire	2,625
35	New Jersey	2,218
42	New Mexico	1,992
31	New York	2,352
30	North Carolina	2,358
3	North Dakota	3,002
11	Ohio	2,710
32	Oklahoma	2,349
40	Oregon	2,080
9	Pennsylvania	2,747
8	Rhode Island	2,756
37	South Carolina	2,196
2	South Dakota	3,021
12	Tennessee	2,708
41	Texas	2,031
48	Utah	1,823
17	Vermont	2,610
36	Virginia	2,198
39	Washington	2,088
13	West Virginia	2,696
14	Wisconsin	2,646
33	Wyoming	2,282

RANK ORDER

RANK	STATE	RATE
1	Massachusetts	3,337
2	South Dakota	3,021
3	North Dakota	3,002
4	Minnesota	2,884
5	Nebraska	2,858
6	Delaware	2,854
7	Missouri	2,789
8	Rhode Island	2,756
9	Pennsylvania	2,747
10	Maine	2,739
11	Ohio	2,710
12	Tennessee	2,708
13	West Virginia	2,696
14	Wisconsin	2,646
15	New Hampshire	2,625
16	Connecticut	2,615
17	Vermont	2,610
18	Indiana	2,569
19	Kansas	2,536
20	Kentucky	2,535
21	Maryland	2,525
22	Iowa	2,507
23	Louisiana	2,461
24	Montana	2,435
25	Illinois	2,423
26	Michigan	2,383
27	Arkansas	2,380
28	Mississippi	2,377
29	Alabama	2,376
30	North Carolina	2,358
31	New York	2,352
32	Oklahoma	2,349
33	Wyoming	2,282
34	Florida	2,236
35	New Jersey	2,218
36	Virginia	2,198
37	South Carolina	2,196
38	Colorado	2,159
39	Washington	2,088
40	Oregon	2,080
41	Texas	2,031
42	New Mexico	1,992
43	Alaska	1,981
44	Georgia	1,948
45	Idaho	1,907
46	Hawaii	1,903
47	Arizona	1,844
48	Utah	1,823
49	California	1,736
50	Nevada	1,622

District of Columbia   4,207

Source: CQ Press using data from U.S. Department of Labor, Bureau of Labor Statistics
   "Occupational Employment and Wages, 2009" (http://www.bls.gov/oes/)
*Does not include self-employed. Includes various doctors, dentists, nurses, therapists, optometrists, paramedics, and technicians. Does not include assistants and aides listed under health care support occupations. Veterinarians and veterinarian technicians have been subtracted from the totals.

Average Annual Wages of Health Care Practitioners and Technicians in 2009

National Average = $69,690*

ALPHA ORDER				RANK ORDER		
RANK	STATE	WAGES		RANK	STATE	WAGES
43	Alabama	$59,740		1	Hawaii	$83,150
9	Alaska	77,100		2	California	82,880
19	Arizona	69,890		3	New Jersey	80,580
41	Arkansas	60,150		4	Maryland	80,490
2	California	82,880		5	Nevada	79,510
15	Colorado	71,520		6	Massachusetts	78,390
10	Connccticut	76,310		7	Oregon	77,990
13	Delaware	75,360		8	New York	77,460
26	Florida	66,410		9	Alaska	77,100
33	Georgia	65,060		10	Connecticut	76,310
1	Hawaii	83,150		11	Minnesota	76,220
31	Idaho	65,200		12	Washington	76,070
24	Illinois	68,000		13	Delaware	75,360
34	Indiana	63,390		14	Rhode Island	71,820
45	Iowa	58,780		15	Colorado	71,520
36	Kansas	62,370		16	New Hampshire	71,470
38	Kentucky	61,280		17	Maine	70,760
41	Louisiana	60,150		18	Wisconsin	70,610
17	Maine	70,760		19	Arizona	69,890
4	Maryland	80,490		20	Vermont	69,500
6	Massachusetts	78,390		21	New Mexico	69,230
22	Michigan	69,070		22	Michigan	69,070
11	Minnesota	76,220		23	Virginia	68,960
47	Mississippi	57,920		24	Illinois	68,000
44	Missouri	59,550		25	Wyoming	66,850
37	Montana	62,210		26	Florida	66,410
40	Nebraska	60,310		27	Ohio	66,170
5	Nevada	79,510		28	North Carolina	65,890
16	New Hampshire	71,470		29	Texas	65,820
3	New Jersey	80,580		30	Utah	65,600
21	New Mexico	69,230		31	Idaho	65,200
8	New York	77,460		32	Pennsylvania	65,100
28	North Carolina	65,890		33	Georgia	65,060
46	North Dakota	58,470		34	Indiana	63,390
27	Ohio	66,170		35	South Carolina	63,250
50	Oklahoma	57,550		36	Kansas	62,370
7	Oregon	77,990		37	Montana	62,210
32	Pennsylvania	65,100		38	Kentucky	61,280
14	Rhode Island	71,820		39	Tcnnessee	60,860
35	South Carolina	63,250		40	Nebraska	60,310
48	South Dakota	57,790		41	Arkansas	60,150
39	Tennessee	60,860		41	Louisiana	60,150
29	Texas	65,820		43	Alabama	59,740
30	Utah	65,600		44	Missouri	59,550
20	Vermont	69,500		45	Iowa	58,780
23	Virginia	68,960		46	North Dakota	58,470
12	Washington	76,070		47	Mississippi	57,920
49	West Virginia	57,670		48	South Dakota	57,790
18	Wisconsin	70,610		49	West Virginia	57,670
25	Wyoming	66,850		50	Oklahoma	57,550
					District of Columbia	76,990

Source: U.S. Department of Labor, Bureau of Labor Statistics
   "Occupational Employment and Wages, 2009" (http://www.bls.gov/oes/)
*Does not include self-employed. Includes various doctors, dentists, nurses, therapists, optometrists, paramedics, and
technicians. Does not include assistants and aides listed under health care support occupations.

Physicians in 2009

National Total = 958,335 Physicians*

ALPHA ORDER

ALPHA ORDER

RANK	STATE	PHYSICIANS	% of USA
27	Alabama	11,507	1.2%
49	Alaska	1,769	0.2%
19	Arizona	16,608	1.7%
31	Arkansas	6,749	0.7%
1	California	116,489	12.2%
22	Colorado	15,222	1.6%
23	Connecticut	15,170	1.6%
46	Delaware	2,488	0.3%
4	Florida	57,066	6.0%
14	Georgia	24,092	2.5%
39	Hawaii	4,800	0.5%
43	Idaho	3,159	0.3%
6	Illinois	40,963	4.3%
21	Indiana	15,790	1.6%
33	Iowa	6,591	0.7%
30	Kansas	7,474	0.8%
28	Kentucky	11,325	1.2%
24	Louisiana	13,323	1.4%
42	Maine	4,380	0.5%
12	Maryland	27,153	2.8%
8	Massachusetts	34,612	3.6%
10	Michigan	29,133	3.0%
17	Minnesota	17,767	1.9%
34	Mississippi	6,078	0.6%
20	Missouri	16,445	1.7%
45	Montana	2,641	0.3%
37	Nebraska	5,143	0.5%
35	Nevada	5,829	0.6%
41	New Hampshire	4,515	0.5%
9	New Jersey	31,081	3.2%
36	New Mexico	5,688	0.6%
2	New York	86,506	9.0%
11	North Carolina	27,407	2.9%
48	North Dakota	1,831	0.2%
7	Ohio	35,465	3.7%
29	Oklahoma	7,476	0.8%
25	Oregon	12,777	1.3%
5	Pennsylvania	44,336	4.6%
40	Rhode Island	4,530	0.5%
26	South Carolina	11,928	1.2%
47	South Dakota	2,104	0.2%
16	Tennessee	18,839	2.0%
3	Texas	59,482	6.2%
32	Utah	6,701	0.7%
44	Vermont	2,750	0.3%
13	Virginia	25,291	2.6%
15	Washington	21,337	2.2%
38	West Virginia	4,894	0.5%
18	Wisconsin	17,024	1.8%
50	Wyoming	1,235	0.1%

RANK ORDER

RANK	STATE	PHYSICIANS	% of USA
1	California	116,489	12.2%
2	New York	86,506	9.0%
3	Texas	59,482	6.2%
4	Florida	57,066	6.0%
5	Pennsylvania	44,336	4.6%
6	Illinois	40,963	4.3%
7	Ohio	35,465	3.7%
8	Massachusetts	34,612	3.6%
9	New Jersey	31,081	3.2%
10	Michigan	29,133	3.0%
11	North Carolina	27,407	2.9%
12	Maryland	27,153	2.8%
13	Virginia	25,291	2.6%
14	Georgia	24,092	2.5%
15	Washington	21,337	2.2%
16	Tennessee	18,839	2.0%
17	Minnesota	17,767	1.9%
18	Wisconsin	17,024	1.8%
19	Arizona	16,608	1.7%
20	Missouri	16,445	1.7%
21	Indiana	15,790	1.6%
22	Colorado	15,222	1.6%
23	Connecticut	15,170	1.6%
24	Louisiana	13,323	1.4%
25	Oregon	12,777	1.3%
26	South Carolina	11,928	1.2%
27	Alabama	11,507	1.2%
28	Kentucky	11,325	1.2%
29	Oklahoma	7,476	0.8%
30	Kansas	7,474	0.8%
31	Arkansas	6,749	0.7%
32	Utah	6,701	0.7%
33	Iowa	6,591	0.7%
34	Mississippi	6,078	0.6%
35	Nevada	5,829	0.6%
36	New Mexico	5,688	0.6%
37	Nebraska	5,143	0.5%
38	West Virginia	4,894	0.5%
39	Hawaii	4,800	0.5%
40	Rhode Island	4,530	0.5%
41	New Hampshire	4,515	0.5%
42	Maine	4,380	0.5%
43	Idaho	3,159	0.3%
44	Vermont	2,750	0.3%
45	Montana	2,641	0.3%
46	Delaware	2,488	0.3%
47	South Dakota	2,104	0.2%
48	North Dakota	1,831	0.2%
49	Alaska	1,769	0.2%
50	Wyoming	1,235	0.1%
	District of Columbia	5,372	0.6%

Source: American Medical Association (Chicago, Illinois)
   "Physician Characteristics and Distribution in the U.S." (2011 Edition)
*As of December 31, 2009. Total does not include 14,041 physicians in the U.S. territories and possessions, at APOs and FPOs, or whose addresses are unknown.

Rate of Physicians in 2009

National Rate = 312 Physicians per 100,000 Population*

ALPHA ORDER

RANK	STATE	RATE
41	Alabama	244
37	Alaska	253
38	Arizona	252
44	Arkansas	234
17	California	315
20	Colorado	303
5	Connecticut	431
29	Delaware	281
18	Florida	308
40	Georgia	245
7	Hawaii	371
49	Idaho	204
16	Illinois	317
39	Indiana	246
47	Iowa	219
33	Kansas	265
34	Kentucky	263
23	Louisiana	297
13	Maine	332
2	Maryland	476
1	Massachusetts	525
24	Michigan	292
11	Minnesota	337
48	Mississippi	206
30	Missouri	275
31	Montana	271
26	Nebraska	286
46	Nevada	221
10	New Hampshire	341
8	New Jersey	357
27	New Mexico	283
3	New York	443
24	North Carolina	292
27	North Dakota	283
19	Ohio	307
50	Oklahoma	203
12	Oregon	334
9	Pennsylvania	352
6	Rhode Island	430
35	South Carolina	262
36	South Dakota	259
22	Tennessee	299
43	Texas	240
42	Utah	241
4	Vermont	442
14	Virginia	321
15	Washington	320
32	West Virginia	269
21	Wisconsin	301
45	Wyoming	227

RANK ORDER

RANK	STATE	RATE
1	Massachusetts	525
2	Maryland	476
3	New York	443
4	Vermont	442
5	Connecticut	431
6	Rhode Island	430
7	Hawaii	371
8	New Jersey	357
9	Pennsylvania	352
10	New Hampshire	341
11	Minnesota	337
12	Oregon	334
13	Maine	332
14	Virginia	321
15	Washington	320
16	Illinois	317
17	California	315
18	Florida	308
19	Ohio	307
20	Colorado	303
21	Wisconsin	301
22	Tennessee	299
23	Louisiana	297
24	Michigan	292
24	North Carolina	292
26	Nebraska	286
27	New Mexico	283
27	North Dakota	283
29	Delaware	281
30	Missouri	275
31	Montana	271
32	West Virginia	269
33	Kansas	265
34	Kentucky	263
35	South Carolina	262
36	South Dakota	259
37	Alaska	253
38	Arizona	252
39	Indiana	246
40	Georgia	245
41	Alabama	244
42	Utah	241
43	Texas	240
44	Arkansas	234
45	Wyoming	227
46	Nevada	221
47	Iowa	219
48	Mississippi	206
49	Idaho	204
50	Oklahoma	203

	District of Columbia	896

Source: CQ Press using data from American Medical Association (Chicago, Illinois)
"Physician Characteristics and Distribution in the U.S." (2011 Edition)
*As of December 31, 2009. National rate does not include physicians in the U.S. territories and possessions, at APOs and FPOs, or whose addresses are unknown.

Percent of Physicians Who Are Female: 2009

National Percent = 29.5% of Physicians*

ALPHA ORDER

RANK	STATE	PERCENT
41	Alabama	23.6
9	Alaska	31.9
30	Arizona	26.7
42	Arkansas	23.5
14	California	30.1
13	Colorado	30.7
11	Connecticut	31.3
10	Delaware	31.5
45	Florida	23.2
25	Georgia	28.6
23	Hawaii	28.7
50	Idaho	19.6
5	Illinois	33.5
31	Indiana	26.6
36	Iowa	24.6
29	Kansas	26.9
33	Kentucky	26.0
32	Louisiana	26.3
28	Maine	27.9
2	Maryland	34.2
1	Massachusetts	36.0
14	Michigan	30.1
17	Minnesota	30.0
49	Mississippi	21.1
23	Missouri	28.7
46	Montana	23.1
33	Nebraska	26.0
38	Nevada	24.0
26	New Hampshire	28.4
7	New Jersey	32.7
6	New Mexico	32.9
4	New York	33.7
22	North Carolina	28.8
42	North Dakota	23.5
20	Ohio	29.5
40	Oklahoma	23.7
18	Oregon	29.9
14	Pennsylvania	30.1
3	Rhode Island	33.8
36	South Carolina	24.6
44	South Dakota	23.3
35	Tennessee	24.9
21	Texas	29.0
48	Utah	21.4
8	Vermont	32.4
12	Virginia	31.1
19	Washington	29.6
39	West Virginia	23.9
27	Wisconsin	28.1
47	Wyoming	22.0

RANK ORDER

RANK	STATE	PERCENT
1	Massachusetts	36.0
2	Maryland	34.2
3	Rhode Island	33.8
4	New York	33.7
5	Illinois	33.5
6	New Mexico	32.9
7	New Jersey	32.7
8	Vermont	32.4
9	Alaska	31.9
10	Delaware	31.5
11	Connecticut	31.3
12	Virginia	31.1
13	Colorado	30.7
14	California	30.1
14	Michigan	30.1
14	Pennsylvania	30.1
17	Minnesota	30.0
18	Oregon	29.9
19	Washington	29.6
20	Ohio	29.5
21	Texas	29.0
22	North Carolina	28.8
23	Hawaii	28.7
23	Missouri	28.7
25	Georgia	28.6
26	New Hampshire	28.4
27	Wisconsin	28.1
28	Maine	27.9
29	Kansas	26.9
30	Arizona	26.7
31	Indiana	26.6
32	Louisiana	26.3
33	Kentucky	26.0
33	Nebraska	26.0
35	Tennessee	24.9
36	Iowa	24.6
36	South Carolina	24.6
38	Nevada	24.0
39	West Virginia	23.9
40	Oklahoma	23.7
41	Alabama	23.6
42	Arkansas	23.5
42	North Dakota	23.5
44	South Dakota	23.3
45	Florida	23.2
46	Montana	23.1
47	Wyoming	22.0
48	Utah	21.4
49	Mississippi	21.1
50	Idaho	19.6

	District of Columbia	39.4

Source: CQ Press using data from American Medical Association (Chicago, Illinois)
"Physician Characteristics and Distribution in the U.S." (2011 Edition)

*As of December 31, 2009. National percent does not include physicians in the U.S. territories and possessions, at APOs and FPOs, or whose addresses are unknown.

Percent of Physicians under 35 Years Old in 2009

National Percent = 15.0% of Physicians*

ALPHA ORDER

RANK	STATE	PERCENT
17	Alabama	15.0
47	Alaska	7.2
37	Arizona	11.2
23	Arkansas	14.5
33	California	12.2
40	Colorado	11.0
11	Connecticut	10.5
27	Delaware	13.4
44	Florida	9.4
31	Georgia	12.8
39	Hawaii	11.1
48	Idaho	6.2
5	Illinois	19.1
29	Indiana	13.2
23	Iowa	14.5
21	Kansas	14.6
16	Kentucky	15.1
10	Louisiana	17.2
46	Maine	7.5
17	Maryland	15.0
6	Massachusetts	19.0
4	Michigan	19.2
13	Minnesota	15.8
34	Mississippi	12.0
1	Missouri	19.6
50	Montana	4.5
9	Nebraska	18.4
45	Nevada	8.3
37	New Hampshire	11.2
30	New Jersey	12.9
36	New Mexico	11.3
1	New York	19.6
15	North Carolina	15.4
35	North Dakota	11.7
7	Ohio	18.6
27	Oklahoma	13.4
42	Oregon	10.6
8	Pennsylvania	18.5
1	Rhode Island	19.6
19	South Carolina	14.7
43	South Dakota	9.7
19	Tennessee	14.7
12	Texas	16.2
21	Utah	14.6
32	Vermont	12.3
26	Virginia	13.9
41	Washington	10.9
14	West Virginia	15.7
25	Wisconsin	14.1
49	Wyoming	5.5

RANK ORDER

RANK	STATE	PERCENT
1	Missouri	19.6
1	New York	19.6
1	Rhode Island	19.6
4	Michigan	19.2
5	Illinois	19.1
6	Massachusetts	19.0
7	Ohio	18.6
8	Pennsylvania	18.5
9	Nebraska	18.4
10	Louisiana	17.2
11	Connecticut	16.5
12	Texas	16.2
13	Minnesota	15.8
14	West Virginia	15.7
15	North Carolina	15.4
16	Kentucky	15.1
17	Alabama	15.0
17	Maryland	15.0
19	South Carolina	14.7
19	Tennessee	14.7
21	Kansas	14.6
21	Utah	14.6
23	Arkansas	14.5
23	Iowa	14.5
25	Wisconsin	14.1
26	Virginia	13.9
27	Delaware	13.4
27	Oklahoma	13.4
29	Indiana	13.2
30	New Jersey	12.9
31	Georgia	12.8
32	Vermont	12.3
33	California	12.2
34	Mississippi	12.0
35	North Dakota	11.7
36	New Mexico	11.3
37	Arizona	11.2
37	New Hampshire	11.2
39	Hawaii	11.1
40	Colorado	11.0
41	Washington	10.9
42	Oregon	10.6
43	South Dakota	9.7
44	Florida	9.4
45	Nevada	8.3
46	Maine	7.5
47	Alaska	7.2
48	Idaho	6.2
49	Wyoming	5.5
50	Montana	4.5
	District of Columbia	26.2

Source: CQ Press using data from American Medical Association (Chicago, Illinois)
"Physician Characteristics and Distribution in the U.S." (2011 Edition)
*As of December 31, 2009. National percent does not include physicians in the U.S. territories and possessions, at APOs and FPOs, or whose addresses are unknown.

Percent of Physicians 65 Years Old and Older in 2009

National Percent = 20.7% of Physicians*

ALPHA ORDER

RANK	STATE	PERCENT
37	Alabama	18.1
50	Alaska	16.7
9	Arizona	22.5
29	Arkansas	19.6
3	California	24.7
24	Colorado	20.4
23	Connecticut	20.8
15	Delaware	21.5
1	Florida	27.3
38	Georgia	18.0
6	Hawaii	23.6
12	Idaho	21.8
35	Illinois	18.5
40	Indiana	17.7
31	Iowa	19.1
19	Kansas	21.2
40	Kentucky	17.7
33	Louisiana	18.8
4	Maine	24.6
19	Maryland	21.2
38	Massachusetts	18.0
30	Michigan	19.5
48	Minnesota	17.4
22	Mississippi	20.9
48	Missouri	17.4
2	Montana	26.3
45	Nebraska	17.6
10	Nevada	22.3
16	New Hampshire	21.4
17	New Jersey	21.3
14	New Mexico	21.7
17	New York	21.3
40	North Carolina	17.7
40	North Dakota	17.7
34	Ohio	18.6
21	Oklahoma	21.1
11	Oregon	21.9
26	Pennsylvania	20.0
26	Rhode Island	20.0
28	South Carolina	19.7
31	South Dakota	19.1
45	Tennessee	17.6
45	Texas	17.6
40	Utah	17.7
5	Vermont	23.9
25	Virginia	20.2
12	Washington	21.8
8	West Virginia	22.7
36	Wisconsin	18.3
7	Wyoming	23.4

RANK ORDER

RANK	STATE	PERCENT
1	Florida	27.3
2	Montana	26.3
3	California	24.7
4	Maine	24.6
5	Vermont	23.9
6	Hawaii	23.6
7	Wyoming	23.4
8	West Virginia	22.7
9	Arizona	22.5
10	Nevada	22.3
11	Oregon	21.9
12	Idaho	21.8
12	Washington	21.8
14	New Mexico	21.7
15	Delaware	21.5
16	New Hampshire	21.4
17	New Jersey	21.3
17	New York	21.3
19	Kansas	21.2
19	Maryland	21.2
21	Oklahoma	21.1
22	Mississippi	20.9
23	Connecticut	20.8
24	Colorado	20.4
25	Virginia	20.2
26	Pennsylvania	20.0
26	Rhode Island	20.0
28	South Carolina	19.7
29	Arkansas	19.6
30	Michigan	19.5
31	Iowa	19.1
31	South Dakota	19.1
33	Louisiana	18.8
34	Ohio	18.6
35	Illinois	18.5
36	Wisconsin	18.3
37	Alabama	18.1
38	Georgia	18.0
38	Massachusetts	18.0
40	Indiana	17.7
40	Kentucky	17.7
40	North Carolina	17.7
40	North Dakota	17.7
40	Utah	17.7
45	Nebraska	17.6
45	Tennessee	17.6
45	Texas	17.6
48	Minnesota	17.4
48	Missouri	17.4
50	Alaska	16.7

District of Columbia 20.8

Source: CQ Press using data from American Medical Association (Chicago, Illinois)
"Physician Characteristics and Distribution in the U.S." (2011 Edition)
*As of December 31, 2009. National percent does not include physicians in the U.S. territories and possessions, at APOs and FPOs, or whose addresses are unknown.

Physicians in Patient Care in 2009

National Total = 739,218 Physicians*

RANK	STATE	PHYSICIANS	% of USA
27	Alabama	9,347	1.3%
49	Alaska	1,461	0.2%
21	Arizona	12,620	1.7%
31	Arkansas	5,408	0.7%
1	California	87,943	11.9%
22	Colorado	11,781	1.6%
23	Connecticut	11,604	1.6%
46	Delaware	1,969	0.3%
4	Florida	42,403	5.7%
14	Georgia	19,013	2.6%
39	Hawaii	3,690	0.5%
43	Idaho	2,516	0.3%
6	Illinois	32,001	4.3%
20	Indiana	12,863	1.7%
33	Iowa	5,069	0.7%
30	Kansas	5,835	0.8%
28	Kentucky	9,189	1.2%
24	Louisiana	10,789	1.5%
42	Maine	3,311	0.4%
13	Maryland	19,647	2.7%
8	Massachusetts	25,667	3.5%
10	Michigan	22,735	3.1%
17	Minnesota	13,938	1.9%
34	Mississippi	4,871	0.7%
19	Missouri	13,017	1.8%
44	Montana	2,026	0.3%
37	Nebraska	4,088	0.6%
35	Nevada	4,548	0.6%
41	New Hampshire	3,469	0.5%
9	New Jersey	24,147	3.3%
36	New Mexico	4,299	0.6%
2	New York	65,676	8.9%
11	North Carolina	21,365	2.9%
48	North Dakota	1,512	0.2%
7	Ohio	27,586	3.7%
29	Oklahoma	5,954	0.8%
25	Oregon	9,609	1.3%
5	Pennsylvania	33,434	4.5%
40	Rhode Island	3,498	0.5%
26	South Carolina	9,559	1.3%
47	South Dakota	1,717	0.2%
16	Tennessee	15,167	2.1%
3	Texas	47,715	6.5%
32	Utah	5,219	0.7%
45	Vermont	2,025	0.3%
12	Virginia	19,651	2.7%
15	Washington	16,077	2.2%
38	West Virginia	3,841	0.5%
18	Wisconsin	13,518	1.8%
50	Wyoming	970	0.1%

RANK	STATE	PHYSICIANS	% of USA
1	California	87,943	11.9%
2	New York	65,676	8.9%
3	Texas	47,715	6.5%
4	Florida	42,403	5.7%
5	Pennsylvania	33,434	4.5%
6	Illinois	32,001	4.3%
7	Ohio	27,586	3.7%
8	Massachusetts	25,667	3.5%
9	New Jersey	24,147	3.3%
10	Michigan	22,735	3.1%
11	North Carolina	21,365	2.9%
12	Virginia	19,651	2.7%
13	Maryland	19,647	2.7%
14	Georgia	19,013	2.6%
15	Washington	16,077	2.2%
16	Tennessee	15,167	2.1%
17	Minnesota	13,938	1.9%
18	Wisconsin	13,518	1.8%
19	Missouri	13,017	1.8%
20	Indiana	12,863	1.7%
21	Arizona	12,620	1.7%
22	Colorado	11,781	1.6%
23	Connecticut	11,604	1.6%
24	Louisiana	10,789	1.5%
25	Oregon	9,609	1.3%
26	South Carolina	9,559	1.3%
27	Alabama	9,347	1.3%
28	Kentucky	9,189	1.2%
29	Oklahoma	5,954	0.8%
30	Kansas	5,835	0.8%
31	Arkansas	5,408	0.7%
32	Utah	5,219	0.7%
33	Iowa	5,069	0.7%
34	Mississippi	4,871	0.7%
35	Nevada	4,548	0.6%
36	New Mexico	4,299	0.6%
37	Nebraska	4,088	0.6%
38	West Virginia	3,841	0.5%
39	Hawaii	3,690	0.5%
40	Rhode Island	3,498	0.5%
41	New Hampshire	3,469	0.5%
42	Maine	3,311	0.4%
43	Idaho	2,516	0.3%
44	Montana	2,026	0.3%
45	Vermont	2,025	0.3%
46	Delaware	1,969	0.3%
47	South Dakota	1,717	0.2%
48	North Dakota	1,512	0.2%
49	Alaska	1,461	0.2%
50	Wyoming	970	0.1%
	District of Columbia	3,861	0.5%

Source: American Medical Association (Chicago, Illinois)
"Physician Characteristics and Distribution in the U.S." (2011 Edition)
*As of December 31, 2009. Total does not include 10,348 physicians in U.S. territories and possessions.

Rate of Physicians in Patient Care in 2009

National Rate = 241 Physicians per 100,000 Population*

ALPHA ORDER

RANK	STATE	RATE
39	Alabama	199
35	Alaska	209
42	Arizona	191
43	Arkansas	187
21	California	238
22	Colorado	234
5	Connecticut	330
28	Delaware	222
24	Florida	229
40	Georgia	193
7	Hawaii	285
49	Idaho	163
15	Illinois	248
38	Indiana	200
47	Iowa	169
37	Kansas	207
31	Kentucky	213
18	Louisiana	240
12	Maine	251
2	Maryland	345
1	Massachusetts	389
25	Michigan	228
9	Minnesota	265
48	Mississippi	165
29	Missouri	217
36	Montana	208
25	Nebraska	228
46	Nevada	172
11	New Hampshire	262
8	New Jersey	277
30	New Mexico	214
3	New York	336
25	North Carolina	228
22	North Dakota	234
19	Ohio	239
50	Oklahoma	161
12	Oregon	251
9	Pennsylvania	265
4	Rhode Island	332
34	South Carolina	210
32	South Dakota	211
16	Tennessee	241
40	Texas	193
43	Utah	187
6	Vermont	326
14	Virginia	249
16	Washington	241
32	West Virginia	211
19	Wisconsin	239
45	Wyoming	178

RANK ORDER

RANK	STATE	RATE
1	Massachusetts	389
2	Maryland	345
3	New York	336
4	Rhode Island	332
5	Connecticut	330
6	Vermont	326
7	Hawaii	285
8	New Jersey	277
9	Minnesota	265
9	Pennsylvania	265
11	New Hampshire	262
12	Maine	251
12	Oregon	251
14	Virginia	249
15	Illinois	248
16	Tennessee	241
16	Washington	241
18	Louisiana	240
19	Ohio	239
19	Wisconsin	239
21	California	238
22	Colorado	234
22	North Dakota	234
24	Florida	229
25	Michigan	228
25	Nebraska	228
25	North Carolina	228
28	Delaware	222
29	Missouri	217
30	New Mexico	214
31	Kentucky	213
32	South Dakota	211
32	West Virginia	211
34	South Carolina	210
35	Alaska	209
36	Montana	208
37	Kansas	207
38	Indiana	200
39	Alabama	199
40	Georgia	193
40	Texas	193
42	Arizona	191
43	Arkansas	187
43	Utah	187
45	Wyoming	178
46	Nevada	172
47	Iowa	169
48	Mississippi	165
49	Idaho	163
50	Oklahoma	161

| | District of Columbia | 644 |

Source: CQ Press using data from American Medical Association (Chicago, Illinois)
"Physician Characteristics and Distribution in the U.S." (2011 Edition)
*As of December 31, 2009. National rate does not include physicians in the U.S. territories and possessions.

Physicians in Primary Care in 2009

National Total = 302,266 Physicians*

ALPHA ORDER				RANK ORDER			
RANK	STATE	PHYSICIANS	% of USA	RANK	STATE	PHYSICIANS	% of USA
27	Alabama	3,912	1.3%	1	California	36,852	12.2%
49	Alaska	705	0.2%	2	New York	26,180	8.7%
20	Arizona	5,019	1.7%	3	Texas	19,044	6.3%
31	Arkansas	2,392	0.8%	4	Florida	16,377	5.4%
1	California	36,852	12.2%	5	Illinois	13,775	4.6%
22	Colorado	4,811	1.6%	6	Pennsylvania	12,573	4.2%
23	Connecticut	4,599	1.5%	7	Ohio	11,199	3.7%
47	Delaware	745	0.2%	8	New Jersey	9,930	3.3%
4	Florida	16,377	5.4%	9	Michigan	9,546	3.2%
13	Georgia	8,180	2.7%	10	Massachusetts	9,501	3.1%
38	Hawaii	1,637	0.5%	11	North Carolina	8,759	2.9%
43	Idaho	1,061	0.4%	12	Virginia	8,323	2.8%
5	Illinois	13,775	4.6%	13	Georgia	8,180	2.7%
19	Indiana	5,375	1.8%	14	Maryland	7,860	2.6%
32	Iowa	2,158	0.7%	15	Washington	6,911	2.3%
30	Kansas	2,411	0.8%	16	Tennessee	6,185	2.0%
28	Kentucky	3,673	1.2%	17	Minnesota	6,002	2.0%
24	Louisiana	4,343	1.4%	18	Wisconsin	5,720	1.9%
41	Maine	1,458	0.5%	19	Indiana	5,375	1.8%
14	Maryland	7,860	2.6%	20	Arizona	5,019	1.7%
10	Massachusetts	9,501	3.1%	21	Missouri	5,018	1.7%
9	Michigan	9,546	3.2%	22	Colorado	4,811	1.6%
17	Minnesota	6,002	2.0%	23	Connecticut	4,599	1.5%
34	Mississippi	2,031	0.7%	24	Louisiana	4,343	1.4%
21	Missouri	5,018	1.7%	25	Oregon	4,155	1.4%
45	Montana	851	0.3%	26	South Carolina	4,016	1.3%
37	Nebraska	1,812	0.6%	27	Alabama	3,912	1.3%
36	Nevada	1,894	0.6%	28	Kentucky	3,673	1.2%
40	New Hampshire	1,464	0.5%	29	Oklahoma	2,496	0.8%
8	New Jersey	9,930	3.3%	30	Kansas	2,411	0.8%
35	New Mexico	1,932	0.6%	31	Arkansas	2,392	0.8%
2	New York	26,180	8.7%	32	Iowa	2,158	0.7%
11	North Carolina	8,759	2.9%	33	Utah	2,048	0.7%
48	North Dakota	706	0.2%	34	Mississippi	2,031	0.7%
7	Ohio	11,199	3.7%	35	New Mexico	1,932	0.6%
29	Oklahoma	2,496	0.8%	36	Nevada	1,894	0.6%
25	Oregon	4,155	1.4%	37	Nebraska	1,812	0.6%
6	Pennsylvania	12,573	4.2%	38	Hawaii	1,637	0.5%
42	Rhode Island	1,388	0.5%	39	West Virginia	1,633	0.5%
26	South Carolina	4,016	1.3%	40	New Hampshire	1,464	0.5%
46	South Dakota	775	0.3%	41	Maine	1,458	0.5%
16	Tennessee	6,185	2.0%	42	Rhode Island	1,388	0.5%
3	Texas	19,044	6.3%	43	Idaho	1,061	0.4%
33	Utah	2,048	0.7%	44	Vermont	908	0.3%
44	Vermont	908	0.3%	45	Montana	851	0.3%
12	Virginia	8,323	2.8%	46	South Dakota	775	0.3%
15	Washington	6,911	2.3%	47	Delaware	745	0.2%
39	West Virginia	1,633	0.5%	48	North Dakota	706	0.2%
18	Wisconsin	5,720	1.9%	49	Alaska	705	0.2%
50	Wyoming	468	0.2%	50	Wyoming	468	0.2%
					District of Columbia	1,455	0.5%

Source: American Medical Association (Chicago, Illinois)
"Physician Characteristics and Distribution in the U.S." (2011 Edition)
*As of December 31, 2009. National total does not include 5,320 physicians in U.S. territories and possessions. Primary Care Specialties include Family Practice, General Practice, Internal Medicine, Obstetrics/Gynecology, and Pediatrics excluding subspecialties within each category.

Rate of Physicians in Primary Care in 2009

National Rate = 98 Physicians per 100,000 Population*

ALPHA ORDER				RANK ORDER		
RANK	STATE	RATE		RANK	STATE	RATE
40	Alabama	83		1	Vermont	146
17	Alaska	101		2	Massachusetts	144
44	Arizona	76		3	Maryland	138
40	Arkansas	83		4	New York	134
20	California	100		5	Rhode Island	132
25	Colorado	96		6	Connecticut	131
6	Connecticut	131		7	Hawaii	126
37	Delaware	84		8	Minnesota	114
31	Florida	88		8	New Jersey	114
40	Georgia	83		10	Maine	111
7	Hawaii	126		10	New Hampshire	111
48	Idaho	69		12	North Dakota	109
14	Illinois	107		12	Oregon	109
37	Indiana	84		14	Illinois	107
46	Iowa	72		15	Virginia	106
34	Kansas	86		16	Washington	104
36	Kentucky	85		17	Alaska	101
23	Louisiana	97		17	Nebraska	101
10	Maine	111		17	Wisconsin	101
3	Maryland	138		20	California	100
2	Massachusetts	144		20	Pennsylvania	100
25	Michigan	96		22	Tennessee	98
8	Minnesota	114		23	Louisiana	97
48	Mississippi	69		23	Ohio	97
37	Missouri	84		25	Colorado	96
33	Montana	87		25	Michigan	96
17	Nebraska	101		25	New Mexico	96
46	Nevada	72		28	South Dakota	95
10	New Hampshire	111		29	North Carolina	93
8	New Jersey	114		30	West Virginia	90
25	New Mexico	96		31	Florida	88
4	New York	134		31	South Carolina	88
29	North Carolina	93		33	Montana	87
12	North Dakota	109		34	Kansas	86
23	Ohio	97		34	Wyoming	86
50	Oklahoma	68		36	Kentucky	85
12	Oregon	109		37	Delaware	84
20	Pennsylvania	100		37	Indiana	84
5	Rhode Island	132		37	Missouri	84
31	South Carolina	88		40	Alabama	83
28	South Dakota	95		40	Arkansas	83
22	Tennessee	98		40	Georgia	83
43	Texas	77		43	Texas	77
45	Utah	74		44	Arizona	76
1	Vermont	146		45	Utah	74
15	Virginia	106		46	Iowa	72
16	Washington	104		46	Nevada	72
30	West Virginia	90		48	Idaho	69
17	Wisconsin	101		48	Mississippi	69
34	Wyoming	86		50	Oklahoma	68

District of Columbia   243

Source: CQ Press using data from American Medical Association (Chicago, Illinois)
        "Physician Characteristics and Distribution in the U.S." (2011 Edition)
*As of December 31, 2009. National rate does not include physicians in U.S. territories and possessions. Primary Care Specialties include Family Practice, General Practice, Internal Medicine, Obstetrics/Gynecology, and Pediatrics excluding subspecialties within each category.

Percent of Physicians in Primary Care in 2009

National Percent = 31.5% of Physicians*

ALPHA ORDER				RANK ORDER		
RANK	STATE	PERCENT		RANK	STATE	PERCENT
8	Alabama	34.0		1	Alaska	39.9
1	Alaska	39.9		2	North Dakota	38.6
45	Arizona	30.2		3	Wyoming	37.9
5	Arkansas	35.4		4	South Dakota	36.8
37	California	31.6		5	Arkansas	35.4
37	Colorado	31.6		6	Nebraska	35.2
43	Connecticut	30.3		7	Hawaii	34.1
46	Delaware	29.9		8	Alabama	34.0
48	Florida	28.7		8	Georgia	34.0
8	Georgia	34.0		8	Indiana	34.0
7	Hawaii	34.1		8	New Mexico	34.0
14	Idaho	33.6		12	Minnesota	33.8
14	Illinois	33.6		13	South Carolina	33.7
8	Indiana	34.0		14	Idaho	33.6
25	Iowa	32.7		14	Illinois	33.6
32	Kansas	32.3		14	Wisconsin	33.6
29	Kentucky	32.4		17	Mississippi	33.4
26	Louisiana	32.6		17	Oklahoma	33.4
20	Maine	33.3		17	West Virginia	33.4
47	Maryland	28.9		20	Maine	33.3
50	Massachusetts	27.5		21	Vermont	33.0
23	Michigan	32.8		22	Virginia	32.9
12	Minnesota	33.8		23	Michigan	32.8
17	Mississippi	33.4		23	Tennessee	32.8
42	Missouri	30.5		25	Iowa	32.7
33	Montana	32.2		26	Louisiana	32.6
6	Nebraska	35.2		27	Nevada	32.5
27	Nevada	32.5		27	Oregon	32.5
29	New Hampshire	32.4		29	Kentucky	32.4
36	New Jersey	31.9		29	New Hampshire	32.4
8	New Mexico	34.0		29	Washington	32.4
43	New York	30.3		32	Kansas	32.3
34	North Carolina	32.0		33	Montana	32.2
2	North Dakota	38.6		34	North Carolina	32.0
37	Ohio	31.6		34	Texas	32.0
17	Oklahoma	33.4		36	New Jersey	31.9
27	Oregon	32.5		37	California	31.6
49	Pennsylvania	28.4		37	Colorado	31.6
40	Rhode Island	30.6		37	Ohio	31.6
13	South Carolina	33.7		40	Rhode Island	30.6
4	South Dakota	36.8		40	Utah	30.6
23	Tennessee	32.8		42	Missouri	30.5
34	Texas	32.0		43	Connecticut	30.3
40	Utah	30.6		43	New York	30.3
21	Vermont	33.0		45	Arizona	30.2
22	Virginia	32.9		46	Delaware	29.9
29	Washington	32.4		47	Maryland	28.9
17	West Virginia	33.4		48	Florida	28.7
14	Wisconsin	33.6		49	Pennsylvania	28.4
3	Wyoming	37.9		50	Massachusetts	27.5
					District of Columbia	27.1

Source: CQ Press using data from American Medical Association (Chicago, Illinois)
     "Physician Characteristics and Distribution in the U.S." (2011 Edition)
*As of December 31, 2009. National percent does not include physicians in U.S. territories and possessions. Primary Care Specialties include Family Practice, General Practice, Internal Medicine, Obstetrics/Gynecology, and Pediatrics excluding subspecialties within each category.

Percent of Population Lacking Access to Primary Care in 2011

National Percent = 11.8% of Population*

ALPHA ORDER

RANK	STATE	PERCENT
10	Alabama	18.7
11	Alaska	17.6
14	Arizona	16.3
28	Arkansas	10.8
32	California	10.2
24	Colorado	11.6
33	Connecticut	9.0
17	Delaware	13.9
15	Florida	15.0
16	Georgia	14.0
49	Hawaii	2.8
13	Idaho	16.8
12	Illinois	17.3
39	Indiana	6.7
23	Iowa	11.9
20	Kansas	12.7
26	Kentucky	11.2
2	Louisiana	32.2
45	Maine	5.1
35	Maryland	8.3
38	Massachusetts	6.9
28	Michigan	10.8
44	Minnesota	5.4
1	Mississippi	32.4
6	Missouri	23.2
6	Montana	23.2
46	Nebraska	4.8
21	Nevada	12.5
47	New Hampshire	4.1
50	New Jersey	1.7
3	New Mexico	30.6
22	New York	12.1
40	North Carolina	6.5
8	North Dakota	22.0
41	Ohio	6.4
9	Oklahoma	21.6
25	Oregon	11.4
43	Pennsylvania	5.9
42	Rhode Island	6.3
19	South Carolina	12.9
4	South Dakota	26.7
31	Tennessee	10.3
18	Texas	13.0
33	Utah	9.0
48	Vermont	2.9
35	Virginia	8.3
27	Washington	10.9
35	West Virginia	8.3
30	Wisconsin	10.6
5	Wyoming	23.6

RANK ORDER

RANK	STATE	PERCENT
1	Mississippi	32.4
2	Louisiana	32.2
3	New Mexico	30.6
4	South Dakota	26.7
5	Wyoming	23.6
6	Missouri	23.2
6	Montana	23.2
8	North Dakota	22.0
9	Oklahoma	21.6
10	Alabama	18.7
11	Alaska	17.6
12	Illinois	17.3
13	Idaho	16.8
14	Arizona	16.3
15	Florida	15.0
16	Georgia	14.0
17	Delaware	13.9
18	Texas	13.0
19	South Carolina	12.9
20	Kansas	12.7
21	Nevada	12.5
22	New York	12.1
23	Iowa	11.9
24	Colorado	11.6
25	Oregon	11.4
26	Kentucky	11.2
27	Washington	10.9
28	Arkansas	10.8
28	Michigan	10.8
30	Wisconsin	10.6
31	Tennessee	10.3
32	California	10.2
33	Connecticut	9.0
33	Utah	9.0
35	Maryland	8.3
35	Virginia	8.3
35	West Virginia	8.3
38	Massachusetts	6.9
39	Indiana	6.7
40	North Carolina	6.5
41	Ohio	6.4
42	Rhode Island	6.3
43	Pennsylvania	5.9
44	Minnesota	5.4
45	Maine	5.1
46	Nebraska	4.8
47	New Hampshire	4.1
48	Vermont	2.9
49	Hawaii	2.8
50	New Jersey	1.7

	District of Columbia	25.3

Source: CQ Press using data from U.S. Department of Health and Human Services, Division of Shortage Designation
"State Population and HPSA Designation Population Statistics" (as of January 20, 2011)
(http://datawarehouse.hrsa.gov/hpsadetail.aspx)

*Percent of population considered under-served by primary medical practitioners (Family and General Practice doctors, Internists, Ob/Gyns, and Pediatricians). An under-served population does not have primary medical care within reasonable economic and geographic bounds.

Physicians in General/Family Practice in 2009

National Total = 93,591 Physicians*

ALPHA ORDER

RANK	STATE	PHYSICIANS	% of USA
27	Alabama	1,347	1.4%
45	Alaska	408	0.4%
20	Arizona	1,566	1.7%
28	Arkansas	1,285	1.4%
1	California	11,072	11.8%
17	Colorado	1,903	2.0%
38	Connecticut	605	0.6%
49	Delaware	257	0.3%
3	Florida	5,120	5.5%
15	Georgia	2,411	2.6%
43	Hawaii	440	0.5%
39	Idaho	590	0.6%
4	Illinois	3,966	4.2%
14	Indiana	2,420	2.6%
30	Iowa	1,165	1.2%
29	Kansas	1,170	1.3%
26	Kentucky	1,366	1.5%
23	Louisiana	1,406	1.5%
37	Maine	630	0.7%
25	Maryland	1,379	1.5%
24	Massachusetts	1,387	1.5%
10	Michigan	2,942	3.1%
11	Minnesota	2,889	3.1%
33	Mississippi	806	0.9%
22	Missouri	1,421	1.5%
42	Montana	453	0.5%
32	Nebraska	885	0.9%
40	Nevada	579	0.6%
41	New Hampshire	507	0.5%
19	New Jersey	1,611	1.7%
34	New Mexico	805	0.9%
5	New York	3,900	4.2%
9	North Carolina	3,020	3.2%
46	North Dakota	396	0.4%
7	Ohio	3,534	3.8%
31	Oklahoma	1,110	1.2%
21	Oregon	1,488	1.6%
6	Pennsylvania	3,800	4.1%
50	Rhode Island	215	0.2%
18	South Carolina	1,651	1.8%
44	South Dakota	422	0.5%
16	Tennessee	1,986	2.1%
2	Texas	6,607	7.1%
35	Utah	785	0.8%
47	Vermont	334	0.4%
12	Virginia	2,847	3.0%
8	Washington	3,078	3.3%
36	West Virginia	684	0.7%
13	Wisconsin	2,477	2.6%
48	Wyoming	269	0.3%

RANK ORDER

RANK	STATE	PHYSICIANS	% of USA
1	California	11,072	11.8%
2	Texas	6,607	7.1%
3	Florida	5,120	5.5%
4	Illinois	3,966	4.2%
5	New York	3,900	4.2%
6	Pennsylvania	3,800	4.1%
7	Ohio	3,534	3.8%
8	Washington	3,078	3.3%
9	North Carolina	3,020	3.2%
10	Michigan	2,942	3.1%
11	Minnesota	2,889	3.1%
12	Virginia	2,847	3.0%
13	Wisconsin	2,477	2.6%
14	Indiana	2,420	2.6%
15	Georgia	2,411	2.6%
16	Tennessee	1,986	2.1%
17	Colorado	1,903	2.0%
18	South Carolina	1,651	1.8%
19	New Jersey	1,611	1.7%
20	Arizona	1,566	1.7%
21	Oregon	1,488	1.6%
22	Missouri	1,421	1.5%
23	Louisiana	1,406	1.5%
24	Massachusetts	1,387	1.5%
25	Maryland	1,379	1.5%
26	Kentucky	1,366	1.5%
27	Alabama	1,347	1.4%
28	Arkansas	1,285	1.4%
29	Kansas	1,170	1.3%
30	Iowa	1,165	1.2%
31	Oklahoma	1,110	1.2%
32	Nebraska	885	0.9%
33	Mississippi	806	0.9%
34	New Mexico	805	0.9%
35	Utah	785	0.8%
36	West Virginia	684	0.7%
37	Maine	630	0.7%
38	Connecticut	605	0.6%
39	Idaho	590	0.6%
40	Nevada	579	0.6%
41	New Hampshire	507	0.5%
42	Montana	453	0.5%
43	Hawaii	440	0.5%
44	South Dakota	422	0.5%
45	Alaska	408	0.4%
46	North Dakota	396	0.4%
47	Vermont	334	0.4%
48	Wyoming	269	0.3%
49	Delaware	257	0.3%
50	Rhode Island	215	0.2%
	District of Columbia	197	0.2%

Source: American Medical Association (Chicago, Illinois)
    "Physician Characteristics and Distribution in the U.S." (2011 Edition)
*As of December 31, 2009. Total does not include 2,163 physicians in U.S. territories and possessions.

Rate of Physicians in General/Family Practice in 2009

National Rate = 30 Physicians per 100,000 Population*

ALPHA ORDER

ALPHA ORDER

RANK	STATE	RATE
35	Alabama	29
2	Alaska	58
42	Arizona	24
11	Arkansas	44
31	California	30
17	Colorado	38
50	Connecticut	17
35	Delaware	29
37	Florida	28
41	Georgia	25
24	Hawaii	34
17	Idaho	38
28	Illinois	31
17	Indiana	38
15	Iowa	39
13	Kansas	42
25	Kentucky	32
28	Louisiana	31
8	Maine	48
42	Maryland	24
46	Massachusetts	21
31	Michigan	30
3	Minnesota	55
39	Mississippi	27
42	Missouri	24
9	Montana	46
6	Nebraska	49
45	Nevada	22
17	New Hampshire	38
49	New Jersey	19
14	New Mexico	40
47	New York	20
25	North Carolina	32
1	North Dakota	61
28	Ohio	31
31	Oklahoma	30
15	Oregon	39
31	Pennsylvania	30
47	Rhode Island	20
22	South Carolina	36
5	South Dakota	52
25	Tennessee	32
39	Texas	27
37	Utah	28
4	Vermont	54
22	Virginia	36
9	Washington	46
17	West Virginia	38
11	Wisconsin	44
6	Wyoming	49

RANK ORDER

RANK	STATE	RATE
1	North Dakota	61
2	Alaska	58
3	Minnesota	55
4	Vermont	54
5	South Dakota	52
6	Nebraska	49
6	Wyoming	49
8	Maine	48
9	Montana	46
9	Washington	46
11	Arkansas	44
11	Wisconsin	44
13	Kansas	42
14	New Mexico	40
15	Iowa	39
15	Oregon	39
17	Colorado	38
17	Idaho	38
17	Indiana	38
17	New Hampshire	38
17	West Virginia	38
22	South Carolina	36
22	Virginia	36
24	Hawaii	34
25	Kentucky	32
25	North Carolina	32
25	Tennessee	32
28	Illinois	31
28	Louisiana	31
28	Ohio	31
31	California	30
31	Michigan	30
31	Oklahoma	30
31	Pennsylvania	30
35	Alabama	29
35	Delaware	29
37	Florida	28
37	Utah	28
39	Mississippi	27
39	Texas	27
41	Georgia	25
42	Arizona	24
42	Maryland	24
42	Missouri	24
45	Nevada	22
46	Massachusetts	21
47	New York	20
47	Rhode Island	20
49	New Jersey	19
50	Connecticut	17

| | District of Columbia | 33 |

Source: CQ Press using data from American Medical Association (Chicago, Illinois)
   "Physician Characteristics and Distribution in the U.S." (2011 Edition)
*As of December 31, 2009. National rate does not include physicians in the U.S. territories and possessions.

Average Annual Wages of Family and General Practitioners in 2009

National Average = $168,550*

ALPHA ORDER

RANK	STATE	WAGES
46	Alabama	$142,850
43	Alaska	149,470
37	Arizona	158,990
1	Arkansas	206,030
28	California	164,290
10	Colorado	184,290
33	Connecticut	161,420
42	Delaware	152,520
47	Florida	137,820
5	Georgia	188,620
39	Hawaii	154,930
15	Idaho	180,410
24	Illinois	166,920
32	Indiana	161,440
8	Iowa	185,920
6	Kansas	187,110
29	Kentucky	164,160
13	Louisiana	182,730
45	Maine	143,990
38	Maryland	155,330
7	Massachusetts	187,070
18	Michigan	178,160
20	Minnesota	174,610
21	Mississippi	173,730
40	Missouri	154,590
48	Montana	137,580
26	Nebraska	165,490
16	Nevada	180,390
41	New Hampshire	153,500
34	New Jersey	160,260
19	New Mexico	176,090
49	New York	137,000
9	North Carolina	185,050
12	North Dakota	183,600
30	Ohio	163,870
27	Oklahoma	165,270
36	Oregon	159,490
22	Pennsylvania	172,840
23	Rhode Island	172,430
31	South Carolina	162,880
11	South Dakota	183,830
35	Tennessee	159,580
14	Texas	181,000
4	Utah	191,600
50	Vermont	133,020
25	Virginia	165,980
44	Washington	146,660
17	West Virginia	178,710
2	Wisconsin	203,040
3	Wyoming	194,680

RANK ORDER

RANK	STATE	WAGES
1	Arkansas	$206,030
2	Wisconsin	203,040
3	Wyoming	194,680
4	Utah	191,600
5	Georgia	188,620
6	Kansas	187,110
7	Massachusetts	187,070
8	Iowa	185,920
9	North Carolina	185,050
10	Colorado	184,290
11	South Dakota	183,830
12	North Dakota	183,600
13	Louisiana	182,730
14	Texas	181,000
15	Idaho	180,410
16	Nevada	180,390
17	West Virginia	178,710
18	Michigan	178,160
19	New Mexico	176,090
20	Minnesota	174,610
21	Mississippi	173,730
22	Pennsylvania	172,840
23	Rhode Island	172,430
24	Illinois	166,920
25	Virginia	165,980
26	Nebraska	165,490
27	Oklahoma	165,270
28	California	164,290
29	Kentucky	164,160
30	Ohio	163,870
31	South Carolina	162,880
32	Indiana	161,440
33	Connecticut	161,420
34	New Jersey	160,260
35	Tennessee	159,580
36	Oregon	159,490
37	Arizona	158,990
38	Maryland	155,330
39	Hawaii	154,930
40	Missouri	154,590
41	New Hampshire	153,500
42	Delaware	152,520
43	Alaska	149,470
44	Washington	146,660
45	Maine	143,990
46	Alabama	142,850
47	Florida	137,820
48	Montana	137,580
49	New York	137,000
50	Vermont	133,020

District of Columbia	160,080

Source: U.S. Department of Labor, Bureau of Labor Statistics
"Occupational Employment and Wages, 2009" (http://www.bls.gov/oes/)
*Does not include self-employed.

Percent of Physicians Who Are Specialists in 2009

National Percent = 71.8% of Physicians*

RANK	STATE	PERCENT		RANK	STATE	PERCENT
12	Alabama	72.8		1	Connecticut	78.2
47	Alaska	63.5		2	New Jersey	77.3
24	Arizona	70.5		3	Rhode Island	76.9
43	Arkansas	64.6		4	Massachusetts	76.7
24	California	70.5		5	New York	76.4
29	Colorado	69.4		6	Maryland	76.2
1	Connecticut	78.2		7	Missouri	74.9
13	Delaware	72.6		8	Louisiana	73.8
32	Florida	68.6		8	Tennessee	73.8
10	Georgia	73.5		10	Georgia	73.5
16	Hawaii	72.2		11	Texas	72.9
48	Idaho	63.0		12	Alabama	72.8
14	Illinois	72.4		13	Delaware	72.6
26	Indiana	69.9		14	Illinois	72.4
46	Iowa	63.7		14	Kentucky	72.4
40	Kansas	66.0		16	Hawaii	72.2
14	Kentucky	72.4		17	Pennsylvania	72.1
8	Louisiana	73.8		18	Michigan	72.0
40	Maine	66.0		19	Ohio	71.7
6	Maryland	76.2		20	North Carolina	71.5
4	Massachusetts	76.7		21	Utah	70.8
18	Michigan	72.0		22	Nevada	70.7
37	Minnesota	66.4		23	Virginia	70.6
26	Mississippi	69.9		24	Arizona	70.5
7	Missouri	74.9		24	California	70.5
49	Montana	62.2		26	Indiana	69.9
39	Nebraska	66.3		26	Mississippi	69.9
22	Nevada	70.7		28	South Carolina	69.7
30	New Hampshire	69.2		29	Colorado	69.4
2	New Jersey	77.3		30	New Hampshire	69.2
37	New Mexico	66.4		31	Wisconsin	68.8
5	New York	76.4		32	Florida	68.6
20	North Carolina	71.5		33	Oklahoma	68.4
45	North Dakota	64.2		34	West Virginia	68.3
19	Ohio	71.7		35	Oregon	67.5
33	Oklahoma	68.4		36	Vermont	66.9
35	Oregon	67.5		37	Minnesota	66.4
17	Pennsylvania	72.1		37	New Mexico	66.4
3	Rhode Island	76.9		39	Nebraska	66.3
28	South Carolina	69.7		40	Kansas	66.0
44	South Dakota	64.4		40	Maine	66.0
8	Tennessee	73.8		40	Washington	66.0
11	Texas	72.9		43	Arkansas	64.6
21	Utah	70.8		44	South Dakota	64.4
36	Vermont	66.9		45	North Dakota	64.2
23	Virginia	70.6		46	Iowa	63.7
40	Washington	66.0		47	Alaska	63.5
34	West Virginia	68.3		48	Idaho	63.0
31	Wisconsin	68.8		49	Montana	62.2
50	Wyoming	59.4		50	Wyoming	59.4
					District of Columbia	77.5

ALPHA ORDER

RANK ORDER

Source: CQ Press using data from American Medical Association (Chicago, Illinois)
        "Physician Characteristics and Distribution in the U.S." (2011 Edition)
*As of December 31, 2009. National percent does not include physicians in the U.S. territories and possessions. Includes
physicians in medical, surgical, and other specialties.

Physicians in Medical Specialties in 2009

National Total = 299,255 Physicians*

ALPHA ORDER

RANK	STATE	PHYSICIANS	% of USA
25	Alabama	3,566	1.2%
49	Alaska	357	0.1%
20	Arizona	4,917	1.6%
33	Arkansas	1,736	0.6%
1	California	35,158	11.7%
23	Colorado	4,184	1.4%
17	Connecticut	5,594	1.9%
43	Delaware	767	0.3%
4	Florida	17,208	5.8%
13	Georgia	7,646	2.6%
38	Hawaii	1,475	0.5%
45	Idaho	639	0.2%
6	Illinois	13,564	4.5%
22	Indiana	4,467	1.5%
36	Iowa	1,570	0.5%
30	Kansas	1,854	0.6%
27	Kentucky	3,377	1.1%
24	Louisiana	4,148	1.4%
42	Maine	1,140	0.4%
10	Maryland	9,532	3.2%
7	Massachusetts	12,567	4.2%
11	Michigan	9,171	3.1%
19	Minnesota	5,022	1.7%
34	Mississippi	1,693	0.6%
18	Missouri	5,486	1.8%
46	Montana	561	0.2%
40	Nebraska	1,343	0.4%
32	Nevada	1,737	0.6%
41	New Hampshire	1,322	0.4%
8	New Jersey	11,758	3.9%
37	New Mexico	1,539	0.5%
2	New York	31,158	10.4%
12	North Carolina	8,388	2.8%
48	North Dakota	452	0.2%
9	Ohio	11,183	3.7%
29	Oklahoma	2,034	0.7%
26	Oregon	3,511	1.2%
5	Pennsylvania	13,869	4.6%
35	Rhode Island	1,681	0.6%
28	South Carolina	3,296	1.1%
47	South Dakota	514	0.2%
15	Tennessee	6,109	2.0%
3	Texas	18,063	6.0%
31	Utah	1,802	0.6%
44	Vermont	761	0.3%
14	Virginia	7,431	2.5%
16	Washington	5,630	1.9%
39	West Virginia	1,367	0.5%
21	Wisconsin	4,733	1.6%
50	Wyoming	218	0.1%

RANK ORDER

RANK	STATE	PHYSICIANS	% of USA
1	California	35,158	11.7%
2	New York	31,158	10.4%
3	Texas	18,063	6.0%
4	Florida	17,208	5.8%
5	Pennsylvania	13,869	4.6%
6	Illinois	13,564	4.5%
7	Massachusetts	12,567	4.2%
8	New Jersey	11,758	3.9%
9	Ohio	11,183	3.7%
10	Maryland	9,532	3.2%
11	Michigan	9,171	3.1%
12	North Carolina	8,388	2.8%
13	Georgia	7,646	2.6%
14	Virginia	7,431	2.5%
15	Tennessee	6,109	2.0%
16	Washington	5,630	1.9%
17	Connecticut	5,594	1.9%
18	Missouri	5,486	1.8%
19	Minnesota	5,022	1.7%
20	Arizona	4,917	1.6%
21	Wisconsin	4,733	1.6%
22	Indiana	4,467	1.5%
23	Colorado	4,184	1.4%
24	Louisiana	4,148	1.4%
25	Alabama	3,566	1.2%
26	Oregon	3,511	1.2%
27	Kentucky	3,377	1.1%
28	South Carolina	3,296	1.1%
29	Oklahoma	2,034	0.7%
30	Kansas	1,854	0.6%
31	Utah	1,802	0.6%
32	Nevada	1,737	0.6%
33	Arkansas	1,736	0.6%
34	Mississippi	1,693	0.6%
35	Rhode Island	1,681	0.6%
36	Iowa	1,570	0.5%
37	New Mexico	1,539	0.5%
38	Hawaii	1,475	0.5%
39	West Virginia	1,367	0.5%
40	Nebraska	1,343	0.4%
41	New Hampshire	1,322	0.4%
42	Maine	1,140	0.4%
43	Delaware	767	0.3%
44	Vermont	761	0.3%
45	Idaho	639	0.2%
46	Montana	561	0.2%
47	South Dakota	514	0.2%
48	North Dakota	452	0.2%
49	Alaska	357	0.1%
50	Wyoming	218	0.1%
	District of Columbia	1,957	0.7%

Source: American Medical Association (Chicago, Illinois)
   "Physician Characteristics and Distribution in the U.S." (2011 Edition)
*As of December 31, 2009. Total does not include 3,276 physicians in U.S. territories and possessions. Medical Specialties are Allergy/Immunology, Cardiovascular Diseases, Dermatology, Gastroenterology, Internal Medicine, Pediatrics, Pediatric Cardiology, and Pulmonary Diseases.

Rate of Nonfederal Physicians in Medical Specialties in 2009

National Rate = 97 Physicians per 100,000 Population*

ALPHA ORDER

RANK	STATE	RATE
31	Alabama	76
48	Alaska	51
32	Arizona	75
43	Arkansas	60
14	California	95
27	Colorado	83
4	Connecticut	159
23	Delaware	87
17	Florida	93
28	Georgia	78
8	Hawaii	114
49	Idaho	41
10	Illinois	105
37	Indiana	70
47	Iowa	52
39	Kansas	66
28	Kentucky	78
18	Louisiana	92
24	Maine	86
2	Maryland	167
1	Massachusetts	191
18	Michigan	92
14	Minnesota	95
45	Mississippi	57
18	Missouri	92
44	Montana	58
32	Nebraska	75
39	Nevada	66
11	New Hampshire	100
6	New Jersey	135
30	New Mexico	77
4	New York	159
22	North Carolina	89
37	North Dakota	70
12	Ohio	97
46	Oklahoma	55
18	Oregon	92
9	Pennsylvania	110
3	Rhode Island	160
36	South Carolina	72
42	South Dakota	63
12	Tennessee	97
35	Texas	73
41	Utah	65
7	Vermont	122
16	Virginia	94
25	Washington	84
32	West Virginia	75
25	Wisconsin	84
50	Wyoming	40

RANK ORDER

RANK	STATE	RATE
1	Massachusetts	191
2	Maryland	167
3	Rhode Island	160
4	Connecticut	159
4	New York	159
6	New Jersey	135
7	Vermont	122
8	Hawaii	114
9	Pennsylvania	110
10	Illinois	105
11	New Hampshire	100
12	Ohio	97
12	Tennessee	97
14	California	95
14	Minnesota	95
16	Virginia	94
17	Florida	93
18	Louisiana	92
18	Michigan	92
18	Missouri	92
18	Oregon	92
22	North Carolina	89
23	Delaware	87
24	Maine	86
25	Washington	84
25	Wisconsin	84
27	Colorado	83
28	Georgia	78
28	Kentucky	78
30	New Mexico	77
31	Alabama	76
32	Arizona	75
32	Nebraska	75
32	West Virginia	75
35	Texas	73
36	South Carolina	72
37	Indiana	70
37	North Dakota	70
39	Kansas	66
39	Nevada	66
41	Utah	65
42	South Dakota	63
43	Arkansas	60
44	Montana	58
45	Mississippi	57
46	Oklahoma	55
47	Iowa	52
48	Alaska	51
49	Idaho	41
50	Wyoming	40

District of Columbia 326

Source: CQ Press using data from American Medical Association (Chicago, Illinois)
   "Physician Characteristics and Distribution in the U.S." (2011 Edition)
*As of December 31, 2009. National rate does not include physicians in U.S. territories and possessions. Medical Specialties are Allergy/Immunology, Cardiovascular Diseases, Dermatology, Gastroenterology, Internal Medicine, Pediatrics, Pediatric Cardiology, and Pulmonary Diseases.

Physicians in Internal Medicine in 2009

National Total = 160,715 Physicians*

ALPHA ORDER					RANK ORDER			

RANK	STATE	PHYSICIANS	% of USA		RANK	STATE	PHYSICIANS	% of USA
26	Alabama	1,914	1.2%		1	California	18,761	11.7%
49	Alaska	167	0.1%		2	New York	17,824	11.1%
20	Arizona	2,596	1.6%		3	Florida	8,906	5.5%
36	Arkansas	780	0.5%		4	Texas	8,833	5.5%
1	California	18,761	11.7%		5	Illinois	7,738	4.8%
23	Colorado	2,139	1.3%		6	Pennsylvania	7,573	4.7%
15	Connecticut	3,293	2.0%		7	Massachusetts	7,334	4.6%
44	Delaware	356	0.2%		8	New Jersey	6,344	3.9%
3	Florida	8,906	5.5%		9	Ohio	5,904	3.7%
13	Georgia	4,029	2.5%		10	Maryland	5,389	3.4%
35	Hawaii	838	0.5%		11	Michigan	5,184	3.2%
45	Idaho	321	0.2%		12	North Carolina	4,320	2.7%
5	Illinois	7,738	4.8%		13	Georgia	4,029	2.5%
22	Indiana	2,251	1.4%		14	Virginia	3,869	2.4%
38	Iowa	770	0.5%		15	Connecticut	3,293	2.0%
32	Kansas	930	0.6%		16	Tennessee	3,157	2.0%
27	Kentucky	1,671	1.0%		17	Washington	3,031	1.9%
25	Louisiana	2,036	1.3%		18	Missouri	2,822	1.8%
42	Maine	641	0.4%		19	Minnesota	2,641	1.6%
10	Maryland	5,389	3.4%		20	Arizona	2,596	1.6%
7	Massachusetts	7,334	4.6%		21	Wisconsin	2,515	1.6%
11	Michigan	5,184	3.2%		22	Indiana	2,251	1.4%
19	Minnesota	2,641	1.6%		23	Colorado	2,139	1.3%
33	Mississippi	875	0.5%		24	Oregon	2,078	1.3%
18	Missouri	2,822	1.8%		25	Louisiana	2,036	1.3%
46	Montana	299	0.2%		26	Alabama	1,914	1.2%
41	Nebraska	703	0.4%		27	Kentucky	1,671	1.0%
30	Nevada	1,019	0.6%		28	South Carolina	1,627	1.0%
39	New Hampshire	741	0.5%		29	Oklahoma	1,049	0.7%
8	New Jersey	6,344	3.9%		30	Nevada	1,019	0.6%
34	New Mexico	850	0.5%		31	Rhode Island	932	0.6%
2	New York	17,824	11.1%		32	Kansas	930	0.6%
12	North Carolina	4,320	2.7%		33	Mississippi	875	0.5%
48	North Dakota	281	0.2%		34	New Mexico	850	0.5%
9	Ohio	5,904	3.7%		35	Hawaii	838	0.5%
29	Oklahoma	1,049	0.7%		36	Arkansas	780	0.5%
24	Oregon	2,078	1.3%		36	Utah	780	0.5%
6	Pennsylvania	7,573	4.7%		38	Iowa	770	0.5%
31	Rhode Island	932	0.6%		39	New Hampshire	741	0.5%
28	South Carolina	1,627	1.0%		40	West Virginia	728	0.5%
47	South Dakota	290	0.2%		41	Nebraska	703	0.4%
16	Tennessee	3,157	2.0%		42	Maine	641	0.4%
4	Texas	8,833	5.5%		43	Vermont	427	0.3%
36	Utah	780	0.5%		44	Delaware	356	0.2%
43	Vermont	427	0.3%		45	Idaho	321	0.2%
14	Virginia	3,869	2.4%		46	Montana	299	0.2%
17	Washington	3,031	1.9%		47	South Dakota	290	0.2%
40	West Virginia	728	0.5%		48	North Dakota	281	0.2%
21	Wisconsin	2,515	1.6%		49	Alaska	167	0.1%
50	Wyoming	119	0.1%		50	Wyoming	119	0.1%
						District of Columbia	1,040	0.6%

Source: American Medical Association (Chicago, Illinois)
   "Physician Characteristics and Distribution in the U.S." (2011 Edition)
*As of December 31, 2009. Total does not include 1,635 physicians in U.S. territories and possessions. Internal Medicine includes Diabetes, Endocrinology, Geriatrics, Hematology, Infectious Diseases, Nephrology, Nutrition, Medical Oncology, and Rheumatology.

Rate of Physicians in Internal Medicine in 2009

National Rate = 52 Physicians per 100,000 Population*

<table>
<tr><td colspan="3">ALPHA ORDER</td><td colspan="3">RANK ORDER</td></tr>
<tr><th>RANK</th><th>STATE</th><th>RATE</th><th>RANK</th><th>STATE</th><th>RATE</th></tr>
<tr><td>29</td><td>Alabama</td><td>41</td><td>1</td><td>Massachusetts</td><td>111</td></tr>
<tr><td>48</td><td>Alaska</td><td>24</td><td>2</td><td>Maryland</td><td>95</td></tr>
<tr><td>33</td><td>Arizona</td><td>39</td><td>3</td><td>Connecticut</td><td>94</td></tr>
<tr><td>46</td><td>Arkansas</td><td>27</td><td>4</td><td>New York</td><td>91</td></tr>
<tr><td>14</td><td>California</td><td>51</td><td>5</td><td>Rhode Island</td><td>88</td></tr>
<tr><td>26</td><td>Colorado</td><td>43</td><td>6</td><td>New Jersey</td><td>73</td></tr>
<tr><td>3</td><td>Connecticut</td><td>94</td><td>7</td><td>Vermont</td><td>69</td></tr>
<tr><td>31</td><td>Delaware</td><td>40</td><td>8</td><td>Hawaii</td><td>65</td></tr>
<tr><td>20</td><td>Florida</td><td>48</td><td>9</td><td>Illinois</td><td>60</td></tr>
<tr><td>29</td><td>Georgia</td><td>41</td><td>9</td><td>Pennsylvania</td><td>60</td></tr>
<tr><td>8</td><td>Hawaii</td><td>65</td><td>11</td><td>New Hampshire</td><td>56</td></tr>
<tr><td>50</td><td>Idaho</td><td>21</td><td>12</td><td>Oregon</td><td>54</td></tr>
<tr><td>9</td><td>Illinois</td><td>60</td><td>13</td><td>Michigan</td><td>52</td></tr>
<tr><td>40</td><td>Indiana</td><td>35</td><td>14</td><td>California</td><td>51</td></tr>
<tr><td>47</td><td>Iowa</td><td>26</td><td>14</td><td>Ohio</td><td>51</td></tr>
<tr><td>41</td><td>Kansas</td><td>33</td><td>16</td><td>Minnesota</td><td>50</td></tr>
<tr><td>33</td><td>Kentucky</td><td>39</td><td>16</td><td>Tennessee</td><td>50</td></tr>
<tr><td>23</td><td>Louisiana</td><td>45</td><td>18</td><td>Maine</td><td>49</td></tr>
<tr><td>18</td><td>Maine</td><td>49</td><td>18</td><td>Virginia</td><td>49</td></tr>
<tr><td>2</td><td>Maryland</td><td>95</td><td>20</td><td>Florida</td><td>48</td></tr>
<tr><td>1</td><td>Massachusetts</td><td>111</td><td>21</td><td>Missouri</td><td>47</td></tr>
<tr><td>13</td><td>Michigan</td><td>52</td><td>22</td><td>North Carolina</td><td>46</td></tr>
<tr><td>16</td><td>Minnesota</td><td>50</td><td>23</td><td>Louisiana</td><td>45</td></tr>
<tr><td>43</td><td>Mississippi</td><td>30</td><td>23</td><td>Washington</td><td>45</td></tr>
<tr><td>21</td><td>Missouri</td><td>47</td><td>25</td><td>Wisconsin</td><td>44</td></tr>
<tr><td>42</td><td>Montana</td><td>31</td><td>26</td><td>Colorado</td><td>43</td></tr>
<tr><td>33</td><td>Nebraska</td><td>39</td><td>26</td><td>North Dakota</td><td>43</td></tr>
<tr><td>33</td><td>Nevada</td><td>39</td><td>28</td><td>New Mexico</td><td>42</td></tr>
<tr><td>11</td><td>New Hampshire</td><td>56</td><td>29</td><td>Alabama</td><td>41</td></tr>
<tr><td>6</td><td>New Jersey</td><td>73</td><td>29</td><td>Georgia</td><td>41</td></tr>
<tr><td>28</td><td>New Mexico</td><td>42</td><td>31</td><td>Delaware</td><td>40</td></tr>
<tr><td>4</td><td>New York</td><td>91</td><td>31</td><td>West Virginia</td><td>40</td></tr>
<tr><td>22</td><td>North Carolina</td><td>46</td><td>33</td><td>Arizona</td><td>39</td></tr>
<tr><td>26</td><td>North Dakota</td><td>43</td><td>33</td><td>Kentucky</td><td>39</td></tr>
<tr><td>14</td><td>Ohio</td><td>51</td><td>33</td><td>Nebraska</td><td>39</td></tr>
<tr><td>44</td><td>Oklahoma</td><td>28</td><td>33</td><td>Nevada</td><td>39</td></tr>
<tr><td>12</td><td>Oregon</td><td>54</td><td>37</td><td>South Carolina</td><td>36</td></tr>
<tr><td>9</td><td>Pennsylvania</td><td>60</td><td>37</td><td>South Dakota</td><td>36</td></tr>
<tr><td>5</td><td>Rhode Island</td><td>88</td><td>37</td><td>Texas</td><td>36</td></tr>
<tr><td>37</td><td>South Carolina</td><td>36</td><td>40</td><td>Indiana</td><td>35</td></tr>
<tr><td>37</td><td>South Dakota</td><td>36</td><td>41</td><td>Kansas</td><td>33</td></tr>
<tr><td>16</td><td>Tennessee</td><td>50</td><td>42</td><td>Montana</td><td>31</td></tr>
<tr><td>37</td><td>Texas</td><td>36</td><td>43</td><td>Mississippi</td><td>30</td></tr>
<tr><td>44</td><td>Utah</td><td>28</td><td>44</td><td>Oklahoma</td><td>28</td></tr>
<tr><td>7</td><td>Vermont</td><td>69</td><td>44</td><td>Utah</td><td>28</td></tr>
<tr><td>18</td><td>Virginia</td><td>49</td><td>46</td><td>Arkansas</td><td>27</td></tr>
<tr><td>23</td><td>Washington</td><td>45</td><td>47</td><td>Iowa</td><td>26</td></tr>
<tr><td>31</td><td>West Virginia</td><td>40</td><td>48</td><td>Alaska</td><td>24</td></tr>
<tr><td>25</td><td>Wisconsin</td><td>44</td><td>49</td><td>Wyoming</td><td>22</td></tr>
<tr><td>49</td><td>Wyoming</td><td>22</td><td>50</td><td>Idaho</td><td>21</td></tr>
<tr><td></td><td></td><td></td><td></td><td>District of Columbia</td><td>173</td></tr>
</table>

Source: CQ Press using data from American Medical Association (Chicago, Illinois)
"Physician Characteristics and Distribution in the U.S." (2011 Edition)
*As of December 31, 2009. National rate does not include physicians in U.S. territories and possessions. Internal Medicine includes Diabetes, Endocrinology, Geriatrics, Hematology, Infectious Diseases, Nephrology, Nutrition, Medical Oncology, and Rheumatology.

Physicians in Pediatrics in 2009

National Total = 74,919 Physicians*

ALPHA ORDER					RANK ORDER			
RANK	STATE	PHYSICIANS	% of USA		RANK	STATE	PHYSICIANS	% of USA
27	Alabama	861	1.1%		1	California	9,110	12.2%
46	Alaska	124	0.2%		2	New York	7,270	9.7%
19	Arizona	1,209	1.6%		3	Texas	5,170	6.9%
30	Arkansas	537	0.7%		4	Florida	3,998	5.3%
1	California	9,110	12.2%		5	Illinois	3,204	4.3%
24	Colorado	1,114	1.5%		6	Ohio	3,065	4.1%
22	Connecticut	1,160	1.5%		7	Pennsylvania	3,028	4.0%
43	Delaware	243	0.3%		8	New Jersey	2,979	4.0%
4	Florida	3,998	5.3%		9	Massachusetts	2,791	3.7%
13	Georgia	2,034	2.7%		10	Maryland	2,293	3.1%
35	Hawaii	401	0.5%		11	Michigan	2,257	3.0%
45	Idaho	145	0.2%		12	North Carolina	2,184	2.9%
5	Illinois	3,204	4.3%		13	Georgia	2,034	2.7%
20	Indiana	1,202	1.6%		14	Virginia	2,021	2.7%
37	Iowa	384	0.5%		15	Tennessee	1,629	2.2%
32	Kansas	486	0.6%		16	Missouri	1,423	1.9%
25	Kentucky	930	1.2%		17	Washington	1,409	1.9%
23	Louisiana	1,124	1.5%		18	Minnesota	1,217	1.6%
42	Maine	268	0.4%		19	Arizona	1,209	1.6%
10	Maryland	2,293	3.1%		20	Indiana	1,202	1.6%
9	Massachusetts	2,791	3.7%		21	Wisconsin	1,193	1.6%
11	Michigan	2,257	3.0%		22	Connecticut	1,160	1.5%
18	Minnesota	1,217	1.6%		23	Louisiana	1,124	1.5%
33	Mississippi	422	0.6%		24	Colorado	1,114	1.5%
16	Missouri	1,423	1.9%		25	Kentucky	930	1.2%
47	Montana	120	0.2%		26	South Carolina	895	1.2%
39	Nebraska	350	0.5%		27	Alabama	861	1.1%
38	Nevada	372	0.5%		28	Oregon	759	1.0%
41	New Hampshire	300	0.4%		29	Utah	594	0.8%
8	New Jersey	2,979	4.0%		30	Arkansas	537	0.7%
36	New Mexico	400	0.5%		31	Oklahoma	509	0.7%
2	New York	7,270	9.7%		32	Kansas	486	0.6%
12	North Carolina	2,184	2.9%		33	Mississippi	422	0.6%
49	North Dakota	90	0.1%		34	Rhode Island	420	0.6%
6	Ohio	3,065	4.1%		35	Hawaii	401	0.5%
31	Oklahoma	509	0.7%		36	New Mexico	400	0.5%
28	Oregon	759	1.0%		37	Iowa	384	0.5%
7	Pennsylvania	3,028	4.0%		38	Nevada	372	0.5%
34	Rhode Island	420	0.6%		39	Nebraska	350	0.5%
26	South Carolina	895	1.2%		40	West Virginia	336	0.4%
48	South Dakota	107	0.1%		41	New Hampshire	300	0.4%
15	Tennessee	1,629	2.2%		42	Maine	268	0.4%
3	Texas	5,170	6.9%		43	Delaware	243	0.3%
29	Utah	594	0.8%		44	Vermont	191	0.3%
44	Vermont	191	0.3%		45	Idaho	145	0.2%
14	Virginia	2,021	2.7%		46	Alaska	124	0.2%
17	Washington	1,409	1.9%		47	Montana	120	0.2%
40	West Virginia	336	0.4%		48	South Dakota	107	0.1%
21	Wisconsin	1,193	1.6%		49	North Dakota	90	0.1%
50	Wyoming	58	0.1%		50	Wyoming	58	0.1%
						District of Columbia	533	0.7%

Source: American Medical Association (Chicago, Illinois)
  "Physician Characteristics and Distribution in the U.S." (2011 Edition)
*As of December 31, 2009. Total does not include 1,087 physicians in U.S. territories and possessions. Pediatrics includes
Adolescent Medicine, Neonatal-Perinatal, Pediatric Allergy, Pediatric Endocrinology, Pediatric Pulmonology, Pediatric
Hematology-Oncology, and Pediatric Nephrology.

Rate of Physicians in Pediatrics in 2009

National Rate = 100 Physicians per 100,000 Population 17 Years and Younger*

	ALPHA ORDER			RANK ORDER	
RANK	STATE	RATE	RANK	STATE	RATE
34	Alabama	76	1	Massachusetts	195
40	Alaska	68	2	Rhode Island	185
38	Arizona	70	3	Maryland	170
34	Arkansas	76	4	New York	164
20	California	97	5	Vermont	151
25	Colorado	91	6	New Jersey	146
7	Connecticut	144	7	Connecticut	144
9	Delaware	117	8	Hawaii	138
17	Florida	99	9	Delaware	117
31	Georgia	79	10	Ohio	113
8	Hawaii	138	11	Pennsylvania	109
50	Idaho	35	11	Tennessee	109
15	Illinois	101	11	Virginia	109
34	Indiana	76	14	New Hampshire	104
47	Iowa	54	15	Illinois	101
39	Kansas	69	16	Louisiana	100
24	Kentucky	92	17	Florida	99
16	Louisiana	100	17	Maine	99
17	Maine	99	17	Missouri	99
3	Maryland	170	20	California	97
1	Massachusetts	195	20	Minnesota	97
22	Michigan	96	22	Michigan	96
20	Minnesota	97	22	North Carolina	96
43	Mississippi	55	24	Kentucky	92
17	Missouri	99	25	Colorado	91
43	Montana	55	25	Wisconsin	91
33	Nebraska	77	27	Washington	90
43	Nevada	55	28	Oregon	87
14	New Hampshire	104	28	West Virginia	87
6	New Jersey	146	30	South Carolina	83
32	New Mexico	78	31	Georgia	79
4	New York	164	32	New Mexico	78
22	North Carolina	96	33	Nebraska	77
42	North Dakota	63	34	Alabama	76
10	Ohio	113	34	Arkansas	76
43	Oklahoma	55	34	Indiana	76
28	Oregon	87	37	Texas	75
11	Pennsylvania	109	38	Arizona	70
2	Rhode Island	185	39	Kansas	69
30	South Carolina	83	40	Alaska	68
47	South Dakota	54	40	Utah	68
11	Tennessee	109	42	North Dakota	63
37	Texas	75	43	Mississippi	55
40	Utah	68	43	Montana	55
5	Vermont	151	43	Nevada	55
11	Virginia	109	43	Oklahoma	55
27	Washington	90	47	Iowa	54
28	West Virginia	87	47	South Dakota	54
25	Wisconsin	91	49	Wyoming	44
49	Wyoming	44	50	Idaho	35
				District of Columbia	467

Source: CQ Press using data from American Medical Association (Chicago, Illinois)
    "Physician Characteristics and Distribution in the U.S." (2011 Edition)
*As of December 31, 2009. National rate does not include physicians in U.S. territories and possessions. Pediatrics includes Adolescent Medicine, Neonatal-Perinatal, Pediatric Allergy, Pediatric Endocrinology, Pediatric Pulmonology, Pediatric Hematology-Oncology, and Pediatric Nephrology.

Physicians in Surgical Specialties in 2009

National Total = 162,037 Physicians*

ALPHA ORDER					RANK ORDER			
RANK	STATE	PHYSICIANS	% of USA		RANK	STATE	PHYSICIANS	% of USA
25	Alabama	2,299	1.4%		1	California	18,841	11.6%
48	Alaska	338	0.2%		2	New York	13,710	8.5%
21	Arizona	2,729	1.7%		3	Texas	11,050	6.8%
34	Arkansas	1,154	0.7%		4	Florida	9,571	5.9%
1	California	18,841	11.6%		5	Pennsylvania	7,274	4.5%
23	Colorado	2,583	1.6%		6	Illinois	6,556	4.0%
24	Connecticut	2,540	1.6%		7	Ohio	6,100	3.8%
46	Delaware	413	0.3%		8	New Jersey	5,168	3.2%
4	Florida	9,571	5.9%		9	Michigan	4,956	3.1%
12	Georgia	4,503	2.8%		10	North Carolina	4,879	3.0%
39	Hawaii	813	0.5%		11	Massachusetts	4,811	3.0%
43	Idaho	609	0.4%		12	Georgia	4,503	2.8%
6	Illinois	6,556	4.0%		13	Virginia	4,350	2.7%
22	Indiana	2,721	1.7%		14	Maryland	4,278	2.6%
33	Iowa	1,164	0.7%		15	Tennessee	3,642	2.2%
30	Kansas	1,320	0.8%		16	Washington	3,289	2.0%
27	Kentucky	2,134	1.3%		17	Missouri	2,936	1.8%
19	Louisiana	2,786	1.7%		18	Wisconsin	2,850	1.8%
42	Maine	708	0.4%		19	Louisiana	2,786	1.7%
14	Maryland	4,278	2.6%		20	Minnesota	2,771	1.7%
11	Massachusetts	4,811	3.0%		21	Arizona	2,729	1.7%
9	Michigan	4,956	3.1%		22	Indiana	2,721	1.7%
20	Minnesota	2,771	1.7%		23	Colorado	2,583	1.6%
31	Mississippi	1,240	0.8%		24	Connecticut	2,540	1.6%
17	Missouri	2,936	1.8%		25	Alabama	2,299	1.4%
44	Montana	488	0.3%		26	South Carolina	2,273	1.4%
36	Nebraska	937	0.6%		27	Kentucky	2,134	1.3%
35	Nevada	982	0.6%		28	Oregon	2,122	1.3%
40	New Hampshire	784	0.5%		29	Oklahoma	1,391	0.9%
8	New Jersey	5,168	3.2%		30	Kansas	1,320	0.8%
38	New Mexico	849	0.5%		31	Mississippi	1,240	0.8%
2	New York	13,710	8.5%		32	Utah	1,237	0.8%
10	North Carolina	4,879	3.0%		33	Iowa	1,164	0.7%
49	North Dakota	309	0.2%		34	Arkansas	1,154	0.7%
7	Ohio	6,100	3.8%		35	Nevada	982	0.6%
29	Oklahoma	1,391	0.9%		36	Nebraska	937	0.6%
28	Oregon	2,122	1.3%		37	West Virginia	910	0.6%
5	Pennsylvania	7,274	4.5%		38	New Mexico	849	0.5%
41	Rhode Island	752	0.5%		39	Hawaii	813	0.5%
26	South Carolina	2,273	1.4%		40	New Hampshire	784	0.5%
47	South Dakota	399	0.2%		41	Rhode Island	752	0.5%
15	Tennessee	3,642	2.2%		42	Maine	708	0.4%
3	Texas	11,050	6.8%		43	Idaho	609	0.4%
32	Utah	1,237	0.8%		44	Montana	488	0.3%
45	Vermont	422	0.3%		45	Vermont	422	0.3%
13	Virginia	4,350	2.7%		46	Delaware	413	0.3%
16	Washington	3,289	2.0%		47	South Dakota	399	0.2%
37	West Virginia	910	0.6%		48	Alaska	338	0.2%
18	Wisconsin	2,850	1.8%		49	North Dakota	309	0.2%
50	Wyoming	249	0.2%		50	Wyoming	249	0.2%
						District of Columbia	847	0.5%

Source: American Medical Association (Chicago, Illinois)
"Physician Characteristics and Distribution in the U.S." (2011 Edition)
*As of December 31, 2009. Total does not include 1,533 physicians in U.S. territories and possessions. Surgical Specialties include Colon and Rectal, General, Neurological, Obstetrics and Gynecology, Ophthalmology, Orthopedic, Otolaryngology, Plastic, Thoracic, and Urological Surgeries.

Rate of Physicians in Surgical Specialties in 2009

National Rate = 53 Physicians per 100,000 Population*

RANK	STATE	RATE
29	Alabama	49
34	Alaska	48
45	Arizona	41
46	Arkansas	40
21	California	51
21	Colorado	51
3	Connecticut	72
36	Delaware	47
18	Florida	52
38	Georgia	46
7	Hawaii	63
47	Idaho	39
21	Illinois	51
42	Indiana	42
47	Iowa	39
36	Kansas	47
29	Kentucky	49
8	Louisiana	62
15	Maine	54
1	Maryland	75
2	Massachusetts	73
24	Michigan	50
16	Minnesota	53
42	Mississippi	42
29	Missouri	49
24	Montana	50
18	Nebraska	52
50	Nevada	37
9	New Hampshire	59
9	New Jersey	59
42	New Mexico	42
5	New York	70
18	North Carolina	52
34	North Dakota	48
16	Ohio	53
49	Oklahoma	38
13	Oregon	55
11	Pennsylvania	58
4	Rhode Island	71
24	South Carolina	50
29	South Dakota	49
11	Tennessee	58
40	Texas	45
41	Utah	44
6	Vermont	68
13	Virginia	55
29	Washington	49
24	West Virginia	50
24	Wisconsin	50
38	Wyoming	46

RANK	STATE	RATE
1	Maryland	75
2	Massachusetts	73
3	Connecticut	72
4	Rhode Island	71
5	New York	70
6	Vermont	68
7	Hawaii	63
8	Louisiana	62
9	New Hampshire	59
9	New Jersey	59
11	Pennsylvania	58
11	Tennessee	58
13	Oregon	55
13	Virginia	55
15	Maine	54
16	Minnesota	53
16	Ohio	53
18	Florida	52
18	Nebraska	52
18	North Carolina	52
21	California	51
21	Colorado	51
21	Illinois	51
24	Michigan	50
24	Montana	50
24	South Carolina	50
24	West Virginia	50
24	Wisconsin	50
29	Alabama	49
29	Kentucky	49
29	Missouri	49
29	South Dakota	49
29	Washington	49
34	Alaska	48
34	North Dakota	48
36	Delaware	47
36	Kansas	47
38	Georgia	46
38	Wyoming	46
40	Texas	45
41	Utah	44
42	Indiana	42
42	Mississippi	42
42	New Mexico	42
45	Arizona	41
46	Arkansas	40
47	Idaho	39
47	Iowa	39
49	Oklahoma	38
50	Nevada	37

	District of Columbia	141

Source: CQ Press using data from American Medical Association (Chicago, Illinois)
"Physician Characteristics and Distribution in the U.S." (2011 Edition)

*As of December 31, 2009. National rate does not include physicians in U.S. territories and possessions. Surgical Specialties include Colon and Rectal, General, Neurological, Obstetrics and Gynecology, Ophthalmology, Orthopedic, Otolaryngology, Plastic, Thoracic, and Urological Surgeries.

Average Annual Wages of Surgeons in 2009

National Average = $219,770*

ALPHA ORDER			RANK ORDER		
RANK	STATE	WAGES	RANK	STATE	WAGES
9	Alabama	$227,290	1	North Carolina	$233,560
NA	Alaska**	NA	2	Rhode Island	233,470
32	Arizona	197,670	3	Nebraska	232,990
13	Arkansas	223,970	4	Iowa	230,530
21	California	222,370	5	Ohio	230,310
11	Colorado	226,410	6	Kansas	230,090
28	Connecticut	207,410	7	Florida	228,530
24	Delaware	212,020	8	Montana	228,520
7	Florida	228,530	9	Alabama	227,290
14	Georgia	223,810	10	Nevada	226,890
33	Hawaii	196,200	11	Colorado	226,410
15	Idaho	223,450	12	Washington	225,250
23	Illinois	213,950	13	Arkansas	223,970
NA	Indiana**	NA	14	Georgia	223,810
4	Iowa	230,530	15	Idaho	223,450
6	Kansas	230,090	16	Utah	223,050
25	Kentucky	211,920	17	South Dakota	222,980
NA	Louisiana**	NA	18	North Dakota	222,730
NA	Maine**	NA	19	New Mexico	222,530
NA	Maryland**	NA	20	Massachusetts	222,420
20	Massachusetts	222,420	21	California	222,370
NA	Michigan**	NA	22	Tennessee	218,150
NA	Minnesota**	NA	23	Illinois	213,950
34	Mississippi	192,890	24	Delaware	212,020
NA	Missouri**	NA	25	Kentucky	211,920
8	Montana	228,520	26	Oklahoma	210,760
3	Nebraska	232,990	27	Virginia	210,180
10	Nevada	226,890	28	Connecticut	207,410
NA	New Hampshire**	NA	29	West Virginia	205,620
NA	New Jersey**	NA	30	Texas	198,280
19	New Mexico	222,530	31	Vermont	197,940
36	New York	185,360	32	Arizona	197,670
1	North Carolina	233,560	33	Hawaii	196,200
18	North Dakota	222,730	34	Mississippi	192,890
5	Ohio	230,310	35	Pennsylvania	191,060
26	Oklahoma	210,760	36	New York	185,360
NA	Oregon**	NA	NA	Alaska**	NA
35	Pennsylvania	191,060	NA	Indiana**	NA
2	Rhode Island	233,470	NA	Louisiana**	NA
NA	South Carolina**	NA	NA	Maine**	NA
17	South Dakota	222,980	NA	Maryland**	NA
22	Tennessee	218,150	NA	Michigan**	NA
30	Texas	198,280	NA	Minnesota**	NA
16	Utah	223,050	NA	Missouri**	NA
31	Vermont	197,940	NA	New Hampshire**	NA
27	Virginia	210,180	NA	New Jersey**	NA
12	Washington	225,250	NA	Oregon**	NA
29	West Virginia	205,620	NA	South Carolina**	NA
NA	Wisconsin**	NA	NA	Wisconsin**	NA
NA	Wyoming**	NA	NA	Wyoming**	NA
				District of Columbia**	NA

Source: U.S. Department of Labor, Bureau of Labor Statistics
"Occupational Employment and Wages, 2009" (http://www.bls.gov/oes/)
*Does not include self-employed.
**Not available.

Physicians in General Surgery in 2009

National Total = 37,338 Physicians*

ALPHA ORDER					RANK ORDER			
RANK	STATE	PHYSICIANS	% of USA		RANK	STATE	PHYSICIANS	% of USA
27	Alabama	525	1.4%		1	California	4,026	10.8%
49	Alaska	76	0.2%		2	New York	3,248	8.7%
20	Arizona	646	1.7%		3	Texas	2,369	6.3%
32	Arkansas	273	0.7%		4	Florida	1,974	5.3%
1	California	4,026	10.8%		5	Pennsylvania	1,865	5.0%
25	Colorado	561	1.5%		6	Ohio	1,534	4.1%
24	Connecticut	563	1.5%		7	Illinois	1,496	4.0%
47	Delaware	97	0.3%		8	Michigan	1,254	3.4%
4	Florida	1,974	5.3%		9	Massachusetts	1,251	3.4%
12	Georgia	1,050	2.8%		10	New Jersey	1,165	3.1%
42	Hawaii	177	0.5%		11	North Carolina	1,115	3.0%
43	Idaho	136	0.4%		12	Georgia	1,050	2.8%
7	Illinois	1,496	4.0%		13	Maryland	953	2.6%
22	Indiana	583	1.6%		14	Virginia	930	2.5%
31	Iowa	284	0.8%		15	Tennessee	918	2.5%
30	Kansas	292	0.8%		16	Washington	776	2.1%
23	Kentucky	568	1.5%		17	Missouri	664	1.8%
21	Louisiana	604	1.6%		18	Wisconsin	656	1.8%
40	Maine	194	0.5%		19	Minnesota	649	1.7%
13	Maryland	953	2.6%		20	Arizona	646	1.7%
9	Massachusetts	1,251	3.4%		21	Louisiana	604	1.6%
8	Michigan	1,254	3.4%		22	Indiana	583	1.6%
19	Minnesota	649	1.7%		23	Kentucky	568	1.5%
33	Mississippi	266	0.7%		24	Connecticut	563	1.5%
17	Missouri	664	1.8%		25	Colorado	561	1.5%
46	Montana	102	0.3%		26	South Carolina	538	1.4%
36	Nebraska	241	0.6%		27	Alabama	525	1.4%
37	Nevada	219	0.6%		28	Oregon	501	1.3%
39	New Hampshire	196	0.5%		29	Oklahoma	316	0.8%
10	New Jersey	1,165	3.1%		30	Kansas	292	0.8%
38	New Mexico	209	0.6%		31	Iowa	284	0.8%
2	New York	3,248	8.7%		32	Arkansas	273	0.7%
11	North Carolina	1,115	3.0%		33	Mississippi	266	0.7%
48	North Dakota	92	0.2%		34	West Virginia	247	0.7%
6	Ohio	1,534	4.1%		35	Utah	246	0.7%
29	Oklahoma	316	0.8%		36	Nebraska	241	0.6%
28	Oregon	501	1.3%		37	Nevada	219	0.6%
5	Pennsylvania	1,865	5.0%		38	New Mexico	209	0.6%
41	Rhode Island	181	0.5%		39	New Hampshire	196	0.5%
26	South Carolina	538	1.4%		40	Maine	194	0.5%
45	South Dakota	104	0.3%		41	Rhode Island	181	0.5%
15	Tennessee	918	2.5%		42	Hawaii	177	0.5%
3	Texas	2,369	6.3%		43	Idaho	136	0.4%
35	Utah	246	0.7%		44	Vermont	116	0.3%
44	Vermont	116	0.3%		45	South Dakota	104	0.3%
14	Virginia	930	2.5%		46	Montana	102	0.3%
16	Washington	776	2.1%		47	Delaware	97	0.3%
34	West Virginia	247	0.7%		48	North Dakota	92	0.2%
18	Wisconsin	656	1.8%		49	Alaska	76	0.2%
50	Wyoming	59	0.2%		50	Wyoming	59	0.2%
						District of Columbia	233	0.6%

Source: American Medical Association (Chicago, Illinois)
"Physician Characteristics and Distribution in the U.S." (2011 Edition)
*As of December 31, 2009. Total does not include 384 physicians in U.S. territories and possessions. General Surgery includes Abdominal, Cardiovascular, Hand, Head and Neck, Pediatric, Traumatic, and Vascular Surgeries.

Rate of Physicians in General Surgery in 2009

National Rate = 12 Physicians per 100,000 Population*

ALPHA ORDER

RANK	STATE	RATE
29	Alabama	11
29	Alaska	11
38	Arizona	10
43	Arkansas	9
29	California	11
29	Colorado	11
6	Connecticut	16
29	Delaware	11
29	Florida	11
29	Georgia	11
11	Hawaii	14
43	Idaho	9
22	Illinois	12
43	Indiana	9
43	Iowa	9
38	Kansas	10
14	Kentucky	13
14	Louisiana	13
7	Maine	15
3	Maryland	17
1	Massachusetts	19
14	Michigan	13
22	Minnesota	12
43	Mississippi	9
29	Missouri	11
38	Montana	10
14	Nebraska	13
50	Nevada	8
7	New Hampshire	15
14	New Jersey	13
38	New Mexico	10
3	New York	17
22	North Carolina	12
11	North Dakota	14
14	Ohio	13
43	Oklahoma	9
14	Oregon	13
7	Pennsylvania	15
3	Rhode Island	17
22	South Carolina	12
14	South Dakota	13
7	Tennessee	15
38	Texas	10
43	Utah	9
1	Vermont	19
22	Virginia	12
22	Washington	12
11	West Virginia	14
22	Wisconsin	12
29	Wyoming	11

RANK ORDER

RANK	STATE	RATE
1	Massachusetts	19
1	Vermont	19
3	Maryland	17
3	New York	17
3	Rhode Island	17
6	Connecticut	16
7	Maine	15
7	New Hampshire	15
7	Pennsylvania	15
7	Tennessee	15
11	Hawaii	14
11	North Dakota	14
11	West Virginia	14
14	Kentucky	13
14	Louisiana	13
14	Michigan	13
14	Nebraska	13
14	New Jersey	13
14	Ohio	13
14	Oregon	13
14	South Dakota	13
22	Illinois	12
22	Minnesota	12
22	North Carolina	12
22	South Carolina	12
22	Virginia	12
22	Washington	12
22	Wisconsin	12
29	Alabama	11
29	Alaska	11
29	California	11
29	Colorado	11
29	Delaware	11
29	Florida	11
29	Georgia	11
29	Missouri	11
29	Wyoming	11
38	Arizona	10
38	Kansas	10
38	Montana	10
38	New Mexico	10
38	Texas	10
43	Arkansas	9
43	Idaho	9
43	Indiana	9
43	Iowa	9
43	Mississippi	9
43	Oklahoma	9
43	Utah	9
50	Nevada	8

District of Columbia 39

Source: CQ Press using data from American Medical Association (Chicago, Illinois)
      "Physician Characteristics and Distribution in the U.S." (2011 Edition)
*As of December 31, 2009. National rate does not include physicians in U.S. territories and possessions. General Surgery
includes Abdominal, Cardiovascular, Hand, Head and Neck, Pediatric, Traumatic, and Vascular Surgeries.

Physicians in Obstetrics and Gynecology in 2009

National Total = 42,233 Physicians*

<table>
<tr><td colspan="4">ALPHA ORDER</td><td colspan="4">RANK ORDER</td></tr>
<tr><th>RANK</th><th>STATE</th><th>PHYSICIANS</th><th>% of USA</th><th>RANK</th><th>STATE</th><th>PHYSICIANS</th><th>% of USA</th></tr>
<tr><td>26</td><td>Alabama</td><td>572</td><td>1.4%</td><td>1</td><td>California</td><td>5,051</td><td>12.0%</td></tr>
<tr><td>47</td><td>Alaska</td><td>80</td><td>0.2%</td><td>2</td><td>New York</td><td>3,642</td><td>8.6%</td></tr>
<tr><td>17</td><td>Arizona</td><td>738</td><td>1.7%</td><td>3</td><td>Texas</td><td>3,073</td><td>7.3%</td></tr>
<tr><td>34</td><td>Arkansas</td><td>272</td><td>0.6%</td><td>4</td><td>Florida</td><td>2,305</td><td>5.5%</td></tr>
<tr><td>1</td><td>California</td><td>5,051</td><td>12.0%</td><td>5</td><td>Illinois</td><td>1,825</td><td>4.3%</td></tr>
<tr><td>22</td><td>Colorado</td><td>706</td><td>1.7%</td><td>6</td><td>Pennsylvania</td><td>1,702</td><td>4.0%</td></tr>
<tr><td>20</td><td>Connecticut</td><td>711</td><td>1.7%</td><td>7</td><td>New Jersey</td><td>1,502</td><td>3.6%</td></tr>
<tr><td>46</td><td>Delaware</td><td>102</td><td>0.2%</td><td>8</td><td>Ohio</td><td>1,485</td><td>3.5%</td></tr>
<tr><td>4</td><td>Florida</td><td>2,305</td><td>5.5%</td><td>9</td><td>Georgia</td><td>1,372</td><td>3.2%</td></tr>
<tr><td>9</td><td>Georgia</td><td>1,372</td><td>3.2%</td><td>10</td><td>Michigan</td><td>1,362</td><td>3.2%</td></tr>
<tr><td>35</td><td>Hawaii</td><td>245</td><td>0.6%</td><td>11</td><td>North Carolina</td><td>1,323</td><td>3.1%</td></tr>
<tr><td>43</td><td>Idaho</td><td>145</td><td>0.3%</td><td>12</td><td>Virginia</td><td>1,261</td><td>3.0%</td></tr>
<tr><td>5</td><td>Illinois</td><td>1,825</td><td>4.3%</td><td>13</td><td>Maryland</td><td>1,174</td><td>2.8%</td></tr>
<tr><td>21</td><td>Indiana</td><td>709</td><td>1.7%</td><td>14</td><td>Massachusetts</td><td>1,144</td><td>2.7%</td></tr>
<tr><td>37</td><td>Iowa</td><td>215</td><td>0.5%</td><td>15</td><td>Tennessee</td><td>932</td><td>2.2%</td></tr>
<tr><td>32</td><td>Kansas</td><td>301</td><td>0.7%</td><td>16</td><td>Washington</td><td>787</td><td>1.9%</td></tr>
<tr><td>27</td><td>Kentucky</td><td>528</td><td>1.3%</td><td>17</td><td>Arizona</td><td>738</td><td>1.7%</td></tr>
<tr><td>18</td><td>Louisiana</td><td>728</td><td>1.7%</td><td>18</td><td>Louisiana</td><td>728</td><td>1.7%</td></tr>
<tr><td>42</td><td>Maine</td><td>165</td><td>0.4%</td><td>19</td><td>Missouri</td><td>726</td><td>1.7%</td></tr>
<tr><td>13</td><td>Maryland</td><td>1,174</td><td>2.8%</td><td>20</td><td>Connecticut</td><td>711</td><td>1.7%</td></tr>
<tr><td>14</td><td>Massachusetts</td><td>1,144</td><td>2.7%</td><td>21</td><td>Indiana</td><td>709</td><td>1.7%</td></tr>
<tr><td>10</td><td>Michigan</td><td>1,362</td><td>3.2%</td><td>22</td><td>Colorado</td><td>706</td><td>1.7%</td></tr>
<tr><td>24</td><td>Minnesota</td><td>641</td><td>1.5%</td><td>23</td><td>Wisconsin</td><td>658</td><td>1.6%</td></tr>
<tr><td>30</td><td>Mississippi</td><td>324</td><td>0.8%</td><td>24</td><td>Minnesota</td><td>641</td><td>1.5%</td></tr>
<tr><td>19</td><td>Missouri</td><td>726</td><td>1.7%</td><td>25</td><td>South Carolina</td><td>598</td><td>1.4%</td></tr>
<tr><td>45</td><td>Montana</td><td>104</td><td>0.2%</td><td>26</td><td>Alabama</td><td>572</td><td>1.4%</td></tr>
<tr><td>38</td><td>Nebraska</td><td>210</td><td>0.5%</td><td>27</td><td>Kentucky</td><td>528</td><td>1.3%</td></tr>
<tr><td>33</td><td>Nevada</td><td>289</td><td>0.7%</td><td>27</td><td>Oregon</td><td>528</td><td>1.3%</td></tr>
<tr><td>41</td><td>New Hampshire</td><td>196</td><td>0.5%</td><td>29</td><td>Oklahoma</td><td>343</td><td>0.8%</td></tr>
<tr><td>7</td><td>New Jersey</td><td>1,502</td><td>3.6%</td><td>30</td><td>Mississippi</td><td>324</td><td>0.8%</td></tr>
<tr><td>36</td><td>New Mexico</td><td>234</td><td>0.6%</td><td>31</td><td>Utah</td><td>303</td><td>0.7%</td></tr>
<tr><td>2</td><td>New York</td><td>3,642</td><td>8.6%</td><td>32</td><td>Kansas</td><td>301</td><td>0.7%</td></tr>
<tr><td>11</td><td>North Carolina</td><td>1,323</td><td>3.1%</td><td>33</td><td>Nevada</td><td>289</td><td>0.7%</td></tr>
<tr><td>50</td><td>North Dakota</td><td>54</td><td>0.1%</td><td>34</td><td>Arkansas</td><td>272</td><td>0.6%</td></tr>
<tr><td>8</td><td>Ohio</td><td>1,485</td><td>3.5%</td><td>35</td><td>Hawaii</td><td>245</td><td>0.6%</td></tr>
<tr><td>29</td><td>Oklahoma</td><td>343</td><td>0.8%</td><td>36</td><td>New Mexico</td><td>234</td><td>0.6%</td></tr>
<tr><td>27</td><td>Oregon</td><td>528</td><td>1.3%</td><td>37</td><td>Iowa</td><td>215</td><td>0.5%</td></tr>
<tr><td>6</td><td>Pennsylvania</td><td>1,702</td><td>4.0%</td><td>38</td><td>Nebraska</td><td>210</td><td>0.5%</td></tr>
<tr><td>39</td><td>Rhode Island</td><td>205</td><td>0.5%</td><td>39</td><td>Rhode Island</td><td>205</td><td>0.5%</td></tr>
<tr><td>25</td><td>South Carolina</td><td>598</td><td>1.4%</td><td>40</td><td>West Virginia</td><td>203</td><td>0.5%</td></tr>
<tr><td>48</td><td>South Dakota</td><td>79</td><td>0.2%</td><td>41</td><td>New Hampshire</td><td>196</td><td>0.5%</td></tr>
<tr><td>15</td><td>Tennessee</td><td>932</td><td>2.2%</td><td>42</td><td>Maine</td><td>165</td><td>0.4%</td></tr>
<tr><td>3</td><td>Texas</td><td>3,073</td><td>7.3%</td><td>43</td><td>Idaho</td><td>145</td><td>0.3%</td></tr>
<tr><td>31</td><td>Utah</td><td>303</td><td>0.7%</td><td>44</td><td>Vermont</td><td>107</td><td>0.3%</td></tr>
<tr><td>44</td><td>Vermont</td><td>107</td><td>0.3%</td><td>45</td><td>Montana</td><td>104</td><td>0.2%</td></tr>
<tr><td>12</td><td>Virginia</td><td>1,261</td><td>3.0%</td><td>46</td><td>Delaware</td><td>102</td><td>0.2%</td></tr>
<tr><td>16</td><td>Washington</td><td>787</td><td>1.9%</td><td>47</td><td>Alaska</td><td>80</td><td>0.2%</td></tr>
<tr><td>40</td><td>West Virginia</td><td>203</td><td>0.5%</td><td>48</td><td>South Dakota</td><td>79</td><td>0.2%</td></tr>
<tr><td>23</td><td>Wisconsin</td><td>658</td><td>1.6%</td><td>49</td><td>Wyoming</td><td>64</td><td>0.2%</td></tr>
<tr><td>49</td><td>Wyoming</td><td>64</td><td>0.2%</td><td>50</td><td>North Dakota</td><td>54</td><td>0.1%</td></tr>
<tr><td></td><td></td><td></td><td></td><td></td><td>District of Columbia</td><td>210</td><td>0.5%</td></tr>
</table>

Source: American Medical Association (Chicago, Illinois)
    "Physician Characteristics and Distribution in the U.S." (2011 Edition)
*As of December 31, 2009. Total does not include 571 physicians in U.S. territories and possessions. Obstetrics and Gynecology includes Gynecology and Oncology, Maternal and Fetal Medicine, and Reproductive Endocrinology.

Rate of Physicians in Obstetrics and Gynecology in 2009

National Rate = 27 Physicians per 100,000 Female Population*

ALPHA ORDER

RANK	STATE	RATE
24	Alabama	24
24	Alaska	24
36	Arizona	22
47	Arkansas	18
16	California	27
13	Colorado	28
2	Connecticut	39
36	Delaware	22
24	Florida	24
16	Georgia	27
3	Hawaii	38
45	Idaho	19
13	Illinois	28
36	Indiana	22
50	Iowa	14
42	Kansas	21
24	Kentucky	24
9	Louisiana	32
24	Maine	24
1	Maryland	40
6	Massachusetts	34
16	Michigan	27
24	Minnesota	24
42	Mississippi	21
24	Missouri	24
42	Montana	21
33	Nebraska	23
36	Nevada	22
11	New Hampshire	29
6	New Jersey	34
33	New Mexico	23
5	New York	36
13	North Carolina	28
49	North Dakota	17
22	Ohio	25
47	Oklahoma	18
16	Oregon	27
20	Pennsylvania	26
3	Rhode Island	38
20	South Carolina	26
45	South Dakota	19
11	Tennessee	29
22	Texas	25
36	Utah	22
6	Vermont	34
10	Virginia	31
24	Washington	24
36	West Virginia	22
33	Wisconsin	23
24	Wyoming	24

RANK ORDER

RANK	STATE	RATE
1	Maryland	40
2	Connecticut	39
3	Hawaii	38
3	Rhode Island	38
5	New York	36
6	Massachusetts	34
6	New Jersey	34
6	Vermont	34
9	Louisiana	32
10	Virginia	31
11	New Hampshire	29
11	Tennessee	29
13	Colorado	28
13	Illinois	28
13	North Carolina	28
16	California	27
16	Georgia	27
16	Michigan	27
16	Oregon	27
20	Pennsylvania	26
20	South Carolina	26
22	Ohio	25
22	Texas	25
24	Alabama	24
24	Alaska	24
24	Florida	24
24	Kentucky	24
24	Maine	24
24	Minnesota	24
24	Missouri	24
24	Washington	24
24	Wyoming	24
33	Nebraska	23
33	New Mexico	23
33	Wisconsin	23
36	Arizona	22
36	Delaware	22
36	Indiana	22
36	Nevada	22
36	Utah	22
36	West Virginia	22
42	Kansas	21
42	Mississippi	21
42	Montana	21
45	Idaho	19
45	South Dakota	19
47	Arkansas	18
47	Oklahoma	18
49	North Dakota	17
50	Iowa	14
	District of Columbia	66

Source: CQ Press using data from American Medical Association (Chicago, Illinois)
"Physician Characteristics and Distribution in the U.S." (2011 Edition)
*As of December 31, 2009. National rate does not include physicians in U.S. territories and possessions. Obstetrics and Gynecology includes Gynecology and Oncology, Maternal and Fetal Medicine, and Reproductive Endocrinology.

Physicians in Ophthalmology in 2009

National Total = 18,128 Physicians*

RANK	STATE	PHYSICIANS	% of USA
27	Alabama	224	1.2%
49	Alaska	30	0.2%
24	Arizona	274	1.5%
34	Arkansas	130	0.7%
1	California	2,255	12.4%
22	Colorado	277	1.5%
20	Connecticut	303	1.7%
44	Delaware	50	0.3%
3	Florida	1,209	6.7%
14	Georgia	426	2.3%
36	Hawaii	102	0.6%
43	Idaho	59	0.3%
6	Illinois	740	4.1%
22	Indiana	277	1.5%
29	Iowa	161	0.9%
30	Kansas	149	0.8%
28	Kentucky	191	1.1%
19	Louisiana	313	1.7%
40	Maine	75	0.4%
11	Maryland	522	2.9%
10	Massachusetts	545	3.0%
9	Michigan	565	3.1%
21	Minnesota	300	1.7%
33	Mississippi	132	0.7%
18	Missouri	326	1.8%
44	Montana	50	0.3%
38	Nebraska	95	0.5%
37	Nevada	100	0.6%
42	New Hampshire	67	0.4%
8	New Jersey	597	3.3%
39	New Mexico	76	0.4%
2	New York	1,714	9.5%
12	North Carolina	501	2.8%
48	North Dakota	31	0.2%
7	Ohio	633	3.5%
31	Oklahoma	144	0.8%
25	Oregon	247	1.4%
5	Pennsylvania	843	4.7%
41	Rhode Island	71	0.4%
26	South Carolina	246	1.4%
47	South Dakota	38	0.2%
16	Tennessee	337	1.9%
4	Texas	1,158	6.4%
32	Utah	134	0.7%
46	Vermont	41	0.2%
13	Virginia	458	2.5%
15	Washington	353	1.9%
35	West Virginia	104	0.6%
17	Wisconsin	330	1.8%
50	Wyoming	17	0.1%

RANK	STATE	PHYSICIANS	% of USA
1	California	2,255	12.4%
2	New York	1,714	9.5%
3	Florida	1,209	6.7%
4	Texas	1,158	6.4%
5	Pennsylvania	843	4.7%
6	Illinois	740	4.1%
7	Ohio	633	3.5%
8	New Jersey	597	3.3%
9	Michigan	565	3.1%
10	Massachusetts	545	3.0%
11	Maryland	522	2.9%
12	North Carolina	501	2.8%
13	Virginia	458	2.5%
14	Georgia	426	2.3%
15	Washington	353	1.9%
16	Tennessee	337	1.9%
17	Wisconsin	330	1.8%
18	Missouri	326	1.8%
19	Louisiana	313	1.7%
20	Connecticut	303	1.7%
21	Minnesota	300	1.7%
22	Colorado	277	1.5%
22	Indiana	277	1.5%
24	Arizona	274	1.5%
25	Oregon	247	1.4%
26	South Carolina	246	1.4%
27	Alabama	224	1.2%
28	Kentucky	191	1.1%
29	Iowa	161	0.9%
30	Kansas	149	0.8%
31	Oklahoma	144	0.8%
32	Utah	134	0.7%
33	Mississippi	132	0.7%
34	Arkansas	130	0.7%
35	West Virginia	104	0.6%
36	Hawaii	102	0.6%
37	Nevada	100	0.6%
38	Nebraska	95	0.5%
39	New Mexico	76	0.4%
40	Maine	75	0.4%
41	Rhode Island	71	0.4%
42	New Hampshire	67	0.4%
43	Idaho	59	0.3%
44	Delaware	50	0.3%
44	Montana	50	0.3%
46	Vermont	41	0.2%
47	South Dakota	38	0.2%
48	North Dakota	31	0.2%
49	Alaska	30	0.2%
50	Wyoming	17	0.1%
	District of Columbia	108	0.6%

Source: American Medical Association (Chicago, Illinois)
"Physician Characteristics and Distribution in the U.S." (2011 Edition)
*As of December 31, 2009. Total does not include 166 physicians in U.S. territories and possessions. Ophthalmology is the branch of medicine dealing with the anatomy, functions, and diseases of the eye.

Rate of Physicians in Ophthalmology in 2009

National Rate = 6 Physicians per 100,000 Population*

<table>
<tr><td colspan="3">ALPHA ORDER</td><td colspan="3">RANK ORDER</td></tr>
<tr><th>RANK</th><th>STATE</th><th>RATE</th><th>RANK</th><th>STATE</th><th>RATE</th></tr>
<tr><td>23</td><td>Alabama</td><td>5</td><td>1</td><td>Connecticut</td><td>9</td></tr>
<tr><td>39</td><td>Alaska</td><td>4</td><td>1</td><td>Maryland</td><td>9</td></tr>
<tr><td>39</td><td>Arizona</td><td>4</td><td>1</td><td>New York</td><td>9</td></tr>
<tr><td>39</td><td>Arkansas</td><td>4</td><td>4</td><td>Hawaii</td><td>8</td></tr>
<tr><td>12</td><td>California</td><td>6</td><td>4</td><td>Massachusetts</td><td>8</td></tr>
<tr><td>12</td><td>Colorado</td><td>6</td><td>6</td><td>Florida</td><td>7</td></tr>
<tr><td>1</td><td>Connecticut</td><td>9</td><td>6</td><td>Louisiana</td><td>7</td></tr>
<tr><td>12</td><td>Delaware</td><td>6</td><td>6</td><td>New Jersey</td><td>7</td></tr>
<tr><td>6</td><td>Florida</td><td>7</td><td>6</td><td>Pennsylvania</td><td>7</td></tr>
<tr><td>39</td><td>Georgia</td><td>4</td><td>6</td><td>Rhode Island</td><td>7</td></tr>
<tr><td>4</td><td>Hawaii</td><td>8</td><td>6</td><td>Vermont</td><td>7</td></tr>
<tr><td>39</td><td>Idaho</td><td>4</td><td>12</td><td>California</td><td>6</td></tr>
<tr><td>12</td><td>Illinois</td><td>6</td><td>12</td><td>Colorado</td><td>6</td></tr>
<tr><td>39</td><td>Indiana</td><td>4</td><td>12</td><td>Delaware</td><td>6</td></tr>
<tr><td>23</td><td>Iowa</td><td>5</td><td>12</td><td>Illinois</td><td>6</td></tr>
<tr><td>23</td><td>Kansas</td><td>5</td><td>12</td><td>Maine</td><td>6</td></tr>
<tr><td>39</td><td>Kentucky</td><td>4</td><td>12</td><td>Michigan</td><td>6</td></tr>
<tr><td>6</td><td>Louisiana</td><td>7</td><td>12</td><td>Minnesota</td><td>6</td></tr>
<tr><td>12</td><td>Maine</td><td>6</td><td>12</td><td>Oregon</td><td>6</td></tr>
<tr><td>1</td><td>Maryland</td><td>9</td><td>12</td><td>Virginia</td><td>6</td></tr>
<tr><td>4</td><td>Massachusetts</td><td>8</td><td>12</td><td>West Virginia</td><td>6</td></tr>
<tr><td>12</td><td>Michigan</td><td>6</td><td>12</td><td>Wisconsin</td><td>6</td></tr>
<tr><td>12</td><td>Minnesota</td><td>6</td><td>23</td><td>Alabama</td><td>5</td></tr>
<tr><td>39</td><td>Mississippi</td><td>4</td><td>23</td><td>Iowa</td><td>5</td></tr>
<tr><td>23</td><td>Missouri</td><td>5</td><td>23</td><td>Kansas</td><td>5</td></tr>
<tr><td>23</td><td>Montana</td><td>5</td><td>23</td><td>Missouri</td><td>5</td></tr>
<tr><td>23</td><td>Nebraska</td><td>5</td><td>23</td><td>Montana</td><td>5</td></tr>
<tr><td>39</td><td>Nevada</td><td>4</td><td>23</td><td>Nebraska</td><td>5</td></tr>
<tr><td>23</td><td>New Hampshire</td><td>5</td><td>23</td><td>New Hampshire</td><td>5</td></tr>
<tr><td>6</td><td>New Jersey</td><td>7</td><td>23</td><td>North Carolina</td><td>5</td></tr>
<tr><td>39</td><td>New Mexico</td><td>4</td><td>23</td><td>North Dakota</td><td>5</td></tr>
<tr><td>1</td><td>New York</td><td>9</td><td>23</td><td>Ohio</td><td>5</td></tr>
<tr><td>23</td><td>North Carolina</td><td>5</td><td>23</td><td>South Carolina</td><td>5</td></tr>
<tr><td>23</td><td>North Dakota</td><td>5</td><td>23</td><td>South Dakota</td><td>5</td></tr>
<tr><td>23</td><td>Ohio</td><td>5</td><td>23</td><td>Tennessee</td><td>5</td></tr>
<tr><td>39</td><td>Oklahoma</td><td>4</td><td>23</td><td>Texas</td><td>5</td></tr>
<tr><td>12</td><td>Oregon</td><td>6</td><td>23</td><td>Utah</td><td>5</td></tr>
<tr><td>6</td><td>Pennsylvania</td><td>7</td><td>23</td><td>Washington</td><td>5</td></tr>
<tr><td>6</td><td>Rhode Island</td><td>7</td><td>39</td><td>Alaska</td><td>4</td></tr>
<tr><td>23</td><td>South Carolina</td><td>5</td><td>39</td><td>Arizona</td><td>4</td></tr>
<tr><td>23</td><td>South Dakota</td><td>5</td><td>39</td><td>Arkansas</td><td>4</td></tr>
<tr><td>23</td><td>Tennessee</td><td>5</td><td>39</td><td>Georgia</td><td>4</td></tr>
<tr><td>23</td><td>Texas</td><td>5</td><td>39</td><td>Idaho</td><td>4</td></tr>
<tr><td>23</td><td>Utah</td><td>5</td><td>39</td><td>Indiana</td><td>4</td></tr>
<tr><td>6</td><td>Vermont</td><td>7</td><td>39</td><td>Kentucky</td><td>4</td></tr>
<tr><td>12</td><td>Virginia</td><td>6</td><td>39</td><td>Mississippi</td><td>4</td></tr>
<tr><td>23</td><td>Washington</td><td>5</td><td>39</td><td>Nevada</td><td>4</td></tr>
<tr><td>12</td><td>West Virginia</td><td>6</td><td>39</td><td>New Mexico</td><td>4</td></tr>
<tr><td>12</td><td>Wisconsin</td><td>6</td><td>39</td><td>Oklahoma</td><td>4</td></tr>
<tr><td>50</td><td>Wyoming</td><td>3</td><td>50</td><td>Wyoming</td><td>3</td></tr>
<tr><td></td><td></td><td></td><td></td><td>District of Columbia</td><td>18</td></tr>
</table>

Source: CQ Press using data from American Medical Association (Chicago, Illinois)
"Physician Characteristics and Distribution in the U.S." (2011 Edition)
*As of December 31, 2009. National rate does not include physicians in U.S. territories and possessions. Ophthalmology is the branch of medicine dealing with the anatomy, functions, and diseases of the eye.

Physicians in Orthopedic Surgery in 2009

National Total = 24,858 Physicians*

RANK	STATE	PHYSICIANS	% of USA
24	Alabama	392	1.6%
46	Alaska	74	0.3%
23	Arizona	405	1.6%
33	Arkansas	180	0.7%
1	California	2,888	11.6%
21	Colorado	443	1.8%
25	Connecticut	380	1.5%
49	Delaware	60	0.2%
4	Florida	1,400	5.6%
13	Georgia	638	2.6%
40	Hawaii	127	0.5%
42	Idaho	125	0.5%
6	Illinois	973	3.9%
20	Indiana	457	1.8%
32	Iowa	201	0.8%
30	Kansas	235	0.9%
28	Kentucky	327	1.3%
22	Louisiana	409	1.6%
43	Maine	124	0.5%
14	Maryland	614	2.5%
9	Massachusetts	752	3.0%
11	Michigan	653	2.6%
17	Minnesota	521	2.1%
34	Mississippi	178	0.7%
19	Missouri	471	1.9%
44	Montana	112	0.5%
35	Nebraska	168	0.7%
38	Nevada	138	0.6%
36	New Hampshire	154	0.6%
10	New Jersey	724	2.9%
37	New Mexico	148	0.6%
2	New York	1,893	7.6%
8	North Carolina	780	3.1%
50	North Dakota	50	0.2%
7	Ohio	932	3.7%
29	Oklahoma	236	0.9%
27	Oregon	333	1.3%
5	Pennsylvania	1,099	4.4%
39	Rhode Island	129	0.5%
26	South Carolina	366	1.5%
47	South Dakota	71	0.3%
16	Tennessee	565	2.3%
3	Texas	1,628	6.5%
31	Utah	207	0.8%
45	Vermont	83	0.3%
12	Virginia	645	2.6%
15	Washington	580	2.3%
41	West Virginia	126	0.5%
18	Wisconsin	507	2.0%
48	Wyoming	63	0.3%

RANK	STATE	PHYSICIANS	% of USA
1	California	2,888	11.6%
2	New York	1,893	7.6%
3	Texas	1,628	6.5%
4	Florida	1,400	5.6%
5	Pennsylvania	1,099	4.4%
6	Illinois	973	3.9%
7	Ohio	932	3.7%
8	North Carolina	780	3.1%
9	Massachusetts	752	3.0%
10	New Jersey	724	2.9%
11	Michigan	653	2.6%
12	Virginia	645	2.6%
13	Georgia	638	2.6%
14	Maryland	614	2.5%
15	Washington	580	2.3%
16	Tennessee	565	2.3%
17	Minnesota	521	2.1%
18	Wisconsin	507	2.0%
19	Missouri	471	1.9%
20	Indiana	457	1.8%
21	Colorado	443	1.8%
22	Louisiana	409	1.6%
23	Arizona	405	1.6%
24	Alabama	392	1.6%
25	Connecticut	380	1.5%
26	South Carolina	366	1.5%
27	Oregon	333	1.3%
28	Kentucky	327	1.3%
29	Oklahoma	236	0.9%
30	Kansas	235	0.9%
31	Utah	207	0.8%
32	Iowa	201	0.8%
33	Arkansas	180	0.7%
34	Mississippi	178	0.7%
35	Nebraska	168	0.7%
36	New Hampshire	154	0.6%
37	New Mexico	148	0.6%
38	Nevada	138	0.6%
39	Rhode Island	129	0.5%
40	Hawaii	127	0.5%
41	West Virginia	126	0.5%
42	Idaho	125	0.5%
43	Maine	124	0.5%
44	Montana	112	0.5%
45	Vermont	83	0.3%
46	Alaska	74	0.3%
47	South Dakota	71	0.3%
48	Wyoming	63	0.3%
49	Delaware	60	0.2%
50	North Dakota	50	0.2%
	District of Columbia	94	0.4%

Source: American Medical Association (Chicago, Illinois)
    "Physician Characteristics and Distribution in the U.S." (2011 Edition)
*As of December 31, 2009. Total does not include 140 physicians in U.S. territories and possessions. Orthopedics is the branch of medicine dealing with the skeletal system.

Rate of Physicians in Orthopedic Surgery in 2009

National Rate = 8 Physicians per 100,000 Population*

ALPHA ORDER

RANK	STATE	RATE
23	Alabama	8
5	Alaska	11
45	Arizona	6
45	Arkansas	6
23	California	8
13	Colorado	9
5	Connecticut	11
37	Delaware	7
23	Florida	8
45	Georgia	6
10	Hawaii	10
23	Idaho	8
23	Illinois	8
37	Indiana	7
37	Iowa	7
23	Kansas	8
23	Kentucky	8
13	Louisiana	9
13	Maine	9
5	Maryland	11
5	Massachusetts	11
37	Michigan	7
10	Minnesota	10
45	Mississippi	6
23	Missouri	8
5	Montana	11
13	Nebraska	9
50	Nevada	5
2	New Hampshire	12
23	New Jersey	8
37	New Mexico	7
10	New York	10
23	North Carolina	8
23	North Dakota	8
23	Ohio	8
45	Oklahoma	6
13	Oregon	9
13	Pennsylvania	9
2	Rhode Island	12
23	South Carolina	8
13	South Dakota	9
13	Tennessee	9
37	Texas	7
37	Utah	7
1	Vermont	13
23	Virginia	8
13	Washington	9
37	West Virginia	7
13	Wisconsin	9
2	Wyoming	12

RANK ORDER

RANK	STATE	RATE
1	Vermont	13
2	New Hampshire	12
2	Rhode Island	12
2	Wyoming	12
5	Alaska	11
5	Connecticut	11
5	Maryland	11
5	Massachusetts	11
5	Montana	11
10	Hawaii	10
10	Minnesota	10
10	New York	10
13	Colorado	9
13	Louisiana	9
13	Maine	9
13	Nebraska	9
13	Oregon	9
13	Pennsylvania	9
13	South Dakota	9
13	Tennessee	9
13	Washington	9
13	Wisconsin	9
23	Alabama	8
23	California	8
23	Florida	8
23	Idaho	8
23	Illinois	8
23	Kansas	8
23	Kentucky	8
23	Missouri	8
23	New Jersey	8
23	North Carolina	8
23	North Dakota	8
23	Ohio	8
23	South Carolina	8
23	Virginia	8
37	Delaware	7
37	Indiana	7
37	Iowa	7
37	Michigan	7
37	New Mexico	7
37	Texas	7
37	Utah	7
37	West Virginia	7
45	Arizona	6
45	Arkansas	6
45	Georgia	6
45	Mississippi	6
45	Oklahoma	6
50	Nevada	5

District of Columbia	16

Source: CQ Press using data from American Medical Association (Chicago, Illinois)
"Physician Characteristics and Distribution in the U.S." (2011 Edition)
*As of December 31, 2009. National rate does not include physicians in U.S. territories and possessions. Orthopedics is the branch of medicine dealing with the skeletal system.

Physicians in Plastic Surgery in 2009

National Total = 7,260 Physicians*

ALPHA ORDER

RANK	STATE	PHYSICIANS	% of USA
27	Alabama	82	1.1%
49	Alaska	7	0.1%
15	Arizona	146	2.0%
34	Arkansas	32	0.4%
1	California	1,124	15.5%
19	Colorado	109	1.5%
20	Connecticut	102	1.4%
42	Delaware	23	0.3%
2	Florida	619	8.5%
11	Georgia	191	2.6%
39	Hawaii	28	0.4%
43	Idaho	21	0.3%
5	Illinois	270	3.7%
20	Indiana	102	1.4%
34	Iowa	32	0.4%
30	Kansas	65	0.9%
24	Kentucky	97	1.3%
26	Louisiana	88	1.2%
44	Maine	16	0.2%
11	Maryland	191	2.6%
10	Massachusetts	201	2.8%
9	Michigan	212	2.9%
23	Minnesota	98	1.3%
32	Mississippi	49	0.7%
18	Missouri	136	1.9%
45	Montana	14	0.2%
34	Nebraska	32	0.4%
31	Nevada	54	0.7%
40	New Hampshire	27	0.4%
7	New Jersey	225	3.1%
37	New Mexico	29	0.4%
3	New York	617	8.5%
14	North Carolina	184	2.5%
47	North Dakota	11	0.2%
8	Ohio	221	3.0%
32	Oklahoma	49	0.7%
29	Oregon	69	1.0%
6	Pennsylvania	261	3.6%
37	Rhode Island	29	0.4%
25	South Carolina	93	1.3%
46	South Dakota	12	0.2%
15	Tennessee	146	2.0%
4	Texas	568	7.8%
28	Utah	79	1.1%
48	Vermont	10	0.1%
13	Virginia	186	2.6%
17	Washington	137	1.9%
40	West Virginia	27	0.4%
22	Wisconsin	100	1.4%
50	Wyoming	3	0.0%

RANK ORDER

RANK	STATE	PHYSICIANS	% of USA
1	California	1,124	15.5%
2	Florida	619	8.5%
3	New York	617	8.5%
4	Texas	568	7.8%
5	Illinois	270	3.7%
6	Pennsylvania	261	3.6%
7	New Jersey	225	3.1%
8	Ohio	221	3.0%
9	Michigan	212	2.9%
10	Massachusetts	201	2.8%
11	Georgia	191	2.6%
11	Maryland	191	2.6%
13	Virginia	186	2.6%
14	North Carolina	184	2.5%
15	Arizona	146	2.0%
15	Tennessee	146	2.0%
17	Washington	137	1.9%
18	Missouri	136	1.9%
19	Colorado	109	1.5%
20	Connecticut	102	1.4%
20	Indiana	102	1.4%
22	Wisconsin	100	1.4%
23	Minnesota	98	1.3%
24	Kentucky	97	1.3%
25	South Carolina	93	1.3%
26	Louisiana	88	1.2%
27	Alabama	82	1.1%
28	Utah	79	1.1%
29	Oregon	69	1.0%
30	Kansas	65	0.9%
31	Nevada	54	0.7%
32	Mississippi	49	0.7%
32	Oklahoma	49	0.7%
34	Arkansas	32	0.4%
34	Iowa	32	0.4%
34	Nebraska	32	0.4%
37	New Mexico	29	0.4%
37	Rhode Island	29	0.4%
39	Hawaii	28	0.4%
40	New Hampshire	27	0.4%
40	West Virginia	27	0.4%
42	Delaware	23	0.3%
43	Idaho	21	0.3%
44	Maine	16	0.2%
45	Montana	14	0.2%
46	South Dakota	12	0.2%
47	North Dakota	11	0.2%
48	Vermont	10	0.1%
49	Alaska	7	0.1%
50	Wyoming	3	0.0%
	District of Columbia	36	0.5%

Source: American Medical Association (Chicago, Illinois)
   "Physician Characteristics and Distribution in the U.S." (2011 Edition)
*As of December 31, 2009. Total does not include 37 physicians in U.S. territories and possessions.

Rate of Physicians in Plastic Surgery in 2009

National Rate = 2 Physicians per 100,000 Population*

<table>
<tr><td colspan="3">ALPHA ORDER</td><td colspan="3">RANK ORDER</td></tr>
<tr><th>RANK</th><th>STATE</th><th>RATE</th><th>RANK</th><th>STATE</th><th>RATE</th></tr>
<tr><td>11</td><td>Alabama</td><td>2</td><td>1</td><td>California</td><td>3</td></tr>
<tr><td>40</td><td>Alaska</td><td>1</td><td>1</td><td>Connecticut</td><td>3</td></tr>
<tr><td>11</td><td>Arizona</td><td>2</td><td>1</td><td>Delaware</td><td>3</td></tr>
<tr><td>40</td><td>Arkansas</td><td>1</td><td>1</td><td>Florida</td><td>3</td></tr>
<tr><td>1</td><td>California</td><td>3</td><td>1</td><td>Maryland</td><td>3</td></tr>
<tr><td>11</td><td>Colorado</td><td>2</td><td>1</td><td>Massachusetts</td><td>3</td></tr>
<tr><td>1</td><td>Connecticut</td><td>3</td><td>1</td><td>New Jersey</td><td>3</td></tr>
<tr><td>1</td><td>Delaware</td><td>3</td><td>1</td><td>New York</td><td>3</td></tr>
<tr><td>1</td><td>Florida</td><td>3</td><td>1</td><td>Rhode Island</td><td>3</td></tr>
<tr><td>11</td><td>Georgia</td><td>2</td><td>1</td><td>Utah</td><td>3</td></tr>
<tr><td>11</td><td>Hawaii</td><td>2</td><td>11</td><td>Alabama</td><td>2</td></tr>
<tr><td>40</td><td>Idaho</td><td>1</td><td>11</td><td>Arizona</td><td>2</td></tr>
<tr><td>11</td><td>Illinois</td><td>2</td><td>11</td><td>Colorado</td><td>2</td></tr>
<tr><td>11</td><td>Indiana</td><td>2</td><td>11</td><td>Georgia</td><td>2</td></tr>
<tr><td>40</td><td>Iowa</td><td>1</td><td>11</td><td>Hawaii</td><td>2</td></tr>
<tr><td>11</td><td>Kansas</td><td>2</td><td>11</td><td>Illinois</td><td>2</td></tr>
<tr><td>11</td><td>Kentucky</td><td>2</td><td>11</td><td>Indiana</td><td>2</td></tr>
<tr><td>11</td><td>Louisiana</td><td>2</td><td>11</td><td>Kansas</td><td>2</td></tr>
<tr><td>40</td><td>Maine</td><td>1</td><td>11</td><td>Kentucky</td><td>2</td></tr>
<tr><td>1</td><td>Maryland</td><td>3</td><td>11</td><td>Louisiana</td><td>2</td></tr>
<tr><td>1</td><td>Massachusetts</td><td>3</td><td>11</td><td>Michigan</td><td>2</td></tr>
<tr><td>11</td><td>Michigan</td><td>2</td><td>11</td><td>Minnesota</td><td>2</td></tr>
<tr><td>11</td><td>Minnesota</td><td>2</td><td>11</td><td>Mississippi</td><td>2</td></tr>
<tr><td>11</td><td>Mississippi</td><td>2</td><td>11</td><td>Missouri</td><td>2</td></tr>
<tr><td>11</td><td>Missouri</td><td>2</td><td>11</td><td>Nebraska</td><td>2</td></tr>
<tr><td>40</td><td>Montana</td><td>1</td><td>11</td><td>Nevada</td><td>2</td></tr>
<tr><td>11</td><td>Nebraska</td><td>2</td><td>11</td><td>New Hampshire</td><td>2</td></tr>
<tr><td>11</td><td>Nevada</td><td>2</td><td>11</td><td>North Carolina</td><td>2</td></tr>
<tr><td>11</td><td>New Hampshire</td><td>2</td><td>11</td><td>North Dakota</td><td>2</td></tr>
<tr><td>1</td><td>New Jersey</td><td>3</td><td>11</td><td>Ohio</td><td>2</td></tr>
<tr><td>40</td><td>New Mexico</td><td>1</td><td>11</td><td>Oregon</td><td>2</td></tr>
<tr><td>1</td><td>New York</td><td>3</td><td>11</td><td>Pennsylvania</td><td>2</td></tr>
<tr><td>11</td><td>North Carolina</td><td>2</td><td>11</td><td>South Carolina</td><td>2</td></tr>
<tr><td>11</td><td>North Dakota</td><td>2</td><td>11</td><td>Tennessee</td><td>2</td></tr>
<tr><td>11</td><td>Ohio</td><td>2</td><td>11</td><td>Texas</td><td>2</td></tr>
<tr><td>40</td><td>Oklahoma</td><td>1</td><td>11</td><td>Vermont</td><td>2</td></tr>
<tr><td>11</td><td>Oregon</td><td>2</td><td>11</td><td>Virginia</td><td>2</td></tr>
<tr><td>11</td><td>Pennsylvania</td><td>2</td><td>11</td><td>Washington</td><td>2</td></tr>
<tr><td>1</td><td>Rhode Island</td><td>3</td><td>11</td><td>Wisconsin</td><td>2</td></tr>
<tr><td>11</td><td>South Carolina</td><td>2</td><td>40</td><td>Alaska</td><td>1</td></tr>
<tr><td>40</td><td>South Dakota</td><td>1</td><td>40</td><td>Arkansas</td><td>1</td></tr>
<tr><td>11</td><td>Tennessee</td><td>2</td><td>40</td><td>Idaho</td><td>1</td></tr>
<tr><td>11</td><td>Texas</td><td>2</td><td>40</td><td>Iowa</td><td>1</td></tr>
<tr><td>1</td><td>Utah</td><td>3</td><td>40</td><td>Maine</td><td>1</td></tr>
<tr><td>11</td><td>Vermont</td><td>2</td><td>40</td><td>Montana</td><td>1</td></tr>
<tr><td>11</td><td>Virginia</td><td>2</td><td>40</td><td>New Mexico</td><td>1</td></tr>
<tr><td>11</td><td>Washington</td><td>2</td><td>40</td><td>Oklahoma</td><td>1</td></tr>
<tr><td>40</td><td>West Virginia</td><td>1</td><td>40</td><td>South Dakota</td><td>1</td></tr>
<tr><td>11</td><td>Wisconsin</td><td>2</td><td>40</td><td>West Virginia</td><td>1</td></tr>
<tr><td>40</td><td>Wyoming</td><td>1</td><td>40</td><td>Wyoming</td><td>1</td></tr>
<tr><td></td><td></td><td></td><td></td><td>District of Columbia</td><td>6</td></tr>
</table>

Source: CQ Press using data from American Medical Association (Chicago, Illinois)
"Physician Characteristics and Distribution in the U.S." (2011 Edition)
*As of December 31, 2009. National rate does not include physicians in U.S. territories and possessions.

Physicians in Other Specialties in 2009

National Total = 227,090 Physicians*

ALPHA ORDER

RANK	STATE	PHYSICIANS	% of USA
28	Alabama	2,510	1.1%
48	Alaska	428	0.2%
18	Arizona	4,060	1.8%
32	Arkansas	1,468	0.6%
1	California	28,079	12.4%
22	Colorado	3,801	1.7%
23	Connecticut	3,727	1.6%
45	Delaware	626	0.3%
4	Florida	12,356	5.4%
14	Georgia	5,556	2.4%
37	Hawaii	1,176	0.5%
43	Idaho	741	0.3%
6	Illinois	9,518	4.2%
21	Indiana	3,843	1.7%
33	Iowa	1,464	0.6%
29	Kansas	1,756	0.8%
27	Kentucky	2,683	1.2%
25	Louisiana	2,900	1.3%
41	Maine	1,043	0.5%
10	Maryland	6,884	3.0%
7	Massachusetts	9,164	4.0%
11	Michigan	6,855	3.0%
19	Minnesota	4,009	1.8%
36	Mississippi	1,317	0.6%
20	Missouri	3,890	1.7%
46	Montana	593	0.3%
38	Nebraska	1,131	0.5%
34	Nevada	1,405	0.6%
42	New Hampshire	1,018	0.4%
9	New Jersey	7,111	3.1%
35	New Mexico	1,387	0.6%
2	New York	21,186	9.3%
12	North Carolina	6,323	2.8%
49	North Dakota	414	0.2%
8	Ohio	8,135	3.6%
31	Oklahoma	1,687	0.7%
24	Oregon	2,996	1.3%
5	Pennsylvania	10,810	4.8%
40	Rhode Island	1,050	0.5%
26	South Carolina	2,739	1.2%
47	South Dakota	443	0.2%
16	Tennessee	4,144	1.8%
3	Texas	14,250	6.3%
30	Utah	1,707	0.8%
44	Vermont	657	0.3%
13	Virginia	6,066	2.7%
15	Washington	5,165	2.3%
39	West Virginia	1,068	0.5%
17	Wisconsin	4,124	1.8%
50	Wyoming	267	0.1%

RANK ORDER

RANK	STATE	PHYSICIANS	% of USA
1	California	28,079	12.4%
2	New York	21,186	9.3%
3	Texas	14,250	6.3%
4	Florida	12,356	5.4%
5	Pennsylvania	10,810	4.8%
6	Illinois	9,518	4.2%
7	Massachusetts	9,164	4.0%
8	Ohio	8,135	3.6%
9	New Jersey	7,111	3.1%
10	Maryland	6,884	3.0%
11	Michigan	6,855	3.0%
12	North Carolina	6,323	2.8%
13	Virginia	6,066	2.7%
14	Georgia	5,556	2.4%
15	Washington	5,165	2.3%
16	Tennessee	4,144	1.8%
17	Wisconsin	4,124	1.8%
18	Arizona	4,060	1.8%
19	Minnesota	4,009	1.8%
20	Missouri	3,890	1.7%
21	Indiana	3,843	1.7%
22	Colorado	3,801	1.7%
23	Connecticut	3,727	1.6%
24	Oregon	2,996	1.3%
25	Louisiana	2,900	1.3%
26	South Carolina	2,739	1.2%
27	Kentucky	2,683	1.2%
28	Alabama	2,510	1.1%
29	Kansas	1,756	0.8%
30	Utah	1,707	0.8%
31	Oklahoma	1,687	0.7%
32	Arkansas	1,468	0.6%
33	Iowa	1,464	0.6%
34	Nevada	1,405	0.6%
35	New Mexico	1,387	0.6%
36	Mississippi	1,317	0.6%
37	Hawaii	1,176	0.5%
38	Nebraska	1,131	0.5%
39	West Virginia	1,068	0.5%
40	Rhode Island	1,050	0.5%
41	Maine	1,043	0.5%
42	New Hampshire	1,018	0.4%
43	Idaho	741	0.3%
44	Vermont	657	0.3%
45	Delaware	626	0.3%
46	Montana	593	0.3%
47	South Dakota	443	0.2%
48	Alaska	428	0.2%
49	North Dakota	414	0.2%
50	Wyoming	267	0.1%
	District of Columbia	1,360	0.6%

Source: American Medical Association (Chicago, Illinois)
   "Physician Characteristics and Distribution in the U.S." (2011 Edition)
*As of December 31, 2009. Total does not include 2,991 physicians in U.S. territories and possessions. Other Specialties include Aerospace Medicine, Anatomic/Clinical Pathology, Anesthesiology, Child Psychiatry, Diagnostic Radiology, Emergency Medicine, Forensic Pathology, Nuclear Medicine, Occupational Medicine, Neurology, Psychiatry, Public Health, Radiation Oncology, Radiology, and other specialties.

Rate of Physicians in Other Specialties in 2009

National Rate = 74 Physicians per 100,000 Population*

RANK	STATE	RATE
43	Alabama	53
34	Alaska	61
31	Arizona	62
45	Arkansas	51
15	California	76
15	Colorado	76
4	Connecticut	106
20	Delaware	71
24	Florida	67
41	Georgia	57
7	Hawaii	91
48	Idaho	48
18	Illinois	74
37	Indiana	60
46	Iowa	49
31	Kansas	62
31	Kentucky	62
27	Louisiana	65
10	Maine	79
2	Maryland	121
1	Massachusetts	139
22	Michigan	69
15	Minnesota	76
50	Mississippi	45
27	Missouri	65
34	Montana	61
30	Nebraska	63
43	Nevada	53
13	New Hampshire	77
9	New Jersey	82
22	New Mexico	69
3	New York	108
24	North Carolina	67
29	North Dakota	64
21	Ohio	70
49	Oklahoma	46
11	Oregon	78
8	Pennsylvania	86
6	Rhode Island	100
37	South Carolina	60
42	South Dakota	55
26	Tennessee	66
40	Texas	58
34	Utah	61
4	Vermont	106
13	Virginia	77
11	Washington	78
39	West Virginia	59
19	Wisconsin	73
46	Wyoming	49

RANK	STATE	RATE
1	Massachusetts	139
2	Maryland	121
3	New York	108
4	Connecticut	106
4	Vermont	106
6	Rhode Island	100
7	Hawaii	91
8	Pennsylvania	86
9	New Jersey	82
10	Maine	79
11	Oregon	78
11	Washington	78
13	New Hampshire	77
13	Virginia	77
15	California	76
15	Colorado	76
15	Minnesota	76
18	Illinois	74
19	Wisconsin	73
20	Delaware	71
21	Ohio	70
22	Michigan	69
22	New Mexico	69
24	Florida	67
24	North Carolina	67
26	Tennessee	66
27	Louisiana	65
27	Missouri	65
29	North Dakota	64
30	Nebraska	63
31	Arizona	62
31	Kansas	62
31	Kentucky	62
34	Alaska	61
34	Montana	61
34	Utah	61
37	Indiana	60
37	South Carolina	60
39	West Virginia	59
40	Texas	58
41	Georgia	57
42	South Dakota	55
43	Alabama	53
43	Nevada	53
45	Arkansas	51
46	Iowa	49
46	Wyoming	49
48	Idaho	48
49	Oklahoma	46
50	Mississippi	45

| | District of Columbia | 227 |

Source: CQ Press using data from American Medical Association (Chicago, Illinois)
   "Physician Characteristics and Distribution in the U.S." (2011 Edition)
*As of December 31, 2009. National rate does not include physicians in U.S. territories and possessions. Other Specialties include Aerospace Medicine, Anatomic/Clinical Pathology, Anesthesiology, Child Psychiatry, Diagnostic Radiology, Emergency Medicine, Forensic Pathology, Nuclear Medicine, Occupational Medicine, Neurology, Psychiatry, Public Health, Radiation Oncology, Radiology, and other specialties.

Physicians in Anesthesiology in 2009

National Total = 42,390 Physicians*

ALPHA ORDER

RANK	STATE	PHYSICIANS	% of USA
27	Alabama	507	1.2%
47	Alaska	85	0.2%
17	Arizona	943	2.2%
34	Arkansas	285	0.7%
1	California	5,369	12.7%
20	Colorado	771	1.8%
23	Connecticut	593	1.4%
46	Delaware	94	0.2%
4	Florida	2,655	6.3%
15	Georgia	995	2.3%
40	Hawaii	157	0.4%
45	Idaho	105	0.2%
5	Illinois	1,861	4.4%
16	Indiana	977	2.3%
33	Iowa	306	0.7%
32	Kansas	343	0.8%
25	Kentucky	553	1.3%
26	Louisiana	529	1.2%
39	Maine	180	0.4%
10	Maryland	1,094	2.6%
9	Massachusetts	1,368	3.2%
12	Michigan	1,009	2.4%
23	Minnesota	593	1.4%
35	Mississippi	261	0.6%
21	Missouri	709	1.7%
42	Montana	136	0.3%
36	Nebraska	243	0.6%
30	Nevada	379	0.9%
38	New Hampshire	194	0.5%
7	New Jersey	1,544	3.6%
37	New Mexico	213	0.5%
2	New York	3,545	8.4%
11	North Carolina	1,016	2.4%
49	North Dakota	62	0.1%
8	Ohio	1,518	3.6%
31	Oklahoma	375	0.9%
22	Oregon	594	1.4%
6	Pennsylvania	1,792	4.2%
43	Rhode Island	125	0.3%
28	South Carolina	483	1.1%
48	South Dakota	73	0.2%
19	Tennessee	784	1.8%
3	Texas	3,290	7.8%
29	Utah	383	0.9%
44	Vermont	107	0.3%
13	Virginia	1,007	2.4%
14	Washington	1,006	2.4%
41	West Virginia	151	0.4%
18	Wisconsin	857	2.0%
50	Wyoming	55	0.1%

RANK ORDER

RANK	STATE	PHYSICIANS	% of USA
1	California	5,369	12.7%
2	New York	3,545	8.4%
3	Texas	3,290	7.8%
4	Florida	2,655	6.3%
5	Illinois	1,861	4.4%
6	Pennsylvania	1,792	4.2%
7	New Jersey	1,544	3.6%
8	Ohio	1,518	3.6%
9	Massachusetts	1,368	3.2%
10	Maryland	1,094	2.6%
11	North Carolina	1,016	2.4%
12	Michigan	1,009	2.4%
13	Virginia	1,007	2.4%
14	Washington	1,006	2.4%
15	Georgia	995	2.3%
16	Indiana	977	2.3%
17	Arizona	943	2.2%
18	Wisconsin	857	2.0%
19	Tennessee	784	1.8%
20	Colorado	771	1.8%
21	Missouri	709	1.7%
22	Oregon	594	1.4%
23	Connecticut	593	1.4%
23	Minnesota	593	1.4%
25	Kentucky	553	1.3%
26	Louisiana	529	1.2%
27	Alabama	507	1.2%
28	South Carolina	483	1.1%
29	Utah	383	0.9%
30	Nevada	379	0.9%
31	Oklahoma	375	0.9%
32	Kansas	343	0.8%
33	Iowa	306	0.7%
34	Arkansas	285	0.7%
35	Mississippi	261	0.6%
36	Nebraska	243	0.6%
37	New Mexico	213	0.5%
38	New Hampshire	194	0.5%
39	Maine	180	0.4%
40	Hawaii	157	0.4%
41	West Virginia	151	0.4%
42	Montana	136	0.3%
43	Rhode Island	125	0.3%
44	Vermont	107	0.3%
45	Idaho	105	0.2%
46	Delaware	94	0.2%
47	Alaska	85	0.2%
48	South Dakota	73	0.2%
49	North Dakota	62	0.1%
50	Wyoming	55	0.1%
	District of Columbia	116	0.3%

Source: American Medical Association (Chicago, Illinois)
   "Physician Characteristics and Distribution in the U.S." (2011 Edition)
*As of December 31, 2009. Total does not include 213 physicians in U.S. territories and possessions.

Rate of Physicians in Anesthesiology in 2009

National Rate = 14 Physicians per 100,000 Population*

ALPHA ORDER			RANK ORDER		
RANK	STATE	RATE	RANK	STATE	RATE
34	Alabama	11	1	Massachusetts	21
27	Alaska	12	2	Maryland	19
14	Arizona	14	3	New Jersey	18
40	Arkansas	10	3	New York	18
8	California	15	5	Connecticut	17
8	Colorado	15	5	Vermont	17
5	Connocticut	17	7	Oregon	16
34	Delaware	11	8	California	15
14	Florida	14	8	Colorado	15
40	Georgia	10	8	Indiana	15
27	Hawaii	12	8	New Hampshire	15
50	Idaho	7	8	Washington	15
14	Illinois	14	8	Wisconsin	15
8	Indiana	15	14	Arizona	14
40	Iowa	10	14	Florida	14
27	Kansas	12	14	Illinois	14
23	Kentucky	13	14	Maine	14
27	Louisiana	12	14	Montana	14
14	Maine	14	14	Nebraska	14
2	Maryland	19	14	Nevada	14
1	Massachusetts	21	14	Pennsylvania	14
40	Michigan	10	14	Utah	14
34	Minnesota	11	23	Kentucky	13
47	Mississippi	9	23	Ohio	13
27	Missouri	12	23	Texas	13
14	Montana	14	23	Virginia	13
14	Nebraska	14	27	Alaska	12
14	Nevada	14	27	Hawaii	12
8	New Hampshire	15	27	Kansas	12
3	New Jersey	18	27	Louisiana	12
34	New Mexico	11	27	Missouri	12
3	New York	18	27	Rhode Island	12
34	North Carolina	11	27	Tennessee	12
40	North Dakota	10	34	Alabama	11
23	Ohio	13	34	Delaware	11
40	Oklahoma	10	34	Minnesota	11
7	Oregon	16	34	New Mexico	11
14	Pennsylvania	14	34	North Carolina	11
27	Rhode Island	12	34	South Carolina	11
34	South Carolina	11	40	Arkansas	10
47	South Dakota	9	40	Georgia	10
27	Tennessee	12	40	Iowa	10
23	Texas	13	40	Michigan	10
14	Utah	14	40	North Dakota	10
5	Vermont	17	40	Oklahoma	10
23	Virginia	13	40	Wyoming	10
8	Washington	15	47	Mississippi	9
49	West Virginia	8	47	South Dakota	9
8	Wisconsin	15	49	West Virginia	8
40	Wyoming	10	50	Idaho	7
				District of Columbia	19

Source: CQ Press using data from American Medical Association (Chicago, Illinois)
"Physician Characteristics and Distribution in the U.S." (2011 Edition)
*As of December 31, 2009. National rate does not include physicians in U.S. territories and possessions.

Physicians in Psychiatry in 2009

National Total = 40,128 Physicians*

<table>
<tr><td colspan="4">ALPHA ORDER</td><td colspan="4">RANK ORDER</td></tr>
<tr><td>RANK</td><td>STATE</td><td>PHYSICIANS</td><td>% of USA</td><td>RANK</td><td>STATE</td><td>PHYSICIANS</td><td>% of USA</td></tr>
<tr><td>28</td><td>Alabama</td><td>349</td><td>0.9%</td><td>1</td><td>California</td><td>5,630</td><td>14.0%</td></tr>
<tr><td>48</td><td>Alaska</td><td>72</td><td>0.2%</td><td>2</td><td>New York</td><td>5,332</td><td>13.3%</td></tr>
<tr><td>22</td><td>Arizona</td><td>574</td><td>1.4%</td><td>3</td><td>Massachusetts</td><td>2,094</td><td>5.2%</td></tr>
<tr><td>33</td><td>Arkansas</td><td>241</td><td>0.6%</td><td>4</td><td>Pennsylvania</td><td>1,949</td><td>4.9%</td></tr>
<tr><td>1</td><td>California</td><td>5,630</td><td>14.0%</td><td>5</td><td>Texas</td><td>1,911</td><td>4.8%</td></tr>
<tr><td>17</td><td>Colorado</td><td>610</td><td>1.5%</td><td>6</td><td>Florida</td><td>1,756</td><td>4.4%</td></tr>
<tr><td>15</td><td>Connecticut</td><td>893</td><td>2.2%</td><td>7</td><td>Illinois</td><td>1,494</td><td>3.7%</td></tr>
<tr><td>44</td><td>Delaware</td><td>98</td><td>0.2%</td><td>8</td><td>New Jersey</td><td>1,382</td><td>3.4%</td></tr>
<tr><td>6</td><td>Florida</td><td>1,756</td><td>4.4%</td><td>9</td><td>Maryland</td><td>1,325</td><td>3.3%</td></tr>
<tr><td>14</td><td>Georgia</td><td>901</td><td>2.2%</td><td>10</td><td>Ohio</td><td>1,157</td><td>2.9%</td></tr>
<tr><td>32</td><td>Hawaii</td><td>249</td><td>0.6%</td><td>11</td><td>North Carolina</td><td>1,129</td><td>2.8%</td></tr>
<tr><td>46</td><td>Idaho</td><td>81</td><td>0.2%</td><td>12</td><td>Virginia</td><td>1,067</td><td>2.7%</td></tr>
<tr><td>7</td><td>Illinois</td><td>1,494</td><td>3.7%</td><td>13</td><td>Michigan</td><td>1,045</td><td>2.6%</td></tr>
<tr><td>26</td><td>Indiana</td><td>450</td><td>1.1%</td><td>14</td><td>Georgia</td><td>901</td><td>2.2%</td></tr>
<tr><td>37</td><td>Iowa</td><td>208</td><td>0.5%</td><td>15</td><td>Connecticut</td><td>893</td><td>2.2%</td></tr>
<tr><td>30</td><td>Kansas</td><td>288</td><td>0.7%</td><td>16</td><td>Washington</td><td>789</td><td>2.0%</td></tr>
<tr><td>27</td><td>Kentucky</td><td>385</td><td>1.0%</td><td>17</td><td>Colorado</td><td>610</td><td>1.5%</td></tr>
<tr><td>24</td><td>Louisiana</td><td>464</td><td>1.2%</td><td>18</td><td>Tennessee</td><td>603</td><td>1.5%</td></tr>
<tr><td>35</td><td>Maine</td><td>219</td><td>0.5%</td><td>19</td><td>Missouri</td><td>594</td><td>1.5%</td></tr>
<tr><td>9</td><td>Maryland</td><td>1,325</td><td>3.3%</td><td>20</td><td>Minnesota</td><td>591</td><td>1.5%</td></tr>
<tr><td>3</td><td>Massachusetts</td><td>2,094</td><td>5.2%</td><td>21</td><td>Wisconsin</td><td>584</td><td>1.5%</td></tr>
<tr><td>13</td><td>Michigan</td><td>1,045</td><td>2.6%</td><td>22</td><td>Arizona</td><td>574</td><td>1.4%</td></tr>
<tr><td>20</td><td>Minnesota</td><td>591</td><td>1.5%</td><td>23</td><td>Oregon</td><td>485</td><td>1.2%</td></tr>
<tr><td>38</td><td>Mississippi</td><td>195</td><td>0.5%</td><td>24</td><td>Louisiana</td><td>464</td><td>1.2%</td></tr>
<tr><td>19</td><td>Missouri</td><td>594</td><td>1.5%</td><td>25</td><td>South Carolina</td><td>463</td><td>1.2%</td></tr>
<tr><td>47</td><td>Montana</td><td>77</td><td>0.2%</td><td>26</td><td>Indiana</td><td>450</td><td>1.1%</td></tr>
<tr><td>41</td><td>Nebraska</td><td>172</td><td>0.4%</td><td>27</td><td>Kentucky</td><td>385</td><td>1.0%</td></tr>
<tr><td>40</td><td>Nevada</td><td>178</td><td>0.4%</td><td>28</td><td>Alabama</td><td>349</td><td>0.9%</td></tr>
<tr><td>39</td><td>New Hampshire</td><td>182</td><td>0.5%</td><td>29</td><td>Oklahoma</td><td>300</td><td>0.7%</td></tr>
<tr><td>8</td><td>New Jersey</td><td>1,382</td><td>3.4%</td><td>30</td><td>Kansas</td><td>288</td><td>0.7%</td></tr>
<tr><td>31</td><td>New Mexico</td><td>278</td><td>0.7%</td><td>31</td><td>New Mexico</td><td>278</td><td>0.7%</td></tr>
<tr><td>2</td><td>New York</td><td>5,332</td><td>13.3%</td><td>32</td><td>Hawaii</td><td>249</td><td>0.6%</td></tr>
<tr><td>11</td><td>North Carolina</td><td>1,129</td><td>2.8%</td><td>33</td><td>Arkansas</td><td>241</td><td>0.6%</td></tr>
<tr><td>45</td><td>North Dakota</td><td>83</td><td>0.2%</td><td>34</td><td>Rhode Island</td><td>227</td><td>0.6%</td></tr>
<tr><td>10</td><td>Ohio</td><td>1,157</td><td>2.9%</td><td>35</td><td>Maine</td><td>219</td><td>0.5%</td></tr>
<tr><td>29</td><td>Oklahoma</td><td>300</td><td>0.7%</td><td>36</td><td>Utah</td><td>209</td><td>0.5%</td></tr>
<tr><td>23</td><td>Oregon</td><td>485</td><td>1.2%</td><td>37</td><td>Iowa</td><td>208</td><td>0.5%</td></tr>
<tr><td>4</td><td>Pennsylvania</td><td>1,949</td><td>4.9%</td><td>38</td><td>Mississippi</td><td>195</td><td>0.5%</td></tr>
<tr><td>34</td><td>Rhode Island</td><td>227</td><td>0.6%</td><td>39</td><td>New Hampshire</td><td>182</td><td>0.5%</td></tr>
<tr><td>25</td><td>South Carolina</td><td>463</td><td>1.2%</td><td>40</td><td>Nevada</td><td>178</td><td>0.4%</td></tr>
<tr><td>49</td><td>South Dakota</td><td>65</td><td>0.2%</td><td>41</td><td>Nebraska</td><td>172</td><td>0.4%</td></tr>
<tr><td>18</td><td>Tennessee</td><td>603</td><td>1.5%</td><td>42</td><td>West Virginia</td><td>168</td><td>0.4%</td></tr>
<tr><td>5</td><td>Texas</td><td>1,911</td><td>4.8%</td><td>43</td><td>Vermont</td><td>163</td><td>0.4%</td></tr>
<tr><td>36</td><td>Utah</td><td>209</td><td>0.5%</td><td>44</td><td>Delaware</td><td>98</td><td>0.2%</td></tr>
<tr><td>43</td><td>Vermont</td><td>163</td><td>0.4%</td><td>45</td><td>North Dakota</td><td>83</td><td>0.2%</td></tr>
<tr><td>12</td><td>Virginia</td><td>1,067</td><td>2.7%</td><td>46</td><td>Idaho</td><td>81</td><td>0.2%</td></tr>
<tr><td>16</td><td>Washington</td><td>789</td><td>2.0%</td><td>47</td><td>Montana</td><td>77</td><td>0.2%</td></tr>
<tr><td>42</td><td>West Virginia</td><td>168</td><td>0.4%</td><td>48</td><td>Alaska</td><td>72</td><td>0.2%</td></tr>
<tr><td>21</td><td>Wisconsin</td><td>584</td><td>1.5%</td><td>49</td><td>South Dakota</td><td>65</td><td>0.2%</td></tr>
<tr><td>50</td><td>Wyoming</td><td>48</td><td>0.1%</td><td>50</td><td>Wyoming</td><td>48</td><td>0.1%</td></tr>
<tr><td></td><td></td><td></td><td></td><td></td><td>District of Columbia</td><td>321</td><td>0.8%</td></tr>
</table>

Source: American Medical Association (Chicago, Illinois)
   "Physician Characteristics and Distribution in the U.S." (2011 Edition)
*As of December 31, 2009. Total does not include 452 physicians in U.S. territories and possessions. Psychiatry includes psychoanalysis.

Rate of Physicians in Psychiatry in 2009

National Rate = 13 Physicians per 100,000 Population*

<table>
<tr><td colspan="3">ALPHA ORDER</td><td colspan="3">RANK ORDER</td></tr>
<tr><td>RANK</td><td>STATE</td><td>RATE</td><td>RANK</td><td>STATE</td><td>RATE</td></tr>
<tr><td>45</td><td>Alabama</td><td>7</td><td>1</td><td>Massachusetts</td><td>32</td></tr>
<tr><td>23</td><td>Alaska</td><td>10</td><td>2</td><td>New York</td><td>27</td></tr>
<tr><td>33</td><td>Arizona</td><td>9</td><td>3</td><td>Vermont</td><td>26</td></tr>
<tr><td>39</td><td>Arkansas</td><td>8</td><td>4</td><td>Connecticut</td><td>25</td></tr>
<tr><td>10</td><td>California</td><td>15</td><td>5</td><td>Maryland</td><td>23</td></tr>
<tr><td>17</td><td>Colorado</td><td>12</td><td>6</td><td>Rhode Island</td><td>22</td></tr>
<tr><td>4</td><td>Connecticut</td><td>25</td><td>7</td><td>Hawaii</td><td>19</td></tr>
<tr><td>21</td><td>Delaware</td><td>11</td><td>8</td><td>Maine</td><td>17</td></tr>
<tr><td>33</td><td>Florida</td><td>9</td><td>9</td><td>New Jersey</td><td>16</td></tr>
<tr><td>33</td><td>Georgia</td><td>9</td><td>10</td><td>California</td><td>15</td></tr>
<tr><td>7</td><td>Hawaii</td><td>19</td><td>10</td><td>Pennsylvania</td><td>15</td></tr>
<tr><td>50</td><td>Idaho</td><td>5</td><td>12</td><td>New Hampshire</td><td>14</td></tr>
<tr><td>17</td><td>Illinois</td><td>12</td><td>12</td><td>New Mexico</td><td>14</td></tr>
<tr><td>45</td><td>Indiana</td><td>7</td><td>12</td><td>Virginia</td><td>14</td></tr>
<tr><td>45</td><td>Iowa</td><td>7</td><td>15</td><td>North Dakota</td><td>13</td></tr>
<tr><td>23</td><td>Kansas</td><td>10</td><td>15</td><td>Oregon</td><td>13</td></tr>
<tr><td>33</td><td>Kentucky</td><td>9</td><td>17</td><td>Colorado</td><td>12</td></tr>
<tr><td>23</td><td>Louisiana</td><td>10</td><td>17</td><td>Illinois</td><td>12</td></tr>
<tr><td>8</td><td>Maine</td><td>17</td><td>17</td><td>North Carolina</td><td>12</td></tr>
<tr><td>5</td><td>Maryland</td><td>23</td><td>17</td><td>Washington</td><td>12</td></tr>
<tr><td>1</td><td>Massachusetts</td><td>32</td><td>21</td><td>Delaware</td><td>11</td></tr>
<tr><td>23</td><td>Michigan</td><td>10</td><td>21</td><td>Minnesota</td><td>11</td></tr>
<tr><td>21</td><td>Minnesota</td><td>11</td><td>23</td><td>Alaska</td><td>10</td></tr>
<tr><td>45</td><td>Mississippi</td><td>7</td><td>23</td><td>Kansas</td><td>10</td></tr>
<tr><td>23</td><td>Missouri</td><td>10</td><td>23</td><td>Louisiana</td><td>10</td></tr>
<tr><td>39</td><td>Montana</td><td>8</td><td>23</td><td>Michigan</td><td>10</td></tr>
<tr><td>23</td><td>Nebraska</td><td>10</td><td>23</td><td>Missouri</td><td>10</td></tr>
<tr><td>45</td><td>Nevada</td><td>7</td><td>23</td><td>Nebraska</td><td>10</td></tr>
<tr><td>12</td><td>New Hampshire</td><td>14</td><td>23</td><td>Ohio</td><td>10</td></tr>
<tr><td>9</td><td>New Jersey</td><td>16</td><td>23</td><td>South Carolina</td><td>10</td></tr>
<tr><td>12</td><td>New Mexico</td><td>14</td><td>23</td><td>Tennessee</td><td>10</td></tr>
<tr><td>2</td><td>New York</td><td>27</td><td>23</td><td>Wisconsin</td><td>10</td></tr>
<tr><td>17</td><td>North Carolina</td><td>12</td><td>33</td><td>Arizona</td><td>9</td></tr>
<tr><td>15</td><td>North Dakota</td><td>13</td><td>33</td><td>Florida</td><td>9</td></tr>
<tr><td>23</td><td>Ohio</td><td>10</td><td>33</td><td>Georgia</td><td>9</td></tr>
<tr><td>39</td><td>Oklahoma</td><td>8</td><td>33</td><td>Kentucky</td><td>9</td></tr>
<tr><td>15</td><td>Oregon</td><td>13</td><td>33</td><td>West Virginia</td><td>9</td></tr>
<tr><td>10</td><td>Pennsylvania</td><td>15</td><td>33</td><td>Wyoming</td><td>9</td></tr>
<tr><td>6</td><td>Rhode Island</td><td>22</td><td>39</td><td>Arkansas</td><td>8</td></tr>
<tr><td>23</td><td>South Carolina</td><td>10</td><td>39</td><td>Montana</td><td>8</td></tr>
<tr><td>39</td><td>South Dakota</td><td>8</td><td>39</td><td>Oklahoma</td><td>8</td></tr>
<tr><td>23</td><td>Tennessee</td><td>10</td><td>39</td><td>South Dakota</td><td>8</td></tr>
<tr><td>39</td><td>Texas</td><td>8</td><td>39</td><td>Texas</td><td>8</td></tr>
<tr><td>39</td><td>Utah</td><td>8</td><td>39</td><td>Utah</td><td>8</td></tr>
<tr><td>3</td><td>Vermont</td><td>26</td><td>45</td><td>Alabama</td><td>7</td></tr>
<tr><td>12</td><td>Virginia</td><td>14</td><td>45</td><td>Indiana</td><td>7</td></tr>
<tr><td>17</td><td>Washington</td><td>12</td><td>45</td><td>Iowa</td><td>7</td></tr>
<tr><td>33</td><td>West Virginia</td><td>9</td><td>45</td><td>Mississippi</td><td>7</td></tr>
<tr><td>23</td><td>Wisconsin</td><td>10</td><td>45</td><td>Nevada</td><td>7</td></tr>
<tr><td>33</td><td>Wyoming</td><td>9</td><td>50</td><td>Idaho</td><td>5</td></tr>
<tr><td></td><td></td><td></td><td></td><td>District of Columbia</td><td>54</td></tr>
</table>

Source: CQ Press using data from American Medical Association (Chicago, Illinois)
"Physician Characteristics and Distribution in the U.S." (2011 Edition)
*As of December 31, 2009. National rate does not include physicians in U.S. territories and possessions. Psychiatry includes psychoanalysis.

Percent of Population Lacking Access to Mental Health Care in 2011

National Percent = 19.8% of Population*

ALPHA ORDER

RANK	STATE	PERCENT
9	Alabama	41.7
13	Alaska	35.3
30	Arizona	17.3
5	Arkansas	45.8
39	California	10.0
34	Colorado	13.7
35	Connecticut	13.0
50	Delaware	0.0
41	Florida	8.9
21	Georgia	28.3
46	Hawaii	5.9
2	Idaho	61.5
17	Illinois	34.0
31	Indiana	15.6
7	Iowa	43.3
12	Kansas	35.7
23	Kentucky	26.7
3	Louisiana	59.3
36	Maine	12.0
43	Maryland	7.3
47	Massachusetts	5.8
36	Michigan	12.0
24	Minnesota	26.5
16	Mississippi	34.5
11	Missouri	36.0
8	Montana	43.0
10	Nebraska	41.5
43	Nevada	7.3
48	New Hampshire	4.3
49	New Jersey	1.3
6	New Mexico	44.6
43	New York	7.3
40	North Carolina	9.9
18	North Dakota	33.5
29	Ohio	18.6
14	Oklahoma	34.8
28	Oregon	22.3
38	Pennsylvania	11.3
31	Rhode Island	15.6
27	South Carolina	24.4
4	South Dakota	48.8
19	Tennessee	33.0
26	Texas	24.9
20	Utah	31.6
42	Vermont	7.4
31	Virginia	15.6
22	Washington	28.1
25	West Virginia	25.7
15	Wisconsin	34.6
1	Wyoming	69.2

RANK ORDER

RANK	STATE	PERCENT
1	Wyoming	69.2
2	Idaho	61.5
3	Louisiana	59.3
4	South Dakota	48.8
5	Arkansas	45.8
6	New Mexico	44.6
7	Iowa	43.3
8	Montana	43.0
9	Alabama	41.7
10	Nebraska	41.5
11	Missouri	36.0
12	Kansas	35.7
13	Alaska	35.3
14	Oklahoma	34.8
15	Wisconsin	34.6
16	Mississippi	34.5
17	Illinois	34.0
18	North Dakota	33.5
19	Tennessee	33.0
20	Utah	31.6
21	Georgia	28.3
22	Washington	28.1
23	Kentucky	26.7
24	Minnesota	26.5
25	West Virginia	25.7
26	Texas	24.9
27	South Carolina	24.4
28	Oregon	22.3
29	Ohio	18.6
30	Arizona	17.3
31	Indiana	15.6
31	Rhode Island	15.6
31	Virginia	15.6
34	Colorado	13.7
35	Connecticut	13.0
36	Maine	12.0
36	Michigan	12.0
38	Pennsylvania	11.3
39	California	10.0
40	North Carolina	9.9
41	Florida	8.9
42	Vermont	7.4
43	Maryland	7.3
43	Nevada	7.3
43	New York	7.3
46	Hawaii	5.9
47	Massachusetts	5.8
48	New Hampshire	4.3
49	New Jersey	1.3
50	Delaware	0.0

District of Columbia 13.1

Source: CQ Press using data from U.S. Department of Health and Human Services, Division of Shortage Designation
"State Population and HPSA Designation Population Statistics" (as of January 20, 2011)
(http://datawarehouse.hrsa.gov/hpsadetail.aspx)
*Percent of population considered under-served by mental health practitioners. An under-served population does not have primary medical care within reasonable economic and geographic bounds.

International Medical School Graduates in 2009

National Total = 245,137 Nonfederal Physicians*

ALPHA ORDER

RANK	STATE	PHYSICIANS	% of USA
25	Alabama	1,871	0.8%
50	Alaska	117	0.0%
15	Arizona	3,819	1.6%
35	Arkansas	1,090	0.4%
2	California	27,271	11.1%
34	Colorado	1,136	0.5%
14	Connecticut	4,495	1.8%
38	Delaware	776	0.3%
3	Florida	21,225	8.7%
13	Georgia	4,905	2.0%
40	Hawaii	732	0.3%
48	Idaho	138	0.1%
5	Illinois	13,938	5.7%
18	Indiana	3,348	1.4%
31	Iowa	1,347	0.5%
30	Kansas	1,437	0.6%
24	Kentucky	2,389	1.0%
22	Louisiana	2,681	1.1%
42	Maine	635	0.3%
11	Maryland	7,428	3.0%
10	Massachusetts	7,688	3.1%
9	Michigan	10,118	4.1%
23	Minnesota	2,676	1.1%
37	Mississippi	821	0.3%
16	Missouri	3,769	1.5%
49	Montana	121	0.0%
39	Nebraska	762	0.3%
26	Nevada	1,805	0.7%
41	New Hampshire	713	0.3%
6	New Jersey	13,907	5.7%
36	New Mexico	995	0.4%
1	New York	35,900	14.6%
17	North Carolina	3,726	1.5%
44	North Dakota	497	0.2%
8	Ohio	10,358	4.2%
29	Oklahoma	1,515	0.6%
33	Oregon	1,178	0.5%
7	Pennsylvania	11,616	4.7%
32	Rhode Island	1,197	0.5%
28	South Carolina	1,613	0.7%
45	South Dakota	296	0.1%
19	Tennessee	3,189	1.3%
4	Texas	14,642	6.0%
43	Utah	593	0.2%
46	Vermont	245	0.1%
12	Virginia	5,505	2.2%
21	Washington	2,774	1.1%
27	West Virginia	1,728	0.7%
20	Wisconsin	3,142	1.3%
47	Wyoming	141	0.1%

RANK ORDER

RANK	STATE	PHYSICIANS	% of USA
1	New York	35,900	14.6%
2	California	27,271	11.1%
3	Florida	21,225	8.7%
4	Texas	14,642	6.0%
5	Illinois	13,938	5.7%
6	New Jersey	13,907	5.7%
7	Pennsylvania	11,616	4.7%
8	Ohio	10,358	4.2%
9	Michigan	10,118	4.1%
10	Massachusetts	7,688	3.1%
11	Maryland	7,428	3.0%
12	Virginia	5,505	2.2%
13	Georgia	4,905	2.0%
14	Connecticut	4,495	1.8%
15	Arizona	3,819	1.6%
16	Missouri	3,769	1.5%
17	North Carolina	3,726	1.5%
18	Indiana	3,348	1.4%
19	Tennessee	3,189	1.3%
20	Wisconsin	3,142	1.3%
21	Washington	2,774	1.1%
22	Louisiana	2,681	1.1%
23	Minnesota	2,676	1.1%
24	Kentucky	2,389	1.0%
25	Alabama	1,871	0.8%
26	Nevada	1,805	0.7%
27	West Virginia	1,728	0.7%
28	South Carolina	1,613	0.7%
29	Oklahoma	1,515	0.6%
30	Kansas	1,437	0.6%
31	Iowa	1,347	0.5%
32	Rhode Island	1,197	0.5%
33	Oregon	1,178	0.5%
34	Colorado	1,136	0.5%
35	Arkansas	1,090	0.4%
36	New Mexico	995	0.4%
37	Mississippi	821	0.3%
38	Delaware	776	0.3%
39	Nebraska	762	0.3%
40	Hawaii	732	0.3%
41	New Hampshire	713	0.3%
42	Maine	635	0.3%
43	Utah	593	0.2%
44	North Dakota	497	0.2%
45	South Dakota	296	0.1%
46	Vermont	245	0.1%
47	Wyoming	141	0.1%
48	Idaho	138	0.1%
49	Montana	121	0.0%
50	Alaska	117	0.0%
	District of Columbia	1,129	0.5%

Source: American Medical Association (Chicago, Illinois)
"Physician Characteristics and Distribution in the U.S." (2011 Edition)
*As of December 31, 2009. Total does not include 6,960 physicians in U.S. territories and possessions.

International Medical School Graduates as a Percent of Physicians in 2009

National Percent = 25.6% of Physicians*

ALPHA ORDER

RANK	STATE	PERCENT
31	Alabama	16.3
48	Alaska	6.6
17	Arizona	23.0
32	Arkansas	16.2
16	California	23.4
47	Colorado	7.5
9	Connecticut	29.6
7	Delaware	31.2
3	Florida	37.2
23	Georgia	20.4
34	Hawaii	15.3
50	Idaho	4.4
6	Illinois	34.0
21	Indiana	21.2
23	Iowa	20.4
27	Kansas	19.2
22	Kentucky	21.1
26	Louisiana	20.1
37	Maine	14.5
11	Maryland	27.4
19	Massachusetts	22.2
5	Michigan	34.7
35	Minnesota	15.1
40	Mississippi	13.5
18	Missouri	22.9
49	Montana	4.6
36	Nebraska	14.8
8	Nevada	31.0
33	New Hampshire	15.8
1	New Jersey	44.7
29	New Mexico	17.5
2	New York	41.5
39	North Carolina	13.6
12	North Dakota	27.1
10	Ohio	29.2
25	Oklahoma	20.3
44	Oregon	9.2
14	Pennsylvania	26.2
13	Rhode Island	26.4
40	South Carolina	13.5
38	South Dakota	14.1
30	Tennessee	16.9
15	Texas	24.6
46	Utah	8.8
45	Vermont	8.9
20	Virginia	21.8
42	Washington	13.0
4	West Virginia	35.3
28	Wisconsin	18.5
43	Wyoming	11.4

RANK ORDER

RANK	STATE	PERCENT
1	New Jersey	44.7
2	New York	41.5
3	Florida	37.2
4	West Virginia	35.3
5	Michigan	34.7
6	Illinois	34.0
7	Delaware	31.2
8	Nevada	31.0
9	Connecticut	29.6
10	Ohio	29.2
11	Maryland	27.4
12	North Dakota	27.1
13	Rhode Island	26.4
14	Pennsylvania	26.2
15	Texas	24.6
16	California	23.4
17	Arizona	23.0
18	Missouri	22.9
19	Massachusetts	22.2
20	Virginia	21.8
21	Indiana	21.2
22	Kentucky	21.1
23	Georgia	20.4
23	Iowa	20.4
25	Oklahoma	20.3
26	Louisiana	20.1
27	Kansas	19.2
28	Wisconsin	18.5
29	New Mexico	17.5
30	Tennessee	16.9
31	Alabama	16.3
32	Arkansas	16.2
33	New Hampshire	15.8
34	Hawaii	15.3
35	Minnesota	15.1
36	Nebraska	14.8
37	Maine	14.5
38	South Dakota	14.1
39	North Carolina	13.6
40	Mississippi	13.5
40	South Carolina	13.5
42	Washington	13.0
43	Wyoming	11.4
44	Oregon	9.2
45	Vermont	8.9
46	Utah	8.8
47	Colorado	7.5
48	Alaska	6.6
49	Montana	4.6
50	Idaho	4.4

District of Columbia   21.0

Source: CQ Press using data from American Medical Association (Chicago, Illinois)
"Physician Characteristics and Distribution in the U.S." (2011 Edition)
*As of December 31, 2009. National percent does not include physicians in the U.S. territories and possessions.

Osteopathic Physicians in 2010

National Total = 62,871 Osteopathic Physicians*

ALPHA ORDER

RANK	STATE	OSTEOPATHS	% of USA
33	Alabama	420	0.7%
46	Alaska	161	0.3%
11	Arizona	1,706	2.7%
38	Arkansas	267	0.4%
3	California	4,562	7.3%
15	Colorado	1,038	1.7%
31	Connecticut	491	0.8%
37	Delaware	269	0.4%
5	Florida	4,157	6.6%
18	Georgia	887	1.4%
41	Hawaii	229	0.4%
36	Idaho	280	0.4%
9	Illinois	2,635	4.2%
19	Indiana	881	1.4%
13	Iowa	1,182	1.9%
24	Kansas	720	1.1%
30	Kentucky	550	0.9%
44	Louisiana	167	0.3%
25	Maine	676	1.1%
21	Maryland	778	1.2%
23	Massachusetts	728	1.2%
2	Michigan	5,296	8.4%
28	Minnesota	558	0.9%
35	Mississippi	345	0.5%
10	Missouri	1,953	3.1%
45	Montana	166	0.3%
43	Nebraska	201	0.3%
28	Nevada	558	0.9%
39	New Hampshire	264	0.4%
8	New Jersey	3,218	5.1%
40	New Mexico	241	0.4%
4	New York	4,297	6.8%
17	North Carolina	910	1.4%
50	North Dakota	61	0.1%
6	Ohio	4,131	6.6%
12	Oklahoma	1,678	2.7%
27	Oregon	646	1.0%
1	Pennsylvania	6,165	9.8%
42	Rhode Island	227	0.4%
32	South Carolina	471	0.7%
47	South Dakota	112	0.2%
26	Tennessee	647	1.0%
7	Texas	3,739	5.9%
34	Utah	351	0.6%
49	Vermont	67	0.1%
14	Virginia	1,082	1.7%
16	Washington	936	1.5%
22	West Virginia	769	1.2%
20	Wisconsin	824	1.3%
48	Wyoming	87	0.1%

RANK ORDER

RANK	STATE	OSTEOPATHS	% of USA
1	Pennsylvania	6,165	9.8%
2	Michigan	5,296	8.4%
3	California	4,562	7.3%
4	New York	4,297	6.8%
5	Florida	4,157	6.6%
6	Ohio	4,131	6.6%
7	Texas	3,739	5.9%
8	New Jersey	3,218	5.1%
9	Illinois	2,635	4.2%
10	Missouri	1,953	3.1%
11	Arizona	1,706	2.7%
12	Oklahoma	1,678	2.7%
13	Iowa	1,182	1.9%
14	Virginia	1,082	1.7%
15	Colorado	1,038	1.7%
16	Washington	936	1.5%
17	North Carolina	910	1.4%
18	Georgia	887	1.4%
19	Indiana	881	1.4%
20	Wisconsin	824	1.3%
21	Maryland	778	1.2%
22	West Virginia	769	1.2%
23	Massachusetts	728	1.2%
24	Kansas	720	1.1%
25	Maine	676	1.1%
26	Tennessee	647	1.0%
27	Oregon	646	1.0%
28	Minnesota	558	0.9%
28	Nevada	558	0.9%
30	Kentucky	550	0.9%
31	Connecticut	491	0.8%
32	South Carolina	471	0.7%
33	Alabama	420	0.7%
34	Utah	351	0.6%
35	Mississippi	345	0.5%
36	Idaho	280	0.4%
37	Delaware	269	0.4%
38	Arkansas	267	0.4%
39	New Hampshire	264	0.4%
40	New Mexico	241	0.4%
41	Hawaii	229	0.4%
42	Rhode Island	227	0.4%
43	Nebraska	201	0.3%
44	Louisiana	167	0.3%
45	Montana	166	0.3%
46	Alaska	161	0.3%
47	South Dakota	112	0.2%
48	Wyoming	87	0.1%
49	Vermont	67	0.1%
50	North Dakota	61	0.1%
	District of Columbia	87	0.1%

Source: American Osteopathic Association
   "Osteopathic Medical Profession Report" (www.osteopathic.org/inside-aoa/about/who-we-are/pages/aoa-annual-statistics.aspx)
*Active osteopaths under age 65 as of May 31, 2010. National total does not include 250 osteopaths not shown by state.
Osteopaths practice a system of medicine based on the theory that disturbances in the musculoskeletal system affect other
body parts, causing many disorders that can be corrected by various manipulative techniques in conjunction with conventional
medical, surgical, pharmacological, and other therapeutic procedures.

Rate of Osteopathic Physicians in 2010

National Rate = 20 Osteopaths per 100,000 Population*

ALPHA ORDER

RANK	STATE	RATE
46	Alabama	9
13	Alaska	23
11	Arizona	26
46	Arkansas	9
36	California	12
17	Colorado	21
28	Connecticut	14
10	Delaware	30
14	Florida	22
46	Georgia	9
21	Hawaii	18
21	Idaho	18
19	Illinois	20
28	Indiana	14
6	Iowa	39
11	Kansas	26
34	Kentucky	13
50	Louisiana	4
2	Maine	51
28	Maryland	14
39	Massachusetts	11
1	Michigan	53
39	Minnesota	11
36	Mississippi	12
9	Missouri	33
23	Montana	17
39	Nebraska	11
17	Nevada	21
19	New Hampshire	20
7	New Jersey	37
36	New Mexico	12
14	New York	22
43	North Carolina	10
46	North Dakota	9
8	Ohio	36
4	Oklahoma	46
23	Oregon	17
3	Pennsylvania	49
14	Rhode Island	22
43	South Carolina	10
28	South Dakota	14
43	Tennessee	10
26	Texas	15
34	Utah	13
39	Vermont	11
28	Virginia	14
28	Washington	14
5	West Virginia	42
26	Wisconsin	15
25	Wyoming	16

RANK ORDER

RANK	STATE	RATE
1	Michigan	53
2	Maine	51
3	Pennsylvania	49
4	Oklahoma	46
5	West Virginia	42
6	Iowa	39
7	New Jersey	37
8	Ohio	36
9	Missouri	33
10	Delaware	30
11	Arizona	26
11	Kansas	26
13	Alaska	23
14	Florida	22
14	New York	22
14	Rhode Island	22
17	Colorado	21
17	Nevada	21
19	Illinois	20
19	New Hampshire	20
21	Hawaii	18
21	Idaho	18
23	Montana	17
23	Oregon	17
25	Wyoming	16
26	Texas	15
26	Wisconsin	15
28	Connecticut	14
28	Indiana	14
28	Maryland	14
28	South Dakota	14
28	Virginia	14
28	Washington	14
34	Kentucky	13
34	Utah	13
36	California	12
36	Mississippi	12
36	New Mexico	12
39	Massachusetts	11
39	Minnesota	11
39	Nebraska	11
39	Vermont	11
43	North Carolina	10
43	South Carolina	10
43	Tennessee	10
46	Alabama	9
46	Arkansas	9
46	Georgia	9
46	North Dakota	9
50	Louisiana	4

District of Columbia 15

Source: CQ Press using data from American Osteopathic Association
   "Osteopathic Medical Profession Report" (www.osteopathic.org/inside-aoa/about/who-we-are/pages/aoa-annual-statistics.aspx)
*Active osteopaths under age 65 as of May 31, 2010. National rate does not include osteopaths not shown by state.
Osteopaths practice a system of medicine based on the theory that disturbances in the musculoskeletal system affect other
body parts, causing many disorders that can be corrected by various manipulative techniques in conjunction with conventional
medical, surgical, pharmacological, and other therapeutic procedures.

Podiatrists in 2009

National Total = 9,720 Podiatrists*

ALPHA ORDER					RANK ORDER			
RANK	STATE	PODIATRISTS	% of USA		RANK	STATE	PODIATRISTS	% of USA
24	Alabama	120	1.2%		1	New York	1,070	11.0%
NA	Alaska**	NA	NA		2	California	830	8.5%
9	Arizona	420	4.3%		3	Florida	660	6.8%
36	Arkansas	40	0.4%		4	Ohio	570	5.9%
2	California	830	8.5%		5	Texas	560	5.8%
26	Colorado	100	1.0%		6	Pennsylvania	550	5.7%
22	Connecticut	130	1.3%		7	New Jersey	450	4.6%
29	Delaware	80	0.8%		8	Illinois	430	4.4%
3	Florida	660	6.8%		9	Arizona	420	4.3%
18	Georgia	140	1.4%		10	Maryland	390	4.0%
NA	Hawaii**	NA	NA		11	Virginia	360	3.7%
NA	Idaho**	NA	NA		12	Michigan	320	3.3%
8	Illinois	430	4.4%		13	Massachusetts	250	2.6%
15	Indiana	160	1.6%		14	North Carolina	180	1.9%
31	Iowa	70	0.7%		15	Indiana	160	1.6%
28	Kansas	90	0.9%		15	Utah	160	1.6%
29	Kentucky	80	0.8%		17	Washington	150	1.5%
31	Louisiana	70	0.7%		18	Georgia	140	1.4%
NA	Maine**	NA	NA		18	Minnesota	140	1.4%
10	Maryland	390	4.0%		18	Missouri	140	1.4%
13	Massachusetts	250	2.6%		18	Wisconsin	140	1.4%
12	Michigan	320	3.3%		22	Connecticut	130	1.3%
18	Minnesota	140	1.4%		22	Tennessee	130	1.3%
39	Mississippi	30	0.3%		24	Alabama	120	1.2%
18	Missouri	140	1.4%		24	Nebraska	120	1.2%
34	Montana	60	0.6%		26	Colorado	100	1.0%
24	Nebraska	120	1.2%		26	Oklahoma	100	1.0%
36	Nevada	40	0.4%		28	Kansas	90	0.9%
39	New Hampshire	30	0.3%		29	Delaware	80	0.8%
7	New Jersey	450	4.6%		29	Kentucky	80	0.8%
36	New Mexico	40	0.4%		31	Iowa	70	0.7%
1	New York	1,070	11.0%		31	Louisiana	70	0.7%
14	North Carolina	180	1.9%		31	South Carolina	70	0.7%
NA	North Dakota**	NA	NA		34	Montana	60	0.6%
4	Ohio	570	5.9%		35	Oregon	50	0.5%
26	Oklahoma	100	1.0%		36	Arkansas	40	0.4%
35	Oregon	50	0.5%		36	Nevada	40	0.4%
6	Pennsylvania	550	5.7%		36	New Mexico	40	0.4%
NA	Rhode Island**	NA	NA		39	Mississippi	30	0.3%
31	South Carolina	70	0.7%		39	New Hampshire	30	0.3%
NA	South Dakota**	NA	NA		39	Wyoming	30	0.3%
22	Tennessee	130	1.3%		NA	Alaska**	NA	NA
5	Texas	560	5.8%		NA	Hawaii**	NA	NA
15	Utah	160	1.6%		NA	Idaho**	NA	NA
NA	Vermont**	NA	NA		NA	Maine**	NA	NA
11	Virginia	360	3.7%		NA	North Dakota**	NA	NA
17	Washington	150	1.5%		NA	Rhode Island**	NA	NA
NA	West Virginia**	NA	NA		NA	South Dakota**	NA	NA
18	Wisconsin	140	1.4%		NA	Vermont**	NA	NA
39	Wyoming	30	0.3%		NA	West Virginia**	NA	NA
					District of Columbia**		NA	NA

Source: U.S. Department of Labor, Bureau of Labor Statistics
    "Occupational Employment and Wages, 2009" (http://www.bls.gov/oes/)
*Does not include self-employed.
**Not available.

Rate of Podiatrists in 2009

National Rate = 3 Podiatrists per 100,000 Population*

<table>
<tr><td colspan="3">ALPHA ORDER</td><td colspan="3">RANK ORDER</td></tr>
<tr><td>RANK</td><td>STATE</td><td>RATE</td><td>RANK</td><td>STATE</td><td>RATE</td></tr>
<tr><td>16</td><td>Alabama</td><td>3</td><td>1</td><td>Delaware</td><td>9</td></tr>
<tr><td>NA</td><td>Alaska**</td><td>NA</td><td>2</td><td>Maryland</td><td>7</td></tr>
<tr><td>4</td><td>Arizona</td><td>6</td><td>2</td><td>Nebraska</td><td>7</td></tr>
<tr><td>38</td><td>Arkansas</td><td>1</td><td>4</td><td>Arizona</td><td>6</td></tr>
<tr><td>22</td><td>California</td><td>2</td><td>4</td><td>Montana</td><td>6</td></tr>
<tr><td>22</td><td>Colorado</td><td>2</td><td>4</td><td>Utah</td><td>6</td></tr>
<tr><td>12</td><td>Connecticut</td><td>4</td><td>4</td><td>Wyoming</td><td>6</td></tr>
<tr><td>1</td><td>Delaware</td><td>9</td><td>8</td><td>New Jersey</td><td>5</td></tr>
<tr><td>12</td><td>Florida</td><td>4</td><td>8</td><td>New York</td><td>5</td></tr>
<tr><td>38</td><td>Georgia</td><td>1</td><td>8</td><td>Ohio</td><td>5</td></tr>
<tr><td>NA</td><td>Hawaii**</td><td>NA</td><td>8</td><td>Virginia</td><td>5</td></tr>
<tr><td>NA</td><td>Idaho**</td><td>NA</td><td>12</td><td>Connecticut</td><td>4</td></tr>
<tr><td>16</td><td>Illinois</td><td>3</td><td>12</td><td>Florida</td><td>4</td></tr>
<tr><td>22</td><td>Indiana</td><td>2</td><td>12</td><td>Massachusetts</td><td>4</td></tr>
<tr><td>22</td><td>Iowa</td><td>2</td><td>12</td><td>Pennsylvania</td><td>4</td></tr>
<tr><td>16</td><td>Kansas</td><td>3</td><td>16</td><td>Alabama</td><td>3</td></tr>
<tr><td>22</td><td>Kentucky</td><td>2</td><td>16</td><td>Illinois</td><td>3</td></tr>
<tr><td>22</td><td>Louisiana</td><td>2</td><td>16</td><td>Kansas</td><td>3</td></tr>
<tr><td>NA</td><td>Maine**</td><td>NA</td><td>16</td><td>Michigan</td><td>3</td></tr>
<tr><td>2</td><td>Maryland</td><td>7</td><td>16</td><td>Minnesota</td><td>3</td></tr>
<tr><td>12</td><td>Massachusetts</td><td>4</td><td>16</td><td>Oklahoma</td><td>3</td></tr>
<tr><td>16</td><td>Michigan</td><td>3</td><td>22</td><td>California</td><td>2</td></tr>
<tr><td>16</td><td>Minnesota</td><td>3</td><td>22</td><td>Colorado</td><td>2</td></tr>
<tr><td>38</td><td>Mississippi</td><td>1</td><td>22</td><td>Indiana</td><td>2</td></tr>
<tr><td>22</td><td>Missouri</td><td>2</td><td>22</td><td>Iowa</td><td>2</td></tr>
<tr><td>4</td><td>Montana</td><td>6</td><td>22</td><td>Kentucky</td><td>2</td></tr>
<tr><td>2</td><td>Nebraska</td><td>7</td><td>22</td><td>Louisiana</td><td>2</td></tr>
<tr><td>22</td><td>Nevada</td><td>2</td><td>22</td><td>Missouri</td><td>2</td></tr>
<tr><td>22</td><td>New Hampshire</td><td>2</td><td>22</td><td>Nevada</td><td>2</td></tr>
<tr><td>8</td><td>New Jersey</td><td>5</td><td>22</td><td>New Hampshire</td><td>2</td></tr>
<tr><td>22</td><td>New Mexico</td><td>2</td><td>22</td><td>New Mexico</td><td>2</td></tr>
<tr><td>8</td><td>New York</td><td>5</td><td>22</td><td>North Carolina</td><td>2</td></tr>
<tr><td>22</td><td>North Carolina</td><td>2</td><td>22</td><td>South Carolina</td><td>2</td></tr>
<tr><td>NA</td><td>North Dakota**</td><td>NA</td><td>22</td><td>Tennessee</td><td>2</td></tr>
<tr><td>8</td><td>Ohio</td><td>5</td><td>22</td><td>Texas</td><td>2</td></tr>
<tr><td>16</td><td>Oklahoma</td><td>3</td><td>22</td><td>Washington</td><td>2</td></tr>
<tr><td>38</td><td>Oregon</td><td>1</td><td>22</td><td>Wisconsin</td><td>2</td></tr>
<tr><td>12</td><td>Pennsylvania</td><td>4</td><td>38</td><td>Arkansas</td><td>1</td></tr>
<tr><td>NA</td><td>Rhode Island**</td><td>NA</td><td>38</td><td>Georgia</td><td>1</td></tr>
<tr><td>22</td><td>South Carolina</td><td>2</td><td>38</td><td>Mississippi</td><td>1</td></tr>
<tr><td>NA</td><td>South Dakota**</td><td>NA</td><td>38</td><td>Oregon</td><td>1</td></tr>
<tr><td>22</td><td>Tennessee</td><td>2</td><td>NA</td><td>Alaska**</td><td>NA</td></tr>
<tr><td>22</td><td>Texas</td><td>2</td><td>NA</td><td>Hawaii**</td><td>NA</td></tr>
<tr><td>4</td><td>Utah</td><td>6</td><td>NA</td><td>Idaho**</td><td>NA</td></tr>
<tr><td>NA</td><td>Vermont**</td><td>NA</td><td>NA</td><td>Maine**</td><td>NA</td></tr>
<tr><td>8</td><td>Virginia</td><td>5</td><td>NA</td><td>North Dakota**</td><td>NA</td></tr>
<tr><td>22</td><td>Washington</td><td>2</td><td>NA</td><td>Rhode Island**</td><td>NA</td></tr>
<tr><td>NA</td><td>West Virginia**</td><td>NA</td><td>NA</td><td>South Dakota**</td><td>NA</td></tr>
<tr><td>22</td><td>Wisconsin</td><td>2</td><td>NA</td><td>Vermont**</td><td>NA</td></tr>
<tr><td>4</td><td>Wyoming</td><td>6</td><td>NA</td><td>West Virginia**</td><td>NA</td></tr>
<tr><td></td><td></td><td></td><td></td><td>District of Columbia**</td><td>NA</td></tr>
</table>

Source: CQ Press using data from U.S. Department of Labor, Bureau of Labor Statistics
    "Occupational Employment and Wages, 2009" (http://www.bls.gov/oes/)
*Does not include self-employed.
**Not available.

Average Annual Wages of Podiatrists in 2009

National Average = $131,730*

<table>
<tr><td colspan="3">ALPHA ORDER</td><td colspan="3">RANK ORDER</td></tr>
<tr><th>RANK</th><th>STATE</th><th>WAGES</th><th>RANK</th><th>STATE</th><th>WAGES</th></tr>
<tr><td>35</td><td>Alabama</td><td>$116,710</td><td>1</td><td>Michigan</td><td>$173,730</td></tr>
<tr><td>NA</td><td>Alaska**</td><td>NA</td><td>2</td><td>Texas</td><td>166,220</td></tr>
<tr><td>28</td><td>Arizona</td><td>124,420</td><td>3</td><td>Wisconsin</td><td>165,990</td></tr>
<tr><td>4</td><td>Arkansas</td><td>163,950</td><td>4</td><td>Arkansas</td><td>163,950</td></tr>
<tr><td>20</td><td>California</td><td>136,440</td><td>5</td><td>Kansas</td><td>161,660</td></tr>
<tr><td>13</td><td>Colorado</td><td>141,520</td><td>6</td><td>Idaho</td><td>160,000</td></tr>
<tr><td>10</td><td>Connecticut</td><td>149,160</td><td>7</td><td>Washington</td><td>158,000</td></tr>
<tr><td>33</td><td>Delaware</td><td>120,020</td><td>8</td><td>Wyoming</td><td>157,610</td></tr>
<tr><td>19</td><td>Florida</td><td>137,140</td><td>9</td><td>Nevada</td><td>156,820</td></tr>
<tr><td>17</td><td>Georgia</td><td>137,660</td><td>10</td><td>Connecticut</td><td>149,160</td></tr>
<tr><td>NA</td><td>Hawaii**</td><td>NA</td><td>11</td><td>Kentucky</td><td>146,050</td></tr>
<tr><td>6</td><td>Idaho</td><td>160,000</td><td>12</td><td>Louisiana</td><td>145,340</td></tr>
<tr><td>39</td><td>Illinois</td><td>107,980</td><td>13</td><td>Colorado</td><td>141,520</td></tr>
<tr><td>24</td><td>Indiana</td><td>132,270</td><td>14</td><td>Maryland</td><td>140,700</td></tr>
<tr><td>25</td><td>Iowa</td><td>130,460</td><td>15</td><td>Missouri</td><td>139,830</td></tr>
<tr><td>5</td><td>Kansas</td><td>161,660</td><td>16</td><td>Minnesota</td><td>138,660</td></tr>
<tr><td>11</td><td>Kentucky</td><td>146,050</td><td>17</td><td>Georgia</td><td>137,660</td></tr>
<tr><td>12</td><td>Louisiana</td><td>145,340</td><td>18</td><td>Montana</td><td>137,530</td></tr>
<tr><td>NA</td><td>Maine**</td><td>NA</td><td>19</td><td>Florida</td><td>137,140</td></tr>
<tr><td>14</td><td>Maryland</td><td>140,700</td><td>20</td><td>California</td><td>136,440</td></tr>
<tr><td>23</td><td>Massachusetts</td><td>132,630</td><td>21</td><td>North Carolina</td><td>136,070</td></tr>
<tr><td>1</td><td>Michigan</td><td>173,730</td><td>22</td><td>New Hampshire</td><td>134,600</td></tr>
<tr><td>16</td><td>Minnesota</td><td>138,660</td><td>23</td><td>Massachusetts</td><td>132,630</td></tr>
<tr><td>36</td><td>Mississippi</td><td>111,550</td><td>24</td><td>Indiana</td><td>132,270</td></tr>
<tr><td>15</td><td>Missouri</td><td>139,830</td><td>25</td><td>Iowa</td><td>130,460</td></tr>
<tr><td>18</td><td>Montana</td><td>137,530</td><td>26</td><td>Ohio</td><td>127,820</td></tr>
<tr><td>38</td><td>Nebraska</td><td>108,650</td><td>27</td><td>New Mexico</td><td>127,810</td></tr>
<tr><td>9</td><td>Nevada</td><td>156,820</td><td>28</td><td>Arizona</td><td>124,420</td></tr>
<tr><td>22</td><td>New Hampshire</td><td>134,600</td><td>29</td><td>Virginia</td><td>124,350</td></tr>
<tr><td>32</td><td>New Jersey</td><td>120,340</td><td>30</td><td>Oregon</td><td>122,660</td></tr>
<tr><td>27</td><td>New Mexico</td><td>127,810</td><td>31</td><td>New York</td><td>120,480</td></tr>
<tr><td>31</td><td>New York</td><td>120,480</td><td>32</td><td>New Jersey</td><td>120,340</td></tr>
<tr><td>21</td><td>North Carolina</td><td>136,070</td><td>33</td><td>Delaware</td><td>120,020</td></tr>
<tr><td>NA</td><td>North Dakota**</td><td>NA</td><td>34</td><td>South Carolina</td><td>119,720</td></tr>
<tr><td>26</td><td>Ohio</td><td>127,820</td><td>35</td><td>Alabama</td><td>116,710</td></tr>
<tr><td>41</td><td>Oklahoma</td><td>99,840</td><td>36</td><td>Mississippi</td><td>111,550</td></tr>
<tr><td>30</td><td>Oregon</td><td>122,660</td><td>37</td><td>Tennessee</td><td>109,710</td></tr>
<tr><td>40</td><td>Pennsylvania</td><td>102,530</td><td>38</td><td>Nebraska</td><td>108,650</td></tr>
<tr><td>NA</td><td>Rhode Island**</td><td>NA</td><td>39</td><td>Illinois</td><td>107,980</td></tr>
<tr><td>34</td><td>South Carolina</td><td>119,720</td><td>40</td><td>Pennsylvania</td><td>102,530</td></tr>
<tr><td>NA</td><td>South Dakota**</td><td>NA</td><td>41</td><td>Oklahoma</td><td>99,840</td></tr>
<tr><td>37</td><td>Tennessee</td><td>109,710</td><td>42</td><td>Utah</td><td>99,740</td></tr>
<tr><td>2</td><td>Texas</td><td>166,220</td><td>NA</td><td>Alaska**</td><td>NA</td></tr>
<tr><td>42</td><td>Utah</td><td>99,740</td><td>NA</td><td>Hawaii**</td><td>NA</td></tr>
<tr><td>NA</td><td>Vermont**</td><td>NA</td><td>NA</td><td>Maine**</td><td>NA</td></tr>
<tr><td>29</td><td>Virginia</td><td>124,350</td><td>NA</td><td>North Dakota**</td><td>NA</td></tr>
<tr><td>7</td><td>Washington</td><td>158,000</td><td>NA</td><td>Rhode Island**</td><td>NA</td></tr>
<tr><td>NA</td><td>West Virginia**</td><td>NA</td><td>NA</td><td>South Dakota**</td><td>NA</td></tr>
<tr><td>3</td><td>Wisconsin</td><td>165,990</td><td>NA</td><td>Vermont**</td><td>NA</td></tr>
<tr><td>8</td><td>Wyoming</td><td>157,610</td><td>NA</td><td>West Virginia**</td><td>NA</td></tr>
<tr><td></td><td></td><td></td><td></td><td>District of Columbia**</td><td>NA</td></tr>
</table>

Source: U.S. Department of Labor, Bureau of Labor Statistics
"Occupational Employment and Wages, 2009" (http://www.bls.gov/oes/)
*Does not include self-employed.
**Not available.

Doctors of Chiropractic in 2009

National Total = 88,314 Chiropractors*

ALPHA ORDER

RANK	STATE	CHIROPRACTORS	% of USA
29	Alabama	807	0.9%
48	Alaska	245	0.3%
11	Arizona	2,415	2.7%
36	Arkansas	512	0.6%
1	California	13,812	15.6%
13	Colorado	2,237	2.5%
25	Connecticut	1,029	1.2%
43	Delaware	340	0.4%
3	Florida	4,923	5.6%
8	Georgia	2,997	3.4%
38	Hawaii	501	0.6%
35	Idaho	558	0.6%
6	Illinois	4,106	4.6%
23	Indiana	1,149	1.3%
19	Iowa	1,645	1.9%
26	Kansas	946	1.1%
27	Kentucky	874	1.0%
33	Louisiana	638	0.7%
40	Maine	389	0.4%
31	Maryland	723	0.8%
17	Massachusetts	2,123	2.4%
9	Michigan	2,909	3.3%
10	Minnesota	2,563	2.9%
44	Mississippi	334	0.4%
16	Missouri	2,139	2.4%
41	Montana	374	0.4%
34	Nebraska	565	0.6%
32	Nevada	641	0.7%
39	New Hampshire	421	0.5%
7	New Jersey	3,244	3.7%
37	New Mexico	508	0.6%
2	New York	5,400	6.1%
18	North Carolina	1,997	2.3%
46	North Dakota	296	0.3%
14	Ohio	2,235	2.5%
30	Oklahoma	790	0.9%
21	Oregon	1,417	1.6%
5	Pennsylvania	4,168	4.7%
47	Rhode Island	282	0.3%
20	South Carolina	1,569	1.8%
42	South Dakota	352	0.4%
24	Tennessee	1,034	1.2%
4	Texas	4,722	5.3%
28	Utah	846	1.0%
49	Vermont	243	0.3%
22	Virginia	1,212	1.4%
12	Washington	2,288	2.6%
45	West Virginia	331	0.4%
15	Wisconsin	2,181	2.5%
50	Wyoming	203	0.2%

RANK ORDER

RANK	STATE	CHIROPRACTORS	% of USA
1	California	13,812	15.6%
2	New York	5,400	6.1%
3	Florida	4,923	5.6%
4	Texas	4,722	5.3%
5	Pennsylvania	4,168	4.7%
6	Illinois	4,106	4.6%
7	New Jersey	3,244	3.7%
8	Georgia	2,997	3.4%
9	Michigan	2,909	3.3%
10	Minnesota	2,563	2.9%
11	Arizona	2,415	2.7%
12	Washington	2,288	2.6%
13	Colorado	2,237	2.5%
14	Ohio	2,235	2.5%
15	Wisconsin	2,181	2.5%
16	Missouri	2,139	2.4%
17	Massachusetts	2,123	2.4%
18	North Carolina	1,997	2.3%
19	Iowa	1,645	1.9%
20	South Carolina	1,569	1.8%
21	Oregon	1,417	1.6%
22	Virginia	1,212	1.4%
23	Indiana	1,149	1.3%
24	Tennessee	1,034	1.2%
25	Connecticut	1,029	1.2%
26	Kansas	946	1.1%
27	Kentucky	874	1.0%
28	Utah	846	1.0%
29	Alabama	807	0.9%
30	Oklahoma	790	0.9%
31	Maryland	723	0.8%
32	Nevada	641	0.7%
33	Louisiana	638	0.7%
34	Nebraska	565	0.6%
35	Idaho	558	0.6%
36	Arkansas	512	0.6%
37	New Mexico	508	0.6%
38	Hawaii	501	0.6%
39	New Hampshire	421	0.5%
40	Maine	389	0.4%
41	Montana	374	0.4%
42	South Dakota	352	0.4%
43	Delaware	340	0.4%
44	Mississippi	334	0.4%
45	West Virginia	331	0.4%
46	North Dakota	296	0.3%
47	Rhode Island	282	0.3%
48	Alaska	245	0.3%
49	Vermont	243	0.3%
50	Wyoming	203	0.2%
	District of Columbia	81	0.1%

Source: Federation of Chiropractic Licensing Boards
"Official Directory" (http://directory.fclb.org/)
*As of December 2009. Licensed active doctors. There is some duplication as some doctors are licensed in more than one state.

Rate of Doctors of Chiropractic in 2009

National Rate = 29 Chiropractors per 100,000 Population*

ALPHA ORDER				RANK ORDER		
RANK	STATE	RATE		RANK	STATE	RATE
45	Alabama	17		1	Iowa	55
18	Alaska	35		2	Minnesota	49
11	Arizona	37		3	North Dakota	46
42	Arkansas	18		4	Colorado	45
11	California	37		5	South Dakota	43
4	Colorado	45		6	Hawaii	39
30	Connecticut	29		6	Vermont	39
9	Delaware	38		6	Wisconsin	39
33	Florida	27		9	Delaware	38
27	Georgia	30		9	Montana	38
6	Hawaii	39		11	Arizona	37
16	Idaho	36		11	California	37
23	Illinois	32		11	New Jersey	37
42	Indiana	18		11	Oregon	37
1	Iowa	55		11	Wyoming	37
19	Kansas	34		16	Idaho	36
39	Kentucky	20		16	Missouri	36
48	Louisiana	14		18	Alaska	35
27	Maine	30		19	Kansas	34
49	Maryland	13		19	South Carolina	34
23	Massachusetts	32		19	Washington	34
30	Michigan	29		22	Pennsylvania	33
2	Minnesota	49		23	Illinois	32
50	Mississippi	11		23	Massachusetts	32
16	Missouri	36		23	New Hampshire	32
9	Montana	38		26	Nebraska	31
26	Nebraska	31		27	Georgia	30
36	Nevada	24		27	Maine	30
23	New Hampshire	32		27	Utah	30
11	New Jersey	37		30	Connecticut	29
35	New Mexico	25		30	Michigan	29
32	New York	28		32	New York	28
37	North Carolina	21		33	Florida	27
3	North Dakota	46		33	Rhode Island	27
40	Ohio	19		35	New Mexico	25
37	Oklahoma	21		36	Nevada	24
11	Oregon	37		37	North Carolina	21
22	Pennsylvania	33		37	Oklahoma	21
33	Rhode Island	27		39	Kentucky	20
19	South Carolina	34		40	Ohio	19
5	South Dakota	43		40	Texas	19
46	Tennessee	16		42	Arkansas	18
40	Texas	19		42	Indiana	18
27	Utah	30		42	West Virginia	18
6	Vermont	39		45	Alabama	17
47	Virginia	15		46	Tennessee	16
19	Washington	34		47	Virginia	15
42	West Virginia	18		48	Louisiana	14
6	Wisconsin	39		49	Maryland	13
11	Wyoming	37		50	Mississippi	11
					District of Columbia	14

Source: CQ Press using data from Federation of Chiropractic Licensing Boards
"Official Directory" (http://directory.fclb.org/)
*As of December 2009. Licensed active doctors. There is some duplication as some doctors are licensed in more than one state.

Average Annual Wages of Chiropractors in 2009

National Average = $80,390*

ALPHA ORDER

RANK	STATE	WAGES
11	Alabama	$94,150
8	Alaska	98,310
41	Arizona	67,390
15	Arkansas	88,240
29	California	76,960
48	Colorado	47,620
14	Connecticut	89,260
2	Delaware	111,190
16	Florida	87,250
46	Georgia	51,360
45	Hawaii	59,650
42	Idaho	64,140
23	Illinois	82,160
22	Indiana	85,200
25	Iowa	81,260
33	Kansas	74,520
6	Kentucky	101,200
37	Louisiana	73,180
34	Maine	74,380
31	Maryland	74,920
19	Massachusetts	86,360
43	Michigan	61,830
20	Minnesota	85,810
44	Mississippi	59,970
35	Missouri	74,370
47	Montana	48,340
26	Nebraska	81,020
4	Nevada	103,430
9	New Hampshire	97,710
27	New Jersey	80,720
38	New Mexico	72,060
18	New York	86,590
3	North Carolina	109,240
24	North Dakota	81,700
7	Ohio	100,940
21	Oklahoma	85,310
NA	Oregon**	NA
39	Pennsylvania	71,180
28	Rhode Island	77,910
36	South Carolina	73,190
NA	South Dakota**	NA
1	Tennessee	112,060
32	Texas	74,590
40	Utah	68,910
13	Vermont	90,570
17	Virginia	86,970
10	Washington	96,520
12	West Virginia	92,530
5	Wisconsin	102,030
30	Wyoming	76,380

RANK ORDER

RANK	STATE	WAGES
1	Tennessee	$112,060
2	Delaware	111,190
3	North Carolina	109,240
4	Nevada	103,430
5	Wisconsin	102,030
6	Kentucky	101,200
7	Ohio	100,940
8	Alaska	98,310
9	New Hampshire	97,710
10	Washington	96,520
11	Alabama	94,150
12	West Virginia	92,530
13	Vermont	90,570
14	Connecticut	89,260
15	Arkansas	88,240
16	Florida	87,250
17	Virginia	86,970
18	New York	86,590
19	Massachusetts	86,360
20	Minnesota	85,810
21	Oklahoma	85,310
22	Indiana	85,200
23	Illinois	82,160
24	North Dakota	81,700
25	Iowa	81,260
26	Nebraska	81,020
27	New Jersey	80,720
28	Rhode Island	77,910
29	California	76,960
30	Wyoming	76,380
31	Maryland	74,920
32	Texas	74,590
33	Kansas	74,520
34	Maine	74,380
35	Missouri	74,370
36	South Carolina	73,190
37	Louisiana	73,180
38	New Mexico	72,060
39	Pennsylvania	71,180
40	Utah	68,910
41	Arizona	67,390
42	Idaho	64,140
43	Michigan	61,830
44	Mississippi	59,970
45	Hawaii	59,650
46	Georgia	51,360
47	Montana	48,340
48	Colorado	47,620
NA	Oregon**	NA
NA	South Dakota**	NA
	District of Columbia**	NA

Source: U.S. Department of Labor, Bureau of Labor Statistics
   "Occupational Employment and Wages, 2009" (http://www.bls.gov/oes/)
*Does not include self-employed.
**Not available.

Physician Assistants in Clinical Practice in 2008

National Total = 73,506 Physician Assistants*

ALPHA ORDER					RANK ORDER			
RANK	STATE	PAs	% of USA		RANK	STATE	PAs	% of USA
38	Alabama	485	0.7%		1	New York	7,916	10.8%
41	Alaska	376	0.5%		2	California	7,115	9.7%
15	Arizona	1,668	2.3%		3	Texas	4,696	6.4%
49	Arkansas	155	0.2%		4	Pennsylvania	4,357	5.9%
2	California	7,115	9.7%		5	Florida	4,324	5.9%
13	Colorado	1,792	2.4%		6	North Carolina	3,586	4.9%
19	Connecticut	1,375	1.9%		7	Michigan	3,015	4.1%
46	Delaware	215	0.3%		8	Georgia	2,369	3.2%
5	Florida	4,324	5.9%		9	Maryland	1,978	2.7%
8	Georgia	2,369	3.2%		10	Washington	1,967	2.7%
48	Hawaii	158	0.2%		11	Ohio	1,960	2.7%
37	Idaho	511	0.7%		12	Illinois	1,950	2.7%
12	Illinois	1,950	2.7%		13	Colorado	1,792	2.4%
32	Indiana	621	0.8%		14	Massachusetts	1,725	2.3%
26	Iowa	765	1.0%		15	Arizona	1,668	2.3%
25	Kansas	796	1.1%		16	Virginia	1,611	2.2%
23	Kentucky	866	1.2%		17	Wisconsin	1,557	2.1%
34	Louisiana	545	0.7%		18	New Jersey	1,434	2.0%
33	Maine	555	0.8%		19	Connecticut	1,375	1.9%
9	Maryland	1,978	2.7%		20	Minnesota	1,251	1.7%
14	Massachusetts	1,725	2.3%		21	Oklahoma	1,072	1.5%
7	Michigan	3,015	4.1%		22	Tennessee	954	1.3%
20	Minnesota	1,251	1.7%		23	Kentucky	866	1.2%
50	Mississippi	86	0.1%		24	Oregon	853	1.2%
31	Missouri	635	0.9%		25	Kansas	796	1.1%
42	Montana	353	0.5%		26	Iowa	765	1.0%
28	Nebraska	731	1.0%		27	South Carolina	743	1.0%
35	Nevada	517	0.7%		28	Nebraska	731	1.0%
39	New Hampshire	420	0.6%		29	West Virginia	719	1.0%
18	New Jersey	1,434	2.0%		30	Utah	693	0.9%
36	New Mexico	516	0.7%		31	Missouri	635	0.9%
1	New York	7,916	10.8%		32	Indiana	621	0.8%
6	North Carolina	3,586	4.9%		33	Maine	555	0.8%
43	North Dakota	243	0.3%		34	Louisiana	545	0.7%
11	Ohio	1,960	2.7%		35	Nevada	517	0.7%
21	Oklahoma	1,072	1.5%		36	New Mexico	516	0.7%
24	Oregon	853	1.2%		37	Idaho	511	0.7%
4	Pennsylvania	4,357	5.9%		38	Alabama	485	0.7%
44	Rhode Island	226	0.3%		39	New Hampshire	420	0.6%
27	South Carolina	743	1.0%		40	South Dakota	409	0.6%
40	South Dakota	409	0.6%		41	Alaska	376	0.5%
22	Tennessee	954	1.3%		42	Montana	353	0.5%
3	Texas	4,696	6.4%		43	North Dakota	243	0.3%
30	Utah	693	0.9%		44	Rhode Island	226	0.3%
45	Vermont	219	0.3%		45	Vermont	219	0.3%
16	Virginia	1,611	2.2%		46	Delaware	215	0.3%
10	Washington	1,967	2.7%		47	Wyoming	192	0.3%
29	West Virginia	719	1.0%		48	Hawaii	158	0.2%
17	Wisconsin	1,557	2.1%		49	Arkansas	155	0.2%
47	Wyoming	192	0.3%		50	Mississippi	86	0.1%
						District of Columbia	231	0.3%

Source: The American Academy of Physician Assistants
"Projected Number of People in Clinical Practice as PAs as of December 31, 2008" (http://www.aapa.org/research/)
*Projected. National total does not include 387 physician assistants who work outside the United States or whose location is unknown.

Rate of Physician Assistants in Clinical Practice in 2008

National Rate = 24 PAs per 100,000 Population*

ALPHA ORDER

RANK	STATE	RATE
47	Alabama	10
1	Alaska	55
24	Arizona	26
49	Arkansas	5
37	California	19
10	Colorado	36
7	Connecticut	39
26	Delaware	25
29	Florida	24
29	Georgia	24
44	Hawaii	12
16	Idaho	34
42	Illinois	15
47	Indiana	10
26	Iowa	25
21	Kansas	28
35	Kentucky	20
44	Louisiana	12
3	Maine	42
13	Maryland	35
23	Massachusetts	27
18	Michigan	30
29	Minnesota	24
50	Mississippi	3
46	Missouri	11
10	Montana	36
4	Nebraska	41
35	Nevada	20
17	New Hampshire	32
39	New Jersey	17
24	New Mexico	26
4	New York	41
7	North Carolina	39
9	North Dakota	38
39	Ohio	17
20	Oklahoma	29
32	Oregon	23
13	Pennsylvania	35
33	Rhode Island	22
39	South Carolina	17
2	South Dakota	51
42	Tennessee	15
37	Texas	19
26	Utah	25
13	Vermont	35
34	Virginia	21
18	Washington	30
6	West Virginia	40
21	Wisconsin	28
10	Wyoming	36

RANK ORDER

RANK	STATE	RATE
1	Alaska	55
2	South Dakota	51
3	Maine	42
4	Nebraska	41
4	New York	41
6	West Virginia	40
7	Connecticut	39
7	North Carolina	39
9	North Dakota	38
10	Colorado	36
10	Montana	36
10	Wyoming	36
13	Maryland	35
13	Pennsylvania	35
13	Vermont	35
16	Idaho	34
17	New Hampshire	32
18	Michigan	30
18	Washington	30
20	Oklahoma	29
21	Kansas	28
21	Wisconsin	28
23	Massachusetts	27
24	Arizona	26
24	New Mexico	26
26	Delaware	25
26	Iowa	25
26	Utah	25
29	Florida	24
29	Georgia	24
29	Minnesota	24
32	Oregon	23
33	Rhode Island	22
34	Virginia	21
35	Kentucky	20
35	Nevada	20
37	California	19
37	Texas	19
39	New Jersey	17
39	Ohio	17
39	South Carolina	17
42	Illinois	15
42	Tennessee	15
44	Hawaii	12
44	Louisiana	12
46	Missouri	11
47	Alabama	10
47	Indiana	10
49	Arkansas	5
50	Mississippi	3

District of Columbia	39

Source: CQ Press using data from The American Academy of Physician Assistants
   "Projected Number of People in Clinical Practice as PAs as of December 31, 2008" (http://www.aapa.org/research/)
*Projected. Rates calculated using 2008 Census population figures.

Average Annual Wages of Physician Assistants in 2009

National Average = $84,830*

<table>
<tr><td colspan="3">ALPHA ORDER</td><td colspan="3">RANK ORDER</td></tr>
<tr><td>RANK</td><td>STATE</td><td>WAGES</td><td>RANK</td><td>STATE</td><td>WAGES</td></tr>
<tr><td>37</td><td>Alabama</td><td>$79,750</td><td>1</td><td>Nevada</td><td>$103,500</td></tr>
<tr><td>4</td><td>Alaska</td><td>92,180</td><td>2</td><td>Washington</td><td>98,880</td></tr>
<tr><td>25</td><td>Arizona</td><td>84,460</td><td>3</td><td>Connecticut</td><td>96,380</td></tr>
<tr><td>49</td><td>Arkansas</td><td>64,120</td><td>4</td><td>Alaska</td><td>92,180</td></tr>
<tr><td>6</td><td>California</td><td>91,670</td><td>5</td><td>New Jersey</td><td>92,100</td></tr>
<tr><td>33</td><td>Colorado</td><td>81,650</td><td>6</td><td>California</td><td>91,670</td></tr>
<tr><td>3</td><td>Connecticut</td><td>96,380</td><td>7</td><td>Maryland</td><td>90,920</td></tr>
<tr><td>8</td><td>Delaware</td><td>90,760</td><td>8</td><td>Delaware</td><td>90,760</td></tr>
<tr><td>17</td><td>Florida</td><td>87,590</td><td>9</td><td>New Hampshire</td><td>90,100</td></tr>
<tr><td>23</td><td>Georgia</td><td>84,590</td><td>10</td><td>Oregon</td><td>89,760</td></tr>
<tr><td>36</td><td>Hawaii</td><td>79,760</td><td>11</td><td>Texas</td><td>88,670</td></tr>
<tr><td>35</td><td>Idaho</td><td>81,310</td><td>12</td><td>Massachusetts</td><td>88,310</td></tr>
<tr><td>43</td><td>Illinois</td><td>71,200</td><td>13</td><td>Utah</td><td>88,190</td></tr>
<tr><td>39</td><td>Indiana</td><td>77,270</td><td>14</td><td>New York</td><td>87,740</td></tr>
<tr><td>28</td><td>Iowa</td><td>82,580</td><td>15</td><td>Minnesota</td><td>87,720</td></tr>
<tr><td>31</td><td>Kansas</td><td>82,100</td><td>16</td><td>Wisconsin</td><td>87,620</td></tr>
<tr><td>30</td><td>Kentucky</td><td>82,230</td><td>17</td><td>Florida</td><td>87,590</td></tr>
<tr><td>44</td><td>Louisiana</td><td>70,420</td><td>18</td><td>Rhode Island</td><td>87,360</td></tr>
<tr><td>21</td><td>Maine</td><td>85,950</td><td>19</td><td>Tennessee</td><td>87,330</td></tr>
<tr><td>7</td><td>Maryland</td><td>90,920</td><td>20</td><td>Michigan</td><td>86,960</td></tr>
<tr><td>12</td><td>Massachusetts</td><td>88,310</td><td>21</td><td>Maine</td><td>85,950</td></tr>
<tr><td>20</td><td>Michigan</td><td>86,960</td><td>22</td><td>Montana</td><td>85,720</td></tr>
<tr><td>15</td><td>Minnesota</td><td>87,720</td><td>23</td><td>Georgia</td><td>84,590</td></tr>
<tr><td>50</td><td>Mississippi</td><td>54,570</td><td>24</td><td>Wyoming</td><td>84,580</td></tr>
<tr><td>46</td><td>Missouri</td><td>68,390</td><td>25</td><td>Arizona</td><td>84,460</td></tr>
<tr><td>22</td><td>Montana</td><td>85,720</td><td>26</td><td>Ohio</td><td>83,890</td></tr>
<tr><td>27</td><td>Nebraska</td><td>82,770</td><td>27</td><td>Nebraska</td><td>82,770</td></tr>
<tr><td>1</td><td>Nevada</td><td>103,500</td><td>28</td><td>Iowa</td><td>82,580</td></tr>
<tr><td>9</td><td>New Hampshire</td><td>90,100</td><td>29</td><td>Vermont</td><td>82,300</td></tr>
<tr><td>5</td><td>New Jersey</td><td>92,100</td><td>30</td><td>Kentucky</td><td>82,230</td></tr>
<tr><td>48</td><td>New Mexico</td><td>66,020</td><td>31</td><td>Kansas</td><td>82,100</td></tr>
<tr><td>14</td><td>New York</td><td>87,740</td><td>32</td><td>North Carolina</td><td>81,850</td></tr>
<tr><td>32</td><td>North Carolina</td><td>81,850</td><td>33</td><td>Colorado</td><td>81,650</td></tr>
<tr><td>41</td><td>North Dakota</td><td>76,260</td><td>34</td><td>South Dakota</td><td>81,530</td></tr>
<tr><td>26</td><td>Ohio</td><td>83,890</td><td>35</td><td>Idaho</td><td>81,310</td></tr>
<tr><td>40</td><td>Oklahoma</td><td>76,770</td><td>36</td><td>Hawaii</td><td>79,760</td></tr>
<tr><td>10</td><td>Oregon</td><td>89,760</td><td>37</td><td>Alabama</td><td>79,750</td></tr>
<tr><td>47</td><td>Pennsylvania</td><td>68,170</td><td>38</td><td>West Virginia</td><td>77,560</td></tr>
<tr><td>18</td><td>Rhode Island</td><td>87,360</td><td>39</td><td>Indiana</td><td>77,270</td></tr>
<tr><td>45</td><td>South Carolina</td><td>69,080</td><td>40</td><td>Oklahoma</td><td>76,770</td></tr>
<tr><td>34</td><td>South Dakota</td><td>81,530</td><td>41</td><td>North Dakota</td><td>76,260</td></tr>
<tr><td>19</td><td>Tennessee</td><td>87,330</td><td>42</td><td>Virginia</td><td>74,000</td></tr>
<tr><td>11</td><td>Texas</td><td>88,670</td><td>43</td><td>Illinois</td><td>71,200</td></tr>
<tr><td>13</td><td>Utah</td><td>88,190</td><td>44</td><td>Louisiana</td><td>70,420</td></tr>
<tr><td>29</td><td>Vermont</td><td>82,300</td><td>45</td><td>South Carolina</td><td>69,080</td></tr>
<tr><td>42</td><td>Virginia</td><td>74,000</td><td>46</td><td>Missouri</td><td>68,390</td></tr>
<tr><td>2</td><td>Washington</td><td>98,880</td><td>47</td><td>Pennsylvania</td><td>68,170</td></tr>
<tr><td>38</td><td>West Virginia</td><td>77,560</td><td>48</td><td>New Mexico</td><td>66,020</td></tr>
<tr><td>16</td><td>Wisconsin</td><td>87,620</td><td>49</td><td>Arkansas</td><td>64,120</td></tr>
<tr><td>24</td><td>Wyoming</td><td>84,580</td><td>50</td><td>Mississippi</td><td>54,570</td></tr>
<tr><td></td><td></td><td></td><td></td><td>District of Columbia</td><td>95,610</td></tr>
</table>

Source: U.S. Department of Labor, Bureau of Labor Statistics
  "Occupational Employment and Wages, 2009" (http://www.bls.gov/oes/)
*Does not include self-employed.

Registered Nurses in 2009

National Total = 2,583,770 Registered Nurses*

ALPHA ORDER

RANK	STATE	NURSES	% of USA
22	Alabama	42,880	1.7%
49	Alaska	5,010	0.2%
25	Arizona	38,570	1.5%
33	Arkansas	23,050	0.9%
1	California	233,030	9.0%
23	Colorado	41,750	1.6%
27	Connecticut	35,790	1.4%
44	Delaware	10,220	0.4%
4	Florida	150,940	5.8%
12	Georgia	65,370	2.5%
45	Hawaii	8,930	0.3%
42	Idaho	10,540	0.4%
7	Illinois	116,340	4.5%
16	Indiana	57,880	2.2%
28	Iowa	30,750	1.2%
32	Kansas	26,320	1.0%
21	Kentucky	43,250	1.7%
24	Louisiana	39,560	1.5%
38	Maine	14,410	0.6%
20	Maryland	51,620	2.0%
10	Massachusetts	83,060	3.2%
9	Michigan	84,620	3.3%
17	Minnesota	57,560	2.2%
30	Mississippi	28,030	1.1%
13	Missouri	62,130	2.4%
46	Montana	8,340	0.3%
34	Nebraska	18,930	0.7%
37	Nevada	16,100	0.6%
39	New Hampshire	13,330	0.5%
11	New Jersey	74,730	2.9%
40	New Mexico	12,340	0.5%
3	New York	165,730	6.4%
8	North Carolina	88,190	3.4%
47	North Dakota	6,260	0.2%
6	Ohio	117,870	4.6%
31	Oklahoma	27,340	1.1%
29	Oregon	30,730	1.2%
5	Pennsylvania	129,810	5.0%
41	Rhode Island	11,630	0.5%
26	South Carolina	38,020	1.5%
43	South Dakota	10,530	0.4%
14	Tennessee	61,980	2.4%
2	Texas	168,020	6.5%
35	Utah	17,670	0.7%
48	Vermont	5,680	0.2%
15	Virginia	60,230	2.3%
18	Washington	54,260	2.1%
36	West Virginia	17,340	0.7%
19	Wisconsin	53,510	2.1%
50	Wyoming	4,700	0.2%

RANK ORDER

RANK	STATE	NURSES	% of USA
1	California	233,030	9.0%
2	Texas	168,020	6.5%
3	New York	165,730	6.4%
4	Florida	150,940	5.8%
5	Pennsylvania	129,810	5.0%
6	Ohio	117,870	4.6%
7	Illinois	116,340	4.5%
8	North Carolina	88,190	3.4%
9	Michigan	84,620	3.3%
10	Massachusetts	83,060	3.2%
11	New Jersey	74,730	2.9%
12	Georgia	65,370	2.5%
13	Missouri	62,130	2.4%
14	Tennessee	61,980	2.4%
15	Virginia	60,230	2.3%
16	Indiana	57,880	2.2%
17	Minnesota	57,560	2.2%
18	Washington	54,260	2.1%
19	Wisconsin	53,510	2.1%
20	Maryland	51,620	2.0%
21	Kentucky	43,250	1.7%
22	Alabama	42,880	1.7%
23	Colorado	41,750	1.6%
24	Louisiana	39,560	1.5%
25	Arizona	38,570	1.5%
26	South Carolina	38,020	1.5%
27	Connecticut	35,790	1.4%
28	Iowa	30,750	1.2%
29	Oregon	30,730	1.2%
30	Mississippi	28,030	1.1%
31	Oklahoma	27,340	1.1%
32	Kansas	26,320	1.0%
33	Arkansas	23,050	0.9%
34	Nebraska	18,930	0.7%
35	Utah	17,670	0.7%
36	West Virginia	17,340	0.7%
37	Nevada	16,100	0.6%
38	Maine	14,410	0.6%
39	New Hampshire	13,330	0.5%
40	New Mexico	12,340	0.5%
41	Rhode Island	11,630	0.5%
42	Idaho	10,540	0.4%
43	South Dakota	10,530	0.4%
44	Delaware	10,220	0.4%
45	Hawaii	8,930	0.3%
46	Montana	8,340	0.3%
47	North Dakota	6,260	0.2%
48	Vermont	5,680	0.2%
49	Alaska	5,010	0.2%
50	Wyoming	4,700	0.2%
	District of Columbia	8,890	0.3%

Source: U.S. Department of Labor, Bureau of Labor Statistics
   "Occupational Employment and Wages, 2009" (http://www.bls.gov/oes/)
*Does not include self-employed.

Rate of Registered Nurses in 2009

National Rate = 842 Nurses per 100,000 Population*

ALPHA ORDER

RANK	STATE	RATE
23	Alabama	911
41	Alaska	717
50	Arizona	585
38	Arkansas	798
47	California	630
34	Colorado	831
12	Connecticut	1,017
3	Delaware	1,155
35	Florida	814
45	Georgia	665
42	Hawaii	689
43	Idaho	682
25	Illinois	901
25	Indiana	901
10	Iowa	1,022
21	Kansas	934
14	Kentucky	1,003
27	Louisiana	881
5	Maine	1,093
24	Maryland	906
2	Massachusetts	1,260
31	Michigan	849
5	Minnesota	1,093
18	Mississippi	950
8	Missouri	1,038
30	Montana	855
7	Nebraska	1,054
49	Nevada	609
13	New Hampshire	1,006
29	New Jersey	858
48	New Mexico	614
32	New York	848
20	North Carolina	940
16	North Dakota	968
11	Ohio	1,021
40	Oklahoma	742
37	Oregon	803
9	Pennsylvania	1,030
4	Rhode Island	1,104
33	South Carolina	834
1	South Dakota	1,296
15	Tennessee	984
44	Texas	678
46	Utah	635
22	Vermont	914
39	Virginia	764
35	Washington	814
17	West Virginia	953
19	Wisconsin	946
28	Wyoming	864

RANK ORDER

RANK	STATE	RATE
1	South Dakota	1,296
2	Massachusetts	1,260
3	Delaware	1,155
4	Rhode Island	1,104
5	Maine	1,093
5	Minnesota	1,093
7	Nebraska	1,054
8	Missouri	1,038
9	Pennsylvania	1,030
10	Iowa	1,022
11	Ohio	1,021
12	Connecticut	1,017
13	New Hampshire	1,006
14	Kentucky	1,003
15	Tennessee	984
16	North Dakota	968
17	West Virginia	953
18	Mississippi	950
19	Wisconsin	946
20	North Carolina	940
21	Kansas	934
22	Vermont	914
23	Alabama	911
24	Maryland	906
25	Illinois	901
25	Indiana	901
27	Louisiana	881
28	Wyoming	864
29	New Jersey	858
30	Montana	855
31	Michigan	849
32	New York	848
33	South Carolina	834
34	Colorado	831
35	Florida	814
35	Washington	814
37	Oregon	803
38	Arkansas	798
39	Virginia	764
40	Oklahoma	742
41	Alaska	717
42	Hawaii	689
43	Idaho	682
44	Texas	678
45	Georgia	665
46	Utah	635
47	California	630
48	New Mexico	614
49	Nevada	609
50	Arizona	585

| | District of Columbia | 1,483 |

Source: CQ Press using data from U.S. Department of Labor, Bureau of Labor Statistics
"Occupational Employment and Wages, 2009" (http://www.bls.gov/oes/)
*Does not include self-employed.

Average Annual Wages of Registered Nurses in 2009

National Average = $66,530*

RANK	STATE	WAGES		RANK	STATE	WAGES
39	Alabama	$57,860		1	California	$85,080
6	Alaska	74,970		2	Massachusetts	81,780
15	Arizona	67,130		3	Hawaii	80,020
42	Arkansas	57,040		4	Maryland	76,330
1	California	85,080		5	New Jersey	74,990
16	Colorado	66,800		6	Alaska	74,970
12	Connecticut	71,930		7	Oregon	73,300
13	Delaware	70,770		8	Nevada	72,940
26	Florida	62,270		9	New York	72,790
29	Georgia	60,940		10	Minnesota	72,760
3	Hawaii	80,020		11	Washington	72,450
28	Idaho	61,320		12	Connecticut	71,930
17	Illinois	65,440		13	Delaware	70,770
38	Indiana	57,910		14	Rhode Island	68,830
50	Iowa	51,930		15	Arizona	67,130
45	Kansas	55,730		16	Colorado	66,800
36	Kentucky	58,110		17	Illinois	65,440
30	Louisiana	60,290		18	Maine	65,240
18	Maine	65,240		19	Texas	64,670
4	Maryland	76,330		20	Michigan	64,100
2	Massachusetts	81,780		21	Pennsylvania	63,600
20	Michigan	64,100		22	New Mexico	63,550
10	Minnesota	72,760		23	Virginia	63,270
40	Mississippi	57,630		24	Vermont	63,230
41	Missouri	57,460		25	Wisconsin	63,200
43	Montana	56,380		26	Florida	62,270
46	Nebraska	55,040		27	New Hampshire	62,060
8	Nevada	72,940		28	Idaho	61,320
27	New Hampshire	62,060		29	Georgia	60,940
5	New Jersey	74,990		30	Louisiana	60,290
22	New Mexico	63,550		31	Ohio	59,740
9	New York	72,790		32	South Carolina	59,680
35	North Carolina	58,880		33	Tennessee	59,520
44	North Dakota	56,110		34	Utah	59,370
31	Ohio	59,740		35	North Carolina	58,880
48	Oklahoma	53,210		36	Kentucky	58,110
7	Oregon	73,300		37	Wyoming	58,060
21	Pennsylvania	63,600		38	Indiana	57,910
14	Rhode Island	68,830		39	Alabama	57,860
32	South Carolina	59,680		40	Mississippi	57,630
47	South Dakota	53,520		41	Missouri	57,460
33	Tennessee	59,520		42	Arkansas	57,040
19	Texas	64,670		43	Montana	56,380
34	Utah	59,370		44	North Dakota	56,110
24	Vermont	63,230		45	Kansas	55,730
23	Virginia	63,270		46	Nebraska	55,040
11	Washington	72,450		47	South Dakota	53,520
49	West Virginia	53,030		48	Oklahoma	53,210
25	Wisconsin	63,200		49	West Virginia	53,030
37	Wyoming	58,060		50	Iowa	51,930

ALPHA ORDER (left) / RANK ORDER (right)

District of Columbia 74,040

Source: U.S. Department of Labor, Bureau of Labor Statistics
   "Occupational Employment and Wages, 2009" (http://www.bls.gov/oes/)
*Does not include self-employed.

Licensed Practical and Licensed Vocational Nurses in 2009

National Total = 728,670 LPN/LVNs*

ALPHA ORDER

RANK	STATE	NURSES	% of USA
19	Alabama	15,210	2.1%
50	Alaska	590	0.1%
25	Arizona	10,180	1.4%
21	Arkansas	11,590	1.6%
2	California	62,300	8.5%
32	Colorado	6,970	1.0%
29	Connecticut	8,730	1.2%
41	Delaware	2,360	0.3%
4	Florida	43,350	5.9%
7	Georgia	25,110	3.4%
48	Hawaii	1,410	0.2%
37	Idaho	2,920	0.4%
9	Illinois	24,390	3.3%
10	Indiana	20,610	2.8%
30	Iowa	7,480	1.0%
31	Kansas	7,130	1.0%
24	Kentucky	10,220	1.4%
12	Louisiana	19,950	2.7%
45	Maine	1,820	0.2%
22	Maryland	10,960	1.5%
17	Massachusetts	16,780	2.3%
15	Michigan	18,720	2.6%
13	Minnesota	19,220	2.6%
26	Mississippi	10,140	1.4%
14	Missouri	18,880	2.6%
38	Montana	2,800	0.4%
34	Nebraska	5,610	0.8%
43	Nevada	2,170	0.3%
40	New Hampshire	2,490	0.3%
18	New Jersey	15,530	2.1%
35	New Mexico	4,840	0.7%
3	New York	45,130	6.2%
16	North Carolina	17,280	2.4%
36	North Dakota	3,300	0.5%
5	Ohio	40,860	5.6%
20	Oklahoma	14,270	2.0%
39	Oregon	2,520	0.3%
6	Pennsylvania	37,700	5.2%
47	Rhode Island	1,510	0.2%
27	South Carolina	9,960	1.4%
44	South Dakota	1,960	0.3%
8	Tennessee	24,950	3.4%
1	Texas	65,850	9.0%
42	Utah	2,240	0.3%
46	Vermont	1,520	0.2%
11	Virginia	19,980	2.7%
28	Washington	9,710	1.3%
33	West Virginia	6,320	0.9%
23	Wisconsin	10,710	1.5%
49	Wyoming	730	0.1%

RANK ORDER

RANK	STATE	NURSES	% of USA
1	Texas	65,850	9.0%
2	California	62,300	8.5%
3	New York	45,130	6.2%
4	Florida	43,350	5.9%
5	Ohio	40,860	5.6%
6	Pennsylvania	37,700	5.2%
7	Georgia	25,110	3.4%
8	Tennessee	24,950	3.4%
9	Illinois	24,390	3.3%
10	Indiana	20,610	2.8%
11	Virginia	19,980	2.7%
12	Louisiana	19,950	2.7%
13	Minnesota	19,220	2.6%
14	Missouri	18,880	2.6%
15	Michigan	18,720	2.6%
16	North Carolina	17,280	2.4%
17	Massachusetts	16,780	2.3%
18	New Jersey	15,530	2.1%
19	Alabama	15,210	2.1%
20	Oklahoma	14,270	2.0%
21	Arkansas	11,590	1.6%
22	Maryland	10,960	1.5%
23	Wisconsin	10,710	1.5%
24	Kentucky	10,220	1.4%
25	Arizona	10,180	1.4%
26	Mississippi	10,140	1.4%
27	South Carolina	9,960	1.4%
28	Washington	9,710	1.3%
29	Connecticut	8,730	1.2%
30	Iowa	7,480	1.0%
31	Kansas	7,130	1.0%
32	Colorado	6,970	1.0%
33	West Virginia	6,320	0.9%
34	Nebraska	5,610	0.8%
35	New Mexico	4,840	0.7%
36	North Dakota	3,300	0.5%
37	Idaho	2,920	0.4%
38	Montana	2,800	0.4%
39	Oregon	2,520	0.3%
40	New Hampshire	2,490	0.3%
41	Delaware	2,360	0.3%
42	Utah	2,240	0.3%
43	Nevada	2,170	0.3%
44	South Dakota	1,960	0.3%
45	Maine	1,820	0.2%
46	Vermont	1,520	0.2%
47	Rhode Island	1,510	0.2%
48	Hawaii	1,410	0.2%
49	Wyoming	730	0.1%
50	Alaska	590	0.1%
	District of Columbia	1,700	0.2%

Source: U.S. Department of Labor, Bureau of Labor Statistics
"Occupational Employment and Wages, 2009" (http://www.bls.gov/oes/)
*Does not include self-employed.

Rate of Licensed Practical and Licensed Vocational Nurses in 2009

National Rate = 237 LPN/LVNs per 100,000 Population*

ALPHA ORDER

RANK	STATE	RATE
10	Alabama	323
47	Alaska	84
40	Arizona	154
3	Arkansas	401
39	California	169
43	Colorado	139
23	Connecticut	248
16	Delaware	267
28	Florida	234
18	Georgia	255
46	Hawaii	109
32	Idaho	189
32	Illinois	189
11	Indiana	321
22	Iowa	249
20	Kansas	253
27	Kentucky	237
2	Louisiana	444
44	Maine	138
31	Maryland	192
19	Massachusetts	254
35	Michigan	188
6	Minnesota	365
9	Mississippi	343
12	Missouri	315
15	Montana	287
13	Nebraska	312
48	Nevada	82
35	New Hampshire	188
38	New Jersey	178
25	New Mexico	241
29	New York	231
37	North Carolina	184
1	North Dakota	510
7	Ohio	354
5	Oklahoma	387
50	Oregon	66
14	Pennsylvania	299
42	Rhode Island	143
30	South Carolina	218
25	South Dakota	241
4	Tennessee	396
17	Texas	266
49	Utah	80
24	Vermont	244
20	Virginia	253
41	Washington	146
8	West Virginia	347
32	Wisconsin	189
45	Wyoming	134

RANK ORDER

RANK	STATE	RATE
1	North Dakota	510
2	Louisiana	444
3	Arkansas	401
4	Tennessee	396
5	Oklahoma	387
6	Minnesota	365
7	Ohio	354
8	West Virginia	347
9	Mississippi	343
10	Alabama	323
11	Indiana	321
12	Missouri	315
13	Nebraska	312
14	Pennsylvania	299
15	Montana	287
16	Delaware	267
17	Texas	266
18	Georgia	255
19	Massachusetts	254
20	Kansas	253
20	Virginia	253
22	Iowa	249
23	Connecticut	248
24	Vermont	244
25	New Mexico	241
25	South Dakota	241
27	Kentucky	237
28	Florida	234
29	New York	231
30	South Carolina	218
31	Maryland	192
32	Idaho	189
32	Illinois	189
32	Wisconsin	189
35	Michigan	188
35	New Hampshire	188
37	North Carolina	184
38	New Jersey	178
39	California	169
40	Arizona	154
41	Washington	146
42	Rhode Island	143
43	Colorado	139
44	Maine	138
45	Wyoming	134
46	Hawaii	109
47	Alaska	84
48	Nevada	82
49	Utah	80
50	Oregon	66

District of Columbia	283

Source: CQ Press using data from U.S. Department of Labor, Bureau of Labor Statistics
    "Occupational Employment and Wages, 2009" (http://www.bls.gov/oes/)
*Does not include self-employed.

Average Annual Wages of Licensed Practical and Licensed Vocational Nurses in 2009
National Average = $40,900*

ALPHA ORDER

RANK	STATE	WAGES
47	Alabama	$33,490
10	Alaska	46,500
11	Arizona	45,650
46	Arkansas	33,750
4	California	49,940
17	Colorado	42,100
1	Connecticut	52,300
9	Delaware	47,210
24	Florida	39,910
38	Georgia	36,170
12	Hawaii	45,000
33	Idaho	37,860
21	Illinois	41,240
32	Indiana	37,920
37	Iowa	36,300
36	Kansas	36,600
39	Kentucky	36,150
35	Louisiana	37,390
28	Maine	39,660
7	Maryland	49,310
5	Massachusetts	49,760
16	Michigan	42,540
30	Minnesota	38,840
45	Mississippi	34,490
42	Missouri	35,100
43	Montana	34,910
41	Nebraska	35,810
8	Nevada	47,900
15	New Hampshire	43,610
2	New Jersey	50,350
5	New Mexico	49,760
18	New York	41,910
27	North Carolina	39,710
44	North Dakota	34,810
24	Ohio	39,910
49	Oklahoma	32,790
13	Oregon	44,830
20	Pennsylvania	41,300
3	Rhode Island	50,010
34	South Carolina	37,450
48	South Dakota	33,390
40	Tennessee	35,990
23	Texas	40,710
26	Utah	39,840
19	Vermont	41,430
31	Virginia	37,950
14	Washington	44,400
50	West Virginia	32,250
22	Wisconsin	41,080
29	Wyoming	39,380

RANK ORDER

RANK	STATE	WAGES
1	Connecticut	$52,300
2	New Jersey	50,350
3	Rhode Island	50,010
4	California	49,940
5	Massachusetts	49,760
5	New Mexico	49,760
7	Maryland	49,310
8	Nevada	47,900
9	Delaware	47,210
10	Alaska	46,500
11	Arizona	45,650
12	Hawaii	45,000
13	Oregon	44,830
14	Washington	44,400
15	New Hampshire	43,610
16	Michigan	42,540
17	Colorado	42,100
18	New York	41,910
19	Vermont	41,430
20	Pennsylvania	41,300
21	Illinois	41,240
22	Wisconsin	41,080
23	Texas	40,710
24	Florida	39,910
24	Ohio	39,910
26	Utah	39,840
27	North Carolina	39,710
28	Maine	39,660
29	Wyoming	39,380
30	Minnesota	38,840
31	Virginia	37,950
32	Indiana	37,920
33	Idaho	37,860
34	South Carolina	37,450
35	Louisiana	37,390
36	Kansas	36,600
37	Iowa	36,300
38	Georgia	36,170
39	Kentucky	36,150
40	Tennessee	35,990
41	Nebraska	35,810
42	Missouri	35,100
43	Montana	34,910
44	North Dakota	34,810
45	Mississippi	34,490
46	Arkansas	33,750
47	Alabama	33,490
48	South Dakota	33,390
49	Oklahoma	32,790
50	West Virginia	32,250
	District of Columbia	47,990

Source: U.S. Department of Labor, Bureau of Labor Statistics
   "Occupational Employment and Wages, 2009" (http://www.bls.gov/oes/)
*Does not include self-employed.

Physical Therapists in 2009

National Total = 174,490 Physical Therapists*

ALPHA ORDER					RANK ORDER			
RANK	STATE	THERAPISTS	% of USA		RANK	STATE	THERAPISTS	% of USA
29	Alabama	1,750	1.0%		1	California	14,250	8.2%
49	Alaska	410	0.2%		2	New York	13,320	7.6%
23	Arizona	2,760	1.6%		3	Texas	11,230	6.4%
31	Arkansas	1,640	0.9%		4	Florida	11,010	6.3%
1	California	14,250	8.2%		5	Pennsylvania	9,200	5.3%
21	Colorado	3,290	1.9%		6	Illinois	7,740	4.4%
20	Connecticut	3,510	2.0%		7	Ohio	7,100	4.1%
46	Delaware	600	0.3%		8	Michigan	6,550	3.8%
4	Florida	11,010	6.3%		9	Massachusetts	6,320	3.6%
17	Georgia	3,820	2.2%		10	New Jersey	6,080	3.5%
39	Hawaii	1,000	0.6%		11	North Carolina	4,340	2.5%
40	Idaho	870	0.5%		12	Indiana	4,170	2.4%
6	Illinois	7,740	4.4%		13	Wisconsin	4,100	2.3%
12	Indiana	4,170	2.4%		14	Missouri	4,030	2.3%
32	Iowa	1,630	0.9%		15	Virginia	3,930	2.3%
30	Kansas	1,690	1.0%		16	Washington	3,840	2.2%
26	Kentucky	2,200	1.3%		17	Georgia	3,820	2.2%
27	Louisiana	2,180	1.2%		18	Tennessee	3,810	2.2%
37	Maine	1,090	0.6%		19	Maryland	3,700	2.1%
19	Maryland	3,700	2.1%		20	Connecticut	3,510	2.0%
9	Massachusetts	6,320	3.6%		21	Colorado	3,290	1.9%
8	Michigan	6,550	3.8%		22	Minnesota	2,980	1.7%
22	Minnesota	2,980	1.7%		23	Arizona	2,760	1.6%
33	Mississippi	1,480	0.8%		24	Oregon	2,430	1.4%
14	Missouri	4,030	2.3%		25	South Carolina	2,300	1.3%
43	Montana	820	0.5%		26	Kentucky	2,200	1.3%
36	Nebraska	1,180	0.7%		27	Louisiana	2,180	1.2%
34	Nevada	1,280	0.7%		28	Oklahoma	1,820	1.0%
35	New Hampshire	1,250	0.7%		29	Alabama	1,750	1.0%
10	New Jersey	6,080	3.5%		30	Kansas	1,690	1.0%
42	New Mexico	850	0.5%		31	Arkansas	1,640	0.9%
2	New York	13,320	7.6%		32	Iowa	1,630	0.9%
11	North Carolina	4,340	2.5%		33	Mississippi	1,480	0.8%
48	North Dakota	420	0.2%		34	Nevada	1,280	0.7%
7	Ohio	7,100	4.1%		35	New Hampshire	1,250	0.7%
28	Oklahoma	1,820	1.0%		36	Nebraska	1,180	0.7%
24	Oregon	2,430	1.4%		37	Maine	1,090	0.6%
5	Pennsylvania	9,200	5.3%		38	Utah	1,080	0.6%
45	Rhode Island	620	0.4%		39	Hawaii	1,000	0.6%
25	South Carolina	2,300	1.3%		40	Idaho	870	0.5%
47	South Dakota	570	0.3%		41	West Virginia	860	0.5%
18	Tennessee	3,810	2.2%		42	New Mexico	850	0.5%
3	Texas	11,230	6.4%		43	Montana	820	0.5%
38	Utah	1,080	0.6%		44	Vermont	700	0.4%
44	Vermont	700	0.4%		45	Rhode Island	620	0.4%
15	Virginia	3,930	2.3%		46	Delaware	600	0.3%
16	Washington	3,840	2.2%		47	South Dakota	570	0.3%
41	West Virginia	860	0.5%		48	North Dakota	420	0.2%
13	Wisconsin	4,100	2.3%		49	Alaska	410	0.2%
50	Wyoming	400	0.2%		50	Wyoming	400	0.2%
					District of Columbia	280	0.2%

Source: U.S. Department of Labor, Bureau of Labor Statistics
   "Occupational Employment and Wages, 2009" (http://www.bls.gov/oes/)
*Does not include self-employed.

Rate of Physical Therapists in 2009

National Rate = 57 Physical Therapists per 100,000 Population*

ALPHA ORDER

RANK	STATE	RATE
50	Alabama	37
27	Alaska	59
45	Arizona	42
31	Arkansas	57
47	California	39
18	Colorado	65
2	Connecticut	100
13	Delaware	68
27	Florida	59
47	Georgia	39
7	Hawaii	77
33	Idaho	56
25	Illinois	60
18	Indiana	65
34	Iowa	54
25	Kansas	60
35	Kentucky	51
39	Louisiana	49
6	Maine	83
18	Maryland	65
3	Massachusetts	96
16	Michigan	66
31	Minnesota	57
36	Mississippi	50
15	Missouri	67
5	Montana	84
16	Nebraska	66
41	Nevada	48
4	New Hampshire	94
11	New Jersey	70
45	New Mexico	42
13	New York	68
43	North Carolina	46
18	North Dakota	65
23	Ohio	62
39	Oklahoma	49
22	Oregon	64
8	Pennsylvania	73
27	Rhode Island	59
36	South Carolina	50
11	South Dakota	70
24	Tennessee	61
44	Texas	45
47	Utah	39
1	Vermont	113
36	Virginia	50
30	Washington	58
42	West Virginia	47
8	Wisconsin	73
8	Wyoming	73

RANK ORDER

RANK	STATE	RATE
1	Vermont	113
2	Connecticut	100
3	Massachusetts	96
4	New Hampshire	94
5	Montana	84
6	Maine	83
7	Hawaii	77
8	Pennsylvania	73
8	Wisconsin	73
8	Wyoming	73
11	New Jersey	70
11	South Dakota	70
13	Delaware	68
13	New York	68
15	Missouri	67
16	Michigan	66
16	Nebraska	66
18	Colorado	65
18	Indiana	65
18	Maryland	65
18	North Dakota	65
22	Oregon	64
23	Ohio	62
24	Tennessee	61
25	Illinois	60
25	Kansas	60
27	Alaska	59
27	Florida	59
27	Rhode Island	59
30	Washington	58
31	Arkansas	57
31	Minnesota	57
33	Idaho	56
34	Iowa	54
35	Kentucky	51
36	Mississippi	50
36	South Carolina	50
36	Virginia	50
39	Louisiana	49
39	Oklahoma	49
41	Nevada	48
42	West Virginia	47
43	North Carolina	46
44	Texas	45
45	Arizona	42
45	New Mexico	42
47	California	39
47	Georgia	39
47	Utah	39
50	Alabama	37
	District of Columbia	47

Source: CQ Press using data from U.S. Department of Labor, Bureau of Labor Statistics
"Occupational Employment and Wages, 2009" (http://www.bls.gov/oes/)
*Does not include self-employed.

Average Annual Wages of Physical Therapists in 2009

National Average = $76,220*

RANK	STATE	WAGES
16	Alabama	$76,260
1	Alaska	87,410
30	Arizona	72,550
23	Arkansas	74,310
5	California	83,740
38	Colorado	69,780
11	Connecticut	79,250
7	Delaware	82,450
9	Florida	79,670
14	Georgia	76,530
50	Hawaii	56,990
34	Idaho	70,780
8	Illinois	80,000
41	Indiana	69,340
36	Iowa	70,100
32	Kansas	72,380
18	Kentucky	75,590
12	Louisiana	77,910
37	Maine	70,020
2	Maryland	86,190
26	Massachusetts	73,320
23	Michigan	74,310
39	Minnesota	69,760
27	Mississippi	73,160
47	Missouri	65,060
49	Montana	64,400
42	Nebraska	68,870
3	Nevada	85,360
35	New Hampshire	70,370
4	New Jersey	83,780
44	New Mexico	67,210
20	New York	74,920
22	North Carolina	74,450
48	North Dakota	64,750
19	Ohio	75,340
40	Oklahoma	69,630
28	Oregon	72,880
21	Pennsylvania	74,630
10	Rhode Island	79,520
31	South Carolina	72,490
45	South Dakota	66,490
15	Tennessee	76,270
6	Texas	83,020
43	Utah	67,540
46	Vermont	65,390
17	Virginia	75,880
25	Washington	73,690
13	West Virginia	76,970
29	Wisconsin	72,580
33	Wyoming	71,310

RANK	STATE	WAGES
1	Alaska	$87,410
2	Maryland	86,190
3	Nevada	85,360
4	New Jersey	83,780
5	California	83,740
6	Texas	83,020
7	Delaware	82,450
8	Illinois	80,000
9	Florida	79,670
10	Rhode Island	79,520
11	Connecticut	79,250
12	Louisiana	77,910
13	West Virginia	76,970
14	Georgia	76,530
15	Tennessee	76,270
16	Alabama	76,260
17	Virginia	75,880
18	Kentucky	75,590
19	Ohio	75,340
20	New York	74,920
21	Pennsylvania	74,630
22	North Carolina	74,450
23	Arkansas	74,310
23	Michigan	74,310
25	Washington	73,690
26	Massachusetts	73,320
27	Mississippi	73,160
28	Oregon	72,880
29	Wisconsin	72,580
30	Arizona	72,550
31	South Carolina	72,490
32	Kansas	72,380
33	Wyoming	71,310
34	Idaho	70,780
35	New Hampshire	70,370
36	Iowa	70,100
37	Maine	70,020
38	Colorado	69,780
39	Minnesota	69,760
40	Oklahoma	69,630
41	Indiana	69,340
42	Nebraska	68,870
43	Utah	67,540
44	New Mexico	67,210
45	South Dakota	66,490
46	Vermont	65,390
47	Missouri	65,060
48	North Dakota	64,750
49	Montana	64,400
50	Hawaii	56,990
	District of Columbia	83,300

Source: U.S. Department of Labor, Bureau of Labor Statistics
   "Occupational Employment and Wages, 2009" (http://www.bls.gov/oes/)
*Does not include self-employed.

Dentists in 2008

National Total = 181,774 Dentists*

ALPHA ORDER

RANK	STATE	DENTISTS	% of USA
28	Alabama	2,032	1.1%
45	Alaska	505	0.3%
16	Arizona	3,302	1.8%
35	Arkansas	1,125	0.6%
1	California	27,922	15.4%
17	Colorado	3,212	1.8%
23	Connecticut	2,610	1.4%
47	Delaware	403	0.2%
4	Florida	9,741	5.4%
13	Georgia	4,260	2.3%
37	Hawaii	1,039	0.6%
39	Idaho	890	0.5%
5	Illinois	8,192	4.5%
21	Indiana	3,009	1.7%
31	Iowa	1,600	0.9%
32	Kansas	1,413	0.8%
25	Kentucky	2,388	1.3%
26	Louisiana	2,066	1.1%
42	Maine	657	0.4%
15	Maryland	4,138	2.3%
10	Massachusetts	5,442	3.0%
8	Michigan	6,060	3.3%
19	Minnesota	3,174	1.7%
34	Mississippi	1,160	0.6%
22	Missouri	2,803	1.5%
44	Montana	548	0.3%
36	Nebraska	1,105	0.6%
33	Nevada	1,330	0.7%
41	New Hampshire	817	0.4%
7	New Jersey	6,925	3.8%
38	New Mexico	916	0.5%
2	New York	14,980	8.2%
14	North Carolina	4,183	2.3%
49	North Dakota	329	0.2%
9	Ohio	6,029	3.3%
29	Oklahoma	1,805	1.0%
24	Oregon	2,574	1.4%
6	Pennsylvania	7,756	4.3%
43	Rhode Island	573	0.3%
27	South Carolina	2,065	1.1%
46	South Dakota	406	0.2%
20	Tennessee	3,015	1.7%
3	Texas	10,936	6.0%
30	Utah	1,743	1.0%
48	Vermont	360	0.2%
11	Virginia	4,640	2.6%
12	Washington	4,579	2.5%
40	West Virginia	844	0.5%
18	Wisconsin	3,208	1.8%
50	Wyoming	266	0.1%

RANK ORDER

RANK	STATE	DENTISTS	% of USA
1	California	27,922	15.4%
2	New York	14,980	8.2%
3	Texas	10,936	6.0%
4	Florida	9,741	5.4%
5	Illinois	8,192	4.5%
6	Pennsylvania	7,756	4.3%
7	New Jersey	6,925	3.8%
8	Michigan	6,060	3.3%
9	Ohio	6,029	3.3%
10	Massachusetts	5,442	3.0%
11	Virginia	4,640	2.6%
12	Washington	4,579	2.5%
13	Georgia	4,260	2.3%
14	North Carolina	4,183	2.3%
15	Maryland	4,138	2.3%
16	Arizona	3,302	1.8%
17	Colorado	3,212	1.8%
18	Wisconsin	3,208	1.8%
19	Minnesota	3,174	1.7%
20	Tennessee	3,015	1.7%
21	Indiana	3,009	1.7%
22	Missouri	2,803	1.5%
23	Connecticut	2,610	1.4%
24	Oregon	2,574	1.4%
25	Kentucky	2,388	1.3%
26	Louisiana	2,066	1.1%
27	South Carolina	2,065	1.1%
28	Alabama	2,032	1.1%
29	Oklahoma	1,805	1.0%
30	Utah	1,743	1.0%
31	Iowa	1,600	0.9%
32	Kansas	1,413	0.8%
33	Nevada	1,330	0.7%
34	Mississippi	1,160	0.6%
35	Arkansas	1,125	0.6%
36	Nebraska	1,105	0.6%
37	Hawaii	1,039	0.6%
38	New Mexico	916	0.5%
39	Idaho	890	0.5%
40	West Virginia	844	0.5%
41	New Hampshire	817	0.4%
42	Maine	657	0.4%
43	Rhode Island	573	0.3%
44	Montana	548	0.3%
45	Alaska	505	0.3%
46	South Dakota	406	0.2%
47	Delaware	403	0.2%
48	Vermont	360	0.2%
49	North Dakota	329	0.2%
50	Wyoming	266	0.1%
	District of Columbia	634	0.3%

Source: American Dental Association
    "Distribution of Dentists, by Region and State, 2008"
*Professionally active dentists. Total includes 65 dentists for whom state is not known.

Rate of Dentists in 2008

National Rate = 60 Dentists per 100,000 Population*

ALPHA ORDER

RANK	STATE	RATE
48	Alabama	43
7	Alaska	73
29	Arizona	51
49	Arkansas	39
5	California	76
11	Colorado	65
6	Connecticut	75
41	Delaware	46
26	Florida	53
47	Georgia	44
2	Hawaii	81
20	Idaho	58
12	Illinois	64
38	Indiana	47
26	Iowa	53
29	Kansas	51
24	Kentucky	56
41	Louisiana	46
33	Maine	50
7	Maryland	73
1	Massachusetts	83
17	Michigan	61
17	Minnesota	61
49	Mississippi	39
38	Missouri	47
22	Montana	57
14	Nebraska	62
29	Nevada	51
14	New Hampshire	62
3	New Jersey	80
41	New Mexico	46
4	New York	77
45	North Carolina	45
29	North Dakota	51
28	Ohio	52
33	Oklahoma	50
10	Oregon	68
14	Pennsylvania	62
25	Rhode Island	54
41	South Carolina	46
33	South Dakota	50
37	Tennessee	48
45	Texas	45
12	Utah	64
20	Vermont	58
19	Virginia	60
9	Washington	70
38	West Virginia	47
22	Wisconsin	57
33	Wyoming	50

RANK ORDER

RANK	STATE	RATE
1	Massachusetts	83
2	Hawaii	81
3	New Jersey	80
4	New York	77
5	California	76
6	Connecticut	75
7	Alaska	73
7	Maryland	73
9	Washington	70
10	Oregon	68
11	Colorado	65
12	Illinois	64
12	Utah	64
14	Nebraska	62
14	New Hampshire	62
14	Pennsylvania	62
17	Michigan	61
17	Minnesota	61
19	Virginia	60
20	Idaho	58
20	Vermont	58
22	Montana	57
22	Wisconsin	57
24	Kentucky	56
25	Rhode Island	54
26	Florida	53
26	Iowa	53
28	Ohio	52
29	Arizona	51
29	Kansas	51
29	Nevada	51
29	North Dakota	51
33	Maine	50
33	Oklahoma	50
33	South Dakota	50
33	Wyoming	50
37	Tennessee	48
38	Indiana	47
38	Missouri	47
38	West Virginia	47
41	Delaware	46
41	Louisiana	46
41	New Mexico	46
41	South Carolina	46
45	North Carolina	45
45	Texas	45
47	Georgia	44
48	Alabama	43
49	Arkansas	39
49	Mississippi	39
	District of Columbia	107

Source: CQ Press using data from American Dental Association
   "Distribution of Dentists, by Region and State, 2008"
*Professionally active dentists. National figure includes 65 dentists for whom state is not known.

Average Annual Wages of Dentists in 2009

National Average = $156,850*

ALPHA ORDER				RANK ORDER		
RANK	STATE	WAGES		RANK	STATE	WAGES
11	Alabama	$177,810		1	Maine	$205,960
2	Alaska	199,720		2	Alaska	199,720
27	Arizona	160,410		3	Delaware	198,770
9	Arkansas	186,710		4	North Dakota	196,450
38	California	148,650		5	Vermont	195,800
34	Colorado	149,560		6	North Carolina	193,600
25	Connecticut	165,090		7	Rhode Island	189,640
3	Delaware	198,770		8	Virginia	187,200
39	Florida	144,680		9	Arkansas	186,710
24	Georgia	167,060		10	New Hampshire	182,720
44	Hawaii	141,020		11	Alabama	177,810
22	Idaho	168,310		12	Oregon	177,680
43	Illinois	142,850		12	Washington	177,680
19	Indiana	170,570		14	New Mexico	174,560
17	Iowa	172,320		15	South Carolina	173,530
30	Kansas	157,930		16	Minnesota	172,560
36	Kentucky	149,430		17	Iowa	172,320
47	Louisiana	134,810		18	Wisconsin	170,660
1	Maine	205,960		19	Indiana	170,570
40	Maryland	144,320		20	Massachusetts	169,340
20	Massachusetts	169,340		21	Nevada	168,940
31	Michigan	157,810		22	Idaho	168,310
16	Minnesota	172,560		23	Tennessee	167,840
26	Mississippi	162,050		24	Georgia	167,060
41	Missouri	143,080		25	Connecticut	165,090
49	Montana	123,230		26	Mississippi	162,050
29	Nebraska	158,630		27	Arizona	160,410
21	Nevada	168,940		28	Ohio	160,250
10	New Hampshire	182,720		29	Nebraska	158,630
32	New Jersey	154,130		30	Kansas	157,930
14	New Mexico	174,560		31	Michigan	157,810
37	New York	149,370		32	New Jersey	154,130
6	North Carolina	193,600		33	Texas	153,630
4	North Dakota	196,450		34	Colorado	149,560
28	Ohio	160,250		35	Wyoming	149,500
46	Oklahoma	134,900		36	Kentucky	149,430
12	Oregon	177,680		37	New York	149,370
45	Pennsylvania	139,400		38	California	148,650
7	Rhode Island	189,640		39	Florida	144,680
15	South Carolina	173,530		40	Maryland	144,320
42	South Dakota	142,900		41	Missouri	143,080
23	Tennessee	167,840		42	South Dakota	142,900
33	Texas	153,630		43	Illinois	142,850
50	Utah	109,440		44	Hawaii	141,020
5	Vermont	195,800		45	Pennsylvania	139,400
8	Virginia	187,200		46	Oklahoma	134,900
12	Washington	177,680		47	Louisiana	134,810
48	West Virginia	133,290		48	West Virginia	133,290
18	Wisconsin	170,660		49	Montana	123,230
35	Wyoming	149,500		50	Utah	109,440
					District of Columbia	164,430

Source: U.S. Department of Labor, Bureau of Labor Statistics
"Occupational Employment and Wages, 2009" (http://www.bls.gov/oes/)
*Does not include self-employed.

Percent of Population Lacking Access to Dental Care in 2011

National Percent = 10.3% of Population*

ALPHA ORDER

RANK	STATE	PERCENT
4	Alabama	23.6
20	Alaska	11.4
18	Arizona	12.5
38	Arkansas	6.5
45	California	3.8
41	Colorado	6.0
27	Connecticut	9.7
12	Delaware	16.2
11	Florida	16.6
25	Georgia	10.0
16	Hawaii	13.0
10	Idaho	16.7
16	Illinois	13.0
46	Indiana	3.0
28	Iowa	9.6
12	Kansas	16.2
38	Kentucky	6.5
2	Louisiana	31.7
9	Maine	16.9
36	Maryland	7.3
32	Massachusetts	8.3
26	Michigan	9.9
43	Minnesota	5.7
1	Mississippi	32.9
8	Missouri	17.7
5	Montana	23.3
49	Nebraska	1.6
14	Nevada	14.3
48	New Hampshire	2.1
50	New Jersey	0.9
3	New Mexico	25.6
40	New York	6.3
22	North Carolina	10.8
33	North Dakota	8.2
35	Ohio	7.4
44	Oklahoma	5.3
15	Oregon	14.1
29	Pennsylvania	9.5
23	Rhode Island	10.7
6	South Carolina	21.1
19	South Dakota	11.9
7	Tennessee	20.1
21	Texas	11.2
41	Utah	6.0
47	Vermont	2.5
30	Virginia	8.6
24	Washington	10.3
34	West Virginia	7.5
31	Wisconsin	8.5
37	Wyoming	7.1

RANK ORDER

RANK	STATE	PERCENT
1	Mississippi	32.9
2	Louisiana	31.7
3	New Mexico	25.6
4	Alabama	23.6
5	Montana	23.3
6	South Carolina	21.1
7	Tennessee	20.1
8	Missouri	17.7
9	Maine	16.9
10	Idaho	16.7
11	Florida	16.6
12	Delaware	16.2
12	Kansas	16.2
14	Nevada	14.3
15	Oregon	14.1
16	Hawaii	13.0
16	Illinois	13.0
18	Arizona	12.5
19	South Dakota	11.9
20	Alaska	11.4
21	Texas	11.2
22	North Carolina	10.8
23	Rhode Island	10.7
24	Washington	10.3
25	Georgia	10.0
26	Michigan	9.9
27	Connecticut	9.7
28	Iowa	9.6
29	Pennsylvania	9.5
30	Virginia	8.6
31	Wisconsin	8.5
32	Massachusetts	8.3
33	North Dakota	8.2
34	West Virginia	7.5
35	Ohio	7.4
36	Maryland	7.3
37	Wyoming	7.1
38	Arkansas	6.5
38	Kentucky	6.5
40	New York	6.3
41	Colorado	6.0
41	Utah	6.0
43	Minnesota	5.7
44	Oklahoma	5.3
45	California	3.8
46	Indiana	3.0
47	Vermont	2.5
48	New Hampshire	2.1
49	Nebraska	1.6
50	New Jersey	0.9
	District of Columbia	3.7

Source: CQ Press using data from U.S. Department of Health and Human Services, Division of Shortage Designation
"State Population and HPSA Designation Population Statistics" (as of January 20, 2011)
(http://datawarehouse.hrsa.gov/hpsadetail.aspx)

*Percent of population considered under-served by dental practitioners. An under-served population does not have primary medical care within reasonable economic and geographic bounds.

Pharmacists in 2009

National Total = 267,870 Pharmacists*

ALPHA ORDER

RANK	STATE	PHARMACISTS	% of USA
22	Alabama	4,550	1.7%
50	Alaska	390	0.1%
21	Arizona	4,830	1.8%
30	Arkansas	2,820	1.1%
1	California	23,060	8.6%
24	Colorado	4,320	1.6%
32	Connecticut	2,670	1.0%
47	Delaware	730	0.3%
3	Florida	16,890	6.3%
10	Georgia	8,060	3.0%
45	Hawaii	920	0.3%
40	Idaho	1,280	0.5%
7	Illinois	9,910	3.7%
13	Indiana	6,900	2.6%
29	Iowa	3,180	1.2%
31	Kansas	2,730	1.0%
26	Kentucky	4,280	1.6%
25	Louisiana	4,290	1.6%
42	Maine	1,190	0.4%
20	Maryland	5,150	1.9%
14	Massachusetts	6,560	2.4%
8	Michigan	9,060	3.4%
17	Minnesota	5,550	2.1%
33	Mississippi	2,330	0.9%
18	Missouri	5,510	2.1%
43	Montana	1,060	0.4%
35	Nebraska	2,240	0.8%
34	Nevada	2,280	0.9%
38	New Hampshire	1,920	0.7%
9	New Jersey	8,300	3.1%
39	New Mexico	1,540	0.6%
4	New York	16,290	6.1%
11	North Carolina	8,030	3.0%
46	North Dakota	880	0.3%
5	Ohio	11,790	4.4%
28	Oklahoma	3,200	1.2%
27	Oregon	3,510	1.3%
6	Pennsylvania	11,580	4.3%
41	Rhode Island	1,240	0.5%
23	South Carolina	4,480	1.7%
44	South Dakota	960	0.4%
15	Tennessee	6,530	2.4%
2	Texas	20,570	7.7%
36	Utah	2,050	0.8%
48	Vermont	460	0.2%
12	Virginia	7,700	2.9%
16	Washington	5,880	2.2%
37	West Virginia	1,950	0.7%
19	Wisconsin	5,190	1.9%
48	Wyoming	460	0.2%

RANK ORDER

RANK	STATE	PHARMACISTS	% of USA
1	California	23,060	8.6%
2	Texas	20,570	7.7%
3	Florida	16,890	6.3%
4	New York	16,290	6.1%
5	Ohio	11,790	4.4%
6	Pennsylvania	11,580	4.3%
7	Illinois	9,910	3.7%
8	Michigan	9,060	3.4%
9	New Jersey	8,300	3.1%
10	Georgia	8,060	3.0%
11	North Carolina	8,030	3.0%
12	Virginia	7,700	2.9%
13	Indiana	6,900	2.6%
14	Massachusetts	6,560	2.4%
15	Tennessee	6,530	2.4%
16	Washington	5,880	2.2%
17	Minnesota	5,550	2.1%
18	Missouri	5,510	2.1%
19	Wisconsin	5,190	1.9%
20	Maryland	5,150	1.9%
21	Arizona	4,830	1.8%
22	Alabama	4,550	1.7%
23	South Carolina	4,480	1.7%
24	Colorado	4,320	1.6%
25	Louisiana	4,290	1.6%
26	Kentucky	4,280	1.6%
27	Oregon	3,510	1.3%
28	Oklahoma	3,200	1.2%
29	Iowa	3,180	1.2%
30	Arkansas	2,820	1.1%
31	Kansas	2,730	1.0%
32	Connecticut	2,670	1.0%
33	Mississippi	2,330	0.9%
34	Nevada	2,280	0.9%
35	Nebraska	2,240	0.8%
36	Utah	2,050	0.8%
37	West Virginia	1,950	0.7%
38	New Hampshire	1,920	0.7%
39	New Mexico	1,540	0.6%
40	Idaho	1,280	0.5%
41	Rhode Island	1,240	0.5%
42	Maine	1,190	0.4%
43	Montana	1,060	0.4%
44	South Dakota	960	0.4%
45	Hawaii	920	0.3%
46	North Dakota	880	0.3%
47	Delaware	730	0.3%
48	Vermont	460	0.2%
48	Wyoming	460	0.2%
50	Alaska	390	0.1%
	District of Columbia	620	0.2%

Source: U.S. Department of Labor, Bureau of Labor Statistics
"Occupational Employment and Wages, 2009" (http://www.bls.gov/oes/)
*Does not include self-employed.

Rate of Pharmacists in 2009

National Rate = 87 Pharmacists per 100,000 Population*

ALPHA ORDER

RANK ORDER

RANK	STATE	RATE		RANK	STATE	RATE
18	Alabama	97		1	New Hampshire	145
50	Alaska	56		2	North Dakota	136
47	Arizona	73		3	Nebraska	125
15	Arkansas	98		4	Rhode Island	118
49	California	62		4	South Dakota	118
32	Colorado	86		6	Montana	109
44	Connecticut	76		7	Indiana	107
39	Delaware	82		7	West Virginia	107
26	Florida	91		9	Iowa	106
39	Georgia	82		10	Minnesota	105
48	Hawaii	71		11	Tennessee	104
36	Idaho	83		12	Ohio	102
42	Illinois	77		13	Kentucky	99
7	Indiana	107		13	Massachusetts	99
9	Iowa	106		15	Arkansas	98
18	Kansas	97		15	South Carolina	98
13	Kentucky	99		15	Virginia	98
20	Louisiana	96		18	Alabama	97
28	Maine	90		18	Kansas	97
28	Maryland	90		20	Louisiana	96
13	Massachusetts	99		21	New Jersey	95
26	Michigan	91		22	Missouri	92
10	Minnesota	105		22	Oregon	92
41	Mississippi	79		22	Pennsylvania	92
22	Missouri	92		22	Wisconsin	92
6	Montana	109		26	Florida	91
3	Nebraska	125		26	Michigan	91
32	Nevada	86		28	Maine	90
1	New Hampshire	145		28	Maryland	90
21	New Jersey	95		30	Washington	88
42	New Mexico	77		31	Oklahoma	87
36	New York	83		32	Colorado	86
32	North Carolina	86		32	Nevada	86
2	North Dakota	136		32	North Carolina	86
12	Ohio	102		35	Wyoming	85
31	Oklahoma	87		36	Idaho	83
22	Oregon	92		36	New York	83
22	Pennsylvania	92		36	Texas	83
4	Rhode Island	118		39	Delaware	82
15	South Carolina	98		39	Georgia	82
4	South Dakota	118		41	Mississippi	79
11	Tennessee	104		42	Illinois	77
36	Texas	83		42	New Mexico	77
45	Utah	74		44	Connecticut	76
45	Vermont	74		45	Utah	74
15	Virginia	98		45	Vermont	74
30	Washington	88		47	Arizona	73
7	West Virginia	107		48	Hawaii	71
22	Wisconsin	92		49	California	62
35	Wyoming	85		50	Alaska	56
					District of Columbia	103

Source: CQ Press using data from U.S. Department of Labor, Bureau of Labor Statistics
   "Occupational Employment and Wages, 2009" (http://www.bls.gov/oes/)
*Does not include self-employed.

Average Annual Wages of Pharmacists in 2009

National Average = $106,630*

ALPHA ORDER

RANK	STATE	WAGES
3	Alabama	$115,060
5	Alaska	113,460
21	Arizona	106,870
45	Arkansas	96,110
1	California	117,080
18	Colorado	107,670
9	Connecticut	111,360
12	Delaware	110,400
22	Florida	106,250
30	Georgia	103,730
23	Hawaii	106,230
44	Idaho	96,710
31	Illinois	103,590
28	Indiana	104,220
48	Iowa	92,380
34	Kansas	103,270
26	Kentucky	105,780
38	Louisiana	102,130
2	Maine	115,760
32	Maryland	103,440
40	Massachusetts	98,690
32	Michigan	103,440
4	Minnesota	113,500
29	Mississippi	103,940
15	Missouri	108,770
47	Montana	93,780
49	Nebraska	91,500
19	Nevada	107,350
7	New Hampshire	112,500
27	New Jersey	104,970
37	New Mexico	102,150
24	New York	106,170
11	North Carolina	110,820
50	North Dakota	90,610
36	Ohio	102,350
43	Oklahoma	97,110
14	Oregon	110,040
42	Pennsylvania	98,170
41	Rhode Island	98,300
17	South Carolina	108,030
46	South Dakota	93,850
8	Tennessee	111,460
13	Texas	110,260
39	Utah	101,370
16	Vermont	108,620
10	Virginia	111,310
25	Washington	105,840
20	West Virginia	107,270
6	Wisconsin	113,210
35	Wyoming	102,880

RANK ORDER

RANK	STATE	WAGES
1	California	$117,080
2	Maine	115,760
3	Alabama	115,060
4	Minnesota	113,500
5	Alaska	113,460
6	Wisconsin	113,210
7	New Hampshire	112,500
8	Tennessee	111,460
9	Connecticut	111,360
10	Virginia	111,310
11	North Carolina	110,820
12	Delaware	110,400
13	Texas	110,260
14	Oregon	110,040
15	Missouri	108,770
16	Vermont	108,620
17	South Carolina	108,030
18	Colorado	107,670
19	Nevada	107,350
20	West Virginia	107,270
21	Arizona	106,870
22	Florida	106,250
23	Hawaii	106,230
24	New York	106,170
25	Washington	105,840
26	Kentucky	105,780
27	New Jersey	104,970
28	Indiana	104,220
29	Mississippi	103,940
30	Georgia	103,730
31	Illinois	103,590
32	Maryland	103,440
32	Michigan	103,440
34	Kansas	103,270
35	Wyoming	102,880
36	Ohio	102,350
37	New Mexico	102,150
38	Louisiana	102,130
39	Utah	101,370
40	Massachusetts	98,690
41	Rhode Island	98,300
42	Pennsylvania	98,170
43	Oklahoma	97,110
44	Idaho	96,710
45	Arkansas	96,110
46	South Dakota	93,850
47	Montana	93,780
48	Iowa	92,380
49	Nebraska	91,500
50	North Dakota	90,610
	District of Columbia	110,020

Source: U.S. Department of Labor, Bureau of Labor Statistics
   "Occupational Employment and Wages, 2009" (http://www.bls.gov/oes/)
*Does not include self-employed.

Optometrists in 2009

National Total = 26,480 Optometrists*

ALPHA ORDER

ALPHA ORDER

RANK	STATE	OPTOMETRISTS	% of USA
32	Alabama	270	1.0%
49	Alaska	60	0.2%
9	Arizona	800	3.0%
29	Arkansas	300	1.1%
1	California	2,620	9.9%
10	Colorado	740	2.8%
38	Connecticut	150	0.6%
43	Delaware	110	0.4%
6	Florida	1,100	4.2%
15	Georgia	600	2.3%
30	Hawaii	290	1.1%
36	Idaho	170	0.6%
2	Illinois	1,800	6.8%
14	Indiana	610	2.3%
26	Iowa	360	1.4%
24	Kansas	380	1.4%
28	Kentucky	320	1.2%
33	Louisiana	250	0.9%
41	Maine	120	0.5%
23	Maryland	420	1.6%
12	Massachusetts	650	2.5%
7	Michigan	900	3.4%
18	Minnesota	540	2.0%
31	Mississippi	280	1.1%
13	Missouri	630	2.4%
46	Montana	90	0.3%
34	Nebraska	230	0.9%
39	Nevada	140	0.5%
43	New Hampshire	110	0.4%
19	New Jersey	510	1.9%
36	New Mexico	170	0.6%
3	New York	1,790	6.8%
11	North Carolina	700	2.6%
43	North Dakota	110	0.4%
8	Ohio	890	3.4%
21	Oklahoma	490	1.9%
20	Oregon	500	1.9%
5	Pennsylvania	1,560	5.9%
47	Rhode Island	80	0.3%
25	South Carolina	370	1.4%
41	South Dakota	120	0.5%
27	Tennessee	330	1.2%
4	Texas	1,680	6.3%
35	Utah	200	0.8%
50	Vermont	50	0.2%
15	Virginia	600	2.3%
22	Washington	440	1.7%
40	West Virginia	130	0.5%
17	Wisconsin	570	2.2%
47	Wyoming	80	0.3%

RANK ORDER

RANK	STATE	OPTOMETRISTS	% of USA
1	California	2,620	9.9%
2	Illinois	1,800	6.8%
3	New York	1,790	6.8%
4	Texas	1,680	6.3%
5	Pennsylvania	1,560	5.9%
6	Florida	1,100	4.2%
7	Michigan	900	3.4%
8	Ohio	890	3.4%
9	Arizona	800	3.0%
10	Colorado	740	2.8%
11	North Carolina	700	2.6%
12	Massachusetts	650	2.5%
13	Missouri	630	2.4%
14	Indiana	610	2.3%
15	Georgia	600	2.3%
15	Virginia	600	2.3%
17	Wisconsin	570	2.2%
18	Minnesota	540	2.0%
19	New Jersey	510	1.9%
20	Oregon	500	1.9%
21	Oklahoma	490	1.9%
22	Washington	440	1.7%
23	Maryland	420	1.6%
24	Kansas	380	1.4%
25	South Carolina	370	1.4%
26	Iowa	360	1.4%
27	Tennessee	330	1.2%
28	Kentucky	320	1.2%
29	Arkansas	300	1.1%
30	Hawaii	290	1.1%
31	Mississippi	280	1.1%
32	Alabama	270	1.0%
33	Louisiana	250	0.9%
34	Nebraska	230	0.9%
35	Utah	200	0.8%
36	Idaho	170	0.6%
36	New Mexico	170	0.6%
38	Connecticut	150	0.6%
39	Nevada	140	0.5%
40	West Virginia	130	0.5%
41	Maine	120	0.5%
41	South Dakota	120	0.5%
43	Delaware	110	0.4%
43	New Hampshire	110	0.4%
43	North Dakota	110	0.4%
46	Montana	90	0.3%
47	Rhode Island	80	0.3%
47	Wyoming	80	0.3%
49	Alaska	60	0.2%
50	Vermont	50	0.2%
	District of Columbia	70	0.3%

Source: U.S. Department of Labor, Bureau of Labor Statistics
   "Occupational Employment and Wages, 2009" (http://www.bls.gov/oes/)
*Does not include self-employed.

Rate of Optometrists in 2009

National Rate = 9 Optometrists per 100,000 Population*

<table>
<tr><td colspan="3">ALPHA ORDER</td><td colspan="3">RANK ORDER</td></tr>
<tr><td>RANK</td><td>STATE</td><td>RATE</td><td>RANK</td><td>STATE</td><td>RATE</td></tr>
<tr><td>43</td><td>Alabama</td><td>6</td><td>1</td><td>Hawaii</td><td>22</td></tr>
<tr><td>21</td><td>Alaska</td><td>9</td><td>2</td><td>North Dakota</td><td>17</td></tr>
<tr><td>11</td><td>Arizona</td><td>12</td><td>3</td><td>Colorado</td><td>15</td></tr>
<tr><td>17</td><td>Arkansas</td><td>10</td><td>3</td><td>South Dakota</td><td>15</td></tr>
<tr><td>35</td><td>California</td><td>7</td><td>3</td><td>Wyoming</td><td>15</td></tr>
<tr><td>3</td><td>Colorado</td><td>15</td><td>6</td><td>Illinois</td><td>14</td></tr>
<tr><td>50</td><td>Connecticut</td><td>4</td><td>7</td><td>Kansas</td><td>13</td></tr>
<tr><td>11</td><td>Delaware</td><td>12</td><td>7</td><td>Nebraska</td><td>13</td></tr>
<tr><td>43</td><td>Florida</td><td>6</td><td>7</td><td>Oklahoma</td><td>13</td></tr>
<tr><td>43</td><td>Georgia</td><td>6</td><td>7</td><td>Oregon</td><td>13</td></tr>
<tr><td>1</td><td>Hawaii</td><td>22</td><td>11</td><td>Arizona</td><td>12</td></tr>
<tr><td>15</td><td>Idaho</td><td>11</td><td>11</td><td>Delaware</td><td>12</td></tr>
<tr><td>6</td><td>Illinois</td><td>14</td><td>11</td><td>Iowa</td><td>12</td></tr>
<tr><td>21</td><td>Indiana</td><td>9</td><td>11</td><td>Pennsylvania</td><td>12</td></tr>
<tr><td>11</td><td>Iowa</td><td>12</td><td>15</td><td>Idaho</td><td>11</td></tr>
<tr><td>7</td><td>Kansas</td><td>13</td><td>15</td><td>Missouri</td><td>11</td></tr>
<tr><td>35</td><td>Kentucky</td><td>7</td><td>17</td><td>Arkansas</td><td>10</td></tr>
<tr><td>43</td><td>Louisiana</td><td>6</td><td>17</td><td>Massachusetts</td><td>10</td></tr>
<tr><td>21</td><td>Maine</td><td>9</td><td>17</td><td>Minnesota</td><td>10</td></tr>
<tr><td>35</td><td>Maryland</td><td>7</td><td>17</td><td>Wisconsin</td><td>10</td></tr>
<tr><td>17</td><td>Massachusetts</td><td>10</td><td>21</td><td>Alaska</td><td>9</td></tr>
<tr><td>21</td><td>Michigan</td><td>9</td><td>21</td><td>Indiana</td><td>9</td></tr>
<tr><td>17</td><td>Minnesota</td><td>10</td><td>21</td><td>Maine</td><td>9</td></tr>
<tr><td>21</td><td>Mississippi</td><td>9</td><td>21</td><td>Michigan</td><td>9</td></tr>
<tr><td>15</td><td>Missouri</td><td>11</td><td>21</td><td>Mississippi</td><td>9</td></tr>
<tr><td>21</td><td>Montana</td><td>9</td><td>21</td><td>Montana</td><td>9</td></tr>
<tr><td>7</td><td>Nebraska</td><td>13</td><td>21</td><td>New York</td><td>9</td></tr>
<tr><td>48</td><td>Nevada</td><td>5</td><td>28</td><td>New Hampshire</td><td>8</td></tr>
<tr><td>28</td><td>New Hampshire</td><td>8</td><td>28</td><td>New Mexico</td><td>8</td></tr>
<tr><td>43</td><td>New Jersey</td><td>6</td><td>28</td><td>Ohio</td><td>8</td></tr>
<tr><td>28</td><td>New Mexico</td><td>8</td><td>28</td><td>Rhode Island</td><td>8</td></tr>
<tr><td>21</td><td>New York</td><td>9</td><td>28</td><td>South Carolina</td><td>8</td></tr>
<tr><td>35</td><td>North Carolina</td><td>7</td><td>28</td><td>Vermont</td><td>8</td></tr>
<tr><td>2</td><td>North Dakota</td><td>17</td><td>28</td><td>Virginia</td><td>8</td></tr>
<tr><td>28</td><td>Ohio</td><td>8</td><td>35</td><td>California</td><td>7</td></tr>
<tr><td>7</td><td>Oklahoma</td><td>13</td><td>35</td><td>Kentucky</td><td>7</td></tr>
<tr><td>7</td><td>Oregon</td><td>13</td><td>35</td><td>Maryland</td><td>7</td></tr>
<tr><td>11</td><td>Pennsylvania</td><td>12</td><td>35</td><td>North Carolina</td><td>7</td></tr>
<tr><td>28</td><td>Rhode Island</td><td>8</td><td>35</td><td>Texas</td><td>7</td></tr>
<tr><td>28</td><td>South Carolina</td><td>8</td><td>35</td><td>Utah</td><td>7</td></tr>
<tr><td>3</td><td>South Dakota</td><td>15</td><td>35</td><td>Washington</td><td>7</td></tr>
<tr><td>48</td><td>Tennessee</td><td>5</td><td>35</td><td>West Virginia</td><td>7</td></tr>
<tr><td>35</td><td>Texas</td><td>7</td><td>43</td><td>Alabama</td><td>6</td></tr>
<tr><td>35</td><td>Utah</td><td>7</td><td>43</td><td>Florida</td><td>6</td></tr>
<tr><td>28</td><td>Vermont</td><td>8</td><td>43</td><td>Georgia</td><td>6</td></tr>
<tr><td>28</td><td>Virginia</td><td>8</td><td>43</td><td>Louisiana</td><td>6</td></tr>
<tr><td>35</td><td>Washington</td><td>7</td><td>43</td><td>New Jersey</td><td>6</td></tr>
<tr><td>35</td><td>West Virginia</td><td>7</td><td>48</td><td>Nevada</td><td>5</td></tr>
<tr><td>17</td><td>Wisconsin</td><td>10</td><td>48</td><td>Tennessee</td><td>5</td></tr>
<tr><td>3</td><td>Wyoming</td><td>15</td><td>50</td><td>Connecticut</td><td>4</td></tr>
<tr><td colspan="3"></td><td colspan="2">District of Columbia</td><td>12</td></tr>
</table>

Source: CQ Press using data from U.S. Department of Labor, Bureau of Labor Statistics
    "Occupational Employment and Wages, 2009" (http://www.bls.gov/oes/)
*Does not include self-employed.

Average Annual Wages of Optometrists in 2009

National Average = $106,960*

ALPHA ORDER				RANK ORDER		
RANK	STATE	WAGES		RANK	STATE	WAGES
38	Alabama	$93,870		1	Louisiana	$142,550
13	Alaska	114,120		2	Tennessee	137,220
8	Arizona	119,380		3	Kansas	129,420
46	Arkansas	75,000		4	Washington	128,880
29	California	101,750		5	Ohio	127,040
44	Colorado	86,640		6	North Carolina	125,490
24	Connecticut	107,430		7	Minnesota	121,830
47	Delaware	74,270		8	Arizona	119,380
17	Florida	112,260		9	Texas	118,300
42	Georgia	89,730		10	Kentucky	117,880
40	Hawaii	92,120		11	New Hampshire	117,460
49	Idaho	70,170		12	West Virginia	116,070
30	Illinois	101,300		13	Alaska	114,120
33	Indiana	99,690		14	Michigan	113,580
37	Iowa	95,270		15	New York	113,220
3	Kansas	129,420		16	North Dakota	112,610
10	Kentucky	117,880		17	Florida	112,260
1	Louisiana	142,550		18	South Dakota	111,830
22	Maine	108,430		19	Virginia	111,430
25	Maryland	105,250		20	New Jersey	111,210
21	Massachusetts	110,670		21	Massachusetts	110,670
14	Michigan	113,580		22	Maine	108,430
7	Minnesota	121,830		23	Rhode Island	108,000
43	Mississippi	89,390		24	Connecticut	107,430
34	Missouri	98,810		25	Maryland	105,250
50	Montana	61,380		26	Wisconsin	103,680
28	Nebraska	102,370		27	Pennsylvania	103,230
41	Nevada	91,130		28	Nebraska	102,370
11	New Hampshire	117,460		29	California	101,750
20	New Jersey	111,210		30	Illinois	101,300
32	New Mexico	99,940		31	Utah	100,980
15	New York	113,220		32	New Mexico	99,940
6	North Carolina	125,490		33	Indiana	99,690
16	North Dakota	112,610		34	Missouri	98,810
5	Ohio	127,040		35	South Carolina	97,480
39	Oklahoma	93,110		36	Vermont	96,390
45	Oregon	76,190		37	Iowa	95,270
27	Pennsylvania	103,230		38	Alabama	93,870
23	Rhode Island	108,000		39	Oklahoma	93,110
35	South Carolina	97,480		40	Hawaii	92,120
18	South Dakota	111,830		41	Nevada	91,130
2	Tennessee	137,220		42	Georgia	89,730
9	Texas	118,300		43	Mississippi	89,390
31	Utah	100,980		44	Colorado	86,640
36	Vermont	96,390		45	Oregon	76,190
19	Virginia	111,430		46	Arkansas	75,000
4	Washington	128,880		47	Delaware	74,270
12	West Virginia	116,070		48	Wyoming	73,310
26	Wisconsin	103,680		49	Idaho	70,170
48	Wyoming	73,310		50	Montana	61,380
					District of Columbia	97,220

Source: U.S. Department of Labor, Bureau of Labor Statistics
    "Occupational Employment and Wages, 2009" (http://www.bls.gov/oes/)
*Does not include self-employed.

Emergency Medical Technicians and Paramedics in 2009

National Total = 217,920 Technicians and Paramedics*

ALPHA ORDER

RANK	STATE	PARAMEDICS	% of USA
23	Alabama	3,290	1.5%
49	Alaska	350	0.2%
22	Arizona	3,760	1.7%
34	Arkansas	1,840	0.8%
1	California	14,790	6.8%
24	Colorado	3,180	1.5%
25	Connecticut	3,040	1.4%
41	Delaware	760	0.3%
6	Florida	9,000	4.1%
11	Georgia	7,380	3.4%
48	Hawaii	510	0.2%
46	Idaho	560	0.3%
5	Illinois	10,590	4.9%
16	Indiana	5,670	2.6%
30	Iowa	2,390	1.1%
29	Kansas	2,660	1.2%
17	Kentucky	4,580	2.1%
26	Louisiana	3,020	1.4%
37	Maine	1,360	0.6%
21	Maryland	3,900	1.8%
14	Massachusetts	6,310	2.9%
12	Michigan	6,950	3.2%
18	Minnesota	4,350	2.0%
35	Mississippi	1,570	0.7%
9	Missouri	8,400	3.9%
40	Montana	800	0.4%
NA	Nebraska**	NA	NA
38	Nevada	1,200	0.6%
36	New Hampshire	1,390	0.6%
10	New Jersey	7,470	3.4%
39	New Mexico	950	0.4%
3	New York	13,580	6.2%
7	North Carolina	8,930	4.1%
44	North Dakota	670	0.3%
8	Ohio	8,770	4.0%
28	Oklahoma	2,720	1.2%
31	Oregon	2,360	1.1%
4	Pennsylvania	12,850	5.9%
43	Rhode Island	680	0.3%
19	South Carolina	4,310	2.0%
41	South Dakota	760	0.3%
13	Tennessee	6,510	3.0%
2	Texas	13,820	6.3%
33	Utah	1,860	0.9%
47	Vermont	540	0.2%
20	Virginia	4,270	2.0%
27	Washington	2,960	1.4%
32	West Virginia	2,080	1.0%
15	Wisconsin	5,720	2.6%
45	Wyoming	620	0.3%

RANK ORDER

RANK	STATE	PARAMEDICS	% of USA
1	California	14,790	6.8%
2	Texas	13,820	6.3%
3	New York	13,580	6.2%
4	Pennsylvania	12,850	5.9%
5	Illinois	10,590	4.9%
6	Florida	9,000	4.1%
7	North Carolina	8,930	4.1%
8	Ohio	8,770	4.0%
9	Missouri	8,400	3.9%
10	New Jersey	7,470	3.4%
11	Georgia	7,380	3.4%
12	Michigan	6,950	3.2%
13	Tennessee	6,510	3.0%
14	Massachusetts	6,310	2.9%
15	Wisconsin	5,720	2.6%
16	Indiana	5,670	2.6%
17	Kentucky	4,580	2.1%
18	Minnesota	4,350	2.0%
19	South Carolina	4,310	2.0%
20	Virginia	4,270	2.0%
21	Maryland	3,900	1.8%
22	Arizona	3,760	1.7%
23	Alabama	3,290	1.5%
24	Colorado	3,180	1.5%
25	Connecticut	3,040	1.4%
26	Louisiana	3,020	1.4%
27	Washington	2,960	1.4%
28	Oklahoma	2,720	1.2%
29	Kansas	2,660	1.2%
30	Iowa	2,390	1.1%
31	Oregon	2,360	1.1%
32	West Virginia	2,080	1.0%
33	Utah	1,860	0.9%
34	Arkansas	1,840	0.8%
35	Mississippi	1,570	0.7%
36	New Hampshire	1,390	0.6%
37	Maine	1,360	0.6%
38	Nevada	1,200	0.6%
39	New Mexico	950	0.4%
40	Montana	800	0.4%
41	Delaware	760	0.3%
41	South Dakota	760	0.3%
43	Rhode Island	680	0.3%
44	North Dakota	670	0.3%
45	Wyoming	620	0.3%
46	Idaho	560	0.3%
47	Vermont	540	0.2%
48	Hawaii	510	0.2%
49	Alaska	350	0.2%
NA	Nebraska**	NA	NA
	District of Columbia**	NA	NA

Source: U.S. Department of Labor, Bureau of Labor Statistics
"Occupational Employment and Wages, 2009" (http://www.bls.gov/oes/)
*Does not include self-employed.
**Not available.

Rate of Emergency Medical Technicians and Paramedics in 2009

National Rate = 71 Technicians and Paramedics per 100,000 Population*

ALPHA ORDER

RANK	STATE	RATE
28	Alabama	70
42	Alaska	50
38	Arizona	57
35	Arkansas	64
47	California	40
36	Colorado	63
18	Connecticut	86
18	Delaware	86
43	Florida	49
26	Georgia	75
48	Hawaii	39
49	Idaho	36
22	Illinois	82
16	Indiana	88
24	Iowa	79
13	Kansas	94
4	Kentucky	106
32	Louisiana	67
7	Maine	103
31	Maryland	68
11	Massachusetts	96
28	Michigan	70
21	Minnesota	83
41	Mississippi	53
1	Missouri	140
22	Montana	82
NA	Nebraska**	NA
45	Nevada	45
5	New Hampshire	105
18	New Jersey	86
44	New Mexico	47
30	New York	69
12	North Carolina	95
6	North Dakota	104
25	Ohio	76
27	Oklahoma	74
37	Oregon	62
9	Pennsylvania	102
34	Rhode Island	65
13	South Carolina	94
13	South Dakota	94
7	Tennessee	103
39	Texas	56
32	Utah	67
17	Vermont	87
40	Virginia	54
46	Washington	44
2	West Virginia	114
10	Wisconsin	101
2	Wyoming	114

RANK ORDER

RANK	STATE	RATE
1	Missouri	140
2	West Virginia	114
2	Wyoming	114
4	Kentucky	106
5	New Hampshire	105
6	North Dakota	104
7	Maine	103
7	Tennessee	103
9	Pennsylvania	102
10	Wisconsin	101
11	Massachusetts	96
12	North Carolina	95
13	Kansas	94
13	South Carolina	94
13	South Dakota	94
16	Indiana	88
17	Vermont	87
18	Connecticut	86
18	Delaware	86
18	New Jersey	86
21	Minnesota	83
22	Illinois	82
22	Montana	82
24	Iowa	79
25	Ohio	76
26	Georgia	75
27	Oklahoma	74
28	Alabama	70
28	Michigan	70
30	New York	69
31	Maryland	68
32	Louisiana	67
32	Utah	67
34	Rhode Island	65
35	Arkansas	64
36	Colorado	63
37	Oregon	62
38	Arizona	57
39	Texas	56
40	Virginia	54
41	Mississippi	53
42	Alaska	50
43	Florida	49
44	New Mexico	47
45	Nevada	45
46	Washington	44
47	California	40
48	Hawaii	39
49	Idaho	36
NA	Nebraska**	NA
	District of Columbia**	NA

Source: CQ Press using data from U.S. Department of Labor, Bureau of Labor Statistics
   "Occupational Employment and Wages, 2009" (http://www.bls.gov/oes/)
*Does not include self-employed.
**Not available.

Average Annual Wages of
Emergency Medical Technicians and Paramedics in 2009
National Average = $33,020*

	ALPHA ORDER				RANK ORDER	
RANK	STATE	WAGES		RANK	STATE	WAGES
22	Alabama	$32,120		1	Hawaii	$47,380
2	Alaska	46,630		2	Alaska	46,630
35	Arizona	30,020		3	Oregon	43,220
41	Arkansas	28,630		4	Washington	41,830
14	California	35,090		5	Maryland	41,150
13	Colorado	36,080		6	New York	38,830
11	Connecticut	36,470		7	Illinois	38,670
9	Delaware	37,470		8	Idaho	38,380
24	Florida	31,900		9	Delaware	37,470
28	Georgia	31,580		10	Massachusetts	37,070
1	Hawaii	47,380		11	Connecticut	36,470
8	Idaho	38,380		11	Nevada	36,470
7	Illinois	38,670		13	Colorado	36,080
37	Indiana	29,690		14	California	35,090
38	Iowa	29,240		15	New Jersey	34,950
42	Kansas	28,110		16	New Hampshire	34,920
43	Kentucky	28,080		17	Wyoming	34,670
19	Louisiana	33,700		18	Virginia	34,650
34	Maine	30,210		19	Louisiana	33,700
5	Maryland	41,150		20	Rhode Island	33,440
10	Massachusetts	37,070		21	Missouri	32,630
25	Michigan	31,730		22	Alabama	32,120
23	Minnesota	31,910		23	Minnesota	31,910
47	Mississippi	26,210		24	Florida	31,900
21	Missouri	32,630		25	Michigan	31,730
49	Montana	25,470		26	South Carolina	31,720
45	Nebraska	27,560		27	North Carolina	31,620
11	Nevada	36,470		28	Georgia	31,580
16	New Hampshire	34,920		29	Tennessee	31,230
15	New Jersey	34,950		30	Utah	30,800
33	New Mexico	30,330		31	Vermont	30,730
6	New York	38,830		32	Texas	30,650
27	North Carolina	31,620		33	New Mexico	30,330
39	North Dakota	29,070		34	Maine	30,210
44	Ohio	27,980		35	Arizona	30,020
46	Oklahoma	26,980		36	Pennsylvania	29,900
3	Oregon	43,220		37	Indiana	29,690
36	Pennsylvania	29,900		38	Iowa	29,240
20	Rhode Island	33,440		39	North Dakota	29,070
26	South Carolina	31,720		40	Wisconsin	29,060
48	South Dakota	25,930		41	Arkansas	28,630
29	Tennessee	31,230		42	Kansas	28,110
32	Texas	30,650		43	Kentucky	28,080
30	Utah	30,800		44	Ohio	27,980
31	Vermont	30,730		45	Nebraska	27,560
18	Virginia	34,650		46	Oklahoma	26,980
4	Washington	41,830		47	Mississippi	26,210
50	West Virginia	23,860		48	South Dakota	25,930
40	Wisconsin	29,060		49	Montana	25,470
17	Wyoming	34,670		50	West Virginia	23,860
					District of Columbia**	NA

Source: U.S. Department of Labor, Bureau of Labor Statistics
    "Occupational Employment and Wages, 2009" (http://www.bls.gov/oes/)
*Does not include self-employed.
**Not available.

Employment in Health Care Support Industries in 2009

National Total = 3,886,690 Aides and Assistants*

ALPHA ORDER

RANK	STATE	EMPLOYEES	% of USA
24	Alabama	50,790	1.3%
48	Alaska	7,430	0.2%
20	Arizona	67,170	1.7%
33	Arkansas	31,600	0.8%
1	California	358,000	9.2%
27	Colorado	49,850	1.3%
23	Connecticut	55,230	1.4%
46	Delaware	10,940	0.3%
4	Florida	211,660	5.4%
15	Georgia	84,290	2.2%
44	Hawaii	13,550	0.3%
41	Idaho	17,630	0.5%
8	Illinois	144,910	3.7%
17	Indiana	81,510	2.1%
28	Iowa	46,690	1.2%
31	Kansas	41,210	1.1%
26	Kentucky	50,050	1.3%
22	Louisiana	58,540	1.5%
38	Maine	23,730	0.6%
21	Maryland	66,650	1.7%
11	Massachusetts	96,820	2.5%
9	Michigan	137,130	3.5%
12	Minnesota	94,660	2.4%
32	Mississippi	34,450	0.9%
16	Missouri	82,110	2.1%
43	Montana	14,490	0.4%
36	Nebraska	25,810	0.7%
37	Nevada	23,840	0.6%
42	New Hampshire	16,780	0.4%
10	New Jersey	122,420	3.1%
35	New Mexico	26,380	0.7%
2	New York	310,510	8.0%
7	North Carolina	146,130	3.8%
45	North Dakota	12,560	0.3%
6	Ohio	198,220	5.1%
29	Oklahoma	45,710	1.2%
30	Oregon	43,980	1.1%
5	Pennsylvania	204,250	5.3%
40	Rhode Island	19,690	0.5%
25	South Carolina	50,440	1.3%
47	South Dakota	10,400	0.3%
18	Tennessee	72,140	1.9%
3	Texas	299,960	7.7%
34	Utah	29,480	0.8%
49	Vermont	6,910	0.2%
14	Virginia	86,080	2.2%
19	Washington	71,420	1.8%
39	West Virginia	23,540	0.6%
13	Wisconsin	92,720	2.4%
50	Wyoming	6,500	0.2%

RANK ORDER

RANK	STATE	EMPLOYEES	% of USA
1	California	358,000	9.2%
2	New York	310,510	8.0%
3	Texas	299,960	7.7%
4	Florida	211,660	5.4%
5	Pennsylvania	204,250	5.3%
6	Ohio	198,220	5.1%
7	North Carolina	146,130	3.8%
8	Illinois	144,910	3.7%
9	Michigan	137,130	3.5%
10	New Jersey	122,420	3.1%
11	Massachusetts	96,820	2.5%
12	Minnesota	94,660	2.4%
13	Wisconsin	92,720	2.4%
14	Virginia	86,080	2.2%
15	Georgia	84,290	2.2%
16	Missouri	82,110	2.1%
17	Indiana	81,510	2.1%
18	Tennessee	72,140	1.9%
19	Washington	71,420	1.8%
20	Arizona	67,170	1.7%
21	Maryland	66,650	1.7%
22	Louisiana	58,540	1.5%
23	Connecticut	55,230	1.4%
24	Alabama	50,790	1.3%
25	South Carolina	50,440	1.3%
26	Kentucky	50,050	1.3%
27	Colorado	49,850	1.3%
28	Iowa	46,690	1.2%
29	Oklahoma	45,710	1.2%
30	Oregon	43,980	1.1%
31	Kansas	41,210	1.1%
32	Mississippi	34,450	0.9%
33	Arkansas	31,600	0.8%
34	Utah	29,480	0.8%
35	New Mexico	26,380	0.7%
36	Nebraska	25,810	0.7%
37	Nevada	23,840	0.6%
38	Maine	23,730	0.6%
39	West Virginia	23,540	0.6%
40	Rhode Island	19,690	0.5%
41	Idaho	17,630	0.5%
42	New Hampshire	16,780	0.4%
43	Montana	14,490	0.4%
44	Hawaii	13,550	0.3%
45	North Dakota	12,560	0.3%
46	Delaware	10,940	0.3%
47	South Dakota	10,400	0.3%
48	Alaska	7,430	0.2%
49	Vermont	6,910	0.2%
50	Wyoming	6,500	0.2%
	District of Columbia	9,740	0.3%

Source: U.S. Department of Labor, Bureau of Labor Statistics
    "Occupational Employment and Wages, 2009" (http://www.bls.gov/oes/)
*Does not include self-employed. Includes various health care assistants and aides not included in the category of health care practitioners and technicians. Among the included occupations are home health aides, nursing aides, psychiatric aides, dental assistants, and pharmacy aides.

Rate of Employees in Health Care Support Industries in 2009

National Rate = 1,266 Aides and Assistants per 100,000 Population*

ALPHA ORDER

RANK	STATE	RATE
41	Alabama	1,079
43	Alaska	1,064
46	Arizona	1,018
39	Arkansas	1,094
48	California	969
47	Colorado	992
9	Connecticut	1,570
26	Delaware	1,236
34	Florida	1,142
50	Georgia	858
45	Hawaii	1,046
35	Idaho	1,141
36	Illinois	1,122
23	Indiana	1,269
11	Iowa	1,552
14	Kansas	1,462
31	Kentucky	1,160
20	Louisiana	1,303
3	Maine	1,800
29	Maryland	1,169
13	Massachusetts	1,468
17	Michigan	1,375
4	Minnesota	1,797
30	Mississippi	1,167
18	Missouri	1,371
12	Montana	1,486
15	Nebraska	1,437
49	Nevada	902
24	New Hampshire	1,267
16	New Jersey	1,406
19	New Mexico	1,313
8	New York	1,589
10	North Carolina	1,558
1	North Dakota	1,942
5	Ohio	1,717
25	Oklahoma	1,240
32	Oregon	1,150
7	Pennsylvania	1,620
2	Rhode Island	1,870
38	South Carolina	1,106
22	South Dakota	1,280
33	Tennessee	1,146
27	Texas	1,210
44	Utah	1,059
37	Vermont	1,111
40	Virginia	1,092
42	Washington	1,072
21	West Virginia	1,294
6	Wisconsin	1,640
28	Wyoming	1,194

RANK ORDER

RANK	STATE	RATE
1	North Dakota	1,942
2	Rhode Island	1,870
3	Maine	1,800
4	Minnesota	1,797
5	Ohio	1,717
6	Wisconsin	1,640
7	Pennsylvania	1,620
8	New York	1,589
9	Connecticut	1,570
10	North Carolina	1,558
11	Iowa	1,552
12	Montana	1,486
13	Massachusetts	1,468
14	Kansas	1,462
15	Nebraska	1,437
16	New Jersey	1,406
17	Michigan	1,375
18	Missouri	1,371
19	New Mexico	1,313
20	Louisiana	1,303
21	West Virginia	1,294
22	South Dakota	1,280
23	Indiana	1,269
24	New Hampshire	1,267
25	Oklahoma	1,240
26	Delaware	1,236
27	Texas	1,210
28	Wyoming	1,194
29	Maryland	1,169
30	Mississippi	1,167
31	Kentucky	1,160
32	Oregon	1,150
33	Tennessee	1,146
34	Florida	1,142
35	Idaho	1,141
36	Illinois	1,122
37	Vermont	1,111
38	South Carolina	1,106
39	Arkansas	1,094
40	Virginia	1,092
41	Alabama	1,079
42	Washington	1,072
43	Alaska	1,064
44	Utah	1,059
45	Hawaii	1,046
46	Arizona	1,018
47	Colorado	992
48	California	969
49	Nevada	902
50	Georgia	858

| | District of Columbia | 1,624 |

Source: CQ Press using data from U.S. Department of Labor, Bureau of Labor Statistics
"Occupational Employment and Wages, 2009" (http://www.bls.gov/oes/)
*Does not include self-employed. Includes various health care assistants and aides not included in the category of health care practitioners and technicians. Among the included occupations are home health aides, nursing aides, psychiatric aides, dental assistants, and pharmacy aides.

Average Annual Wages of Employees in Health Care Support Industries in 2009

National Average = $26,710*

ALPHA ORDER				RANK ORDER		
RANK	**STATE**	**WAGES**		**RANK**	**STATE**	**WAGES**
46	Alabama	$22,560		1	Alaska	$35,670
1	Alaska	35,670		2	Massachusetts	31,990
19	Arizona	27,150		3	Connecticut	31,850
47	Arkansas	22,280		4	Hawaii	30,960
6	California	30,050		5	Washington	30,700
10	Colorado	29,550		6	California	30,050
3	Connecticut	31,850		7	New Hampshire	29,870
13	Delaware	29,400		8	Maryland	29,830
24	Florida	26,140		9	Rhode Island	29,680
35	Georgia	24,610		10	Colorado	29,550
4	Hawaii	30,960		11	Nevada	29,490
37	Idaho	24,410		12	Oregon	29,450
17	Illinois	27,910		13	Delaware	29,400
27	Indiana	25,790		14	New York	28,640
28	Iowa	25,630		15	Vermont	28,450
34	Kansas	24,620		16	New Jersey	28,380
30	Kentucky	25,310		17	Illinois	27,910
49	Louisiana	21,950		18	Minnesota	27,810
26	Maine	25,830		19	Arizona	27,150
8	Maryland	29,830		20	Wyoming	27,140
2	Massachusetts	31,990		21	Wisconsin	26,910
22	Michigan	26,520		22	Michigan	26,520
18	Minnesota	27,810		23	Pennsylvania	26,430
50	Mississippi	21,150		24	Florida	26,140
41	Missouri	24,170		25	Virginia	25,850
40	Montana	24,240		26	Maine	25,830
29	Nebraska	25,330		27	Indiana	25,790
11	Nevada	29,490		28	Iowa	25,630
7	New Hampshire	29,870		29	Nebraska	25,330
16	New Jersey	28,380		30	Kentucky	25,310
43	New Mexico	23,920		31	Ohio	25,110
14	New York	28,640		32	Tennessee	24,930
42	North Carolina	23,990		33	Utah	24,760
36	North Dakota	24,420		34	Kansas	24,620
31	Ohio	25,110		35	Georgia	24,610
45	Oklahoma	23,240		36	North Dakota	24,420
12	Oregon	29,450		37	Idaho	24,410
23	Pennsylvania	26,430		38	South Dakota	24,370
9	Rhode Island	29,680		39	South Carolina	24,260
39	South Carolina	24,260		40	Montana	24,240
38	South Dakota	24,370		41	Missouri	24,170
32	Tennessee	24,930		42	North Carolina	23,990
44	Texas	23,630		43	New Mexico	23,920
33	Utah	24,760		44	Texas	23,630
15	Vermont	28,450		45	Oklahoma	23,240
25	Virginia	25,850		46	Alabama	22,560
5	Washington	30,700		47	Arkansas	22,280
48	West Virginia	22,060		48	West Virginia	22,060
21	Wisconsin	26,910		49	Louisiana	21,950
20	Wyoming	27,140		50	Mississippi	21,150
					District of Columbia	29,920

Source: U.S. Department of Labor, Bureau of Labor Statistics
   "Occupational Employment and Wages, 2009" (http://www.bls.gov/oes/)
*Does not include self-employed. Includes various health care assistants and aides not included in the category of health care practitioners and technicians. Among the included occupations are home health aides, nursing aides, psychiatric aides, dental assistants, and pharmacy aides.

VII. Physical Fitness

Users of Exercise Equipment in 2009. 497
Participants in Golf in 2009 498
Participants in Running/Jogging in 2009 499
Participants in Swimming in 2009 500
Participants in Tennis in 2009. 501
Alcohol Consumption in 2007 502
Adult Per Capita Alcohol Consumption in 2007 503
Apparent Beer Consumption in 2007 504
Adult Per Capita Beer Consumption in 2007 505
Wine Consumption in 2007 506
Adult Per Capita Wine Consumption in 2007 507
Distilled Spirits Consumption in 2007 508
Adult Per Capita Distilled Spirits Consumption in 2007 . . 509
Percent of Adults Who Do Not Drink Alcohol: 2009. 510
Percent of Adults Who Are Binge Drinkers: 2009 511
Percent of Adults Who Smoke: 2009 512
Percent of Men Who Smoke: 2009. 513
Percent of Women Who Smoke: 2009 514
Percent of Adults Who Are Former Smokers: 2009 515

Percent of Adults Who Have Never Smoked: 2009 516
Percent of Population Who Are Illicit Drug Users: 2008. . 517
Percent of Adults Overweight: 2009. 518
Percent of Adults Obese: 2009 519
Percent of Adults Overweight or Obese: 2009 520
Percent of Adults Who Do Not Exercise: 2009 521
Percent of Adults Who Exercise Vigorously: 2009 522
Percent of Adults Who Are Disabled: 2009 523
Percent of Adults with High Blood Pressure: 2009 524
Percent of Adults with High Cholesterol: 2009 525
Percent of Adults Who Have Visited a Dentist or Dental
  Clinic: 2008 526
Percent of Adults 65 Years Old and Older Who Have
  Lost All Their Natural Teeth: 2008 527
Percent of Adults Who Average Five or More Servings
  of Fruits and Vegetables Each Day: 2009 528
Percent of Adults Rating Their Health as Fair or Poor
  in 2009 529
Safety Belt Usage Rate in 2009 530

Users of Exercise Equipment in 2009

National Total = 57,206,000 Users

ALPHA ORDER					RANK ORDER			
RANK	STATE	USERS	% of USA		RANK	STATE	USERS	% of USA
25	Alabama	794,000	1.4%		1	California	7,568,000	13.2%
NA	Alaska*	NA	NA		2	Texas	4,971,000	8.7%
21	Arizona	989,000	1.7%		3	New York	4,025,000	7.0%
38	Arkansas	260,000	0.5%		4	Florida	3,056,000	5.3%
1	California	7,568,000	13.2%		5	Virginia	2,345,000	4.1%
18	Colorado	1,084,000	1.9%		6	Ohio	2,112,000	3.7%
29	Connecticut	557,000	1.0%		7	Illinois	2,077,000	3.6%
48	Delaware	23,000	0.0%		8	North Carolina	2,025,000	3.5%
4	Florida	3,056,000	5.3%		9	Pennsylvania	1,955,000	3.4%
11	Georgia	1,639,000	2.9%		10	Michigan	1,852,000	3.2%
NA	Hawaii*	NA	NA		11	Georgia	1,639,000	2.9%
36	Idaho	359,000	0.6%		12	New Jersey	1,546,000	2.7%
7	Illinois	2,077,000	3.6%		13	Massachusetts	1,367,000	2.4%
22	Indiana	907,000	1.6%		14	Minnesota	1,285,000	2.2%
35	Iowa	384,000	0.7%		15	Washington	1,272,000	2.2%
30	Kansas	541,000	0.9%		16	Missouri	1,135,000	2.0%
24	Kentucky	894,000	1.6%		17	Maryland	1,124,000	2.0%
23	Louisiana	898,000	1.6%		18	Colorado	1,084,000	1.9%
44	Maine	183,000	0.3%		19	Wisconsin	1,046,000	1.8%
17	Maryland	1,124,000	2.0%		20	Tennessee	1,000,000	1.7%
13	Massachusetts	1,367,000	2.4%		21	Arizona	989,000	1.7%
10	Michigan	1,852,000	3.2%		22	Indiana	907,000	1.6%
14	Minnesota	1,285,000	2.2%		23	Louisiana	898,000	1.6%
42	Mississippi	188,000	0.3%		24	Kentucky	894,000	1.6%
16	Missouri	1,135,000	2.0%		25	Alabama	794,000	1.4%
46	Montana	169,000	0.3%		26	Oregon	778,000	1.4%
41	Nebraska	205,000	0.4%		27	New Mexico	691,000	1.2%
33	Nevada	420,000	0.7%		28	Utah	602,000	1.1%
34	New Hampshire	387,000	0.7%		29	Connecticut	557,000	1.0%
12	New Jersey	1,546,000	2.7%		30	Kansas	541,000	0.9%
27	New Mexico	691,000	1.2%		30	South Carolina	541,000	0.9%
3	New York	4,025,000	7.0%		32	Oklahoma	507,000	0.9%
8	North Carolina	2,025,000	3.5%		33	Nevada	420,000	0.7%
40	North Dakota	223,000	0.4%		34	New Hampshire	387,000	0.7%
6	Ohio	2,112,000	3.7%		35	Iowa	384,000	0.7%
32	Oklahoma	507,000	0.9%		36	Idaho	359,000	0.6%
26	Oregon	778,000	1.4%		37	Rhode Island	278,000	0.5%
9	Pennsylvania	1,955,000	3.4%		38	Arkansas	260,000	0.5%
37	Rhode Island	278,000	0.5%		39	Vermont	230,000	0.4%
30	South Carolina	541,000	0.9%		40	North Dakota	223,000	0.4%
45	South Dakota	171,000	0.3%		41	Nebraska	205,000	0.4%
20	Tennessee	1,000,000	1.7%		42	Mississippi	188,000	0.3%
2	Texas	4,971,000	8.7%		43	West Virginia	184,000	0.3%
28	Utah	602,000	1.1%		44	Maine	183,000	0.3%
39	Vermont	230,000	0.4%		45	South Dakota	171,000	0.3%
5	Virginia	2,345,000	4.1%		46	Montana	169,000	0.3%
15	Washington	1,272,000	2.2%		47	Wyoming	143,000	0.2%
43	West Virginia	184,000	0.3%		48	Delaware	23,000	0.0%
19	Wisconsin	1,046,000	1.8%		NA	Alaska*	NA	NA
47	Wyoming	143,000	0.2%		NA	Hawaii*	NA	NA
						District of Columbia*	NA	NA

Source: The National Sporting Goods Association
   "NSGA Sports Participation Survey, January-December 2009" (Copyright 2010, reprinted with permission)
*Not available.

Participants in Golf in 2009

National Total = 22,317,000 Golfers

RANK	STATE	GOLFERS	% of USA		RANK	STATE	GOLFERS	% of USA
14	Alabama	549,000	2.5%		1	California	2,374,000	10.6%
NA	Alaska*	NA	NA		2	Texas	1,513,000	6.8%
13	Arizona	634,000	2.8%		3	New York	1,420,000	6.4%
35	Arkansas	175,000	0.8%		4	Virginia	1,183,000	5.3%
1	California	2,374,000	10.6%		5	Illinois	1,116,000	5.0%
21	Colorado	358,000	1.6%		6	Florida	1,052,000	4.7%
27	Connecticut	285,000	1.3%		7	Ohio	938,000	4.2%
NA	Delaware*	NA	NA		8	Michigan	899,000	4.0%
6	Florida	1,052,000	4.7%		9	Pennsylvania	820,000	3.7%
33	Georgia	203,000	0.9%		10	Massachusetts	728,000	3.3%
NA	Hawaii*	NA	NA		11	Washington	699,000	3.1%
32	Idaho	210,000	0.9%		12	Wisconsin	671,000	3.0%
5	Illinois	1,116,000	5.0%		13	Arizona	634,000	2.8%
20	Indiana	361,000	1.6%		14	Alabama	549,000	2.5%
22	Iowa	354,000	1.6%		15	Maryland	523,000	2.3%
37	Kansas	165,000	0.7%		16	Minnesota	519,000	2.3%
17	Kentucky	510,000	2.3%		17	Kentucky	510,000	2.3%
34	Louisiana	188,000	0.8%		18	North Carolina	480,000	2.2%
41	Maine	66,000	0.3%		19	Missouri	373,000	1.7%
15	Maryland	523,000	2.3%		20	Indiana	361,000	1.6%
10	Massachusetts	728,000	3.3%		21	Colorado	358,000	1.6%
8	Michigan	899,000	4.0%		22	Iowa	354,000	1.6%
16	Minnesota	519,000	2.3%		23	South Carolina	315,000	1.4%
39	Mississippi	129,000	0.6%		24	Utah	311,000	1.4%
19	Missouri	373,000	1.7%		25	New Jersey	303,000	1.4%
42	Montana	57,000	0.3%		26	Tennessee	297,000	1.3%
40	Nebraska	91,000	0.4%		27	Connecticut	285,000	1.3%
30	Nevada	260,000	1.2%		28	Oregon	276,000	1.2%
31	New Hampshire	252,000	1.1%		29	New Mexico	273,000	1.2%
25	New Jersey	303,000	1.4%		30	Nevada	260,000	1.2%
29	New Mexico	273,000	1.2%		31	New Hampshire	252,000	1.1%
3	New York	1,420,000	6.4%		32	Idaho	210,000	0.9%
18	North Carolina	480,000	2.2%		33	Georgia	203,000	0.9%
36	North Dakota	171,000	0.8%		34	Louisiana	188,000	0.8%
7	Ohio	938,000	4.2%		35	Arkansas	175,000	0.8%
38	Oklahoma	132,000	0.6%		36	North Dakota	171,000	0.8%
28	Oregon	276,000	1.2%		37	Kansas	165,000	0.7%
9	Pennsylvania	820,000	3.7%		38	Oklahoma	132,000	0.6%
46	Rhode Island	0	0.0%		39	Mississippi	129,000	0.6%
23	South Carolina	315,000	1.4%		40	Nebraska	91,000	0.4%
43	South Dakota	32,000	0.1%		41	Maine	66,000	0.3%
26	Tennessee	297,000	1.3%		42	Montana	57,000	0.3%
2	Texas	1,513,000	6.8%		43	South Dakota	32,000	0.1%
24	Utah	311,000	1.4%		44	Wyoming	28,000	0.1%
45	Vermont	25,000	0.1%		45	Vermont	25,000	0.1%
4	Virginia	1,183,000	5.3%		46	Rhode Island	0	0.0%
11	Washington	699,000	3.1%		46	West Virginia	0	0.0%
46	West Virginia	0	0.0%		NA	Alaska*	NA	NA
12	Wisconsin	671,000	3.0%		NA	Delaware*	NA	NA
44	Wyoming	28,000	0.1%		NA	Hawaii*	NA	NA
						District of Columbia*	NA	NA

ALPHA ORDER

RANK ORDER

Source: The National Sporting Goods Association
"NSGA Sports Participation Survey, January-December 2009" (Copyright 2010, reprinted with permission)
*Not available.

Participants in Running/Jogging in 2009

National Total = 32,212,000 Runners/Joggers

ALPHA ORDER				RANK ORDER			
RANK	STATE	RUNNERS	% of USA	RANK	STATE	RUNNERS	% of USA
23	Alabama	514,000	1.6%	1	California	5,281,000	16.4%
NA	Alaska*	NA	NA	2	Texas	2,409,000	7.5%
27	Arizona	392,000	1.2%	3	New York	2,183,000	6.8%
41	Arkansas	84,000	0.3%	4	Illinois	1,552,000	4.8%
1	California	5,281,000	16.4%	5	North Carolina	1,195,000	3.7%
20	Colorado	549,000	1.7%	6	Michigan	1,158,000	3.6%
18	Connecticut	623,000	1.9%	7	New Jersey	1,154,000	3.6%
45	Delaware	39,000	0.1%	8	Florida	1,136,000	3.5%
8	Florida	1,136,000	3.5%	9	Georgia	1,073,000	3.3%
9	Georgia	1,073,000	3.3%	10	Pennsylvania	981,000	3.0%
NA	Hawaii*	NA	NA	11	Washington	959,000	3.0%
32	Idaho	245,000	0.8%	12	Ohio	931,000	2.9%
4	Illinois	1,552,000	4.8%	13	Tennessee	864,000	2.7%
24	Indiana	492,000	1.5%	14	South Carolina	770,000	2.4%
34	Iowa	179,000	0.6%	15	Minnesota	758,000	2.4%
33	Kansas	194,000	0.6%	16	Virginia	757,000	2.4%
28	Kentucky	344,000	1.1%	17	Missouri	681,000	2.1%
39	Louisiana	106,000	0.3%	18	Connecticut	623,000	1.9%
35	Maine	178,000	0.6%	19	Massachusetts	583,000	1.8%
25	Maryland	480,000	1.5%	20	Colorado	549,000	1.7%
19	Massachusetts	583,000	1.8%	21	Wisconsin	527,000	1.6%
6	Michigan	1,158,000	3.6%	22	Utah	516,000	1.6%
15	Minnesota	758,000	2.4%	23	Alabama	514,000	1.6%
38	Mississippi	135,000	0.4%	24	Indiana	492,000	1.5%
17	Missouri	681,000	2.1%	25	Maryland	480,000	1.5%
43	Montana	71,000	0.2%	26	Oklahoma	444,000	1.4%
36	Nebraska	171,000	0.5%	27	Arizona	392,000	1.2%
31	Nevada	279,000	0.9%	28	Kentucky	344,000	1.1%
40	New Hampshire	105,000	0.3%	29	New Mexico	336,000	1.0%
7	New Jersey	1,154,000	3.6%	30	Oregon	281,000	0.9%
29	New Mexico	336,000	1.0%	31	Nevada	279,000	0.9%
3	New York	2,183,000	6.8%	32	Idaho	245,000	0.8%
5	North Carolina	1,195,000	3.7%	33	Kansas	194,000	0.6%
42	North Dakota	82,000	0.3%	34	Iowa	179,000	0.6%
12	Ohio	931,000	2.9%	35	Maine	178,000	0.6%
26	Oklahoma	444,000	1.4%	36	Nebraska	171,000	0.5%
30	Oregon	281,000	0.9%	37	Rhode Island	147,000	0.5%
10	Pennsylvania	981,000	3.0%	38	Mississippi	135,000	0.4%
37	Rhode Island	147,000	0.5%	39	Louisiana	106,000	0.3%
14	South Carolina	770,000	2.4%	40	New Hampshire	105,000	0.3%
46	South Dakota	28,000	0.1%	41	Arkansas	84,000	0.3%
13	Tennessee	864,000	2.7%	42	North Dakota	82,000	0.3%
2	Texas	2,409,000	7.5%	43	Montana	71,000	0.2%
22	Utah	516,000	1.6%	44	Vermont	46,000	0.1%
44	Vermont	46,000	0.1%	45	Delaware	39,000	0.1%
16	Virginia	757,000	2.4%	46	South Dakota	28,000	0.1%
11	Washington	959,000	3.0%	46	Wyoming	28,000	0.1%
48	West Virginia	19,000	0.1%	48	West Virginia	19,000	0.1%
21	Wisconsin	527,000	1.6%	NA	Alaska*	NA	NA
46	Wyoming	28,000	0.1%	NA	Hawaii*	NA	NA
					District of Columbia*	NA	NA

Source: The National Sporting Goods Association
 "NSGA Sports Participation Survey, January-December 2009" (Copyright 2010, reprinted with permission)
*Not available.

Participants in Swimming in 2009

National Total = 50,226,000 Swimmers

ALPHA ORDER

RANK	STATE	SWIMMERS	% of USA
21	Alabama	777,000	1.5%
NA	Alaska*	NA	NA
23	Arizona	719,000	1.4%
31	Arkansas	400,000	0.8%
1	California	6,562,000	13.1%
20	Colorado	801,000	1.6%
22	Connecticut	774,000	1.5%
47	Delaware	80,000	0.2%
2	Florida	3,434,000	6.8%
6	Georgia	2,352,000	4.7%
NA	Hawaii*	NA	NA
35	Idaho	301,000	0.6%
9	Illinois	1,721,000	3.4%
17	Indiana	1,006,000	2.0%
34	Iowa	324,000	0.6%
44	Kansas	115,000	0.2%
19	Kentucky	829,000	1.7%
32	Louisiana	369,000	0.7%
42	Maine	176,000	0.4%
25	Maryland	672,000	1.3%
16	Massachusetts	1,140,000	2.3%
7	Michigan	1,970,000	3.9%
24	Minnesota	692,000	1.4%
36	Mississippi	287,000	0.6%
13	Missouri	1,364,000	2.7%
45	Montana	102,000	0.2%
41	Nebraska	186,000	0.4%
26	Nevada	571,000	1.1%
37	New Hampshire	283,000	0.6%
8	New Jersey	1,883,000	3.7%
29	New Mexico	514,000	1.0%
4	New York	3,096,000	6.2%
10	North Carolina	1,720,000	3.4%
43	North Dakota	140,000	0.3%
11	Ohio	1,713,000	3.4%
30	Oklahoma	490,000	1.0%
28	Oregon	542,000	1.1%
5	Pennsylvania	2,392,000	4.8%
39	Rhode Island	215,000	0.4%
27	South Carolina	557,000	1.1%
46	South Dakota	81,000	0.2%
12	Tennessee	1,408,000	2.8%
3	Texas	3,280,000	6.5%
33	Utah	339,000	0.7%
40	Vermont	195,000	0.4%
15	Virginia	1,170,000	2.3%
14	Washington	1,182,000	2.4%
38	West Virginia	239,000	0.5%
18	Wisconsin	998,000	2.0%
48	Wyoming	28,000	0.1%

RANK ORDER

RANK	STATE	SWIMMERS	% of USA
1	California	6,562,000	13.1%
2	Florida	3,434,000	6.8%
3	Texas	3,280,000	6.5%
4	New York	3,096,000	6.2%
5	Pennsylvania	2,392,000	4.8%
6	Georgia	2,352,000	4.7%
7	Michigan	1,970,000	3.9%
8	New Jersey	1,883,000	3.7%
9	Illinois	1,721,000	3.4%
10	North Carolina	1,720,000	3.4%
11	Ohio	1,713,000	3.4%
12	Tennessee	1,408,000	2.8%
13	Missouri	1,364,000	2.7%
14	Washington	1,182,000	2.4%
15	Virginia	1,170,000	2.3%
16	Massachusetts	1,140,000	2.3%
17	Indiana	1,006,000	2.0%
18	Wisconsin	998,000	2.0%
19	Kentucky	829,000	1.7%
20	Colorado	801,000	1.6%
21	Alabama	777,000	1.5%
22	Connecticut	774,000	1.5%
23	Arizona	719,000	1.4%
24	Minnesota	692,000	1.4%
25	Maryland	672,000	1.3%
26	Nevada	571,000	1.1%
27	South Carolina	557,000	1.1%
28	Oregon	542,000	1.1%
29	New Mexico	514,000	1.0%
30	Oklahoma	490,000	1.0%
31	Arkansas	400,000	0.8%
32	Louisiana	369,000	0.7%
33	Utah	339,000	0.7%
34	Iowa	324,000	0.6%
35	Idaho	301,000	0.6%
36	Mississippi	287,000	0.6%
37	New Hampshire	283,000	0.6%
38	West Virginia	239,000	0.5%
39	Rhode Island	215,000	0.4%
40	Vermont	195,000	0.4%
41	Nebraska	186,000	0.4%
42	Maine	176,000	0.4%
43	North Dakota	140,000	0.3%
44	Kansas	115,000	0.2%
45	Montana	102,000	0.2%
46	South Dakota	81,000	0.2%
47	Delaware	80,000	0.2%
48	Wyoming	28,000	0.1%
NA	Alaska*	NA	NA
NA	Hawaii*	NA	NA
	District of Columbia*	NA	NA

Source: The National Sporting Goods Association
   "NSGA Sports Participation Survey, January-December 2009" (Copyright 2010, reprinted with permission)
*Not available.

Participants in Tennis in 2009

National Total = 10,818,000 Tennis Players

ALPHA ORDER

RANK	STATE	PLAYERS	% of USA
30	Alabama	53,000	0.5%
NA	Alaska*	NA	NA
34	Arizona	37,000	0.3%
32	Arkansas	46,000	0.4%
1	California	1,278,000	11.8%
16	Colorado	265,000	2.4%
12	Connocticut	324,000	3.0%
43	Delaware	10,000	0.1%
4	Florida	630,000	5.8%
8	Georgia	532,000	4.9%
NA	Hawaii*	NA	NA
24	Idaho	139,000	1.3%
7	Illinois	553,000	5.1%
28	Indiana	89,000	0.8%
35	Iowa	35,000	0.3%
44	Kansas	0	0.0%
21	Kentucky	165,000	1.5%
40	Louisiana	27,000	0.2%
41	Maine	22,000	0.2%
20	Maryland	173,000	1.6%
29	Massachusetts	56,000	0.5%
13	Michigan	293,000	2.7%
11	Minnesota	341,000	3.2%
26	Mississippi	100,000	0.9%
17	Missouri	259,000	2.4%
33	Montana	43,000	0.4%
44	Nebraska	0	0.0%
35	Nevada	35,000	0.3%
19	New Hampshire	180,000	1.7%
9	New Jersey	450,000	4.2%
27	New Mexico	94,000	0.9%
2	New York	899,000	8.3%
10	North Carolina	418,000	3.9%
39	North Dakota	29,000	0.3%
18	Ohio	255,000	2.4%
42	Oklahoma	14,000	0.1%
25	Oregon	111,000	1.0%
6	Pennsylvania	564,000	5.2%
44	Rhode Island	0	0.0%
23	South Carolina	144,000	1.3%
31	South Dakota	52,000	0.5%
15	Tennessee	286,000	2.6%
5	Texas	589,000	5.4%
44	Utah	0	0.0%
44	Vermont	0	0.0%
14	Virginia	290,000	2.7%
3	Washington	726,000	6.7%
38	West Virginia	32,000	0.3%
22	Wisconsin	145,000	1.3%
37	Wyoming	33,000	0.3%

RANK ORDER

RANK	STATE	PLAYERS	% of USA
1	California	1,278,000	11.8%
2	New York	899,000	8.3%
3	Washington	726,000	6.7%
4	Florida	630,000	5.8%
5	Texas	589,000	5.4%
6	Pennsylvania	564,000	5.2%
7	Illinois	553,000	5.1%
8	Georgia	532,000	4.9%
9	New Jersey	450,000	4.2%
10	North Carolina	418,000	3.9%
11	Minnesota	341,000	3.2%
12	Connecticut	324,000	3.0%
13	Michigan	293,000	2.7%
14	Virginia	290,000	2.7%
15	Tennessee	286,000	2.6%
16	Colorado	265,000	2.4%
17	Missouri	259,000	2.4%
18	Ohio	255,000	2.4%
19	New Hampshire	180,000	1.7%
20	Maryland	173,000	1.6%
21	Kentucky	165,000	1.5%
22	Wisconsin	145,000	1.3%
23	South Carolina	144,000	1.3%
24	Idaho	139,000	1.3%
25	Oregon	111,000	1.0%
26	Mississippi	100,000	0.9%
27	New Mexico	94,000	0.9%
28	Indiana	89,000	0.8%
29	Massachusetts	56,000	0.5%
30	Alabama	53,000	0.5%
31	South Dakota	52,000	0.5%
32	Arkansas	46,000	0.4%
33	Montana	43,000	0.4%
34	Arizona	37,000	0.3%
35	Iowa	35,000	0.3%
35	Nevada	35,000	0.3%
37	Wyoming	33,000	0.3%
38	West Virginia	32,000	0.3%
39	North Dakota	29,000	0.3%
40	Louisiana	27,000	0.2%
41	Maine	22,000	0.2%
42	Oklahoma	14,000	0.1%
43	Delaware	10,000	0.1%
44	Kansas	0	0.0%
44	Nebraska	0	0.0%
44	Rhode Island	0	0.0%
44	Utah	0	0.0%
44	Vermont	0	0.0%
NA	Alaska*	NA	NA
NA	Hawaii*	NA	NA
	District of Columbia*	NA	NA

Source: The National Sporting Goods Association
"NSGA Sports Participation Survey, January-December 2009" (Copyright 2010, reprinted with permission)
*Not available.

Alcohol Consumption in 2007

National Total = 564,410,000 Gallons*

ALPHA ORDER

RANK	STATE	GALLONS	% of USA
26	Alabama	7,602,000	1.3%
47	Alaska	1,540,000	0.3%
16	Arizona	12,366,000	2.2%
35	Arkansas	4,204,000	0.7%
1	California	68,375,000	12.1%
18	Colorado	10,789,000	1.9%
28	Connecticut	6,747,000	1.2%
43	Delaware	2,275,000	0.4%
3	Florida	41,098,000	7.3%
10	Georgia	15,576,000	2.8%
39	Hawaii	2,769,000	0.5%
38	Idaho	3,051,000	0.5%
5	Illinois	24,506,000	4.3%
19	Indiana	10,750,000	1.9%
31	Iowa	5,464,000	1.0%
34	Kansas	4,379,000	0.8%
29	Kentucky	6,414,000	1.1%
23	Louisiana	9,365,000	1.7%
40	Maine	2,764,000	0.5%
21	Maryland	10,167,000	1.8%
14	Massachusetts	13,357,000	2.4%
8	Michigan	17,962,000	3.2%
20	Minnesota	10,354,000	1.8%
32	Mississippi	5,275,000	0.9%
17	Missouri	11,528,000	2.0%
45	Montana	2,214,000	0.4%
37	Nebraska	3,325,000	0.6%
27	Nevada	7,362,000	1.3%
33	New Hampshire	4,603,000	0.8%
9	New Jersey	16,532,000	2.9%
36	New Mexico	3,836,000	0.7%
4	New York	33,159,000	5.9%
11	North Carolina	14,656,000	2.6%
48	North Dakota	1,526,000	0.3%
7	Ohio	19,019,000	3.4%
30	Oklahoma	5,614,000	1.0%
25	Oregon	7,983,000	1.4%
6	Pennsylvania	22,350,000	4.0%
44	Rhode Island	2,251,000	0.4%
24	South Carolina	8,782,000	1.6%
46	South Dakota	1,669,000	0.3%
22	Tennessee	9,494,000	1.7%
2	Texas	41,921,000	7.4%
41	Utah	2,696,000	0.5%
49	Vermont	1,403,000	0.2%
13	Virginia	13,386,000	2.4%
15	Washington	12,403,000	2.2%
42	West Virginia	2,675,000	0.5%
12	Wisconsin	13,689,000	2.4%
50	Wyoming	1,205,000	0.2%

RANK ORDER

RANK	STATE	GALLONS	% of USA
1	California	68,375,000	12.1%
2	Texas	41,921,000	7.4%
3	Florida	41,098,000	7.3%
4	New York	33,159,000	5.9%
5	Illinois	24,506,000	4.3%
6	Pennsylvania	22,350,000	4.0%
7	Ohio	19,019,000	3.4%
8	Michigan	17,962,000	3.2%
9	New Jersey	16,532,000	2.9%
10	Georgia	15,576,000	2.8%
11	North Carolina	14,656,000	2.6%
12	Wisconsin	13,689,000	2.4%
13	Virginia	13,386,000	2.4%
14	Massachusetts	13,357,000	2.4%
15	Washington	12,403,000	2.2%
16	Arizona	12,366,000	2.2%
17	Missouri	11,528,000	2.0%
18	Colorado	10,789,000	1.9%
19	Indiana	10,750,000	1.9%
20	Minnesota	10,354,000	1.8%
21	Maryland	10,167,000	1.8%
22	Tennessee	9,494,000	1.7%
23	Louisiana	9,365,000	1.7%
24	South Carolina	8,782,000	1.6%
25	Oregon	7,983,000	1.4%
26	Alabama	7,602,000	1.3%
27	Nevada	7,362,000	1.3%
28	Connecticut	6,747,000	1.2%
29	Kentucky	6,414,000	1.1%
30	Oklahoma	5,614,000	1.0%
31	Iowa	5,464,000	1.0%
32	Mississippi	5,275,000	0.9%
33	New Hampshire	4,603,000	0.8%
34	Kansas	4,379,000	0.8%
35	Arkansas	4,204,000	0.7%
36	New Mexico	3,836,000	0.7%
37	Nebraska	3,325,000	0.6%
38	Idaho	3,051,000	0.5%
39	Hawaii	2,769,000	0.5%
40	Maine	2,764,000	0.5%
41	Utah	2,696,000	0.5%
42	West Virginia	2,675,000	0.5%
43	Delaware	2,275,000	0.4%
44	Rhode Island	2,251,000	0.4%
45	Montana	2,214,000	0.4%
46	South Dakota	1,669,000	0.3%
47	Alaska	1,540,000	0.3%
48	North Dakota	1,526,000	0.3%
49	Vermont	1,403,000	0.2%
50	Wyoming	1,205,000	0.2%
	District of Columbia	1,981,000	0.4%

Source: U.S. Department of Health and Human Services, National Institute on Alcohol Abuse and Alcoholism
"Volume Beverage and Ethanol Consumption for States" (http://www.niaaa.nih.gov/Resources/)

*This is apparent consumption of actual alcohol, not entire volume of an alcoholic beverage (for example, wine is roughly 11% absolute alcohol content). Apparent consumption is based on several sources which together approximate sales but do not actually measure consumption. Accordingly, figures for some states may be skewed by purchases by nonresidents.

Adult Per Capita Alcohol Consumption in 2007

National Per Capita = 2.6 Gallons Consumed per Adult 21 Years and Older*

ALPHA ORDER

RANK	STATE	PER CAPITA
40	Alabama	2.3
5	Alaska	3.3
18	Arizona	2.8
46	Arkansas	2.1
24	California	2.7
9	Colorado	3.1
24	Connecticut	2.7
3	Delaware	3.7
10	Florida	3.0
37	Georgia	2.4
15	Hawaii	2.9
10	Idaho	3.0
24	Illinois	2.7
37	Indiana	2.4
30	Iowa	2.6
44	Kansas	2.2
46	Kentucky	2.1
10	Louisiana	3.0
18	Maine	2.8
34	Maryland	2.5
18	Massachusetts	2.8
34	Michigan	2.5
18	Minnesota	2.8
30	Mississippi	2.6
24	Missouri	2.7
7	Montana	3.2
24	Nebraska	2.7
2	Nevada	4.1
1	New Hampshire	4.8
30	New Jersey	2.6
18	New Mexico	2.8
40	New York	2.3
40	North Carolina	2.3
5	North Dakota	3.3
40	Ohio	2.3
44	Oklahoma	2.2
15	Oregon	2.9
34	Pennsylvania	2.5
15	Rhode Island	2.9
18	South Carolina	2.8
10	South Dakota	3.0
46	Tennessee	2.1
30	Texas	2.6
50	Utah	1.6
10	Vermont	3.0
37	Virginia	2.4
24	Washington	2.7
49	West Virginia	2.0
4	Wisconsin	3.4
7	Wyoming	3.2

RANK ORDER

RANK	STATE	PER CAPITA
1	New Hampshire	4.8
2	Nevada	4.1
3	Delaware	3.7
4	Wisconsin	3.4
5	Alaska	3.3
5	North Dakota	3.3
7	Montana	3.2
7	Wyoming	3.2
9	Colorado	3.1
10	Florida	3.0
10	Idaho	3.0
10	Louisiana	3.0
10	South Dakota	3.0
10	Vermont	3.0
15	Hawaii	2.9
15	Oregon	2.9
15	Rhode Island	2.9
18	Arizona	2.8
18	Maine	2.8
18	Massachusetts	2.8
18	Minnesota	2.8
18	New Mexico	2.8
18	South Carolina	2.8
24	California	2.7
24	Connecticut	2.7
24	Illinois	2.7
24	Missouri	2.7
24	Nebraska	2.7
24	Washington	2.7
30	Iowa	2.6
30	Mississippi	2.6
30	New Jersey	2.6
30	Texas	2.6
34	Maryland	2.5
34	Michigan	2.5
34	Pennsylvania	2.5
37	Georgia	2.4
37	Indiana	2.4
37	Virginia	2.4
40	Alabama	2.3
40	New York	2.3
40	North Carolina	2.3
40	Ohio	2.3
44	Kansas	2.2
44	Oklahoma	2.2
46	Arkansas	2.1
46	Kentucky	2.1
46	Tennessee	2.1
49	West Virginia	2.0
50	Utah	1.6

District of Columbia 4.5

Source: CQ Press using data from U.S. Dept of Health and Human Services, National Institute on Alcohol Abuse and Alcoholism
"Volume Beverage and Ethanol Consumption for States" (http://www.niaaa.nih.gov/Resources/)
*This is apparent consumption of actual alcohol, not entire volume of an alcoholic beverage (for example, wine is roughly 11% absolute alcohol content). Apparent consumption is based on several sources which together approximate sales but do not actually measure consumption. Accordingly, figures for some states may be skewed by purchases by nonresidents.

Apparent Beer Consumption in 2007

National Total = 6,550,633,000 Gallons of Beer Consumed*

ALPHA ORDER

RANK	STATE	GALLONS	% of USA
24	Alabama	103,905,000	1.6%
49	Alaska	15,930,000	0.2%
13	Arizona	152,116,000	2.3%
34	Arkansas	54,473,000	0.8%
1	California	694,575,000	10.6%
22	Colorado	112,196,000	1.7%
32	Connecticut	59,186,000	0.9%
45	Delaware	21,735,000	0.3%
3	Florida	436,764,000	6.7%
9	Georgia	195,525,000	3.0%
40	Hawaii	31,358,000	0.5%
42	Idaho	30,810,000	0.5%
6	Illinois	282,149,000	4.3%
17	Indiana	129,115,000	2.0%
30	Iowa	75,735,000	1.2%
33	Kansas	58,017,000	0.9%
27	Kentucky	80,559,000	1.2%
19	Louisiana	122,963,000	1.9%
41	Maine	31,275,000	0.5%
25	Maryland	103,401,000	1.6%
20	Massachusetts	121,219,000	1.9%
8	Michigan	202,770,000	3.1%
23	Minnesota	108,608,000	1.7%
31	Mississippi	75,600,000	1.2%
15	Missouri	141,305,000	2.2%
43	Montana	27,900,000	0.4%
36	Nebraska	46,013,000	0.7%
28	Nevada	77,411,000	1.2%
37	New Hampshire	42,075,000	0.6%
14	New Jersey	145,932,000	2.2%
35	New Mexico	49,608,000	0.8%
4	New York	328,061,000	5.0%
10	North Carolina	189,055,000	2.9%
47	North Dakota	18,427,000	0.3%
7	Ohio	277,088,000	4.2%
29	Oklahoma	76,208,000	1.2%
26	Oregon	88,380,000	1.3%
5	Pennsylvania	306,675,000	4.7%
44	Rhode Island	22,005,000	0.3%
21	South Carolina	114,300,000	1.7%
46	South Dakota	21,668,000	0.3%
18	Tennessee	126,428,000	1.9%
2	Texas	585,365,000	8.9%
39	Utah	33,615,000	0.5%
48	Vermont	15,975,000	0.2%
11	Virginia	158,732,000	2.4%
16	Washington	130,388,000	2.0%
38	West Virginia	41,648,000	0.6%
12	Wisconsin	157,185,000	2.4%
50	Wyoming	14,147,000	0.2%

RANK ORDER

RANK	STATE	GALLONS	% of USA
1	California	694,575,000	10.6%
2	Texas	585,365,000	8.9%
3	Florida	436,764,000	6.7%
4	New York	328,061,000	5.0%
5	Pennsylvania	306,675,000	4.7%
6	Illinois	282,149,000	4.3%
7	Ohio	277,088,000	4.2%
8	Michigan	202,770,000	3.1%
9	Georgia	195,525,000	3.0%
10	North Carolina	189,055,000	2.9%
11	Virginia	158,732,000	2.4%
12	Wisconsin	157,185,000	2.4%
13	Arizona	152,116,000	2.3%
14	New Jersey	145,932,000	2.2%
15	Missouri	141,305,000	2.2%
16	Washington	130,388,000	2.0%
17	Indiana	129,115,000	2.0%
18	Tennessee	126,428,000	1.9%
19	Louisiana	122,963,000	1.9%
20	Massachusetts	121,219,000	1.9%
21	South Carolina	114,300,000	1.7%
22	Colorado	112,196,000	1.7%
23	Minnesota	108,608,000	1.7%
24	Alabama	103,905,000	1.6%
25	Maryland	103,401,000	1.6%
26	Oregon	88,380,000	1.3%
27	Kentucky	80,559,000	1.2%
28	Nevada	77,411,000	1.2%
29	Oklahoma	76,208,000	1.2%
30	Iowa	75,735,000	1.2%
31	Mississippi	75,600,000	1.2%
32	Connecticut	59,186,000	0.9%
33	Kansas	58,017,000	0.9%
34	Arkansas	54,473,000	0.8%
35	New Mexico	49,608,000	0.8%
36	Nebraska	46,013,000	0.7%
37	New Hampshire	42,075,000	0.6%
38	West Virginia	41,648,000	0.6%
39	Utah	33,615,000	0.5%
40	Hawaii	31,358,000	0.5%
41	Maine	31,275,000	0.5%
42	Idaho	30,810,000	0.5%
43	Montana	27,900,000	0.4%
44	Rhode Island	22,005,000	0.3%
45	Delaware	21,735,000	0.3%
46	South Dakota	21,668,000	0.3%
47	North Dakota	18,427,000	0.3%
48	Vermont	15,975,000	0.2%
49	Alaska	15,930,000	0.2%
50	Wyoming	14,147,000	0.2%
	District of Columbia	15,053,000	0.2%

Source: U.S. Department of Health and Human Services, National Institute on Alcohol Abuse and Alcoholism
"Volume Beverage and Ethanol Consumption for States" (http://www.niaaa.nih.gov/Resources/)
*This is apparent consumption and is based on several sources which together approximate sales but do not actually measure consumption. Reported state volumes reflect only in-state purchases. Accordingly, figures for some states may be skewed by purchases by nonresidents.

Adult Per Capita Beer Consumption in 2007

National Per Capita = 30.5 Gallons Consumed per Adult 21 Years and Older*

ALPHA ORDER

RANK	STATE	PER CAPITA
27	Alabama	31.4
18	Alaska	33.9
17	Arizona	34.3
43	Arkansas	27.0
42	California	27.4
23	Colorado	32.3
47	Connecticut	23.4
15	Delaware	35.1
23	Florida	32.3
33	Georgia	29.5
22	Hawaii	33.3
30	Idaho	30.0
28	Illinois	31.1
36	Indiana	28.8
14	Iowa	35.5
32	Kansas	29.7
44	Kentucky	26.2
4	Louisiana	40.0
26	Maine	31.7
45	Maryland	25.7
46	Massachusetts	25.6
40	Michigan	28.2
34	Minnesota	29.3
9	Mississippi	37.4
21	Missouri	33.5
4	Montana	40.0
10	Nebraska	36.9
2	Nevada	42.6
1	New Hampshire	43.8
48	New Jersey	23.3
13	New Mexico	36.0
49	New York	23.2
34	North Carolina	29.3
3	North Dakota	40.1
20	Ohio	33.6
31	Oklahoma	29.8
23	Oregon	32.3
19	Pennsylvania	33.7
37	Rhode Island	28.7
11	South Carolina	36.2
7	South Dakota	38.5
39	Tennessee	28.4
12	Texas	36.1
50	Utah	19.6
16	Vermont	34.7
38	Virginia	28.6
41	Washington	27.9
29	West Virginia	30.8
6	Wisconsin	38.9
8	Wyoming	37.7

RANK ORDER

RANK	STATE	PER CAPITA
1	New Hampshire	43.8
2	Nevada	42.6
3	North Dakota	40.1
4	Louisiana	40.0
4	Montana	40.0
6	Wisconsin	38.9
7	South Dakota	38.5
8	Wyoming	37.7
9	Mississippi	37.4
10	Nebraska	36.9
11	South Carolina	36.2
12	Texas	36.1
13	New Mexico	36.0
14	Iowa	35.5
15	Delaware	35.1
16	Vermont	34.7
17	Arizona	34.3
18	Alaska	33.9
19	Pennsylvania	33.7
20	Ohio	33.6
21	Missouri	33.5
22	Hawaii	33.3
23	Colorado	32.3
23	Florida	32.3
23	Oregon	32.3
26	Maine	31.7
27	Alabama	31.4
28	Illinois	31.1
29	West Virginia	30.8
30	Idaho	30.0
31	Oklahoma	29.8
32	Kansas	29.7
33	Georgia	29.5
34	Minnesota	29.3
34	North Carolina	29.3
36	Indiana	28.8
37	Rhode Island	28.7
38	Virginia	28.6
39	Tennessee	28.4
40	Michigan	28.2
41	Washington	27.9
42	California	27.4
43	Arkansas	27.0
44	Kentucky	26.2
45	Maryland	25.7
46	Massachusetts	25.6
47	Connecticut	23.4
48	New Jersey	23.3
49	New York	23.2
50	Utah	19.6

District of Columbia — 33.9

Source: CQ Press using data from U.S. Dept of Health and Human Services, National Institute on Alcohol Abuse and Alcoholism "Volume Beverage and Ethanol Consumption for States" (http://www.niaaa.nih.gov/Resources/)

*This is apparent consumption and is based on several sources which together approximate sales but do not actually measure consumption. Reported state volumes reflect only in-state purchases. Accordingly, figures for some states may be skewed by purchases by nonresidents.

Wine Consumption in 2007

National Total = 711,788,000 Gallons of Wine Consumed*

ALPHA ORDER

RANK	STATE	GALLONS	% of USA
29	Alabama	6,381,000	0.9%
46	Alaska	1,874,000	0.3%
16	Arizona	13,032,000	1.8%
39	Arkansas	3,008,000	0.4%
1	California	125,250,000	17.6%
15	Colorado	14,120,000	2.0%
17	Connecticut	12,827,000	1.8%
37	Delaware	3,250,000	0.5%
3	Florida	57,313,000	8.1%
14	Georgia	14,995,000	2.1%
32	Hawaii	4,008,000	0.6%
28	Idaho	6,735,000	0.9%
5	Illinois	32,742,000	4.6%
24	Indiana	9,699,000	1.4%
38	Iowa	3,220,000	0.5%
40	Kansas	2,560,000	0.4%
31	Kentucky	4,679,000	0.7%
26	Louisiana	7,531,000	1.1%
36	Maine	3,668,000	0.5%
18	Maryland	12,738,000	1.8%
7	Massachusetts	25,546,000	3.6%
11	Michigan	19,018,000	2.7%
22	Minnesota	10,520,000	1.5%
44	Mississippi	2,171,000	0.3%
21	Missouri	11,017,000	1.5%
45	Montana	2,165,000	0.3%
43	Nebraska	2,272,000	0.3%
23	Nevada	10,061,000	1.4%
30	New Hampshire	6,252,000	0.9%
6	New Jersey	30,240,000	4.2%
34	New Mexico	3,784,000	0.5%
2	New York	57,880,000	8.1%
13	North Carolina	15,636,000	2.2%
49	North Dakota	959,000	0.1%
12	Ohio	18,121,000	2.5%
33	Oklahoma	3,936,000	0.6%
19	Oregon	11,794,000	1.7%
10	Pennsylvania	19,176,000	2.7%
35	Rhode Island	3,669,000	0.5%
27	South Carolina	6,825,000	1.0%
48	South Dakota	1,092,000	0.2%
25	Tennessee	7,784,000	1.1%
4	Texas	39,223,000	5.5%
41	Utah	2,490,000	0.3%
42	Vermont	2,462,000	0.3%
9	Virginia	20,053,000	2.8%
8	Washington	20,435,000	2.9%
47	West Virginia	1,215,000	0.2%
20	Wisconsin	11,758,000	1.7%
50	Wyoming	766,000	0.1%

RANK ORDER

RANK	STATE	GALLONS	% of USA
1	California	125,250,000	17.6%
2	New York	57,880,000	8.1%
3	Florida	57,313,000	8.1%
4	Texas	39,223,000	5.5%
5	Illinois	32,742,000	4.6%
6	New Jersey	30,240,000	4.2%
7	Massachusetts	25,546,000	3.6%
8	Washington	20,435,000	2.9%
9	Virginia	20,053,000	2.8%
10	Pennsylvania	19,176,000	2.7%
11	Michigan	19,018,000	2.7%
12	Ohio	18,121,000	2.5%
13	North Carolina	15,636,000	2.2%
14	Georgia	14,995,000	2.1%
15	Colorado	14,120,000	2.0%
16	Arizona	13,032,000	1.8%
17	Connecticut	12,827,000	1.8%
18	Maryland	12,738,000	1.8%
19	Oregon	11,794,000	1.7%
20	Wisconsin	11,758,000	1.7%
21	Missouri	11,017,000	1.5%
22	Minnesota	10,520,000	1.5%
23	Nevada	10,061,000	1.4%
24	Indiana	9,699,000	1.4%
25	Tennessee	7,784,000	1.1%
26	Louisiana	7,531,000	1.1%
27	South Carolina	6,825,000	1.0%
28	Idaho	6,735,000	0.9%
29	Alabama	6,381,000	0.9%
30	New Hampshire	6,252,000	0.9%
31	Kentucky	4,679,000	0.7%
32	Hawaii	4,008,000	0.6%
33	Oklahoma	3,936,000	0.6%
34	New Mexico	3,784,000	0.5%
35	Rhode Island	3,669,000	0.5%
36	Maine	3,668,000	0.5%
37	Delaware	3,250,000	0.5%
38	Iowa	3,220,000	0.5%
39	Arkansas	3,008,000	0.4%
40	Kansas	2,560,000	0.4%
41	Utah	2,490,000	0.3%
42	Vermont	2,462,000	0.3%
43	Nebraska	2,272,000	0.3%
44	Mississippi	2,171,000	0.3%
45	Montana	2,165,000	0.3%
46	Alaska	1,874,000	0.3%
47	West Virginia	1,215,000	0.2%
48	South Dakota	1,092,000	0.2%
49	North Dakota	959,000	0.1%
50	Wyoming	766,000	0.1%
	District of Columbia	3,836,000	0.5%

Source: U.S. Department of Health and Human Services, National Institute on Alcohol Abuse and Alcoholism
"Volume Beverage and Ethanol Consumption for States" (http://www.niaaa.nih.gov/Resources/)
*This is apparent consumption and is based on several sources which together approximate sales but do not actually measure consumption. Reported state volumes reflect only in-state purchases. Accordingly, figures for some states may be skewed by purchases by nonresidents.

Adult Per Capita Wine Consumption in 2007

National Per Capita = 3.3 Gallons Consumed per Adult 21 Years and Older*

ALPHA ORDER				RANK ORDER		
RANK	STATE	PER CAPITA		RANK	STATE	PER CAPITA
39	Alabama	1.9		1	Idaho	6.6
17	Alaska	4.0		2	New Hampshire	6.5
23	Arizona	2.9		3	Nevada	5.5
43	Arkansas	1.5		4	Massachusetts	5.4
8	California	4.9		5	Vermont	5.3
15	Colorado	4.1		6	Delaware	5.2
7	Connecticut	5.1		7	Connecticut	5.1
6	Delaware	5.2		8	California	4.9
14	Florida	4.2		9	New Jersey	4.8
32	Georgia	2.3		9	Rhode Island	4.8
12	Hawaii	4.3		11	Washington	4.4
1	Idaho	6.6		12	Hawaii	4.3
19	Illinois	3.6		12	Oregon	4.3
33	Indiana	2.2		14	Florida	4.2
43	Iowa	1.5		15	Colorado	4.1
48	Kansas	1.3		15	New York	4.1
43	Kentucky	1.5		17	Alaska	4.0
29	Louisiana	2.5		18	Maine	3.7
18	Maine	3.7		19	Illinois	3.6
21	Maryland	3.2		19	Virginia	3.6
4	Massachusetts	5.4		21	Maryland	3.2
27	Michigan	2.6		22	Montana	3.1
25	Minnesota	2.8		23	Arizona	2.9
49	Mississippi	1.1		23	Wisconsin	2.9
27	Missouri	2.6		25	Minnesota	2.8
22	Montana	3.1		26	New Mexico	2.7
41	Nebraska	1.8		27	Michigan	2.6
3	Nevada	5.5		27	Missouri	2.6
2	New Hampshire	6.5		29	Louisiana	2.5
9	New Jersey	4.8		30	North Carolina	2.4
26	New Mexico	2.7		30	Texas	2.4
15	New York	4.1		32	Georgia	2.3
30	North Carolina	2.4		33	Indiana	2.2
36	North Dakota	2.1		33	Ohio	2.2
33	Ohio	2.2		33	South Carolina	2.2
43	Oklahoma	1.5		36	North Dakota	2.1
12	Oregon	4.3		36	Pennsylvania	2.1
36	Pennsylvania	2.1		38	Wyoming	2.0
9	Rhode Island	4.8		39	Alabama	1.9
33	South Carolina	2.2		39	South Dakota	1.9
39	South Dakota	1.9		41	Nebraska	1.8
42	Tennessee	1.7		42	Tennessee	1.7
30	Texas	2.4		43	Arkansas	1.5
47	Utah	1.4		43	Iowa	1.5
5	Vermont	5.3		43	Kentucky	1.5
19	Virginia	3.6		43	Oklahoma	1.5
11	Washington	4.4		47	Utah	1.4
50	West Virginia	0.9		48	Kansas	1.3
23	Wisconsin	2.9		49	Mississippi	1.1
38	Wyoming	2.0		50	West Virginia	0.9
					District of Columbia	8.6

Source: CQ Press using data from U.S. Dept of Health and Human Services, National Institute on Alcohol Abuse and Alcoholism
"Volume Beverage and Ethanol Consumption for States" (http://www.niaaa.nih.gov/Resources/)

*This is apparent consumption and is based on several sources which together approximate sales but do not actually measure consumption. Reported state volumes reflect only in-state purchases. Accordingly, figures for some states may be skewed by purchases by nonresidents.

Distilled Spirits Consumption in 2007

National Total = 432,629,000 Gallons of Distilled Spirits Consumed*

ALPHA ORDER

RANK	STATE	GALLONS	% of USA
29	Alabama	5,117,000	1.2%
46	Alaska	1,415,000	0.3%
18	Arizona	9,341,000	2.2%
35	Arkansas	3,320,000	0.8%
1	California	51,001,000	11.8%
15	Colorado	9,535,000	2.2%
27	Connecticut	5,909,000	1.4%
39	Delaware	2,135,000	0.5%
2	Florida	34,186,000	7.9%
10	Georgia	11,784,000	2.7%
41	Hawaii	2,046,000	0.5%
42	Idaho	1,935,000	0.4%
5	Illinois	18,455,000	4.3%
20	Indiana	8,975,000	2.1%
32	Iowa	3,992,000	0.9%
34	Kansas	3,500,000	0.8%
28	Kentucky	5,318,000	1.2%
22	Louisiana	6,959,000	1.6%
38	Maine	2,149,000	0.5%
17	Maryland	9,418,000	2.2%
11	Massachusetts	11,210,000	2.6%
6	Michigan	15,532,000	3.6%
14	Minnesota	9,999,000	2.3%
33	Mississippi	3,876,000	0.9%
19	Missouri	9,118,000	2.1%
44	Montana	1,652,000	0.4%
37	Nebraska	2,339,000	0.5%
25	Nevada	6,280,000	1.5%
30	New Hampshire	4,631,000	1.1%
8	New Jersey	14,754,000	3.4%
36	New Mexico	2,714,000	0.6%
3	New York	26,594,000	6.1%
13	North Carolina	10,052,000	2.3%
47	North Dakota	1,394,000	0.3%
12	Ohio	10,249,000	2.4%
31	Oklahoma	4,080,000	0.9%
26	Oregon	6,045,000	1.4%
7	Pennsylvania	14,784,000	3.4%
43	Rhode Island	1,916,000	0.4%
24	South Carolina	6,711,000	1.6%
48	South Dakota	1,346,000	0.3%
23	Tennessee	6,814,000	1.6%
4	Texas	25,595,000	5.9%
40	Utah	2,097,000	0.5%
50	Vermont	891,000	0.2%
21	Virginia	8,897,000	2.1%
16	Washington	9,488,000	2.2%
45	West Virginia	1,566,000	0.4%
9	Wisconsin	12,405,000	2.9%
49	Wyoming	1,142,000	0.3%

RANK ORDER

RANK	STATE	GALLONS	% of USA
1	California	51,001,000	11.8%
2	Florida	34,186,000	7.9%
3	New York	26,594,000	6.1%
4	Texas	25,595,000	5.9%
5	Illinois	18,455,000	4.3%
6	Michigan	15,532,000	3.6%
7	Pennsylvania	14,784,000	3.4%
8	New Jersey	14,754,000	3.4%
9	Wisconsin	12,405,000	2.9%
10	Georgia	11,784,000	2.7%
11	Massachusetts	11,210,000	2.6%
12	Ohio	10,249,000	2.4%
13	North Carolina	10,052,000	2.3%
14	Minnesota	9,999,000	2.3%
15	Colorado	9,535,000	2.2%
16	Washington	9,488,000	2.2%
17	Maryland	9,418,000	2.2%
18	Arizona	9,341,000	2.2%
19	Missouri	9,118,000	2.1%
20	Indiana	8,975,000	2.1%
21	Virginia	8,897,000	2.1%
22	Louisiana	6,959,000	1.6%
23	Tennessee	6,814,000	1.6%
24	South Carolina	6,711,000	1.6%
25	Nevada	6,280,000	1.5%
26	Oregon	6,045,000	1.4%
27	Connecticut	5,909,000	1.4%
28	Kentucky	5,318,000	1.2%
29	Alabama	5,117,000	1.2%
30	New Hampshire	4,631,000	1.1%
31	Oklahoma	4,080,000	0.9%
32	Iowa	3,992,000	0.9%
33	Mississippi	3,876,000	0.9%
34	Kansas	3,500,000	0.8%
35	Arkansas	3,320,000	0.8%
36	New Mexico	2,714,000	0.6%
37	Nebraska	2,339,000	0.5%
38	Maine	2,149,000	0.5%
39	Delaware	2,135,000	0.5%
40	Utah	2,097,000	0.5%
41	Hawaii	2,046,000	0.5%
42	Idaho	1,935,000	0.4%
43	Rhode Island	1,916,000	0.4%
44	Montana	1,652,000	0.4%
45	West Virginia	1,566,000	0.4%
46	Alaska	1,415,000	0.3%
47	North Dakota	1,394,000	0.3%
48	South Dakota	1,346,000	0.3%
49	Wyoming	1,142,000	0.3%
50	Vermont	891,000	0.2%
	District of Columbia	1,967,000	0.5%

Source: U.S. Department of Health and Human Services, National Institute on Alcohol Abuse and Alcoholism
"Volume Beverage and Ethanol Consumption for States" (http://www.niaaa.nih.gov/Resources/)

*This is apparent consumption and is based on several sources which together approximate sales but do not actually measure consumption. Reported state volumes reflect only in-state purchases. Accordingly, figures for some states may be skewed by purchases by nonresidents.

Adult Per Capita Distilled Spirits Consumption in 2007

National Per Capita = 2.0 Gallons Consumed per Adult 21 Years and Older*

ALPHA ORDER

RANK	STATE	PER CAPITA
46	Alabama	1.5
5	Alaska	3.0
24	Arizona	2.1
40	Arkansas	1.6
26	California	2.0
8	Colorado	2.7
16	Connecticut	2.3
3	Delaware	3.4
10	Florida	2.5
37	Georgia	1.8
19	Hawaii	2.2
31	Idaho	1.9
26	Illinois	2.0
26	Indiana	2.0
31	Iowa	1.9
37	Kansas	1.8
39	Kentucky	1.7
16	Louisiana	2.3
19	Maine	2.2
16	Maryland	2.3
12	Massachusetts	2.4
19	Michigan	2.2
8	Minnesota	2.7
31	Mississippi	1.9
19	Missouri	2.2
12	Montana	2.4
31	Nebraska	1.9
2	Nevada	3.5
1	New Hampshire	4.8
12	New Jersey	2.4
26	New Mexico	2.0
31	New York	1.9
40	North Carolina	1.6
5	North Dakota	3.0
48	Ohio	1.2
40	Oklahoma	1.6
19	Oregon	2.2
40	Pennsylvania	1.6
10	Rhode Island	2.5
24	South Carolina	2.1
12	South Dakota	2.4
46	Tennessee	1.5
40	Texas	1.6
48	Utah	1.2
31	Vermont	1.9
40	Virginia	1.6
26	Washington	2.0
48	West Virginia	1.2
4	Wisconsin	3.1
5	Wyoming	3.0

RANK ORDER

RANK	STATE	PER CAPITA
1	New Hampshire	4.8
2	Nevada	3.5
3	Delaware	3.4
4	Wisconsin	3.1
5	Alaska	3.0
5	North Dakota	3.0
5	Wyoming	3.0
8	Colorado	2.7
8	Minnesota	2.7
10	Florida	2.5
10	Rhode Island	2.5
12	Massachusetts	2.4
12	Montana	2.4
12	New Jersey	2.4
12	South Dakota	2.4
16	Connecticut	2.3
16	Louisiana	2.3
16	Maryland	2.3
19	Hawaii	2.2
19	Maine	2.2
19	Michigan	2.2
19	Missouri	2.2
19	Oregon	2.2
24	Arizona	2.1
24	South Carolina	2.1
26	California	2.0
26	Illinois	2.0
26	Indiana	2.0
26	New Mexico	2.0
26	Washington	2.0
31	Idaho	1.9
31	Iowa	1.9
31	Mississippi	1.9
31	Nebraska	1.9
31	New York	1.9
31	Vermont	1.9
37	Georgia	1.8
37	Kansas	1.8
39	Kentucky	1.7
40	Arkansas	1.6
40	North Carolina	1.6
40	Oklahoma	1.6
40	Pennsylvania	1.6
40	Texas	1.6
40	Virginia	1.6
46	Alabama	1.5
46	Tennessee	1.5
48	Ohio	1.2
48	Utah	1.2
48	West Virginia	1.2

District of Columbia 4.4

Source: CQ Press using data from U.S. Dept of Health and Human Services, National Institute on Alcohol Abuse and Alcoholism
"Volume Beverage and Ethanol Consumption for States" (http://www.niaaa.nih.gov/Resources/)
*This is apparent consumption and is based on several sources which together approximate sales but do not actually measure consumption. Reported state volumes reflect only in-state purchases. Accordingly, figures for some states may be skewed by purchases by nonresidents.

Percent of Adults Who Do Not Drink Alcohol: 2009

National Median = 45.6% of Adults*

ALPHA ORDER				RANK ORDER		
RANK	**STATE**	**PERCENT**		**RANK**	**STATE**	**PERCENT**
5	Alabama	62.9		1	Tennessee	74.9
28	Alaska	44.8		2	Utah	74.2
22	Arizona	47.6		3	West Virginia	71.7
7	Arkansas	59.2		4	Mississippi	63.3
23	California	47.1		5	Alabama	62.9
42	Colorado	39.6		6	Kentucky	60.8
50	Connecticut	33.0		7	Arkansas	59.2
35	Delaware	42.2		8	Oklahoma	57.3
19	Florida	48.7		9	South Carolina	56.6
11	Georgia	54.6		10	Idaho	55.4
18	Hawaii	49.5		11	Georgia	54.6
10	Idaho	55.4		12	North Carolina	54.5
32	Illinois	43.5		13	Indiana	52.5
13	Indiana	52.5		14	Louisiana	51.9
33	Iowa	42.6		15	New Mexico	50.5
16	Kansas	50.0		16	Kansas	50.0
6	Kentucky	60.8		17	Missouri	49.9
14	Louisiana	51.9		18	Hawaii	49.5
36	Maine	42.1		19	Florida	48.7
31	Maryland	43.9		19	Texas	48.7
45	Massachusetts	37.0		21	Virginia	48.0
29	Michigan	44.6		22	Arizona	47.6
44	Minnesota	38.5		23	California	47.1
4	Mississippi	63.3		24	Ohio	46.3
17	Missouri	49.9		25	Nevada	46.0
37	Montana	41.5		26	Wyoming	45.6
39	Nebraska	40.9		27	Pennsylvania	45.4
25	Nevada	46.0		28	Alaska	44.8
48	New Hampshire	35.3		29	Michigan	44.6
34	New Jersey	42.4		30	New York	44.2
15	New Mexico	50.5		31	Maryland	43.9
30	New York	44.2		32	Illinois	43.5
12	North Carolina	54.5		33	Iowa	42.6
43	North Dakota	39.5		34	New Jersey	42.4
24	Ohio	46.3		35	Delaware	42.2
8	Oklahoma	57.3		36	Maine	42.1
38	Oregon	41.2		37	Montana	41.5
27	Pennsylvania	45.4		38	Oregon	41.2
46	Rhode Island	36.0		39	Nebraska	40.9
9	South Carolina	56.6		39	Washington	40.9
41	South Dakota	40.4		41	South Dakota	40.4
1	Tennessee	74.9		42	Colorado	39.6
19	Texas	48.7		43	North Dakota	39.5
2	Utah	74.2		44	Minnesota	38.5
47	Vermont	35.5		45	Massachusetts	37.0
21	Virginia	48.0		46	Rhode Island	36.0
39	Washington	40.9		47	Vermont	35.5
3	West Virginia	71.7		48	New Hampshire	35.3
49	Wisconsin	33.2		49	Wisconsin	33.2
26	Wyoming	45.6		50	Connecticut	33.0
					District of Columbia	31.9

Source: U.S. Department of Health and Human Services, Centers for Disease Control and Prevention
"2009 Behavioral Risk Factor Surveillance Summary Prevalence Data" (http://apps.nccd.cdc.gov/brfss/)
*Persons 18 and older reporting not having at least one drink of alcohol in the past 30 days.

Percent of Adults Who Are Binge Drinkers: 2009

National Median = 15.8% of Adults*

ALPHA ORDER

RANK	STATE	PERCENT
45	Alabama	10.7
9	Alaska	17.9
29	Arizona	14.9
44	Arkansas	11.3
23	California	15.8
20	Colorado	16.3
5	Connecticut	19.0
6	Delaware	18.5
36	Florida	13.3
46	Georgia	10.5
16	Hawaii	17.1
37	Idaho	13.0
11	Illinois	17.7
34	Indiana	14.2
6	Iowa	18.5
31	Kansas	14.5
43	Kentucky	12.4
32	Louisiana	14.4
27	Maine	15.1
42	Maryland	12.6
12	Massachusetts	17.6
16	Michigan	17.1
3	Minnesota	20.2
47	Mississippi	10.1
15	Missouri	17.2
14	Montana	17.3
9	Nebraska	17.9
13	Nevada	17.5
23	New Hampshire	15.8
33	New Jersey	14.3
39	New Mexico	12.8
20	New York	16.3
39	North Carolina	12.8
2	North Dakota	21.4
22	Ohio	16.1
37	Oklahoma	13.0
28	Oregon	15.0
19	Pennsylvania	16.6
8	Rhode Island	18.2
41	South Carolina	12.7
4	South Dakota	19.3
50	Tennessee	6.8
29	Texas	14.9
49	Utah	8.8
16	Vermont	17.1
35	Virginia	13.5
26	Washington	15.2
48	West Virginia	9.2
1	Wisconsin	23.9
23	Wyoming	15.8

RANK ORDER

RANK	STATE	PERCENT
1	Wisconsin	23.9
2	North Dakota	21.4
3	Minnesota	20.2
4	South Dakota	19.3
5	Connecticut	19.0
6	Delaware	18.5
6	Iowa	18.5
8	Rhode Island	18.2
9	Alaska	17.9
9	Nebraska	17.9
11	Illinois	17.7
12	Massachusetts	17.6
13	Nevada	17.5
14	Montana	17.3
15	Missouri	17.2
16	Hawaii	17.1
16	Michigan	17.1
16	Vermont	17.1
19	Pennsylvania	16.6
20	Colorado	16.3
20	New York	16.3
22	Ohio	16.1
23	California	15.8
23	New Hampshire	15.8
23	Wyoming	15.8
26	Washington	15.2
27	Maine	15.1
28	Oregon	15.0
29	Arizona	14.9
29	Texas	14.9
31	Kansas	14.5
32	Louisiana	14.4
33	New Jersey	14.3
34	Indiana	14.2
35	Virginia	13.5
36	Florida	13.3
37	Idaho	13.0
37	Oklahoma	13.0
39	New Mexico	12.8
39	North Carolina	12.8
41	South Carolina	12.7
42	Maryland	12.6
43	Kentucky	12.4
44	Arkansas	11.3
45	Alabama	10.7
46	Georgia	10.5
47	Mississippi	10.1
48	West Virginia	9.2
49	Utah	8.8
50	Tennessee	6.8
	District of Columbia	20.1

Source: U.S. Department of Health and Human Services, Centers for Disease Control and Prevention
"2009 Behavioral Risk Factor Surveillance Summary Prevalence Data" (http://apps.nccd.cdc.gov/brfss/)
*Males having five or more alcoholic drinks and females having four or more alcoholic drinks on one occasion during the previous month.

Percent of Adults Who Smoke: 2009

National Median = 17.9% of Adults*

ALPHA ORDER

RANK	STATE	PERCENT
7	Alabama	22.5
12	Alaska	20.6
40	Arizona	16.1
11	Arkansas	21.5
49	California	12.9
33	Colorado	17.1
43	Connecticut	15.4
23	Delaware	18.3
33	Florida	17.1
29	Georgia	17.7
43	Hawaii	15.4
39	Idaho	16.3
21	Illinois	18.6
5	Indiana	23.1
32	Iowa	17.2
28	Kansas	17.8
1	Kentucky	25.6
8	Louisiana	22.1
31	Maine	17.3
45	Maryland	15.2
47	Massachusetts	15.0
18	Michigan	19.6
36	Minnesota	16.8
4	Mississippi	23.3
5	Missouri	23.1
36	Montana	16.8
38	Nebraska	16.7
9	Nevada	22.0
41	New Hampshire	15.8
41	New Jersey	15.8
25	New Mexico	17.9
24	New York	18.0
14	North Carolina	20.3
21	North Dakota	18.6
14	Ohio	20.3
3	Oklahoma	25.5
25	Oregon	17.9
16	Pennsylvania	20.2
46	Rhode Island	15.1
13	South Carolina	20.4
30	South Dakota	17.5
9	Tennessee	22.0
25	Texas	17.9
50	Utah	9.8
33	Vermont	17.1
19	Virginia	19.0
48	Washington	14.9
1	West Virginia	25.6
20	Wisconsin	18.8
17	Wyoming	19.9

RANK ORDER

RANK	STATE	PERCENT
1	Kentucky	25.6
1	West Virginia	25.6
3	Oklahoma	25.5
4	Mississippi	23.3
5	Indiana	23.1
5	Missouri	23.1
7	Alabama	22.5
8	Louisiana	22.1
9	Nevada	22.0
9	Tennessee	22.0
11	Arkansas	21.5
12	Alaska	20.6
13	South Carolina	20.4
14	North Carolina	20.3
14	Ohio	20.3
16	Pennsylvania	20.2
17	Wyoming	19.9
18	Michigan	19.6
19	Virginia	19.0
20	Wisconsin	18.8
21	Illinois	18.6
21	North Dakota	18.6
23	Delaware	18.3
24	New York	18.0
25	New Mexico	17.9
25	Oregon	17.9
25	Texas	17.9
28	Kansas	17.8
29	Georgia	17.7
30	South Dakota	17.5
31	Maine	17.3
32	Iowa	17.2
33	Colorado	17.1
33	Florida	17.1
33	Vermont	17.1
36	Minnesota	16.8
36	Montana	16.8
38	Nebraska	16.7
39	Idaho	16.3
40	Arizona	16.1
41	New Hampshire	15.8
41	New Jersey	15.8
43	Connecticut	15.4
43	Hawaii	15.4
45	Maryland	15.2
46	Rhode Island	15.1
47	Massachusetts	15.0
48	Washington	14.9
49	California	12.9
50	Utah	9.8

District of Columbia	15.3

Source: U.S. Department of Health and Human Services, Centers for Disease Control and Prevention
"2009 Behavioral Risk Factor Surveillance Summary Prevalence Data" (http://apps.nccd.cdc.gov/brfss/)
*Persons 18 and older who have smoked more than 100 cigarettes during their lifetime and who currently smoke every day or some days.

Percent of Men Who Smoke: 2009

National Median = 19.6% of Men*

ALPHA ORDER			RANK ORDER		
RANK	**STATE**	**PERCENT**	**RANK**	**STATE**	**PERCENT**
5	Alabama	25.7	1	West Virginia	27.7
19	Alaska	20.7	2	Mississippi	27.2
37	Arizona	18.0	3	Kentucky	27.1
17	Arkansas	21.0	3	Oklahoma	27.1
48	California	15.6	5	Alabama	25.7
27	Colorado	19.5	6	Louisiana	25.1
45	Connecticut	16.2	7	Indiana	24.9
21	Delaware	20.2	8	Tennessee	24.6
37	Florida	18.0	9	Missouri	24.3
24	Georgia	20.0	10	North Carolina	23.1
42	Hawaii	16.8	11	Nevada	22.7
32	Idaho	18.7	12	Virginia	22.5
20	Illinois	20.6	13	Texas	22.1
7	Indiana	24.9	14	Pennsylvania	21.5
26	Iowa	19.6	14	South Carolina	21.5
33	Kansas	18.6	16	Ohio	21.2
3	Kentucky	27.1	17	Arkansas	21.0
6	Louisiana	25.1	17	Michigan	21.0
31	Maine	18.9	19	Alaska	20.7
43	Maryland	16.7	20	Illinois	20.6
46	Massachusetts	16.1	21	Delaware	20.2
17	Michigan	21.0	21	Wisconsin	20.2
33	Minnesota	18.6	23	Wyoming	20.1
2	Mississippi	27.2	24	Georgia	20.0
9	Missouri	24.3	25	New Mexico	19.8
44	Montana	16.4	26	Iowa	19.6
35	Nebraska	18.5	27	Colorado	19.5
11	Nevada	22.7	28	Vermont	19.4
40	New Hampshire	17.3	29	New York	19.3
39	New Jersey	17.6	29	North Dakota	19.3
25	New Mexico	19.8	31	Maine	18.9
29	New York	19.3	32	Idaho	18.7
10	North Carolina	23.1	33	Kansas	18.6
29	North Dakota	19.3	33	Minnesota	18.6
16	Ohio	21.2	35	Nebraska	18.5
3	Oklahoma	27.1	35	Oregon	18.5
35	Oregon	18.5	37	Arizona	18.0
14	Pennsylvania	21.5	37	Florida	18.0
49	Rhode Island	15.2	39	New Jersey	17.6
14	South Carolina	21.5	40	New Hampshire	17.3
41	South Dakota	16.9	41	South Dakota	16.9
8	Tennessee	24.6	42	Hawaii	16.8
13	Texas	22.1	43	Maryland	16.7
50	Utah	11.9	44	Montana	16.4
28	Vermont	19.4	45	Connecticut	16.2
12	Virginia	22.5	46	Massachusetts	16.1
46	Washington	16.1	46	Washington	16.1
1	West Virginia	27.7	48	California	15.6
21	Wisconsin	20.2	49	Rhode Island	15.2
23	Wyoming	20.1	50	Utah	11.9
				District of Columbia	15.8

Source: U.S. Department of Health and Human Services, Centers for Disease Control and Prevention
"2009 Behavioral Risk Factor Surveillance Summary Prevalence Data" (http://apps.nccd.cdc.gov/brfss/)
*Males 18 and older who have smoked more than 100 cigarettes during their lifetime and who currently smoke every day or some days.

Percent of Women Who Smoke: 2009

National Median = 16.7% of Women*

ALPHA ORDER				RANK ORDER		
RANK	STATE	PERCENT		RANK	STATE	PERCENT
10	Alabama	19.7		1	Kentucky	24.2
8	Alaska	20.5		2	Oklahoma	24.0
40	Arizona	14.3		3	West Virginia	23.6
5	Arkansas	21.9		4	Missouri	22.0
49	California	10.2		5	Arkansas	21.9
39	Colorado	14.6		6	Indiana	21.4
38	Connecticut	14.7		7	Nevada	21.3
27	Delaware	16.6		8	Alaska	20.5
28	Florida	16.3		9	Mississippi	19.8
32	Georgia	15.5		10	Alabama	19.7
44	Hawaii	13.9		10	Wyoming	19.7
44	Idaho	13.9		12	Tennessee	19.6
26	Illinois	16.7		13	Ohio	19.5
6	Indiana	21.4		14	Louisiana	19.3
37	Iowa	14.8		14	South Carolina	19.3
24	Kansas	17.1		16	Pennsylvania	19.1
1	Kentucky	24.2		17	Michigan	18.2
14	Louisiana	19.3		18	South Dakota	18.1
30	Maine	15.8		19	North Dakota	17.9
46	Maryland	13.8		20	North Carolina	17.7
43	Massachusetts	14.0		21	Montana	17.3
17	Michigan	18.2		21	Wisconsin	17.3
35	Minnesota	14.9		23	Oregon	17.2
9	Mississippi	19.8		24	Kansas	17.1
4	Missouri	22.0		25	New York	16.8
21	Montana	17.3		26	Illinois	16.7
33	Nebraska	15.0		27	Delaware	16.6
7	Nevada	21.3		28	Florida	16.3
40	New Hampshire	14.3		29	New Mexico	16.1
42	New Jersey	14.2		30	Maine	15.8
29	New Mexico	16.1		30	Virginia	15.8
25	New York	16.8		32	Georgia	15.5
20	North Carolina	17.7		33	Nebraska	15.0
19	North Dakota	17.9		33	Vermont	15.0
13	Ohio	19.5		35	Minnesota	14.9
2	Oklahoma	24.0		35	Rhode Island	14.9
23	Oregon	17.2		37	Iowa	14.8
16	Pennsylvania	19.1		38	Connecticut	14.7
35	Rhode Island	14.9		39	Colorado	14.6
14	South Carolina	19.3		40	Arizona	14.3
18	South Dakota	18.1		40	New Hampshire	14.3
12	Tennessee	19.6		42	New Jersey	14.2
46	Texas	13.8		43	Massachusetts	14.0
50	Utah	7.7		44	Hawaii	13.9
33	Vermont	15.0		44	Idaho	13.9
30	Virginia	15.8		46	Maryland	13.8
46	Washington	13.8		46	Texas	13.8
3	West Virginia	23.6		46	Washington	13.8
21	Wisconsin	17.3		49	California	10.2
10	Wyoming	19.7		50	Utah	7.7

District of Columbia	14.8

Source: U.S. Department of Health and Human Services, Centers for Disease Control and Prevention
"2009 Behavioral Risk Factor Surveillance Summary Prevalence Data" (http://apps.nccd.cdc.gov/brfss/)
*Females 18 and older who have smoked more than 100 cigarettes during their lifetime and who currently smoke every day or some days.

Percent of Adults Who Are Former Smokers: 2009

National Median = 25.5% of Adults*

<table>
<tr><td colspan="3">ALPHA ORDER</td><td colspan="3">RANK ORDER</td></tr>
<tr><td>RANK</td><td>STATE</td><td>PERCENT</td><td>RANK</td><td>STATE</td><td>PERCENT</td></tr>
<tr><td>45</td><td>Alabama</td><td>22.8</td><td>1</td><td>Vermont</td><td>31.6</td></tr>
<tr><td>8</td><td>Alaska</td><td>28.1</td><td>2</td><td>Maine</td><td>31.1</td></tr>
<tr><td>22</td><td>Arizona</td><td>26.0</td><td>3</td><td>Rhode Island</td><td>29.6</td></tr>
<tr><td>8</td><td>Arkansas</td><td>28.1</td><td>4</td><td>New Hampshire</td><td>29.4</td></tr>
<tr><td>42</td><td>California</td><td>23.2</td><td>5</td><td>Massachusetts</td><td>28.5</td></tr>
<tr><td>26</td><td>Colorado</td><td>25.5</td><td>6</td><td>Delaware</td><td>28.4</td></tr>
<tr><td>7</td><td>Connecticut</td><td>28.2</td><td>7</td><td>Connecticut</td><td>28.2</td></tr>
<tr><td>6</td><td>Delaware</td><td>28.4</td><td>8</td><td>Alaska</td><td>28.1</td></tr>
<tr><td>10</td><td>Florida</td><td>27.6</td><td>8</td><td>Arkansas</td><td>28.1</td></tr>
<tr><td>48</td><td>Georgia</td><td>22.0</td><td>10</td><td>Florida</td><td>27.6</td></tr>
<tr><td>13</td><td>Hawaii</td><td>26.9</td><td>10</td><td>Oregon</td><td>27.6</td></tr>
<tr><td>46</td><td>Idaho</td><td>22.1</td><td>12</td><td>South Dakota</td><td>27.2</td></tr>
<tr><td>44</td><td>Illinois</td><td>23.1</td><td>13</td><td>Hawaii</td><td>26.9</td></tr>
<tr><td>39</td><td>Indiana</td><td>23.7</td><td>13</td><td>Wisconsin</td><td>26.9</td></tr>
<tr><td>37</td><td>Iowa</td><td>24.2</td><td>15</td><td>Washington</td><td>26.7</td></tr>
<tr><td>41</td><td>Kansas</td><td>23.3</td><td>16</td><td>Nevada</td><td>26.5</td></tr>
<tr><td>29</td><td>Kentucky</td><td>25.3</td><td>17</td><td>Minnesota</td><td>26.4</td></tr>
<tr><td>42</td><td>Louisiana</td><td>23.2</td><td>17</td><td>Montana</td><td>26.4</td></tr>
<tr><td>2</td><td>Maine</td><td>31.1</td><td>19</td><td>New York</td><td>26.3</td></tr>
<tr><td>40</td><td>Maryland</td><td>23.4</td><td>20</td><td>North Carolina</td><td>26.2</td></tr>
<tr><td>5</td><td>Massachusetts</td><td>28.5</td><td>21</td><td>Wyoming</td><td>26.1</td></tr>
<tr><td>26</td><td>Michigan</td><td>25.5</td><td>22</td><td>Arizona</td><td>26.0</td></tr>
<tr><td>17</td><td>Minnesota</td><td>26.4</td><td>22</td><td>Pennsylvania</td><td>26.0</td></tr>
<tr><td>46</td><td>Mississippi</td><td>22.1</td><td>24</td><td>New Mexico</td><td>25.8</td></tr>
<tr><td>30</td><td>Missouri</td><td>24.8</td><td>24</td><td>Ohio</td><td>25.8</td></tr>
<tr><td>17</td><td>Montana</td><td>26.4</td><td>26</td><td>Colorado</td><td>25.5</td></tr>
<tr><td>32</td><td>Nebraska</td><td>24.6</td><td>26</td><td>Michigan</td><td>25.5</td></tr>
<tr><td>16</td><td>Nevada</td><td>26.5</td><td>28</td><td>New Jersey</td><td>25.4</td></tr>
<tr><td>4</td><td>New Hampshire</td><td>29.4</td><td>29</td><td>Kentucky</td><td>25.3</td></tr>
<tr><td>28</td><td>New Jersey</td><td>25.4</td><td>30</td><td>Missouri</td><td>24.8</td></tr>
<tr><td>24</td><td>New Mexico</td><td>25.8</td><td>31</td><td>Tennessee</td><td>24.7</td></tr>
<tr><td>19</td><td>New York</td><td>26.3</td><td>32</td><td>Nebraska</td><td>24.6</td></tr>
<tr><td>20</td><td>North Carolina</td><td>26.2</td><td>33</td><td>Oklahoma</td><td>24.5</td></tr>
<tr><td>38</td><td>North Dakota</td><td>24.0</td><td>33</td><td>South Carolina</td><td>24.5</td></tr>
<tr><td>24</td><td>Ohio</td><td>25.8</td><td>33</td><td>West Virginia</td><td>24.5</td></tr>
<tr><td>33</td><td>Oklahoma</td><td>24.5</td><td>36</td><td>Virginia</td><td>24.4</td></tr>
<tr><td>10</td><td>Oregon</td><td>27.6</td><td>37</td><td>Iowa</td><td>24.2</td></tr>
<tr><td>22</td><td>Pennsylvania</td><td>26.0</td><td>38</td><td>North Dakota</td><td>24.0</td></tr>
<tr><td>3</td><td>Rhode Island</td><td>29.6</td><td>39</td><td>Indiana</td><td>23.7</td></tr>
<tr><td>33</td><td>South Carolina</td><td>24.5</td><td>40</td><td>Maryland</td><td>23.4</td></tr>
<tr><td>12</td><td>South Dakota</td><td>27.2</td><td>41</td><td>Kansas</td><td>23.3</td></tr>
<tr><td>31</td><td>Tennessee</td><td>24.7</td><td>42</td><td>California</td><td>23.2</td></tr>
<tr><td>49</td><td>Texas</td><td>21.6</td><td>42</td><td>Louisiana</td><td>23.2</td></tr>
<tr><td>50</td><td>Utah</td><td>15.1</td><td>44</td><td>Illinois</td><td>23.1</td></tr>
<tr><td>1</td><td>Vermont</td><td>31.6</td><td>45</td><td>Alabama</td><td>22.8</td></tr>
<tr><td>36</td><td>Virginia</td><td>24.4</td><td>46</td><td>Idaho</td><td>22.1</td></tr>
<tr><td>15</td><td>Washington</td><td>26.7</td><td>46</td><td>Mississippi</td><td>22.1</td></tr>
<tr><td>33</td><td>West Virginia</td><td>24.5</td><td>48</td><td>Georgia</td><td>22.0</td></tr>
<tr><td>13</td><td>Wisconsin</td><td>26.9</td><td>49</td><td>Texas</td><td>21.6</td></tr>
<tr><td>21</td><td>Wyoming</td><td>26.1</td><td>50</td><td>Utah</td><td>15.1</td></tr>
<tr><td></td><td></td><td></td><td></td><td>District of Columbia</td><td>24.2</td></tr>
</table>

Source: U.S. Department of Health and Human Services, Centers for Disease Control and Prevention
  "2009 Behavioral Risk Factor Surveillance Summary Prevalence Data" (http://apps.nccd.cdc.gov/brfss/)
*Persons 18 and older who have smoked more than 100 cigarettes during their lifetime and who currently do not smoke.

Percent of Adults Who Have Never Smoked: 2009

National Median = 55.3% of Adults*

ALPHA ORDER

RANK	STATE	PERCENT
31	Alabama	54.6
45	Alaska	51.3
13	Arizona	57.8
47	Arkansas	50.4
2	California	63.9
15	Colorado	57.4
21	Connecticut	56.3
39	Delaware	53.4
25	Florida	55.3
6	Georgia	60.3
14	Hawaii	57.7
3	Idaho	61.6
12	Illinois	58.3
41	Indiana	53.2
9	Iowa	58.7
7	Kansas	58.8
50	Kentucky	49.1
30	Louisiana	54.7
43	Maine	51.6
4	Maryland	61.5
19	Massachusetts	56.6
28	Michigan	54.9
17	Minnesota	56.8
31	Mississippi	54.6
42	Missouri	52.1
17	Montana	56.8
9	Nebraska	58.7
44	Nevada	51.4
28	New Hampshire	54.9
7	New Jersey	58.8
22	New Mexico	56.2
23	New York	55.7
38	North Carolina	53.5
15	North Dakota	57.4
36	Ohio	53.8
48	Oklahoma	50.0
33	Oregon	54.5
37	Pennsylvania	53.7
24	Rhode Island	55.4
27	South Carolina	55.2
25	South Dakota	55.3
40	Tennessee	53.3
5	Texas	60.5
1	Utah	75.1
45	Vermont	51.3
20	Virginia	56.5
11	Washington	58.4
49	West Virginia	49.9
34	Wisconsin	54.3
35	Wyoming	54.0

RANK ORDER

RANK	STATE	PERCENT
1	Utah	75.1
2	California	63.9
3	Idaho	61.6
4	Maryland	61.5
5	Texas	60.5
6	Georgia	60.3
7	Kansas	58.8
7	New Jersey	58.8
9	Iowa	58.7
9	Nebraska	58.7
11	Washington	58.4
12	Illinois	58.3
13	Arizona	57.8
14	Hawaii	57.7
15	Colorado	57.4
15	North Dakota	57.4
17	Minnesota	56.8
17	Montana	56.8
19	Massachusetts	56.6
20	Virginia	56.5
21	Connecticut	56.3
22	New Mexico	56.2
23	New York	55.7
24	Rhode Island	55.4
25	Florida	55.3
25	South Dakota	55.3
27	South Carolina	55.2
28	Michigan	54.9
28	New Hampshire	54.9
30	Louisiana	54.7
31	Alabama	54.6
31	Mississippi	54.6
33	Oregon	54.5
34	Wisconsin	54.3
35	Wyoming	54.0
36	Ohio	53.8
37	Pennsylvania	53.7
38	North Carolina	53.5
39	Delaware	53.4
40	Tennessee	53.3
41	Indiana	53.2
42	Missouri	52.1
43	Maine	51.6
44	Nevada	51.4
45	Alaska	51.3
45	Vermont	51.3
47	Arkansas	50.4
48	Oklahoma	50.0
49	West Virginia	49.9
50	Kentucky	49.1
	District of Columbia	60.6

Source: U.S. Department of Health and Human Services, Centers for Disease Control and Prevention
"2009 Behavioral Risk Factor Surveillance Summary Prevalence Data" (http://apps.nccd.cdc.gov/brfss/)
*Persons 18 and older who have not smoked more than 100 cigarettes during their lifetime.

Percent of Population Who Are Illicit Drug Users: 2008

National Percent = 8.0% of Population*

ALPHA ORDER

RANK	STATE	PERCENT
40	Alabama	6.7
3	Alaska	11.8
14	Arizona	9.0
26	Arkansas	8.0
11	California	9.1
4	Colorado	11.7
22	Connecticut	8.2
11	Delaware	9.1
28	Florida	7.8
32	Georgia	7.3
8	Hawaii	9.9
26	Idaho	8.0
35	Illinois	7.2
18	Indiana	8.8
50	Iowa	4.1
37	Kansas	6.8
21	Kentucky	8.4
35	Louisiana	7.2
11	Maine	9.1
32	Maryland	7.3
17	Massachusetts	8.9
14	Michigan	9.0
22	Minnesota	8.2
43	Mississippi	6.4
31	Missouri	7.4
7	Montana	10.0
43	Nebraska	6.4
10	Nevada	9.4
6	New Hampshire	10.7
43	New Jersey	6.4
19	New Mexico	8.7
14	New York	9.0
28	North Carolina	7.8
49	North Dakota	5.9
30	Ohio	7.6
25	Oklahoma	8.1
2	Oregon	12.2
42	Pennsylvania	6.6
1	Rhode Island	13.3
40	South Carolina	6.7
46	South Dakota	6.3
22	Tennessee	8.2
46	Texas	6.3
48	Utah	6.2
5	Vermont	11.6
32	Virginia	7.3
9	Washington	9.6
37	West Virginia	6.8
19	Wisconsin	8.7
37	Wyoming	6.8

RANK ORDER

RANK	STATE	PERCENT
1	Rhode Island	13.3
2	Oregon	12.2
3	Alaska	11.8
4	Colorado	11.7
5	Vermont	11.6
6	New Hampshire	10.7
7	Montana	10.0
8	Hawaii	9.9
9	Washington	9.6
10	Nevada	9.4
11	California	9.1
11	Delaware	9.1
11	Maine	9.1
14	Arizona	9.0
14	Michigan	9.0
14	New York	9.0
17	Massachusetts	8.9
18	Indiana	8.8
19	New Mexico	8.7
19	Wisconsin	8.7
21	Kentucky	8.4
22	Connecticut	8.2
22	Minnesota	8.2
22	Tennessee	8.2
25	Oklahoma	8.1
26	Arkansas	8.0
26	Idaho	8.0
28	Florida	7.8
28	North Carolina	7.8
30	Ohio	7.6
31	Missouri	7.4
32	Georgia	7.3
32	Maryland	7.3
32	Virginia	7.3
35	Illinois	7.2
35	Louisiana	7.2
37	Kansas	6.8
37	West Virginia	6.8
37	Wyoming	6.8
40	Alabama	6.7
40	South Carolina	6.7
42	Pennsylvania	6.6
43	Mississippi	6.4
43	Nebraska	6.4
43	New Jersey	6.4
46	South Dakota	6.3
46	Texas	6.3
48	Utah	6.2
49	North Dakota	5.9
50	Iowa	4.1

District of Columbia	12.1

Source: U.S. Department of Health and Human Services, Substance Abuse and Mental Health Services Administration
"2007-2008 National Surveys on Drug Use and Health" (June 2010, http://www.oas.samhsa.gov/2k8state/toc.cfm)
*Population 12 years and older who used any illicit drug at least once within month of survey.

Percent of Adults Overweight: 2009

National Median = 36.2% of Adults*

ALPHA ORDER

RANK	STATE	PERCENT
21	Alabama	36.6
6	Alaska	37.9
3	Arizona	38.3
42	Arkansas	35.1
31	California	35.8
19	Colorado	36.7
4	Connecticut	38.0
27	Delaware	36.1
15	Florida	36.9
10	Georgia	37.6
45	Hawaii	34.9
25	Idaho	36.2
12	Illinois	37.1
41	Indiana	35.2
1	Iowa	38.7
31	Kansas	35.8
48	Kentucky	34.7
50	Louisiana	33.7
8	Maine	37.8
27	Maryland	36.1
35	Massachusetts	35.7
39	Michigan	35.3
6	Minnesota	37.9
45	Mississippi	34.9
44	Missouri	35.0
2	Montana	38.4
17	Nebraska	36.8
21	Nevada	36.6
23	New Hampshire	36.5
4	New Jersey	38.0
25	New Mexico	36.2
36	New York	35.6
39	North Carolina	35.3
8	North Dakota	37.8
13	Ohio	37.0
38	Oklahoma	35.4
13	Oregon	37.0
30	Pennsylvania	36.0
19	Rhode Island	36.7
31	South Carolina	35.8
15	South Dakota	36.9
27	Tennessee	36.1
11	Texas	37.3
49	Utah	34.0
47	Vermont	34.8
42	Virginia	35.1
37	Washington	35.5
31	West Virginia	35.8
24	Wisconsin	36.4
17	Wyoming	36.8

RANK ORDER

RANK	STATE	PERCENT
1	Iowa	38.7
2	Montana	38.4
3	Arizona	38.3
4	Connecticut	38.0
4	New Jersey	38.0
6	Alaska	37.9
6	Minnesota	37.9
8	Maine	37.8
8	North Dakota	37.8
10	Georgia	37.6
11	Texas	37.3
12	Illinois	37.1
13	Ohio	37.0
13	Oregon	37.0
15	Florida	36.9
15	South Dakota	36.9
17	Nebraska	36.8
17	Wyoming	36.8
19	Colorado	36.7
19	Rhode Island	36.7
21	Alabama	36.6
21	Nevada	36.6
23	New Hampshire	36.5
24	Wisconsin	36.4
25	Idaho	36.2
25	New Mexico	36.2
27	Delaware	36.1
27	Maryland	36.1
27	Tennessee	36.1
30	Pennsylvania	36.0
31	California	35.8
31	Kansas	35.8
31	South Carolina	35.8
31	West Virginia	35.8
35	Massachusetts	35.7
36	New York	35.6
37	Washington	35.5
38	Oklahoma	35.4
39	Michigan	35.3
39	North Carolina	35.3
41	Indiana	35.2
42	Arkansas	35.1
42	Virginia	35.1
44	Missouri	35.0
45	Hawaii	34.9
45	Mississippi	34.9
47	Vermont	34.8
48	Kentucky	34.7
49	Utah	34.0
50	Louisiana	33.7

District of Columbia	31.6

Source: U.S. Department of Health and Human Services, Centers for Disease Control and Prevention
"2009 Behavioral Risk Factor Surveillance Summary Prevalence Data" (http://apps.nccd.cdc.gov/brfss/)
*Persons 18 and older. Does not include obese adults. Overweight is defined as a Body Mass Index (BMI) of 25.0 to 29.9 regardless of sex. BMI is a ratio of height to weight. As an example, a person 5' 8" and weighing 171 pounds has a BMI of 26. See http://www.cdc.gov/healthyweight/assessing/bmi/index.html.

Percent of Adults Obese: 2009

National Median = 26.9% of Adults*

ALPHA ORDER

RANK	STATE	PERCENT
7	Alabama	31.6
36	Alaska	25.4
32	Arizona	25.9
8	Arkansas	31.5
34	California	25.5
50	Colorado	19.0
49	Connecticut	21.0
24	Delaware	27.6
28	Florida	26.5
23	Georgia	27.7
47	Hawaii	22.9
39	Idaho	25.1
25	Illinois	27.4
14	Indiana	30.0
19	Iowa	28.5
18	Kansas	28.8
4	Kentucky	32.4
2	Louisiana	33.9
29	Maine	26.4
27	Maryland	26.8
48	Massachusetts	21.8
10	Michigan	30.3
36	Minnesota	25.4
1	Mississippi	35.4
9	Missouri	30.6
44	Montana	23.7
21	Nebraska	28.1
29	Nevada	26.4
31	New Hampshire	26.3
43	New Jersey	23.9
33	New Mexico	25.6
41	New York	24.6
12	North Carolina	30.1
20	North Dakota	28.4
15	Ohio	29.8
5	Oklahoma	32.0
45	Oregon	23.6
21	Pennsylvania	28.1
40	Rhode Island	24.9
12	South Carolina	30.1
10	South Dakota	30.3
3	Tennessee	32.9
16	Texas	29.5
42	Utah	24.0
46	Vermont	23.4
34	Virginia	25.5
26	Washington	26.9
6	West Virginia	31.7
17	Wisconsin	29.2
36	Wyoming	25.4

RANK ORDER

RANK	STATE	PERCENT
1	Mississippi	35.4
2	Louisiana	33.9
3	Tennessee	32.9
4	Kentucky	32.4
5	Oklahoma	32.0
6	West Virginia	31.7
7	Alabama	31.6
8	Arkansas	31.5
9	Missouri	30.6
10	Michigan	30.3
10	South Dakota	30.3
12	North Carolina	30.1
12	South Carolina	30.1
14	Indiana	30.0
15	Ohio	29.8
16	Texas	29.5
17	Wisconsin	29.2
18	Kansas	28.8
19	Iowa	28.5
20	North Dakota	28.4
21	Nebraska	28.1
21	Pennsylvania	28.1
23	Georgia	27.7
24	Delaware	27.6
25	Illinois	27.4
26	Washington	26.9
27	Maryland	26.8
28	Florida	26.5
29	Maine	26.4
29	Nevada	26.4
31	New Hampshire	26.3
32	Arizona	25.9
33	New Mexico	25.6
34	California	25.5
34	Virginia	25.5
36	Alaska	25.4
36	Minnesota	25.4
36	Wyoming	25.4
39	Idaho	25.1
40	Rhode Island	24.9
41	New York	24.6
42	Utah	24.0
43	New Jersey	23.9
44	Montana	23.7
45	Oregon	23.6
46	Vermont	23.4
47	Hawaii	22.9
48	Massachusetts	21.8
49	Connecticut	21.0
50	Colorado	19.0

	District of Columbia	20.1

Source: U.S. Department of Health and Human Services, Centers for Disease Control and Prevention
   "2009 Behavioral Risk Factor Surveillance Summary Prevalence Data" (http://apps.nccd.cdc.gov/brfss/)
*Persons 18 and older.   Obese is defined as a Body Mass Index (BMI) of 30.0 or more regardless of sex. BMI is a ratio of
height to weight. As an example, a person 5' 8" and weighing 197 pounds has a BMI of 30. See
http://www.cdc.gov/healthyweight/assessing/bmi/index.html.

Percent of Adults Overweight or Obese: 2009

National Median = 63.1% of Adults*

ALPHA ORDER

RANK	STATE	PERCENT
3	Alabama	68.2
29	Alaska	63.3
24	Arizona	64.2
12	Arkansas	66.6
40	California	61.3
50	Colorado	55.7
45	Connecticut	59.0
27	Delaware	63.7
28	Florida	63.4
19	Georgia	65.3
48	Hawaii	57.8
40	Idaho	61.3
23	Illinois	64.5
20	Indiana	65.2
7	Iowa	67.2
22	Kansas	64.6
9	Kentucky	67.1
4	Louisiana	67.6
24	Maine	64.2
32	Maryland	62.9
49	Massachusetts	57.5
15	Michigan	65.6
29	Minnesota	63.3
1	Mississippi	70.3
15	Missouri	65.6
36	Montana	62.1
21	Nebraska	64.9
31	Nevada	63.0
33	New Hampshire	62.8
37	New Jersey	61.9
38	New Mexico	61.8
44	New York	60.2
18	North Carolina	65.4
13	North Dakota	66.2
10	Ohio	66.8
6	Oklahoma	67.4
42	Oregon	60.6
26	Pennsylvania	64.1
39	Rhode Island	61.6
14	South Carolina	65.9
7	South Dakota	67.2
2	Tennessee	69.0
10	Texas	66.8
47	Utah	58.0
46	Vermont	58.2
42	Virginia	60.6
34	Washington	62.4
5	West Virginia	67.5
15	Wisconsin	65.6
35	Wyoming	62.2

RANK ORDER

RANK	STATE	PERCENT
1	Mississippi	70.3
2	Tennessee	69.0
3	Alabama	68.2
4	Louisiana	67.6
5	West Virginia	67.5
6	Oklahoma	67.4
7	Iowa	67.2
7	South Dakota	67.2
9	Kentucky	67.1
10	Ohio	66.8
10	Texas	66.8
12	Arkansas	66.6
13	North Dakota	66.2
14	South Carolina	65.9
15	Michigan	65.6
15	Missouri	65.6
15	Wisconsin	65.6
18	North Carolina	65.4
19	Georgia	65.3
20	Indiana	65.2
21	Nebraska	64.9
22	Kansas	64.6
23	Illinois	64.5
24	Arizona	64.2
24	Maine	64.2
26	Pennsylvania	64.1
27	Delaware	63.7
28	Florida	63.4
29	Alaska	63.3
29	Minnesota	63.3
31	Nevada	63.0
32	Maryland	62.9
33	New Hampshire	62.8
34	Washington	62.4
35	Wyoming	62.2
36	Montana	62.1
37	New Jersey	61.9
38	New Mexico	61.8
39	Rhode Island	61.6
40	California	61.3
40	Idaho	61.3
42	Oregon	60.6
42	Virginia	60.6
44	New York	60.2
45	Connecticut	59.0
46	Vermont	58.2
47	Utah	58.0
48	Hawaii	57.8
49	Massachusetts	57.5
50	Colorado	55.7

| | District of Columbia | 51.7 |

Source: CQ Press using data from U.S. Department of Health and Human Services, Centers for Disease Control and Prevention "2009 Behavioral Risk Factor Surveillance Summary Prevalence Data" (http://apps.nccd.cdc.gov/brfss/)

*Persons 18 and older. Overweight is defined as a Body Mass Index (BMI) of 25.0 to 29.9 regardless of sex. Obese is a BMI of 30.0 or greater. BMI is a ratio of height to weight. As an example, a person 5' 8" and weighing 165 pounds has a BMI of 25. The same height at 197 pounds has a BMI of 30. See http://www.cdc.gov/healthyweight/assessing/bmi/index.html.

Percent of Adults Who Do Not Exercise: 2009

National Median = 23.8% of Adults*

ALPHA ORDER				RANK ORDER		
RANK	STATE	PERCENT		RANK	STATE	PERCENT
4	Alabama	31.0		1	West Virginia	33.2
31	Alaska	22.4		2	Mississippi	32.3
46	Arizona	19.0		3	Oklahoma	31.4
6	Arkansas	29.8		4	Alabama	31.0
33	California	22.1		4	Tennessee	31.0
47	Colorado	17.7		6	Arkansas	29.8
38	Connecticut	21.6		7	Kentucky	29.7
36	Delaware	21.9		8	Louisiana	28.6
20	Florida	24.7		9	Texas	27.3
23	Georgia	24.2		10	Indiana	27.2
44	Hawaii	19.6		11	North Dakota	26.8
41	Idaho	21.0		12	Missouri	26.7
27	Illinois	23.6		13	New York	26.4
10	Indiana	27.2		13	North Carolina	26.4
23	Iowa	24.2		13	Ohio	26.4
29	Kansas	23.2		16	New Jersey	26.2
7	Kentucky	29.7		16	South Carolina	26.2
8	Louisiana	28.6		18	Pennsylvania	25.7
39	Maine	21.2		19	Rhode Island	24.9
26	Maryland	23.8		20	Florida	24.7
42	Massachusetts	20.9		21	South Dakota	24.5
27	Michigan	23.6		22	Nevada	24.4
50	Minnesota	15.8		23	Georgia	24.2
2	Mississippi	32.3		23	Iowa	24.2
12	Missouri	26.7		23	Nebraska	24.2
34	Montana	22.0		26	Maryland	23.8
23	Nebraska	24.2		27	Illinois	23.6
22	Nevada	24.4		27	Michigan	23.6
39	New Hampshire	21.2		29	Kansas	23.2
16	New Jersey	26.2		30	Wyoming	22.5
31	New Mexico	22.4		31	Alaska	22.4
13	New York	26.4		31	New Mexico	22.4
13	North Carolina	26.4		33	California	22.1
11	North Dakota	26.8		34	Montana	22.0
13	Ohio	26.4		34	Wisconsin	22.0
3	Oklahoma	31.4		36	Delaware	21.9
47	Oregon	17.7		36	Virginia	21.9
18	Pennsylvania	25.7		38	Connecticut	21.6
19	Rhode Island	24.9		39	Maine	21.2
16	South Carolina	26.2		39	New Hampshire	21.2
21	South Dakota	24.5		41	Idaho	21.0
4	Tennessee	31.0		42	Massachusetts	20.9
9	Texas	27.3		43	Vermont	20.2
47	Utah	17.7		44	Hawaii	19.6
43	Vermont	20.2		45	Washington	19.5
36	Virginia	21.9		46	Arizona	19.0
45	Washington	19.5		47	Colorado	17.7
1	West Virginia	33.2		47	Oregon	17.7
34	Wisconsin	22.0		47	Utah	17.7
30	Wyoming	22.5		50	Minnesota	15.8
					District of Columbia	19.6

Source: U.S. Department of Health and Human Services, Centers for Disease Control and Prevention
   "2009 Behavioral Risk Factor Surveillance Summary Prevalence Data" (http://apps.nccd.cdc.gov/brfss/)
*Persons 18 and older who, in the previous month, did not participate in any physical activities.

Percent of Adults Who Exercise Vigorously: 2009

National Median = 29.4% of Adults*

ALPHA ORDER				RANK ORDER		
RANK	STATE	PERCENT		RANK	STATE	PERCENT
47	Alabama	21.1		1	Alaska	40.1
1	Alaska	40.1		2	Utah	38.1
21	Arizona	30.1		3	Montana	36.3
42	Arkansas	25.3		4	Idaho	36.0
10	California	32.9		5	Wyoming	35.3
6	Colorado	34.6		6	Colorado	34.6
14	Connecticut	32.0		7	Hawaii	34.5
26	Delaware	29.3		7	Vermont	34.5
41	Florida	25.6		9	Oregon	33.7
35	Georgia	27.5		10	California	32.9
7	Hawaii	34.5		10	New Hampshire	32.9
4	Idaho	36.0		12	Maine	32.7
15	Illinois	31.8		13	New Mexico	32.3
31	Indiana	28.2		14	Connecticut	32.0
37	Iowa	26.9		15	Illinois	31.8
35	Kansas	27.5		15	Virginia	31.8
45	Kentucky	23.6		17	Michigan	31.3
46	Louisiana	22.0		18	Wisconsin	31.1
12	Maine	32.7		19	Massachusetts	30.8
22	Maryland	29.9		20	Washington	30.4
19	Massachusetts	30.8		21	Arizona	30.1
17	Michigan	31.3		22	Maryland	29.9
25	Minnesota	29.4		22	Nevada	29.9
48	Mississippi	19.7		24	Nebraska	29.7
33	Missouri	27.8		25	Minnesota	29.4
3	Montana	36.3		26	Delaware	29.3
24	Nebraska	29.7		27	North Dakota	29.2
22	Nevada	29.9		28	Rhode Island	29.0
10	New Hampshire	32.9		29	Texas	28.6
38	New Jersey	26.8		30	New York	28.4
13	New Mexico	32.3		31	Indiana	28.2
30	New York	28.4		32	Pennsylvania	27.9
39	North Carolina	25.9		33	Missouri	27.8
27	North Dakota	29.2		34	Ohio	27.6
34	Ohio	27.6		35	Georgia	27.5
40	Oklahoma	25.8		35	Kansas	27.5
9	Oregon	33.7		37	Iowa	26.9
32	Pennsylvania	27.9		38	New Jersey	26.8
28	Rhode Island	29.0		39	North Carolina	25.9
43	South Carolina	24.4		40	Oklahoma	25.8
44	South Dakota	23.9		41	Florida	25.6
49	Tennessee	17.2		42	Arkansas	25.3
29	Texas	28.6		43	South Carolina	24.4
2	Utah	38.1		44	South Dakota	23.9
7	Vermont	34.5		45	Kentucky	23.6
15	Virginia	31.8		46	Louisiana	22.0
20	Washington	30.4		47	Alabama	21.1
50	West Virginia	15.6		48	Mississippi	19.7
18	Wisconsin	31.1		49	Tennessee	17.2
5	Wyoming	35.3		50	West Virginia	15.6
					District of Columbia	34.1

Source: U.S. Department of Health and Human Services, Centers for Disease Control and Prevention
   "2009 Behavioral Risk Factor Surveillance Summary Prevalence Data" (http://apps.nccd.cdc.gov/brfss/)
*Persons 18 and older.   Vigorous exercise is activity that caused large increases in breathing or heart rate at least 20 minutes
three or more times per week (such as running, aerobics, or heavy yard work).

Percent of Adults Who Are Disabled: 2009

National Median = 18.9%*

<table>
<tr><td colspan="3">ALPHA ORDER</td><td colspan="3">RANK ORDER</td></tr>
<tr><th>RANK</th><th>STATE</th><th>PERCENT</th><th>RANK</th><th>STATE</th><th>PERCENT</th></tr>
<tr><td>5</td><td>Alabama</td><td>23.5</td><td>1</td><td>West Virginia</td><td>27.1</td></tr>
<tr><td>13</td><td>Alaska</td><td>21.4</td><td>2</td><td>Oklahoma</td><td>25.0</td></tr>
<tr><td>29</td><td>Arizona</td><td>18.6</td><td>3</td><td>Kentucky</td><td>24.8</td></tr>
<tr><td>6</td><td>Arkansas</td><td>22.8</td><td>4</td><td>Mississippi</td><td>24.1</td></tr>
<tr><td>37</td><td>California</td><td>17.2</td><td>5</td><td>Alabama</td><td>23.5</td></tr>
<tr><td>34</td><td>Colorado</td><td>18.0</td><td>6</td><td>Arkansas</td><td>22.8</td></tr>
<tr><td>46</td><td>Connecticut</td><td>16.1</td><td>7</td><td>Washington</td><td>22.5</td></tr>
<tr><td>31</td><td>Delaware</td><td>18.3</td><td>8</td><td>Missouri</td><td>22.1</td></tr>
<tr><td>14</td><td>Florida</td><td>20.9</td><td>9</td><td>Tennessee</td><td>21.8</td></tr>
<tr><td>47</td><td>Georgia</td><td>16.0</td><td>10</td><td>Maine</td><td>21.7</td></tr>
<tr><td>50</td><td>Hawaii</td><td>14.9</td><td>10</td><td>South Carolina</td><td>21.7</td></tr>
<tr><td>20</td><td>Idaho</td><td>20.1</td><td>12</td><td>Oregon</td><td>21.5</td></tr>
<tr><td>47</td><td>Illinois</td><td>16.0</td><td>13</td><td>Alaska</td><td>21.4</td></tr>
<tr><td>21</td><td>Indiana</td><td>20.0</td><td>14</td><td>Florida</td><td>20.9</td></tr>
<tr><td>45</td><td>Iowa</td><td>16.4</td><td>15</td><td>New Mexico</td><td>20.8</td></tr>
<tr><td>25</td><td>Kansas</td><td>18.9</td><td>16</td><td>Montana</td><td>20.7</td></tr>
<tr><td>3</td><td>Kentucky</td><td>24.8</td><td>16</td><td>Ohio</td><td>20.7</td></tr>
<tr><td>18</td><td>Louisiana</td><td>20.3</td><td>18</td><td>Louisiana</td><td>20.3</td></tr>
<tr><td>10</td><td>Maine</td><td>21.7</td><td>19</td><td>North Carolina</td><td>20.2</td></tr>
<tr><td>37</td><td>Maryland</td><td>17.2</td><td>20</td><td>Idaho</td><td>20.1</td></tr>
<tr><td>35</td><td>Massachusetts</td><td>17.9</td><td>21</td><td>Indiana</td><td>20.0</td></tr>
<tr><td>22</td><td>Michigan</td><td>19.9</td><td>22</td><td>Michigan</td><td>19.9</td></tr>
<tr><td>41</td><td>Minnesota</td><td>17.1</td><td>23</td><td>Vermont</td><td>19.2</td></tr>
<tr><td>4</td><td>Mississippi</td><td>24.1</td><td>24</td><td>Pennsylvania</td><td>19.0</td></tr>
<tr><td>8</td><td>Missouri</td><td>22.1</td><td>25</td><td>Kansas</td><td>18.9</td></tr>
<tr><td>16</td><td>Montana</td><td>20.7</td><td>25</td><td>Nevada</td><td>18.9</td></tr>
<tr><td>35</td><td>Nebraska</td><td>17.9</td><td>27</td><td>Utah</td><td>18.7</td></tr>
<tr><td>25</td><td>Nevada</td><td>18.9</td><td>27</td><td>Wyoming</td><td>18.7</td></tr>
<tr><td>31</td><td>New Hampshire</td><td>18.3</td><td>29</td><td>Arizona</td><td>18.6</td></tr>
<tr><td>49</td><td>New Jersey</td><td>15.0</td><td>30</td><td>New York</td><td>18.5</td></tr>
<tr><td>15</td><td>New Mexico</td><td>20.8</td><td>31</td><td>Delaware</td><td>18.3</td></tr>
<tr><td>30</td><td>New York</td><td>18.5</td><td>31</td><td>New Hampshire</td><td>18.3</td></tr>
<tr><td>19</td><td>North Carolina</td><td>20.2</td><td>33</td><td>Wisconsin</td><td>18.1</td></tr>
<tr><td>37</td><td>North Dakota</td><td>17.2</td><td>34</td><td>Colorado</td><td>18.0</td></tr>
<tr><td>16</td><td>Ohio</td><td>20.7</td><td>35</td><td>Massachusetts</td><td>17.9</td></tr>
<tr><td>2</td><td>Oklahoma</td><td>25.0</td><td>35</td><td>Nebraska</td><td>17.9</td></tr>
<tr><td>12</td><td>Oregon</td><td>21.5</td><td>37</td><td>California</td><td>17.2</td></tr>
<tr><td>24</td><td>Pennsylvania</td><td>19.0</td><td>37</td><td>Maryland</td><td>17.2</td></tr>
<tr><td>37</td><td>Rhode Island</td><td>17.2</td><td>37</td><td>North Dakota</td><td>17.2</td></tr>
<tr><td>10</td><td>South Carolina</td><td>21.7</td><td>37</td><td>Rhode Island</td><td>17.2</td></tr>
<tr><td>41</td><td>South Dakota</td><td>17.1</td><td>41</td><td>Minnesota</td><td>17.1</td></tr>
<tr><td>9</td><td>Tennessee</td><td>21.8</td><td>41</td><td>South Dakota</td><td>17.1</td></tr>
<tr><td>41</td><td>Texas</td><td>17.1</td><td>41</td><td>Texas</td><td>17.1</td></tr>
<tr><td>27</td><td>Utah</td><td>18.7</td><td>44</td><td>Virginia</td><td>16.8</td></tr>
<tr><td>23</td><td>Vermont</td><td>19.2</td><td>45</td><td>Iowa</td><td>16.4</td></tr>
<tr><td>44</td><td>Virginia</td><td>16.8</td><td>46</td><td>Connecticut</td><td>16.1</td></tr>
<tr><td>7</td><td>Washington</td><td>22.5</td><td>47</td><td>Georgia</td><td>16.0</td></tr>
<tr><td>1</td><td>West Virginia</td><td>27.1</td><td>47</td><td>Illinois</td><td>16.0</td></tr>
<tr><td>33</td><td>Wisconsin</td><td>18.1</td><td>49</td><td>New Jersey</td><td>15.0</td></tr>
<tr><td>27</td><td>Wyoming</td><td>18.7</td><td>50</td><td>Hawaii</td><td>14.9</td></tr>
<tr><td></td><td></td><td></td><td></td><td>District of Columbia</td><td>16.1</td></tr>
</table>

Source: U.S. Department of Health and Human Services, Centers for Disease Control and Prevention
"2009 Behavioral Risk Factor Surveillance Summary Prevalence Data" (http://apps.nccd.cdc.gov/brfss/)
*Persons 18 and older. Adults who are limited in any activities because of physical, mental, or emotional problems.

Percent of Adults with High Blood Pressure: 2009

National Median = 28.7% of Adults*

ALPHA ORDER

RANK	STATE	PERCENT
3	Alabama	37.2
43	Alaska	26.4
41	Arizona	26.6
6	Arkansas	34.4
46	California	25.7
49	Colorado	22.4
37	Connecticut	27.1
16	Delaware	30.8
10	Florida	32.1
14	Georgia	31.3
18	Hawaii	30.2
45	Idaho	25.9
25	Illinois	28.9
14	Indiana	31.3
30	Iowa	28.0
26	Kansas	28.7
4	Kentucky	36.4
5	Louisiana	35.7
20	Maine	30.0
23	Maryland	29.4
46	Massachusetts	25.7
22	Michigan	29.8
50	Minnesota	21.6
2	Mississippi	37.4
17	Missouri	30.6
32	Montana	27.7
37	Nebraska	27.1
34	Nevada	27.5
27	New Hampshire	28.6
29	New Jersey	28.1
41	New Mexico	26.6
28	New York	28.5
12	North Carolina	31.5
40	North Dakota	26.8
11	Ohio	31.7
6	Oklahoma	34.4
36	Oregon	27.2
13	Pennsylvania	31.4
18	Rhode Island	30.2
8	South Carolina	32.7
21	South Dakota	29.9
9	Tennessee	32.6
24	Texas	29.1
48	Utah	23.1
39	Vermont	27.0
34	Virginia	27.5
30	Washington	28.0
1	West Virginia	37.6
32	Wisconsin	27.7
44	Wyoming	26.1

RANK ORDER

RANK	STATE	PERCENT
1	West Virginia	37.6
2	Mississippi	37.4
3	Alabama	37.2
4	Kentucky	36.4
5	Louisiana	35.7
6	Arkansas	34.4
6	Oklahoma	34.4
8	South Carolina	32.7
9	Tennessee	32.6
10	Florida	32.1
11	Ohio	31.7
12	North Carolina	31.5
13	Pennsylvania	31.4
14	Georgia	31.3
14	Indiana	31.3
16	Delaware	30.8
17	Missouri	30.6
18	Hawaii	30.2
18	Rhode Island	30.2
20	Maine	30.0
21	South Dakota	29.9
22	Michigan	29.8
23	Maryland	29.4
24	Texas	29.1
25	Illinois	28.9
26	Kansas	28.7
27	New Hampshire	28.6
28	New York	28.5
29	New Jersey	28.1
30	Iowa	28.0
30	Washington	28.0
32	Montana	27.7
32	Wisconsin	27.7
34	Nevada	27.5
34	Virginia	27.5
36	Oregon	27.2
37	Connecticut	27.1
37	Nebraska	27.1
39	Vermont	27.0
40	North Dakota	26.8
41	Arizona	26.6
41	New Mexico	26.6
43	Alaska	26.4
44	Wyoming	26.1
45	Idaho	25.9
46	California	25.7
46	Massachusetts	25.7
48	Utah	23.1
49	Colorado	22.4
50	Minnesota	21.6
	District of Columbia	26.1

Source: U.S. Department of Health and Human Services, Centers for Disease Control and Prevention
"2009 Behavioral Risk Factor Surveillance Summary Prevalence Data" (http://apps.nccd.cdc.gov/brfss/)
*Persons 18 and older who have been told by a doctor, nurse, or other health professional that they have high blood pressure.

Percent of Adults with High Cholesterol: 2009

National Median = 37.5% of Adults*

ALPHA ORDER

RANK	STATE	PERCENT
8	Alabama	39.9
45	Alaska	35.0
4	Arizona	40.9
16	Arkansas	38.7
36	California	36.5
43	Colorado	35.3
29	Connecticut	37.3
23	Delaware	38.2
10	Florida	39.7
31	Georgia	37.0
12	Hawaii	38.9
30	Idaho	37.2
25	Illinois	37.5
8	Indiana	39.9
25	Iowa	37.5
18	Kansas	38.6
2	Kentucky	41.6
33	Louisiana	36.9
15	Maine	38.8
27	Maryland	37.4
42	Massachusetts	35.6
18	Michigan	38.6
48	Minnesota	33.9
3	Mississippi	41.4
23	Missouri	38.2
36	Montana	36.5
27	Nebraska	37.4
18	Nevada	38.6
18	New Hampshire	38.6
31	New Jersey	37.0
47	New Mexico	34.2
12	New York	38.9
7	North Carolina	40.0
46	North Dakota	34.8
11	Ohio	39.6
6	Oklahoma	40.3
43	Oregon	35.3
12	Pennsylvania	38.9
38	Rhode Island	36.4
1	South Carolina	41.8
38	South Dakota	36.4
50	Tennessee	32.9
4	Texas	40.9
49	Utah	33.6
41	Vermont	35.7
35	Virginia	36.7
16	Washington	38.7
22	West Virginia	38.5
40	Wisconsin	35.8
33	Wyoming	36.9

RANK ORDER

RANK	STATE	PERCENT
1	South Carolina	41.8
2	Kentucky	41.6
3	Mississippi	41.4
4	Arizona	40.9
4	Texas	40.9
6	Oklahoma	40.3
7	North Carolina	40.0
8	Alabama	39.9
8	Indiana	39.9
10	Florida	39.7
11	Ohio	39.6
12	Hawaii	38.9
12	New York	38.9
12	Pennsylvania	38.9
15	Maine	38.8
16	Arkansas	38.7
16	Washington	38.7
18	Kansas	38.6
18	Michigan	38.6
18	Nevada	38.6
18	New Hampshire	38.6
22	West Virginia	38.5
23	Delaware	38.2
23	Missouri	38.2
25	Illinois	37.5
25	Iowa	37.5
27	Maryland	37.4
27	Nebraska	37.4
29	Connecticut	37.3
30	Idaho	37.2
31	Georgia	37.0
31	New Jersey	37.0
33	Louisiana	36.9
33	Wyoming	36.9
35	Virginia	36.7
36	California	36.5
36	Montana	36.5
38	Rhode Island	36.4
38	South Dakota	36.4
40	Wisconsin	35.8
41	Vermont	35.7
42	Massachusetts	35.6
43	Colorado	35.3
43	Oregon	35.3
45	Alaska	35.0
46	North Dakota	34.8
47	New Mexico	34.2
48	Minnesota	33.9
49	Utah	33.6
50	Tennessee	32.9
	District of Columbia	34.6

Source: U.S. Department of Health and Human Services, Centers for Disease Control and Prevention
"2009 Behavioral Risk Factor Surveillance Summary Prevalence Data" (http://apps.nccd.cdc.gov/brfss/)
*Persons 18 and older who have had their cholesterol checked and have been told that they have high blood cholesterol.

Percent of Adults Who Have Visited a Dentist or Dental Clinic: 2008

National Median = 71.3%*

<table>
<tr><td colspan="3">ALPHA ORDER</td><td colspan="3">RANK ORDER</td></tr>
<tr><th>RANK</th><th>STATE</th><th>PERCENT</th><th>RANK</th><th>STATE</th><th>PERCENT</th></tr>
<tr><td>42</td><td>Alabama</td><td>65.0</td><td>1</td><td>Connecticut</td><td>80.3</td></tr>
<tr><td>39</td><td>Alaska</td><td>66.3</td><td>2</td><td>Massachusetts</td><td>79.3</td></tr>
<tr><td>34</td><td>Arizona</td><td>68.3</td><td>3</td><td>Rhode Island</td><td>79.0</td></tr>
<tr><td>45</td><td>Arkansas</td><td>63.5</td><td>4</td><td>Delaware</td><td>76.9</td></tr>
<tr><td>27</td><td>California</td><td>70.3</td><td>5</td><td>New Hampshire</td><td>76.8</td></tr>
<tr><td>32</td><td>Colorado</td><td>68.5</td><td>6</td><td>Michigan</td><td>76.0</td></tr>
<tr><td>1</td><td>Connecticut</td><td>80.3</td><td>7</td><td>New Jersey</td><td>75.9</td></tr>
<tr><td>4</td><td>Delaware</td><td>76.9</td><td>8</td><td>Vermont</td><td>75.5</td></tr>
<tr><td>30</td><td>Florida</td><td>69.1</td><td>9</td><td>Hawaii</td><td>75.4</td></tr>
<tr><td>22</td><td>Georgia</td><td>71.8</td><td>10</td><td>Minnesota</td><td>75.3</td></tr>
<tr><td>9</td><td>Hawaii</td><td>75.4</td><td>11</td><td>Virginia</td><td>75.2</td></tr>
<tr><td>29</td><td>Idaho</td><td>69.5</td><td>12</td><td>New York</td><td>74.2</td></tr>
<tr><td>31</td><td>Illinois</td><td>68.9</td><td>13</td><td>North Dakota</td><td>74.1</td></tr>
<tr><td>34</td><td>Indiana</td><td>68.3</td><td>14</td><td>Iowa</td><td>73.4</td></tr>
<tr><td>14</td><td>Iowa</td><td>73.4</td><td>15</td><td>Washington</td><td>73.3</td></tr>
<tr><td>21</td><td>Kansas</td><td>71.9</td><td>15</td><td>Wisconsin</td><td>73.3</td></tr>
<tr><td>43</td><td>Kentucky</td><td>64.4</td><td>17</td><td>Utah</td><td>72.7</td></tr>
<tr><td>28</td><td>Louisiana</td><td>69.8</td><td>18</td><td>Maryland</td><td>72.6</td></tr>
<tr><td>23</td><td>Maine</td><td>71.5</td><td>18</td><td>South Dakota</td><td>72.6</td></tr>
<tr><td>18</td><td>Maryland</td><td>72.6</td><td>20</td><td>Ohio</td><td>72.2</td></tr>
<tr><td>2</td><td>Massachusetts</td><td>79.3</td><td>21</td><td>Kansas</td><td>71.9</td></tr>
<tr><td>6</td><td>Michigan</td><td>76.0</td><td>22</td><td>Georgia</td><td>71.8</td></tr>
<tr><td>10</td><td>Minnesota</td><td>75.3</td><td>23</td><td>Maine</td><td>71.5</td></tr>
<tr><td>49</td><td>Mississippi</td><td>59.5</td><td>24</td><td>Oregon</td><td>71.4</td></tr>
<tr><td>46</td><td>Missouri</td><td>62.7</td><td>25</td><td>Nebraska</td><td>71.3</td></tr>
<tr><td>40</td><td>Montana</td><td>66.0</td><td>26</td><td>Pennsylvania</td><td>71.1</td></tr>
<tr><td>25</td><td>Nebraska</td><td>71.3</td><td>27</td><td>California</td><td>70.3</td></tr>
<tr><td>44</td><td>Nevada</td><td>63.7</td><td>28</td><td>Louisiana</td><td>69.8</td></tr>
<tr><td>5</td><td>New Hampshire</td><td>76.8</td><td>29</td><td>Idaho</td><td>69.5</td></tr>
<tr><td>7</td><td>New Jersey</td><td>75.9</td><td>30</td><td>Florida</td><td>69.1</td></tr>
<tr><td>40</td><td>New Mexico</td><td>66.0</td><td>31</td><td>Illinois</td><td>68.9</td></tr>
<tr><td>12</td><td>New York</td><td>74.2</td><td>32</td><td>Colorado</td><td>68.5</td></tr>
<tr><td>32</td><td>North Carolina</td><td>68.5</td><td>32</td><td>North Carolina</td><td>68.5</td></tr>
<tr><td>13</td><td>North Dakota</td><td>74.1</td><td>34</td><td>Arizona</td><td>68.3</td></tr>
<tr><td>20</td><td>Ohio</td><td>72.2</td><td>34</td><td>Indiana</td><td>68.3</td></tr>
<tr><td>50</td><td>Oklahoma</td><td>57.9</td><td>36</td><td>Wyoming</td><td>68.0</td></tr>
<tr><td>24</td><td>Oregon</td><td>71.4</td><td>37</td><td>South Carolina</td><td>67.7</td></tr>
<tr><td>26</td><td>Pennsylvania</td><td>71.1</td><td>38</td><td>Tennessee</td><td>66.8</td></tr>
<tr><td>3</td><td>Rhode Island</td><td>79.0</td><td>39</td><td>Alaska</td><td>66.3</td></tr>
<tr><td>37</td><td>South Carolina</td><td>67.7</td><td>40</td><td>Montana</td><td>66.0</td></tr>
<tr><td>18</td><td>South Dakota</td><td>72.6</td><td>40</td><td>New Mexico</td><td>66.0</td></tr>
<tr><td>38</td><td>Tennessee</td><td>66.8</td><td>42</td><td>Alabama</td><td>65.0</td></tr>
<tr><td>47</td><td>Texas</td><td>62.6</td><td>43</td><td>Kentucky</td><td>64.4</td></tr>
<tr><td>17</td><td>Utah</td><td>72.7</td><td>44</td><td>Nevada</td><td>63.7</td></tr>
<tr><td>8</td><td>Vermont</td><td>75.5</td><td>45</td><td>Arkansas</td><td>63.5</td></tr>
<tr><td>11</td><td>Virginia</td><td>75.2</td><td>46</td><td>Missouri</td><td>62.7</td></tr>
<tr><td>15</td><td>Washington</td><td>73.3</td><td>47</td><td>Texas</td><td>62.6</td></tr>
<tr><td>48</td><td>West Virginia</td><td>60.7</td><td>48</td><td>West Virginia</td><td>60.7</td></tr>
<tr><td>15</td><td>Wisconsin</td><td>73.3</td><td>49</td><td>Mississippi</td><td>59.5</td></tr>
<tr><td>36</td><td>Wyoming</td><td>68.0</td><td>50</td><td>Oklahoma</td><td>57.9</td></tr>
<tr><td></td><td></td><td></td><td></td><td>District of Columbia</td><td>72.6</td></tr>
</table>

Source: U.S. Department of Health and Human Services, Centers for Disease Control and Prevention
"2008 Behavioral Risk Factor Surveillance Summary Prevalence Data" (http://apps.nccd.cdc.gov/brfss/)
*Persons 18 and older who have visited a dentist within the past year for any reason.

Percent of Adults 65 Years Old and Older
Who Have Lost All Their Natural Teeth: 2008
National Median = 18.5%*

ALPHA ORDER

RANK	STATE	PERCENT
6	Alabama	26.0
17	Alaska	20.7
45	Arizona	13.5
9	Arkansas	23.1
49	California	10.1
40	Colorado	15.0
46	Connecticut	13.2
36	Delaware	16.7
36	Florida	16.7
9	Georgia	23.1
50	Hawaii	9.6
32	Idaho	17.3
21	Illinois	19.1
13	Indiana	21.7
25	Iowa	18.5
18	Kansas	20.5
7	Kentucky	23.7
8	Louisiana	23.2
12	Maine	21.9
48	Maryland	12.4
27	Massachusetts	18.3
39	Michigan	15.6
47	Minnesota	13.0
3	Mississippi	27.3
5	Missouri	26.2
23	Montana	18.7
33	Nebraska	17.2
29	Nevada	17.7
25	New Hampshire	18.5
33	New Jersey	17.2
28	New Mexico	18.1
35	New York	17.0
15	North Carolina	21.3
19	North Dakota	20.1
16	Ohio	20.8
4	Oklahoma	26.8
38	Oregon	16.0
14	Pennsylvania	21.5
29	Rhode Island	17.7
11	South Carolina	22.7
24	South Dakota	18.6
2	Tennessee	31.5
31	Texas	17.5
43	Utah	13.9
20	Vermont	19.8
41	Virginia	14.6
44	Washington	13.8
1	West Virginia	37.8
42	Wisconsin	14.5
21	Wyoming	19.1

RANK ORDER

RANK	STATE	PERCENT
1	West Virginia	37.8
2	Tennessee	31.5
3	Mississippi	27.3
4	Oklahoma	26.8
5	Missouri	26.2
6	Alabama	26.0
7	Kentucky	23.7
8	Louisiana	23.2
9	Arkansas	23.1
9	Georgia	23.1
11	South Carolina	22.7
12	Maine	21.9
13	Indiana	21.7
14	Pennsylvania	21.5
15	North Carolina	21.3
16	Ohio	20.8
17	Alaska	20.7
18	Kansas	20.5
19	North Dakota	20.1
20	Vermont	19.8
21	Illinois	19.1
21	Wyoming	19.1
23	Montana	18.7
24	South Dakota	18.6
25	Iowa	18.5
25	New Hampshire	18.5
27	Massachusetts	18.3
28	New Mexico	18.1
29	Nevada	17.7
29	Rhode Island	17.7
31	Texas	17.5
32	Idaho	17.3
33	Nebraska	17.2
33	New Jersey	17.2
35	New York	17.0
36	Delaware	16.7
36	Florida	16.7
38	Oregon	16.0
39	Michigan	15.6
40	Colorado	15.0
41	Virginia	14.6
42	Wisconsin	14.5
43	Utah	13.9
44	Washington	13.8
45	Arizona	13.5
46	Connecticut	13.2
47	Minnesota	13.0
48	Maryland	12.4
49	California	10.1
50	Hawaii	9.6
	District of Columbia	15.9

Source: U.S. Department of Health and Human Services, Centers for Disease Control and Prevention
   "2008 Behavioral Risk Factor Surveillance Summary Prevalence Data" (http://apps.nccd.cdc.gov/brfss/)
*Those who have had all their natural teeth extracted.

Percent of Adults Who Average Five or More Servings of Fruits and Vegetables Each Day: 2009
National Median = 23.4%*

ALPHA ORDER

RANK	STATE	PERCENT
41	Alabama	20.3
25	Alaska	23.4
20	Arizona	24.1
40	Arkansas	20.4
5	California	27.7
16	Colorado	24.8
2	Connecticut	28.3
15	Delaware	25.0
19	Florida	24.4
18	Georgia	24.5
24	Hawaii	23.5
17	Idaho	24.6
32	Illinois	22.5
38	Indiana	20.6
44	Iowa	18.5
43	Kansas	18.6
35	Kentucky	21.1
46	Louisiana	16.9
3	Maine	28.0
6	Maryland	27.6
11	Massachusetts	26.2
31	Michigan	22.6
34	Minnesota	21.9
47	Mississippi	16.8
42	Missouri	19.9
13	Montana	25.7
37	Nebraska	20.9
23	Nevada	23.7
4	New Hampshire	27.9
9	New Jersey	26.4
29	New Mexico	23.2
8	New York	26.8
38	North Carolina	20.6
32	North Dakota	22.5
36	Ohio	21.0
50	Oklahoma	14.6
10	Oregon	26.3
20	Pennsylvania	24.1
12	Rhode Island	26.1
45	South Carolina	17.4
49	South Dakota	15.7
26	Tennessee	23.3
22	Texas	23.8
26	Utah	23.3
1	Vermont	29.3
7	Virginia	27.3
14	Washington	25.1
48	West Virginia	16.2
30	Wisconsin	22.7
26	Wyoming	23.3

RANK ORDER

RANK	STATE	PERCENT
1	Vermont	29.3
2	Connecticut	28.3
3	Maine	28.0
4	New Hampshire	27.9
5	California	27.7
6	Maryland	27.6
7	Virginia	27.3
8	New York	26.8
9	New Jersey	26.4
10	Oregon	26.3
11	Massachusetts	26.2
12	Rhode Island	26.1
13	Montana	25.7
14	Washington	25.1
15	Delaware	25.0
16	Colorado	24.8
17	Idaho	24.6
18	Georgia	24.5
19	Florida	24.4
20	Arizona	24.1
20	Pennsylvania	24.1
22	Texas	23.8
23	Nevada	23.7
24	Hawaii	23.5
25	Alaska	23.4
26	Tennessee	23.3
26	Utah	23.3
26	Wyoming	23.3
29	New Mexico	23.2
30	Wisconsin	22.7
31	Michigan	22.6
32	Illinois	22.5
32	North Dakota	22.5
34	Minnesota	21.9
35	Kentucky	21.1
36	Ohio	21.0
37	Nebraska	20.9
38	Indiana	20.6
38	North Carolina	20.6
40	Arkansas	20.4
41	Alabama	20.3
42	Missouri	19.9
43	Kansas	18.6
44	Iowa	18.5
45	South Carolina	17.4
46	Louisiana	16.9
47	Mississippi	16.8
48	West Virginia	16.2
49	South Dakota	15.7
50	Oklahoma	14.6

District of Columbia	31.5

Source: U.S. Department of Health and Human Services, Centers for Disease Control and Prevention
"2009 Behavioral Risk Factor Surveillance Summary Prevalence Data" (http://apps.nccd.cdc.gov/brfss/)
*Persons 18 and older.

Percent of Adults Rating Their Health as Fair or Poor in 2009

National Median = 14.5% of Adults*

ALPHA ORDER				RANK ORDER		
RANK	STATE	PERCENT		RANK	STATE	PERCENT
3	Alabama	21.6		1	West Virginia	23.7
46	Alaska	11.3		2	Kentucky	22.8
26	Arizona	14.5		3	Alabama	21.6
7	Arkansas	19.7		4	Mississippi	21.4
8	California	19.6		5	Tennessee	21.3
41	Colorado	12.0		6	Louisiana	20.8
49	Connecticut	10.3		7	Arkansas	19.7
34	Delaware	12.9		8	California	19.6
12	Florida	16.5		8	Oklahoma	19.6
19	Georgia	15.4		10	North Carolina	18.1
29	Hawaii	13.8		11	New Mexico	17.1
20	Idaho	15.2		12	Florida	16.5
20	Illinois	15.2		13	Indiana	16.4
13	Indiana	16.4		14	South Carolina	16.3
45	Iowa	11.4		15	Missouri	16.1
38	Kansas	12.3		16	Texas	16.0
2	Kentucky	22.8		17	Nevada	15.9
6	Louisiana	20.8		17	Ohio	15.9
31	Maine	13.4		19	Georgia	15.4
34	Maryland	12.9		20	Idaho	15.2
41	Massachusetts	12.0		20	Illinois	15.2
22	Michigan	14.8		22	Michigan	14.8
50	Minnesota	10.1		22	New York	14.8
4	Mississippi	21.4		22	Pennsylvania	14.8
15	Missouri	16.1		25	New Jersey	14.6
26	Montana	14.5		26	Arizona	14.5
32	Nebraska	13.1		26	Montana	14.5
17	Nevada	15.9		28	Virginia	14.2
40	New Hampshire	12.1		29	Hawaii	13.8
25	New Jersey	14.6		30	Washington	13.6
11	New Mexico	17.1		31	Maine	13.4
22	New York	14.8		32	Nebraska	13.1
10	North Carolina	18.1		32	Oregon	13.1
44	North Dakota	11.6		34	Delaware	12.9
17	Ohio	15.9		34	Maryland	12.9
8	Oklahoma	19.6		36	Rhode Island	12.7
32	Oregon	13.1		37	Wyoming	12.4
22	Pennsylvania	14.8		38	Kansas	12.3
36	Rhode Island	12.7		39	South Dakota	12.2
14	South Carolina	16.3		40	New Hampshire	12.1
39	South Dakota	12.2		41	Colorado	12.0
5	Tennessee	21.3		41	Massachusetts	12.0
16	Texas	16.0		43	Wisconsin	11.9
48	Utah	10.8		44	North Dakota	11.6
47	Vermont	10.9		45	Iowa	11.4
28	Virginia	14.2		46	Alaska	11.3
30	Washington	13.6		47	Vermont	10.9
1	West Virginia	23.7		48	Utah	10.8
43	Wisconsin	11.9		49	Connecticut	10.3
37	Wyoming	12.4		50	Minnesota	10.1
					District of Columbia	10.9

Source: U.S. Department of Health and Human Services, Centers for Disease Control and Prevention
"2009 Behavioral Risk Factor Surveillance Summary Prevalence Data" (http://apps.nccd.cdc.gov/brfss/)
*Persons 18 and older.

Safety Belt Usage Rate in 2009

National Rate = 84.0% Use Safety Belts

RANK	STATE	PERCENT
15	Alabama	90.0
22	Alaska	86.1
35	Arizona	80.8
45	Arkansas	74.4
5	California	95.3
34	Colorado	81.1
24	Connecticut	85.9
18	Delaware	88.4
26	Florida	85.2
17	Georgia	88.9
2	Hawaii	97.9
38	Idaho	79.2
11	Illinois	91.7
10	Indiana	92.6
7	Iowa	93.1
41	Kansas	77.0
37	Kentucky	79.7
44	Louisiana	74.5
30	Maine	82.6
6	Maryland	94.0
47	Massachusetts	73.6
1	Michigan	98.0
13	Minnesota	90.2
42	Mississippi	76.0
40	Missouri	77.2
38	Montana	79.2
27	Nebraska	84.8
12	Nevada	91.0
49	New Hampshire	68.9
9	New Jersey	92.7
14	New Mexico	90.1
19	New York	88.0
16	North Carolina	89.5
32	North Dakota	81.5
29	Ohio	83.6
28	Oklahoma	84.2
3	Oregon	96.6
20	Pennsylvania	87.9
43	Rhode Island	74.7
32	South Carolina	81.5
48	South Dakota	72.1
36	Tennessee	80.6
8	Texas	92.9
22	Utah	86.1
25	Vermont	85.3
31	Virginia	82.3
4	Washington	96.4
21	West Virginia	87.0
46	Wisconsin	73.8
50	Wyoming	67.6

RANK	STATE	PERCENT
1	Michigan	98.0
2	Hawaii	97.9
3	Oregon	96.6
4	Washington	96.4
5	California	95.3
6	Maryland	94.0
7	Iowa	93.1
8	Texas	92.9
9	New Jersey	92.7
10	Indiana	92.6
11	Illinois	91.7
12	Nevada	91.0
13	Minnesota	90.2
14	New Mexico	90.1
15	Alabama	90.0
16	North Carolina	89.5
17	Georgia	88.9
18	Delaware	88.4
19	New York	88.0
20	Pennsylvania	87.9
21	West Virginia	87.0
22	Alaska	86.1
22	Utah	86.1
24	Connecticut	85.9
25	Vermont	85.3
26	Florida	85.2
27	Nebraska	84.8
28	Oklahoma	84.2
29	Ohio	83.6
30	Maine	82.6
31	Virginia	82.3
32	North Dakota	81.5
32	South Carolina	81.5
34	Colorado	81.1
35	Arizona	80.8
36	Tennessee	80.6
37	Kentucky	79.7
38	Idaho	79.2
38	Montana	79.2
40	Missouri	77.2
41	Kansas	77.0
42	Mississippi	76.0
43	Rhode Island	74.7
44	Louisiana	74.5
45	Arkansas	74.4
46	Wisconsin	73.8
47	Massachusetts	73.6
48	South Dakota	72.1
49	New Hampshire	68.9
50	Wyoming	67.6
	District of Columbia	93.0

Source: U.S. Department of Transportation, National Highway Traffic Safety Administration
"Seat Belt Use in 2009" (http://www-nrd.nhtsa.dot.gov/Pubs/811324.pdf)

VIII. Appendix

Population in 2009 532
Population in 2008 533
Male Population in 2009 534
Female Population in 2009 535

Population in 2009

National Total = 307,006,550*

ALPHA ORDER

RANK	STATE	POPULATION	% of USA
23	Alabama	4,708,708	1.5%
47	Alaska	698,473	0.2%
14	Arizona	6,595,778	2.1%
32	Arkansas	2,889,450	0.9%
1	California	36,961,664	12.0%
22	Colorado	5,024,748	1.6%
29	Connecticut	3,518,288	1.1%
45	Delaware	885,122	0.3%
4	Florida	18,537,969	6.0%
9	Georgia	9,829,211	3.2%
42	Hawaii	1,295,178	0.4%
39	Idaho	1,545,801	0.5%
5	Illinois	12,910,409	4.2%
16	Indiana	6,423,113	2.1%
30	Iowa	3,007,856	1.0%
33	Kansas	2,818,747	0.9%
26	Kentucky	4,314,113	1.4%
25	Louisiana	4,492,076	1.5%
41	Maine	1,318,301	0.4%
19	Maryland	5,699,478	1.9%
15	Massachusetts	6,593,587	2.1%
8	Michigan	9,969,727	3.2%
21	Minnesota	5,266,214	1.7%
31	Mississippi	2,951,996	1.0%
18	Missouri	5,987,580	2.0%
44	Montana	974,989	0.3%
38	Nebraska	1,796,619	0.6%
35	Nevada	2,643,085	0.9%
40	New Hampshire	1,324,575	0.4%
11	New Jersey	8,707,739	2.8%
36	New Mexico	2,009,671	0.7%
3	New York	19,541,453	6.4%
10	North Carolina	9,380,884	3.1%
48	North Dakota	646,844	0.2%
7	Ohio	11,542,645	3.8%
28	Oklahoma	3,687,050	1.2%
27	Oregon	3,825,657	1.2%
6	Pennsylvania	12,604,767	4.1%
43	Rhode Island	1,053,209	0.3%
24	South Carolina	4,561,242	1.5%
46	South Dakota	812,383	0.3%
17	Tennessee	6,296,254	2.1%
2	Texas	24,782,302	8.1%
34	Utah	2,784,572	0.9%
49	Vermont	621,760	0.2%
12	Virginia	7,882,590	2.6%
13	Washington	6,664,195	2.2%
37	West Virginia	1,819,777	0.6%
20	Wisconsin	5,654,774	1.8%
50	Wyoming	544,270	0.2%

RANK ORDER

RANK	STATE	POPULATION	% of USA
1	California	36,961,664	12.0%
2	Texas	24,782,302	8.1%
3	New York	19,541,453	6.4%
4	Florida	18,537,969	6.0%
5	Illinois	12,910,409	4.2%
6	Pennsylvania	12,604,767	4.1%
7	Ohio	11,542,645	3.8%
8	Michigan	9,969,727	3.2%
9	Georgia	9,829,211	3.2%
10	North Carolina	9,380,884	3.1%
11	New Jersey	8,707,739	2.8%
12	Virginia	7,882,590	2.6%
13	Washington	6,664,195	2.2%
14	Arizona	6,595,778	2.1%
15	Massachusetts	6,593,587	2.1%
16	Indiana	6,423,113	2.1%
17	Tennessee	6,296,254	2.1%
18	Missouri	5,987,580	2.0%
19	Maryland	5,699,478	1.9%
20	Wisconsin	5,654,774	1.8%
21	Minnesota	5,266,214	1.7%
22	Colorado	5,024,748	1.6%
23	Alabama	4,708,708	1.5%
24	South Carolina	4,561,242	1.5%
25	Louisiana	4,492,076	1.5%
26	Kentucky	4,314,113	1.4%
27	Oregon	3,825,657	1.2%
28	Oklahoma	3,687,050	1.2%
29	Connecticut	3,518,288	1.1%
30	Iowa	3,007,856	1.0%
31	Mississippi	2,951,996	1.0%
32	Arkansas	2,889,450	0.9%
33	Kansas	2,818,747	0.9%
34	Utah	2,784,572	0.9%
35	Nevada	2,643,085	0.9%
36	New Mexico	2,009,671	0.7%
37	West Virginia	1,819,777	0.6%
38	Nebraska	1,796,619	0.6%
39	Idaho	1,545,801	0.5%
40	New Hampshire	1,324,575	0.4%
41	Maine	1,318,301	0.4%
42	Hawaii	1,295,178	0.4%
43	Rhode Island	1,053,209	0.3%
44	Montana	974,989	0.3%
45	Delaware	885,122	0.3%
46	South Dakota	812,383	0.3%
47	Alaska	698,473	0.2%
48	North Dakota	646,844	0.2%
49	Vermont	621,760	0.2%
50	Wyoming	544,270	0.2%
	District of Columbia	599,657	0.2%

Source: U.S. Bureau of the Census
    "Population Estimates" (December 23, 2009, http://www.census.gov/popest/estimates.php)
*Resident population.

Population in 2008

National Total = 304,374,846*

ALPHA ORDER

RANK	STATE	POPULATION	% of USA
23	Alabama	4,677,464	1.5%
47	Alaska	688,125	0.2%
15	Arizona	6,499,377	2.1%
32	Arkansas	2,867,764	0.9%
1	California	36,580,371	12.0%
22	Colorado	4,935,213	1.6%
29	Connecticut	3,502,932	1.2%
45	Delaware	876,211	0.3%
4	Florida	18,423,878	6.1%
9	Georgia	9,697,838	3.2%
42	Hawaii	1,287,481	0.4%
39	Idaho	1,527,506	0.5%
5	Illinois	12,842,954	4.2%
16	Indiana	6,388,309	2.1%
30	Iowa	2,993,987	1.0%
33	Kansas	2,797,375	0.9%
26	Kentucky	4,287,931	1.4%
25	Louisiana	4,451,513	1.5%
41	Maine	1,319,691	0.4%
19	Maryland	5,658,655	1.9%
14	Massachusetts	6,543,595	2.1%
8	Michigan	10,002,486	3.3%
21	Minnesota	5,230,567	1.7%
31	Mississippi	2,940,212	1.0%
18	Missouri	5,956,335	2.0%
44	Montana	968,035	0.3%
38	Nebraska	1,781,949	0.6%
35	Nevada	2,615,772	0.9%
40	New Hampshire	1,321,872	0.4%
11	New Jersey	8,663,398	2.8%
36	New Mexico	1,986,763	0.7%
3	New York	19,467,789	6.4%
10	North Carolina	9,247,134	3.0%
48	North Dakota	641,421	0.2%
7	Ohio	11,528,072	3.8%
28	Oklahoma	3,644,025	1.2%
27	Oregon	3,782,991	1.2%
6	Pennsylvania	12,566,368	4.1%
43	Rhode Island	1,053,502	0.3%
24	South Carolina	4,503,280	1.5%
46	South Dakota	804,532	0.3%
17	Tennessee	6,240,456	2.1%
2	Texas	24,304,290	8.0%
34	Utah	2,727,343	0.9%
49	Vermont	621,049	0.2%
12	Virginia	7,795,424	2.6%
13	Washington	6,566,073	2.2%
37	West Virginia	1,814,873	0.6%
20	Wisconsin	5,627,610	1.8%
50	Wyoming	532,981	0.2%

RANK ORDER

RANK	STATE	POPULATION	% of USA
1	California	36,580,371	12.0%
2	Texas	24,304,290	8.0%
3	New York	19,467,789	6.4%
4	Florida	18,423,878	6.1%
5	Illinois	12,842,954	4.2%
6	Pennsylvania	12,566,368	4.1%
7	Ohio	11,528,072	3.8%
8	Michigan	10,002,486	3.3%
9	Georgia	9,697,838	3.2%
10	North Carolina	9,247,134	3.0%
11	New Jersey	8,663,398	2.8%
12	Virginia	7,795,424	2.6%
13	Washington	6,566,073	2.2%
14	Massachusetts	6,543,595	2.1%
15	Arizona	6,499,377	2.1%
16	Indiana	6,388,309	2.1%
17	Tennessee	6,240,456	2.1%
18	Missouri	5,956,335	2.0%
19	Maryland	5,658,655	1.9%
20	Wisconsin	5,627,610	1.8%
21	Minnesota	5,230,567	1.7%
22	Colorado	4,935,213	1.6%
23	Alabama	4,677,464	1.5%
24	South Carolina	4,503,280	1.5%
25	Louisiana	4,451,513	1.5%
26	Kentucky	4,287,931	1.4%
27	Oregon	3,782,991	1.2%
28	Oklahoma	3,644,025	1.2%
29	Connecticut	3,502,932	1.2%
30	Iowa	2,993,987	1.0%
31	Mississippi	2,940,212	1.0%
32	Arkansas	2,867,764	0.9%
33	Kansas	2,797,375	0.9%
34	Utah	2,727,343	0.9%
35	Nevada	2,615,772	0.9%
36	New Mexico	1,986,763	0.7%
37	West Virginia	1,814,873	0.6%
38	Nebraska	1,781,949	0.6%
39	Idaho	1,527,506	0.5%
40	New Hampshire	1,321,872	0.4%
41	Maine	1,319,691	0.4%
42	Hawaii	1,287,481	0.4%
43	Rhode Island	1,053,502	0.3%
44	Montana	968,035	0.3%
45	Delaware	876,211	0.3%
46	South Dakota	804,532	0.3%
47	Alaska	688,125	0.2%
48	North Dakota	641,421	0.2%
49	Vermont	621,049	0.2%
50	Wyoming	532,981	0.2%
	District of Columbia	590,074	0.2%

Source: U.S. Bureau of the Census
   "Population Estimates" (December 23, 2009, http://www.census.gov/popest/estimates.php)
*Resident population.

Male Population in 2009

National Total = 151,449,490 Males

<table>
<tr><td colspan="4">ALPHA ORDER</td><td colspan="4">RANK ORDER</td></tr>
<tr><td>RANK</td><td>STATE</td><td>MALES</td><td>% of USA</td><td>RANK</td><td>STATE</td><td>MALES</td><td>% of USA</td></tr>
<tr><td>23</td><td>Alabama</td><td>2,281,612</td><td>1.5%</td><td>1</td><td>California</td><td>18,505,202</td><td>12.2%</td></tr>
<tr><td>47</td><td>Alaska</td><td>362,225</td><td>0.2%</td><td>2</td><td>Texas</td><td>12,378,092</td><td>8.2%</td></tr>
<tr><td>14</td><td>Arizona</td><td>3,306,841</td><td>2.2%</td><td>3</td><td>New York</td><td>9,499,163</td><td>6.3%</td></tr>
<tr><td>32</td><td>Arkansas</td><td>1,415,500</td><td>0.9%</td><td>4</td><td>Florida</td><td>9,123,926</td><td>6.0%</td></tr>
<tr><td>1</td><td>California</td><td>18,505,202</td><td>12.2%</td><td>5</td><td>Illinois</td><td>6,359,626</td><td>4.2%</td></tr>
<tr><td>22</td><td>Colorado</td><td>2,531,085</td><td>1.7%</td><td>6</td><td>Pennsylvania</td><td>6,138,709</td><td>4.1%</td></tr>
<tr><td>29</td><td>Connecticut</td><td>1,717,636</td><td>1.1%</td><td>7</td><td>Ohio</td><td>5,633,403</td><td>3.7%</td></tr>
<tr><td>45</td><td>Delaware</td><td>429,662</td><td>0.3%</td><td>8</td><td>Michigan</td><td>4,902,854</td><td>3.2%</td></tr>
<tr><td>4</td><td>Florida</td><td>9,123,926</td><td>6.0%</td><td>9</td><td>Georgia</td><td>4,835,262</td><td>3.2%</td></tr>
<tr><td>9</td><td>Georgia</td><td>4,835,262</td><td>3.2%</td><td>10</td><td>North Carolina</td><td>4,590,185</td><td>3.0%</td></tr>
<tr><td>40</td><td>Hawaii</td><td>654,421</td><td>0.4%</td><td>11</td><td>New Jersey</td><td>4,268,344</td><td>2.8%</td></tr>
<tr><td>39</td><td>Idaho</td><td>775,918</td><td>0.5%</td><td>12</td><td>Virginia</td><td>3,874,865</td><td>2.6%</td></tr>
<tr><td>5</td><td>Illinois</td><td>6,359,626</td><td>4.2%</td><td>13</td><td>Washington</td><td>3,328,953</td><td>2.2%</td></tr>
<tr><td>16</td><td>Indiana</td><td>3,164,688</td><td>2.1%</td><td>14</td><td>Arizona</td><td>3,306,841</td><td>2.2%</td></tr>
<tr><td>30</td><td>Iowa</td><td>1,485,609</td><td>1.0%</td><td>15</td><td>Massachusetts</td><td>3,204,983</td><td>2.1%</td></tr>
<tr><td>34</td><td>Kansas</td><td>1,399,823</td><td>0.9%</td><td>16</td><td>Indiana</td><td>3,164,688</td><td>2.1%</td></tr>
<tr><td>26</td><td>Kentucky</td><td>2,117,406</td><td>1.4%</td><td>17</td><td>Tennessee</td><td>3,069,243</td><td>2.0%</td></tr>
<tr><td>25</td><td>Louisiana</td><td>2,185,135</td><td>1.4%</td><td>18</td><td>Missouri</td><td>2,926,002</td><td>1.9%</td></tr>
<tr><td>42</td><td>Maine</td><td>643,580</td><td>0.4%</td><td>19</td><td>Wisconsin</td><td>2,809,066</td><td>1.9%</td></tr>
<tr><td>20</td><td>Maryland</td><td>2,763,806</td><td>1.8%</td><td>20</td><td>Maryland</td><td>2,763,806</td><td>1.8%</td></tr>
<tr><td>15</td><td>Massachusetts</td><td>3,204,983</td><td>2.1%</td><td>21</td><td>Minnesota</td><td>2,620,570</td><td>1.7%</td></tr>
<tr><td>8</td><td>Michigan</td><td>4,902,854</td><td>3.2%</td><td>22</td><td>Colorado</td><td>2,531,085</td><td>1.7%</td></tr>
<tr><td>21</td><td>Minnesota</td><td>2,620,570</td><td>1.7%</td><td>23</td><td>Alabama</td><td>2,281,612</td><td>1.5%</td></tr>
<tr><td>31</td><td>Mississippi</td><td>1,431,040</td><td>0.9%</td><td>24</td><td>South Carolina</td><td>2,221,134</td><td>1.5%</td></tr>
<tr><td>18</td><td>Missouri</td><td>2,926,002</td><td>1.9%</td><td>25</td><td>Louisiana</td><td>2,185,135</td><td>1.4%</td></tr>
<tr><td>44</td><td>Montana</td><td>487,981</td><td>0.3%</td><td>26</td><td>Kentucky</td><td>2,117,406</td><td>1.4%</td></tr>
<tr><td>38</td><td>Nebraska</td><td>891,652</td><td>0.6%</td><td>27</td><td>Oregon</td><td>1,897,054</td><td>1.3%</td></tr>
<tr><td>35</td><td>Nevada</td><td>1,346,046</td><td>0.9%</td><td>28</td><td>Oklahoma</td><td>1,821,974</td><td>1.2%</td></tr>
<tr><td>41</td><td>New Hampshire</td><td>652,948</td><td>0.4%</td><td>29</td><td>Connecticut</td><td>1,717,636</td><td>1.1%</td></tr>
<tr><td>11</td><td>New Jersey</td><td>4,268,344</td><td>2.8%</td><td>30</td><td>Iowa</td><td>1,485,609</td><td>1.0%</td></tr>
<tr><td>36</td><td>New Mexico</td><td>994,635</td><td>0.7%</td><td>31</td><td>Mississippi</td><td>1,431,040</td><td>0.9%</td></tr>
<tr><td>3</td><td>New York</td><td>9,499,163</td><td>6.3%</td><td>32</td><td>Arkansas</td><td>1,415,500</td><td>0.9%</td></tr>
<tr><td>10</td><td>North Carolina</td><td>4,590,185</td><td>3.0%</td><td>33</td><td>Utah</td><td>1,400,974</td><td>0.9%</td></tr>
<tr><td>48</td><td>North Dakota</td><td>325,000</td><td>0.2%</td><td>34</td><td>Kansas</td><td>1,399,823</td><td>0.9%</td></tr>
<tr><td>7</td><td>Ohio</td><td>5,633,403</td><td>3.7%</td><td>35</td><td>Nevada</td><td>1,346,046</td><td>0.9%</td></tr>
<tr><td>28</td><td>Oklahoma</td><td>1,821,974</td><td>1.2%</td><td>36</td><td>New Mexico</td><td>994,635</td><td>0.7%</td></tr>
<tr><td>27</td><td>Oregon</td><td>1,897,054</td><td>1.3%</td><td>37</td><td>West Virginia</td><td>892,120</td><td>0.6%</td></tr>
<tr><td>6</td><td>Pennsylvania</td><td>6,138,709</td><td>4.1%</td><td>38</td><td>Nebraska</td><td>891,652</td><td>0.6%</td></tr>
<tr><td>43</td><td>Rhode Island</td><td>511,490</td><td>0.3%</td><td>39</td><td>Idaho</td><td>775,918</td><td>0.5%</td></tr>
<tr><td>24</td><td>South Carolina</td><td>2,221,134</td><td>1.5%</td><td>40</td><td>Hawaii</td><td>654,421</td><td>0.4%</td></tr>
<tr><td>46</td><td>South Dakota</td><td>405,920</td><td>0.3%</td><td>41</td><td>New Hampshire</td><td>652,948</td><td>0.4%</td></tr>
<tr><td>17</td><td>Tennessee</td><td>3,069,243</td><td>2.0%</td><td>42</td><td>Maine</td><td>643,580</td><td>0.4%</td></tr>
<tr><td>2</td><td>Texas</td><td>12,378,092</td><td>8.2%</td><td>43</td><td>Rhode Island</td><td>511,490</td><td>0.3%</td></tr>
<tr><td>33</td><td>Utah</td><td>1,400,974</td><td>0.9%</td><td>44</td><td>Montana</td><td>487,981</td><td>0.3%</td></tr>
<tr><td>49</td><td>Vermont</td><td>306,024</td><td>0.2%</td><td>45</td><td>Delaware</td><td>429,662</td><td>0.3%</td></tr>
<tr><td>12</td><td>Virginia</td><td>3,874,865</td><td>2.6%</td><td>46</td><td>South Dakota</td><td>405,920</td><td>0.3%</td></tr>
<tr><td>13</td><td>Washington</td><td>3,328,953</td><td>2.2%</td><td>47</td><td>Alaska</td><td>362,225</td><td>0.2%</td></tr>
<tr><td>37</td><td>West Virginia</td><td>892,120</td><td>0.6%</td><td>48</td><td>North Dakota</td><td>325,000</td><td>0.2%</td></tr>
<tr><td>19</td><td>Wisconsin</td><td>2,809,066</td><td>1.9%</td><td>49</td><td>Vermont</td><td>306,024</td><td>0.2%</td></tr>
<tr><td>50</td><td>Wyoming</td><td>277,040</td><td>0.2%</td><td>50</td><td>Wyoming</td><td>277,040</td><td>0.2%</td></tr>
<tr><td></td><td></td><td></td><td></td><td></td><td>District of Columbia</td><td>283,063</td><td>0.2%</td></tr>
</table>

Source: CQ Press using data from U.S. Bureau of the Census
"SC-EST2009-AGESEX_RES - State Characteristic Estimates" (http://www.census.gov/popest/datasets.html)

Female Population in 2009

National Total = 155,557,060 Females

ALPHA ORDER

RANK	STATE	FEMALES	% of USA
23	Alabama	2,427,096	1.6%
47	Alaska	336,248	0.2%
15	Arizona	3,288,937	2.1%
32	Arkansas	1,473,950	0.9%
1	California	18,456,462	11.9%
22	Colorado	2,493,663	1.6%
29	Connecticut	1,800,652	1.2%
45	Delaware	455,460	0.3%
4	Florida	9,414,043	6.1%
9	Georgia	4,993,949	3.2%
42	Hawaii	640,757	0.4%
39	Idaho	769,883	0.5%
5	Illinois	6,550,783	4.2%
16	Indiana	3,258,425	2.1%
30	Iowa	1,522,247	1.0%
33	Kansas	1,418,924	0.9%
26	Kentucky	2,196,707	1.4%
25	Louisiana	2,306,941	1.5%
40	Maine	674,721	0.4%
19	Maryland	2,935,672	1.9%
13	Massachusetts	3,388,604	2.2%
8	Michigan	5,066,873	3.3%
21	Minnesota	2,645,644	1.7%
31	Mississippi	1,520,956	1.0%
18	Missouri	3,061,578	2.0%
44	Montana	487,008	0.3%
38	Nebraska	904,967	0.6%
35	Nevada	1,297,039	0.8%
41	New Hampshire	671,627	0.4%
11	New Jersey	4,439,395	2.9%
36	New Mexico	1,015,036	0.7%
3	New York	10,042,290	6.5%
10	North Carolina	4,790,699	3.1%
48	North Dakota	321,844	0.2%
7	Ohio	5,909,242	3.8%
28	Oklahoma	1,865,076	1.2%
27	Oregon	1,928,603	1.2%
6	Pennsylvania	6,466,058	4.2%
43	Rhode Island	541,719	0.3%
24	South Carolina	2,340,108	1.5%
46	South Dakota	406,463	0.3%
17	Tennessee	3,227,011	2.1%
2	Texas	12,404,210	8.0%
34	Utah	1,383,598	0.9%
49	Vermont	315,736	0.2%
12	Virginia	4,007,725	2.6%
14	Washington	3,335,242	2.1%
37	West Virginia	927,657	0.6%
20	Wisconsin	2,845,708	1.8%
50	Wyoming	267,230	0.2%

RANK ORDER

RANK	STATE	FEMALES	% of USA
1	California	18,456,462	11.9%
2	Texas	12,404,210	8.0%
3	New York	10,042,290	6.5%
4	Florida	9,414,043	6.1%
5	Illinois	6,550,783	4.2%
6	Pennsylvania	6,466,058	4.2%
7	Ohio	5,909,242	3.8%
8	Michigan	5,066,873	3.3%
9	Georgia	4,993,949	3.2%
10	North Carolina	4,790,699	3.1%
11	New Jersey	4,439,395	2.9%
12	Virginia	4,007,725	2.6%
13	Massachusetts	3,388,604	2.2%
14	Washington	3,335,242	2.1%
15	Arizona	3,288,937	2.1%
16	Indiana	3,258,425	2.1%
17	Tennessee	3,227,011	2.1%
18	Missouri	3,061,578	2.0%
19	Maryland	2,935,672	1.9%
20	Wisconsin	2,845,708	1.8%
21	Minnesota	2,645,644	1.7%
22	Colorado	2,493,663	1.6%
23	Alabama	2,427,096	1.6%
24	South Carolina	2,340,108	1.5%
25	Louisiana	2,306,941	1.5%
26	Kentucky	2,196,707	1.4%
27	Oregon	1,928,603	1.2%
28	Oklahoma	1,865,076	1.2%
29	Connecticut	1,800,652	1.2%
30	Iowa	1,522,247	1.0%
31	Mississippi	1,520,956	1.0%
32	Arkansas	1,473,950	0.9%
33	Kansas	1,418,924	0.9%
34	Utah	1,383,598	0.9%
35	Nevada	1,297,039	0.8%
36	New Mexico	1,015,036	0.7%
37	West Virginia	927,657	0.6%
38	Nebraska	904,967	0.6%
39	Idaho	769,883	0.5%
40	Maine	674,721	0.4%
41	New Hampshire	671,627	0.4%
42	Hawaii	640,757	0.4%
43	Rhode Island	541,719	0.3%
44	Montana	487,008	0.3%
45	Delaware	455,460	0.3%
46	South Dakota	406,463	0.3%
47	Alaska	336,248	0.2%
48	North Dakota	321,844	0.2%
49	Vermont	315,736	0.2%
50	Wyoming	267,230	0.2%
	District of Columbia	316,594	0.2%

Source: CQ Press using data from U.S. Bureau of the Census
"SC-EST2009-AGESEX_RES - State Characteristic Estimates" (http://www.census.gov/popest/datasets.html)

Sources

American Academy of Physicians Assistants
950 North Washington Street
Alexandria, VA   22314-1552
703-836-2272
www.aapa.org

American Cancer Society, Inc.
1599 Clifton Road, NE.
Atlanta, GA   30329-4251
800-227-2345
www.cancer.org

American Dental Association
211 E. Chicago Ave.
Chicago, IL   60611-2678
312-440-2500
www.ada.org

American Hospital Association
155 N. Wacker Drive
Chicago, IL   60606
312-422-3000
www.aha.org

American Medical Association
515 North State Street
Chicago, IL   60610
800-621-8335
www.ama-assn.org

American Osteopathic Association
142 East Ontario Street
Chicago, IL   60611
800-621-1773
www.osteopathic.org

Bureau of Labor Statistics
2 Massachusetts Ave., NE
Washington, DC   20212-0001
202-691-5200
www.bls.gov

Bureau of the Census
4600 Silver Hill Road
Washington, DC   20233-0001
800-923-8282
www.census.gov

Centers for Disease Control and Prevention
1600 Clifton Road
Atlanta, GA   30333
800-232-4636
www.cdc.gov

Centers for Medicare and Medicaid Services
7500 Security Boulevard
Baltimore, MD   21244-1850
877-267-2323
www.cms.hhs.gov

Federation of Chiropractic Licensing Boards
5401 W 10th Street, Ste 101
Greeley, CO   80634
970-356-3500
www.fclb.org

Health Resources and Services Administration
Division of Practitioner Data Banks
5600 Fishers Lane
Rockville MD 20857
800-767-6732
www.hrsa.gov

HealthLeaders/InterStudy
One Vantage Way, B-300
Nashville TN 37228
800-643-7600
http://home.healthleaders-interstudy.com

Medical Expenditure Panel Survey
Agency for Healthcare Research and Quality
540 Gaither Road
Rockville MD   20850
301-427-1364
www.meps.ahrq.gov

National Association of State Budget Officers
444 N Capitol St., NW, Ste 642
Washington DC   20001-1551
202-624-5382
www.nasbo.org

National Center for Health Statistics
U.S. Department of Health and Human Services
3311 Toledo Road
Hyattsville, MD   20782
800-232-4636
www.cdc.gov/nchs/

National Highway Traffic Safety Administration
1200 New Jersey Ave., SE
West Building
Washington, DC   20590
888-327-4236
www.nhtsa.gov

**National Institute on Alcohol Abuse
and Alcoholism**
National Institutes of Health
5635 Fishers Lane, MSC 9304
Bethesda, MD   20892-9304
301-443-3860
www.niaaa.nih.gov/

National Sporting Goods Association
1601 Feehanville Drive, Ste 300
Mt. Prospect, IL   60056
800-815-5422
www.nsga.org

**Substance Abuse and Mental Health Services
Administration**
U.S. Department of Health and Human Services
1 Choke Cherry Road
Rockville MD   20857
877-SAMHSA-7
www.samhsa.gov

Index

A

Abortion
    by age of woman, 79–83
    by stage of gestation, 84–87
    first time, percent, 73
    numbers of, 68
    rate of, 71
    ratio of, 70
    to out-of-state residents, 72
    to teenagers, 79–83
Accidents, deaths by, 164–166
Admissions to community hospitals, 202
AIDS
    cases, 364–367
    children cases, 367
    deaths, 131–133
Alcohol consumption, 502, 503
Alcohol-induced deaths, 179–181
Anesthesiologists, 452, 453
Alzheimer's Disease, deaths by, 134–136
Assisted reproductive technology
    births from, 62–65
    multiple births from, 65
    procedures, 61
Arthritis, percent with, 408
Asthma, percent with, 407

B

Beds, hospital
    average number per hospital, 201
    children's hospital, 213
    community hospital, 199–21
    nursing home, 226, 227
    psychiatric hospital, 217
    rehabilitation hospital, 215
Beer consumption, 504, 505
Binge drinkers, 511
Births
    by age of mother, 33–46
    by assisted reproductive technology,
      62–65
    by method of delivery, 48–52
    by race of mother, 8–10, 16–19
    Hispanic, 11, 12, 20, 21

    low birthweight, 23–27
    number of, 3, 13
    pre-term 22
    rates, 4, 14
    to teenagers, 33–44
    to unmarried women, 28–32
    to young teens, 43, 44
Bladder cancer, cases, 340, 341
Blood pressure, percent with high, 524
Brain cancer, deaths by, 111, 112
Breast cancer
    cases, 342, 343
    deaths, 113, 114

C

Cancer
    bladder cases, 340, 341
    brain deaths, 111, 112
    breast (female), 113, 114, 342, 343
    cases, total and by cause, 336–363
    cervical cases, 359, 360
    colon and rectum, 115, 116, 345, 346
    deaths by, 107–110
    leukemia, 117, 118
    liver deaths, 119, 120
    lung, 121, 122, 350, 351
    lymphoma, 123, 124, 352, 353
    ovarian deaths, 125, 126
    pancreatic deaths, 127, 128
    prostate, 129, 130, 354, 355
    skin melanoma cases, 357, 358
    uterine cases, 362, 363
Cerebrovascular disease, deaths by, 138,
    139
Cervical cancer cases, 359, 360
Cesarean births, 50–52
Children's hospitals, 212, 213
Children's insurance (CHIP), 264–269
Chiropractors, 464, 465
Chlamydia cases, 401, 402
Cholesterol, percent with high, 525
Chronic liver disease, deaths by, 140–142
Chronic lower respiratory disease, deaths
    by, 143–145

Colon and rectum cancer
    cases, 345, 346
    deaths, 115, 116
Community hospitals
    beds in, 199–201
    number of, 189
    per square miles, 191
    rate of, 190
Community mental health centers, 219

D

Deaths
    by cause, 107–184
    infant, 99–102
    neonatal, 103–106
    numbers of, 90, 92, 96
    occupational, 185, 186
    rates, 91, 93–95, 97, 98
Dentists
    access to, 482
    expenditures for, 315–318
    number of, 479
    rate of, 480
    visits to, 526
Diabetes mellitus
    deaths by, 146–148
    percent of adults with, 409
Distilled spirits, consumption of, 508, 509
Doctors (see physicians)
Drinkers, binge, 511
Drug-induced deaths, 182–184
Drugs
    expenditures for, 327–329
    use of illicit, 517

E

Emergency medical technicians, 489–491
Emergency outpatient visits, 208
Expenditures, personal health care,
    305–307
Employment, health industries, 413, 414,
    492, 493
Exercise, 521, 522
Exercise equipment, use of, 497

F

Fatalities, occupational, 185, 186
Fertility, rate of, 6, 15
Finance, health care, 232–333
Firearm injury, deaths from, 170–172
For-profit hospitals, 197

G

General surgeons, 440, 441
General/family practice physicians, 427, 428
Golf, participants in, 498
Gonorrhea, cases and rates, 403, 404
Government health insurance, 255, 261
Government health expenditures, 297–302
Graduates of international medical schools, 457, 458
Gynecologists and obstetricians, 442, 443

H

Health insurance (see insurance)
Health Maintenance Organizations (HMOs), 270–274
Health practitioners
    employment, 413, 414
    wages of, 415
Health programs, government expenditures for, 300–302
Health care support industries
    employment, 492, 493
    wages, 494
Heart disease, deaths by, 149–151
Hepatitis, cases and rates, 372–375
HMOs, 270–274
Home health agencies, 222
Homicide, deaths by, 173–175
Hospices, 223, 224
Hospital
    admissions, 202
    average stay in, 205
    beds, 199–201, 211, 213, 215, 217, 226, 227
    community, 189–208
    expenditures for care in, 309–311
    for profit, 197
    government expenditures for, 297–299
    in rural areas, 194, 195
    in urban areas, 192, 193
    non-government not-for-profit, 196
    number of, 189, 196–198, 210, 212, 214, 216, 218–223, 225
    occupancy rate, 206
    psychiatric, 216, 217
    state and local government-owned, 198

I

Immunizations, 396
Infant deaths, 99–102
Influenza and pneumonia, deaths by, 158–160
Injury, deaths by, 161–163
Inpatient days, community hospitals, 203

Insurance
    children's health, 264–269
    coverage, 244–263
    employment-based, 253, 259
    government, 255, 261
    Medicaid, 263, 285–296
    Medicare, 275–284
    military health, 256, 262
    premiums, 238–243
    private health, 252, 258
    uninsured, 244–249
Internal medicine physicians, 433, 434
International medical school graduates, 457, 458
Investor-owned hospitals, 197

J

Jogging/running, participants in, 499

K

Kidney disease, deaths from, 155–157

L

Legionellosis, cases and rates, 376, 377
Leukemia, 117, 118, 348, 349
Licensed practical and vocational nurses, 473, 475
Liquor, consumption of, 508, 509
Liver cancer, deaths, 119, 120
Liver disease, deaths by, 140, 142
Low birth weight births, 13, 14, 23–27
Lung cancer
    cases, 350, 351
    deaths, 121, 122
Lyme disease, cases and rates, 378, 379

M

Malaria, cases and rates, 380, 381
Malignant neoplasms (cancers) deaths, 152–154
Malpractice, medical payments, 234
Managed health care, 270–274, 278, 287, 288
Mammograms, prevalence of, 344
Medicaid
    children covered by, 263
    enrollees, 285, 287
    expenditures, 289–295
    facilities, 209–227
    federal match, 296
Medicare
    enrollees, 275–278
    facilities, 209–227
    managed care enrollees, 278
    payments, 282–284
    prescription drug program, 280, 281
    physicians, 281
Melanoma (skin cancer) cases, 357, 358
Meningitis, cases and rates, 382, 383
Mental health
    access to, 456
    community centers, 219

percent with serious psychological distress, 410
Military health insurance, 256, 262
Mortality, 90–186
Mothers, teenage, 33–44
Motor vehicle accidents, deaths by, 167–169

N

Natality, 3–67
Neonatal deaths
    by race, 103–106
    number of, 103
    rate of, 104–106
Nephritis, deaths by, 155–157
Nondrinkers, 510
Non-government not-for-profit hospitals, 196
Nurses, 470–475
Nursing homes
    beds, 226, 227
    expenditures for care, 321–323
    numbers of, 225
    occupancy rate, 228
    resident rate, 229
    population, 230
Nutrition, fruits and vegetables intake, 528

O

Obese adults, 519, 520
Obstetricians and gynecologists, 442, 443
Occupancy rates, hospital, 206
Occupational fatalities, 185, 186
Ophthalmologists, 444, 445
Optometrists, 486–488
Osteopathic physicians, 459, 460
Outpatient visits, 207
Ovarian cancer deaths, 125, 126
Overweight or obese
    percent of adults, 518, 520

P

Pap smears, frequency, of 361
Paramedics, 489–491
Pediatric physicians, 435, 436
Pertussis, cases and rates, 394, 395
Pharmacists, 483–485
Physical therapists, 476–478
Physical therapy facilities, 220
Physician assistants, 467–469
Physicians
    expenditures for services, 312–314
    Chiropractic, 464–466
    M.D. by age, 419, 420
    M.D. by sex, 418
    M.D. by specialty, 427–4553
    M.D. in patient care, 421, 422
    M.D. in primary care, 423–425
    Medicare participation, 279
    Osteopathic, 459, 460
    Podiatric, 460–463
Plastic surgeons, 448, 449

Pneumonia and influenza, deaths by, 158–160
Pneumonia vaccinations, 398
Podiatrists, 461–463
Pregnancy rate
    overall, 66
    teenage, 67
Premiums, average for health insurance, 238, 241
Prenatal care, 57–60
Prescription drugs, expenditures, for 327–329
Pre-term births, 22
Primary care
    access to, 426
    physicians in, 423–425
Private health insurance, 252, 258
Prostate cancer
    cases, 354, 355
    deaths, 129, 130
Providers, health care, 413–494
PSA test, percent receiving, 356
Psychiatric hospitals, 216, 217
Psychiatrists, 454, 455

R

Rabies (animal), cases and rates, 384, 385
Rectum and colon cancer
    cases, 345, 346
    deaths, 115, 116

Rehabilitation hospitals, 214, 215
Respiratory diseases, deaths from, 143–145
Registered nurses, 470–472
Running/jogging, participants, 499
Rural health clinics, 221

S

Salmonellosis, cases and rates, 388, 389
SCHIP (see Children's insurance)
Sexually transmitted diseases, 399–406
Seatbelt use, 530
Shigellosis, cases and rates, 390, 391
Skin melanoma cases, 357, 358
Smoking, costs of, 304
Smokers
    by sex, 513, 514
    former, 515
    never have smoked, 516
    percent of adult population, 512
Specialists, medical, 431–455
Sports participation, 497–501
State and local government expenditures for health, 300–302
State and local government expenditures for hospitals, 297–299
State and local government-owned hospitals, 198
Suicide, deaths by, 176–178
Surgeons, 437–449
Surgery centers, 218

Swimming, participants, 500
Syphilis, cases and rates, 405, 406

T

Teenage births
    by race, 37–42
    number of, 33, 43
    percent, 34, 39, 42
    rate of, 35, 38, 41
    to young teens, 43, 44
Tennis, participants, 501
Tobacco settlement, state funds from, 303
Tooth loss, 527

U

Uninsured, 244–249
Unmarried women, births to, 28–32

V

Vaccinations, 396–398
Vaginal births, 48, 49

W

West Nile Disease, cases and rates, 392, 393
Whooping cough, cases and rates, 394, 395
Wine consumption, 506, 507

Y

Young teens, births to, 43, 44